MYLES

FIFTEENTH EDITION

TEXTBOOK FOR

MIDWIVES

For Elsevier:

Commissioning Editor: Mairi McCubbin
Development Editor: Sheila Black
Project Manager: Nancy Arnott
Designer: Charles Gray
Illustration Manager: Merlyn Harvey
Illustrators: Amanda Williams and Ian Ramsden

MYLES

FIFTEENTH EDITION

TEXTBOOK FOR

MIDWIVES

Edited by

Diane M. Fraser

BEd MPhil PhD MTD RM RGN
Professor of Midwifery and Head of Academic Division of Midwifery, Faculty of Medicine and Health Sciences,
University of Nottingham, Queen's Medical Centre, Nottingham, UK

Margaret A. Cooper

BA RGN RM MTD
Pre-registration Midwifery Programme Director, Academic Division of Midwifery,
Faculty of Medicine and Health Sciences,
University of Nottingham, Queen's Medical Centre, Nottingham, UK

Foreword by

Jill Crawford

NMC Council member 2002–2008;
NMC President 2008

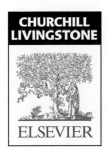

CHURCHILL
LIVINGSTONE

ELSEVIER

EDINBURGH LONDON NEW YORK OXFORD PHILADELPHIA ST LOUIS SYDNEY TORONTO 2009

CHURCHILL
LIVINGSTONE
ELSEVIER

First edition 1953	Ninth edition 1981
Second edition 1956	Tenth edition 1985
Third edition 1958	Eleventh edition 1989
Fourth edition 1961	Twelfth edition 1993
Fifth edition 1964	Thirteenth edition 1999
Sixth edition 1968	Fourteenth edition 2003
Seventh edition 1971	Fifteenth edition 2009
Eighth edition 1975	

ISBN: 978-0-443-06939-0 (Main Edition)
ISBN: 978-0-443-06844-7 (International Edition)

British Library Cataloguing in Publication Data
A catalogue record for this book is available from the British Library

Library of Congress Cataloging in Publication Data
A catalog record for this book is available from the Library of Congress

Notice
Knowledge and best practice in this field are constantly changing. As new
research and experience broaden our knowledge, changes in practice, treatment
and drug therapy may become necessary or appropriate. Readers are advised to
check the most current information provided (i) on procedures featured or (ii) by
the manufacturer of each product to be administered, to verify the recommended
dose or formula, the method and duration of administration, and contraindications.
It is the responsibility of the practitioner, relying on their own experience and
knowledge of the patient, to make diagnoses, to determine dosages and the
best treatment for each individual patient, and to take all appropriate safety
precautions. To the fullest extent of the law, neither the Publisher nor the Editors
assume any liability for any injury and/or damage to persons or property arising
out or related to any use of the material contained in this book.

The Publisher

ELSEVIER your source for books,
journals and multimedia
in the health sciences
www.elsevierhealth.com

Working together to grow
libraries in developing countries

www.elsevier.com | www.bookaid.org | www.sabre.org

ELSEVIER   BOOK AID International   Sabre Foundation

The
Publisher's
policy is to use
**paper manufactured
from sustainable forests**

Printed in China

Contents

Contributors

Robina Aslam MSc PGCEA RGN RM ADM
Midwife teacher, Academic Division of Midwifery,
Lincoln Centre, Faculty of Medicine and Health
Sciences, University of Nottingham, Lincoln, UK

53 Risk Management in midwifery

Jean E. Bain BN RN
Neonatal Transport Coordinator, Neonatal Unit,
Ninewells Hospital, Dundee, UK

43 Recognizing the ill baby

Diane Barrowclough Ed D MMedSci BA(Hons)
RN RM ADM
Senior Lecturer, School of Health Studies,
Division of Midwifery and Women's Health,
University of Bradford, Bradford, UK

13 Preparing for pregnancy

Kuldip Kaur Bharj BSc MSc DipN(Lond) RN RM MTD
IHSM RSA
Senior Lecturer, Midwifery Department, School of
Healthcare Studies, University of Leeds, Leeds, UK

3 The social context of childbirth and motherhood

Susan Brydon MSc RM RGN
Midwife, Supervisor of Midwives, Maternity Unit,
Queen's Medical Centre, Nottingham, UK

53 Risk management in midwifery

Terri Coates MSc ADM DipEd RM RN CIM
Freelance Lecturer and Writer; Clinical Midwife,
Salisbury NHS Trust, Salisbury, UK

*31 Malpositions of the occiput and
   malpresentations*
33 Midwifery and obstetric emergencies

Margaret A. Cooper BA RGN RM MTD
Pre-registration Midwifery Programme Director,
Academic Division of Midwifery, Faculty of Medicine
and Health Sciences, University of Nottingham,
Queens Medical Centre, Nottingham, UK

1 The midwife
3 The social context of childbirth and motherhood

Helen Crafter MSc FPCert ADM PGCEA RGN RM
Senior Lecturer in Midwifery, Faculty of Health
and Human Sciences, Thames Valley University,
London, UK

20 Problems of pregnancy

Susan Dapaah DHSc BSc(Hons)MA ADM CertEd RM
Senior Lecturer in Midwifery, Faculty of Health,
Staffordshire University, Stafford, UK

*23 Sexually transmissible and reproductive tract infections
   in pregnancy*

Victor E. Dapaah MD FFFP FRCOG
Consultant Obstetrician and Gynaecologist,
Department of Obstetrics and Gynaecology,
Staffordshire General Hospital, Stafford, UK

*23 Sexually transmissible and reproductive tract
   infections in pregnancy*

Margie Davies RGN RM
Midwifery Liaison Officer, Multiple Births
Foundation, London, UK

24 Multiple pregnancy

Soo Downe BA(Hons) MSc PhD RM
Professor of Midwifery Studies, School of Public
Health & Clinical Sciences, University of Central
Lancashire, Preston, UK

*28 The transition and the second stage of labour:
   physiology and the role of the midwife*

Jean Duerden MBA DMS RGN RM RSCN
Formerly LSA Midwifery Officer for Yorkshire and
Northern Lincolnshire, Leeds, UK

52 Midwifery supervision and clinical governance

Carole England BSc(Hons) CertEd(FE) RGN RM
Midwife Teacher, Academic Division of Midwifery,
Derby Centre, University of Nottingham,
Derby, UK

42 The healthy low birthweight baby

Philomena Farrell RN RM
Clinical Midwife Manager, Regional Neonatal
Intensive Care Unit, Royal Jubilee Maternity Service,
Belfast, UK

39 The baby at birth

Diane M. Fraser BEd MPhil PhD MTD RM RGN
Professor and Head of Academic Division of
Midwifery, Faculty of Medicine and Health Sciences,
Queen's Medical Centre, University of Nottingham,
Nottingham, UK

1 The midwife

Alison Gibbs MSc RGN
Matron, Children's Services, Lincoln County Hospital,
Lincoln, UK

44 Respiratory problems

Claire Greig PhD BN MSc ADM NCert RGN MTD SCM
Senior Lecturer, Napier University, Edinburgh, UK

45 Trauma during birth, haemorrhage and convulsions

Adela Hamilton BSC(Hons) MA CertMgt CertTch SRN SCM
Senior Lecturer in Midwifery, School of Community
and Health Sciences, City University,
London, UK

27 Comfort and support in labour
32 Assisted births

Jenny Hassall BSc MSc PGCert RM RN
Senior Midwifery Lecturer, School of Nursing
and Midwifery, University of Brighton,
Eastbourne, UK

14 Change and adaptation in pregnancy

Pauline Hudson Med PGCE RM ADM
Visiting Lecturer, Academic Division of Midwifery,
University of Nottingham, Nottingham, UK; formerly
Sexual Health Nurse Practitioner, Bassetlaw Primary
Care Trust, Retford Hospital, Retford, UK

37 Contraception and sexual health

Billie Hunter PhD BN PGDip DNCert PGCE HV RN RM
Professor of Midwifery, School of Health Science,
University of Swansea, Swansea, UK

2 The emotional context of midwifery

Sally Inch RN RM
Infant Feeding Specialist, Women's Centre Breast-
feeding Clinic and Human Milk Bank, The John
Radcliffe Hospital, Oxford, UK

41 Infant feeding

Beverley Kirk BA(Hons) PGCE
English Teacher/Associate Assistant Head, Ashfield
School, Kirkby-in-Ashfield, UK

18 Specialized antenatal investigations

Judith Lee MCSP
Clinical Lead Women's Health Physiotherapist,
Physiotherapy Department, Nottingham University
Hospitals NHS Trust, Nottingham, UK

16 Special exercises for pregnancy and the puerperium

Carmel Lloyd MA ADM PGCEA RN RM
Midwifery Advisor, Nursing and Midwifery Council,
London, UK

21 Medical disorders associated with pregnancy
22 Hypertensive disorders of pregnancy

Rosemary Mander MSc PhD MTD RGN SCM
Professor of Midwifery, University of Edinburgh,
Nursing Studies, School of Health in Social Science,
Edinburgh, UK

6 Evidence-based practice
38 Bereavement and loss in maternity care

Sally Marchant DipEd PhD RM RN
Editor, *MIDIRS Midwifery Digest*, Bristol, UK

34 Physiology and care in the puerperium
35 Physical problems and complications in the puerperium

Carol McCormick BSc(Hons) PGDL ADM RN RM
Consultant Midwife, Maternity Unit, Nottingham
University Hospitals NHS Trust, Nottingham, UK

25 *The first stage of labour: physiology and early care*
26 *Active first stage of labour*

Christine McCourt BA PhD
Professor of Anthropology and Health, Centre for
Research in Midwifery and Childbirth, Thames
Valley University, Brentford, UK

51 *Community, public health and social services*

Sue McDonald BAppSc PhD CHN RN RM FACM
Professor of Midwifery and Women's Health,
Mercy Hospital for Women, Heidelberg, Australia

29 *Physiology and management of the third stage of labour*

Christina McKenzie MSc RM ADM RGN PGCEA DipPSGD
Head of Midwifery, Nursing and Midwifery Council,
London, UK

7 *Midwifery regulation in the United Kingdom*

Alison Miller DipHMS RM RN
Programme Director and Midwifery Lead,
Confidential Enquiry into Maternal and Child Health
(CEMACH), London, UK

56 *Maternal and perinatal health, mortality and statistics*

Irene Murray BSc(Hons) MTD RN RM
Teaching Fellow (Midwifery), Department of Nursing
and Midwifery, University of Stirling, Centre for
Health Science, Raigmore Hospital, Inverness, UK

14 *Change and adaptation in pregnancy*

Mary L. Nolan BA(Hons) MA PhD RGN
Professor of Perinatal Education, Institute of Health,
Social Care and Psychology, University of Worcester;
Senior Tutor, The National Childbirth Trust,
London, UK

15 *Antenatal education: principles and practice*

Margaret R. Oates MB ChB DPM FRCPsych
Senior Lecturer in Psychiatry, University of
Nottingham; Honorary Consultant, Nottingham
Health Care Trust, Nottingham, UK

36 *Perinatal mental health*

Salmon Omokanye MB BS FMCOG FRCOG FFSRH
Consultant and Lead Clinician,
Central Health Clinic, Sheffield Contraception
and Sexual Health, Sheffield, UK

37 *Contraception and sexual health*

Lesley Page BA MSc PhD RM RN
Visiting Professor of Midwifery, Nightingale
School of Nursing and Midwifery, King's College,
London, UK

4 *Woman-centred, midwife-friendly care: principles,
patterns and culture of practice*

Patricia Percival BAppSc MAppSc PhD RN RM
Registered Nurse and Midwife, Ascot, Australia

47 *Jaundice and infection*

Maureen D. Raynor MA PGCEA ADM RMN RN RM
Midwife Teacher, Post Graduate Education Centre,
Academic Division of Midwifery, University of
Nottingham, Nottingham, UK

36 *Perinatal mental health*

Lindsay Reid BA DipEd PhD ADM
Midwife writer and researcher, Fife, UK

54 *Organization of the health services in the UK*

Nancy M. Riddick-Thomas MA ADM CertEd RM RGN
Professional Head of Midwifery Education,
Faculty of Health, Sport & Science, University of
Glamorgan, Pontypridd, UK

5 *Ethics in midwifery*

Annie Rimmer BEd(Hons) RM RN ADM
Senior Lecturer/Course Leader, School of
Nursing and Midwifery, University of Brighton,
Eastbourne, UK

30 *Prolonged pregnancy and disorders of
uterine action*

Jane M. Rutherford DM MRCOG
Consultant in Fetomaternal Medicine,
Department of Obstetrics and Gynaecology,
Queen's Medical Centre, Nottingham, UK

49 *Pharmacology and childbirth*

Iolanda G. J. Serci BSc MSc PgDipNurs PgCertNutrn RN RM
Midwife Lecturer, School of Nursing and Midwifery,
The Robert Gordon University, Aberdeen, UK

10 Hormonal cycles: fertilization and early development
12 The fetus

Della Sherratt BEd(Hons) MA RN RM MTD
NDNCert FETCert
Independent International Midwifery Advisor
and Trainer

55 International midwifery

Judith Simpson MD MRCPCH
Consultant Neonatologist, Paediatric Department,
Queen Mother's Hospital, Glasgow, UK

46 Congenital abnormalities

Norma Sittlington BSc(Hons) MSc RN RSCN RM ANNP
Royal Jubilee Maternity Service, Regional Neonatal
Unit, Belfast, Ireland

39 The baby at birth
40 The normal baby

Nina Smith BA(Hons) MA
Manager, BA and Diploma Programmes for NCT spe-
cialist workers and senior Tutor, National Childbirth
Trust, London, UK

15 Antenatal education: principles and practice

Amanda Sullivan BA(Hons) PGDip PhD RM RGN
Director of Nursing and Integrated Governance
(Formerly Midwife Consultant, Antenatal Screening),
Nottinghamshire County Teaching Primary Care
Trust, Nottingham, UK

18 Specialized antenatal investigations

Ian M. Symonds MMedSci DM MRCOG FRANZCOG
Professor/Senior Staff Specialist in Obstetrics and
Gynaecology, Department of Obstetrics and
Gynaecology, School of Medicine and Public Health,
Faculty of Health, John Hunter Hospital, Newcastle,
Australia

19 Abnormalities of early pregnancy

Ros Thomas MCSP PGCert
Formerly Advanced Practioner Physiotherapist in
Womens Health, Royal United Hospital, Bath, UK;
Freelance Clinical Lecturer, Corsham, UK

16 Special exercises for pregnancy and the puerperium

Denise Tiran MSc RM RGN ADM PGCEA
Visiting lecturer, University of Greenwich, London,
UK: Director, Expectancy Ltd, Meopham, UK

50 Complementary therapies in midwifery

Tom Turner MB FRCP FRCPCH
Consultant Paediatrician, Neonatal Unit, Queen
Mother's Hospital, Glasgow, UK

46 Congenital abnormalities

Mary E. Vance BSc(Hons) MPhil PGCert TLT RM
LSA Midwifery Officer - North of Scotland,
LSA Consortium, Inverness, UK

8 The female pelvis and the reproductive organs
9 The female urinary tract
11 The placenta

Anne Viccars BSc(Hons) MA PGDipEd RM RGN
Senior Lecturer in Midwifery, School of Health
and Social Care, Bournemouth University,
Bournemouth, UK

17 Antenatal care

Stephen P. Wardle MB ChB FRCPCH MD
Consultant Neonatologist, Neonatal Intensive Care
Unit, Queen's Medical Centre, Nottingham University
Hospitals, Nottingham, UK

48 Metabolic and endocrine disorders and drug
withdrawal

Foreword

When a midwife cares for a woman, she becomes an integral part of that woman's life story. Years later, women can and do recount the words and acts of the midwives who accompanied them on their journeys to motherhood.

It is not simply that women remember how they were cared for. The care they receive often has a fundamental influence on their sense of themselves as women and mothers.

My own experience of care from a midwife inspired in me a passionate commitment to the profession of midwifery. She came on shift at a point in my labour when I, and others, were losing faith in my ability to give birth. I had been hauled out of the birth pool for assessment and the news was not good. Previously unwanted and unplanned interventions were being mooted and I was ready to agree to anything that would reduce the pain and deliver my baby safely.

At that point, I heard a gentle knock and in she walked. The first thing she did was to look me in the eyes and smile. At that point, I knew I'd be OK.

The second thing she did was to tell me how well I was doing, ask me to get back in the pool and tell me how much she was looking forward to this birth. Her calm, reassuring manner conveyed that she had confidence in me to give birth to my baby. I believed her.

Two hours later, I scooped a funny looking little fellow from the water. I thought he was the most miraculous thing in the world and I was the cleverest woman on the planet. Those feelings carried me through the hardest of times as a new mother and have made me walk taller as a woman since.

By being truly with women, midwives can change the lives of them and their children. My experience, as a mother, antenatal teacher and President of the Nursing and Midwifery Council, is that midwives carry this weight of responsibility well.

For this reason, I am honoured to be writing the Foreword to a text that will support and encourage future and current midwives to be with women.

The breadth and depth of this edition of *Myles Textbook for Midwives* is testimony to the holistic nature of midwifery care. The editors have skilfully interwoven chapters that will help midwives meet the social, emotional and physical needs of childbearing women.

In this edition, the chapter on women's emotional health is divided into two sections. These differentiate clearly between the psychological context of childbearing and perinatal psychiatric disorders. This gives clarity to an important and often neglected area of midwifery.

The text reflects well the changing social and political context of midwifery. Women increasingly want to be involved in decisions about how they and their babies are cared for. To enable this to happen, midwives need to be able to provide women with accessible, evidence-based information. The chapter on *Antenatal Education: Principles and Practice* gives practical ideas for education that liberates rather than encourages conformity.

The current political focus on midwifery services for disadvantaged women is identified in the chapter on 'The Social Context of Childbirth and Motherhood'. This focus is the result of stark evidence that women and babies who are most at risk of a poor outcome are least likely to receive the care they need[1].

The poor outcomes for disadvantaged women are attributable to a number of factors, including inaccessible services and judgemental attitudes. In the course of reviewing maternity services and antenatal teaching, I have repeatedly been told by disadvantaged women about how services have failed them, as a result of staff prejudging them and their wishes or of inadequate service provision.

One example is a teenage mother living in a deprived community who wished to breast-feed but whose partner was given a bottle to feed the baby while she was being stitched. Another is a young non-English speaking woman of Asian origin who said she did not know if she had been given any choices about birth as her husband had interpreted for her throughout her care.

The implications of these examples are obvious. The baby of the teenage mother was denied the many benefits of breast-feeding that would have mitigated his social disadvantage. The woman of Asian origin, as well as being denied any choice, had no means to communicate fundamental issues, such as domestic violence or undisclosed previous pregnancies.

Bharj's and Cooper's chapter eloquently explores the links between social disadvantage and poor health outcomes. It will support midwives to provide appropriate care for the women who need it most.

One of the strengths of this edition of *Myles* is that it addresses the challenges facing midwives and the stress these places on them. The emotional aspect of a midwife's work is rarely recognized. Billie Hunter's exploration of this is a welcome and necessary addition to the text.

A source of frustration to both midwives and women is the fact that the relationships between them often last no more than a shift on labour ward or a couple of antenatal visits. I particularly like Lesley Page's chapter entitled 'Woman-centred, Midwife-friendly Care' for its pragmatic and practical guidance. Page extols midwives to 'do the best you can' and points out that making a small change, such as moving furniture in a birth room, can make a big difference. It is this spirit that makes midwives so invaluable to child-bearing women. Page deals with the conflicting pressures that midwives face from medical and midwifery colleagues, women and their employers. In these circumstances, the professional autonomy of midwives is crucial. This is conferred by regulation.

The role that regulation plays in this autonomy is explored in Christina McKenzie's chapter, 'Midwifery Regulation in the United Kingdom'. McKenzie highlights the mechanisms of regulation, such as supervision, the Nursing and Midwifery Council's (NMC) Code of Professional Conduct and the Midwives Rules. Used wisely, regulation can give more power to a midwife's elbow. This newly extended chapter will support more midwives to use regulation to support women.

Midwives are among the people who have inspired me most, both those who have cared for me and those I have had the privilege to work alongside. These midwives have practised both the art and science of midwifery: listening to and respecting women; helping to keep things normal; involving other professionals when necessary; coordinating care to keep the woman at the centre.

This text will help midwives be confident in their role, skills and knowledge so that they can be truly with the women they care for. On behalf of all the women now and in the future who walk taller because of a midwife's role in their life story, thank you. Enjoy the read.

Jill Crawford

---

[1]Lewis G (ed) 2007. The Confidential Enquiry into Maternal and Child Health (CEMACH). Saving Mothers' Lives: reviewing maternal deaths to make motherhood safer – 2003-2005. The Seventh Report on Confidential Enquiries into Maternal Deaths in the United Kingdom. London, CEMACH.

Preface

This 15th edition of *Myles Textbook for Midwives* remains a substantial textbook, published in response to students and midwives overwhelming demand for such a key text. In acknowledgement of the increase in e-learning, most of the chapter authors have also produced some multiple choice questions that can be accessed electronically for self-assessment. In addition, the illustrations have been reproduced on the web with and without labels to aid student learning and as a resource for university midwife lecturers.

Given the importance of using best evidence to underpin midwifery practice, it has been vital to include sufficient references while ensuring essential content is not lost in a plethora of reference sources. This means that those source materials included can only be examples of the extensive literature available. Research findings and systematic reviews are regularly reported and only those available in the year prior to publication of this edition could be included.

Alongside this comprehensive textbook, Elsevier has published a *Survival Guide to Midwifery* which contains edited material from the *Myles* textbook. This *Survival Guide* does not include references in order to make it easily portable for use in clinical practice and for examination revision. Both books will be invaluable sources of information for students and midwives working in different practice contexts.

We are especially pleased that many chapter authors have continued to contribute to successive editions of this important textbook. A number of new authors are included in the 15th edition and in recognition of the 'emotion' work of midwives, a new chapter has been included. While the majority of expertise to write a book for midwives must come from midwives, the multi-professional and user contributions reflect the imperative to work and learn together to enhance the quality of maternity services for women and their families.

Women expect midwives to provide competent midwifery care and the content of this book is designed with this aim in mind. Equally essential are women's expectations that their care will be individualized and the attitudes and interpersonal skills of midwives will enable a professional/friend relationship to be developed. Specific chapters address the importance of these aspects of midwifery care and include parents' childbirth stories.

Whatever the context and the culture of the setting, this text seeks to convey the importance of woman-centred midwife-friendly care. Childbirth and parenting are life-changing experiences, although for the majority, the physiological process will be normal. When there are complications, the quality of individualized care and being enabled to make informed choices become even more important. The midwife has a key role to play in assisting women to make these choices and feel in control when presented with difficult options and dilemmas. This edition has therefore retained the integrated nature of sections of the 14th edition to continue to reduce the false impression that women fall into a 'low' or 'high' risk category for the whole of the childbearing continuum. Women's care pathway is likely to have episodes of complexity requiring additional care at particular times. This should not mean a total transference of lead carer. Instead the midwife has a key role in ensuring the woman receives the additional care and investigations needed from the most appropriate care provider at the most appropriate time. Midwifery care and support is required throughout. Hence the midwife's communication and teamwork skills and ability to juggle competing priorities and take decisions in complex situations are paramount requirements for competent midwifery practice.

In the UK, the work of the professional regulatory body, the Nursing and Midwifery Council (NMC) has seen rapid developments. The revisions incorporated in Chapter 7 have been essential to enable students and midwives to understand the statutory and guideline responsibilities of the NMC. However, midwives in the UK must though regularly access the NMC website to ensure they are using the most up to date rules and standards for midwifery practice.

Myles textbook has always prioritized the inclusion of clear and easy-to-understand illustrations. Where appropriate new diagrams have been drawn to enhance presentations and incorporate new evidence. This has been particularly important in relation to the anatomy of the pregnant uterus and lactating breast. The colour plate section of the book has also been much appreciated by students and hence has been retained.

The importance of providing women with the best available evidence to assist them make choices appropriate for them and their personal circumstances has been endorsed by the government. This provides midwives with dilemmas as to how much information they ask for and provide at each point in the childbearing period. Too much or too little information or advice at the wrong point can be confusing and hence the relationship between midwife and woman must be paramount, so that potential outcomes and uncertainties can be discussed honestly and good decisions made.

This book cannot provide all the knowledge midwives might need when working with women to make decisions about their care pathway and utilize interventions appropriately. However, we hope it will provide a comprehensive framework to assist in the decision-making process and stimulate midwives' passion for life-long learning.

(*Note:* Whenever the female gender is used the male is also implied and vice versa as appropriate.)

Nottingham 2009

Diane M. Fraser
Maggie A. Cooper

Acknowledgements

The volume editors wish to thank those authors who originated some of the chapters in earlier editions and whose work has provided the foundation for the current volume.

These include:

Jo Alexander
Jean Ball
Thelma Bamfield
Ruth Bennett
Anne Bent
Greta Beresford
Ruth Bevis
Tricia Murphy-Black
Eileen Brayshaw
Linda Brown
Patricia Cassidy
Sarah Das
Chloe Fisher
Liz Floyd
Jocelyn Franey
Annie Halliday
Edith Hillan
Deborah Hughes
Lea Jamieson
Rosemary Jenkins

Margaret Lang
Victoria Lewis
Alison Livingstone
Anne Matthew
Sinead McNally
Maureen Michie
Dora Opoku
Jean Proud
Sarah Rankin
Sarah Roch
Carolyn Roth
Christine Shiers
Jennifer Sleep
Helen Stapleton
Valerie Thomson
Anne Thompson
Valerie Tickner
Elizabeth Torley
Josephine Williams
Jane Winship

They also wish to thank those critical readers, particularly consultant obstetrician Margaret Ramsay, whose constructive comments facilitated the task of editing key chapters. The support of family, friends and colleagues has been much appreciated. Finally, the hard work of the chapter authors must be very warmly acknowledged and particular thanks must go to Lesley Dingley for her invaluable administrative support.

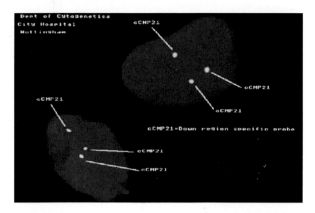

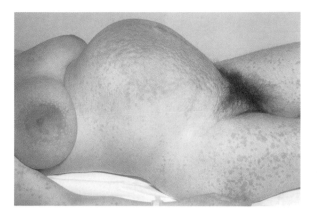

Plate 1 FISH showing Trisomy 21 (Down syndrome). (Reproduced with kind permission from the Department of Cytogenetics, Nottingham City Hospital NHS Trust.) (See text p 305.)

Plate 2 Pemphigoid gestationis (herpes gestationis). The generalised rash appeared at 34 weeks and responded to corticosteroids. This skin disease is rare (1 in 5-10,000 pregnancies), unique to pregnancy and of unknown aetiology. It resolves soon after delivery and may recur in successive pregnancies. Because of the increased risk of intrauterine death, fetal condition must be carefully assessed, and labour induced when the fetus is mature. (Reproduced with kind permission from Beischer, Mackay & Colditz 1997). (See text p 351.)

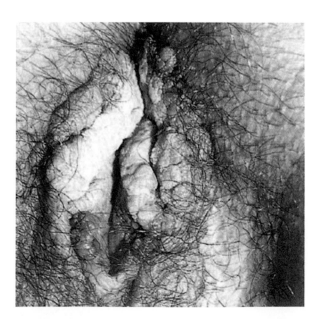

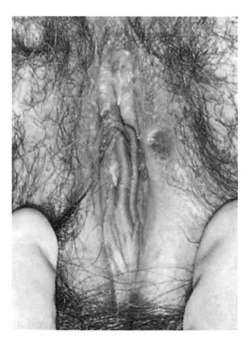

Plate 3 Massive warts in pregnancy. (Reproduced with kind permission from Blackwell Publishing, from Adler et al 2004.) (See text p 424.)

Plate 4 Primary chancre of vulva. (Reproduced with kind permission from Blackwell Publishing, from Adler et al 2004.) (See text p 423.)

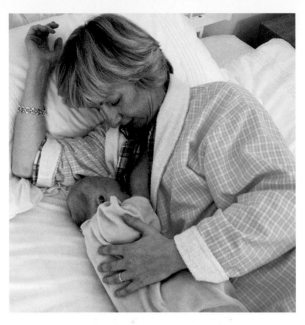

Plate 5 Mother feeding lying down. (Reproduced with kind permission from the Health Education Board for Scotland.) (See text p 794.)

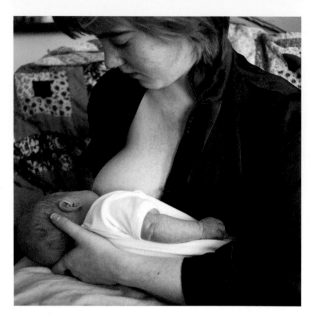

Plate 6 Mother feeding sitting up. (Reproduced with kind permission from the Health Education Board for Scotland.) (See text p 794.)

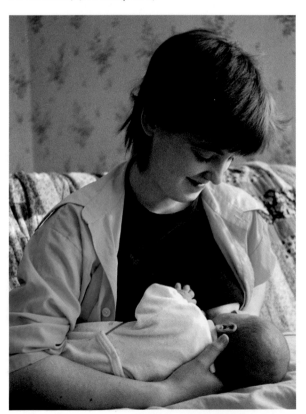

Plate 7 Mother supporting the baby's head with her fingers. (Reproduced with kind permission from the Health Education Board for Scotland.) (See text p 795.)

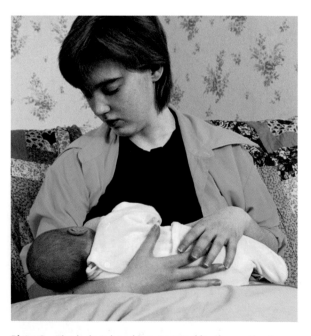

Plate 8 The baby's head is supported by the mother's forearm. (Reproduced with kind permission from the Health Education Board for Scotland.) (See text p 795.)

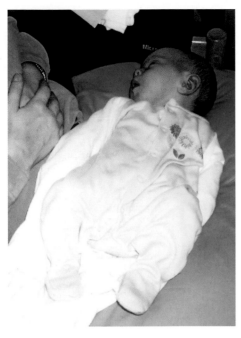

Plate 9 The Vancouver wrap to keep baby's hands by his side. (See text p 795.)

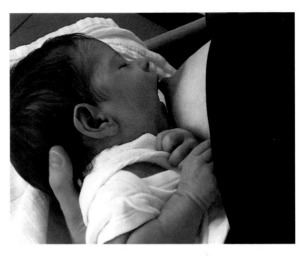

Plate 10 A wide gape. (Photo courtesy of the Health Education Board for Scotland and Mark-it TV *www.markittelevision.com*.) (See text p 795.)

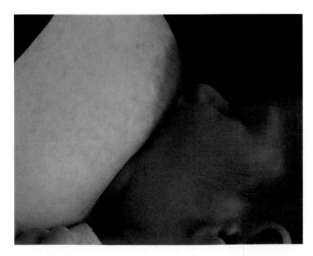

Plate 11 The baby forms a 'teat' from the breast and nipple. (Photo courtesy of the Health Education Board for Scotland and Mark-it TV *www.markittelevision.com*.) (See text p 795.)

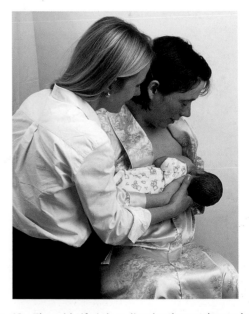

Plate 12 The midwife is kneeling by the mother to help her attach to the baby. (Reproduced with kind permission of Nancy Durrel-McKenna.) (See text p 796.)

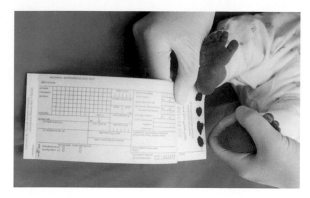

Plate 13   Blood screening. (See text p 779.)

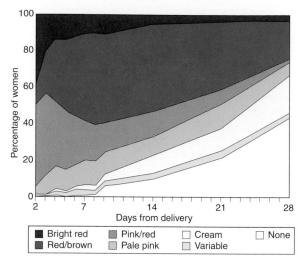

Plate 14   The colour of vaginal loss reported by women for the first 28 days postpartum. (Reproduced with kind permission from Midwifery 1995 15:80.) (See text p 657.)

Plate 15   Stool colour comparator. (Reproduced with kind permission from the Midwifery Department, Ninewells Hospital, Dundee, UK.) (See text p 798.)

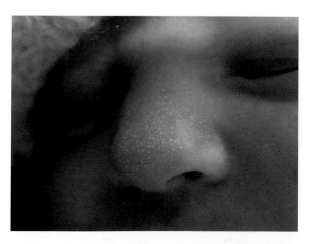

Plate 16   Milia (with thanks to Carl Kuschel 2007). (See text p 836.)

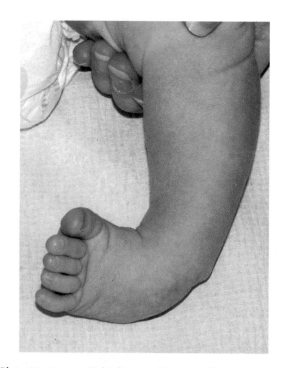

Plate 17   Congenital talipes equinovarus. (See text p 894.)

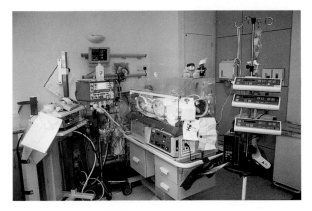

Plate 18 Neonatal intensive care. (See text p 844.)

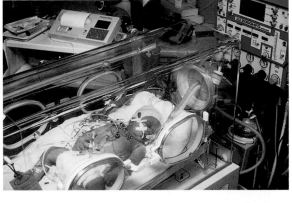

Plate 19 A baby requiring intensive care. (See text p 844.)

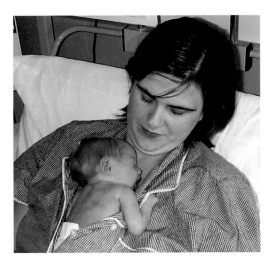

Plate 20 Kangaroo care. (See text p 828.)

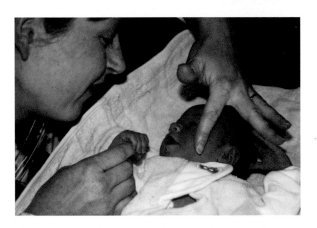

Plate 21 A jaundiced baby with its mother. Note the contrast in colour between the jaundiced skin of the baby and the mother's unjaundiced skin. (See text p 902.)

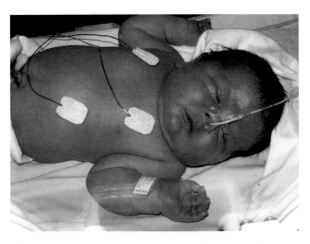

Plate 22 The baby of a diabetic mother. (See text p 931.)

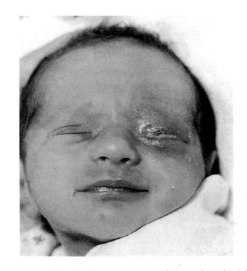

Plate 23 Ophthalmia neonatorum. (Reproduced with kind permission from Blackwell Publishing, from Adler et al 2004.) (See text p 421.)

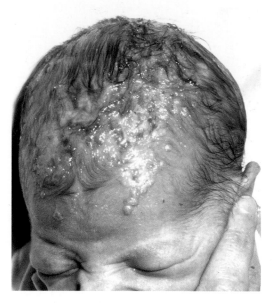

Plate 24 A rash produced by the herpes simplex virus. (See text p 837.)

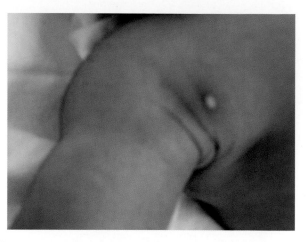

Plate 25 Staphylococcal pustule (with thanks to Carl Kuschel 2007). (See text p 837.)

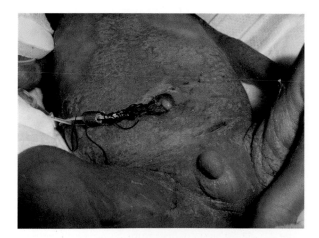

Plate 26 Staphylococcal abdomen (with thanks to Carl Kuschel 2007). (See text p 837.)

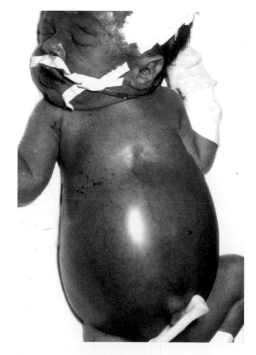

Plate 27 A distended abdomen in necrotising enterocolities. (See text p 842.)

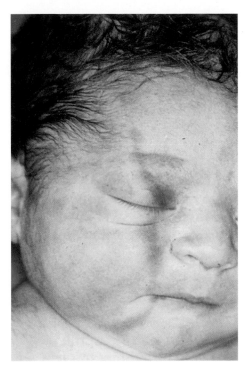

Plate 28 Forceps abrasion on cheek. (Reproduced by permission from Thomas and Harvey 1997.) (See text p 860.)

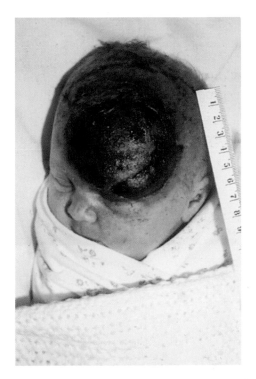

Plate 29 Scalp abrasion during vacuum-assisted birth; note the chignon. (Reproduced by permission from Thomas and Harvey 1997.) (See text p 860.)

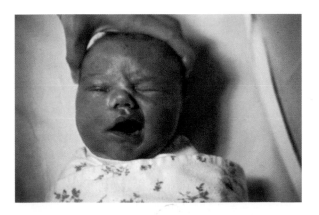

Plate 30 Right-sided facial palsy. Note that the eye is open on the paralysed side and the mouth is drawn over to the non-paralysed side. (Reproduced by permission from Thomas and Harvey 1997.) (See text p 861.)

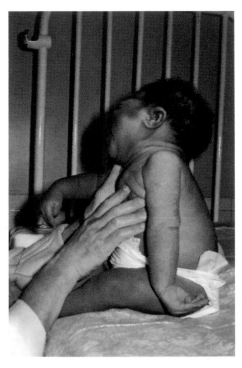

Plate 31 Erb's palsy. (Reproduced by permission from Thomas and Harvey 1997.) (See text p 599, p 862.)

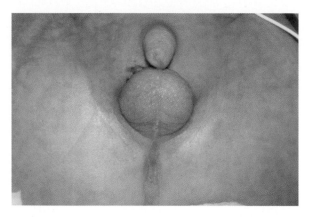

Plate 32 Imperforate anus with recto-vesical fistula (1). (Reproduced with permission of Donna Bain.) (See text p 885.)

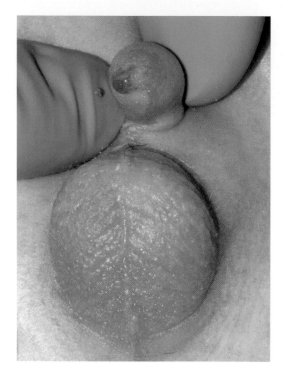

Plate 33 Imperforate anus with recto-vesical fistula (2). (Reproduced with permission of Donna Bain.) (See text p 885.)

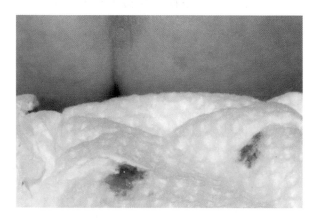

Plate 34 Imperforate anus with recto-vesical fistula and napkin containing meconium stained urine. (Reproduced with permission of Donna Bain.) (See text p 885.)

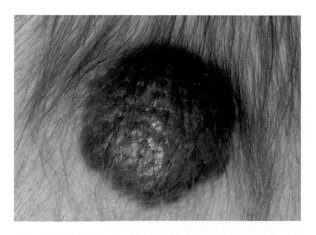

Plate 35 Evolving capillary haemangioma. (Reproduced with permission of Sharon Murphy.) (See text p 896.)

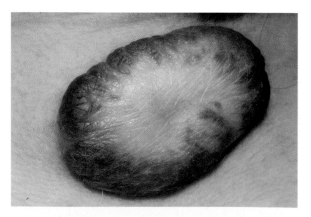

Plate 36 Regressing capillary haemangioma with typical pallor. (Reproduced with permission of Sharon Murphy.) (See text p 896.)

Section 1
Midwifery

SECTION CONTENTS

1 The midwife

Diane M. Fraser   Margaret A. Cooper

The midwife is recognized worldwide as being the person who is alongside and supporting women giving birth. The midwife also has a key role in promoting the health and well-being of childbearing women and their families before conception, antenatally and postnatally, including family planning.

In the UK, midwives are being urged to expand their role even further in the field of public health. Their responsibilities are to diagnose and monitor pregnancies, labours and postpartum progress, to work with childbearing women and other healthcare professionals to achieve the best possible outcomes for each individual family. This demands a wide range of skills, knowledge and personal attributes.

The chapter aims to:

- define the midwife in terms of expectations of her capabilities, from both the perspectives of childbearing women, the UK statutory body; World Health Organization (WHO) and the European Union (EU)
- discuss the continuing education and professional development of practising midwives.

Midwives, women and their birth partners

Midwife means 'with woman' or, in France, 'wise woman'. Throughout the ages, women have depended upon a skilled person, usually another woman, to be with them during childbirth. In the past, men were excluded from the birthing room, being allowed in only once the baby was born.

3

Now pregnant women are encouraged to choose a birth partner, male or female, to support them in labour. Midwives must therefore develop the skills to involve the woman's chosen birth partner(s) as well as supporting the woman. At times, this requires the midwife to stand back, observe, listen and intervene only when invited to do so or when it is in the best interests of the woman, fetus or baby. At other times the midwife will need to ensure that the woman's partner is appropriately informed about childbirth and parenting so that they can make sound decisions together. In the past, midwives have been criticized for neglecting the needs of fathers, ignoring them or pressurizing them to become more involved than they would choose if allowed to make their own decision (Bartels 1999).

On occasions, the midwife might need to act as the woman's advocate when the partner's/friend's/relative's actions are unlikely to enhance, or could harm, the health and safety of mother and child. In the 2003–2005 review of maternal deaths in the UK, over 14% of deaths were to women who reported to a health professional that they were in an abusive relationship (Lewis 2007). To understand and empathize with each woman's individual needs and encourage her to have confidence in her own body and capabilities for parenting, the midwife needs a high level of knowledge and decision-making abilities. It is this thorough grounding in knowledge, experience and personal insight that enables her to refrain from taking control away from the mother, while being at hand to step in when assistance is needed.

Alliances between childbearing women and midwives were pivotal in stemming the tide of technologically dominated, actively managed labours of the 1970s and 1980s (O'Driscoll & Meagher 1980). In 1992, the Government's Select Committee report (known as the Winterton report) on the maternity services was published (House of Commons Health Committee 1992). Evidence from women cited the importance of their having more choice, control and continuity of care when using the maternity services. More recently, Government policy further stated the need for the maternity services to ensure women have choice, access and continuity of care

in a safe service (DH 2007). Chapter 4 discusses some of the ways in which midwives and maternity services have responded.

Midwives and normal childbirth

Alongside the move to provide women with more choice, control and continuity has been the debate about what is 'normal' (Downe 2004) and how much choice should be available to women in a resource-limited National Health Service (NHS) and increasingly litigious society (see Ch. 53 Risk management). A difficulty of definition arises over whether any interventions can be classed as being 'normal' and from whose perspective. For example an ultrasound scan in early pregnancy has become routine but can change an anticipated pleasurable event to a stressful pregnancy (see Chs 18 and 38). At the other extreme, views are polarized as to whether women whose pregnancy is uncomplicated should be able to demand a caesarean rather than a vaginal birth (Kaufman & Liu 2001).

Midwives will find themselves working as independent practitioners with their 'normal' caseload for much of the time yet, perhaps on the same day, participating in a multiprofessional team when complications develop. There are strong arguments for providing women whose care becomes more complicated with as good, if not even better, continuity of midwifery care if it can really be claimed that midwives are 'with woman' (Gould 2002). At times, this will give midwives dilemmas in prioritization and on occasion, their own views will not always coincide with those of the woman or other healthcare professionals. Chapter 5 may help in the resolution of ethical dilemmas, while the book as a whole will assist midwives in diagnosing and providing care both when childbirth is straightforward and when it is less so. No textbook or current best evidence can provide all the answers and midwives need to learn to cope with uncertainty, be knowledgeable about what is known and not known and have the confidence to engage effectively in multiprofessional discussions about best practice, audit and research. Although intellectual and clinical skills and competencies are essential for safe midwifery practice, the midwife's interpersonal skills are likely to be what makes a difference to women's experiences and memories of childbirth.

Definition and capabilities of the midwife

Midwives need to be aware of the legislation and guidelines defining their role, describing their scope of practice and specifying standards of competence or proficiency. Some of the most significant are highlighted in this chapter.

In 1972, a definition of the midwife was developed by the International Confederation of Midwives (ICM). A year later, it was adopted by the International Federation of Gynaecology and Obstetrics (FIGO) followed by the WHO. In 1990, at the Kobe Council meeting, the ICM amended the definition, which was later ratified by FIGO in 1991 and by WHO in 1992. In 2005, it was amended slightly by the ICM Council (Box 1.1).

At the European level, member states of the EU (known at the time as the European Community, EC), prepared a list of activities that midwives should be entitled to take up within its territory (EC Midwives Directive 1980). Although midwives must learn about all of these activities, in the UK it is recognized that it is highly unlikely that midwives would be expected to be proficient in them all – for example the manual removal of the placenta would be carried out by a doctor unless no doctor is available and the mother's life is at risk (Box 1.2).

Fitness for practice, award and purpose

It might be expected that if midwives are fit to practice, they will also be fit to work in any setting and be eligible to receive the appropriate award from the university where they were educated.

Fitness for practice

In the UK, the Nursing and Midwifery Council specify what proficiencies have to be achieved before a student is eligible to register as a practising midwife (NMC 2004a). A list of proficiencies does not

Box 1.1 International definition of the midwife (ICM 2005)

'A midwife is a person who, having been regularly admitted to a midwifery educational programme, duly recognized in the country in which it is located, has successfully completed the prescribed course of studies in midwifery and has acquired the requisite qualifications to be registered and/or legally licensed to practise midwifery.

The midwife is recognized as a responsible and accountable professional who works in partnership with women to give the necessary support, care and advice during pregnancy, labour and the postpartum period, to conduct births on the midwife's own responsibility and to provide care for the newborn and the infant. This care includes preventative measures, the promotion of normal birth, the detection of complications in mother and child, the accessing of medical care or other appropriate assistance and the carrying out of emergency measures.

The midwife has an important task in health counselling and education, not only for the woman, but also within the family and the community. This work should involve antenatal education and preparation for parenthood and may extend to women's health, sexual or reproductive health and child care.

A midwife may practise in any setting including the home, community, hospitals, clinics or health units'.

necessarily capture what should be a holistic definition of a competent midwife. Figure 1.1 demonstrates the outcome of a research study that attempted to do so (Fraser et al 1998). The 'professional/friend' dimension in this model was found to be of most significance to childbearing women (Berg et al 1996, Fraser 1999, Waldenstrom et al 1995). Assessment schemes for fitness for practice must therefore encompass this dimension as well as assessment of clinical proficiencies and the NMC essential skills clusters (2007).

Box 1.2 Activities of a midwife: the European Directive (NMC 2004b, p 36–37)

'Member states shall ensure that midwives are at least entitled to take up and pursue the following activities:

- to provide sound family planning information and advice
- to diagnose pregnancies and monitor normal pregnancies; to carry out examinations necessary for the monitoring of the development of normal pregnancies
- to prescribe or advise on the examinations necessary for the earliest possible diagnosis of pregnancies at risk
- to provide a programme of parenthood preparation and a complete preparation for childbirth including advice on hygiene and nutrition
- to care for and assist the mother during labour and to monitor the condition of the fetus in utero by the appropriate clinical and technical means
- to conduct spontaneous deliveries including where required an episiotomy and in urgent cases a breech delivery
- to recognize the warning signs of abnormality in the mother or infant which necessitate referral to a doctor and to assist the latter where appropriate; to take the necessary emergency measures in the doctor's absence, in particular the manual removal of the placenta, possibly followed by manual examination of the uterus
- to examine and care for the newborn infant; to take all initiatives which are necessary in case of need and to carry out where necessary immediate resuscitation
- to care for and monitor the progress of the mother in the post-natal period and to give all necessary advice to the mother on infant care to enable her to ensure the optimum progress of the new-born infant
- to carry out the treatment prescribed by a doctor
- to maintain all necessary records'.

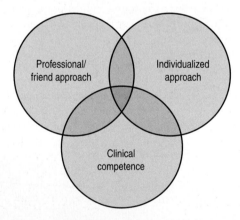

Figure 1.1 An holistic, integrated model of a competent midwife. (From Fraser et al 1998, p 32, reproduced with permission from the English National Board for Nursing, Midwifery and Health Visiting, ENB.)

Fitness for award

In addition to the requirements of the NMC, universities have to demonstrate that their programmes meet Quality Assurance Agency for Higher Education (QAAHE) subject benchmark statements. The QAAHE developed an overarching health professions framework encompassing:

- expectations of the health profession in providing patient/client services
- the application of practice in securing, maintaining or improving health and well-being
- the knowledge, understanding and skills that underpin the education and training of healthcare professionals.

This framework illustrates the academic and practitioner features that are held in common. These are developed more fully in each subject's benchmark statement and standards to describe the profession specific expectations and requirements. A total of 34 midwifery standards have been specified to set out the different expectations of midwives entering their first post immediately on completion of a pre-registration programme of midwifery (QAAHE 2001).

Fitness for purpose

Although NHS Trusts can now refer to national proficiency (NMC 2004a) and benchmark standards (QAAHE 2001) to clarify their expectations of new midwives, there are still likely to be local variations. This might include variations in opportunities, for example to suture perineums (Ch. 28), 'top-up' epidurals (Ch. 27) or assist women to give birth in water. What is more important than small variations in learning opportunities and the development of specific psychomotor skills is a midwife's personal insight including the recognition of her capabilities and when it is necessary to learn new skills.

When taking up employment, it is essential for midwives to discuss their development needs and ensure that they are not expected to undertake activities for which they have not been prepared or are inappropriate for their level of expertise. Each midwife is allocated, or chooses a person to be her supervisor of midwives. This person is invaluable in assisting with a midwife's personal development plan and providing support in difficult contexts (Ch. 52).

Autonomous midwifery practice

Once qualified as a midwife, there are a variety of employment opportunities. However, whichever type of midwifery organization provides employment, the midwife, even at the point of registration, has responsibility for and autonomy within her sphere of practice. Professional autonomy for midwives does not, however, mean that midwives should create professional boundaries and exert powers to protect their territory. Instead autonomy means having freedom to act on behalf of childbearing women, working in partnership with them and having the knowledge and capability to provide continuity of carer for women with straightforward pregnancies as well as working in partnership with other members of the healthcare team (DoH 2001) when this is in the best interests of the woman, fetus or newborn. Chapter 2 discusses how the midwife's responsibilities can be described as 'emotion work'.

The NMC describes seven guiding principles which establish their philosophy and values in relation to expected outcomes of midwifery programmes.

1. Provision of women-centred care

Every woman expects to be treated as though she is special and important. Although at times maternity units and community workloads can be busy, individual women want midwives to be there for them, not for someone else. It is essential that midwives have an understanding of social, cultural and context differences (see Ch. 3) so that they can respond to the needs of women and their families in a variety of care settings and prioritize and manage work appropriately. Of particular importance is working with families to draw up a plan of care and support and then evaluate and modify that care as circumstances warrant. To do this, midwives need knowledge of available resources and expertise so that members of the multidisciplinary team and other organizations can be drawn upon as required to meet the holistic needs of individual women.

2. Ethical and legal obligations

The practice of a midwife is controlled by law (NMC 2004b and Ch. 7). Midwives also need to be familiar with other Acts of Parliament and Statutory Instruments that impact on their practice. Dimond has written extensively on the interpretation and application of law in midwifery in journals and in her own book (Dimond 2002).

The NMC Code (NMC 2008a) sets requirements for the behaviour of midwives and nurses in relation to conduct, performance and ethics (see Ch. 5). Midwives may find themselves expected to care for women who have decided to terminate their pregnancy. Whilst midwives may exercise a conscientious objection in relation to participating in the termination, they cannot refuse to provide care for the woman because they disagree with her decision to terminate. Counselling services are normally provided for women and staff facing these sorts of ethical dilemmas and stressful situations.

3. Respect for individuals and communities

Society is composed of people from many cultural, ethnic and religious backgrounds. Midwifery care must be provided in a non-discriminatory way and without prejudice. Where midwives find they do not have the skills or expertise to provide effective care for individuals or groups then they need to seek assistance. In areas where there are a number of women who do not speak the local language, link workers or an interpreting service can be more appropriate than asking another family member, especially a child, to communicate between the woman and the midwife (see Chs 3 and 55).

4. Quality and excellence

Individual midwives should strive for continual improvement and excellence in midwifery practice. To protect the health and well-being of mothers and babies, supervision of midwives is enshrined in statute. Clinical governance has more recently been established to assure the quality of all the health services provided by an individual NHS Trust and has many principles that mirror statutory supervision of midwives (Ch. 52). Auditing of standards and discussion of difficult maternity care scenarios are ways in which all professional groups can work together to improve the quality of the service. Involvement of mothers in evaluating care and suggestions for areas that need improvement have become even more important in contributing to quality and excellence in the maternity services.

5. The changing nature and context of midwifery practice

The pace of change is likely to increase throughout the new millennium and midwives need to be prepared to adapt accordingly. This is likely to include embracing new technologies, provided they enhance the quality of care, working in new ways as patterns of care change and listening to mothers to understand what matters to them (see Chs 4 and 18). It will be essential for midwives to discriminate between change that is likely to benefit the woman and her family and change that is for administrative or other non-care-related convenience. Midwives need to be flexible and also become agents of change when necessary. This might necessitate learning new skills or further developing existing ones and having the initiative to identify when change is needed.

6. Evidence-based practice and learning

The use of the term 'evidence-based' rather than 'research-based' practice has been growing (Proctor & Renfrew 2000, Renfrew 1997). This is intended to draw practitioners' attention to the need for sound evidence for effective care and not assume that all research is of value but that it must be critically analysed. It is also intended to foster the use of systematic reviews such as *Effective care in pregnancy and childbirth* (Chalmers et al 1989), the regularly updated guides and the electronic Cochrane Library to which most universities and NHS Trusts subscribe. Assistance with accessing the literature can normally be obtained from librarians as well as from journals and books (e.g. Stanton & Fraser 2000).

Chapter 6 provides more information on evidence and research and midwives need to be aware that there are now many good qualitative studies that add to the body of midwifery knowledge and understanding. The midwife has a responsibility to make use of all available resources to inform her practice, including experiential knowledge. She has a duty to weigh up the latest clinical evidence, that elicited by her personal observations, and to take account of her experiences and the woman's wishes.

7. Lifelong learning

Development of different learning styles can aid effective lifelong learning. Laurillard (2002) and Miller et al (1994) believe that it is important to encourage students to vary their learning style according to context or goal. Whereas some might learn best by adopting a surface or memory style of learning, this alone will be inadequate unless students can also develop a deep level of processing information. The 'skills drills' that are suggested to help midwives respond rapidly and effectively to emergency situations (Ch. 33) lend themselves to surface styles of learning, but when situations are complex and require much investigation and reflection then problem-solving and critiquing skills become essential. With so much information available, it can be difficult for midwives to know where to go to keep up-to-date. Databases are useful for searching for topics of relevance and systematic reviews are invaluable in synthesising and evaluating the huge amount of research data.

As well as learning from the literature, midwives also need to grasp opportunities to learn from each other by observing and discussing different ways of practising and, where necessary, seeking out appropriate education or training events.

Continuing professional development (CPD)

All midwives and nurses have to meet PREP (post-registration education and practice) requirements to renew their professional registration (NMC 2008b). Evidence to fulfil these requirements has to be presented in the form of a personal professional profile which demonstrates that practitioners have been developing their knowledge and expertise during the previous 3 years. However, in a rapidly changing maternity service, these minimum requirements are likely to be insufficient for competent midwifery practice.

Professional profiles

There are many commercially produced guides to assist in preparing a professional profile as well as folders that can be purchased to record evidence of CPD. However, a ring binder and set of dividers can equally well fulfil a practitioner's needs and lends itself to being individually stylized. Alternatively, the profile can be maintained electronically but a hard copy will be needed if requested for audit purposes by the Nursing and Midwifery Council.

Midwives are required to record evidence of study and learning relevant to their sphere of practice. The following five categories should cover most fields of professional practice:

- care enhancement, e.g. developments in practice, standard setting, empowering women
- reducing risk, e.g. health promotion and screening, identification of health problems, protection of individuals
- client/patient and colleague support, e.g. counselling, leadership, supervision
- practice development, e.g. personal research and study, change agent, visiting other practice areas
- education development, e.g. mentorship and lecturer/practice educator programmes.

As well as being a mandatory requirement for maintaining professional registration, a personal profile can be useful when applying for a job, providing evidence when claiming non-standard entry or advanced standing for a course of study as well as aiding personal development through reflection and as a basis for discussion at supervisory reviews.

APL and APEL

Accreditation of prior learning (APL) and accreditation of prior experiential learning (APEL) are often possible for a number of post-registration courses. These involve matching what you have done before with the course you are now interested in studying. If there is evidence of equivalence, then exemption from certain modules and units might be permitted. Credit will then be awarded provided there is evidence that prior study or learning is authentic, relevant, had appropriate depth and breadth and was relatively recent. APL/APEL schemes vary between universities and just because one university will allow perhaps a third of the course to be exempt through APL/APEL there is no guarantee that another will allow the same sort of percentage exemption. Normally there will be advisors to guide prospective students through the process.

Career pathways

There are a number of different possibilities for midwives to consider when planning their longer-term careers. Whichever route is intended, all will require evidence of high motivation and lifelong learning. The following nine hallmarks of a lifelong nurse/midwife learner were identified in 1994 and are still relevant (ENB 1994):

- responsible and accountable for their work
- self-reliant in their way of working
- adaptable to changing healthcare needs
- flexible to changing demands
- challenging and creative
- innovative
- resourceful
- able to work as agents of change
- able to share and promote good practice and knowledge.

This can be a helpful framework when identifying training and education needs for development alongside acquiring new skills to meet service needs. Midwives now have an exciting array of career opportunities, which include: caseload practice; a career as expert/leader in specific areas of midwifery practice such as consultant midwife, birth centre lead midwife, neonatal practitioner, hospital labour suite coordinator and ventouse practitioner; a career in management, whether in midwifery or more general management in the NHS; a career as midwife researcher on midwifery and collaborative projects; a career in education as a midwife lecturer in a university; a career in standard setting and audit; a career as the midwife expert in multiprofessional teams such as teenage pregnancy, drug addiction, domestic abuse, fetomaternal medicine and also opportunities to work in developing countries (see Ch. 55). In addition a midwife learns a multitude of valuable transferable skills.

As you pursue your midwifery career it is essential to reflect in and on your practice (some useful guidance can be found in Church & Raynor 2000). By so doing, you will not only understand more about your own learning capabilities, but most importantly will see how you can make a difference to the childbirth experiences of women and their families. Reflection is not, however, sufficient; it needs to be followed by appropriate action and understanding that different actions may be required in different contexts. Chapters 3 and 4 provide a discussion of some of the varying contexts in which a midwife practises.

REFERENCES

Bartels R 1999 Experience of childbirth from the father's perspective. British Journal of Midwifery 7:681–683

Berg M, Lundgren I, Hermansson E et al 1996 Women's experience of the encounter with the midwife during childbirth. Midwifery 12:11–15

Chalmers I, Enkin M, Keirse M J N C (eds) 1989 Effective care in pregnancy and childbirth. Oxford University Press, Oxford

Church P, Raynor M D 2000 Reflection and articulating intuition. In: Fraser D (ed.) Professional studies for midwifery practice. Churchill Livingstone, Edinburgh, p 23–43

Dimond B 2002 Legal aspects of midwifery, 2nd edn. Books for Midwives Press, Hale

DoH (Department of Health) 2001 Working together – learning together. A framework for lifelong learning for the NHS. DoH, London

DH (Department of Health) 2007 Maternity matters: Choice, access and continuity of care in a safe service. DH, London

Downe S 2004 Normal childbirth: Evidence and debate. Churchill Livingstone, Edinburgh

EC Midwives Directive 1980 EC Council Directive 80/155/EEC Article 4. Official Journal of the European Communities L33/28

ENB (English National Board for Nursing Midwifery and Health Visiting) 1994 Creating lifelong learners. Partnerships for care. ENB, London

Fraser D M 1999 Women's perceptions of midwifery care: a longitudinal study to inform curriculum development. Birth, Issues in Perinatal Care 26:99–107

Fraser D, Murphy R, Worth-Butler M 1998 Preparing effective midwives: an outcome evaluation of the effectiveness of pre-registration programmes of education. ENB, London

Gould D 2002 One-to-one midwifery – making it happen. British Journal of Midwifery 10:17

House of Commons Health Committee 1992 Second report, Maternity services, Vol 1. HMSO, London

ICM (International Confederation of Midwives) 2005 Definition of the midwife. ICM, London

Kaufman T, Liu D 2001 Should caesareans be performed only on the basis of medical need? Nursing Times 97:17

Laurillard D 2002 Rethinking university teaching, 2nd edn. Routledge Palmer, London

Lewis G (ed.) 2007 The Confidential Enquiry into Maternal and Child Health (CEMACH). Saving Mothers' Lives: reviewing maternal deaths to make motherhood safer – 2003–2005. The Seventh Report on Confidential Enquiries into Maternal Deaths in the United Kingdom. CEMACH, London

Miller C, Tomlinson A, Jones M 1994 Learning styles and facilitating reflection. ENB, London

NMC (Nursing and Midwifery Council) 2008a The Code: Standards of conduct, performance and ethics for nurses and midwives. NMC, London

NMC (Nursing and Midwifery Council) 2007 Introduction of essential skills clusters for pre-registration midwifery education programmes. NMC circular 23/2007. NMC, London

NMC (Nursing and Midwifery Council) 2008b The PREP handbook. NMC, London

NMC (Nursing and Midwifery Council) 2004a Standards of proficiency for pre-registration midwifery education. NMC, London

NMC (Nursing and Midwifery Council) 2004b Midwives rules and standards. NMC, London

O'Driscoll K, Meagher D 1980 Active management of labour. W B Saunders, London

Proctor S, Renfrew M (eds) 2000 Research and practice in midwifery. A guide to evidence-based practice. Baillière Tindall, Edinburgh

QAAHE (Quality Assurance Agency for Higher Education) 2001 Subject benchmark statements: healthcare programme – midwifery. QAAHE, Gloucester

Renfrew M J 1997 The development of evidence based practice. British Journal of Midwifery 5:100–104

Stanton W, Fraser D 2000 Accessing the literature. In: Fraser D (ed.) Professional studies for midwifery practice. Churchill Livingstone, Edinburgh, p 2–3

Waldenstrom U, Borg I M, Olsson B 1995 The childbirth experience: a study of 295 new mothers. Birth 23:144–153

2

The emotional context of midwifery

Billie Hunter

In this chapter the emotional context of midwifery work is explored. Pregnancy and childbirth are emotional experiences for the woman and her family. Midwives need to work in an emotionally aware and sensitive way, in order to ensure that these feelings are acknowledged and responded to. To do this effectively, midwives also need to be aware of their own feelings. Much of midwifery work is emotionally demanding. Midwives need to understand why this is so, and find ways to manage feelings that are effective and sustainable. How midwives 'feel' about their work and the women they care for is important. It has significant implications for communication and interpersonal relationships with both clients and colleagues. It also has much wider implications for the quality of maternity services in general.

This chapter aims to:

- explore why maternity care requires management of emotions
- define what is meant by 'emotion work'
- identify the sources of emotion work for midwives
- explore how conflicting models of practice may create emotion work
- describe how midwives manage their emotions
- consider how midwives can develop emotional awareness.

> **Box 2.1** Key terms
>
> **Emotion work:** the work undertaken to manage feelings so that they are appropriate for a particular situation.
>
> **Feeling rules:** social norms regarding which emotions are considered appropriate to feel and to display, affected by social setting and culture.

Introduction

By its very nature, midwifery work involves a range of emotions. Midwifery is rarely dull. Even when it entails what may appear to be routine and mundane activities, these are often far from ordinary experiences for those on the receiving end of maternity care. While it is easy to see why birth is a highly charged emotional event; it may be less obvious to appreciate why an antenatal booking or postnatal visit can generate emotions. But women tell us that this can be so (Edwards 2000, Redshaw et al 2007, Wilkins 2000). There is clear evidence from research studies that women do not always receive the emotional support from midwives that they would wish (Beech & Phipps 2004, Berg et al 1996, Redshaw et al 2007).

It may also be less easy to understand how maternity care may be an emotional experience for those providing care – but we also know from research evidence that midwives have just this experience (Begley 2003, Deery 2005, Hunter 2004a, 2005, 2006, Kirkham 1999). In the words of a first year midwifery student:

It can be incredibly stressful, can be emotionally draining or the other way – an absolute high

(Hunter & Deery 2005, p 11)

What is meant by 'emotion work'?

Over the past 25 years there has been growing interest in how emotions affect the work that we do (Fineman 2000). This interest was stimulated by an American study undertaken by Arlie Russell Hochschild in 1983, which drew attention to the importance of emotion in the workplace, and to the work that needs be done when managing emotions. Hochschild's study of American flight attendants identified that a significant aspect of their work was to create a safe and secure environment for passengers, and that in order to do so, they needed to manage the emotions of their customers and themselves.

Hochschild defined emotional labour as: 'The induction or suppression of feeling in order to sustain an outward appearance that produces in others a sense of being cared for in a convivial, safe place' (Hochschild 1983, p 7). In other words, it is the work that is undertaken to manage feelings so that they are appropriate for a particular situation (Hochschild 1983). This is done in accordance with 'feeling rules', social norms regarding which emotions it is considered appropriate to feel and to display. (For example, Hunter and Deery (2005) note how midwives describe suppressing their feelings in order to maintain a reassuring atmosphere for women and their partners.)

Hochschild used the term 'emotional labour' to mean management of emotion within the public domain, as part of the employment contract between employer and employee; 'emotion work' referred to management of emotion in the private domain, i.e. the home. Hochschild's research focused particularly on commercial organizations, where workers are required to provide a veneer of hospitality in order to present a corporate image, with the ultimate aim of profit making (e.g. the 'switch on smile' of the flight attendants or the superficial enjoinders to 'have a nice day' from shop assistants). This requires the use of 'acting' techniques, which Hochschild (1983) argues may estrange workers from what they are really feeling. My research study (Hunter 2004a) suggests that the emotion management of midwives is different to this. Midwives were more able to exercise autonomy in how they controlled emotions, and emotion management was driven by a desire to 'make a difference' based on ideals of caring and service, that Bolton (2005, p 93) describes as 'philanthropic emotion management'. Thus I will use the term 'emotion work' in this chapter.

Emotions and healthcare

Although the emotional aspect of work appears to be as demanding as physical labour, it is often unrecognized, under-reported and under-valued (Hochschild 1983, James 1992). It is particularly common in public service work, and is often part of the 'invisible' work undertaken by women. The idea of emotion work is particularly relevant to healthcare, and there has been growing interest in this issue over the past 15 years (e.g. Bolton 2000, James 1992, Smith 1992). Smith (1992) investigated how student nurses learnt to 'do' emotion work. She observed that they gained emotion management skills 'on the job', using senior nurses as role models. Their emotional responses changed during their education. By the time they reached their final year, most had learnt self-protective coping strategies to manage feelings of distress and grief. These strategies included distancing themselves from patients and using a task-orientated approach to care. There is also evidence that midwives may use similar strategies (Hunt and Symonds 1995, Hunter 2004a).

Sources of emotion work in maternity care

What is it about maternity care that generates emotion work for midwives? On the surface, it could be presumed that midwifery is the 'happy side' of healthcare, and that only positive emotions will usually be felt. While it is often the case that the childbirth experience is a source of joy for all involved, sadly this is not always so.

Research studies suggest that there are various sources of emotion work in midwifery. These can be grouped into three key themes, which are discussed in turn:

1. Midwife–woman relationships
2. Collegial relationships
3. The organization of maternity care.

It is important to note that these themes are often interlinked. For example, the organization of maternity care impacts on both midwife–woman relationships and on collegial relationships.

Midwife–woman relationships

The nature of pregnancy and childbirth means that midwives work with women and their families during some of the most emotionally charged times of human life. The excited anticipation that generally surrounds the announcement of a pregnancy and the birth of a baby may be tempered with anxieties about changes in role identity, altered sexual relationships and fears about pain and altered body image (Raphael Leff 2005). Thus it is important to remember that even the most delighted of new mothers may experience a wide range of feelings about their experiences.

We must also remember that pregnancy and birth are not always joyful experiences: for example, midwives work with women who have unplanned or unwanted pregnancies, who are in unhappy or abusive relationships, and where fetal abnormalities or antenatal problems are detected. In these cases, midwives need to support women and their partners with great sensitivity and emotional awareness. This requires excellent interpersonal skills, particularly the ability to listen. It is easy in such distressing situations to try to help by giving advice and adopting a problem-solving approach. However, the evidence suggests that this is often inappropriate, and that what is much more beneficial is a non-judgemental listening ear (Clement 1995).

Childbirth itself is a time of heightened emotion, and brings with it exposure to pain, bodily fluids and issues of sexuality, all of which may prove challenging to the woman, her partner and also to those caring for her. Attending a woman in childbirth is highly intimate work, and the feelings that this engenders may come as a surprise to new students. For example, undertaking vaginal examinations is an intimate activity, and needs to be acknowledged as such (Bergstrom et al 1992, Stewart 2005). In the past, the emotional aspects of these issues have tended to be ignored within the education of midwives.

Relationships between midwives and women may vary considerably in their quality, level of intimacy and sense of personal connection. Some relationships may be intense and short-lived (e.g. when a midwife and woman meet on the labour ward or birth centre for the first time); intense and long-lived (e.g. when a midwife provides continuity of carer throughout pregnancy, birth and the postnatal period). They may also be relatively superficial, whether the contact is short-lived or longer standing. There is evidence that a key issue in midwife–woman relationships is the level of 'reciprocity' that is experienced (Fleming 1998, Hunter 2006). Reciprocity is defined as 'exchanging things with others for mutual benefit'

(*Oxford Dictionary* 2003). When relationships are experienced as 'reciprocal' or 'balanced', the midwife and woman are in a harmonious situation. Both are able to give to the other and to receive what is given (e.g. the midwife can give support and advice, and the woman is happy to accept this, and in return affirm the value of the midwife's care).

In contrast, relationships may become unbalanced, and in these situations emotion work is needed by the midwife. For example, a woman may be hostile to the midwife's advice, or alternatively, she may expect more in terms of personal friendship than the midwife feels it is appropriate or feasible to offer. Some midwives working in continuity of care schemes have expressed concerns about 'getting the balance right' in their relationships with women, so that they can offer authentic support without overstepping personal boundaries and becoming burnt out (Hunter 2006, Stevens & McCourt 2002a,b).

Establishing and maintaining reciprocal relationships can prove challenging at times. The concept of being a 'professional friend' (Fraser 1999, Pairman 2000, Walsh 1999) can be helpful in these situations, as it describes a model of midwife–woman relationships which is not only warm and supportive, but also sustainable for all concerned. It is also important that midwives pay careful attention to the power dynamics of their relationships with women. Both Leap (2000) and Cronk (2000) provide insights into these dynamics, noting the potential that exists for midwives to assume power over women. In different ways, they suggest practical solutions to help re-balance such relationships.

Collegial relationships

Relationships between midwives and their colleagues, both within midwifery and with other health and social care professionals, are also key sources of emotion work. Much of the existing evidence pertains to relationships between midwifery colleagues. These relationships may be positive or negative experiences.

Positive collegial relationships provide both practical and emotional support (Sandall 1997). Walsh (2007) provides an excellent example of these in his ethnography of a free standing birth centre. He observed a strong 'communitarian ideal' (Walsh 2007, p 77), whereby midwives provided each other

with mutual support built on trust, compassion and solidarity. He attributes this to the birth centre model, with its emphasis on relationships, facilitation and cooperation.

Sadly, however, such experiences are not always universal. There is also evidence that intimidation and bullying exists within contemporary UK midwifery (Hadikin & O'Driscoll 2000, Hunter 2005, Kirkham 1999, Leap 1997). The concept of 'horizontal violence' (Leap 1997) is often used to explain this problem. Kirkham (1999) explains how groups who have been oppressed internalize the values of powerful groups, thereby rejecting their own values. As a result, criticism is directed within the group (hence the term 'horizontal violence'), particularly towards those who are considered to have different views from the norm. This type of workplace conflict inevitably affects the emotional well-being of the midwifery workforce (Hunter 2005).

The organization of maternity care

The way in which maternity care is organized may also be a source of emotion work for midwives. The fragmented, task orientated nature of much hospital-based maternity care creates emotionally difficult situations for midwives (Ball et al 2002, Deery 2005, Dykes 2005, Hunter 2004a, 2005, Kirkham 1999), as it reduces opportunities for establishing meaningful relationships with clients and colleagues, and for doing 'real midwifery'. The study by Ball et al (2002) identified frustration with the organization of maternity care as one of the key reasons why midwives leave the profession. A study by Lavender and Chapple (2004) explored the views of midwives working in different settings. They found that all participants shared a common model of ideal practice, which included autonomy, equity of care for women and job satisfaction. However, midwives varied in how successful they were in achieving this. Advantageous factors were thought to be strong midwifery leadership and a workplace culture that promoted normality. Free-standing birth centres were usually described as being more satisfying and supportive environments, which facilitated the establishing of rewarding relationships with women and their families. Conversely, consultant-led units were often experienced negatively; this was partly the result of a dominant medicalized model of child-birth, a task-orientated approach to care and a culture of 'lots of criticism and no praise' (Lavender and Chapple 2004, p 9).

In general, it would appear that midwives working in community-based practice or in birth centre settings are more emotionally satisfied with their work (Hunter 2004a, Sandall 1997, Walsh 2007). Although there is the potential for continuity of care schemes to increase emotion work as a result of altered boundaries in the midwife–woman relationship, there is also evidence to suggest that when these schemes are organized and managed effectively, they provide emotional rewards for both midwives and clients.

A key reason underpinning these differing emotion work experiences appears to be the co-existence of conflicting models of midwifery practice (Hunter 2004a). Although midwifery as a profession has a strong commitment to providing woman-centred care, this is frequently not achievable in practice, particularly within large institutions. An approach to care which focuses on the needs of individual women may be at odds with an approach which is driven by institutional demands to provide efficient and equitable care to large numbers of women and babies 24 hrs a day, 7 days a week. When midwives are able to work in a 'with woman' way, there is congruence between ideals and reality, and work is experienced as being emotionally rewarding. When it is impossible for midwives to work in this way, as is often the case, midwives experience a sense of disharmony. This may lead to anger, distress and frustration, all of which require emotion work (Hunter 2004a).

Managing emotions in midwifery

So how do midwives learn to manage emotions, and what are the 'feeling rules' within midwifery regarding appropriate emotional display? In my own research study (Hunter 2004a, Hunter and Deery 2005), I found that midwives described two different approaches to emotion management: **'affective neutrality'** and **'affective awareness'**. These different approaches were often in conflict and presented mixed messages to student midwives.

Affective neutrality

Affective neutrality could also be described as 'professional detachment'. From this perspective, emotion must be suppressed in order to get the work done efficiently. By minimizing the emotional content of work, its emotional 'messiness' is reduced and work becomes an emotion-free zone. This approach fits well within a culture that values efficiency, hierarchical relationships, standardization of care and completion of tasks. Personal emotions are managed by the individual, in order to hide them as much as possible from clients and colleagues. Coping strategies, such as distancing, 'toughening up' and impression management are used in order to present an appropriate 'professional performance', i.e. a professional who is neutral and objective. When dealing with clients, there is avoidance of discussing emotional issues and a focus on practical tasks. This is clearly not in the best interests of women.

Although this may appear to be an outdated approach to dealing with emotion in contemporary maternity care, there is ample evidence that this approach continues, particularly within hospital settings. This can be problematic for midwives who wish to work in more emotionally aware ways, and can detract from the quality of care. An example from my research is the experience of a student midwife who, early on in her clinical experience, had cared for a woman whose baby was stillborn (Hunter and Deery 2005). The student was very upset by the experience, and described how she had been shocked and in tears. However, there was no opportunity for her to discuss her feelings with her colleagues; in fact, any possibility of this was effectively squashed by the decision of the senior midwives to send her home early. The impression she received was that personal emotions should be suppressed at all costs and that she should not seek emotional support from her colleagues. This was very different from the approach that she had been encouraged to adopt by her lecturers, and she felt confused and frustrated. Similar experiences have been described by Irish student midwives. Begley (2003, p 25) found that 'student midwives suffered strong feelings of distress when caring for women encountering perinatal loss', and that they lacked support in both clinical and educational areas. An accumulation of unsupportive situations such as this may ultimately result in midwives deciding to leave the profession (Ball et al 2002).

Affective awareness

In contrast, **'affective awareness'** fits well with a 'new midwifery' approach to practice (Page & McCandlish 2006). In this approach, referred to by Copp as 'the professional with a heart' (Copp 1998, p 304), it is considered important to be aware of feelings and express them when possible. This may be in relation to women's emotional experiences, or when dealing with personal emotions. Sharing feelings enables them to be explored and named. It also provides opportunities for developing supportive and nurturing relationships between midwives and women, and between midwives and colleagues. For example, a student midwife in my study described how her mentor encouraged her to talk through her feelings after she had cared for a woman during an obstetric emergency (Hunter & Deery 2005). The student considered that sharing her feelings acted as a 'release valve', which helped her to come to terms with her experience and feel that she was not alone in her reactions.

Affective awareness fits within a wider contemporary Western culture which emphasizes the benefits of the 'talking cure', that is the therapeutic value of talking things through (e.g. via counselling or psychotherapy). However, it is important that midwives recognize the limits of their own expertise, so they do not find themselves out of their depth. Working in partnership with women, particularly in continuity of care schemes, means that midwives are more likely to develop close connections with women and their families. If emotionally difficult events occur, midwives 'feel' more. This was a frequent experience of community-based midwives in my own study (Hunter 2006). We need to be alert to this, so that we do not become so overwhelmed by our clients' experiences that we lose our own personal boundaries. We will be of little effective support to women and colleagues if this happens. It is important to know our limits and make use of agencies who can offer skilled support as appropriate (e.g. Relate, SANDS, MIND. See list of useful addresses below).

Challenges

It is also important not to be overly critical of midwives who adopt an 'affectively neutral' approach, but to try to understand why this may be occurring. In my research study, most participants did not consider this to be the best way of dealing with emotion, believing that 'affective awareness' was the ideal way to practice. But when they felt 'stressed out', they described 'retreating' emotionally and 'putting on an act' to get through the day (Hunter & Deery 2005). Stress may be the result of unsustainable workloads, staff shortages, conflicts with colleagues or difficulties in personal lives. In order to understand emotion work in midwifery, we need to be aware of the broader social and political context in which maternity care is provided. Understanding emotion work requires us to think carefully, not just about individual midwives, but also about the complexities of the maternity services. In order to move away from a blame culture in midwifery, we need to work at developing empathy, in order to better understand each others' behaviour.

It is also important to ensure cultural sensitivity in relation to emotion. The ways that emotions are displayed, and the types of emotion that are considered appropriate for display will vary from culture to culture, as well as within cultures (Fineman 2003). Midwives need to develop skills in reading the emotional language of a situation and avoid ethnocentricity.

Developing emotional awareness

It is possible to develop emotional skills in the same way as it is possible to develop any skills. In other words, we can develop our 'emotional awareness' (Hunter 2004b) or 'emotional intelligence' (Goleman 2005). Goleman (2005) claims that emotionally intelligent people: know their emotions, manage their emotions, motivate themselves, recognize the emotions of others and handle relationships effectively. He suggests ways that emotional intelligence can be developed, so that an individual can have a high 'EQ' (emotional intelligence quotient) in the way that they may have a high IQ (intelligence quotient).

The idea of emotional intelligence has caught the public imagination, although some would argue that Goleman's ideas are rather simplistic and lack a substantive research base (e.g. Fineman 2003, p 52). Instead, Fineman (2003, p 54) prefers the notion of 'emotional sensitivity', which he claims can be developed through 'processes of feminisation, emotionally responsive leadership styles, valuing intuition, and tolerance for a wide range of emotional expression and candour'. Whatever the preferred terminology, it would seem that these ideas have particular relevance to midwifery, given the emotionally demanding nature of this work. Midwives need to develop emotional awareness so that they know what it is they are feeling, why they are feeling it, and how others may be feeling. They also need to develop a language to articulate these feelings, in a manner that is authentic.

So how can midwives develop their emotional awareness? There are a number of options that may be helpful. Attendance on counselling courses and assertiveness courses can help to develop insights into personal feelings, which by extension provide insights into the possible feelings of others. Supervision may also provide opportunities for exploration of the emotions of both self and others, with the aim of recognizing and responding appropriately to these.

It is particularly important that emotional issues are given careful and sensitive attention during pre-registration education. This could take the form of role-play, or by making use of participative theatre. Drama workshops have been used effectively with student midwives (Baker 2000) to explore various aspects of their clinical experience, including a range of emotional issues, in a safe and supportive environment. One advantage of such an approach is that participants realize that they are not alone in their experiences. With a skilled workshop facilitator, difficult situations can be considered in a broader context, so that they are understood as shared rather than personal problems. These methods could also be beneficial for qualified midwives, especially clinical mentors, as part of in-service training.

Emotional issues also need attention within clinical practice, if they are not to be seen as something that is explored only 'in the classroom'. As we have seen, there may be 'mixed messages' about what emotions should be felt and displayed. These mixed messages are not helpful in creating an emotionally attuned environment. Supervision of midwives could have a role to play here. It has the potential to provide a supportive environment for understanding emotion, particularly if a 'clinical supervision' approach is taken. This is a method of peer support and review aimed at creating a safe and non-judgemental space in which the emotional support needs of midwives can be considered (Deery 2005, Kirkham & Stapleton 2000). The importance of 'caring for the carers' is crucial, but often underestimated.

Finally, as Fineman (2003) recommends, those in leadership positions within midwifery need to set the scene by adopting leadership styles which are emotionally responsive. In this way, a ripple effect through the whole workforce could be created.

> **Box 2.2** Key issues
>
> - Midwifery is an emotionally demanding profession, requiring 'emotion work'
> - Key sources of emotion work are: midwife–woman relationships, collegial relationships, organizational issues
> - Excellent communication and interpersonal skills are needed to manage emotion effectively, for the benefit of all
> - 'Caring for the carers' is essential for the provision of good quality maternity care.

Conclusion (see Box 2.2)

Midwives need to develop skills in emotion work in order to manage sensitively and effectively the feelings of women, families, colleagues and also to manage their own personal feelings. Providing a supportive, non-judgemental space for midwives to explore and better understand the emotional demands of work is essential. Understanding emotions helps us to develop empathy, crucial for interpersonal relationships with colleagues and clients. There is much about midwifery practice that is emotionally demanding, so it is imperative that midwives become skilled emotion workers, and that this is valued as much as technical skills. By developing these skills, midwives have the potential to enhance the emotional well-being of the women they care for, and also the emotional well-being of themselves and their colleagues. As a result, the quality of maternity care will also be enhanced.

REFERENCES

Baker K 2000 Acting the part: Using drama to empower student midwives. Practising Midwife 3(1):20–21

Ball L, Curtis P, Kirkham M 2002 Why do midwives leave? Women's Informed Childbearing and Health Research Group, University of Sheffield

Beech B L, Phipps B 2004 Normal birth: women's stories. In: Downe S (ed.) Normal childbirth: evidence and debate. Churchill Livingstone, Edinburgh, p 59–70

Begley C 2003 'I cried...I had to...': Student midwives' experiences of stillbirth, miscarriage and neonatal death. Evidence Based Midwifery 1(1):20–26

Berg M, Lundgren I, Hermansson E, et al 1996 Women's experience of the encounter with the midwife during childbirth. Midwifery 12:11–15

Bergstrom L, Roberts J, Skillman L, et al 1992 'You'll feel me touching you sweetie': Vaginal examinations during the second stage of labour. Birth 1:10–25

Bolton S C 2000 Who cares? Offering emotion work as a 'gift' in the nursing labour process. Journal of Advanced Nursing 32(3):580–586

Bolton S C 2005 Emotion management in the workplace. Palgrave Macmillan, Basingstoke

Clement C 1995 Listening visits in pregnancy: a strategy for preventing postnatal depression? Midwifery 11(2): 75–80

Copp M 1998 When emotion work is doomed to fail: Ideological and structural constraints of emotion management. Symbolic Interaction 21(3):299–328

Cronk M 2000 The midwife: A professional servant? In: Kirkham M (ed.) The midwife–mother relationship. Macmillan, Basingstoke, p 19–27

Deery R 2005 An action research study exploring midwives' support needs and the effect of group clinical supervision. Midwifery 21:161–176

Dykes F 2005 A critical ethnographic study of encounters between midwives and breast-feeding women in postnatal wards in England. Midwifery 21(3): 241–252

Edwards N 2000 Women planning homebirths: Their own views on their relationships with midwives. In: Kirkham M (ed.) The midwife–mother relationship. Macmillan, Basingstoke, p 55–84

Fineman S (ed.) 2000 Emotion in organizations, 2nd edn. SAGE, London

Fineman S 2003 Understanding emotion at work. SAGE, London

Fleming V 1998. Women and midwives in partnership: a problematic relationship? Journal of Advanced Nursing 27:8–14

Fraser D 1999 Women's perceptions of midwifery care: a longitudinal study to inform curriculum development. Birth 26:99–107

Goleman D 2005 Emotional intelligence. Bantam Books, London

Hadikin R, O'Driscoll M 2000 The bullying culture: cause, effect, harm reduction. Books for Midwives Press, Oxford

Hochschild A R 1983 The managed heart. Commercialization of human feeling. University of California Press, Berkeley

Hunt S, Symonds A 1995 The social meaning of midwifery. Macmillan, Basingstoke

Hunter B 2004a Conflicting ideologies as a source of emotion work in midwifery. Midwifery 20:261–272

Hunter B 2004b The importance of emotional intelligence in midwifery. Editorial. British Journal of Midwifery 12(10):1–2

Hunter B 2005 Emotion work and boundary maintenance in hospital-based midwifery. Midwifery 21:253–266

Hunter B 2006 The importance of reciprocity in relationships between community-based midwives and mothers. Midwifery 22(4):308–322

Hunter B, Deery R 2005 Building our knowledge about emotion work in midwifery: combining and comparing findings from two different research studies. Evidence Based Midwifery 3(1):10–15

James N 1992 Care = organisation + physical labour + emotional labour. Sociology of Health and Illness 14(4):489–509

Kirkham M 1999 The culture of midwifery in the National Health Service in England. Journal of Advanced Nursing 30(3):732–739

Kirkham M, Stapleton H 2000 Midwives' support needs as childbirth changes. Journal of Advanced Nursing 32(2): 465–472

Lavender T, Chapple J 2004 An exploration of midwives' views of the current system of maternity care in England. Midwifery 20:324–334

Leap N 1997 Making sense of 'horizontal violence' in midwifery. British Journal of Midwifery 5:689

Leap N 2000 'The less we do, the more we give'. In: Kirkham M (ed.) The midwife–mother relationship. Macmillan, Basingstoke, p 1–17

Page L A, McCandlish R (eds) 2006 The new midwifery. Science and sensitivity in practice, 2nd edn. Churchill Livingstone, Edinburgh

Pairman S 2000. Women-centred midwifery: partnerships or professional friendships? In: Kirkham (ed.) The midwife–mother relationship. Macmillan, Basingstoke, p 207–225

Raphael Leff J 2005 Psychological processes of childbearing. Centre for Psychoanalytic Studies, London

Redshaw M, Rowe R, Hockley C, et al 2007 Recorded delivery: a national survey of women's experience of maternity care. National Perinatal Epidemiology Unit (NPEU), Oxford

Sandall J 1997 Midwives' burnout and continuity of care. British Journal of Midwifery 5(2):106–111

Smith P 1992 The emotional labour of nursing. Macmillan, Basingstoke

Stevens T, McCourt C 2002a. One-to-one midwifery practice part 2: the transition period. British Journal of Midwifery 10 (1):45–50

Stevens T, McCourt C, 2002b. One-to-one midwifery practice part 3: Meaning for midwives. British Journal of Midwifery 10(2):111–115

Stewart M 2005 'I'm just going to wash you down': sanitizing the vaginal examination. Journal of Advanced Nursing 51 (6):587–94

Walsh D 1999 An ethnographic study of women's experience of partnership caseload midwifery practice: the professional as friend. Midwifery 15:165–176

Walsh D 2007 Improving maternity services. Small is beautiful – lessons from a birth centre. Radcliffe Publishing, Oxford

Wilkins R 2000 Poor relations: the paucity of the professional paradigm. In: Kirkham M (ed.) The midwife–mother relationship. Macmillan, Basingstoke, p 28–54

FURTHER READING

Dryden W and Constantinou D 2004 Assertiveness step by step. Sheldon Press, London

This short book is written by well respected authors in the field. It offers practical, evidence-based advice on developing assertiveness and emotional awareness.

Fineman S 2003 Understanding emotion at work. SAGE, London

A lively and readable book that provides additional insights into how emotions impact upon the workplace. Considers issues such as leadership and change, bullying and sexual harassment. Although the book is aimed at those studying the sociology or psychology of work and organizations, there is much here of interest and relevance to midwives.

Goleman D 2005 Emotional intelligence. Bantam Books, London

The key text explaining the concept of emotional intelligence. A popular and easy to read book.

Heron J 2001 Helping the client: a creative practical guide, 6th edn. SAGE, London

A classic text used in many disciplines. Describes six forms of 'helping behaviour' which can be adopted by any practitioner who works in face to face situations with clients. Heron's six stage model is often used as a model for clinical supervision of nurses and midwives.

Hunter B, Deery R (eds) 2009 Emotions in Midwifery and Reproduction. Palgrave Macmillan, Basingstoke.

This new edited book brings together the work of leading international researchers. The book explores the significance of emotions to the day-to-day work of midwives.

Kirkham M. (ed.) 2000 The midwife–mother relationship. Macmillan, Basingstoke

This very useful edited book provides many insights into the emotional aspects of maternity care, from the perspectives of both women and midwives.

USEFUL ADDRESSES

Relate (relationship counselling)
Tel: 01788 573 241
www.relate.org.uk

MIND (mental health charity)
15–19 Broadway, London E15 4BQ
Tel: 020 8519 2122
www.contact@mind.org.uk

SANDS (stillbirth and neonatal death charity)
28 Portland Place, London W1B 1LY
Tel: 020 7436 5881 (helpline); 020 7436 7940 (head office)
www.uk-sands.org

3 The social context of childbirth and motherhood

Kuldip Kaur Bharj   Margaret A. Cooper

This chapter provides a brief overview of the social context within which the twenty-first century maternity services are organized and delivered; it highlights the importance of factors such as ethnicity, culture, religion, disability, sexuality and social exclusion which may impact upon the quality of maternity services. Having an understanding of such issues will enable the midwife to work effectively in partnership with women to ensure that the care that is offered meets individual needs of all women, their babies and families.

The chapter aims to:

- discuss the social context of childbirth in the UK
- consider and explore the issues which disadvantage some women in terms of quality and access to maternity services
- discuss the factors which promote the delivery of responsive maternity services harnessing current philosophies of maternity services
- discuss the strategies that midwives may utilize to provide and deliver maternity care to women from disadvantaged backgrounds.

The context of care

The journey of having a baby is a profound event. Although this journey may be similar for all women in terms of physiological explanations, its meaning to each woman is individual and unique because the social context of her life and experience is shaped by social, cultural, spiritual, emotional and psychological factors. Therefore, maternity services strive to provide care that is not only safe but is easily accessible and is responsive to women's individual linguistic, faith and cultural needs, that communicates effectively and provides the information that facilitates informed choices. Correspondingly, government proposals and recommendations reflect these aspirations, advocating that maternity services must be responsive to the individual needs of women and their families, listen to their views and respect their ethnic, cultural, social and family backgrounds (Department of Health (DH) 2004, 2007a,b, NHS Quality Improvement Scotland 2005, Scottish Executive Health Department (SEHD) 2001, Northern Ireland Department of Health, Social Services and Public Safety (NI DHSSPS) 2002, Welsh Assembly Government (WAG) 2005). The directives reaffirm that women should be the central focus and maternity services should be designed to fit around the woman, her baby and family, with specific emphasis to support normal childbirth and to offer medical intervention only if absolutely necessary. While midwives recognize that meeting individual and unique needs of every woman during childbirth will lead to a fulfilling experience, achieving individualized care remains a challenge particularly when caring for women who are vulnerable or experience disadvantage.

Over the past two decades, a number of policy directives have propelled the NHS to modernize maternity services to meet the needs of women. The policy reforms in the UK have recommended many radical changes in the way maternity services are commissioned and provided (DH 1997, 2000a,b, National Assembly for Wales 2001, 2005, SEHD 2005a,b, DHSSPS 2004, 2005). In particular, they emphasize the need for NHS provider units to be more responsive to the needs of their local population, more sensitive to the needs of all service users, and to offer greater choice, higher standards and better quality of healthcare provision. The need for maternity service re-design is greater than ever before if benefits such as safer care, improving access and outcomes, more choice, promoting normality, local ante- and postnatal services closer to home and home-like birth environment are to be realized (Shribman 2007).

Consequently, the beginnings of the twenty-first century have seen the transformation of the NHS at systems and at organizational level to provide better care, better patient experience and better value for money. The reforms are to deliver a *Patient-led NHS* (DH 2005), where the services are to be provided through stronger commissioning. The direction of travel is to move away from monolithic provider organizations to that of diversity of providers. More and different providers of maternity services is likely to expand community based provision, creating an opportunity for maternity services to be commissioned from a range of providers such as other NHS providers, voluntary sector, private sector and social enterprise. The expansion of providers will inevitably introduce an environment of contestability with explicit competition. The policy desire is to offer women and their families a greater choice in the services they want and need (DH 2007b), guaranteeing a wider choice of type and place of maternity care and birth by the end of 2009 (DH 2007a).

Simultaneously, the NHS has undergone a major restructuring programme, bringing about dramatic changes to the way health and social care is delivered locally. The White Paper: *Our health, Our care, Our say: a new direction for community services* (DH 2006a) and *The NHS in England: the operating framework for 2006/7* (DH 2006b) have been catalysts for these reforms, proposing a shift of services from hospitals into the community, with the provision of care much closer to home and greater integration with local authority services and having shared responsibilities for public health.

Midwives are the cornerstone of delivering maternity service reforms. Their roles and responsibilities will increasingly focus to deliver greater productivity and best value for money, offering real choice and improvement in women's maternity experiences. These reforms are creating opportunities for midwives to work in new ways and undertake new and different roles. Midwives are required to be much more oriented towards public health and the reforms provide increased opportunities to work in more diverse teams to provide integrated services. The working environment is changing where midwives are increasingly accountable for the care they provide creating a new form of ownership.

Disadvantaged groups

In the twentieth century, childbirth was transformed from a social, domestic event into a highly technological, medical procedure. The 1980s saw a rise in concerns about the way maternity services were organized and delivered; this led to campaigns calling for better access to effective and appropriate obstetric and midwifery care and the need for services to be tailored to meet consumer needs. While women from the middle classes were somewhat reluctant to have intervention imposed on them and called for a less clinical environment for intrapartum care, women from vulnerable and disadvantaged backgrounds complained that they were more likely to receive less favourable treatment, asserting that services failed to take account of their linguistic, religious and cultural needs and some, particularly those from the black and minority ethnic (BME) groups claimed that they experienced additional difficulties owing to stereotypes and discrimination (Cartwright 1979, Larbie 1985, Phoenix 1990). (Note: The use of terminology to describe different groups in the community is an extremely sensitive issue and there is no single acceptable term that embraces all members of the minority ethnic groups. The term 'black and minority ethnic communities' has been used here to include all individuals who experience discrimination and disadvantage associated with 'race' and ethnicity.) Many of the reasons given by women for dissatisfaction with maternity services include fragmented care, long waiting times, insensitive care, lack of emotional support, inadequate explanations, lack of information, medical control, inflexibility of hospital routines, and dehumanizing aspects of hospitalization and reproductive technologies (Kitzinger 1978, 1990, Oakley 1979, Reid & Garcia 1989).

Universally, there is no agreed definition of vulnerability, however, the term 'vulnerable groups' is often used to refer to groups of people who are at risk of being marginalized in accessing maternity services and social exclusion. These groups of people or communities are more likely to experience social marginalization as a result of a number of interrelated factors such as unemployment, poor or limited skills, low income, poor housing, poverty, high crime environment, poor or ill health and family breakdown. Women from these vulnerable groups may experience disadvantage either due to mental or physical impairment, or particular characteristics no longer attributed to mental or physical impairment but that have historically led to individuals experiencing prejudice and discrimination, for example

ethnicity or disability. Or it may be concerned with the manner in which individuals or organizations interact with women leading to prejudice and discrimination (Hart et al 2001).

Providing woman-centred care is a complex issue, particularly in a diverse society where individual's and families' health needs are varied and not homogenous. Listening and responding to women's views and respecting their ethnic, cultural, social and family backgrounds is critical to developing responsive maternity services. Persistent concerns have been expressed about the poor neonatal and maternal health outcomes among disadvantaged and socially excluded groups (Lewis 2007, Lewis & Drife 2001, 2004), suggesting not all groups in society enjoy equal access to maternity services (Dixon-Woods 2005, Redshaw et al 2007). The Confidential Enquiry into Maternal and Child Health Report (CEMACH) for the triennium 2003–2005 testified that 'the link between adverse pregnancy outcomes and vulnerability and social exclusion are nowhere more starkly demonstrated than by this enquiry'. The report goes on to state that 'those women who need maternity services most use them least' (Lewis 2007, p 44).

Women may be viewed as disadvantaged not because they have, for example, a disability or are from travelling communities, but because they are more likely to be socially excluded. They are more likely to experience discrimination or be unemployed and it is the detrimental impact of these circumstances on health that is of concern (see Box 3.1). There is strong evidence that disadvantaged groups have poorer health and poorer access to healthcare, with clear links between inequality in social life and inequality in health, demonstrating that inequality exists in both mortality and morbidity (HCHC 2003, Macfarlane & Mugford 2000, Modood et al 1997, Palmer et al 2006). People from these groups have not enjoyed the health gains from wider social and environmental improvements, and are less likely to adopt healthier lifestyles or obtain fair access to services at the same level as the most affluent sectors of the community.

In a broad sense, the government has affirmed its commitment to address issues of inequalities in health, and policy directives are compelling maternity services to readjust themselves and to become conversant with health needs of women from vulnerable and disadvantaged backgrounds. The health

> **Box 3.1** Women who are most likely to experience disadvantage
>
> - The very young
> - Those with disability (physical, sensory or learning)
> - Those living in relative poverty
> - Those from black and minority ethnic backgrounds
> - Those from travelling communities
> - Asylum seekers
> - Those who misuse substances
> - Lesbians.

of those community groups who are at a higher risk of poorer health outcomes has been given a designated priority area (Acheson 1998, DH 1999, 2000a, 2001). Provider units and healthcare professionals are made responsible for development and delivery of maternity services in such a way that they give an important consideration to the needs of people from vulnerable groups as well as eradicate inequality.

To facilitate care that is responsive to the needs of women, health professionals need to understand women's social, cultural and historical backgrounds so that care is tailor-made to meet their needs. A number of models of care have been introduced to deliver culturally congruent care, including some examples of midwifery-led case-loading teams developed around the needs of vulnerable groups, e.g. Blackburn Midwifery Group Practice (Byrom 2006), however the philosophy of 'woman-centred care' is that used to meet individual needs of the women who experience disadvantage.

Women from disadvantaged groups: implications for practice

Young mothers

Britain has the highest rate of teenage pregnancy and teenage parenthood in Europe. Some 90 000 teenagers in England become pregnant every year; of these, nearly 8000 are under the age of 16 years. Approximately three-fifths of teenage conceptions will result in live births (Social Exclusion Unit 1999). Many young mothers do achieve a successful outcome to their pregnancy and parenting; it should, however, also be recognized that mortality and morbidity among babies born to these mothers is increased and that the mothers show a higher risk of developing complications, such as hypertensive disorders and intrapartum complications (Lewis & Drife 2004). Young teenage mothers tend to present late for antenatal care and are disproportionately likely to have some risk factors associated with poor antenatal health (e.g. poverty and smoking).

For many young mothers, pregnancy and parenthood means an early conclusion to their education with consequent reduced career opportunities and increased likelihood that they will find themselves socially excluded and living in poverty. The Government's Social Exclusion Unit report on teenage pregnancy (1999) set two major targets: (1) to halve the pregnancy rate in under 18-year-old teenagers by the year 2010 and (2) to achieve a reduction in the risk of long term exclusion for teenage parents and their children. Midwives have a role to play in the achievement of both these targets through their public health role and the provision of appropriate, accessible services. The Government Action Plan on Social Exclusion describes a 'cycle of disadvantage' with deprivation passing down from one generation to the next; it goes on to suggest that the daughter of a teenage mother is twice as likely as the daughter of an older mother to become pregnant in her teen years (HM Government 2006, p 8).

With appropriate support, young mothers can make an effective transition to parenthood. They can be assisted to develop good parenting and life skills and be helped out of this potential downward spiral. MacKeith & Phillipson (1997), writing about young mothers, argue that being judgemental achieves nothing positive but it reduces self-esteem, engenders resentment and destroys the relationship between the midwife and her client. While some progress has been made towards achieving the 2010 targets, there is still much to do; 'A guide to commissioning and delivering maternity services' offers assistance in developing local strategies (Teenage Pregnancy Unit et al 2004).

Women with disability

Women with disability are increasingly becoming users of the maternity services as they seek to live full and autonomous lives. The midwife needs to allow sufficient time to assess how the disability may impact on the woman's experience of childbirth and parenting and to work with her in identifying any resources that may alleviate perceived difficulties. Assumptions should not be made on visual observation alone. Where possible, the woman should have a named midwife with whom she can build a trusting relationship and have continuity of care. An introduction to other professionals who may be involved in the care should be considered early in pregnancy. Comprehensive record-keeping will reduce the likelihood of repetitive questioning.

The woman will probably be well informed about her disability but may need the midwife to provide advice on the impact that the physiological changes of pregnancy and labour may have on her, for example the increased weight and change in posture. Some women and their partners may raise concerns regarding a genetic condition that could be passed on to their baby and need referral to specialist services such as a genetic counsellor. Midwives and other healthcare professionals should recognize the need to approach antenatal screening in a sensitive manner (see Ch.18). Midwives need to be aware of local information pertaining to professional and voluntary organizations and networks and adopt a multidisciplinary approach to planning and provision of services. The Common Assessment Framework may be an appropriate tool for the midwife to use to ensure a coordinated multi-agency approach to care (DfES 2006).

A birth plan will help the woman to identify her specific needs alongside the issues that most pregnant women are concerned with, such as choice of pain relief and views on interventions. Midwives should empower women with a disability to make informed choices about all aspects of their antenatal, intrapartum and postnatal care (RCM 2000a). If the woman is to give birth in hospital it may be helpful for her to visit the unit, meet some of the staff and assess the environment and resources in relation to her special needs. A single room should be offered to her to facilitate the woman's control over her immediate environment and, where appropriate, to adapt it to accommodate any equipment that she may wish to bring with her. A woman who is blind or partially sighted may prefer to give birth at home where she is familiar with the environment. If she has a guide dog then consideration needs to be given to its presence in the hospital environment.

Women with learning difficulties may need a friend or carer to help with the birth plan but the midwife should not overlook who is the client; she must involve her as much as possible and recognize that she may have feelings and anxieties that she is less able to articulate.

Midwives need to understand the worldview of women with disabilities in order to shape the maternity services to meet the individual needs of these women. They need to value key principles of rights, independence, choice and inclusion. Many women with disability may have been educationally disadvantaged, as they may have had to miss compulsory education in school years because of receiving medical treatment. The disability may have led to social isolation, which in turn could have restricted the woman's awareness of available services. Midwives also need to have knowledge of the potential effect that disability may have on the individual woman as a recipient of maternity care.

Women living in relative poverty

It is well documented that women living in poverty are more likely to suffer health inequalities and have a higher rate of maternal and perinatal mortality (Lewis 2007, Lewis & Drife 2004, Townsend & Davidson 1982, Whitehead 1987).

Tackling inequality is high on the public health agenda and the midwife has an important role in targeting women in need. Sure Start and Sure Start Plus schemes have contributed to bringing services together and addressing the needs of disadvantaged parents; see Box 3.2, Karen's story.

Salmon & Powell (1998) recognize that midwives should be sensitive to the financial difficulties that some women face and should not give inappropriate advice that may reinforce an already vulnerable situation. They also recognize that concepts such as continuity and choice may be viewed as secondary for women struggling with the daily reality of managing poverty.

Box 3.2 Karen's story

'Karen' escaped domestic abuse with her son – so serious that she had to change her name so that she could not be traced. She also has a criminal record for fraud (she forged a name to obtain goods when she was desperate for money). She has now met a new partner and has had a baby. Her life is really improving, they are buying a house through a council partnership scheme and she now has a part-time job. Karen believes her 'success' has been greatly helped by support from Sure Start.

'Hello, my name is Karen, mum to Ethan, 7 years and Chloe, 6 months. We are regular users of the Sure Start services. My son, Ethan has some special needs and has one-to-one support from Claire who gives him the understanding that he needs; she also helps me with trying to help Ethan and it has made a fantastic difference. While I was pregnant with Chloe, I used Maria, the midwife, who came to me as I found it hard to get around; she checked my baby's heartbeat – that was lovely to hear. She also gave me her mobile number and if I ever needed her I could just call and when you have a high risk pregnancy it is such a reassuring feeling to know someone is there for you. On a Friday I go to an art and craft group, we learn new skills, from making purses to painting. I have also run a group on a Monday for mums over 24, as I felt this service was lacking, but without the support of Megan and Nasreen to do this I would not have done it. I moved to this city about three and a half years ago and was very lonely and isolated, but joining the groups at Sure Start I now have a good circle of friends and I have my confidence back. All of the workers at Sure Start do a great job and a lot of people don't realize how much work they do with individuals and in the community. I would like to say a big thank you to you all.'

Women from the black and minority ethnic communities

The UK has continued to see major demographic changes in the profile of its population and is more ethnically diverse now than ever before (Office for National Statistics, ONS 2001). According to the 2001 census, there are approximately 4.6 million people from a BME origin residing in UK, constituting 7.9% of the total population, having risen from a figure of 3 million (or 5.5%) in 1991. Of these, nearly 50% of the population account for South-Asian origin (people of Indian, Pakistani, and Bangladeshi backgrounds) and approximately 2% of the people are from Black backgrounds, that is, Black Caribbean, Black Africans and Black other and 0.4% each of Chinese and of various origins including Arabs and 'mixed' backgrounds.

However, there is considerable variation in the distribution of the BME population within the UK countries and within the regions. The BME population is principally located in England, where the BME population is approximately 9%; in Scotland and Wales the BME composition is of approximately 2% each and in Northern Ireland it is less than 1%. These statistics are important for maternity services, so that they can respond to the demographic composition and diversity of BME populations. However, Britain's BME population not only differs from the majority of the population but also has sub-groups which differ from each other in terms of culture, lifestyle, language and religion.

When referring to multi-ethnic societies, a basic understanding of the culture is often assumed to mean the way of life of a society or a group of people and is used to express social life, food, clothing, music and behaviours. The concept of culture has been defined by many (Helman 1994, Leininger 1978, Lewis 1976), providing a variety of insights into the concept. However, the commonalities are that culture is learned, it is shared and it is passed on from generation to generation. Members of the society learn a set of guidelines through which they attain concepts of role expectancies, values and attitudes of society; it is therefore not genetically inherited but is socially constructed and the behaviour of individuals is shaped by the values and attitudes they hold as well as the physical and geographical surroundings in which they interact. Individuals perceive and respond to stimuli from economic, social and political factors in different ways and they will be affected differently according to age, gender, social class, occupation and many other factors. Culture is very much a dynamic state, it is not a group phenomenon and to treat it as homogeneous can be quite dangerous as it can lead to generalizations. Some aspects can be true for some and not for others belonging to the same cultural group.

An understanding of some of the cultural differences between social groups is essential in ensuring that professional practice is closely matched to meet the needs of individual clients, promoting the delivery of culturally congruent care. An understanding of the role culture plays in determining health, health behaviours and illness is essential when planning and delivering services that meet the health needs of the local population. However, some caution the role of culture in explaining patterns of health and health-related behaviour, arguing that emphasis on culture diverts attention away from the role of broad structural process in discrimination and the role that racism plays in health status (Ahmad 1993, 1996, Stubbs 1993). In practice then, emphasis on culture could lead to attributing inequalities entirely in cultural differences, diverting attention from the real causes of discrimination and racism often faced by women from diverse backgrounds.

Ethnic diversity in the UK has created major challenges for maternity services. In the triennium 2003–2005, more than 20% of births in the UK were to mothers who themselves were born elsewhere (Lewis 2007). CEMACH reports have demonstrated that the inability to respond appropriately to the individual needs of women from different backgrounds is reflected in persistent poor health outcomes for both mother and baby (Lewis 2007, Lewis & Drife 2001, 2004). The last two decades have seen a much more consistent approach to health policy to redress this discrepancy and, coupled with the Race Relations (Amendment) Act of 2000, has propelled widespread transformation underpinned by the duty to promote racial equality, firmly placing the responsibility for responding to ethnic diversity on provider organizations and healthcare professionals (DH 1997, 2000a).

Gerrish et al (1996) found that midwives lacked knowledge of many issues when providing care to women from BME groups but were concerned to learn more. Healthcare professionals who are not equipped with basic information about ethnic groups are more likely to make assumptions about the needs and preferences of women based on inaccurate stereotypes. It is critical that midwives should be equipped with knowledge, enabling them to provide high quality, anti-discriminatory care that is appropriate and responsive to the varied health needs of the diverse population.

Women from the BME population experience disadvantage and are socially excluded for two main reasons. First, some women are more likely to be categorized into lower socioeconomic status; they are predominantly residents of deprived inner city areas, have poor housing, are at risk of high unemployment, and have low paid occupations, poor working conditions, poor social security rights, and low income, all of which lead to poverty. Often factors, such as lifestyle, environmental factors and genetic determinants are cited as indicators of poor health outcomes dismissing key social determinants of poverty, poor housing and poor education (Nazroo 1997, Platt 2007).

Second, because their skin colour and ethnic origin make them visible minorities, they are more likely to experience racial harassment, discrimination and social inequalities (Nazroo 2001). Institutionalized racism and general reluctance by organizations and individuals to address the sensitive issue of ethnicity are likely contributors to inequalities of health and access to maternity services (RCM 2003). It is important to understand concepts of discrimination and racism and how this can marginalize women.

Discrimination is a process whereby one person is treated less favourably than another and occurs when prejudice is brought into action, often to the disadvantage of particular groups or individuals. Discrimination can operate in two forms: (a) Direct discrimination operates at an individual level and (b) indirect discrimination is usually at an institutional level. Direct discrimination arises where an individual is treated less favourably, on the grounds of gender, 'race', disability, sexual orientation, religion, culture or age, than another person would be treated in the same or similar circumstances. An example from the Commission for Racial Equality follows (CRE 1994, p 22):

> *A receptionist at a community health clinic tells a black woman that there are no appointments available for at least 2 weeks. She then proceeds to offer a white woman an appointment for the next day.*

Indirect discrimination occurs when a requirement or condition that applies to everyone has the effect of excluding a significantly greater proportion of people from a particular group than others. An example adapted from the CRE (1994) is:

An antenatal clinic offers classes on breathing and relaxation techniques for expectant mothers. These classes are also open to their partners. Women from some ethnic groups who experience difficulty in discussing childbirth issues in male company often drop out or do not attend. They miss out on these facilities, as there are no classes for women only.

Racism on the other hand, is a doctrine or ideology or dogma that is underpinned by the assumption that some groups are superior to others, and is interpreted as the systematic oppression of individuals or groups based on their skin colour or ethnic origin (Fernando 1991). Racism is associated with power that enables individuals, or institutions to make things happen or prevent them from happening. It is the enactment of prejudice and discrimination, either at an individual or institutional level, by those who are in power either by an act of deliberation or unintentionally.

Racism can operate at an individual and/or institutional level. Individual racism operates through the behaviour of people at a personal level, leading to discrimination. An example of individual racism is where a healthcare practitioner does not offer translating or interpreting services because she believes that while in England, everyone should speak English. This in fact will lead to a poorer quality of service.

Institutional racism, on the other hand, is 'the collective failure of an organization to provide an appropriate and professional service to people because of their colour, culture or ethnic origin. It can be seen or detected in processes, attitudes and behaviour which amount to discrimination, through unwitting prejudice, ignorance, thoughtlessness and racist stereotyping, which disadvantages ethnic minority people' (Macpherson 1999, p 28). This suggests that institutional racism is essentially a situation when racial prejudice becomes part and parcel of institutions and is set in the structures of the society, so that long-standing practices can cause organizations to discriminate unintentionally.

Often the term 'race' is used to refer to people from the BME communities. This term is underpinned by the premise that people are differentiated by specific genetic and physical characteristics (e.g. Caucasian, Negroid, etc.) and are connected by common descent and origin. However, the scientific explanations reject the notion that there is a biological difference in the 'races', arguing that there is little genetic difference between different 'races' and, more so, that genetic differences within 'races' are greater than the differences between 'races' (Rose & Rose 1986). Notwithstanding this, 'race' is widely used in the social and political context and is associated with concepts, such as discrimination and racism.

Ethnicity has largely replaced the term 'race', encompassing all of the ways in which people from one group seek to differentiate themselves from other groups. 'Ethnicity is an indicator of the process by which people create and maintain a sense of group identity and solidarity which they use to distinguish themselves from "others"' (Smaje 1995, p 16). Ethnicity is a self-claimed identity and is socially constructed; people of a particular group have a common sense of belonging, and have shared beliefs, values and cultural traditions as well as biological characteristics. In general, people use these terms to identify the 'other' groups but it must be remembered that all people have a culture and ethnicity.

When people value their own culture more highly, perceiving their cultural ways to be the best, they devalue and belittle other ethnic groups, perceiving 'others' culture as bizarre and strange; this is referred to as *ethnocentrism*. Ethnocentric behaviour, in particular when other individuals' cultural requirements may be ignored or dismissed as unimportant, would do very little to meet the tenets of woman-centred care and hinders the delivery of responsive care. Many maternity services are still based on an ethnocentric model, e.g. education for parenthood is not culturally sensitive where women and their partners are positively encouraged to attend jointly (Katbamna 2000).

BME groups as users of the maternity service: The majority of women from BME groups express satisfaction with maternity services. While some argue that ethnicity is not a marker for good or poor quality (Hirst & Hewison 2001, 2002), others have reported a plausible relationship between ethnicity and women's proficiency in speaking and reading English with poor quality of care (Bharj 2007, Bowes &

Domokos 1996a, 2003). Many women assert that their ability to access maternity services is impaired because they are offered little or no information regarding options of care during pregnancy, childbirth and postnatal period (Bharj 2007, Katbamna 2000). Women are therefore not aware of the range of maternity services and choices available to them. For example, a video plus leaflet on hospital delivery in Bengali will tell only half the story with respect to birth options if the leaflet on home birth is available only in English (CRE 1994). Women who do not have full and appropriate information cannot easily access health services and the consequence is poor uptake of maternity and other preventative services.

Extensive evidence indicates that lack of proficiency to speak and read English adversely impacts on women's experience and their ability to access and utilize maternity services (Bowes & Domokos 1996a, Chan 2000, Katbamna 2000, Woollett & Dosanjh-Matwala 1990a,b), impacting adversely on the quality of maternity services and maternity outcomes (Lewis & Drife 2004). Often lack of interventions to overcome communication and language barriers, such as qualified interpreters is cited as a major challenge in accessing maternity services (Harper-Bulman & McCourt 2002). Use of relatives or friends as interpreters during sensitive consultations is viewed by women to be inappropriate. In some studies, women reported that their requests to see a female doctor were dismissed and they were distressed when treated by a male doctor, particularly when they observed purdah (Sivagnanam 2004).

Some women from the BME communities have reported that midwives are unable to develop positive relationships with them, marring their childbirth experiences (Ellis 2004, Woollett & Dosanjh-Matwala 1990a,b). Midwifery care based on discriminatory attitudes and institutional racism has not only tarnished women's maternity experience but has led to substandard care (Bharj 2007, Bowler 1993a,b, Richens 2003, Sivagnanam 2004).

Consequently, women in such environments feel that the reception and handling they receive is less than adequate and they are left feeling humiliated. Those women who have poor experiences of maternity services are less likely to access maternity and preventative services readily. Often, service provision is inappropriate and insensitive with claims that stereotyping and discrimination within the NHS remain major issues that underpin their experiences of maternity services. The following two key elements can assist in the provision of equitable maternity services:

1. ensuring that women from the BME communities have full evidence based information about maternity services, understand what it offers and when and how they can use it
2. ensuring that all health services, including maternity and preventive services, are appropriate to the healthcare needs of the local population, including those from the BME population, and that they are delivered in a manner that is ethnically sensitive.

Asylum seekers

Midwives need to be aware of the complex needs of this group of vulnerable women who, in addition to the problems described above, have often experienced traumatic events in their home country, may be isolated from their family and friends and face uncertainty regarding their future domicile.

Women from travelling families

It would be wrong to categorize travelling families as a homogeneous group. This umbrella term merely serves to describe the nomadic nature of their lifestyle but fails to recognize their origins or the social context of their lives. Travellers may belong to a distinct social group such as the Romanies, their origins may lie in this country or elsewhere such as Ireland or Eastern Europe, or they may be part of the social grouping loosely termed 'New Age' travellers or part of the Showman's Guild travelling community. As with all social groups, their cultural background will influence their beliefs about and experience of health and childbearing.

A common factor, which may apply to all, is the likelihood of prejudice and marginalization. Midwives need to examine their own beliefs and values and develop their knowledge to address the needs of travelling families with respect and provide a service which is non-judgemental. An informed approach to lifestyle interpretation may stop the midwife identifying the woman as an antenatal defaulter with the negative connotations that accompany that label. Moving on may be through choice related to lifestyle, but equally it may be the result of eviction from unofficial sites.

Some health authorities have designated services for travelling families that contribute to uptake and continuity of care. These carers understand the culture and are aware of specific health needs; they can also access appropriate resources, for example a general practitioner (GP) who is receptive to travellers' needs. A trusting relationship is important to people who are frequently subjected to discrimination. Handheld records contribute to continuity of care and communication between care providers, but the maternity service also needs to address communication challenges for individuals who do not have a postal address or who have low levels of literacy.

Women who are lesbian

Evidence suggests that an increasing number of women are seeking motherhood within a lesbian relationship. The exact numbers are unclear as it is the woman's choice as to whether she makes her sexual orientation known. The midwife can, however, create an environment in which she feels safe to do so. Communication and careful framing of questions can reduce the risk of causing offence and assist the midwife in the provision of woman-centred care.

Wilton & Kaufmann (2001) identify the booking interview as the first time, as a user of the maternity service, that the woman must consider how she will respond to questions such as 'when did you last have sex?' or 'what is the father's name?' Issues such as parenting, sex and contraception may have different meanings for the midwife and the woman and therefore careful use of non-heterosexist language by the midwife will help to promote a climate for open communication (Hastie 2000, p 65). Hastie argues that the 'realities of lesbian experiences are hidden from the mainstream heterosexist society and so stereotypes are rife among health practitioners'; she goes on to say that oppression and invisibility damage health. The RCM (2000b) Position Paper 22 on maternity care for lesbian mothers, states that midwives should take a lead in

challenging discriminatory language and behaviour, both positively and constructively. Wilton & Kaufmann (2001) suggest that this can be achieved by developing awareness and understanding, signaling acceptance and improving service delivery.

Midwives meeting the needs of women from disadvantaged groups

Midwives are in a unique position to exploit the opportunities created by the NHS reforms to deliver equitable services, and to create responsive organizations and practices. They have a moral, ethical, legal and professional responsibility to provide individualized care and to develop equitable service provision and delivery (NMC 2008).

The Race Relations (Amendment) Act 2000, the Disability Discrimination Act (DDA) 2005 and the Equality Act 2006 require all organizations to produce schemes that promote race, disability and gender equality in employment and service provision and delivery.

Midwives have a statutory obligation to provide relevant and responsive maternity services for all women and their families. Organizations and individuals are charged to develop and deliver maternity services in such a way that they give an important consideration to the needs of women from disadvantaged groups as well as reducing inequalities of health.

Midwives play a key role in bringing about change. They have a responsibility to facilitate an environment that provides all women and their families with appropriate information and encourages more active participation in the decision-making process, including ensuring 'informed consent'.

Competence in working with women from disadvantaged groups

Midwives need to be knowledgeable and understand their own values, attitudes, norms and expectations that affect their professional practice. They must understand the backgrounds of the clients, enabling them to respond equitably and appropriately. Midwives also need to be aware of issues of prejudice, discrimination and racism and how these manifest themselves in the provision and delivery of health-care and may act as a barrier to seeking healthcare.

Midwives need to be equipped with knowledge and understanding of cultures and lifestyles of the women for whom they care. It is only then that they can feel confident to plan the services that the women require and deserve. Several texts provide essential background knowledge concerning women who experience disadvantage; although such background information is helpful, midwives should adopt a critical approach to reading such material and applying it to individual women in order to avoid generalizations and stereotypical responses. It is evident that prior knowledge is helpful, however midwives should develop sensitive approaches through which they can ascertain this information from the women which will assist with delivery of responsive care as well as assist the development of relationships between women and midwives.

Meeting information needs

Women from disadvantaged backgrounds often lack knowledge and understanding of the maternity services. They are not always given adequate information about the full range of maternity services and options of care available to them during pregnancy, labour and postnatal period. Often information is not available in appropriate formats to reach women who have visual or hearing impairment or who lack proficiency in speaking and reading English. Therefore, they are unaware of the range of maternity services and choices available to them.

Many women, for example those from lower socioeconomic groups or from the BME groups, feel less confident than others in actively participating in making decisions about the care they receive and indeed are less able to make informed choices. They are unable to give informed consent. These factors leave the women feeling frustrated and isolated, marring their experience of maternity services as well as their relationships with midwives.

Midwives should take account of the difficulties encountered by women who are less familiar with the health services and less confident, and ensure that they create an environment that empowers the woman to explain her views and wishes regarding her maternity care.

Consideration should be given to other service users of maternity services, for example, fathers who are the sole carers for their babies have reported that the majority of information on pregnancy and childbirth is aimed at women and their informational needs are not addressed.

Communication and language needs

Communication is a bedrock on which to promote access and woman-centred services, for two reasons. First, women can access and use services only if they are aware of their existence. Midwives can overcome this issue by communicating appropriately and giving timely information to enable women to access maternity services. Second, many women from disadvantaged backgrounds are not confident and are unable to express their needs and preferences to the midwives and so fail to utilize services effectively (Davies & Bath 2001, Hart et al 2001). Consequently, exercising choice and control over the care they receive becomes a challenge and women-centred care will remain a myth for them (Hunt & Symonds 1995, Neile 1997, Stapleton 1997). Midwives can play an important role in facilitating two-way communication to enable women to participate in making decisions about the care they want, need and receive.

Communication difficulty, due either to linguistic limitations or to other forms of disability remains problematic (Baxter 1997, Bowes and Domokos 1996a, Hart et al 2001, Woollett & Dosanjh-Matwala 1990a). Midwives claim that communication and language difficulties hinder the delivery of effective maternity services and have expressed dissatisfaction with the care they provide when they cannot effectively communicate with women who lack proficiency in speaking English, or women with hearing or visual impairment. They state that inability to understand the women as well as explain themselves leaves them frustrated (Audit Commission 1995). Often midwives unintentionally exhibit these frustrations in their behaviour and attitude, which are negatively perceived by the women, marring their experience of maternity services. Consequently, women are less likely to access maternity and preventative services readily.

Midwives recognize that communication and language difficulties may be addressed by making use of professional qualified interpreters or liaison workers or signers (Hayes 1989). However, despite recognition of the value of qualified interpreters in improving service provision and satisfaction, interpreting services are not adequately meeting the demand (Baxter 1997). In practice, the use of qualified interpreters is intermittent and fragmented. Financial resources, midwives beliefs and attitudes, time constraints and the nature of employment of qualified interpreters determine the availability of qualified interpreters (Bharj 2007).

To overcome communication and language difficulties, often women are encouraged to bring their own interpreters (e.g. adults, family members, neighbours and children) (Katbamna 2000). Relying on such measures leads to 'making do' and 'making the best of the situation'. Five women out of a total of 19 who died as a result of domestic violence could not speak English and in all cases the husband acted as interpreter (Lewis 2007). Although interpreter or translator contributions can be useful in overcoming communication difficulties, they can be major barriers during the consultation process, especially when discussing sensitive and personal issues. Voluntary interpreters or relatives and friends are often untrained in the art of interpreting, have little or no knowledge of the NHS and are often confused themselves by medical terminology.

For many, the use of interpreters will be fundamental in the communication process. To this end, midwives should be adequately prepared to use them effectively, taking into account the need for privacy and dignity. Midwives should also utilize interpersonal skills effectively and be sensitive to the communication process between themselves and women who experience communication difficulties so as to create an opportunity for effective and efficient exchange of information. This would serve to provide women with clear, balanced and evidence-based information that they can understand, enabling them to make appropriate informed choices and exercise control over the care they receive.

In circumstances where women cannot effectively communicate with their midwives, they are unable to fully participate in decisions made about their care. These women feel that professionals and hospitals 'take over' and make decisions about them without first discussing all the options, or informing

---

Box 3.3 Communication and information strategy

- Provide information in appropriate community languages and formats to all consumers regarding choices and the services available
- Explore different mediums of communication, for example audiotapes, videotapes, appropriate and sensitive pictorial information, Braille and large print, language line
- During the translation process, ensure that translators are experienced in the appropriate field, and are familiar with medical terminology used
- Take into consideration sensitivity of cultural/ religious beliefs when presenting information
- Ensure that publicity/information materials project positive images of people from the black and minority ethnic communities, women with disability and other groups who are at risk of being socially excluded
- Explore various channels for the dissemination of information to members of socially excluded groups, for example, local ethnic press, radio, television and local community road shows.

---

them of their rights. Box 3.3 provides suggestions for developing a communication and information strategy.

Midwives play a key role in bringing about change. As advocates of women, they should ensure that the needs and wishes of women, in particular those who may not be able to communicate effectively, are taken into consideration during the planning and delivery of services. As change agents, they will need to utilize skills of adaptability, flexibility and political awareness in the development and implementation of innovatory practices to ensure that they are available equitably to all women. Midwives should actively participate in raising awareness of the available services among all women.

Working in partnership

For midwives to work in partnership with women, they need to develop a meaningful relationship with women. Partnership working and its impact in promoting woman-centred care has been discussed in detail, identifying issues such as trust, power and empowerment need due consideration (Calvert 2002, Kirkham 2000). Issues of trust and confidence between women and midwives contribute to meaningful relationships, facilitating an environment where the midwife can ascertain the needs and preferences of the women as well as providing appropriate information so that the woman can make informed choices and be involved in decision-making about her care. Midwives, however, acknowledge that they have difficulty in developing positive relationships with some women, in particular those from a disadvantaged background (Hart et al 2001). Midwives provide the necessary physical care but not appropriate emotional and psychological care and as a result do not really get to know them (Bowes & Domokos 1996a). Often when there is no feedback from these women, midwives get frustrated and angry.

Stereotyping and discrimination play a major role in hindering the development of meaningful relationships. There is well-documented evidence illustrating the detrimental effect of discrimination and racism on people's health (Virdee 1997). Several studies confirm that midwives commonly use stereotypes of women in determining their needs and preferences and utilize these to make judgements about the kind of care women deserve, as well as what a particular woman is likely to want during labour and birth (Bowler 1993a,b; Green et al 1990, Pope et al 2001). Often these stereotypes and prejudices have detrimental effect on women's maternity experiences (HCHC 2003, Redshaw et al 2007).

Women who are 'more visible' are more likely to be negatively stereotyped and negative experiences may be significant factors in reducing women's confidence and prevent them from exercising choice and control over the care they receive. For example, women with disabilities are cared for in a paternalistic manner, which hinders their empowerment; women from travelling families are viewed by society as a threat, dishonest scroungers and dirty; women from South Asian backgrounds are seen as stupid, smelly, attention-seeking, making too much noise during labour and having low pain threshold (Bowler 1993a,b). When professional practices are based on these stereotypes there can be harrowing consequences, for example, in Bowler's study (1993a,b), based on the assumption that Asian women have low pain threshold it was found that midwives often withheld pain relief from them as they considered they were not in real need nor deserving of such care.

Many organizations and midwives claim that they treat everyone the same; care delivery is based upon individualized practices, informed by normal policies and routine practices and women's backgrounds make no difference. This approach is possibly based upon the premise that equal provision is made for all women and the women are expected to integrate and make use of the pre-existing services. This approach in itself can lead to discriminatory practices, where universal provisions fail to meet specific health requirements of women from disadvantaged groups.

Women from socially excluded groups are often seen to have 'special needs', making extra demands on the service. Emphasis on cultural differences that account for ill health, for example tuberculosis, rickets, hepatitis, has contributed towards pathologizing culture. Hence, government initiatives such as the 'stop the rickets' and the 'Asian mother and baby' campaigns have been criticized by many from the BME who claim their communities are singled out, with the blame on their cultural dietary habits or lifestyles, or even their inability to care for their children (Rocheron 1988, Torkington 1984). These approaches focus on cultural idiosyncrasies with particular emphasis on linguistic or cultural differences and quite effectively obscure power differentials between minority ethnic groups and the majority.

Discriminatory attitudes and hostility coupled with their adverse impact on women will do little towards the development of a meaningful relationship. Consequently, partnership working will be rhetoric for women from disadvantaged background as will issues of continuity, choice and control. Midwives need to consider such issues and where possible draw upon transcultural models to provide anti-oppressive care promoting the tenets of woman-centred care for women from disadvantaged groups.

Conclusion

This chapter has focused on a number of issues that require consideration by organizations and midwives when providing and delivering maternity services to all women and their families, in particular those who are most at risk of being excluded. The NHS reforms coupled with government proposals to modernize maternity services to respond effectively to the contemporary population have created exciting opportunities for healthcare practitioners to develop and implement equitable services. However, midwives cannot achieve this huge agenda on their own; organizations have to create an environment to drive some of these changes at a strategic level. The needs and preferences of women from disadvantaged backgrounds must be brought into the mainstream and integrated into the planning and commissioning processes through effective meaningful engagement. The voices of the members who are most at risk of exclusion should be listened to at every point of the planning and commissioning cycle. It is only then that we can provide responsive and appropriate services to meet the needs of all women and their families.

REFERENCES

Acheson S D 1998 Independent Inquiry into Inequalities and Health. The Acheson Report. The Stationery Office, London

Ahmad W I U (ed.) 1993 'Race' and health in contemporary Britain. Open University Press, Buckingham

Ahmad W I U 1996 The trouble with culture. In: Kelleher D, Hillier S (eds) Researching cultural differences in health. Routledge, London, p 190–219

Audit Commission 1995 What seems to be the matter: communication between hospitals and patients. Audit Commission for Local Authorities and National Health Service for England and Wales, London

Baxter C 1997 The case for bilingual workers within the maternity services. British Journal of Midwifery 5(9): 568–572

Bharj K K 2007 Pakistani Muslim women birthing in northern England; exploration of experiences and context. Doctoral Thesis. Sheffield Hallam University, Sheffield

Bowes A M, Domokos T M 1996a Race, gender and culture in South Asian women's health: a study in Glasgow. In: McKie L (ed.) Researching women's health: methods and process. Quay Books, Dinton

Bowes A, Domokos T M 2003 Your dignity is hung up at the door: Pakistani and White women's experiences of childbirth. In: Earle S, Letherby G (eds) Gender, identity and reproduction. Palgrave Macmillan, Basingstoke

Bowler I 1993a They're not the same as us: midwives' stereotypes of south Asian descent maternity patients. Sociology of Health and Illness 15(2):157–178

Bowler I 1993b Stereotype of women of Asian descent in midwifery, some evidence. Midwifery 9:7–16

Byrom S (2006) Antenatal care in children's centres – making it happen. Midwives 9(11):446–447

Calvert S 2002 Being with women: the midwife–woman relationship. In: Mander R, Fleming V (eds) Failure to progress, the contraction of the midwifery profession. Routledge, London

Cartwright A 1979 The dignity of labour? Tavistock, London

Chan C 2000 A study of health services for the Chinese minority in Manchester. British Journal of Community Nursing 5:140–147

CRE (Commission for Racial Equality) 1994 Race relations code of practice in primary healthcare services. CRE, London, p 22

Davies M M, Bath P A 2001 The maternity information concerns of Somali women in the United Kingdom. Journal of Advanced Nursing 36(2):237–245

DfES (Department for Education and Skills) 2006 Working together to safeguard children. HMSO, London

DH (Department of Health) 1997 The new NHS: modern, dependable. DoH, London

DH (Department of Health) 1999 Saving lives: our healthier nation. White Paper. HMSO, London

DH (Department of Health) 2000a The NHS plan. A plan for investment, a plan for reform. Stationery Office, London

DH (Department of Health) 2000b The vital connections: an equalities framework for the NHS. DH, London

DH (Department of Health) 2001 Shifting the balance of power within the NHS: securing delivery. DH, London

DH (Department of Health) 2004 National service framework for children, young people and maternity services. DH, London

DH (Department of Health) 2005 Creating a patient-led NHS, delivering the NHS Improvement Plan. DH, London

DH (Department of Health) 2006a Our health, our care, our say: a new direction for community services. White Paper. Cm 6737. The Stationery Office, London

DH (Department of Health) 2006b The NHS in England: the operating framework for 2006/7. HMSO, London

DH (Department of Health) 2007a Maternity matters: choice, access and continuity of care in a safe service. DH, London

DH (Department of Health) 2007b Choice matters: 2007–8, putting patients in control. DH, London

DHSSPS (Department of Health, Social Services and Public Safety) 2004 A healthier future. A twenty year vision for health and wellbeing in Northern Ireland. DHSSPS, Belfast

DHSSPS (Department of Health, Social Services and Public Safety) 2005 It's what matters to patients. Northern Ireland Essence of Care Project. DHSSPS, Belfast

Dixon-Woods M 2005 Vulnerable groups and access to healthcare: a critical interpretive review. Report for the National Co-ordinating Centre for NHS Service Delivery and Organization R & D (NCCSDO). University of Leicester, Leicester

Ellis N 2004 Birth experiences of South Asian Muslim women: marginalized choice within the maternity services. In:

Kirkham M (ed.) Informed choice in maternity care. Palgrave Macmillan, Basingstoke

Fernando S 1991 Mental health, race and culture. Macmillan/MIND, London, p 24

Gerrish K, Husband C, MacKenzie J 1996 Nursing for a multi-ethnic society. Open University Press, Buckingham

Green J M, Kitzinger J V, Coupland V A 1990 Stereotype of childbearing women. Midwifery 6(3):125–132

Hastie N 2000 Cultural conceptions. In: Fraser D (ed.) Professional studies for midwifery practice. Churchill Livingstone, Edinburgh, p 63–75

Harper-Bulman K, McCourt C 2002 Somali refugee women's experiences of maternity care in west London: a case study. Critical Public Health 12(4):365–379

Hart A, Lockey R, Henwood F, et al 2001 Addressing inequalities in health: new directions in midwifery education and practice. Research report No. 20. English National Board for Nursing, Midwifery and Health Visiting, London

Hayes L 1989 The role of the interpreter/linkworker in the maternity service. Unpublished MA thesis. University of Warwick, Coventry

HCHC (House of Commons Health Committee) 2003 Inequalities in access to maternity services. Eighth report of Session 2002–03. The Stationery Office, London

Helman C G 1994 Culture, health and illness, 3rd edn. Butterworth-Heinemann, Oxford

Hirst J, Hewison J 2001 Pakistani and indigenous 'white' women's views and the Donabedian–Maxwell grid: a consumer-focused template for assessing the quality of maternity care. International Journal of Healthcare Quality Assurance 14(7):308–316

Hirst J, Hewison J 2002 Hospital postnatal care: obtaining the views of Pakistani and indigenous 'white' women. Clinical Effectiveness in Nursing 6(1):10–18

HM Government 2006 Reaching out: an action plan on social exclusion. Cabinet Office, London

Hunt S, Symonds A 1995 The social meaning of midwifery. MacMillan, Basingstoke

Katbamna S 2000 'Race' and childbirth. Open University Press, Buckingham

Kirkham M (ed.) 2000 The midwife–mother relationship. MacMillan, Basingstoke

Kitzinger J 1990 Strategies of the early childbirth movement: a case study of the National Childbirth Trust. In: Garcia J, Kilpatrick R, Richards M (eds) The politics of maternity care. Oxford University Press, New York, Ch 5, p 92–115

Kitzinger S 1978 Women as mothers. Fontana, London

Larbie J 1985 Black women and the maternity services. Health Education Council and the National Extension College for Training in Health and Race, London

Leininger M M 1978 Trans-cultural nursing: concepts, theories and practice. John Wiley, New York

Lewis G (ed.) 2007 The Confidential Enquiry into Maternal and Child Health (CEMACH). Saving Mothers Lives: reviewing maternal deaths to make motherhood safer – 2003–2005. The Seventh Report on Confidential Enquiries into Maternal Deaths in the United Kingdom. CEMACH, London

Lewis G, Drife J (eds) 2004 Why mothers die. The Sixth Report of the Confidential Enquiries into Maternal Deaths in United Kingdom 2000–2002. The Confidential Enquiries into Maternal and Child Health. RCOG Press, London

Lewis G, Drife J (eds) 2001 Why mothers die. The Fifth Report of the Confidential Enquiries into Maternal Deaths in the United Kingdom 1997–1999. The National Institute of Clinical Excellence. RCOG Press, London

Lewis I M 1976 Social anthropology. Penguin, Harmondsworth

Macfarlane A, Mugford M 2000 Birth counts: statistics of pregnancy and childbirth. The Stationery Office, London

MacKeith P, Phillipson R 1997 Young mothers. In: Kargar I, Hunt S C (eds) Challenges in maternity care. Macmillan, Basingstoke

Macpherson W 1999 The Stephen Lawrence inquiry: report of an inquiry. Home Office, London

Modood T, Berthoud R, Lakey J, et al 1997 Ethnic minorities in Britain: diversity and disadvantage. The Fourth National Survey of Ethnic Minorities. Policies Studies Institute, London

National Assembly for Wales 2001 Improving Health in Wales: A Plan for the NHS and its partners. National Assembly for Wales, Cardiff

National Assembly for Wales 2005 Designed for life – a world class health service for Wales. National Assembly for Wales, Cardiff

Nazroo J 1997 The health of Britain's ethnic minorities: findings from a national survey. Policies Studies Institute, London

Nazroo J 2001 Ethnicity, class and health. Policy Studies Institute, London

Neile E 1997 Control for black and ethnic minority women: a meaningless pursuit. In: Kirkham M J, Perkins E R (eds) Reflections on midwifery. Baillière Tindall, London, Ch 6, p 114–134

NHS Quality Improvement Scotland 2005 Clinical standards – maternity services. NHS Quality Improvement Scotland, Edinburgh

NI DHSSPS (Northern Ireland Department of Health, Social Services and Public Safety) 2002 Developing better services: modernizing hospitals and reforming structures. NI DHSSPS, Belfast

NMC (Nursing and Midwifery Council) 2008 The Code: Standards of conduct, performance and ethics for nurses and midwives. NMC, London

Oakley A 1979 Becoming a mother. Martin Robertson, Oxford

ONS (Office for National Statistics) 2001 Social trends 31. ONS, London

Palmer G, MacInnes T, Kenway P 2006 Monitoring poverty and social exclusion 2006. Joseph Rowntree Foundation, York

Phoenix A 1990 Black women and the maternity services. In: Garcia J, Kilpatrick R, Richards M (eds) The politics of maternity care. Oxford University Press, New York, Ch 15, p 274–299

Platt L 2007 Poverty and ethnicity in the UK. The Policy Press, Bristol

Pope R, Graham L, Patel S 2001 Woman-centred care. International Journal of Nursing Studies 38:227–238

RCM (Royal College of Midwives) 2000a Position Paper 4a: woman-centred care. Reprinted in RCM Midwives Journal 2001 4(2):46–47

RCM (Royal College of Midwives) 2000b Maternity care for lesbian mothers. Position Paper No. 22. RCM, London

RCM 2003 Evidence provided for the House of Commons Health Committee (2003) Inequalities in Access to Maternity Services, Eighth Report of Session 2002–03. The Stationery Office, London, p 17

Redshaw M, Rowe R, Hockley C, et al 2007 Recorded delivery: a national survey of women's experience of maternity care 2006. National Perinatal Epidemiology Unit, Oxford

Reid M, Garcia J 1989 Women's views of care during pregnancy and childbirth. In: Chalmers I, Enkin M, Keirse M J N C (eds) Effective care in pregnancy and childbirth. Clarendon Press, Oxford, p 131–142

Richens Y 2003 Exploring the experiences of women of Pakistani origin of UK maternity services. Report prepared for the 8th Mary Seacole. Online. Available: www.yanarichens.com

Rocheron Y 1988 The Asian mother and baby campaign: the construction of ethnic minorities 'health needs'. Critical Social Policy 22:4–23

Rose S, Rose H 1986 Less than human nature. Race and Class 27(3):47–66

Salmon D, Powell J 1998 Caring for women in poverty: a critical review. British Journal of Midwifery 6(2):108–111

Scottish Executive Health Department (SEHD) 2001 A framework for maternity services in Scotland. Scottish Executive, Scotland

Scottish Executive Health Department (SEHD) 2005a Delivering for health. Scottish Executive, Edinburgh

Scottish Executive Health Department (SEHD) 2005b Building a health service fit for the future. Scottish Executive, Edinburgh

Shribman S 2007 Making it better: for mother and baby. Clinical case for change. Department of Health, London

Sivagnanam R (ed.) 2004 Experiences of maternity services: Muslim women's perspectives. The Maternity Alliance, London

Smaje C 1995 Health, race and ethnicity: making sense of the evidence. King's Fund Institute, London, p 16

Social Exclusion Unit 1999 Teenage pregnancy. Stationery Office, London

Stapleton H 1997 Choice in the face of uncertainty. In: Kirkham M J, Perkins E R (eds) Reflections on midwifery. Baillière Tindall, London, Ch 3, p 47–69

Stubbs P 1993 'Ethnically sensitive' or 'anti-racist'? Models for health research and service delivery. In: Ahmad W I U (ed.) Race and health in contemporary Britain. Open University Press, Buckingham, Ch 3, p 34–47

Teenage Pregnancy Unit 2004 DH Nursing and midwifery policy, Royal College of Midwives. RCM, London

Torkington P 1984 Blaming black women – rickets and racism. In: O'Sullivan S (ed.) 1987 Women's health, a spare rib reader. Pandora, London, Ch 2, p 82–85

Townsend P, Davidson N 1982 Inequalities in health: the Black report. Penguin, Harmondsworth

Virdee S 1997 Racial harassment. In: Modood T, Berthoud R, Lakey J et al (eds) 1997 Ethnic minorities in Britain: diversity and disadvantage; Fourth National Survey of Ethnic Minorities. Policies Studies Institute, London, Ch 8, p 259–289

WAG (Welsh Assembly Government) 2005 NSF for Children, Young People and Maternity Services in Wales. Welsh Assembly Government, Cardiff

Wilton T, Kaufmann T 2001 Lesbian mothers' experiences of maternity care in the UK. Midwifery 17:203–211

Woollett A, Dosanjh-Matwala N 1990a Pregnancy and antenatal care: the attitudes and experiences of Asian women. Child Care, Health and Development 16(1):63–78

Woollett A, Dosanjh-Matwala N 1990b Postnatal care: the attitudes and experiences of Asian women in east London. Midwifery 6:178–184

Whitehead M 1987 The health divide: inequalities in health in the 1980s. Health Education Council, London

4 Woman-centred, midwife-friendly care: principles, patterns and culture of practice

Lesley Page

CHAPTER CONTENTS

Midwives hold an important key to positive care around the time of childbirth that will contribute to a good start for the baby and parents during this critical period of human life. The key to unlocking the potential of midwifery is the appropriate organization and culture of care. Where the organization of care is right, allowing for continuity of care, the exercise of autonomy in practice, good support and a strong community base, midwives may provide more effective, sensitive and appropriate care. Highly centralized, fragmented care in which professional autonomy is not possible, severely restricts the potential of midwives to make their full contribution to the care of childbearing women. This chapter examines the principles of midwifery and the way that the organization of practice and the culture or ethos of care may be developed. This reformed midwifery will be referred to as 'The New Midwifery' (Page & McCandlish 2006).

This chapter aims to examine:

- the background to recent changes to the patterns and culture of practice
- the principles of the new midwifery
- key characteristics of different patterns of practice
- how different patterns of practice may support these principles
- working in different ways
- how to manage situations in which neither midwives nor women have a range of choices about how and where to give birth, or the pattern of practice.

Background

The roots of midwifery lie in the care of childbearing women by other women from their own community or family. Even after the professionalization of midwifery, with the registration of midwives, the majority were community-based. The majority of births were home births, with the balance of home versus hospital births being altered over the last half century in the UK. This brought about a division between hospital and community midwifery; where midwives were hospital-based they were organized on a model of acute care nursing. Thus, care became highly fragmented. In addition, as maternity care became more and more technical and medical in its nature, it became more difficult for midwives to practise autonomously. Thus, the potential for an ongoing relationship between the woman and her midwife was eroded, and the ability for midwives to use all their skills and knowledge and to manage care was diminished.

Since the early 1980s, much work has been undertaken to redevelop continuity in the relationship between women and their midwives, and to enable midwives to practise more autonomously. This work has happened in many parts of the world. It has consisted of changes in midwifery regulation, and in policy at governmental and local level, of developments of innovative practice and of research and evaluation. In some countries, e.g. the Netherlands, New Zealand and Canada, many midwives are not employees of a health service but may work in publicly or insurance-funded independent practices. Ideally, although practising independently, these midwives have access to local health services with mechanisms for consultation, referral and transfer when problems occur. In two of the Provinces of Canada, for example, midwives have admitting privileges to local hospitals where they are part of medical departments (Page 2000, Sandall et al 2001).

The new midwifery

What has arisen from these developments in policy and practice is a reformation of midwifery that takes in some of the historical values and functions of midwifery while adapting it to the needs of the modern world and more complex health services. What has been called the 'new midwifery' has emerged over recent years.

The internationally accepted definition of a midwife is a basis for understanding the scope of practice of midwifery (Nursing and Midwifery Council [NMC] 2004). However, it is only a starting point. This definition provides no ideas on how midwifery is similar to medical maternity practice, and how it differs. There are two aspects of effective midwifery that make it unique. First, midwives are the specialists in normal labour and birth, and hold the potential to support normal healthy outcomes. Second, midwives have the potential to work through a personal relationship with women (the original meaning of midwife) through the whole of pregnancy, birth and the early weeks of life, including labour; this relationship has been described in a number of ways that include one of friendship, of partnership and of skilled companion. Such a relationship is crucial to developing the new midwifery into practice.

Principles of patterns of practice for the new midwifery

The development of the new midwifery contains essential elements. These are:

- working in a positive relationship with women
- being aware of the significance of pregnancy and birth and the early weeks of life as the start of human life and the new family
- avoiding harm by using the best information or evidence in practice
- having adequate skills to deliver effective care and support
- promoting health and well-being.

The principles of patterns of practice that support development of the new midwifery are as follows:

- woman-centred care, including choice, control and continuity for women. Wide access to care is crucial
- the potential for the development of a personal continuous relationship between the woman and her midwife
- community-based care

- midwifery autonomy and a clear expression of the distinct nature of midwifery practice, including the support of normal or physiological birth
- appropriate support for midwives
- a positive organizational culture
- an interface with other professionals, midwives, doctors, nurses and health visitors, and hospitals and mechanisms for consultation, referral and transfer
- cost-effectiveness.

I will discuss each of these principles in detail, then the patterns of practice that will support them.

Woman-centred care, access, choice, control and continuity

The term 'woman-centred care' is often used to describe the philosophy of care promoted in the early 1990s in the UK (House of Commons 1992, DH 1993, SOHHD 1993). This term means that women and their families should be at the heart of everything midwives do in practice. They should be given choice in the place of birth, caregiver and care, and be given control over their own care and experience. Two keys to achieving these principles are the provision of continuity of carer – a professional who they could get to know and trust over time who would provide and manage most care – and the restoration of autonomous midwifery.

The policy document *Maternity Matters: Choice, access and continuity of care in a safe service* (DH 2007) widens the principles of woman-centred care in an important way. While some of the principles of the earlier policy documents remain, *Maternity Matters* also includes the importance of access to care. Widening access to care is important in the light of inequalities in the experience and outcome of care that are influenced by ethnicity and deprivation. *Maternity Matters* also sets out plans for a reconfiguration of services that will centralize more medically led and complex care in larger hospitals, and provide midwifery-led care in community-based services. This will provide a guarantee of:

1. Choice of how to access maternity care
2. Choice of type of antenatal care
3. Choice of place of birth – depending on their circumstances, women and their partners will be able to choose between three different options. These are:

- a home birth
- birth in a local facility, including a hospital, under the care of a midwife
- birth in a hospital supported by a local maternity care team including midwives, anaesthetists and consultant obstetricians. For some women, this will be the safest option.

Choice of place of postnatal care

The exercise of choice is a complex process that is harder than it sounds, but is important. Widening access to maternity care is one of the most important issues of modern day services and may be linked to continuity and choice in care. In this chapter, I argue that whichever way the maternity services are reconfigured the basis of effective, safe and positive care is a continuing relationship with one named professional over the period of care. The named professional should provide most but not all care and should coordinate care.

Choice and control

To my mind the word 'choice' does not do justice to the way in which midwives work with women to help them retain personal autonomy and a sense of being a strong, powerful mother. A more accurate description would be to help women make informed decisions. The best decisions are informed not only by the evidence but also the health, personal circumstances and preferences, beliefs and values of individual women. The midwife is a mediator working with the health service in the interests of the woman and her family, using her experience and the best evidence and information. In Page & McCandlish (2006) a number of experienced midwives have given examples of how they have worked with individual women using the five steps of evidence-based care to help women in making the number of decisions that they face in modern and highly complex maternity services.

The five steps of evidence based midwifery are:

1. Finding out what is important to the woman and her family
2. Using information from the clinical examination
3. Seeking and assessing evidence to inform decisions

4. Talking it through
5. Reflecting on outcomes feelings and consequences.

In many ways, the idea is a simple one. Involving women in making decisions about their own care and that of their baby and having a respectful relationship with them should not be difficult. However, there are a number of things that will make it easier for midwives (and others) to work in this way. First, the choices need to be available. If, for example, the woman wishes to give birth outside of the hospital, this will obviously be difficult if no alternatives are available. Second, decisions are often set against a back drop of a health service in which intervention is the norm, and it is difficult for both midwives and the women they are caring for to make choices that go against this norm. It is particularly difficult to go against this norm if things do not work out as planned. Third, given the amount of information and the number of interventions available, and the diverse nature of many of the communities in which the midwives practise, it is very difficult to have a discussion over time on the basis of a relationship in which the woman and her midwife know and trust each other, unless there is some continuity of care.

The move to give women more personal autonomy and midwives more professional autonomy have paralleled each other over recent decades. Midwives whose scholarly work has been derived from practice have provided rich literature in which this idea of involving women in making decisions about their care and the care of their baby is seen as an important aspect of supporting a positive transition to parenthood in which the woman builds on her own personal strengths and finds confidence in making decisions about her care and the care of her child. This idea, called in shorthand form 'choice', represents one of the most fundamental shifts in values in the maternity services. It represents a shift from a situation in which women have things done to them, to a situation in which professionals work with women, planning care around their needs rather than along routine or institutionally driven lines.

Leap and Edwards (2006), in calling for a more nuanced examination of choice, highlight the context of oppression in maternity services and women's lives, and criticize the idea of informed choice that puts the onus of control on the individual without recognizing that social inequalities are particularly powerful. Genuine choices are often limited by what is available and acceptable to local services and communities. To give women genuine choice requires a change to health services so that choices are actually available. It also requires that all professionals, including medical staff, are encouraged to look their beloved beliefs, practices and rituals in the eye and question them to see if they are genuinely likely to be beneficial to individual women and families. This is not an easy thing for any of us to do.

Working through a relationship with the woman

It is far easier to work with women in helping them make the right decisions for them and their baby and family, if decisions can be talked through, considered over time and in the context of a trusting and respectful relationship. Pairman (2006) describes the relationship as the medium from which midwives practise. Building this relationship requires continuity of care. Freely (1995, p 7) describes the importance of the structure of continuity of care well: 'Midwives can do a better job if their work is structured in such a way as to enable them to become acquainted with and take responsibility for their patients'. Freeley described the care she received from a team of midwives as 'care with a face and a memory and an ever open ear. It made me feel like an active participant' (p 7). In comparison, the care she experienced in the conventional system was from a 'faceless institution'. It is through the development of relationships between caregivers and childbearing women and their families that we make the change from faceless institution to humanistic supportive care.

The relationship between women and their midwives is seen by women as important in itself, and not only as an instrumental means of leading to other outcomes (Wilkins 2000). However, the development of a relationship is also the basis of the ability to give women choice and control, and helps in the support of physiological birth and in the comforting role of the midwife. Importantly, this relationship is the medium for the support the midwife may give the family in their journey to their new roles and responsibility, the transition to parenthood. As the skilled companion (Campbell 1984), the midwife acts as a guide and supporter, helping the woman through rough and difficult terrain, enjoying the pleasures and excitement of the journey, while allowing the woman and her partner to make their own journey and learn the lessons and gather a sense of their own strength from the journey and its completion.

If midwives know and understand the women they are caring for, and where trust has grown between them, they will find it easier to respond to individual needs, to comfort and to encourage women through some of the difficulties, not only of pregnancy and after the birth but also through labour and birth. Women describe the importance of knowing their midwife, particularly during labour and birth, and of the confidence and trust this brings (McCourt et al 2006).

Women who have received 'continuity' of care do not use the term continuity. These women talk about the value of knowing their caregivers and why this is important to them. Women tend to link supportive care with knowing their midwife (McCourt et al 2006).

In the study by McCourt et al (2000, p 282), women who had received one-to-one care described the importance of the availability of the midwife both directly and over time; the words of the women themselves describe the trust that develops and the way that knowing the midwife is reassuring as follows:

I knew exactly what was going to happen, when and how, that was one bit of it. Another thing is you knew the person there, and she was there only herself, no one else.

There is a sense of intimacy, of feeling that the midwife was accessible, on the same level as the woman:

Well I could talk to her about anything and say to her everything, that's how much confidence I had in her.

Women also described the way midwives become a part of the experience:

Well they do know me, they recognize me, but my midwife, she was part of it, part of the birth, the baby.

Women talked about the midwife as a friend, as being like family. They described midwives they had come to know as 'my midwife' in contrast to 'the midwife' or 'they'. There was a sense of closeness to the midwife, of a special relationship.

It is this 'with woman' aspect of midwifery that many midwives have tried to reintroduce to midwifery practice over recent years: the relationship that allows a spirit of 'being with' rather than 'doing to'. Midwives have explained the great lengths they go to in order to develop the relationship that puts women at the heart of care, and seeks and supports their active involvement in their pregnancy and birth (Pairman 2006).

Midwives who describe the relationship, like women, describe it in terms of friendship, partnership, professional friendship and professional servant (Kirkham 2000). It is a relationship in which midwife and woman contribute equally, and is one of sharing, involving trust, shared control and respect, and shared meaning through understanding (Pairman 2000). It acts as a foundation for shared decision-making, and facilitates communication. Although called a friendship, it is not exactly a friendship because the midwife enters as an expert, and the relationship is usually terminated at the end of care. It can be seen as a friendship with a purpose.

The relationship is used intentionally to shift power towards the woman, what Cronk (2000) has described as the professional servant, but midwives cannot empower women unless they themselves are empowered (Kirkham 2000). The trust is not only by the woman from the midwife but requires that the midwife believes in or trusts the woman (Leap 2000). It is recognized that the most powerful help for a woman may come from doing as little as possible, as Leap (2000, p 2) puts it, 'the less we do the more we give'. Although there are times, particularly in labour, when a midwife may need to take charge or take control, this works better when there is a previously formed relationship (Anderson 2000).

Importance of continuity and what it means

It is difficult to form the kind of relationship described unless the pattern of practice allows the provision of what has become known as 'continuity of carer'. The term 'continuity of carer' is a description of the structure that is set up to enable the relationship between the woman and her midwife to develop over time. This structure should organize care so that individual women may receive most of their care from a named midwife. This named midwife provides and manages most of the midwifery care for a woman, and is likely to be available for critical events in the woman's pregnancy including labour and birth. This is not the same as solo practice. In the most effective organizations the midwife has a partner or small number of partners who will stand in for the named midwife when she is unavailable, and who will also have formed a relationship with the woman. Essentially, in this system of care, midwives follow women through the service, rather than having women progress through a number of teams of people. The latter is an assembly line or conveyer belt of sorts.

The development of patterns of practice that allow true continuity of caregiver may require radical change. It will also require a system of on call for a large number of midwives. It is the need for these radical changes that has led to the development of tremendous controversy and debate around the need for continuity of carer, particularly among midwives. It has been claimed that what women really want is continuity of care – a shared philosophy. This denies the importance of the relationship in itself to women, and the use of self that a midwife may give in supporting and comforting and encouraging women. It also denies the difficulty of large numbers of people making complex decisions in the same way as others, given their own personal values and knowledge. In addition, the lack of a real knowledge of the medical history and personal values and preferences of the individual woman makes it very difficult to make personally sensitive and appropriate decisions.

It has also been argued that women have other priorities, such as the health of their baby and good information, as though such desires could be ranked in a hierarchy (Page 1995). Some have interpreted evidence in such a way that they argue women do not really want continuity of carer. In reality, evidence to refute or support the idea that it is important for women to have continuity of caregiver, or that particular outcomes are the direct outcomes of continuity of carer, is not easy to develop or interpret from the dominant paradigm of research: the randomized controlled trial. In addition, finding out about what women want from care around birth is difficult. Women tend to expect what is on offer

(DeVries et al 2001). Even so, when surveys of women who have experienced 'continuity of carer' are undertaken, the majority indicate that it is important to them, and even in surveys of women who have not experienced 'continuity of carer', the majority indicate that it would be helpful to them. Moreover, qualitative research is beginning to explain why it is so important to so many women (McCourt et al 2006).

Much of the debate about whether or not women want continuity and about the interpretation of the outcomes of studies of continuity of care have focused on whether or not it is continuity as a shared philosophy of care that is important or whether or not it is knowing one's midwife that matters. The hierarchy developed by Saulz and adapted for maternity helps clarify the concepts. The following is taken from McCourt et al (2006, p 143–144).

> General reviews of continuity of care have tended to conceptualise continuity in a range of ways (Haggerty et al 2003). All have aimed to develop a common understanding of the concept of continuity in order to understand the impact in different settings. Unless we understand the mechanisms through which care delivered over time improves outcomes, continuity interventions may be misdirected or inappropriately evaluated.
>
> From these various definitions, it appears that continuity can most usefully be defined as a hierarchical concept ranging from the basic availability of information about the woman's past history to a complex interpersonal relationship between provider and woman characterized by trust and a sense of responsibility (Saultz 2003). At the base of this hierarchy is the notion of informational continuity. This concept might be the most important aspect of continuity in preventing medical errors and ensuring safety (Cook et al 2000), but by itself informational continuity might not improve access to, or satisfaction with care. Longitudinal continuity creates a familiar setting in which care can occur and should make it easier for women to access care when needed, but it does not assure a relationship of personal trust between an individual care provider and a recipient of care (Table 4.1).
>
> By arranging these concepts as a hierarchy, it is implied that at least some informational continuity is required for longitudinal continuity to be present and that longitudinal continuity is required for interpersonal continuity to exist in a midwife–woman relationship.
>
> There have been a number of ways of measuring continuity, i.e. who usually provides care, and for how long, normally based on the health record (Saultz 2003). However, these do not take into account the content of the visit and the nature of

Table 4.1 Hierarchical definition of continuity of care

Level of continuity	Description
1. Informational	An organized collection of medical and social information about each woman is readily available to any healthcare professional caring for her. A systematic process also allows accessing and communicating about this information among those involved in the care.
2. Longitudinal	In addition to informational continuity, each woman has a 'place' where she receives most care, which allows the care to occur in an accessible and familiar environment from an organized team of providers. This team assumes responsibility for coordinating the quality of care, including preventive services.
3. Interpersonal	In addition to longitudinal continuity, an ongoing relationship exists between each woman and a midwife. The woman knows the midwife by name and has come to trust the midwife on a personal basis. The woman uses this personal midwife for basic midwifery care and depends on the midwife to assume personal responsibility for her overall care. When the personal midwife is not available, coverage arrangement assures that longitudinal continuity occurs.

Adapted from (Saultz 2003) in McCourt et al 2006, with permission.

the interaction. Multiple definitions and measures have also made it difficult to generalize about the effect of continuity (Donaldson 2001). Research on whether continuity of care is effective has measured outcomes such as behaviours of recipients and caregivers, adherence to advice, use of services, clinical sequelae, clinician knowledge of patient's conditions, costs, and patient and staff satisfaction. Surveys have shown that patients and staff value continuity and that it is positively associated with staff satisfaction, but the causal direction is unknown.

In maternity care, there has been debate about two important and subtly different concepts to examine here – 'continuity of care' and 'continuity of carer'. Continuity of care means ensuring that there is a shared philosophy and approach to care that women experience. As we will show, this is often discussed but difficult to achieve in large fragmented systems of care, even where there is a 'team' approach. Continuity of carer means enabling midwives to organise their practice so that they may form a continuing working relationship with women in their care. It means enabling midwives to work with women through the whole of pregnancy, birth and the early weeks of newborn life, so that they may get to know each other and form a relationship that is based on trust between the two. This relationship, of trust and mutual respect, has been fundamental to the development of midwifery knowledge and wisdom.

The development of a high level of continuity of carer may be the most difficult change to achieve, but is probably the most fundamental or important change to bring about. It is helped tremendously if community and hospital services can be integrated, and if most of a woman's care is moved away from centralized institutions and given in the community.

Community-based care

If the midwife can become a part of the woman's community, getting to know the woman and her family more personally, learning to understand their lives and the nature of the life around them, she will be able to be more responsive to them as individuals, and may be released from the depersonalization of the institution. This is also important in allowing midwives to respond to the needs and characteristics of different neighbourhoods and communities, and to understand the racial and ethnic mix and level of poverty or affluence of 'her' patch. Such knowledge helps in deciding whether the development of different community services, for example a shop-front practice or premises within a housing estate, are appropriate (Davies 2000). It takes healthcare to the community rather than expecting women to visit for healthcare. Increasing accessibility and attractiveness are important parts of good healthcare. Community-based care can be provided either in the home (e.g. antenatal visits at home, or a genuine choice of home birth) or in community centres, midwives' or doctors' surgeries or offices situated in the community. Small hospitals, and out-of-hospital birth centres, will provide care that is both near the woman's own home and less acute care for at least a small group of women.

Second, when the care of childbearing women takes place in an acute care setting, in the main by specialists or consultants, there will be a tendency to use more medical and surgical interventions. Care provided by skilled, confident and experienced primary practitioners (midwives and family doctors or GPs) is more likely to support physiological processes and less likely to lead to unnecessary intervention (Page 2007).

Home birth will lead to a more profound change from hospital birth than any other change in the organization of care. The best evidence on the outcomes of home birth and the experience of home birth for women without complications or real risk factors shows persistently that there is a lower rate of interventions, and that women who ask for a home birth generally enjoy the experience (Page 2006). Birth at home means that the woman can relax in her own environment, and that she is in a different power relationship with professionals, who are invited into her home. Although there are exceptions (Edwards 2000), in general, the relationship is of a higher quality. Home birth brings with it its own pattern of practice, and on the whole it is easier to provide the woman with midwives she can get to know and trust.

Community-based care, if organized effectively, may increase access to care. Ensuring wide access is one of the most important factors in reducing inequalities in health and in increasing choice for the majority of women, not only the most informed or affluent. *Saving Mothers' Lives* (Lewis 2007) reported that vulnerable women with socially complex lives, those from the most deprived areas of England and asylum seekers and refugees had a higher than average risk of maternal mortality (see Ch. 56).

The factors associated with this higher risk were problems with access, lack of follow-up care, inadequate translation, inadequate referrals, poor interagency working. Continuity of care is a way of combating these gaps in the service. Murray and Bachus (2005) describe a multitude of barriers to accessing timely and optimal care, including the lack of information in appropriate formats, negative and stereotypical attitudes of staff, lack of continuity of care, and poor communication and coordination between maternity and other services.

In England the linking of midwifery group practices with 'Sure Start' projects has provided an opportunity to work with other agencies in providing the complex support that more vulnerable and socially excluded and deprived women and their families may need. Sure Start is the government programme to deliver the best start in life for every child. Sure Start brings together, early education, childcare, health and family support in local communities. The One-to-One Midwifery Project at Guy's and St Thomas' Maternity Service serving a deprived community in South London had one midwifery practice working with a Sure Start Centre. There was a reduction in the 'did not attend' rate between the standard service and the One-to-One Service providing continuity of care (Singh et al, personal communication, 2007). The 'did not attend rate' is an important indicator. While the relationship between poor outcomes and failure to attend appointments is unclear, it was found that 17% of the women who died from indirect or direct causes booked for maternity care after 22 weeks' gestation or had missed over four routine antenatal visits (Lewis 2007).

Midwifery autonomy – expressing the unique nature of midwifery in practice

To practise the new midwifery, the midwife needs professional autonomy. This does not mean, however, that the midwife should practise in isolation. She needs to work in an interface with other members of the healthcare team, while knowing that the contribution she makes is unique and cannot be made by any other member of the team. The midwife has specialist approaches and skills that no other member of the healthcare team has, even though some of her role will overlap with that of doctors, both GPs and obstetricians (Page 2001).

Professional autonomy requires that:

- the midwife is responsible for all care unless she makes a referral to another health professional
- any guidelines and policies should have been developed and approved by midwifery after a proper process of consultation.

The worldview of midwifery is to have confidence in normal or physiological processes, rather than feeling that these could fail at any moment. This worldview requires a different knowledge base, research interest and skill set in midwives. During pregnancy and birth, there should be sufficient focus on the woman's experience, and help and support for distressing aspects of pregnancy and birth, as well as sharing the enjoyment and joy. Presence, comfort and appropriate touch, reassurance and encouragement are central aspects of midwife-led care. Particularly during labour and birth, midwifery autonomy allows the midwife to take into account the woman as an individual in making decisions about care, and to provide more flexible care. I have never been able to see how midwife-led care or autonomous midwifery can be effective without some basis of continuity. However, there is considerable debate about this matter and midwife-led care rather than continuity has been the aim of a number of innovations.

Supporting midwives

In most of the Western world, maternity services have been centralized into acute care hospitals. This is despite the fact that pregnancy is a normal part of the life of the majority of women, and that childbearing is in general a healthy life event. Instead it would be more appropriate for care to be given in the primary care sector of the health service, rather than by specialists in an acute care setting.

There are problems with the centralization of birth into acute care, including a tendency, referred to earlier, in all large organizations of people to move towards institutionalization. Kirkham wrote, 'with the centralization of birth into hierarchically organized and increasingly large hospitals, midwifery increasingly adopted the responses and values of those institutions. All these responses served to protect the status quo which reinforced the values of obstetrics not midwifery'. Kirkham drew on the work of Raphael-Leff who 'sees the fragmented care given in maternity hospitals as part of a social defence system ... constructed to help individual professionals avoid experiencing anxiety, guilt, doubt and uncertainty. Both caring and gratitude are diminished in a system where people are treated in a depersonalized way and any activities which threaten the status quo are intensely resisted' (Kirkham 2000, p 157).

The majority of midwives in the economically developed world work in large institutions, usually hospitals. Often, such institutions unconsciously attend to the needs of staff before families. Often, they are arranged in such a way that it is very difficult for staff to provide the best care. Any group of people is likely to develop a life of its own. In many health services there is a rigid hierarchy or an informal power structure that may give some groups like midwives little professional autonomy. This is not simply a matter of a hierarchy in which midwives have less power than other professionals because, although it is the case that midwives are often lower in the health service hierarchy than doctors, much of the oppression of midwifery comes from within midwifery itself.

Deery and Kirkham (2006) describe the cultural context of midwifery in the UK. NHS Midwives have talked about their support needs and their lack of support. They believe that because the culture of NHS midwifery is a female culture of 'service and sacrifice' (Deery & Kirkham 2006, p 125) it is seen as selfish to address personal needs. Yet, as they point out, while support needs have not moved beyond an acknowledgement of stress and burn out, Sandall's work (Sandall 1997) has linked support for midwives with both their job satisfaction and the quality of care they give to women.

Midwives manifest a number of ways of coping with the needs of the organization. Deery and Kirkham draw on the work of Menzies Lyth (1979, 1988), Lipsky (1980) Raphael-Leff (1991) to explain and describe the ways midwives cope with the needs of the institution. Task-oriented care, standard practices and rigid routines provide a defence against stress and anxiety. Midwives are like public service workers who work directly with the public within bureaucracies who in practice must deal with clients on a mass basis. 'At best street level bureaucrats invent benign modes of mass processing that more or less permit them to deal with the public fairly, appropriately and successfully. At worst, they give in to favouritism, stereotyping and routinizing all of which serve private or agency purposes (Lipsky 1980, p xii). Raphael-Leff applies the work of Menzies Lyth to midwifery identifying three defence mechanisms that midwives use to protect themselves against stress and anxiety. These are:

- the splitting up of the midwife–patient relationship
- denial and detachment of feelings
- redistribution of responsibility.

The development of continuity of care, and support for midwives to understand and express some of the anxieties that develop from working with women in a professional relationship (Deery & Kirkham 2006), while enabling autonomous practice, will go a long way to breaking down these defence mechanisms.

Deery and Kirkham (2006) describe the importance of a balance of engagement and detachment in relationships with women. This implies being involved but recognizing limits of what one can and cannot do. The difficulty is that managing the workload often becomes the priority, rather than the needs of women. Social defence systems in the organization that are a dysfunctional form of protecting ourselves from anxiety and distress often involve an evasion of relationship. This evasion inhibits growth. Support for the primary task of midwifery fosters personal and professional growth. It helps to build working structures within which relationships can grow. These need a smaller scale organization of care, and a degree of separation from the obstetrical model, and enhancement of professional autonomy and continuity of care. Positive relationships require higher levels of self awareness and skills in social analysis. Skills of support can be developed and guided reflection and clinical supervision is seen as an important tool (Deery & Kirkham 2006).

Deery and Kirkham (2007) also describe the competing organizational and client demands as a health hazard for midwives. They propose that emotions contribute to health if they are mobilized appropriately, but they become 'toxic' if they reappear unconsciously in ways that are destructive and unhelpful. There is a higher value placed on technology, competence and efficiency but there is little place for emotional work in midwifery (see also Ch. 2). Humane institutions are people-changing institutions with awareness of the potential for positive and negative change.

Supporting midwives helps support women

The development of a 'woman-centred' organization is sometimes seen as being at odds with developing a supportive organization for midwives. Yet this need not be the case. McCourt et al (2006) describe how what provides satisfaction to women can be a mutual source of satisfaction to midwives, in particular the development of a meaningful relationship with women. In the one-to-one service, the midwives' positive views and their comments on strengths focused on:

- enabling the development of relationships with women and families and with other professionals
- greater autonomy of practice
- considerable professional and personal development
- flexibility, variety and mutual support (Stevens & McCourt 2001, p 12).

Sandall (1997) describes the characteristics of occupational autonomy, developing meaningful relationships with women, and social support as important factors in work satisfaction for midwives.

The development of continuity-of-carer schemes and close relationships with women gives midwives a sense of primary loyalty to women and can release a midwife from feeling that her main allegiance is to the profession or her employer (Brodie 1997, Page 1995). This may be one of the most empowering aspects of working with women. Yet the recognition of the prevailing culture of midwifery shows how difficulties may arise in changing patterns of practice and in creating greater midwifery autonomy.

A positive organizational culture

Woman-centred care *need* not be at conflict with the needs of midwives or indeed other staff; neither *should* it be at conflict. Retention of midwives and work satisfaction are crucial to an effective and 'positive' organizational culture. A positive culture is, in other words, a place that 'feels good' and supports good work.

Organizational culture here means the ethos, atmosphere, aims, values and expectations, and relations between people (professionals and those being cared for) within the structure that is the context for practice. Culture is reflected in the priorities we choose, the way we spend our time, our language and behaviour. In the maternity services, the culture should:

- be woman-centred – that is, staff behaviour, policies, guidelines, and buildings are focused on the individual needs of women

- be supportive of staff, with attention to midwives
- support continuous learning and professional and personal development – that is, priority is given to learning and provision of resources, including time; there is evidence of discussion, questioning, reflection, challenge and review; practice is seen as an opportunity to learn; there is comfort in senior staff learning from junior staff and vice versa; care is evidence-based
- accept that physiological pregnancy and birth are the normal base of practice and should be supported (Caesarean Section Working Group of the Ontario Women's Health Council 2000)
- demonstrate relationships between staff that are respectful with an understanding of the strength of the role of each professional group and the distinct contribution to be made by each.

Connection with the health services and mechanisms for consultation and referral

Some of the patterns of care I will review include independent or private practice. Possibly these patterns hold the greatest potential for professional autonomy. However, it is crucial that autonomy is not confused with separation or isolation of practice. In today's world, women are entitled to more complex and medical care if it is needed. Perhaps one of the highest level skills of any midwife is to be able to differentiate between situations in which she can support physiological birth and those when consultation or referral is needed.

Autonomous midwifery needs a strong interface with colleagues and the health service or hospital. I have seen at first hand the results of a hospital service that treats midwives antagonistically, does not recognize them as professionals and where this antagonism results in delays in care for mother and baby. The worst situations are when a mother or baby has to be transferred to hospital because of acute problems at a home birth, and antagonism to home birth or the midwife are allowed to result in emotional responses that affect care. A connective supportive interface will be helped by multiprofessional guidelines and policies for practice, discussion and active negotiation with colleagues, and help in understanding roles, particularly around a time of change. It is recognized in the discussions about

relative safety of home and hospital birth that the safety net of the system is crucial (Olsen 1997). Sometimes guidelines are seen as a hazard to midwifery autonomy, but guidelines such as the 'Kloosterman list' in the Netherlands may serve to protect the autonomy of midwives and the right to home birth (Sandall et al 2001).

Balancing the needs to redevelop a distinct identity and a sense of purpose that goes beyond being a doctor's assistant, yet still working together cooperatively with medical colleagues, may not be easy. It is for this reason that the profession needs strong leaders who can articulate the unique nature of midwifery practice, maintain effective relationships and negotiate a safe environment for midwives who will challenge current boundaries of practice.

Cost-effectiveness

There is no such thing as a health service with unlimited resources, nor will it ever be possible, or even right, to develop innovations that take a disproportionate share of the health service budget. Innovations should be cost-effective – this means that resources should be used appropriately and provide value for money; they should add something to the quality of care. In most healthcare systems, there are choices made between priorities. In today's world it may be that technology or the use of technology will be funded before something like an increase in the number of midwives. This choice reflects the values of the dominant culture. A tool for assessing the number of midwives required is important (Ball & Washbrook 1996).

One problem is that it is often assumed that the current way of organizing things is the most cost-effective, and anything that improves the quality of care of necessity costs more. However, the current system of standard care as it is provided in countries like the UK is actually very wasteful; it is not cost-effective. First, although midwives may not be paid enough for what they do, the numbers are so great, that salaries take up the largest part of the maternity budget. When the role of midwives is restricted, as it is by present culture and structures, this is a huge waste of money and resources. Second, the traditional organization of midwives on shifts is an inflexible system that does not follow the ebb and flow of midwifery workload. Innovations such as one-to-one midwifery have reduced length of stay, have the potential to reduce beds, have reduced the intervention rate and have also increased the number of births per midwife-post (Piercey 1996, Piercey et al 2001). Yet still, even after a thorough evaluation, it is often viewed as being too expensive.

Patterns of practice for the new midwifery

It is important to recognize that the patterns of practice and culture of our midwifery services, whether traditional or innovative, are always a product of the wider social environment and nature of the health service. Thus, for example the nature of midwifery in the Netherlands has arisen because of a number of broad social factors like the nature of the family, the place of women in the family, attitudes to healthcare, and geography. In addition, the structure and culture of the health service, and laws, have established a strong base for the maintenance of midwifery as a profession (Sandall et al 2001). Likewise, the development of midwifery in the UK, its strengths and problems, must be viewed in the light of the nature of the NHS. However, as in all other parts of life, a process of globalization has meant that many of the industrialized countries share similar trends. For example most of these, with the exception of the Netherlands, have centralized maternity services. Many have a very high operative and assisted birth rate. The principles of the new midwifery described earlier require a particular pattern or structure of practice.

Four key characteristics of patterns of practice

The pattern of practice is defined here as the structure or organization of care around four key characteristics. These characteristics are:

1. Employee or independent practitioner
2. Community, integrated or centralized care
3. Continuity or fragmented care
4. Midwifery autonomy or medicalized approaches.

First I will define and describe these key characteristics, and then I will give an example of a different pattern of practice that integrates these characteristics.

Employee or independent practice

In some parts of the world (e.g. the Netherlands, New Zealand and some of the Provinces of Canada), midwives practise as independent practitioners, having their services funded for each course of care either by the health service or health insurance. There is a big difference between publicly funded or privately funded independent midwifery practice because a publicly funded practice, if widely enough available, will give access to the majority of women rather than the small numbers who are able or willing to pay for their midwifery care. In general, publicly funded independent midwives may find it easier than privately funded midwives to form an interface with the maternity services for back-up, consultation, referral and transfer. In the UK, the Independent Midwives Association (IMA) are working to have a community model where midwives who are practising independently (with a contract with individual women and their families) to work under the umbrella of the NHS so that women may use their care as NHS patients (see http://www.independentmidwives.org.uk/s).

Midwives who are an employee of an organization will inevitably find some limitations on practice, as the midwife must follow the policies and guidelines of the institution or employer. However, with enlightened and strong midwifery leadership, this may not be too much of a problem, and there is usually greater security for the midwife in such a position. In services that are not progressive, or where there is not strong and enlightened midwifery leadership, the situation can be very frustrating and will severely limit the ability of any midwife to give of her best.

Community-based, integrated care or centralized care

At one end of the continuum the woman may have all of her care at home, including the birth and care after the birth. Some women will have all of their care in pregnancy and most of the care after the birth in the community – either at home or in the midwife's or doctor's surgery or office. Some services will integrate community and hospital so that the emphasis is on having a midwife follow women through the system of care from start to finish. At the other extreme, women receive all their care in an acute care centralized hospital setting. The place of care and birth will have a profound effect on the nature of care, outcomes of care and the ability of the midwife to use her abilities to the full.

Continuity of caregiver or fragmented care

The highest level of continuity of caregiver is to have one practitioner who provides all the care, including care during labour and birth. A few women receive this from midwives in solo practice. However, this is impractical for many midwives as it places permanent on-call demands on them. Close to this is a system whereby the woman has most of her care from one named midwife who is responsible for all care and provides most hands-on care. This midwife is supported by another midwife, or small number of midwives, who will get to know the women in their partner's caseload and provide cover when the named midwife is unavailable. This is often called a *personal caseload*. Approaches to this pattern of practice are described in detail by McCourt et al (2006).

Some patterns, usually called team midwifery, will offer continuity from a team of midwives. This is often known as a *team caseload* rather than a personal caseload (Page et al 2000). In general, the level of continuity achieved is not so high. Some teams, if they are too large, or extend only to hospital or community care, may even break down continuity.

For a time, in the UK, there was an emphasis on providing *shared care*. This was aimed at making the services of a specialist or consultant obstetrician available to all women. Some use the term 'shared care' differently. Canadian midwives may use the term to describe sharing care with a partner or colleague, another midwife. In the UK, the principle of shared care led to complete fragmentation, and moved much care into the hospital. There are still a number of women who have not met the doctor who is a name on the medical records, and who see a different person at nearly every visit.

Midwifery autonomy versus medicalized midwifery

The upper end of midwifery autonomy will be found in independent midwifery, and in home births and out-of-hospital birth centres. It is important to repeat that this term implies professional control over how the practice is organized, values of the practice and the use of interventions. It does not imply practising in isolation or antagonism with others in the health service. Midwifery, as discussed at length earlier in the chapter, has a distinct and unique approach to childbirth care. Midwifery autonomy allows this to be expressed in practice. However, in many parts of the world, midwifery follows the obstetric model.

Working in different ways

The maternity services in the economically developed world are configured in a number of different ways. They may consist of small to large hospitals, general practice or family doctor care, birth centres, small community hospitals, community services. Here I will focus on a pattern of care called One-to-One Midwifery as an example of a development that increased continuity of carer in a large medicalized maternity service in London. It has been replicated in a number of other services and in different parts of the world.

One-to-one midwifery

This form of practice provides one named midwife who is responsible for the care of individual women. This named midwife works with a midwife partner who gets to know the women in her caseload and provides on-call cover when the named midwife is unavailable. This pattern of practice integrates a high level of continuity with midwifery-led care. Care is organized in group practices of six to eight midwives to provide support, allocation of the caseload and peer review of practice. The pilot (McCourt & Page 1996) was set up to provide for the requirements of the 'Changing Childbirth' report (DH 1993), specifically to provide a service that is sensitive to the needs of individual women and their families, and to give women choice, continuity and control.

Midwives meet the woman at the beginning of pregnancy and provide care throughout. Because it is geographically-based, the midwives are situated in a local community and provide much care in the woman's own home. All women in the local neighbourhood are cared for by the service, including low and high risk women. Where the woman has a low risk pregnancy the midwife is the lead professional and responsible for all care. Where the woman has complications or is high risk the midwife works with the medical team but is still responsible for all midwifery care. Women choose whether to give birth in the home or in the hospital.

Outcomes of one-to-one midwifery

One-to-one midwifery was first implemented in November 1993. Two cohort studies were undertaken to assess one-to-one midwifery and to compare it with standard care (McCourt et al 2006, Page et al 1999, 2001). The first was undertaken soon after implementation, and the second when the service was well established. As far as we know it is the only study of an innovation once it had been running for some time. The study focused on:

- women's responses to their care
- clinical interventions and outcomes for both mothers and babies
- standards of care
- continuity of care
- use of economic resources.

There was a lower rate of clinical intervention associated with one-to-one care, and the differences between the groups were increased in the second cohort. The high level of continuity through all the processes of pregnancy and birth, and after birth, was maintained in the second cohort (Page et al 1999, 2001). Standards of care were also maintained, despite the newness of the service in the first cohort (McCourt & Page 1996).

Women receiving one-to-one care were far more satisfied with their care, and had a closer relationship with those midwives caring for them. In general, the responses to pregnancy and birth were more positive. Many women in both groups felt it was important to have continuity of carer through the whole process including labour and birth; the majority of women who had received one-to-one care felt that it was very important (76%) or quite important (10%) (Beake et al 2001).

Especially if the savings from the reduced interventions are taken into account, one-to-one promises to be a very cost-effective pattern of care. Midwives who chose to practise in this way were highly satisfied with this approach to practice (Beake et al 2001, McCourt & Page 1996, Page et al 2001).

How to work in different patterns of practice: working in one-to-one and continuity of caregiver schemes

In this pattern of practice you will be called on to provide skilled and knowledgeable care through all the periods of pregnancy and birth. Many midwives will feel the need to refresh skills in a particular area. You should talk to an experienced midwife, and look at your job description or requirements of practice carefully, thinking through areas in which you need development. A good orientation and support for the first weeks, plus an orientation manual, are very important for midwives starting out in this pattern of practice (Stevens & McCourt 2001). Having confidence and competence in these clinical skills will reduce the stress of starting out. But remember that one of the advantages of this form of practice is that you will learn very quickly.

You also need to think about time management. There are a number of patterns of on-call and it is important to find one that suits you and your partners. You will need to work flexibly, but ensure that you keep enough time for personal life, family, friends and rest and relaxation. Good administrative support is invaluable. Some times will be very busy, and some very quiet; it is important to use the quiet time for rest and relaxation. Accessories that will allow organization and enhance security include a palm pilot, a mobile phone, a security alarm and a good map or satellite navigator. You will be required to travel for some of your time. It is important to have a good tour of your patch, and learn about one-way streets and parking; about safe and less safe areas and about weather patterns if in more remote or northerly areas. You need to think about how you might safeguard your personal security on the streets and in homes.

There are a number of policies regarding lone worker security that provide useful policy and advice.

Relationships with women

Your skills will be integrated through your relationship with individual women and their families, making them central to the decision-making process and using evidence to inform decisions. This takes considerable experience and good interpersonal skills. You will wish to find out about the groups of people in your area; are there different racial or ethnic groups, and are there pockets of poverty? Although your care will be very important to the women and families in your practice, you will need to recognize that you may not be able to sort out a long or complex background of difficulties, nor may you be able to ameliorate all social situations. Although you should seek to form a supportive relationship that may feel like friendship, it is important to ensure that there are boundaries around your life so you may meet your own needs for a healthy balanced life. Having your own network of support at home and at work is important.

Relationships with other staff

One of the rewards of working in a small practice is the possible camaraderie with your colleagues. These practices can be supportive, stimulating and fun. However, when there are severe tensions between members of the group it can be very difficult. Even if you have chosen your partners, you may find difficulties in working together. It is important to talk through and agree values and practices as far as is possible, and to hold regular meetings (Stevens & McCourt 2001, Sandall et al 2008). Establishing a process of peer review that is both challenging but supportive is important. You will work with a number of other professionals in the health service. As in all relationships, a level of trust is crucial to effective working relationships.

Constraints and how to handle them

When there are no choices

Many maternity services will not offer midwives a choice of patterns of practice and many midwives will not be free to move to find a maternity service of their choice. Some midwifery services will make good care very difficult to achieve; even if you can achieve good care it may take a lot out of you. When practising in less than ideal situations it is important to do the best you can, while recognizing that there are some factors out of your control and accepting that your contribution is limited. It is important, though, not to give up completely. Work out your most important

principles and how to put them into practice. For example, giving women choice and control when you meet them for the first time in active labour is not easy. But still you can make sure you spend even a little 'contracted' time in establishing a relationship, and in finding out about the woman's central values and preferences, even if this has to be done between contractions. Watching body language is more important than ever in this situation.

The politics

Everyone is a potential leader, not just those in management positions. Sometimes suggesting and helping to make a small change can make a big difference. Perhaps you could suggest, for example, moving the furniture in the birth room around so that it is easier for the woman to move. Or you might get furniture, such as rocking chairs and birth balls, in place. Often there is a manager or managers who will feel empowered knowing that midwives at the grass roots are seeking change. Do not be frightened to make suggestions. Enthusiasm among students and staff is infectious and adds more than can be imagined to the work situation. If you find problems, be ready to describe them to the appropriate people, but be ready to propose a solution and if possible to contribute to it.

Doing the best you can

Few midwives practise in a perfect environment. Frustrations may arise in any pattern of practice. When they do it is important to be clear on what is the most important value to you, and that you know that you are doing no harm to those in your care. If circumstances lead you to believe that any situation is unsafe, it is a professional responsibility to seek help and to report the situation.

Conclusion

Midwives have the potential to make a big difference to the start of life for the family. This difference may be good or harmful. The pattern and culture of practice will affect the ability of midwives to give of their best. Careful consideration and development of the most effective, efficient and humane pattern of practice may be the most important part of healthcare.

REFERENCES

Anderson T 2000 Feeling safe enough to let go: the relationship between a woman and her midwife during the second stage of labour. In: Kirkham M (ed.) The midwife–mother relationship. Macmillan, London, p 92–118

Ball J, Washbrook M 1996 Birthrate plus. A framework for workforce planning and decision making for midwifery services. Books for Midwives Press, Cheshire

Beake S, McCourt C, Page L 2001 Evaluation of one-to-one midwifery second cohort study. Hammersmith Hospitals NHS Trust/Thames Valley University, London

Brodie P 1997 Being with women: the experiences of Australian team midwives (thesis). University of Technology, Sydney

Caesarean Section Working Group of the Ontario Women's Health Council 2000 Attaining and maintaining best practices in the use of caesarean sections: an analysis of four Ontario hospitals. Ontario Women's Health Council, Ontario

Campbell A 1984 Moderated love: a theology of professional care. SPCK, London

Cook R I, Render M, Woods D D 2000 Gaps in the continuity of care and progress on patient safety. British Medical Journal 320:791–794

Cronk M 2000 The midwife: a professional servant. In: Kirkham M (ed.) The midwife–mother relationship. MacMillan, London

Davies J 2000 Being with women who are economically without. In: Kirkham M (ed.) The midwife–mother relationship. MacMillan, London, p 120–141

Deery R, Kirkham M 2007 Drained and dumped on: the generation and accumulation of emotional toxic waste in community midwifery. In: Kirkham M (ed.) Exploring the dirty side of women's health. Routledge, London

Deery R, Kirkham M. 2006 Supporting midwives to support women In: Page L A, McCandlish R (eds) The new midwifery: science and sensitivity in practice, 2nd edn. Churchill Livingstone, Edinburgh

DeVries R, Salvelson H B, Wiegers T A et al 2001 What (and why) do women want? The desires of women and the design of maternity care. In: DeVries R B C, Teijlingen E R V, Wrede S (eds) Birth by design: pregnancy, maternity care, and midwifery in North America and Europe. Routledge, New York, p 243–266

DH (Department of Health) 1993 Changing childbirth. The report of the Expert Maternity Group, Vol 1 (the Cumberlege report). DoH, London

DH (Department of Health) 2007 Maternity matters: choice, access and continuity of care in a safe service. DH, London

Donaldson M S 2001 Continuity of care: a reconceptualization. Medical Care Research and Review 58(3):255–290

Edwards N 2000 Women planning homebirths: their own views on their relationships with midwives. In: Kirkham M (ed.) The midwife–mother relationship. MacMillan, London, p 55–84

Freely M 1995 Team midwifery – a personal experience. In: Page L (ed.) Effective group practice in midwifery: working with women. Blackwell Science, Oxford, p 3–11

Haggerty J L, Reid R J, Freeman G K 2003 Continuity of care: a multidisciplinary review. British Medical Journal 327 (425):1219–1221

House of Commons (Winterton report) 1992 Maternity services: the second report from the Health Committee session 1991–92. HMSO, London

Kirkham M 2000 The midwife–mother relationship. MacMillan, London

Leap N 2000 'The less we do, the more we give'. In: Kirkham M (ed.) The midwife–mother relationship. MacMillan, London, p 1–17

Leap N, Edwards N 2006 The politics of involving women in decision making. In: Page L A, McCandlish R (eds) The new midwifery: science and sensitivity in practice, 2nd edn. Churchill Livingstone, Edinburgh

Lewis, G (ed.) (2007) The Confidential Enquiry into Maternal and Child Health (CEMACH). Saving mothers' lives: reviewing maternal deaths to make motherhood safer 2003–2005. The seventh report on Confidential Enquiries into Maternal Deaths in the United Kingdom. CEMACH, London

Lipsky M (1980) Street level bureaucracy: dilemmas of the individual in public services. Russell Sage Foundation, New York.

McCourt C, Page L 1996 Report on the evaluation of one-to-one midwifery. Centre for Midwifery Practice, Thames Valley University, London

McCourt C, Hirst J, Page L A 2000 Dimensions and attributes of caring: women's perceptions. In: Page L A, McCandlish R (eds) The new midwifery: science and sensitivity in practice, 2nd edn. Churchill Livingstone, Edinburgh, p 269–287

McCourt C, Stevens T, Sandall J et al 2006 Working with women, developing continuity of care in practice. In: Page L A, McCandlish R (eds) The new midwifery: science and sensitivity in practice, 2nd edn. Churchill Livingstone, Edinburgh, p 143

Menzies Lyth I 1979 The functioning of social systems as a defence against anxiety. Tavistock Institute of Human Relations, London

Menzies Lyth I 1988 Containing anxiety in institutions. Selected Essays 1. Free Association Books, London

Murray S, Bachus L 2005 Patient safety and adverse maternal health outcomes: the missing social inequalities 'lens'. British Journal of Obstetrics and Gynaecology 112:1139–1343

Nursing and Midwifery Council 2004 Midwives Rules and Standards. NMC, London

Olsen O 1997 Meta-analysis of the safety of home birth. Birth 24:4–13

Page L 1995 Putting principles into practice. In: Page L (ed.) Effective group practice: working with women. Blackwell Science, Oxford

Page L 2000 Midwifery in Canada. International Midwifery 13:6–7

Page L 2001 The midwife's role in pregnancy and labour. In: Chamberlain G S P (ed.) Turnbull's obstetrics. Churchill Livingstone, Edinburgh, p 473–486

Page L A 2006 Being with Jane in childbirth: putting science and sensitivity into practice. In: Page L A, McCandlish R (eds) The new midwifery: science and sensitivity in practice, 2nd edn. Churchill Livingstone, Edinburgh

Page L 2007 Do we have enough evidence to judge midwife led maternity units safe? British Medical Journal 335:642

Page L, Beake S, Vail A et al 2001 Clinical outcomes of one-to-one midwifery practice. British Journal of Midwifery 9:700–706

Page L, Cooke P, Percival P 2000 Providing one-to-one practice and enjoying it. In: Page L A, McCandish R (eds) The new midwifery: science and sensitivity in practice, 2nd edn. Churchill Livingstone, Edinburgh, p 123–140

Page L, McCandlish R (eds) 2006 The new midwifery: science and sensitivity in practice, 2nd edn. Churchill Livingstone, Edinburgh

Page L A, McCourt C, Beake S et al 1999 Clinical interventions and outcomes of one-to-one midwifery practice. Journal of Public Health Medicine 21(3):243–248

Pairman S 2000 Women-centred midwifery: partnerships or professional friendships. In: Kirkham M (ed.) The midwife–mother relationship. MacMillan, London, p 207–225

Pairman S 2006 Midwifery partnership: working 'with' women. In: Page L A, McCandlish R (eds) The new midwifery: science and sensitivity in practice, 2nd edn. Churchill Livingstone, Edinburgh

Piercey J 1996 Report on the evaluation of one-to-one midwifery practice. Thames Valley University, London

Piercey J, Page L A, McCourt C 2001 Evaluation of one-to-one midwifery second cohort study/midwives responses. Hammersmith Hospitals NHS Trust/Thames Valley University, London

Raphael-Leff L 1991 Psychological processes in childbearing. Chapman and Hall, London.

Sandall J 1997 Midwives' burnout and continuity of care. British Journal of Midwifery 5:106–111

Sandall J, Bourgeault I L, Meijer W J et al 2001 Deciding who cares: winners and losers in the late twentieth century. In: DeVries R, Benoit C, Van Teijlingen E R et al (eds) Birth by design: pregnancy, maternity care, and midwifery in North America and Europe. Routledge, New York, p 117–138

Sandall J, Page L, Homer C et al 2008 Continuity of care-what is the evidence. In: Homer C, Brody P, Leap N (eds) Midwifery continuity of care: A practical guide. Churchill Livingstone, Elsevier, Australia

Saultz J W 2003 Defining and measuring interpersonal continuity of care. Annals of Family Medicine 1(3): 134–143

SOHHD (Scottish Office Home and Health Department) 1993 Provision of Maternity Services in Scotland. A policy review. HMSO, Edinburgh

Stevens T, McCourt C 2001 Midwives' responses. In: Beake S, McCourt C, Page L (eds) Evaluation of one-to-one midwifery second cohort study. Hammersmith Hospitals NHS Trust/Thames Valley University, London, p 8–15

Wilkins R 2000 Poor relations: the paucity of the professional paradigm. In: Kirkham M (ed.) The midwife–mother relationship. Macmillan, London, p 28–52

5 Ethics in midwifery

Nancy M. Riddick-Thomas

CHAPTER CONTENTS

Modern midwifery involves many different practices and conflicts. The days of clinical practice being clear-cut, right or wrong are long gone. Increasingly, uncertainties are present, causing midwives to make decisions in the absence of robust evidence. There is a need to explore what it is about current practice that causes these dilemmas and to offer support mechanisms to manage situations when they arise. Changes in society over the last two decades have meant changes in healthcare provision. The publication of the patient's charter (DH 1991), Your Guide to the NHS (DH 2001), along with The NHS Plan (DH 2000) and the NHS Complaints Regulations (2004) have raised public awareness of the choices available as well as raising people's expectations regarding involvement in care decisions.

The chapter aims to:

- raise awareness of ethical theories and their use in supporting clinical practice
- explore aspects of clinical practice that health professionals face on a daily basis
- clarify areas of potential conflict
- offer a degree of direction for further discussion or study.

Introduction

The area of ethics is complex, difficult and could be seen, by some, as off-putting. This need not be so. It should be used as a daily tool to support decision-making and to enable rather than disable practice. If used like this it should be liberating and empowering. Being ethically aware is a step towards being an autonomous practitioner. It means taking responsibility, empowering others and facilitating professional growth and development.

When attempting to explore a new area, one of the initial problems is often the terminology used. Consider for a moment your first experiences within a clinical setting. The language used may have been familiar but the terminology was so new you may have felt lost. Ethics is the same; some of the terminology used is different and the words need greater explanation and understanding. Other parts of the terminology appear, on the surface, to be easier and more commonplace (Box 5.1). Even so, when asked to clarify or explain your understanding of these words, it is often not so easy.

What you will find is there can be more than one interpretation for a word. Different people may understand different things from the same words. So, ethics is often about exploring values and beliefs and clarifying what people understand, think and feel in a given situation, often from what they say as much as what they do.

Beliefs and values are very personal. They are dependent on many things, not least an individual's background, society and personal views developed over time. Time for reflection to explore these issues is important. It is also essential for health professionals to be open and honest about practice dilemmas.

A potential area of conflict is that of law. Law and ethics are often seen as complementary to one another, yet at times they are also seen to be placed on opposite sides of a coin. Any exploration of ethics should also be able to guide the reader to such areas of overlap or conflict. The study of ethics will provide the framework for exploration and aid resolution of dilemmas. However, it has to be remembered that ethics will not provide a quick fix, or an easy answer.

Jones (2000, p 8) has outlined ethics as being 'the basic principles and concepts that guide human beings in thought and action'. The same could be said of philosophy, in that moral philosophy is often the foundation of modern ethical decision making and ethics itself is the application of philosophical principles to everyday situations. To understand this better there is a need to explore the theories surrounding ethics and their supportive philosophical frameworks.

Framework and theories

When first exploring the ethics of a situation it is helpful to have a framework with which to work. There are many ethical frameworks that could be adopted to use in clinical situations. Edwards (1996) advocates a four-level system based on the work of Melia (1989, p 6–7). Edwards believes that there are four levels of moral thinking that can help formulate arguments and discussions and ultimately assist in solving moral dilemmas (Box 5.2).

Level one: judgements

Judgements are frequently made readily, based on information gained. Such judgements may have no real foundation except the belief of the individual who made it.

Throughout our daily lives we make judgements about each other, whether it is on the bus, in the

---

Box 5.1 Terminology

Informed consent	Information regarding options for care/treatment
Rights	Justified claim to a demand
Duty	A requirement to act in a certain manner
Justice	Being treated fairly
Best interests	Deciding on best course for an individual
Utilitarian	Greatest good for greatest number
Deontological	Duty of care
Beneficence	Doing good
Non-maleficence	Avoiding harm

Box 5.2 Edward's levels of ethics

Level one	Judgements
Level two	Rules
Level three	Principles
Level four	Ethical theories

(After Edwards 1996).

supermarket or during a shift on a busy ward. What is important to remember is that it is often an instant judgement that has been made, possibly biased, and it may not necessarily have been well thought through or based on all available evidence. How judgements are made is interesting. What informs a judgement is often linked to personal values and beliefs, society, as well as experiences of similar past events. All these and more shape the decision-making processes and to be aware of them is the first step to understanding yourself and your own moral values. It can be helpful to reflect on past judgements and consider whether, in retrospect, they were well founded or based on personal bias or prejudice.

Level two: rules

Rules govern our daily lives and differ depending on the society or culture in which we live. When looking at ethics, rules are what guide our practice and control our actions. Rules come in many forms and from many sources. Beauchamp & Childress (2001) outline different types of rules. These include *substantive rules* covering such things as privacy, truth telling or confidentiality, *authority rules* determined by those in power and enforced on a country or section of society, and *procedural rules* defining a set course of action or line to be followed. Rules can also be enabling, they can define the limits or boundaries of practice and can allow freedom to act knowing the safe limits of those actions. The Nursing and Midwifery Council (NMC) in the UK sets rules for midwives in the form of the Midwives Rules and Standards (2004). These are statutory rules bound by legal processes, and if used appropriately can guide and enable practice and so ease dilemmas. Supporting rules is the NMC Code (NMC 2008a). Codes are less formal or obligatory than rules and are seen as guidelines to support safe practice.

Level three: principles

Four main principles underpin this level. Beauchamp & Childress (2001) have explained these in considerable detail. The first of these is *respect for autonomy*. This term has been used extensively over the last few years. The focus of modern healthcare has been around the professional's duty to respect individuals' autonomy and whenever possible to promote or enable them to exercise their autonomy. This is especially true in maternity services where women are placed at the centre of care and their views and wishes are seen as key to care delivery. The second principle is *non-maleficence*, interpreted as avoiding harm. It could be said that most healthcare professionals would be trying to do this. Brown et al (1992) advised us that this principle is a strong one and as such should not be taken lightly. Harm may sometimes be a consequence of an action in healthcare; the aim should be to minimize harm as much as possible. The third principle is that of *beneficence* – doing good or balancing the benefits against the harms in a given situation (Beauchamp & Childress 2001). This entails positive action on one person's part to benefit another person. This can be difficult for health professionals when a client/patient chooses a course of action that may not be in their best interests. This may be made more difficult for midwives when there is a need to consider the best interests of both the woman and her fetus/baby. Balancing benefits and harms can in itself cause dilemmas.

The fourth principle, *justice*, means to be treated fairly. In many instances this is all people want. It is important that healthcare professionals are seen to be acting fairly and treating all clients as equals. Gannon (2005) outlines that justice is about people's rights, duties and obligations. It is about the equal sharing of these to the people who are owed them. He feels that people should be able to have equal access to healthcare based on need. Within the maternity services justice is important in that all women should be treated as equals, all should have access to the same level of care and services, all should have the same options for care and choices for such aspects as place of birth, method of delivery, levels of antenatal and postnatal care (NPEU 2007, DH 2007). Justice and fairness will be explored further later in this chapter.

Level four: ethical theories

There are a number of theories that could be explored and applied to midwifery/healthcare. Liberalism, communitarianism and casuistry, are a few that are explained in more depth by Beauchamp & Childress (2001). Feminism is another that some find of use and a classic text for this would be

Tong (1997). Generally, theories are taken to mean the two main ethical theories of utilitarianism and deontology. Many texts outline these two theories in more detail as they are the most widely used and form the foundation of much ethical decision making (Beauchamp & Childress 2001, Jones 2000, Thompson et al 2000).

Utilitarian theory

Utilitarian theory has been widely adapted over the years. It is based on the idea of balancing the consequences of following certain actions or rules. This can be thought of as a very large pair of scales, with the benefits of an action on one side and the harm or consequences of taking the action on the other. There is a need to tip the scales in favour of the benefits over the possible harms that could occur. This theory stems from the work of Jeremy Bentham and later John Stuart Mill in the nineteenth century (Raphael 1989). They believed that pleasure was more desirable than pain and that anything that increased pleasure for the majority of people must be a morally right action. Practically, this theory is attractive in that it can aid decision-making for the masses; an action is good if it provides benefits for the many. Scarce resources within the NHS have meant that very difficult decisions have to be made. Determinations of where the greatest good lies and how to do the least harm in any given situation have become important. Such decision making may be made easier by applying ethical theories (Tschudin 1994).

Many aspects of midwifery care have been organized on utilitarian principles. Antenatal clinics allow many women to be seen by skilled professionals under one roof. Many screening tests are offered to all irrespective of need or individual assessment, and team midwifery often means what fits with the midwives rather than with individual women (Flint 1993, p 59). There may be times when such practices are appropriate; for example for some safety issues everyone should follow set procedures to ensure standards of care are maintained. When you are next called on to make a decision ask yourself how the balance of benefits and harms would weigh on a scale. If you have time try to discuss the range of consequences each option carries before making the final decision.

Deontology theory

Deontology is the second of these theories. Jones (2000) tells us this term is from the Greek word 'deon' meaning duty. As health professionals you would all say you have a duty towards your clients/patients. But there is a need to explore where else your duty lies. This list could be quite long (Box 5.3).

The list could be longer if you added personal duties (i.e. family, friends, etc.). Recognizing that you have a duty of care is one thing, balancing the competing demands of those duties is quite another. Conflicting duties can cause dilemmas in deciding the best course of action. It is often difficult to prioritize such duties, but some prioritization needs to occur to enable decision making to be meaningful.

There are no easy answers here. This work is based on that of Immanuel Kant (Hollis 1985) and there have been a number of interpretations of his writings over time (Edwards 1996). Kant emphasized that to do one's duty is the most important thing, irrespective of any consequences that carrying out this duty may produce. How you interpret your duty may vary depending on your situation, values or beliefs. Some may base their duty on natural laws, others religion and the ten commandments.

This is where a difference is seen between utilitarianism and deontology. In following a utilitarian theory it would be essential to consider the consequences and choose the best course of action – that is, the one that produces the best outcome for the most people. Following a deontological approach on the other hand would require the person to carry out something that is seen as a duty irrespective of any consequences. This would be very hard in practice for most people as it suggests certainties of

---

Box 5.3 Duty of care to...

- Self
- Colleagues
- Clients/patients
- Relatives
- Fetus/baby
- Employer
- Profession (NMC)

actions, and an attitude of irrelevance towards consequences of actions. Life is often more complicated, however, and as such many other factors need to be considered.

Another aspect of Kant's work was the emphasis on *respect for persons*. To this end, he believed that people are individual and should be treated with respect, not merely as a means to an end. Beauchamp & Childress (2001) believe that if an action necessitates treating someone without respect then it is the action that is wrong. Respect for persons is important within maternity care. Each woman is an individual and her experience will be personal to her and respecting women as individuals is a fundamental part of a midwife's role.

Having considered the four levels of judgements, rules, principles and theories, consider the case scenario in Box 5.4 for a few minutes. It may help you apply the framework to your practice. Make a few notes of what ethical issues it raises. It can be seen that in working with Susan, a midwife would call on all four of Edward's levels.

Using Edward's four levels, the midwife supporting Susan during her pregnancy can work through what she should do. On talking to Susan and discovering her wishes for pregnancy and birth it is clear that she holds strong views about the type of experience she wants. It would be easy for the

midwife to make an immediate *judgement* about both Susan and her reasons for wanting a low technology pregnancy and birth. During the course of the meeting between Susan and her midwife it would be important for the ground rules to be set and the midwife would have to outline the legal and moral *rules* that govern her practice. One such moral rule that would be vital is that of truth telling. In order for Susan and her midwife to build a trusting relationship that would be of benefit throughout the pregnancy it is important that honesty is established and both parties are truthful with each other. What the midwife has to acknowledge and promote in this relationship is the *principle of autonomy*. Principles are rather general, but autonomy is based on the understanding of respect for choices made by people.

The midwife needs to establish that what is being asked for is Susan's choice of how she would like events in her pregnancy to be managed; it is important these are informed and rational requests, based on sound judgements and beliefs. This having been established, the midwife then has a duty to uphold that choice if she is to respect Susan's autonomy and earn her trust. As long as this relationship continues to be founded on the above judgements, rules and principles, then the midwife would be seen to be demonstrating aspects of *ethical theories*. The midwife is taking a position that she sees as her duty to care for Susan, acting in the best interests of both her and her unborn child. In moral philosophy, this would be called a deontological stance. She is also utilizing aspects of consequentialism, as she is weighing up the benefits and harms of Susan's requests and will be trying to advocate a position which causes the least harm, but also maximizes the possible benefits. Both these positions have been outlined by Beauchamp & Childress (2001) and Thompson et al (2000).

Having outlined the levels of decision-making (Edwards 1996), it is important that we now explore some other influences on the midwife's role. There are aspects that are either part of or develop from the basic moral frameworks outlined above. These are aspects of ethics that are seen daily in professional life, but they could still cause problems, dilemmas or conflicts in one form or another.

Box 5.4 Case Scenario: Susan

Susan is 23 years old and is pregnant with her second child. She has requested that she have minimal interventions during the pregnancy and a natural birth, no interventions, no vaginal examinations, no drugs and a quiet environment. Her previous pregnancy was complicated by raised blood pressure, which culminated in Susan having a caesarean section. Susan is adamant that nothing will go wrong this time. She is happy to have her baby in hospital, in light of the first pregnancy's events, but would like to maintain more control and feels that provided her blood pressure remains within normal limits there should be no reason a midwife should intervene. Her midwife is anxious to ensure safety of mother and fetus/child, while also building Susan's trust.

Consent/information giving

Informed consent is a relatively recent term; indeed, Beauchamp & Childress (2001, p 77) suggest that it was not until the mid-1970s that the term was explored in any real detail. It has been claimed that within ethics, informed consent means 'giving patients and clients as much information as they need' (Jones 2000, p 104). This is traditionally what ethical consent is held to be. This principle is very different, however, to the legal standpoint in that 'consent' within legal frameworks is taken to be based on the reasonable person standard, or the 'Bolam' test (Dimond 2006, p 245). Consent within ethics means that the client has listened, understood and agreed to the procedure or treatment being proposed. For many reasons this may not be realistic. Johnstone (2000, p 210) outlines some reasons why consent may not be realistic in everyday clinical practice. These are summarized as:

- lack of time
- clients will forget
- most clients do not want to know
- most clients would not understand
- it could be harmful if clients refused treatment based on information given
- considering all these, gaining informed consent is impracticable.

These reasons seem plausible; there will always be situations where a client has said 'what do you think?' or you find the client has asked two or three of your colleagues for the same information after you have spent 10 minutes explaining things. One other important aspect that is not on Johnstone's list is that of the professional's knowledge base. To be able to provide information and then gain a valid consent, the professional attempting to gain that consent has to be at least as knowledgeable as the client from whom consent is being sought. With increasing use of the World Wide Web, this is becoming an almost impossible task. Health professionals have a duty to keep up-to-date and be able to inform their clients to the best of their ability (NMC 2004 point 3, NMC 2008a).

Consider once again the case scenario in Box 5.4. There will be many times during Susan's pregnancy when consent may be required. To ensure that the consent given is valid, the midwife will have to hold wide-ranging discussions on such things as antenatal screening tests, ultrasound scanning, birth choices and birth interventions such as pain relief, positions for birth and active management of the third stage of labour. The midwife must also be sure that Susan understands the options and alternatives open to her. Susan has asked for minimal interventions, so without being judgemental or coercive, the midwife will have to explore Susan's views and recommend what she believes is 'best practice'. Respecting a person's right to exercise choice and decision-making can be difficult. What if Susan was requesting something that did not meet the standards of best practice? How would the midwife be expected to react then? The Midwives Rules and Standards (NMC 2004) can be used in such a situation to inform and enable the midwife to act in the woman's best interests. The midwife would have backup support systems from both her supervisor of midwives (see Ch. 52) and her immediate line manager.

Enabling informed consent to occur and empowering women to decide what is best for them are fundamental parts of 'respect for autonomy' (Brown et al 1992). When attempting to support the midwife in such situations, there is an apparent need to fall back on the legal definition of a 'reasonable person'. However, Brown et al (1992) have explored this issue and advise caution in following a reasonable person standard. They argue that if all reasonable people would choose one procedure but Susan chooses another then Susan could be seen as being unreasonable because she is the only one to choose the other type of procedure. It may be easier and possibly more desirable for some in today's litigation-conscious health service to abide by a legal definition of competence that Maclean (2001, p 46) outlines as an ability to 'comprehend, retain and use information and weigh it in the balance' (see also NMC 2008a.)

For a health professional it can be very difficult to respect a person's autonomy when current evidence tells you their request is not best practice. At times, the courts have been called on to decide; for example in the case of Re S (Savage 1998) both the mother and fetus's lives were at risk, yet the mother refused treatment that could have saved the fetus and lessened the risk of morbidity or mortality for herself. These cases are rare, but they can damage the client–professional relationship if not managed well.

Advocacy and collaborative relationships

When faced with clients who, despite all information, support and encouragement, are still reluctant to act or speak up for themselves, many midwives are finding they need to take on an advocacy role on their behalf. Advocacy is seen as speaking out on another's behalf (Gates 1994). There is, again, a fine dividing line between advocacy and paternalism. Put simplistically, paternalism is acting on another's behalf, whereas advocacy is speaking out on another's behalf.

When taking on the role of advocate there is a need to be clear on a number of points. Acting as an advocate can be difficult and involves putting personal views or values aside. Advocacy means speaking out for someone's rights.

Within any decision-making process there is a need to work with others, to collaborate in attempting to come to the right decision. There have been many calls for health professionals to work together (Audit Commission 1997); such calls are now also being extended to public health and social care (WAG 2005, DH 2007, NPEU 2007).

Law and ethics

The position of law, ethics and reproductive health has been widely explored (Callahan 1995, Dimond 2006, Mason & McCall Smith 2000). There are times when these seem to work together to support each other and when calling on one may clarify the position of the other. There are also times when there appears a great divide between the two and no middle ground can be found.

To examine these issues more closely, there is a need to look towards modern society. Many of the modern laws are developed from and stand firmly in the foundations of society (Mason & McCall Smith 2000). The values and practices of society often inform the development of laws, although Mason & McCall Smith (2000) suggest that the laws

take such a considerable time to change, and that the healthcare professions are often left unsure of their legal position.

A dilemma for the maternity services of today is that of provision of a home birth service. The governmental policies (NMC 2006) and professional advice (www.rcmnormalbirth.org.uk) is that home birth should be a real option for women. Should a woman choose such a birth, she should be supported in her choice and have the appropriate professionals available to be with her during the birth. Yet the midwifery service, like many parts of the NHS, is under funded and many maternity units cannot offer such a service without compromising the care of other women (House of Commons Health Committee Report 2007). Utilitarian principles may have taken priority in this incidence. To provide a home birth service for all who request it could mean harm coming to other users of the maternity services; the greatest good here may be to restrict or not offer a home birth service until it can be fully staffed and safe for all women.

It may be seen that in being supported by the law you may also be constrained by it. Fear of litigation appears to be a guiding principle of modern practice. Risk management and clinical governance are high on most health service agendas (Symon & Kirkham 2006). The underlying reason for the development of these within clinical practice has been improvement in practices and the establishment of common standards and provision of safe care. It is important that midwives are aware of and become involved in these initiatives if collaboration and cooperation between disciplines are to be promoted.

Human rights

One aspect of law that has taken on a more prominent role and gained importance for health professionals in recent years is that of Human Rights. The European Convention of Human Rights (1950) set out to protect fundamental human rights (Caulfield 2005), and the UK was the first signatory to the convention. The principles established at that time have become part of British society's values and norms. So much so, that 1998 saw the introduction of the Human Rights Act (Dimond 2006). It has become important that midwives are aware of and are encouraged to work within the boundaries of this. The following parts are of particular importance for midwives:

- Article 2 – right to life
- Article 5 – right to liberty and security
- Article 12 – right to marry (this article outlines a right to 'found a family' which has implications for discussions surrounding fertility and artificial conception (Dimond 2006, p 669)
- Article 14 – prohibition of discrimination.

Gruskin & Dickens (2006) have outlined how human rights laws clearly place an obligation on governments to protect individual's human rights. One benefit of the Act is that it has placed the patient or client at the centre of healthcare. The patient experience has become an important measure of quality and effectiveness of the health services. Caulfield (2005) believes that such changes have led to a review of the NHS complaints system. Certainly within midwifery services, women's views are becoming stronger and are having an influence in shaping services; this has been seen in the Audit Commission Report (1997) and more recently in the National Perinatal Epidemiology Unit report *Recorded Delivery* (2007). This latest report is reinforced by the Department of Health's (2007) strategic vision for improving choice, access and continuity of care. This strategy for England again attempts to 'put women and their partners at the centre of their local maternity service provision' (DH 2007, p 7). With this in mind, midwives should remember that when someone has a right to something there is usually a corresponding duty on someone else to facilitate the right (Beauchamp & Childress 2001). Women could be said to have a right to safe and competent care when pregnant. This would fit with Article 5 and it would naturally follow that as midwives are educated to provide midwifery care they have an obligation that the care provided is both safe and competent. It may also be argued that the UK Government, via the NMC also has an obligation in regulating its practitioners, to ensure that they are practising safely and competently. The NMC does this via their Post Registration Education and Practice (PREP) system (NMC 2008b),

as well as by setting the Midwives Rules and Standards (2004). The NMC's statutory function in relation to supervision of midwives is also an important part of this process (see Ch. 52).

Justice and fairness

It has already been seen that health service resources are limited and to provide care a degree of rationing needs to take place (Gannon 2005). In providing midwifery care there is a need to ensure justice and fairness in the care being delivered. In ethical terms, justice is taken to mean '*fair, equitable and appropriate treatment in light of what is due or owed to persons*' (Beauchamp & Childress 2001, p 226). If it can be shown that someone is owed something, say a pregnant woman is owed a certain standard of care, then that woman has a right to that standard of care and someone has a corresponding duty to provide the care to the appropriate standard. An injustice is committed if that standard of maternity care is not available and it could be said that the woman has failed to receive the expected standard of maternity care she is entitled to. That duty of care, while owed by the NHS and maternity services, falls ultimately to each and every midwife providing care to the woman.

Edwards (1996) outlines the equity or fairness part of justice in saying that individual treatment should be consistent and equals should be treated equally. A woman asking for information on breastfeeding in the postnatal ward may receive detailed advice and support from the midwife. That same midwife should give any other women asking for help and advice the same level of advice, care and support. Should a woman at home ask for information on baby care, she should be able to expect the same type and quality of information as her friend or neighbour who may have asked the same questions.

A dilemma that arises in attempting to treat all women as equals is that of need. In trying to be equitable, is there a need to determine if all women should be treated equally? A midwife has to weigh up each woman's needs and alter the care accordingly. The woman who asked for breastfeeding advice earlier may have read widely, had previous experience of breastfeeding and have plenty of support available when she returns home. The second woman by contrast may be a first time mother, who has not attended any parent education classes, not read or know much about breastfeeding and have little support at home. Clearly the information, advice and support needs to be different for these two women. On the face of it, their questions may be the same and one would expect the same type of answer, but in finding out a little background information the midwife would be justified in not treating these two women in the same way as their needs are very different. So, it is clear that midwives must be aware of and consider equity and justice in their dealings with women, but they also have to consider women as individuals and be able to justify different practices in the basis of need.

Research

Any examination of ethics would not be complete without also looking into the ethical implications of research in the maternity services. Robson (1997, p 470) has outlined the British Psychological Society's research involving human participants, while Cormack (2000) contains a chapter by Hazel McHaffie that uses two case scenarios to emphasize the issues to be considered. Whichever approach is taken there are some common aspects that most authors emphasize. These can be summarized as the 'five Cs' (Box 5.5).

- **Caring.** Any research that is undertaken should be performed in a caring manner. Those who are subjects of research should be able to expect the highest standards of care and their care would not be adversely affected if they chose not to participate.
- **Consent.** This has to be gained prior to any research being undertaken. Those involved in research should know what the research is about, what it entails and the risks, benefits and alternatives.

Robson (1997) recommends that the subjects must also be clear that they should be able to retain the ability to opt out of the research should they change their minds.

- **Confidentiality.** All research should maintain confidentiality of its subjects. Taking part in research should not put any individual under the spotlight, or highlight the person in any way. If there were any need to disclose information Cormack (2000) advises that permission would have to be sought in advance of any disclosure occurring.
- **Codes.** These are guidelines for practice. They make recommendations about how practice should be governed in certain situations. There are ethical codes related to research on human subjects. The National Patient Safety Agency issues advice on these (NPSA 2007). Thompson et al (2000, p 340) highlighted both the code of practice on the use of fetuses and fetal material in research and treatment, and the World Medical Association Declaration of Helsinki.
- **Committees.** There are statutory committees set up to monitor and control research involving human subjects within healthcare. The National Research Ethics Service (NRES) (NPSA 2007) has combined the previous work of Local (LREC) and Multi-Centred Research Ethics Committees (MREC). The aim is to provide a robust ethical review to protect safety, dignity and well-being of research participants. All health authorities will be required to liaise with this body to review, monitor and control the research carried out within their areas. Any health research carried out must be submitted for consideration by this committee.

The fundamental principle when considering whether research is ethical is that of protection of the vulnerable; this may be the staff, clients or the researchers themselves (Cormack 2000). Although advancement of knowledge is important, it should not be made at the cost of compromising any one group of society. It is not only those involved in carrying out research who should be aware of the research protocols but also those involved in it and those who may simply be working within the same clinical area. To this end, it can be helpful to ask some very simple questions such as those in Box 5.6.

Box 5.5 'Five Cs' of ethical research
1. Caring
2. Consent
3. Confidentiality
4. Codes
5. Committees

> **Box 5.6** Ten questions to ask
>
> 1. What is the scientific background of the research?
> 2. What are the qualifications of the person/s leading the project?
> 3. Are there any circumstances that could cause bias for a researcher?
> 4. Is there any foreseeable effect on health?
> 5. If any hazards or discomforts exist, are there plans to accommodate them?
> 6. How is consent gained? Is it clear and in writing?
> 7. How are confidentiality and anonymity assured for all subjects?
> 8. Is there an information sheet for subjects to read?
> 9. Have subjects been given the opportunity of opting out?
> 10. Are there contact details if staff or subjects require more information or are concerned regarding any aspect of the research?

(Adapted from DH 1992.)

Current ethical issues

When studying ethics you become aware of so many aspects of life that have ethical implications that can and do make working within the maternity services challenging. The media, in their many forms, play an important role in today's society and often force us to become ethically aware of issues we may not have particularly thought about, or that may not have become 'public' until they became headline news.

At times like this it is to professionals that clients turn for answers to their many questions. This has been seen on a number of occasions in the last few years. In France a 62-year-old woman received IVF (Dimond 2006, p 548); this became headline news prompting many discussions on the implications for the child and the rights of older women to access such treatments. A woman recently lost her case to have her embryos implanted because her ex-fiancé did not now wish to become a father (Laurance 2007), this prompted much discussion on the rights of the partner under the Human Fertilisation and Embryology Act (HFEA 1990). These embryos were at the limit allowed for storage under the Act and would then have to be destroyed.

Such events can be very distressing for any health professional involved. Having a structured framework to work through the issues can help. But having open and meaningful discussions with colleagues is vital if a deeper understanding of the situation is to be gained. Such things as rights of individuals, protection of the vulnerable, duty of care and where the best interests lie should be explored openly and safely away from the client's bedside (Dimond 2006). That is not to say that clients should not be involved, but the moment of crisis may not be the best time to explore sensitive issues, and sometimes a client representative may be better placed to speak out in a time of distress.

Conclusion

The area of ethics is growing and the need for health professionals to become more aware of the issues involved is escalating. This chapter has raised the possibility of using a framework (Edwards 1996) to organize your thoughts and decision-making processes.

A starting point must be the clarification of personal values, beliefs and moral principles. Without this it will be difficult to move forward and assist others with their problems and dilemmas. Many things, family, friends, society and professional life (Jones 2000) will have shaped your individual values and beliefs. By examining and reflecting on these you will be able to acknowledge any biases you may hold and start to work through them. Reflection skills have become important in modern professional life as a means of critically reviewing events and learning from them.

Moving forward may not be easy, but it is important if care is to improve and standards are to be maintained. Many reports in recent years have recommended that the midwifery profession include its client group in decision-making. Pregnant women should have an increased number of choices, they should have more control over events and midwives should be providing them with continuity of care (DH 2007). But in providing women with these things midwives are also having to confront the fact that women need more information. The quality of information giving is dependent, in part, on midwives' knowledge base. Midwives must also ensure that once women have the options for care the choices they make are informed and are based on sound research-based evidence (Price 2001, RCM 2000).

Another aspect of moving forward is that of collaborative care. There have been many calls for health professionals to work more closely together (Audit Commission 1997; NMC 2008a). To work together means to resolve any differences between professions. Doctors and midwives might have different starting points, but this should not mean that a middle ground cannot be found. Sharing codes of practice and developing a joint code may be the first step towards closer relationships.

Studying ethics will raise many questions, some of which will not lend themselves to satisfactory answers. Although that is frustrating, sharing of dilemmas and gaining different viewpoints may help. Multidisciplinary case conferences, seminars and study sessions could be one way forward. Medical, midwifery, health visiting and social work professionals are just some of those whose viewpoints could be included to broaden the discussion and add to the overall quality of care provided.

Midwives may find their PREP profile (NMC 2008b) provides a tool to reflect upon many private dilemmas and conflicts. Within the profile there is an opportunity to address a number of ethical questions. Such questions could be: 'who has rights in a situation?', 'was there a duty of care?', 'what was in the client's best interests?', and 'how can one balance the good of one action against any possible harm it could cause?'. These may help you explore the issues and organize your thoughts in preparation for the next time that you are faced with a similar issue.

REFERENCES

Audit Commission 1997 First class delivery: improving maternity services in England and Wales. Audit Commission, London

Beauchamp T L, Childress J F 2001 Principles of biomedical ethics, 5th edn. Oxford University Press, Oxford

Brown J M, Kitson A L, McKnight T J 1992 Challenges in caring. Chapman & Hall, London

Callahan J C 1995 Reproduction ethics and the law: feminist perspectives. Indiana University Press, Bloomington

Caulfield H 2005 Accountability. Blackwell, Oxford

Cormack D 2000 The research process in nursing, 4th edn. Blackwell Science, Oxford

Dimond B 2006 The legal aspects of midwifery, 3rd edn. Books for Midwives, Hale

DH (Department of Health) 1991 The patient's charter. HMSO, London

DH (Department of Health) 1992 Local Research Ethics Committees. HMSO, London, p 2

DH (Department of Health) 2000 The NHS Plan: a plan for reform. HMSO, London

DH (Department of Health) 2001 Your guide to the NHS. HMSO, London

DH (Department of Health) 2007 Maternity matters: Choice, access and continuity of care in a safe service. HMSO, London

Edwards S D 1996 Nursing ethics: a principle based approach. Macmillan, Basingstoke

European Convention for the protection of human rights and fundamental freedoms 1950 Council for Europe, Strasbourg

Flint C 1993 Midwifery teams and caseloads. Butterworth Heinemann, Oxford

Gannon W 2005 Biomedical ethics. Oxford University Press, Oxford

Gates B 1994 Advocacy: a nurses' guide. Scutari, London

Gruskin S, Dickens B 2006 Editorial: Human rights and ethics in public health. American Journal of Public Health 96 (11):1903–1905

HFEA (Human Fertilisation and Embryology Authority) 1990. HMSO, London

Hollis M 1985 Invitation to philosophy. Blackwell Sciences, Oxford

House of Commons Health Committee Report 2007 Workforce planning 4th Report Session 2006–2007, Vol 1. HMSO, London

Human Rights Act 1998. HMSO, London

Johnstone M-J 2000 Bioethics a nursing perspective, 3rd edn. Harcourt Saunders, Sydney

Jones S 2000 Ethics in midwifery, 2nd edn. Mosby, New York

Laurance J 2007 Woman loses final round battle to use frozen embryos. The Independent 11 April. Online. Available: http://news.independent.co.uk/europe/article2439528.ece

Maclean A 2001 Briefcase on medical law. Cavendish, London, p 46

Mason J K, McCall Smith R A 2000 Law and medical ethics. Butterworth, London

Melia K 1989 Everyday nursing ethics. Macmillan, London, p 6–7

National Patient Safety Agency 2007 National Research Ethics Service. Online. Available: www.nres.npsa.nhs.uk/recs/index/htm

National Perinatal Epidemiology Unit (NPEU) 2007 Recorded delivery: a new survey of womens' experience of maternity care. NPEU, Oxford

NHS (Complaints) Regulations 2004 SI 2004 No 1768. HMSO, London

Nursing and Midwifery Council 2004 Midwives Rules and Standards. NMC, London

Nursing and Midwifery Council 2006 Midwives and Home Birth Circular 8–2006 NMC, London

Nursing and Midwifery Council 2008b The PREP handbook. NMC, London

Nursing and Midwifery Council 2008a NMC Code: NMC, London

Price S 2001 Using the MIDIRS informed choice leaflets in clinical practice. MIDIRS Midwifery Digest 11(2):261–263

Raphael D D 1989 Moral philosophy. Oxford University Press, Oxford

RCM (Royal College of Midwives) 2000. Vision 2000. RCM, London

Robson C 1997 Real world research. Blackwell Science, Oxford

Savage W 1998 The right to choose. Nursing Standard 12(35):14

Symon A, Kirkham M 2006 Risk and choice in maternity care: an international perspective Churchill Livingstone, London

Thompson I E, Melia K M, Boyd K M 2000 Nursing ethics, 4th edn. Churchill Livingstone, London

Tong R 1997 Feminist approaches to bioethics. Westview, Oxford

Tschudin V 1994 Deciding ethically: a practical approach to nursing challenges. Baillière Tindall, London

WAG (Welsh Assembly Government) 2005 Designed for Life: creating a world class health and social care for Wales in the 21st Century. WAG, Cardiff

FURTHER READING

Frith L 1996 Ethics and midwifery: issues in contemporary practice. Butterworth Heinemann, Oxford

An interesting book focusing on a variety of aspects related to midwifery practice. Clearly discusses midwifery issues and relates to the ethical theories that underpin them. This is an easy book to read and would be useful as a supportive text for midwifery students.

Beauchamp T L, Childress J F 2001 Principles of biomedical ethics, 5th edn. Oxford University Press, Oxford

An ethical theories book that most readers will find useful to dip into. Not a book for bedtime reading, rather a text that is essential to support any enquiry into ethics. It is nicely linked to healthcare and uses case studies to apply the theories to clinical practice.

Jones S 2000 Ethics in midwifery, 2nd edn. Mosby, London

A good basic introduction to ethics in the midwifery setting. Easy to read and compact enough to carry around. Divided into two sections this book first outlines the main theory standpoints and uses a case study approach in the second section to lead the reader through the process of ethical enquiry and decision-making.

Thompson I E, Melia K M, Boyd K M 2000 Nursing ethics, 4th edn. Churchill Livingstone, London

A comprehensive text written from a nursing perspective but has many good aspects that the student midwife will find useful. Easy to read and navigate, it is a good reference text, which is well referenced.

Bowden P 1997 Caring. Routledge, London

This has a feminist focus and uses the basic ethical theories to examine the issues raised. Highlights the four roles of mothering, friendship, nursing and citizenship.

Ford N 2002 The prenatal person: ethics from conception to birth. Blackwell, Oxford

Explores ethics at a difficult time; reproductive technologies are explored with some background on the technologies, with links to ethical and religious implications.

Freeman M 2004 Human rights. Blackwell, Oxford

Explores the concept of human rights and the moral rules. Leads the reader from the history of the concept to exploring application and cultural differences.

6 Evidence-based practice

Rosemary Mander

When she provides care during childbearing, the midwife does so by virtue of her expert knowledge. This knowledge distinguishes her from all the people who offer opinions to the childbearing woman. The midwife's unique knowledge which determines her practice derives from many sources. Traditionally, the midwife drew on her personal experience of childbearing. More recently, the midwife's occupational experience has assumed greater significance. Precedent has been quoted as an important influence (Thomson A 2000) and this may have been enforced by those in authority. Another factor in influencing midwifery practice has been ritual (Rodgers 2000). It is only relatively recently that research, and more recently still research evidence, have been required to determine midwifery practice.

This chapter aims to:

- examine the meaning of 'research'
- introduce the concepts underpinning research
- discuss the role of the woman consumer in research
- consider the research basis of midwifery practice
- encourage critical reading of research
- indicate the steps needed to implement research in practice.

Research

Although the term 'research' may carry many implications, a dictionary definition is useful: 'systematic investigation towards increasing the sum of knowledge' (Macdonald 1981, p 1148).

Clearly, research is about asking questions, but not in a haphazard way. Systematic questioning is crucial to research. Thus planning, in the form of the 'research process', underpins research activity. The purpose of this activity is encompassed in the definition offered above, in that research aims to improve knowledge by increasing it. In caring situations, knowledge is intended to ensure more effective care.

Evidence

The term 'evidence' refers to a particular form of research. This is what has been referred to by Chalmers as 'strong research' (1993, p 3). The need for 'evidence' was initiated by the observations made by Cochrane (1972). He identified the lack of scientific rigour in medical decisions, and went on to single out obstetricians for merciless criticism because of their want of rigour. A group of obstetricians, with other maternity practitioners, responded to this scathing condemnation by attempting to correct the situation. To develop a resource for practitioners who lacked opportunities to search and evaluate the literature, this group began reviewing research systematically. This resulted, first, in the publication of two significant volumes and, later, the ongoing development of the Cochrane database. Unsurprisingly, evidence should facilitate evidence-based practice, which has been defined as:

The conscientious, explicit and judicious use of current best evidence in making decisions about the care of individual patients.

(Sackett et al 1996, p 71).

Audit

Another term used frequently in the maternity area, 'audit', is widely misunderstood. Unlike research, audit differs in that it has not been subjected to the scrutiny of a research ethics committee (Maresh 1999). Occasionally, one may wonder whether this is the only difference. The more acceptable criteria, however, for audit are:

- well-localized in terms of function, geography, or both
- cyclical activity
- objectives measurable to ensure comparability
- subsequent action, such as change in service provision, intended.

The processes involved in audit also differ from research and have been outlined as:

- identification of elements of care for examination
  - asking questions
  - exploring issues
  - setting standards
  - reviewing criteria
- choice and application of methods to appraise care, include rigorous data analysis
- feedback of results to improve service.

Thus, Hughes (2005) highlights the cyclical nature of audit and its direct application to specific clinical settings. The crucial role of the clinical environment becomes clear when recalling the three traditional aspects of audit – that is, focusing on structure, process or outcome. This role and focus on outcomes is well illustrated by an audit of care of the woman with type 1 diabetes mellitus (Kernaghan et al 2006).

Although it is the *process* that is most frequently addressed by audit, it is, conversely, this aspect that is least likely to be satisfactorily audited (Walsh 1999, p 430). The problem, according to Walsh, is that the audit loop is rarely completely closed; meaning that guidelines are set and data collected, but strategies to correct any shortfall may not be implemented. Additionally, there is no evaluation of changing practice when it is implemented. Thus, the audit process is effectively stalled, and the cycle fails to develop into the audit spiral leading to improved healthcare (Maresh 1999, p 137).

Although numerical approaches are often assumed to be fundamental to audit, Maresh (1999, p 140) maintains that this is not necessarily so. He argues that hard-edged statistical approaches are not always necessary for audit. His idea of this 'softer' approach appears in his example, in which he suggests that obtaining women's views about their care is an 'alternative method of auditing maternal morbidity' (Maresh 1999, p 140). Such data may be obtained through qualitative research, rather than quantitatively, to identify women's perspective on their experience of pregnancy.

Some problems inherent in audit manifested themselves in a study of a change in maternity care following the Changing Childbirth report (Beake et al 1998, DH 1993). One example is that the demarcation between audit, addressing ongoing practice, and research, featuring new interventions, became blurred in this study. Thus, my opening criticism of audit may still be justified, rather than being historical as Walsh states (1999, p 430). Another of the problems that Beake and colleagues encountered in the course of their audit related to data collection. They relied on women's medical case notes to provide the data to be used for audit. These auditors realized that instruments being used for data collection had been developed for a different purpose – that is, to record care. Thus, these researchers could draw limited conclusions about their woman-centred intervention.

Rationale for research-based and evidence-based practice

Research-based practice in nursing and midwifery has long been regarded as a means of ensuring high quality care. Additionally, some consider that the professions' status may be enhanced by such intellectual activity. The introduction of evidence-based practice (EBP), however, began with medical practitioners' response to Cochrane's withering criticism of obstetricians' abysmal research utilization record, mentioned above (1972).

Evidence-based practice has been advocated by many UK policy documents. These recommendations have argued that it may facilitate more appropriate resource allocation in the UK health service, by increasing effectiveness and efficiency. Effectiveness has been defined as how successfully the aim is achieved, whereas efficiency is 'how well one does something' (Paton 1995, p 31). Evidence-based practice forms the mainstay of 'clinical governance', which is a UK government initiative to improve the quality of healthcare (Badham et al 2006). While midwifery has long had access to strong evidence relating to the use of episiotomy (Sleep 1991), other aspects of midwifery care are seriously deficient. These aspects include contentious issues such as where the woman should experience uncomplicated childbirth (Olsen & Jewell 1998). Other examples, involving the midwife, include techniques

contributing to the 'medicalization' of childbearing; these include the questionable benefits of continuous electronic fetal monitoring (CEFM) in labour (Alfirevic et al 2006) and whether the benefits of routine ultrasound examination in pregnancy justify its use (Bricker & Neilson 2000).

As well as the extension of knowledge and more appropriate care, research evidence which is provided by multi-agency, multiprofessional and multidisciplinary teams carries further advantages. These additional benefits include reducing divisions between education, research and clinical practice (McCloughen & O'Brien 2006). Such research has been advocated as one means of lessening the theory-practice gap.

Randomized controlled trial

The strength of the research or quality of the evidence utilized to build evidence-based practice is clearly crucial. For this reason, the research design that is usually regarded as the most powerful, the randomized controlled trial (RCT), is the one most frequently recommended. For a summary of the hierarchy of strength of evidence, see Box 6.1

The RCT overcomes bias inherent when past experience, single case studies or case series without comparison groups are the basis of care (Donnan 2000). The power of the RCT is found in its objectivity or freedom from bias, which is likely to affect the results with other research designs. The bias that

---

Box 6.1 Source of evidence

- Randomized controlled trial (the subjects acting as their own controls)
- Systematic review of randomized trials
- Single randomized trial
- Systematic review of observational studies
- Single observational study
- Physiological study
- Unsystematic clinical studies
- A hierarchy of strength of evidence for treatment decisions, from highest to lowest

(Adapted from McKibbon et al 2002.)

may materialize accidentally is associated with the sampling or selection of subjects for the experimental treatment and the control group, who receive no treatment, a placebo or the standard care. As the name indicates, the allocation to either the intervention or control group is by randomization. In this way all have an equal chance of being in either group and systematic inter-group differences are avoided.

A recent example of randomization is the RCT on correcting an occipito-posterior position of the fetus (Stremler et al 2005). Randomization was by a telephone-based computerized system in which the computer assigned the woman to either the intervention or control group. Such precautions mean that the findings are relevant or generalizable to a wider target population than just the sample involved. Enkin and colleagues (2000, p 10) maintain that the logic underpinning the RCT, if implemented conscientiously, makes this research design 'the gold standard for comparing alternative forms of care'. Bias may be further reduced by ensuring that, as far as possible, the woman and baby, those caring for them and those collecting data are 'blind' or unaware of the treatment group to which allocation has been made.

The principles of conducting a RCT which justify confidence in the results have been listed by Sleep (1991) (Box 6.2).

After data have been collected to measure the outcomes in all treatment groups, the data are subjected to statistical analysis. Thus, an assessment is made of whether differences in outcomes are due to chance, rather than the experimental intervention. This statistical analysis must be rigorous. The published research report includes a full account of the analysis, as well as detailing any deviation from the protocol. Because the researcher follows the research protocol conscientiously, the findings may be checked by other researchers by replicating the study.

Despite the power of the RCT, it is still necessary for the practitioner to scrutinize the research report to ensure that the context and intervention are relevant to the present situation. This scrutiny is vital in maternity care, where systems of care differ greatly and where cultural values are fundamental to the attitudes of women and staff. Such scrutiny is likely to take account of not only the research findings and local context, but also the midwife's knowledge of the woman, her personal and professional experience and her intuition.

The RCT is the research method that underpins evidence-based practice. Other forms of evidence may be utilized in practice, but these other forms are often considered as of lesser value (see Box 6.1). The RCT is one example of the quantitative research approach.

Research methods

Quantitative research

Research mentioned up to this point in this chapter has focused on areas of care amenable to scientific measurement, or quantification. Thus, the methods used are known as quantitative methods (Balnaves & Caputi 2001). In the next section there will be some discussion of another approach, known as qualitative research. If the researcher's area of interest involves phenomena that may be counted, numbered or otherwise measured then a quantitative approach is likely to be the more appropriate.

When I undertook a study examining student midwives' employment decisions and practice, I decided that quantitative methods were suitable (Mander 1994). These methods permitted counting how many students and new midwives planned to practise midwifery and how many had other plans. I also

---

Box 6.2 Principles of conducting a randomized controlled trial

- The number of subjects should be adequate to ensure that differences are not due to chance
- Randomization of the subjects happens before the intervention and there is no withdrawal
- The allocation must not be predictable
- Compliance with the intervention should be complete
- When the data are analysed, each subject is retained in the allocated group, regardless of the actual treatment.

(After Sleep 1991, p 201.)

counted how many and measured for how long the midwives practised. In this research, as in all quantitative research, the researcher sought to maintain objectivity. Thus, the researcher tries to remain impartial and reduce bias by avoiding personal involvement with the data or respondents. The researcher also seeks to limit personal or subjective interpretation of the data, as described in the account of RCTs above. In my research on student midwives I pre-tested the research instrument (a postal questionnaire) to ensure its reliability and validity (see below). A pilot test is used to test the complete research protocol, rather than a pretest of one aspect.

Quantitative research involves a structured format, giving rise to one of its strengths, being easily replicated. This structure invariably begins with a literature search, on the basis of which the researcher formulates a hypothesis and possibly research questions. The researcher then tests the hypothesis and answers the research questions by using the most appropriate research design. Following on from the design are various methods of sampling, data collection and statistical analysis; various possibilities are considered before deciding which will best answer the research questions (Rees 2003).

Reliability and validity

The issues of reliability and validity are crucial to the methods and instruments employed.

- *Reliability* is the constancy or accuracy of a measurement or observation. Simplistically, this might refer to a sphygmomanometer being accurately calibrated.
- *Validity* is whether the research is measuring what it is supposed to be measuring, or perhaps inadvertently measuring something closely related.

In qualitative research quality is equally important but different ways of assessing quality are used.

Quantitative research has been criticized on the grounds of it being reductionist. This is because, in order to make sense of the respondents' behaviour or responses, the researcher must simplify or reduce the events to basic component parts. The researcher must consider carefully the appropriateness of a reductionist approach in a topic as complex as childbearing. A quantitative research approach may neglect some important aspect of the phenomenon under study. This may be because the researcher is unaware of it or perhaps it is too complex, or otherwise challenging, to address.

Qualitative research

Qualitative approaches may be more appropriate to help the midwife find answers to complex and challenging questions (Holloway 2005). Although some critics regard qualitative research as 'soft', it may be more suitable for examining the human aspects of childbearing. A crucial feature of all forms of qualitative research is their ability to understand the person's experience. To achieve this, the researcher must observe the person's actions or listen to or read their thoughts. In this way the perspective of the person experiencing the phenomenon becomes apparent. This is the 'emic' approach, and is clearly different from the 'etic' or quantitative approach. The qualitative researcher does not seek objectivity; the reverse applies, as the researcher interacts personally with the informant and the data. In this way, the researcher seeks a complete understanding of the phenomenon, event or experience.

There are different forms of qualitative research, including grounded theory, phenomenology and ethnography, which differ in their theoretical basis, the researcher's involvement and the degree of structure. The qualitative method chosen will depend on existing knowledge about the topic, as determined by the literature search, and the researcher's expertise.

Qualitative data analysis does not use statistical tests, although computer programmes are available (St John & Johnson 2000). As always, data analysis involves the researcher's profound involvement. This input is challenging, as the topics are sensitive – as in my study of the midwife's care of the mother relinquishing her baby for adoption (Mander 1995).

Qualitative research's exploratory nature makes it ideally suited to areas where knowledge is scanty. Thus, this type of research may be regarded as a building brick of midwifery theory. A further strength of qualitative research is its ability to provide fresh perspectives on familiar phenomena. This matters when the midwife seeks to understand the woman's experience of childbearing or care.

Triangulation and mixed methods

Qualitative and quantitative are the two main approaches to research, which have much to offer midwifery. These approaches may not be discrete entities, though, as they may be combined in one project. This combination is one form of 'triangulation', which may incorporate several or varied methods, theoretical approaches or sources of data. The strengths of each research approach should be considered and they may be combined by triangulation or using a 'mixed methods' approach. Thus the strength of a qualitative study may be enhanced.

To some researchers the gap between these two approaches is unbridgeable (Carr 1994, Clarke 1995), but the situation may be viewed differently. Rather than being 'right' or 'wrong', the reader or consumer of research should look for the appropriateness of the research approach to the question being asked. Perhaps postal questionnaires and significance tests are not suitable for studying intimate matters.

The research process

The systematic approach of research differentiates it from other forms of questioning and is termed 'the research process'. Rees (2003) outlines the stages of the research process, beginning with developing the research question. For Rees this process ends with the 'communication of the findings'. This may take the form of a written report, journal article or verbal presentation to colleagues or conference delegates. Perhaps, though, the process does not end with the dissemination of the findings. Following 'publication', each practitioner has a responsibility to be aware of the research and to take an interest in its utilization. This stage may, subsequently, be followed by evaluation of the implementation and changing practice.

Research ethics

The woman for whom the midwife provides care, seeks her help for that reason – that is, to obtain care. Because this is so obvious, we must question whether researchers should be permitted to recruit the woman and baby for research during that care. This question, and others, raises ethical issues for the midwife (Beauchamp & Childress 2001). These and other ethical issues were addressed in Chapter 5. One fundamentally crucial ethical principle which deserves attention here, though, is autonomy.

Autonomy, meaning 'self-rule', is a most basic and inalienable human right. It means that the woman has the right to decide what does or does not happen to her and her body. A woman seeking midwifery care has no obligation to participate in research associated with her care, but must choose freely whether to do so. Both the researcher and midwife are obliged to ensure that the woman knows that she is not compelled to participate in research and that, if she does agree, she is always free to withdraw.

Pressure on the woman to participate may be subtle, so information must be in writing for her to keep. To enable the woman to decide she must be informed about the details and implications of the study before agreeing. Researchers are usually required to obtain the woman's written consent but the consent form per se is insignificant compared with the information which makes any consent fully informed. The researcher should also allow the woman time to reconsider; over 24 hrs is recommended. This protects women who are especially vulnerable, such as women in labour or who have given birth to a sick baby.

An extension of autonomy is the researcher's responsibility to ensure anonymity and confidentiality for respondents. Thus, not only is the person not named but also she and her data are not identifiable. Confidentiality is more elusive, especially when a small number of participants are involved in a study focusing on an easily recognized activity, such as giving birth to a baby with a disability.

Research critique

The term 'critique' means the careful examination or criticism of research, for example of a report. Unlike criticism's usual meaning, critique carries no negative overtones. Critique does, however, comprise a fair, balanced judgement, seeking strengths as well as any limitations. Having already mentioned its strengths, I here attempt a critique of evidence-based practice.

The evidence base of practice rightly has been criticized for being incomplete. Evidence exists only on those aspects of care that have been subjected to research. One estimate is that only about 12% of midwifery care is supported by evidence. Thus it may be that the evidence base is inadequate to permit the midwife to provide comprehensive care.

This incomplete evidence base is an aspect of evidence-based practice (EBP) being addressed by ongoing research. Such research, though, may produce new evidence that conflicts with or contradicts existing knowledge. It is the practitioner's responsibility to ensure that she utilizes the current best evidence. This requires her to assess research (see below).

Some practitioners consider that EBP may be inappropriate in an activity as uniquely human as childbearing. EBP may reduce the humanity of care. This danger has been referred to as 'routinization' or even as 'cookbook care' (Kim 2000). This argument about reducing care's humanity has been extended to include the effects of EBP on the practitioner's occupational group. So achieving or maintaining professional status among EBP practitioners may be reduced (Bonell 1999). This latter point is the reverse of the truth. This is because, EBP requires the practitioner to employ certain skills in addition to the knowledge, personal experience, occupational experience, empathy and intuition ordinarily used by the midwife. These additional skills include needing to understand the evidence base of practice. She must understand the strengths and weaknesses of research and distinguish the evidence to be utilized as against that to be rejected.

Research utilization by the practitioner

Having established the significance of research to midwifery, and particularly practice, we should consider the reality of midwives' research utilization. This is one of the final stages of the research process and, perhaps for that reason, is neglected. Research utilization has attracted considerable attention in nursing (French 2005, Rodgers 2000). When nurses first examined this problem, Hunt (1981) found that their difficulties related to their education. She identified nurses' lack of knowledge about research findings. Even when this did not apply, the nurse encountered difficulty in understanding and believing the research. Any chance of utilizing research was hampered by nurses' ignorance about its application. A sinister phenomenon highlighted by Hunt was the organization forbidding the nurse from using research.

The problems identified by Hunt among nurses were subsequently endorsed by a study of midwives' attitudes (Meah et al 1996). This study involved 32 midwives participating in group interviews to elicit important themes. Educational deficits again emerged. The midwives could not evaluate research, or interpret statistics or understand methods. Hunt's sinister organizational impediment again emerged; Meah and colleagues found that midwives lacked autonomy in implementing research and they lacked role models from whom to learn research-based practice. Clearly, as these researchers observed, many of these faults are partly researchers' responsibility.

A perplexing phenomenon was found by Hicks (1992) to limit the midwife's use of midwifery research. Using a cross-over technique, 18 midwives were asked to evaluate two research reports. Half were told that the reports were by a midwife and an obstetrician, respectively, and the other half were told that they were by an obstetrician and a midwife respectively. The midwives consistently judged the report thought to be by the midwife as poorer than the other. Thus, Hicks demonstrates midwives' low opinion of midwifery research; such low esteem may further inhibit research utilization.

Another study also illuminated midwives' research utilization (Harris 1992). Using research into perineal pain control as her example, Harris asked 76 staff what research they knew about and what research they utilized. She identified profound ignorance of the plentiful authoritative research on this crucial topic. In contrast, Harris revealed the staff's better knowledge and enthusiastic implementation of research of questionable authority and relevance; research recommending withdrawing air-rings from frail elderly patients was applied to new mothers.

An important intervention study attempted to resolve these problems (Hundley et al 2000). These researchers employed a quasi-experimental research design to assess changes in research awareness and practice among midwives and nurses. The intervention, applied to only the experiment group, involved education on certain policy and practice topics for 'ward sisters'. The researchers found that staff attitudes to research, knowledge of research and involvement in research significantly improved in the 'educated' group. Quite appropriately, however, these researchers mention that changing practice is difficult. The change that they engendered, though, involved a considerable change in the culture of the research sites, as has been identified elsewhere (Rogers et al 2000).

The consumer of research

It may be apparent by now that there is little value in undertaking research – that is, beginning the research process – unless it is completed. The most important aspect of the process is the utilization of research. Although the researcher is crucial in the dissemination of research findings, the utilization decision is made by the research consumer.

We should consider who is the research consumer (Tallon et al 2000). In an otherwise admirable book, Buggins and Nolan (2000) define the consumer simply as the consumer of healthcare. The consumers of research, however, comprise a far wider group.

The ultimate research consumer is the person who receives or participates in care. In midwifery this is the childbearing woman and her family. It is necessary, though, that for the woman to experience evidence-based care, the staff should practice EBP. For this reason, the midwife is also a research consumer. To extend further the range of research consumers, we should also include the midwifery student, because her education provides the foundation for practice.

The midwifery student

The midwifery student learns about research in several ways.

First, research underpins her education (Thomson P 2000). In this way, she learns the techniques that are outlined below to critique relevant studies. The student also learns about research evidence and the areas of practice yet to be researched.

Second, in her clinical experience, the student observes the utilization of research by her mentor, acting as a role model.

Third, the student may become involved in research. This may be by attending journal clubs organized by active researchers and by meeting researchers at seminars and conferences. Additionally the involvement may be associated with participating in ongoing research in her clinical placements.

Finally, the student may find opportunities for undertaking research. Such an immense responsibility is not available to all midwifery students. The rationale is that, for the research to be valuable or at least harmless, the student requires supervision from an experienced researcher with time to invest in this learner (Mander 1988).

The midwifery student may undertake a critique of a research report during her midwifery programme. This is an opportunity to use the research literature as the basis of an informed discussion. The student should welcome this chance to present a reasoned judgement, supported by literature, of a research paper.

The midwife

The midwife is likely to encounter research reports in a wide range of midwifery, nursing and other journals as well as at meetings and conferences. Following the midwife's critical reading of a research report in a journal or elsewhere, certain choices present themselves (Box 6.3):

- The midwife believes that the findings will resolve a problem identified in her clinical setting. On the basis of this, she seeks to implement it and evaluate the outcomes.

- The midwife decides to ignore the study because it is:
  - irrelevant to her workplace
  - too seriously flawed to be of value
  - undertaken in a setting with a different maternity system and is not transferable.

Box 6.3 Actions following reading a research report

- Implementation
- Rejection as inappropriate
- Replication to test appropriateness

- Although the research has limitations or was undertaken elsewhere, some of the issues are relevant to the midwife's clinical area. For these reasons, a researcher will be approached to assist the midwifery staff in further investigating this work by replicating this study locally with a suitable sample.

The woman

The childbearing woman, the ultimate consumer of research, may be involved in a number of ways. Increasingly women are involved in earlier stages of research. This is through the need for the childbearing woman's specialized input into planning and implementing the study. Women have for too long acted just as the subjects of research. It is appropriate now for the woman to be a full partner in the research process as well as in clinical decision-making.

The information and advice that the midwife gives to the woman during her childbearing experience should, as far as possible, be research based. This information may be provided verbally, as a website address or in the form of evidence-based leaflets (O'Mara 2003). With the increasing availability of research evidence the internet helps the woman to find information. The woman, though, may still benefit from help in locating information of a suitable standard on the internet (Stewart 2005).

Critical reading

Any consumer's reading of a research report should involve critical reading; this term means that the report should be judged well, that is fairly, rather than harshly or excessively negatively. Similarly, reading research requires an objective examination, in order to identify strengths and any limitations. Even the best research may have weak points, but the reverse may also be true in that even a weak study has some points from which the consumer can learn (LoBiondo-Wood et al 2002).

As mentioned above, asking questions is fundamental to research. This applies to the researcher, but also to the research consumer such as the clinical midwife. Many of the midwife's questions will relate to practice, especially to routines that have become established as 'unit policy' and over the use of which she has little control. Some of her questions will be answered by the research literature, but whether this is so depends on her critical reading. Thus, the consumer should adopt a questioning approach to care in childbearing, an example of which is her reading of research, including the following points.

The complete research

The consumer should consider the material in its entirety, rather than piecemeal. This complete picture illuminates points that might otherwise be missed; for example, a small sample might be inappropriate to permit conclusions, but in an in-depth qualitative study a small sample is reasonable. Similarly, in a quantitative study, tables and statistical tests may disconcert some readers, but they are crucial to the findings and need to be read alongside the text.

A further advantage of reading the complete report is in the reader finding any points that have been neglected or even omitted. In this way, the reader is able to question the reason why this information is not included. This may be an oversight, but may be because the researcher wishes to minimize some questionable aspect of the study. An example would be when the response rate is not stated. The reader should be cautious about the quality of this work and may even suspect that the rate was unacceptably low. Response rates reflect the instrument's suitability and the importance of the study to participants.

Specific points

While examining the complete report, the midwife should question whether the various parts form a unified whole, whether they are discrete entities or whether there are gaps in the presentation. One problem is that one part does not lead into the next; for example, the research questions may bear little relation to the literature review from which they should have arisen. This would lead the reader to wonder how these questions originated. Another example would be if the conclusions are not well-related to the findings, when the reader might ask whether the researcher chose the conclusions before doing the research.

Author's details or affiliation

The author's name, designation and qualifications are helpful in forming initial impressions. This may be because of knowledge of and respect for this researcher's previous work. Or it may be due to the need for an examination of this particular problem from, for example, a midwifery or organizational viewpoint. The researcher's base or institution may assist in deciding its relevance if, for instance, the report was written in a country where maternity care differs.

Introduction

The introduction should allow the reader to decide whether the report is likely to be helpful.

Literature review

To show why the current project is needed, the literature review outlines the development of knowledge about the topic up to the present time. Gaps in the literature should be highlighted, as they support the current study. If recent research is not mentioned, the reader should question when the research was undertaken in case it is out of date. If important research is omitted, the reason should be sought; the omission may reflect ignorance or perhaps another agenda. The literature review should demonstrate a relevant theoretical framework; based on a high level of knowledge, this framework helps with framing questions and designing the study (Cormack & Benton 2000, p 80). Some research approaches, such as grounded theory, review the literature alongside rather than before the data collection.

Hypothesis/research questions

The hypothesis or research questions, or both, emerge inevitably out of the literature review. These statements or questions are phrased precisely to exclude ambiguity.

Research approach/design

The research approach or design includes discussion of the possibilities that were considered and not employed. The researcher's understanding of the issues relating to research design will demonstrate that this approach will answer the research questions.

Research method

The research method describes the complete research as it was planned. This begins with the subjects and the sample. In a quantitative study it would be necessary to give details of the calculations to produce the sample for findings to be statistically significant. The reader will ask whether the subjects would be able to provide the information to answer the research questions. An example of this not being done is if in certain groups such as children who cannot speak for themselves, the focus is on carers' views.

Details of how the sample was identified and recruited are also necessary. A random sample strengthens a research project, but a convenience sample needs to be identified.

Data collection

The data collection details how the research instrument was chosen, designed, tested and applied. This applies particularly to questionnaires, but also to interview schedules or observation checklists. The reader must consider whether these aspects are appropriate to answer the research questions, considering the various instruments' strengths and limitations. The quality, that is the reliability and validity of the method, is critically discussed here.

Data analysis

The data analysis should be explained, including discussion and an explanation of any statistical tests.

Ethical implications

The research's ethical implications are considered, with discussion of how dilemmas were resolved. Obtaining ethical approval is reported and the possibility of harm to the participant is discussed, including physical or emotional trauma or lowered self esteem. Strategies to maintain participants' anonymity and confidentiality are recounted here.

Research findings

The findings begin with aspects of the research deviating from that described in the method section. Then response rates and other demographic data are provided. The reader notes any omission, which indicates the study was not completed.

This section includes discussion of the findings or this may be separate. The discussion relates the findings to the research questions. The researcher identifies whether there were any unanswered research questions and the reasons.

This discussion includes the researcher's *own* criticism of the research, in the form of a limitations section (Benton & Cormack 2000).

Reading the conclusions

The conclusions present a summary of the main findings and should be well substantiated. This section may include recommendations which are firmly supported by the research.

Conclusion

The need for midwifery practice to be 'evidence-based' is constantly reiterated. The meaning of 'evidence-based' care is less frequently considered. It is important to examine carefully the meaning of evidence and the forms in which evidence may be employed by midwives. The methods used to obtain this evidence also deserve attention. The difference between evaluative research and audit is important in that audit is compared with predetermined standards. Such material will be utilized by students and midwives in their midwifery practice, as well as by childbearing women. It may, thus, encourage some to embark on their own research.

REFERENCES

Alfirevic Z, Devane D, Gyte G M L 2006 Continuous cardiotocography (CTG) as a form of electronic fetal monitoring (EFM) for fetal assessment during labour. Cochrane Database of Systematic Reviews, Issue 3:CD006066

Badham J, Wall D, Sinfield M et al 2006 The essence of care in clinical governance. Clinical Governance: An International Journal 11(1):22–29

Balnaves M, Caputi P 2001 Introduction to quantitative research methods: an investigative approach. SAGE, London

Beake S, McCourt C, Page L et al 1998 The use of clinical audit in evaluating maternity services reform: a clinical reflection. Journal of Evaluation in Clinical Practice 4(1):75–83

Beauchamp T L, Childress J F 2001 Principles of biomedical ethics, 5th edn. Oxford University Press, Oxford

Benton D C, Cormack D F S 2000 Reviewing and evaluating the literature. In: Cormack D F S (ed.) The research process in nursing, 4th edn. Blackwell Science, Oxford, p 103–113

Bonell C 1999 Evidence-based nursing: a stereotyped view of quantitative and experimental research could work against professional autonomy and authority. Journal of Advanced Nursing 30(1):18–23

Bricker L, Neilson J P 2000 Routine Doppler ultrasound in pregnancy. Cochrane Database of Systematic Reviews, Issue 2:CD001450

Buggins E, Nolan M 2000 Involving consumers in research. In: Proctor S, Renfrew M (eds) Linking research and practice in midwifery: a guide to evidence-based practice. Baillière Tindall, New York, p 89–102

Carr L T 1994 Strengths and weaknesses of quantitative and qualitative research: what method for nursing? Journal of Advanced Nursing 20(4):716–721

Chalmers I 1993 Effective care in midwifery: research the professions and the public. Midwives Chronicle 106(1260):3–12

Clarke L 1995 Nursing research: science visions and telling stories. Journal of Advanced Nursing 21(3):584–593

Cochrane A L 1972 Effectiveness and efficiency. Nuffield Provincial Hospitals Trust, London

Cormack D F S, Benton D C 2000 Asking the research questions. In: Cormack D F S (ed.) The research process in nursing, 4th edn. Blackwell Science, Oxford, p 77–88

DH (Department of Health) 1993 Changing childbirth: report of the Expert Maternity Group. DH, London

Donnan P T 2000 Experimental research. In: Cormack D F S (ed.) The research process in nursing, 4th edn. Blackwell Science, Oxford, p 175

Enkin M, Keirse M, Renfrew M et al 2000 A guide to effective care in pregnancy and childbirth, 3rd edn. Oxford University Press, Oxford

French B 2005 The process of research use in nursing. Journal of Advanced Nursing 49(2):125–134

Harris M 1992 The impact of research findings on current practice in relieving postpartum perineal pain in a large district general hospital. Midwifery 8(3):125–131

Hicks C 1992 Research in midwifery: are midwives their own worst enemies? Midwifery 8(1).12–18

Holloway I 2005 (ed.) Qualitative research in healthcare. Open University Press, Maidenhead

Hughes R 2005 Is audit research? The relationships between clinical audit and social-research. International Journal of Healthcare Quality Assurance 18(4–5):289–299

Hundley V, Milne J, Leighton-Beck L et al 2000 Raising research awareness among midwives and nurses: does it work? Journal of Advanced Nursing 31:78–88

Hunt J M 1981 Indicators for nursing practice: the use of research findings. Journal of Advanced Nursing 6(4):189–194

Kernaghan D, Penney G C, Pearson D W M 2006 Pregnancy-related care and outcomes for women with Type 1 diabetes in Scotland: a five-year population-based audit cycle. Clinical Governance: An International Journal 11(2):114–127

Kim M 2000 Evidence-based nursing: connecting knowledge to practice. Chart 97(9):1, 4–6

LoBiondo-Wood G, Haber J, Krainovich-Miller B 2002 Critical reading strategies: overview of the research process. In: LoBiondo-Wood, G, Haber, J (eds) Nursing research:

methods, critical appraisal, and utilization, 5th edn. Mosby, St Louis, Ch. 2

Macdonald A M 1981 Chambers' twentieth century dictionary. Chambers, Edinburgh, p 1148

Mander R 1988 Encouraging students to be research minded. Nurse Education Today 8(1):30–35

Mander R 1994 Midwifery training and the years after qualification. In: Robinson S, Thomson A (eds) Midwives, research and childbirth. Routledge, London, vol 3, p 233–259

Mander R 1995 The care of the mother grieving a baby relinquished for adoption. Avebury, Aldershot

Maresh M 1999 Auditing care. In: Marsh G, Renfrew M (eds) Community-based maternity care. Oxford general practice series. Oxford University Press, Oxford, p137–152

McCloughen A, O'Brien L 2006 Interagency collaborative research projects: Illustrating potential problems, and finding solutions in the nursing literature. International Journal of Mental Health Nursing 15(3):171–180

McKibbon A, Hunt D, Richardson W S et al 2002 Introduction: the philosophy of evidence-based medicine. In: Guyatt G, Rennie D (eds) Users' guides to the medical literature: a manual for evidence-based clinical practice. American Medical Association Press, Chicago, p 3–12

Meah S, Luker K A, Cullum N A 1996 An exploration of midwives' attitudes to research and perceived barriers to research utilisation. Midwifery 12(2):73–84

Olsen O, Jewell M D 1998 Home versus hospital birth. Cochrane Database of Systematic Reviews 3:CD000352.

O'Mara L 2003 Evidence based patient information leaflets in maternity care had limited visibility and did not promote informed choice of childbearing women. Evidence-based Nursing 6(1):27

Paton C 1995 Competition and planning in the NHS. Chapman & Hall, London, p 31

Rees C 2003 An introduction to research for midwives. Books for Midwives, Hale, p 8

Rodgers S E 2000 The extent of nursing research utilization in general medical and surgical wards. Journal of Advanced Nursing 32(1):182–193

Rogers S, Humphrey C, Nazareth I et al 2000 Designing trials of interventions to change professional practice in primary care: lessons from an exploratory study of two change strategies. British Medical Journal 320(7249):1580–1583

Sackett D, Rosenburg W, Gray J A et al 1996 Evidence based medicine: what it is and what it isn't. British Medical Journal 312(7023):71–72

Sleep J 1991 Perineal care: a series of five randomised controlled trials. In: Robinson S, Thomson A M (eds) Midwives research and childbirth. Chapman & Hall, London, p 199–251

St John W, Johnson P 2000 The pros and cons of data analysis software for qualitative research. Journal of Nursing Scholarship 32(4):393–397

Stewart S (2005) Caught in the web: an over view of e-health and midwifery practice. British Journal of Midwifery 13(9):546–550

Stremler R, Hodnett E, Petryshen P et al 2005 Randomized controlled trial of hands-and-knees positioning for occipitoposterior position in labor. Birth 32(4):243–251

Tallon D, Chard J, Dieppe P 2000 Relation between agendas of the research community and the research consumer. The Lancet 355(9220):2037–2040

Thomson A 2000 Is there evidence for the medicalisation of maternity care? MIDIRS Midwifery Digest 10(4):416–420

Thomson P 2000 Implementing evidence-based healthcare: the nurse teachers' role in supporting the dissemination and implementation of the SIGN clinical guidelines. Nurse Education Today 20(3):207–217

Walsh D 1999 Demystifying clinical audit. MIDIRS Midwifery Digest 9(4):430–431

FURTHER READING

General research texts

Parahoo K 2006 Nursing research: principles, process and issues, 2nd edn. Macmillan, London.

This book is at a suitable level for the student or midwife interested in research.

Cormack D F S (ed.) 2000 The research process in nursing, 4th edn. Blackwell Science, Oxford

This authoritative edited book discusses important issues in considerable depth.

Rees C 2003 An introduction to research for midwives, 2nd edn. Butterworth-Heinemann, Edinburgh

This book is highly accessible and utilizes examples of situations and studies that are familiar to the midwife. A useful section on research critique is provided.

Evidence-based research

Brown B, Crawford P, Hicks C 2003 Evidence-based research: dilemmas and debates in healthcare. Open University Press, Maidenhead

A book to help any reader to make sense of the research evidence.

Quantitative research

Balnaves M, Caputi P 2001 Introduction to quantitative research methods. SAGE, London

Relatively challenging topics are addressed in a student-friendly style.

Feminist research

Letherby G 2003 Feminist research in theory and practice. Open University Press, Milton Keynes

The issues relevant to research for and by women are analysed comprehensively.

Implementation of research

Proctor S, Renfrew M 2001 Linking research and practice in midwifery: a guide to evidence-based practice. Baillière Tindall, Edinburgh

The challenges and benefits of evidence-based midwifery practice are addressed by these well-recognized midwife researchers.

Qualitative research

Holliday A 2002 Doing and writing qualitative research. SAGE, London

These methods are highly appropriate in midwifery and are becoming increasingly important. Their significance is clearly demonstrated.

Evidence-based practice

Walsh D (2007) Evidence-based care for normal labour and birth. Routledge, London

A range of issues as well as examples are covered in an accessible style in this series of journal articles.

USEFUL WEBSITES

Bandolier – a bulletin that summarizes RCTs in an easy to access and easy to read format:
http://www.jr2.ox.ac.uk/bandolier/

Cochrane database – often considered the last word in locating evidence:
http://www.mrw.interscience.wiley.com/cochrane/cochrane_search_fs.html

CRD – NHS Centre for Reviews and Dissemination, York University:
http://www.york.ac.uk/inst/crd/

MIDIRS Midwifery Digest – An abstracting service which has an online facility:
http://www.midirs.org/midirs/midweb1.nsf/services?openform

National Electronic Library for Health – an excellent resource with many links and NICE guidelines. It also has a primary care specific site:
http://www.nelh.nhs.uk/midwife/default.asp

7 Midwifery regulation in the United Kingdom

Christina McKenzie

Regulation of healthcare professionals does not stand still and is constantly evolving, albeit in some instances, slowly. The struggles for legislation to control the practice of midwives in the UK prior to the first Midwives Act and since have been well documented (Cowell & Wainwright (1981), Donnison (1988), Heagerty (1996) and Towler & Bramall (1986)), and can be explored in detail in those texts.

The chapter aims to:

describe the current regulatory framework for midwives practising in the UK. This will enable midwives and student midwives to appreciate the structure that supports them in their practice, their responsibilities and the ethos behind the current approach to midwifery regulation. Within this chapter the reader can consider:

- the purpose of regulation of healthcare professionals
- the functions and scope of the current midwifery regulatory body – The Nursing and Midwifery Council
- the legal process that is followed when changing statutory regulation
- the framework for statutory supervision of midwives
- proposed changes to regulation in the twenty-first century.

The purpose of midwifery regulation

Statutory regulation provides structure and boundaries that can be understood and interpreted by both professionals and the public, and it is the basis of a contract of trust between the public and the profession. Although the primary purpose of regulation is protection of the public, the same mechanism protects midwives and supports them in their practice. The UK was not the first country to establish legislation governing the practice of midwives as governments in Austria, Norway and Sweden had taken such an approach as early as 1801.

Regulation of midwifery can and should play a key part in helping to improve women's experiences of the maternity services. Women and their families look to regulation to ensure that they are being cared for by competent and skilled midwives who are properly educated and up to date in their practice. It is important therefore, not to think of regulation in terms of abstract concepts or principles, but what it means in ordinary everyday aspects of healthcare, and how it can support the types of care that women need or we would want for ourselves and our families. Midwifery regulation enables the public to be assured that anyone calling themselves a midwife is competent to practise as a midwife.

In the UK, no-one can call themself a midwife or practise as a midwife unless they are on the Nursing and Midwifery Council's (NMC) Register. This registration must be active, which means that the midwife has met the continuing professional development and practice requirements to stay on the Register and has paid the fee that enables this to happen.

As Frances Blunden stated in 2007, 'Much of the current approach to regulation is far too reactive, with a tendency to focus on serious misdemeanours. We wait for someone to get it wrong dramatically and then very slowly take action. Women should not have to die or to be seriously harmed by the actions of midwives or other professionals before the protection that regulation is supposed to afford them swings into action. That's an approach that lets down women, their babies, and professionals, sometimes very badly.'

There has been a change in the ethos and approach to regulation in the UK during the past 5 years and regulation is moving to a more proactive stance that seeks to prevent harm from happening in the first place. This change will hopefully ensure that midwives, wherever they practise, adopt the values and principles of a woman-centred approach to regulation in all that they do.

Self-regulation

In the UK, midwives are members of a self-regulating profession. Self-regulation is a privilege in many ways, as it means that the standards for education and practice expected of any midwife are set by midwives themselves. Self-regulating professions have regulatory bodies that are funded by the professionals themselves. In the case of midwives and nurses, their initial and subsequent periodic registration payment is the sole funding that pays for all of the functions of their regulatory body, the NMC.

In the UK self-regulation is achieved through a statutory midwifery committee of the NMC, which advises the Nursing and Midwifery Council (The Council) about what is needed to ensure safe and competent midwives. The midwifery committee has powers defined under Section 41 of The Nursing and Midwifery Order (2001). The term 'statutory' means that the role and scope of the committee is set in law and cannot be reduced or the committee disbanded unless there is a change in legislation to allow that to happen. Any rules or standards for midwifery education or practice set by the midwifery committee are subsequently approved by the Council before they can come into effect.

While midwives practise in a wide range of settings, as a profession they are unified by underlying values and responsibilities. Being a midwife is not merely a job, it is a professional responsibility. Each midwife has a personal responsibility for their own practice by being aware of their own strengths and weaknesses in practice. Each is expected to take steps to ensure they develop their skills and knowledge to ensure that they maintain their own competence.

There has been and remains rising public concern in the UK about healthcare professionals regulating themselves as a result of some high profile media cases where patient care was severely compromised (Kennedy 2001).

Midwives have a responsibility to be aware when a colleague's practice is not up to the expected standards and to take appropriate action when this is the case. Self-regulation and professional freedom are based on the assumption that professionals can be trusted to work without supervision and, where necessary, to take action against colleagues (Hogg 2000).

Midwives also share a collective responsibility for how women and their families are treated and cared for. This means that they have a responsibility to highlight both individual instances where practices are compromising safe and appropriate care for women, but also where the systems or processes within organizations providing services for women are compromising safe care.

Although most healthcare professions in the UK set their own standards and codes of conduct, this was not always the case for midwives. When the original Midwives Act came into force in 1902, the body it created, the Central Midwives Board (CMB), had no requirement for even one midwife to be included on its Council. Until 1983, it was the case that the midwifery statutory bodies of the UK were dominated by doctors who also held the chairmanships until the last decade prior to their dissolution.

> This powerful body was not, as was the case with other professional statutory bodies, to be largely constituted of members of the occupation to be regulated, but to be in the hands of medical practitioners (RCM 1991).

At the present time, self-regulation of midwifery does not exist in some countries. In some instances, regulations for midwifery education or practice are set by the national Government, or by another professional group who may be perceived as 'senior'.

The midwifery profession, as are other professions in the UK, is affected to varying extents by national regulations that are set by others who are not part of the profession. Examples of this are legislation to protect vulnerable children or adults (DH 2006, 2007a), medicines legislation (see Ch. 49), employment legislation or health and safety regulations in the workplace. All midwives are bound by these national laws in the same way as others.

Protection of the public cannot be achieved through the Regulatory body alone. It is more likely when the combination of statutory regulation, personal self-regulation, employment practices, professional organizations, education and other means of working with a common purpose achieves a strong framework that enhances protection of the public.

However, as the events at Bristol showed, it can be very difficult for individual professionals to act ethically and raise these issues within their organization for fear of reprisal. It is here that the regulator and regulation can play an active role in supporting the individual midwife by offering guidance to her. The regulator can also work actively with other service regulators such as the local supervising authorities or the Healthcare Commission in England or Quality Improvement Scotland, etc. to ensure early action is taken to prevent unnecessary harm to women or their families.

The NMC code

Midwives and midwifery practice in the UK are bound by a set of rules and standards that set the minimum requirements for anyone wishing to practise midwifery within the four countries. In addition to these requirements, which affect only midwives, there is a further set of ethical and behavioural standards to which all midwives and nurses working in the UK must adhere (NMC 2008a).

This is perhaps the most significant of the standards set by the regulatory body for midwives as it contains the ethical and moral codes that all midwives are expected to comply with. The Code applies to anyone who is on the NMC Register; however the relevance and need for codes of practice and conduct go beyond nurses and midwives and their day-to-day contact with women or patients.

Even when off-duty, midwives must still adhere to the principles and values embodied in The Code, particularly as they directly relate to the women and families that have been in their care. An example of this is respecting women's confidentiality. How easy would it be to breach this should a midwife discuss a difficult day with a woman or her family, to her partner or friend?

The regulator is clear that midwives working as managers also need to abide by The Code and principles of good practice, and have a duty towards women and their families, as well as the wider community. Although they may have minimal direct contact with women, their conduct, practice and professional decisions can fundamentally affect women's care. There is a public expectation that their first consideration in all activities must be the interests and safety of women and families.

Increasingly, women come into contact with support workers who are taking on many roles or tasks that in the past have been undertaken by midwives (NHS Employers 2005). There have been concerns expressed about the increasing role maternity support workers are playing in some hospitals and communities in providing care, and that this might be putting women and babies at risk (Sandall et al 2006). This raises another important question for the midwives who are asking support workers to take on roles that are outside their level of competence, and their personal responsibility for this under The Code.

The Code defines what women and their families have the right to expect in any encounter with a midwife. These can be summarized under the following:

- Act always in the best interest of women and their families
- Practise always in a safe and competent way
- Be personally accountable for maintaining your competency and skills
- Practise only within the scope of your competence
- Do not compromise the safety of the individual woman or her family either by act of commission or omission
- Do not ask someone else to do something that is neither appropriate to their skills or beyond their competence
- Do not forget the skills of midwifery, compassion, interpersonal skills and support for women and their families
- Respect the life, dignity and rights of the individuals you care for.

Although The Code sets out the principles and values for professional midwifery practice, it cannot guarantee high quality care unless the individual midwife internalizes the values that underpin the Code and takes personal responsibility for complying with its requirements.

Public expectations of professionalism and regulation

Women and their families look to regulation and the regulator for protection from 'bad' professionals. They expect effective systems to pick up poor performance and to address the problems effectively, with appropriate sanctions or measures. They also expect effective redress mechanisms if something goes wrong that are timely and easy to access. Unfortunately, many of the public's assumptions about regulation are misguided as there is no coherent regulatory system that guarantees quality and safety across the whole healthcare system.

Most members of the public do not know how midwives or other healthcare professionals are regulated and may not be concerned to know how this is achieved. This is because they receive good treatment from most professionals when they receive healthcare. The fact that a midwife is a member of a professional Register acts as a symbol of quality and competence that women can have trust in.

The public have high expectations of midwives, that they are compassionate, competent and provide safe care. Women allow midwives and the other healthcare professionals involved in their maternity care to have intimate access to their lives, home and property because they trust them to do what they are supposed to do, and to do it right. Trust is fundamental to the healthcare relationship. It is the responsibility of every midwife to maintain and build that public trust and confidence at all times. To betray that trust may not only cause physical or emotional harm, but also potentially undermines the reputation of the whole profession.

When is a midwife not a midwife?

'Midwife' is a title protected in statute in the UK. This means that no-one can call themselves a midwife or indeed imply they are a midwife in a business unless they hold active registration on the midwives part of the NMC register. In practical terms, this means that although a number of individuals may hold a midwifery qualification, they cannot use the title midwife nor provide midwifery care and advice unless they have met all requirements to join *and maintain* their registration as a midwife.

This has important implications for organizations who may wish to employ someone who holds a midwifery qualification but who does not hold midwifery registration, to offer care or advice to pregnant women. Such an approach increases risk to the public as the person would not be competent to provide midwifery care or advice. It would also mean that the individual concerned would be committing a criminal offence.

This most often applies to those who may have trained as a midwife and as a nurse but who have lapsed or not met requirements to maintain the midwife part of their registration. It would also apply to anyone wishing to work in the UK who may have trained as a midwife outside the UK but who is not registered as such with the NMC.

There are also implications for anyone wishing to set up a business with the term midwife or midwifery in the name of the business. In the UK, most types of businesses have to be registered with Companies House. Permission must be sought from the NMC for the title to be used in this context otherwise Companies House will refuse to register the name of the business. This is one way of reducing the risk of misleading the public, as the business title could imply that it relates to midwifery services or products.

A brief history of UK midwifery regulation

The first Midwives Act in the UK was passed in 1902. This Act of Parliament was not initiated by the Government of the time but was promoted by individual Members of Parliament through Private Members' Bills and supported in the House of Lords by others who supported midwife registration. The main provisions of the Midwives Act 1902 were as follows:

1. Prohibition of unqualified practice
2. The establishment of the Central Midwives Board with statutory functions
3. Rules regulating the practice of midwives
4. Local supervising authorities and the supervision of midwives.

The Midwives Act 1902 established the Central Midwives Board (CMB) with jurisdiction over midwives in England and Wales. This was followed by The Midwives (Scotland) Act 1915 and The Midwives Act (Ireland) 1918, which established similar bodies in Scotland and Ireland. In Northern Ireland, the Joint Nurses and Midwives Council (Northern Ireland) Act 1922 made provision for a Joint Council to take over responsibility for nurses and midwives, and the Nurses and Midwives (Northern Ireland) Act 1970 established the Northern Ireland Council for Nurses and Midwives (NICNM).

This meant that prior to 1983, four separate bodies were responsible for the regulation of midwifery in the UK. In the intervening years, the legislation was amended and changed to address the need for improved education of midwives and differences in healthcare and in some instances healthcare policy.

On 1 July 1983, the statutory control of the practice, education and supervision of midwives became the responsibility of the United Kingdom Central Council (The UKCC) and four National Boards for Nursing, Midwifery and Health Visiting, one in each of the four countries of the UK. The primary legislation under the regulatory body previous to the NMC, the UKCC, was the two Nurses, Midwives and Health Visitors Acts 1979 and 1992. These two Acts were consolidated in the Nurses, Midwives and Health Visitors Act 1997.

During the 1990s, the government devolved power away from the UK parliament based in Westminster, to the other three countries of the UK so they could establish their own parliaments or assemblies. This devolution has not impacted greatly on the regulation of midwives as they are one of the established professions. The power to regulate established professions remains with the UK parliament at Westminster, advised by the Department of Health England. Only new health-related professions that may be established in the future will be exempt from this approach.

The NMC was established in 2002 by The Nursing and Midwifery Order 2001 and took over most of the functions of the UKCC and the four national boards. This reunited standards for education with standards for practice and supervision of midwives on a UK basis. The creation of this UK-wide regulatory body the Nursing and Midwifery Council was contrary to the trend of devolving powers to national parliaments.

The Nursing and Midwifery Council

The Nursing and Midwifery Council (NMC) is the UK-wide regulator for two professions, nursing and midwifery. The primary purpose of the NMC is protection of the public and it does this through maintaining a register of all nurses, midwives and specialist community public health nurses eligible to practise within the UK and by setting standards for their education, training and conduct. As of March 2006, the number of midwives and nurses registered with the NMC was over 682 000, of whom approximately 43 000 were midwives (NMC 2007a).

The powers of the NMC are set out within the Nursing and Midwifery Order 2001 (The Order), which is the main legislation that lays out the NMC's role and responsibilities. As was the case with the CMB and UKCC, one of the core functions of the NMC is to establish and improve standards of midwifery and nursing care in order to serve and protect the public.

To achieve its aims the NMC:

- maintains a register that lists all qualified nurses, midwives and specialist community public health nurses
- sets standards and guidelines for nursing and midwifery conduct, performance and ethics
- provides advice for nurses, midwives and the public about professional standards
- quality assures nursing and midwifery education
- sets standards and provides guidance for local supervising authorities for midwives
- considers allegations of misconduct, lack of competence or unfitness to practise because of ill health.

The main purpose of The Order was to provide a stronger framework for public protection and to implement important reforms to the system of professional regulation. This was partially in response to increasing public concern in the UK with regard to health professions self-regulating, as there were

fears in some quarters that professions were protecting themselves rather than protecting the public. The intent behind The Order was to make regulation simple, streamlined and more effective in dealing with the many complex issues affecting the modern day health services, users of the service and the key professions of nursing and midwifery so vital to it. The Order is not perfect however, and there remain anomalies that will need further legislative changes to improve systems. An example of this is the need to consolidate the processes involved in dealing with fitness to practise. At present, this is dealt with through three separate committees, but as a result of policy change that separates the regulators' function of investigation and prosecution from that of hearing evidence and making judgements, there is a need to consolidate processes through one committee in the future.

Although most of the key functions that are needed for regulation of midwives and nurses remain unchanged, some important additions were included in the NMC's remit. These include:

- power for the NMC to design procedures to make and maintain efficiency
- greater representation of public and patient interest and involvement
- increase in lay participation balanced with professional representation
- faster and more transparent procedures
- a wider definition of unfitness to practise for reasons of misconduct or lack of competence
- more powers to deal with these in a fair and effective manner
- greater transparency and accountability to the public
- consistency across professional boundaries
- greater cooperation and partnership with different professions, the NHS and private sectors.

For midwifery, one of the key changes resulting from the Order concerned setting standards and providing advice and guidance for local supervising authorities (LSA) as this had been the responsibility of the four national boards.

The Order does give the NMC the power to delegate some functions should it wish. New standards for the monitoring of quality of education programmes came into effect across the UK in 2006 and responsibility for monitoring and reporting on these has been delegated to an independent monitoring agency. There are however, no provisions under The Order for the delegation of setting standards for the LSAs, a function which is seen by many as an effective mechanism for public protection.

The Register

The Register is the tool that enables the NMC to deliver protection of the public. It acts as a guarantee for the public that only those who are safe and competent to provide care can do so. Any midwife who wishes to practise in the UK must be a member of the NMC register otherwise she would be practising illegally.

At the present time, the Register is made up of three parts covering two professions. These are the Midwives part of the Register, the Nurses part of the Register and the Specialist Community Public Health Nurses part of the Register.

To gain entry to either the midwives' or the nurses' part of the register, an applicant must have completed successfully the relevant pre-registration education programme. They must have demonstrated that they have reached competence by the end of the programme and that they are of good health and good character. Entry to the specialist community public health part of the register cannot be made directly. This can only be achieved by midwives and nurses who hold registration and who have gone on to complete a specialist level qualification related to public health.

Every person holding registration has an individual personal identification number (PIN). This can be used by employers or members of the public to check with the NMC that the person holding the PIN is indeed on the NMC register and as such is fit for practice. The NMC is bound by law to make the register available for inspection by members of the public; however it is up to the Council to maintain and publish the register in a manner it considers appropriate.

Midwives who trained in the UK or in the European Union must apply to join the NMC Register before they can work as a midwife in the UK. Their pre-registration midwifery education programmes must have met the European requirements and as such can be recognized anywhere in the EU (EU 1980, amended 1989).

If a midwife trained outside the UK or European Union, then they must also apply to join the NMC Register before they can work as a midwife in the UK. As part of the application process, they must be able to demonstrate that their original midwifery programme has met the same standards that are required in the UK and that they hold competence in the English language to a high level. They must also have held registration and practised as a midwife in their original training country for a minimum of one year after gaining their original qualification as a midwife.

Once they have demonstrated to the regulator that they have met these requirements, then they will gain approval to complete an adaptation programme. Adaptation programmes are designed to help the midwife to practise in the context, culture and expectations of UK society and give the midwife an opportunity to demonstrate she is competent to provide midwifery care in the UK. When this has been completed successfully the midwife can then be signed off by a supervisor of midwives and a lead midwife for education as fit to join the NMC register.

All midwives wishing to practise in the UK have an additional legal requirement to give notice of their intention to practise (ITP) each year. This is done via statutory organizations called local supervising authorities (LSAs) who are obliged to inform the NMC when they have received notifications from midwives. The ITP notification is linked to the midwife's registration at the NMC and it is illegal for any midwife to practise without having submitted her notification before she practises in any local supervising authority. The only exception to this would be if she had to provide unexpected emergency care to a woman somewhere in the UK, in which circumstance the ITP can be submitted retrospectively to the local supervising authority where the emergency took place. The link between ITP notification and registration means that this is one way of monitoring whether a midwife has met the practice requirements for maintaining her registration. If a midwife has not submitted her notification of intention to practise, anyone checking her registration status will be informed that the legal requirement has not been met.

Statutory instruments

The next section describes the process involved in creating regulatory documents and standards. To aid understanding, specific legislation affecting midwives in the UK has been used as an illustration.

One of the first principles to understand is that there is a hierarchy in both the type of statutory legislation and the language used within legislation. This hierarchy imposes different levels of compulsion on the organizations and individuals affected by the legislation. All legislation is divided into primary and secondary legislation, with differences between the two.

The Nursing and Midwifery Order

This is the main legislation that established the NMC. It is a Statutory Instrument (SI) made under Section 60 of the Health Act 1999 and, within the NMC, is generally referred to as 'The Order'.

The Order sets out what the Council is required to do (*shall*) and provides permissive powers for things that it can choose to do if it so wishes (*may*). The numbered paragraphs within The Order are referred to as Articles (Newton 2006).

Primary legislation is enshrined in Acts of Parliament, which have been debated in the House of Commons and the House of Lords before receiving the Royal Assent. Such legislation is expected to last at least one or two decades before being revised. With the pressure that exists on parliamentary time, Acts of Parliament are frequently designed as 'enabling legislation' in that they provide a framework from which statutory rules may be derived, otherwise known as secondary or subordinate legislation. All secondary legislation is published in statutory instruments (Newton 2006).

Statutory Rules (secondary legislation) do not generally require parliamentary time as they were in the past, when agreed, endorsed by the Secretary of State. This function was transferred to the Privy Council, who lay the Rules before the House of Commons for formal and generally, automatic approval (Box 7.1). Statutory rules can in theory be implemented or amended much more quickly than is the case for primary legislation, though at best this will take several weeks or months.

Box 7.1 Statutory Instruments implementing the Nursing and Midwifery Order 2001

The Statutory Instruments implementing the Nursing and Midwifery Order 2001 are all made by order of the Privy Council and fall into two categories:

1. Orders relating to matters to be determined by the Privy Council

2. Rules made by the NMC in respect of various aspects of its functions.

To make matters more complex however, the Nursing and Midwifery Order 2001 is neither of the above. It came into being under what is known as the affirmative Order procedure. The affirmative Order procedure is an ancient and infrequently used law-making process with its roots going as far back as to Henry VIII. Because of this association, it is sometimes known as the Henry VIII rule. It differs from primary legislation in that although it also receives Royal assent, unlike primary legislation, it is not debated in either the House of Commons or the House of Lords. This procedure is more amenable for rule amendments without the need for a major discussion and passage through the Parliamentary process. Statutory rules can emanate from an Order and this is an important difference between an Order and secondary rules.

Although the affirmative Order procedure shares many similarities with secondary legislation, which as has been noted are published in statutory instruments, there is an important difference between the two: The Nursing and Midwifery Order 2001 has written within it secondary law-making powers, which will be made by statutory instruments. For example, the latest Midwives Rules came about via statutory instruments, as did the NMC Rules and procedures governing fitness to practise. There are a number of other Rules all made by Statutory instruments, such as the rules necessary to establish the professional register and those brought in for election to the Council that took over in 2005 (Newton 2006).

Affirmative Orders have, in common with secondary rules, the facility to adapt, amend and implement rule changes more quickly than an Act of Parliament.

Their appeal for the government of the UK in a time of rapidly changing health and social scene may well lie in their amenability to be changed quickly and bypass lengthy Parliamentary procedures.

The progress of The Order in all other ways was akin to the way statutory rules are made. The draft order was 'laid' before each House of Parliament for a period of one month. Though points for clarification and objections could be raised, there could be no amendments once it was 'laid' and had to be accepted in its entirety (Table 7.1).

Section 60 orders

Amendments to The Order have to be made by means of another order made under Section 60 of the Health Act 1999, known as a Section 60 Order.

A Section 60 Order is drafted by the Department of Health. It is subject to consultation and may be amended before being laid before Parliament. It is then subject to debate in both Houses and, once approved, is presented to Her Majesty in Council for the Order to be made. This is known as the affirmative resolution procedure.

Rules

The Order requires the Council, which is in effect the board of trustees of the NMC, to stipulate various matters. Examples of these are:

* requirements for midwives' education and practice
* requirements for supervision of midwives.

These matters must be included in the Rules and the responsibility for approving these Rules cannot be delegated by the Council. This is why, when the statutory midwifery committee of the NMC makes a decision relating to midwifery education, practice or supervision, it has to be approved by the Council before it comes into effect.

Some rules apply to all nurses as well as all midwives on the NMC Register. Examples of these are:

* fees for registration
* entry requirements to pre-registration education programmes that allow application to the Register
* the number of hours of education and practice needed by every midwife or nurse to stay on the Register
* the time period during which someone who is the subject of a fitness to practise allegation may submit written representations.

The process for making rules

Any underlying policy that may result in amendments to Rules or Standards is developed by NMC staff and overseen by the relevant committee. For midwifery, this work is normally carried out within the midwifery department of the NMC and is overseen by the midwifery committee.

The NMC has a duty to consult on all its policy and standards and this is a requirement on the NMC enshrined within The Order. Consultation is an interesting concept; it can range from discussions, to inform thinking about potential policy change through to seeking advice from experts to define policy.

The NMC uses a variety of methods to consult and in relation to midwifery policy starts consultation at early stages in development work. This is achieved by involving midwives and women using maternity services at the beginning of a piece of work to help shape the broad content of any standards or guidance. The NMC may then go on to invite individuals with acknowledged expertise to participate in working groups to refine this work before then going out to a more formal public consultation if the outcome of work involves significant change to the existing standards of midwifery practice.

Table 7.1	Matters determined by the Privy Council	
SI number	**Title**	**Came into effect**
2004/1762	The Nursing and Midwifery Order 2001 (Transitional Provisions) Order of Council 2004	1 August 2004
2004/1763	Nursing and Midwifery Order 2001 (Legal Assessors) Order of Council 2004	1 August 2004
2004/1765	Nurses and Midwives (Parts of and Entries in the Register) Order of Council 2004	1 August 2004
2004/1766	European Nursing and Midwifery Qualifications Designation Order of Council 2004	1 August 2004
2004/1771	The Health Act 1999 (Consequential Amendments) (Nursing and Midwifery) Order 2004	1 August 2004

Formal consultations can be paper-based question and answer forms, web-based on line questionnaires or via facilitated focus groups. The NMC uses focus groups to ensure that more in depth views are gained on profession-specific matters such as the standards for the preparation and practice of supervisors of midwives. Midwives, members of the public and others can apply to join focus group consultations to discuss and feedback their views on any proposed standards or policy.

Ultimately, any decisions on new standards or policy are made by the regulatory body. The information gained through consultation helps the NMC to understand any impact that its decisions may have, and is likely to influence the content of any standards that may result. Not everyone will be happy about every standard or change that may be required by the NMC. Midwives can influence the outcome of the work of the NMC by participating in its work and by responding to consultations so that their views become known.

Once a consultation is concluded, the NMC considers the feedback from this and then the Rules are drafted by solicitors instructed by the NMC. This can take several drafts to ensure that the intent is not lost when translated into the obligatory legal language.

The proposed rules are then subject to approval by the Privy Council which acts on the advice of solicitors from the Department of Health. The final version of the rules is then 'made' (approved) by the Council. Once that is achieved the rules are signed by the Chief Executive and Registrar of the NMC and the President of the NMC. The official seal of the NMC is then applied to the document, the original copy of which is stored within the NMC vaults (see Table 7.2 for examples of rules).

Amendments to an existing set of rules have to be made by means of another set of Amendment Rules and the process for preparing and making Amendment Rules is the same.

Making rules is a long process which takes many, many months to complete because of the time taken to agree policy, consult and amend policy if needed and draft and lay the rules before parliament. For this reason The Order enabled the NMC to set many of its requirements within standards, and these are developed in a slightly different way to rules in the hierarchy of legislation. Standards are as binding on the education, practice and behaviour of midwives as rules but in theory are easier to amend if change is needed.

Standards

The Order requires the Council to establish standards in relation to various aspects of its functions, for example:

- standards of competence that must be reached before a student midwife can be admitted to the midwives' part of the Register
- standards for supervision of midwives
- standards for the use of supervised practice
- local supervising authority standards.

The NMC is required to consult before establishing any standards in the same way as for Rules and before it publishes the standards. The final version of any standards are agreed by the midwifery

Table 7.2 Rules made by the NMC

Number	Title	Came into effect
2003/1738	Nursing and Midwifery Council (Practice Committees) (Interim Constitution) Rules Order of Council 2003	4 August 2003
2004/1654	Nursing and Midwifery Council (Fees) Rules Order of Council 2004	1 August 2004
2004/1761	Nursing and Midwifery Council (Fitness to Practise) Rules Order of Council 2004	1 August 2004
2004/1764	Nursing and Midwifery Council (Midwives) Rules Order of Council 2004	1 August 2004
2004/1767	Nursing and Midwifery Council (Education, Registration and Registration Appeals) Rules Order of Council 2004	1 August 2004
2005/2250	Nursing and Midwifery Council (Election Scheme) Rules Order of Council 2005	12 September 2005
2005/3353	Nursing and Midwifery Council (Fees) (Amendment) Rules Order of Council 2005	1 January 2006
2005/3354	Nursing and Midwifery Council (Education, Registration and Registration Appeals) (Amendment) Rules Order of Council 2005	1 January 2006

committee and approved by Council before they come into effect. Standards should be considered as 'must do' in terms of midwifery education, practice and supervision.

Guidance

The Order requires the NMC to give guidance on a number of matters, for example:

- completion of intention to practise notifications
- access by women to local supervising authority midwifery officers
- notification of change of correspondence address to the NMC
- professional indemnity insurance.

Again the NMC is required to consult before giving any guidance and to publish that guidance, and similarly, the power to approve and amend guidance rests with the Council. Such guidance gives direction and is considered as a level of practice or behaviour that is expected of all midwives. In regulatory terms it is not something that can be considered as only advisory or useful information. As such NMC guidance can be considered by a conduct panel when assessing a midwife's fitness to remain on the Register should any allegations be made against her.

Advice

In addition to the statutory requirements upon the regulator in the UK to provide guidance for practice, the NMC is also required to provide help and advice to midwives that relates to their professional responsibilities in practice. This may be very different in approach to advice gained from a professional representative organization such as the Royal College of Midwives. Advice from the regulator will be based on the rules and standards for midwifery practice and will include where appropriate ethical consideration of the situations midwives may find themselves in. The regulator would not however, offer advice on employment matters or advice on how maternity services could be provided as this is outwith its remit.

The NMC publishes advice from time to time on a range of subjects that affect regulation, education or practice. Examples of these include:

- exposure prone procedures in midwifery practice
- advertising and sponsorship

- chaperoning
- conscientious objection
- delegation of care
- independent practice
- midwives and home birth.

The content of this type of NMC advice is not required to be consulted on, although in practice it may be in a limited way. One way of achieving this is to develop such advice with input from other organizations or representatives such as the UK-wide local supervising authority midwifery officers' forum, or with representatives of women's groups such as the National Childbirth Trust.

Such advice is published via NMC circulars as is the information to external organizations that changes in standards are about to come into place. Copies of this type of advice can be obtained from the NMC via its website www.nmc-uk.org. If a professional situation is more complex, a midwife can ask for personal advice by using the NMC's professional advisory service.

The Midwives Rules and Standards

The Midwives Rules and Standards are specific to the midwifery profession and are developed through the midwifery committee and approved by the Council. The powers that enable the development of these statutory instruments are set by The Order in Articles 41, 42 and 43.

Article 41 defines the role and scope of the midwifery committee and the obligation that the Council has to consult with the committee on any of its work that affects midwifery. This places the midwifery committee in a very powerful position on behalf of the midwifery profession. At present the committee is made up of two practising midwives from each of the four countries of the UK and two lay members of Council. In addition the committee has co-opted three lay members from women's representative organizations to assist its work and decision-making.

Article 42 relates to midwifery practice and allows the NMC to make rules specifically to regulate midwifery practice beyond those rules that affect all midwives and nurses. The Order empowers the NMC to draw up secondary legislation in the form of rules. Midwives rules are passed under this procedure and the rules referred to in this article were made by Statutory Instrument (NMC 2004).

It was the practice with previous regulatory bodies for the midwives rules to be supplemented by a code of practice. These codes did not have a legal status, although they did provide information intended to assist safe practice. This approach was changed by the NMC, which has included standards and guidance within the statutory instrument known as the Midwives rules and standards.

Article 42 has two parts. Part one empowers Council to regulate the practice of midwifery with rules that may address:

- the circumstances and procedures that may lead to a midwife being suspended from practice
- a requirement for midwives to give notice of their intention to practise (ITP) to the local supervision authority in which they intend to practise
- a requirement for midwives to attend education and training programmes specified by the NMC.

Part two relates to the local supervising authorities and their obligation to inform the Council of any midwives notifying them of their intention to practise.

Article 43 relates to local supervision of midwives and gives the Council the power to set standards in relation to supervision. This is also the section that deals with referral of midwives to the NMC if there are concerns about their fitness to practise and enables the supervising authorities to suspend midwives from practice if there is a significant risk to the public were they to remain able to practise.

The regulator has used the permissive powers it has within The Order to describe rules and more detailed standards on all of these areas that have a significant impact on midwifery. These statutory requirements can be viewed as enabling midwifery practice, so that the scope and input of midwives and midwifery with women can be developed and expanded to meet the changing needs and expectations of society. Conversely, some may choose to use them in a restrictive way to impede practice or healthy change, which was not the intent of the regulatory body.

Offences

There are some interesting inclusions in The Order that mean that anyone breaching the requirements of The Order could be liable for criminal prosecution, and one relates specifically to midwifery.

Article 45 is an important three-part section within The Order and defines who may provide care for a woman during childbirth. Childbirth has a statutory definition within the Midwives rules and standards and therefore includes pregnancy, birth and the postnatal period.

Parts one and two state that only a registered midwife or a registered medical practitioner, or a student midwife or a medical student as part of a statutorily recognized course, may attend a woman in childbirth. There is immunity for anyone acting to help a woman or baby in a sudden emergency. Outside these categories, anyone attending or assuming responsibility for care is committing an offence.

Part three describes the penalty involved if convicted, which is a fine not exceeding level 5 on the standard scale (to a maximum of £5000) to anyone who contravenes this Article. The fine was raised from level 4 in the previous legislation under the UKCC to reflect the seriousness of this issue.

This restriction was retained in spite of representation by women's groups for a fine for this offence to be dropped altogether. The Association for the Improvement in Maternity Services (AIMS) took the view that, given the debate about midwifery attendance at home births in the late 1990s, a woman may at least have the attendance of a partner, or as a last resort a relative, in cases where a woman wanting to give birth at home has no qualified midwife available to attend her. AIMS argued that having someone unqualified is better than having no one in attendance at all. During the House of Lords debate (Hansard 2001), Lord Hunt stated that the point of the offence is to protect the function of midwifery in the interest of public safety, an offence that has been in force in the UK since the first Midwives Act of 1902.

Employers and protection of the public

As has been discussed previously, protection of the public is best achieved through a joint approach to regulation. This means that employers have a vital role in ensuring that midwives working for them have the appropriate skills and knowledge for the job and hold current registration with the NMC. If an employer does not have robust systems in place for ensuring that their midwives have met the statutory requirements including active midwifery registration then they may be putting the women and babies they are providing care for at risk.

The employer's role in protection of the public starts when they recruit staff and good employment practices protect the midwife too. The employer should take up references from any previous employer to ensure that there were no concerns about the safety of practice or good character of the applicant in previous roles. Any employer considering a midwife should also ensure that registration is in place by checking the NMC Register and carry out a criminal records check to ensure that the person is not barred from caring for vulnerable children or adults. New legislation has been created in England through the Safeguarding Vulnerable Groups Act 2006 (DH 2006) and in Scotland through the Protection of Vulnerable Groups (Scotland) Act 2007 (DH 2007a) to strengthen requirements relating to care of vulnerable children and adults.

Finally employment in any area related to midwifery advice or practice should not start until it has been confirmed that the midwife has submitted her notification of intention to practise to the local supervising authority.

Each midwife is personally responsible for keeping herself up-to-date and competent. Although not a statutory requirement upon employers, it is in the employers' interest to support midwives to achieve this. Safe and competent midwives reduce the risk to the employer that poor practice may occur. It also increases the likelihood that the employer is providing a safe system of care to women and their families. Of course this does not just relate to providing midwives with time and access to ongoing professional and personal development. This includes provision of safe working environments and staffing levels that reduce the risk of things going wrong.

Employers who engage with supervision of midwifery in an active and positive way by working collaboratively and supportively with the local supervising authority and supervisors of midwives will reduce risk as this will strengthen their clinical governance systems.

Robust Human Resource systems to ensure regular (at least annual) registration checks will ensure that only those who have met requirements for safe and competent practice are providing care and have continued registration. Human error does occur in relation to maintaining registration and good employment processes will act as 'belt and braces'

for safety for the employer. Any insurance scheme (see Ch. 53) that may protect the organization financially in the event of litigation against poor practice would be invalidated should an individual midwife have allowed her registration to lapse, regardless of why this may have occurred.

This is perhaps the opportunity to consider the matter of personal indemnity insurance. Indemnity insurance protects the midwife herself, and offers a degree of financial security for the woman and her baby should things go wrong. There may be a need for financial compensation to cover the costs of ongoing care if it is needed. As most midwives are employed by organizations this is rarely a problem as the employer usually holds vicarious liability for the midwife's practice and therefore provides indemnity through its insurers. It remains a problem for midwives who practise on a self employed basis, as there is no indemnity insurance cover available to them through existing insurance companies.

While recognizing the dilemma for self-employed midwives, the NMC recommends that all midwives hold professional indemnity insurance. If this proves not to be the case the midwife is expected to inform the woman about the lack of insurance and what the implications of that might be. This will enable the woman to choose to continue care with that midwife or to move to alternative midwifery care where insurance is available. The midwife is expected to record that she has given the information on this matter and its implications, within the woman's maternity records.

Dealing with poor practice

There is a perception among many midwives that the regulator only deals with misconduct. While this is a very important part of the regulator's role, and one which uses the largest part of its annual budget, it is relevant only to a very small minority of midwives on the NMC Register. This is because the majority of midwives practise safely and within the scope of their skills and knowledge to the required standards, often despite restrictions in resources, or increasingly complex caseloads within their employment.

As at 2008, the NMC receives approximately 1600 complaints against nurses and midwives per year and of those, approximately 100 are about midwives. When this is considered against the 43 000 midwives on the Register, it can be seen that the numbers referred

---

Box 7.2 Sources of complaints

- Members of the public (women, relatives, patients etc.)
- Police
- Employers
- Local Supervising Authority (approx. 15% of midwifery referrals)
- Other professional regulators or organizations (GMC, HCC, etc.).

---

to the NMC are actually very small. Allegations against midwives come from a variety of sources (Box 7.2).

The NMC will not deal with allegations against anyone on its Register unless two criteria are fulfilled. The complaint must be made in writing by a named person or representative of an organization and it must be made 'in the form required'. This means that the allegation must contain essential information about where and when an incident or pattern of events took place and who was involved. Further information on what is required can be downloaded from the NMC website on www.nmc-uk.org and is in a slightly different form for employers or the LSA than if an allegation is being made by a member of the public who may not have access to some information, such as PINs or the midwife's name.

Once an allegation is received in the form required, NMC staff carry out further investigation before a case can be brought to a committee who will consider whether there is a case to answer or not. The information from the investigation is collated and will include:

- midwife's name and PIN
- witness statements
- maternity, midwifery and medical care notes
- reports from disciplinary hearings, transcripts, notes of meetings
- reports from supervisory or LSA investigations
- certificate of conviction/ disclosure print.

Previous UK regulators could only deal with allegations of misconduct or ill health that were so serious that they might lead to suspension or removal from the Register. For this reason a number of complaints made about individual midwives were not progressed by the UKCC.

This situation changed on 1 August 2004 as the NMC powers to deal with fitness to practise were extended to include lack of competence. The range of sanctions available to the NMC were also extended, giving conduct panels much more scope to deal with matters of concern than had previously been the case. This increased the number of cases going forward for consideration by a conduct panel. These sanctions are to:

- take no further action or refer to screeners
- impose a conditions of practice order for up to 3 years
- suspend registration for up to 1 year
- impose a caution for not less than 1 year, nor more than 5 years
- strike the midwife off the register.

A significant change that is likely to increase the number of referrals to the NMC relates to the burden of proof that an investigating or conduct panel must consider. Until 2007, this was set at the same level as for criminal cases heard in the UK courts and was that the allegation must have been proved beyond all reasonable doubt.

This is changing and will move in 2008 to what is called a civil standard of proof. This means that the evidence supporting the allegation is judged on a balance of probability that the midwife's care or behaviour did not meet the required practice standards or Code of conduct set by the regulator. While this change has caused some anxiety among the professional organizations representing midwives, it has enhanced the public's belief that a regulator will protect them from poor practice as the priority.

Any midwife who has had an allegation made against her will be made aware that this is the case by the NMC so she can provide her evidence to the investigation or to the conduct panel who are considering any allegations made against her. The midwife's conduct will be measured against the standards of education, practice and conduct required when the incident took place.

Suspension from midwifery practice

It may be appropriate to consider suspension from midwifery practice in the context of dealing with poor practice. There are only two organizations that can suspend a midwife from practice in the UK. These are the NMC or a local supervising authority, and in both cases the suspension means the midwife cannot practise anywhere in the UK whilst the suspension is in place. An employer may suspend a midwife from duty to enable it to conduct an investigation but that would not prevent the midwife from practising elsewhere, however unwise that might be.

Suspension from practice is a very serious matter as it could prevent a midwife from earning a living and is therefore not a step that is taken lightly (NMC 2007b). It would only be used if there was evidence of significant risk to the public were the midwife to continue to practise. This may be for reasons of the midwife's ill health, chronic lack of competence or gross professional misconduct.

If a local supervising authority decides to suspend a midwife from practice, it must make a formal referral to the NMC and include all the information gained from the supervisory or LSA investigation that led to the decision to suspend from practice. The LSA suspension is immediate in effect and the NMC will make a note on the midwife's registration to indicate this is the case. The LSA is also obliged to share this information with the midwife concerned so that she is aware what is happening.

The NMC will set up an interim orders hearing to review the LSA suspension. If it upholds the decision to continue the suspension from practice it will replace the LSA suspension with an interim suspension order. The NMC can also decide on review of the evidence that suspension is not required and may replace it with an interim condition of practice order which will restrict the way the midwife can practice. It can also overturn the suspension from practice if it decides that the risk to the public is not high enough to warrant suspension (Fig. 7.1).

Should new evidence become available to the local supervising authority that imposed the suspension, and it concludes that suspension is no longer warranted, it can lift its suspension and inform the NMC who will take this into account in relation to any interim order for suspension.

Regardless of the outcome from the interim orders hearing, the NMC will continue to investigate the allegations against the midwife until such time as it can make a judgement about whether or not there is a case to answer.

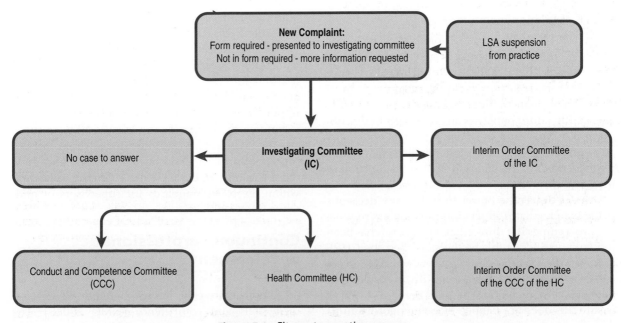

Figure 7.1 Fitness to practise process.

Regulation of midwifery education

The regulatory framework relating to education is enshrined within Articles 15–20 of The Order, and is a key function of the NMC. Monitoring of the quality of education used to sit with the four national boards but is now the remit of the NMC and is known as the quality assurance process. This is one of the areas where The Order allows the Council to delegate its function. The Council has set its rules and standards for the content, length and delivery of pre-registration midwifery education programmes and it contracts with external agencies to monitor that its requirements are being met.

There is no specific requirement under The Order for midwifery education to come under the remit of the midwifery committee. During the consultation phase of the draft Orders, this non-inclusion of midwifery education in the midwifery committee's remit caused a great deal of concern to organizations representing midwifery, such as the RCM. They argued that one of the basics of autonomy of any profession includes having control of educating and training its members. Although the final Order did not reflect this wish, the first Council of the NMC decided that the Midwifery Committee would have included in its remit, matters relating to midwifery education (Newton 2006).

How is regulation monitored?

In the UK, all healthcare regulatory bodies, including the NMC, are monitored by an overarching body called the Council for Healthcare Regulatory Excellence (CHRE). Each regulator has to report on its progress against performance objectives each year to the CHRE. The CHRE in turn publishes an annual report describing and commenting on its findings, highlighting any good practice it finds and recommending any changes it thinks needs to be made to improve the function of the healthcare regulators (www.chre.org.uk).

The CHRE has the power to review any decisions made by a regulator in relation to its fitness to practise proceedings if it thinks that the decision has been too lenient. Should this be the case, then the CHRE can refer the case for judicial review, which is a very costly process for the regulator involved both in financial and reputation terms. The NMC tries to ensure this does not happen by being rigorous in its selection and training of anyone sitting on its conduct panels as well as by setting clear standards about what is expected of midwives on its Register. It also ensures than any conduct panel considering allegations about midwifery practice includes an experienced practising midwife.

Statutory supervision of midwives

The main purpose of statutory supervision of midwives (see Ch. 52) is protection of the public. In this, supervision of midwives reflects the primary purpose of the UK regulatory body. Supervision of midwives was enshrined within statute to reflect its purpose and value in ensuring safe standards of care to women and their families.

Supervision of midwives is independent of any employment situation and all midwives in the UK, regardless of type or place of work, must comply with statutory supervision.

The local supervising authorities (LSAs) are statutory entities that are required to ensure that supervision of midwifery takes place and that midwifery practice is safe, evidence based and meets NMC standards. They are responsible for appointing and ensuring there are enough supervisors of midwives in the area they are responsible for. They also appoint the local supervising authority midwifery officers. The responsibility for the LSA is different in each of the four countries.

The standards expected of all LSAs are set by the NMC, and this power is enabled by Article 43 of The Order. This Article details how LSAs are to exercise general supervision over all midwives practising within their area according to the Council's rules. It also requires them to report to the NMC any situation where the LSA is of the opinion that the fitness to practise of a midwife in its area is impaired.

Part two of this Article requires the NMC to stipulate the qualifications of individuals whom the LSA can appoint as supervisors of midwives, and these are set out in rule 11 of the midwives rules and within the NMC standards for supervisors of midwives (NMC 2007c).

Continuous professional development

All midwives are expected to maintain and develop their skills and competence (NMC 2008b). The Order requires the NMC to make rules regarding the standards midwives need to meet with respect to their continuing professional development, and there are implications of failure to comply with the requirements for their registration status if a midwife does not meet these standards. The current standards for maintaining registration inherited by the NMC are too vague to offer real protection to women and the need for development of a new post-registration framework is one of the major issues passed from the UKCC to the NMC.

The NMC has started to review the requirements that midwives will have to meet in order to stay on the register in future. These will focus on maintaining and demonstrating competence with protecting the woman from possible poor practice as the priority. This is a radical change in approach from one that focuses on the personal development wishes of the individual midwife as the priority; however there is a balance to be achieved between both groups.

The development of this programme of regulation is also likely to result in changes to the format and structure of the Register itself so that it becomes more meaningful in terms of the skills and abilities of those with specialist interests who hold registration. Much of this change has been led by the profession itself, however there are significant political policy changes that are considered in the final section of this chapter.

'Trust, Assurance and Safety – The Regulation of Health Professionals in the 21st Century'

Regulation is not static and for midwives it has evolved continuously since its inception in 1902. Events in the UK during the late 1990s have increased public anxiety about professional self-regulation. Several public enquiries were held and reports published that made recommendations for changes in the regulators and regulation across the UK. This culminated in two government consultations during 2006 that looked at the regulation of medical and non medical health professionals. February 2007 saw the publication of a White Paper, *Trust, Assurance and Safety – The Regulation of Health Professionals in the 21st Century*

(DH 2007b) describing proposed changes to all of the healthcare regulators and regulation in the UK, and two other documents, *Safeguarding Patients* (DH 2007c) and *Learning from Tragedy, Keeping Patients Safe* (DH 2007d). Although the impetus for change was primarily focused on medical regulation, the impact will be felt across all healthcare regulators and will mean significant change for the NMC and the regulation of midwives.

The key principles within the White Paper that will underpin statutory professional regulation for the future were described by Patricia Hewitt MP in 2007 when she was Secretary of State for Health. These are:

- the overriding interest will be the safety and quality of care that patients (and women) receive from health professionals
- professional regulation needs to sustain the confidence of both the public and professionals through demonstrable impartiality. Regulators need to be independent of government, the professionals themselves, employers, educators and all other interest groups involved in healthcare
- professional regulation will be about sustaining, improving and assuring the professional standards of the majority of healthcare professionals as well as identifying and addressing poor practice or bad behaviour
- professional regulation should not create unnecessary burdens and be proportionate to the risk it addresses and benefit it brings
- professional regulatory systems that ensure strength and integrity of health professionals whilst enabling flexibility to meet different health needs and approaches in the four countries of the UK.

These principles underpin significant changes to the concept and process of self-regulation of midwives by midwives and will completely redefine how the NMC is structured and governed. Many of the changes will require primary and secondary legislative changes and as described previously, some will take many years to achieve.

There are seven main areas that will require change for most regulatory bodies:

1. independence, governance and accountability of professional regulators
2. revalidation
3. tackling concerns locally
4. tackling concerns nationally
5. education and the role of the regulator
6. information about health professionals
7. new roles and emerging professions.

It is proposed that all regulators including the NMC increase their independence and impartiality. For the NMC this means that the current balance between lay and registrant Council members will change to an equal number of each and the overall size of the Council reduce. Some have described this change as the Council becoming more board-like although it has proved difficult to determine what this will mean in reality. It is likely to reduce the level of detailed input by Council members to the operational work of the regulator and increase the level of strategic governance of senior executive staff as a result. In future all members of the Council will be independently appointed, rather than the mix of elected registrant members and appointed lay members that exists at present. This may be the greatest challenge for the profession as it brings the whole concept of self-regulation into question for the future.

Regulatory Councils will become more accountable directly to Parliament and devolved administrations rather than as currently to the Department of Health. This will increase the regulators' ability to take an impartial view on standards that may be required to improve practice and safety.

Within the White Paper, there is a large emphasis on all healthcare regulators becoming more consistent in their approach. This would make some sense certainly for the public, who may have to interact with several regulatory bodies should they wish to explore the practice standards of all the healthcare professionals involved in their care. This is likely to impact particularly in areas such as entry requirements for pre-registration programmes, requirements for maintaining registration and inter-regulatory approaches to entries on professional registers denoting specialist level qualifications.

The current NMC registration renewal period is 3 years, however this may change to come in line with the majority of other regulators who have 5-year periods for the same matter. These types of issues are being discussed at the present time within a number of inter-regulatory working groups who will advise on the future pattern for all.

The concept of a licence to practise for doctors has emerged, not entirely alien to midwives with their intention to practise notification and PREP requirement systems. This may be based on an objective process for formatively and summatively appraising continued fitness to practise and may well contain differing elements for those healthcare professionals engaged in areas of care that are considered higher risk than others (Hampton 2006). Examples of this might be midwives or doctors who are working in isolation from peer support and overview. It appears inevitable that the requirements for midwives to demonstrate continued competence and updating to enable them to maintain registration will be strengthened and will need to be consistent in approach with other regulators and professions. This is likely to be a large and thorny area of change in regulation terms and is likely to take several years to develop before change is implemented.

Midwives will recognize elements of the supervision framework in the proposals to create 'medical affiliates' appointed and accountable to the General Medical Council. The intent behind this is closer monitoring of medical practice on a local level and provision of advice and support to employers in managing concerns about medical practice.

As mentioned previously, the standard of proof will change to that of a civil standard and will apply across all regulators in the UK, as will change to the approach when handling allegations against registrants that they are not fit to practise. The NMC has already moved in this direction and its approach has been validated by the contents of the White Paper proposals. There will be a separation between investigations of allegations against midwives and considering and judging a case against a midwife. This means the NMC will move from handling all aspects of the process to one of investigation and prosecution, a system that will seem more akin to the current UK law court system.

Professional indemnity insurance is likely to become mandatory for all health professionals within the next 5 years. It remains to be seen if this marks the end of self-employment opportunities for midwives or whether creative solutions that retain the expertise of midwifery within independent practice can be developed to enable women to continue to have access to this type of care provision.

The NMC will continue to have responsibility for setting the standards and requirements for midwifery education, however there is a greater emphasis on the role of employers in relation to testing for competence in English language amongst applicants for posts.

There will be changes to the Register in terms of entry requirements and the information held on the Register relating to individual midwives and nurses to enhance inter-regulator consistency. One area where work has commenced relates to a single definition of 'good character' that will be applied to all professional registers. This ties into proposals to strengthen links between student midwives and the midwives part of the register and whether there should be a more formal relationship between students and the regulator before qualification.

Regulation of existing healthcare professions is a retained function that sits with the parliament at Westminster and is not devolved to the new administrations in Scotland, Wales or Northern Ireland. There are a number of professional groups who are not statutorily regulated at the present time and some of these are potentially as risky to the public as the established professions. Such groups are likely to have statutory regulation introduced to set and monitor standards in the same way as midwifery experienced in 1902. There is also consideration of emerging professions and whether they should be regulated or not. One decision has been made and that is not to create new regulatory bodies but to use one or more of the existing regulators to take on this function. It remains to be seen whether maternity support workers will be included in such regulation and if so whether they share regulation with midwives or elsewhere with other healthcare professionals.

The White Paper is intended to create a 'lasting settlement' for professional regulation in the UK. Given the rapid and continuous change in society and the expectations of society this is a high aspiration and one, given the history of midwifery regulation over the past 105 years, is unlikely. Midwives need to understand regulation and how it is achieved so they can continue to influence the policy makers about requirements and standards for their profession as they have always done with the needs of women at the centre.

REFERENCES

Blunden F 2007 Extracts from the key speakers address at the NMC Annual Lecture, Cardiff

Cowell B, Wainwright D 1981 Behind the blue door: the history of the Royal College of Midwives. Baillière Tindall, London

Department of Health 2006 Safeguarding Vulnerable Groups Act. The Stationery Office, Norwich

Department of Health 2007a Protection of Vulnerable Groups (Scotland). The Stationery Office, Norwich

Department of Health 2007b Trust, Assurance and Safety – The Regulation of Health Professionals in the 21st Century. The Stationery Office, Norwich

Department of Health 2007c Safeguarding Patients. The Stationery Office, Norwich

Department of Health 2007d Learning from tragedy, keeping patients safe. The Stationery Office, Norwich

Donnison J 1988 Midwives and medical men, a history of the struggle for the control of childbirth, 2nd edn. Historical Publications, Wakefield

EU (European Union) 1980 Midwives Directive 80/155EEC Article 4 amended by the European Union Directive 89/594/EEC. EU, Brussels

Hampton P. 2006 Reducing administrative burdens: effective inspections and enforcement. HM Treasury, London

Health Act 1999. HMSO, London

Heagerty B V 1996. Reassuring the guilty: the Midwives Act and control of English midwives in the early 20th century. In: Kirkham M (ed.) Supervision of midwives. Books for midwives Press, Hale

Hogg C 2000 Professional self-regulation: a patient centred approach. A consultation document. Consumers' Association, London

Kennedy I 2001 Bristol Royal Infirmary Inquiry 2001. Learning from Bristol. The report of the public inquiry into children's heart surgery at the Bristol Royal Infirmary, 1984–1995. TSO, London

Newton J 2006 Overview of current NMC legislation. Council Members Handbook. NMC, London

NHS Employers 2005 Maternity support workers: Enhancing the work of maternity teams. London, NHS

NMC 2004 Midwives rules and standards. NMC, London

NMC 2008b The PREP handbook. NMC, London

NMC 2007a Statistical analysis of the Register April 2005–March 2006. NMC, London

NMC 2007b Fitness to practise annual report 2005–2006. NMC, London

NMC 2007c Standards for supervision of midwives. NMC, London

NMC 2008a The Code: Standards of conduct, performance and ethics for nurses and midwives. NMC, London.

RCM 1991 Report of the Royal College of Midwives commission on legislation relating to midwives. RCM, London

Sandall J, Manthorpe J, Mansfield A et al 2006 Support workers in maternity services: a national scoping study of NHS Trusts providing care in England. Kings College, London

The Midwives Act 1902. HMSO, London

The Midwives (Scotland) Act 1915. HMSO, London

The Midwives Act (Ireland) 1918. HMSO, London

The Nurses, Midwives and Health Visitors Act 1979, 1992, 1997. HMSO, London.

The Nursing and Midwifery Order 2001 (SI2002/253). The Stationery Office, Norwich

Towler J, Bramall J 1986 Midwives in history and society. Croom Helm, England.

2

Section 2
Human anatomy and reproduction

SECTION CONTENTS

8 The female pelvis and the reproductive organs

Mary E. Vance

Midwives need to have knowledge of the anatomical features of the female body and to understand the processes of reproduction but must never forget that a woman's body is unique, personal and private. The anatomy and physiology of the reproductive organs is described in appropriate chapters throughout the book.

The pelvis

Competence in recognizing the anatomy of a normal pelvis is key to midwifery practice as one of the ways to estimate a woman's progress in labour is by assessing the relationship of the fetus to certain pelvic landmarks. Knowledge of pelvic anatomy is also needed in order to be able to detect deviations from normal.

The pelvic girdle

The pelvic girdle, a basin shaped cavity, is a bony ring between the movable vertebrae of the vertebral column which it supports, and the lower limbs that it rests on. It contains and protects the bladder, rectum and internal reproductive organs. Some women experience pelvic girdle pain in pregnancy and need referral to an obstetric physiotherapist (see Ch. 16).

Functions

The primary function of the pelvic girdle is to allow movement of the body, especially walking and running. This makes it necessary for the sacroiliac joint to be immensely strong and virtually immobile. The pelvis also takes the weight of the sitting body onto the ischial tuberosities.

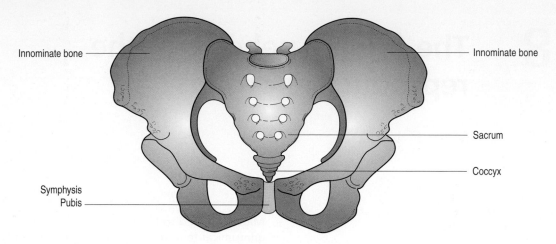

Figure 8.1   The pelvic bones.

Pelvic bones

The pelvic girdle, which is stronger and more massively constructed than the wall of the cranial or thoracic cavities, is composed of four bones: two innominate laterally and anteriorly and the sacrum and coccyx posteriorly (Fig. 8.1).

Innominate bones

Each innominate bone is made up of three bones that have fused together: the ilium, the ischium and the pubis (Fig. 8.2).

The ilium is the large flared-out part. When the hand is placed on the hip, it rests on the iliac crest, which is the upper border. At the front of the iliac crest can be felt a bony prominence known as the anterior superior iliac spine. A short distance below it is the anterior inferior iliac spine. There are two similar points at the other end of the iliac crest, namely the posterior superior and the posterior inferior iliac spines. The concave anterior surface of the ilium is the iliac fossa.

The ischium is the thick lower part. It has a large prominence known as the ischial tuberosity, on which the body rests when sitting. Behind and a little above the tuberosity is an inward projection, the ischial spine. In labour, the station of the fetal head is estimated in relation to the ischial spines.

The pubis forms the anterior part. It has a body and two oar-like projections, the superior ramus and the inferior ramus. The two pubic bones meet

at the symphysis pubis and the two inferior rami form the pubic arch, merging into a similar ramus on the ischium. The space enclosed by the body of the pubic bone, the rami and the ischium is called the obturator foramen.

The innominate bone contains a deep cup to receive the head of the femur termed the acetabulum, which is composed of the three fused bones in the following proportions: two-fifths ilium, two-fifths ischium and one-fifth pubis (Fig. 8.2).

On the lower border of the innominate bone are found two curves. One curve extends from the

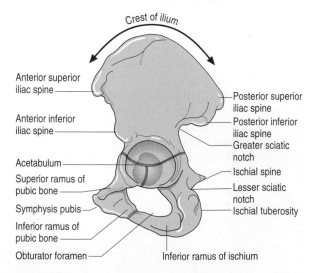

Figure 8.2   Lateral view of the innominate bone showing important landmarks.

posterior inferior iliac spine up to the ischial spine and is called the greater sciatic notch; it is wide and rounded. The other curve lies between the ischial spine and the ischial tuberosity and is known as the lesser sciatic notch (Fig. 8.2).

The sacrum

The sacrum is a wedge-shaped bone consisting of five fused vertebrae. The upper border of the first sacral vertebra, which juts forward, is known as the sacral promontory. The anterior surface of the sacrum is concave and is referred to as the hollow of the sacrum. Laterally the sacrum extends into a wing or ala. Four pairs of holes or foramina pierce the sacrum and, through these, nerves from the cauda equina emerge to supply the pelvic organs. The posterior surface is roughened to receive attachments of muscles.

The coccyx

The coccyx is a vestigial tail. It consists of four fused vertebrae, forming a small triangular bone, which articulates with the fifth sacral segment.

Pelvic joints

There are four pelvic joints: one symphysis pubis, two sacroiliac joints and one sacrococcygeal joint.

The **symphysis pubis** is the midline cartilaginous joint uniting the rami of the left and right pubic bones.

The **sacroiliac joints** are strong, weight-bearing synovial joints with irregular elevations and depressions that produce interlocking of the bones. They join the sacrum to the ilium and as a result connect the spine to the pelvis. The joints allow a limited backward and forward movement of the tip and promontory of the sacrum, sometimes known as 'nodding' of the sacrum.

The **sacrococcygeal** joint is formed where the base of the coccyx articulates with the tip of the sacrum. It permits the coccyx to be deflected backwards during the birth of the fetal head.

Pelvic ligaments

The pelvic joints are held together by very strong ligaments that are designed not to allow movement. However, during pregnancy the hormone relaxin gradually loosens all the pelvic ligaments allowing slight pelvic movement providing more room for the fetal head as it passes through the pelvis. A widening of 2–3mm at the symphysis pubis during pregnancy above the normal gap of 4–5mm is normal but if it widens significantly, the degree of movement permitted may give rise to pain on walking (see Chs 16 and 19).

The ligaments connecting the bones of the pelvis with each other can be divided into four groups:

- those connecting the sacrum and ilium – the sacroiliac ligaments
- those passing between the sacrum and ischium – the sacrotuberous ligaments and the sacrospinous ligaments
- those uniting the sacrum and coccyx – the sacrococcygeal ligaments
- those between the two pubic bones – the interpubic ligaments.

The ligaments that are important to midwifery practice are the sacrotuberous and the sacrospinous ligaments as they form the posterior wall of the pelvic outlet (Fig. 8.3).

The four types of pelvis

The size of the pelvis varies not only in the two sexes, but also in different members of the same sex. The height of the individual does not appear to influence the size of the pelvis in any way as women of short stature, in general, have broad pelves. Nevertheless, the pelvis is occasionally equally contracted in all its dimensions, so much so that all its diameters can measure 1.25cm. less than the average. This type of pelvis, known as a justo minor pelvis, can result in normal labour and birth if the fetal size is consistent with the size of the maternal pelvis. However, if the fetus is large, a degree of cephalopelvic disproportion will result. The same is true when a malpresentation or malposition of the fetus exists.

The principal divergences, however, are found at the brim (Fig. 8.4) and affect the relation of the anteroposterior to the transverse diameter. If one of the measurements is reduced by 1cm or more from the normal, the pelvis is said to be contracted and may give rise to difficulty in labour or necessitate caesarean section. Classically, pelves have been described as falling into four categories: the

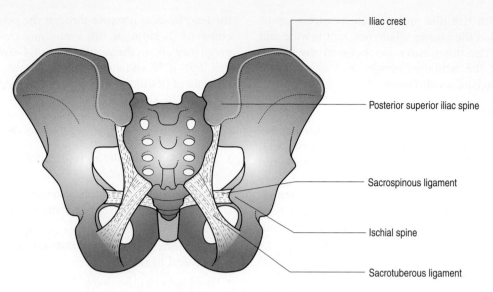

Figure 8.3 Posterior view of the pelvis showing the ligaments.

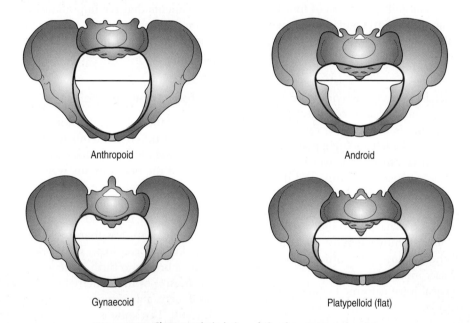

Anthropoid

Android

Gynaecoid

Platypelloid (flat)

Figure 8.4 Characteristic brim of the four types of pelvis.

gynaecoid pelvis, the android pelvis, the anthropoid pelvis and the platypelloid pelvis (Table 8.1).

The gynaecoid pelvis (Fig. 8.5)

This is the best type for childbearing as it has a rounded brim, generous forepelvis, straight side walls, a shallow cavity with a well-curved sacrum and a sub-pubic arch of 90°.

The android pelvis

The android pelvis is so called because it resembles the male pelvis. Its brim is heart-shaped, it has a narrow forepelvis and its transverse diameter is situated towards the back. The side walls converge, making it funnel shaped and it has a deep cavity and a straight sacrum. The ischial spines are prominent and the sciatic notch is narrow. The sub-pubic angle is less

Table 8.1 Features of the four types of pelvis

Features	Gynaecoid	Android	Anthropoid	Platypelloid
Brim	Rounded	Heart-shaped	Long oval	Kidney-shaped
Forepelvis	Generous	Narrow	Narrowed	Wide
Side walls	Straight	Convergent	Divergent	Divergent
Ischial spines	Blunt	Prominent	Blunt	Blunt
Sciatic notch	Rounded	Narrow	Wide	Wide
Sub-pubic angle	90°	<90°	>90°	>90°
Incidence	50%	20%	25% (50% in non-Caucasian)	5%

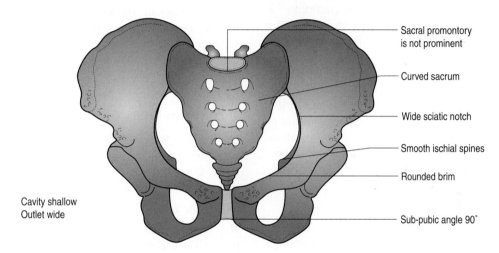

Sacral promontory is not prominent

Curved sacrum

Wide sciatic notch

Smooth ischial spines

Rounded brim

Sub-pubic angle 90°

Cavity shallow
Outlet wide

Figure 8.5 Normal female pelvis (gynaecoid).

than 90°. It is found in short and heavily built women who have a tendency to be hirsute.

Because of the narrow forepelvis and the fact that the greater space lies in the hindpelvis the heart-shaped brim favours an occipitoposterior position. Furthermore, funnelling in the cavity may hinder progress in labour. At the pelvic outlet, the prominent ischial spines sometimes prevent complete internal rotation of the head and the anteroposterior diameter becomes caught on them, causing a deep transverse arrest. The narrowed sub-pubic angle cannot easily accommodate the biparietal diameter (Fig. 8.6) and this displaces the head backwards. Because of these factors, this type of pelvis is the least suited to childbearing.

The anthropoid pelvis

The anthropoid pelvis has a long, oval brim in which the anteroposterior diameter is longer than

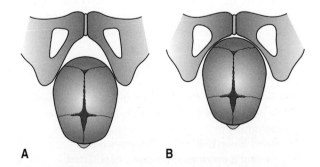

A   B

Figure 8.6 (A) Outlet of android pelvis. The fetal head, which does not fit into the acute pubic arch, is forced backwards onto the perineum. (B) Outlet of the gynaecoid pelvis. The head fits snugly into the pubic arch.

the transverse diameter. The side walls diverge and the sacrum is long and deeply concave. The ischial spines are not prominent and the sciatic notch and the sub-pubic angle are very wide. Women with this type of pelvis tend to be tall, with narrow shoulders. Labour does not usually present any difficulties, but a direct occipitoanterior or direct occipitoposterior position is often a feature and the position adopted for engagement may persist to birth.

The platypelloid pelvis

The platypelloid (flat) pelvis has a kidney-shaped brim in which the anteroposterior diameter is reduced and the transverse diameter increased. The sacrum is flat and the cavity shallow. The ischial spines are blunt, and the sciatic notch and the sub-pubic angle are both wide. The head must engage with the sagittal suture in the transverse diameter, but usually descends through the cavity without difficulty. Engagement may necessitate lateral tilting of the head, known as asynclitism, in order to allow the biparietal diameter to pass the narrowest anteroposterior diameter of the brim (Box 8.1).

Other pelvic variations

High assimilation pelvis occurs when the 5th lumbar vertebra is fused to the sacrum and the angle

of inclination of the pelvic brim is increased. Engagement of the head is difficult but once achieved labour progresses normally.

Deformed pelvis may result from a developmental anomaly, dietary deficiency, injury or disease (Box 8.2).

The pelvis in relation to pregnancy and childbirth

The pelvis is divided by an oblique plane which passes through the prominence of the sacrum, the arcuate line (the smooth rounded border on the internal surface of the ilium), the pectineal line (a ridge on the superior ramus of the pubic bone) and the upper margin of the symphysis pubis, into the true and the false pelvis.

The true pelvis

The true pelvis is the bony canal through which the fetus must pass during birth. It is divided into a brim, a cavity and an outlet.

The pelvic brim

The superior circumference forms the brim of the true pelvis, the included space being called the inlet. The brim is round except where the sacral promontory projects into it.

Midwives need to be familiar with the fixed points on the pelvic brim that are known as its landmarks. Commencing posteriorly these are (see Fig. 8.8 for numbers):

- sacral promontory (1)
- sacral ala or wing (2)
- sacroiliac joint (3)
- iliopectineal line, which is the edge formed at the inward aspect of the ilium (4)
- iliopectineal eminence, which is a roughened area formed where the superior ramus of the pubic bone meets the ilium (5)
- superior ramus of the pubic bone (6)
- upper inner border of the body of the pubic bone (7)
- upper inner border of the symphysis pubis (8).

Box 8.1 Negotiating the pelvic brim in asynclitism

Anterior asynclitism

The anterior parietal bone moves down behind the symphysis pubis until the parietal eminence enters the brim. The movement is then reversed and the head tilts in the opposite direction until the posterior parietal bone negotiates the sacral promontory and the head is engaged.

Posterior asynclitism

The movements of anterior asynclitism are reversed. The posterior parietal bone negotiates the sacral promontory prior to the anterior parietal bone moving down behind the symphysis pubis.

Once the pelvic brim has been negotiated, descent progresses normally accompanied by flexion and internal rotation.

Box 8.2 Deformed pelves

Developmental anomalies

The Naegele's and Robert's pelves are rare malformations caused by a failure in development. In the Naegele's pelvis, one sacral ala is missing and the sacrum is fused to the ilium causing a grossly asymmetric brim. The Robert's pelvis has similar malformations which are bilateral. In both instances, the abnormal brim prevents engagement of the fetal head.

Dietary deficiency

Deficiency of vitamins and minerals necessary for the formation of healthy bones is less frequently seen today than in the past but might still complicate pregnancy and labour to some extent.

A *Rachitic pelvis* is a pelvis deformed by Rickets in early childhood, as a consequence of malnutrition. The weight of the upper body presses downwards on to the softened pelvic bones, the sacral promontory is pushed downwards and forwards and the ilium and ischium are drawn outwards resulting in a flat pelvic brim similar to that of the platypelloid pelvis (Fig. 8.7). The sacrum tends to be straight with the coccyx bending acutely forward. Because the tuberosities are wide apart, the pubic arch is wide. The clinical signs of rickets are bow legs and spinal deformity.

If severe contraction is present caesarean section is required to deliver the baby. The fetal head will attempt to enter the pelvis by asynclitism.

Osteomalacic pelvis. The disease osteomalacia is rarely encountered in the UK. It is due to an acquired deficiency of calcium and occurs in adults. All bones of the skeleton soften because of gross calcium deficiency. The pelvic canal is squashed together until the brim becomes a Y-shaped slit. Labour is impossible. In early pregnancy, incarceration of the gravid uterus may occur because of the gross deformity.

Injury and disease

Trauma. A pelvis that has been fractured will develop callus formation or may fail to unite correctly. This may lead to reduced measurements and therefore to some degree of contraction. Conditions sustained in childhood such as fractures of the pelvis or lower limbs, congenital dislocation of the hip and poliomyelitis may lead to unequal weight-bearing, which will also cause deformity.

Spinal deformity. If kyphosis (forward angulation) or scoliosis (lateral curvature) is evident, or is suggested by a limp or deformity, the midwife must refer the woman to a doctor. Pelvic contraction is likely in these cases.

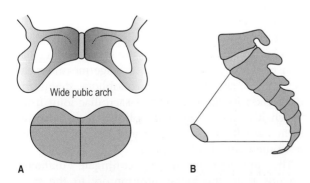

A   **B**

Wide pubic arch

Figure 8.7 Rachitic flat pelvis. (A) Note wide pubic arch and kidney-shaped brim. (B) The lateral view shows the diminished anteroposterior diameter of the brim and the increased anteroposterior diameter of the outlet.

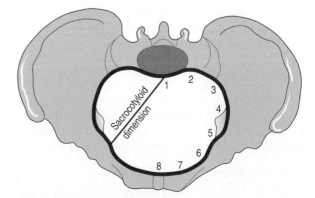

Sacrocotyloid dimension

Figure 8.8 Brim of female pelvis.

The pelvic cavity

The cavity of the true pelvis extends from the brim superiorly to the outlet inferiorly. The anterior wall is formed by the pubic bones and symphysis pubis and its depth is 4 cm. The posterior wall is formed by the curve of the sacrum, which is 12 cm in length. Because there is such a difference in these measurements, the cavity forms a curved canal. Its lateral walls are the sides of the pelvis, which are mainly covered by the obturator internus muscle.

The cavity contains the pelvic colon, rectum, bladder and some of the reproductive organs. The rectum is placed posteriorly, in the curve of the sacrum and coccyx, the bladder is anterior behind the symphysis pubis.

The pelvic outlet

The lower circumference of the true pelvis is very irregular; the space enclosed by it is called the outlet. Two outlets are described: the anatomical and the obstetrical. The anatomical outlet is formed by the lower borders of each of the bones together with the sacrotuberous ligament. The obstetrical outlet is of greater practical significance because it includes the narrow pelvic strait through which the fetus must pass. The narrow pelvic strait lies between the sacrococcygeal joint, the two ischial spines and the lower border of the symphysis pubis. The obstetrical outlet is the space between the narrow pelvic strait and the anatomical outlet. This outlet is diamond-shaped.

The false pelvis

The false pelvis is the part of the pelvis situated above the pelvic brim. It is formed by the upper flared-out portions of the iliac bones and protects the abdominal organs. However, the false pelvis has no significance in midwifery.

Pelvic diameters

Knowledge of the diameters of the normal female pelvis is essential in the practice of midwifery because contraction of any of them can result in malposition or malpresentation of the presenting part of the fetus.

Diameters of the brim

The brim has three principal diameters: the transverse diameter, the oblique diameter and the anteroposterior diameter (Figs. 8.9, 8.10).

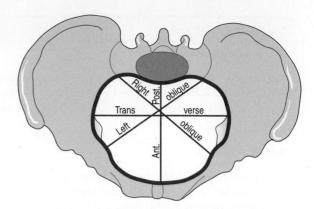

Figure 8.9 View of pelvic brim showing diameters.

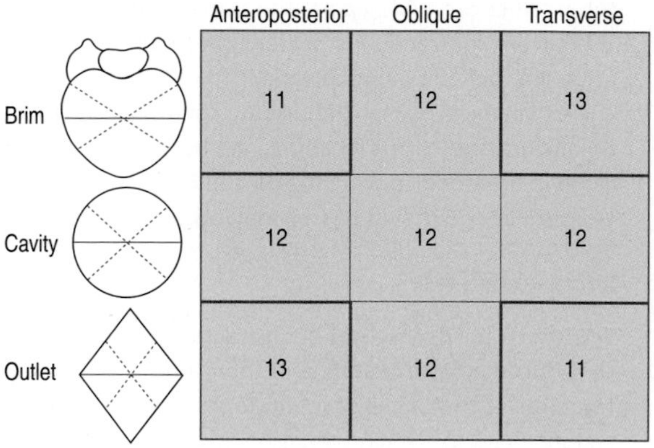

	Anteroposterior	Oblique	Transverse
Brim	11	12	13
Cavity	12	12	12
Outlet	13	12	11

Figure 8.10 Measurements of the pelvic canal in centimetres.

The transverse diameter extends across the greatest width of the brim; its average measurement is about 13 cm.

The oblique diameter extends from the iliopectineal eminence of one side to the sacroiliac articulation of the opposite side; its average measurement is about 12 cm. There are two oblique diameters. Each takes its name from the sacroiliac joint from which it arises, so the left oblique diameter arises from the left sacroiliac joint and the right oblique from the right sacroiliac joint.

The anteroposterior or conjugate diameter extends from the sacral promontory to the symphysis pubis. Three conjugate diameters can be measured: the anatomical conjugate, the obstetrical conjugate and the internal or diagonal conjugate (Fig. 8.11).

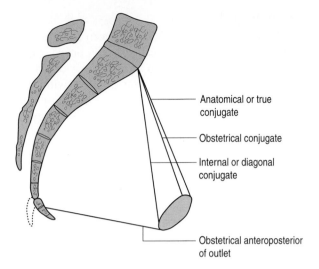

Figure 8.11 Median section of the pelvis showing anteroposterior diameters.

The anatomical conjugate, which averages 12 cm, is measured from the sacral promontory to the uppermost point of the symphysis pubis.

The obstetrical conjugate, which averages 11 cm, is measured from the sacral promontory to the posterior border of the upper surface of the symphysis pubis, which is 1.25 cm lower. This conjugate is of significance to midwives as it represents the available space for passage of the fetal head through the bony pelvis (Fig. 8.12).

The term true conjugate may be used to refer to either of these measurements and the midwife should take care to establish which is intended.

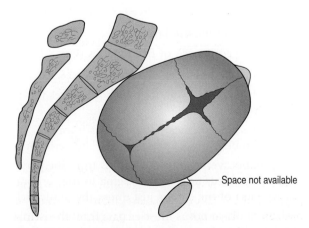

Figure 8.12 Fetal head negotiating the narrow obstetrical conjugate.

The diagonal conjugate is also measured anteroposteriorly from the lower border of the symphysis to the sacral promontory. It may be estimated on vaginal examination as part of a pelvic assessment and should measure 12–13 cm. However, in the UK, this measurement is no longer taken.

Certain structures pass through the pelvic brim, which may affect the space available for the fetus, for instance the descending colon enters the pelvis near the left sacroiliac joint.

Another dimension, the sacrocotyloid (see Fig. 8.8), passes from the sacral promontory to the iliopectineal eminence on each side and measures 9–9.5 cm. Its importance is concerned with posterior positions of the occiput when the parietal eminences of the fetal head may become caught (see Ch. 31).

Diameters of the cavity

The cavity is circular in shape and although it is not possible to measure its diameters exactly, they are all considered to be 12 cm (Fig. 8.10).

Diameters of the outlet

The outlet which is diamond-shaped has three diameters: the anteroposterior diameter, the oblique diameter and the transverse diameter (Fig. 8.10).

The anteroposterior diameter extends from the lower border of the symphysis pubis to the sacrococcygeal joint. It measures 13 cm. As the coccyx may be deflected backwards during labour, this diameter indicates the space available during birth.

The oblique diameter, although there are no fixed points, is said to be between the obturator foramen and the sacrospinous ligament. The measurement is taken as being 12 cm.

The transverse diameter extends between the two ischial spines and measures 10–11 cm. It is the narrowest diameter in the pelvis. The plane of least pelvic dimensions is said to be at the level of the ischial spines.

Orientation

In the standing position, the pelvis is placed such that the anterior superior iliac spine and the front edge of the symphysis pubis are in the same vertical plane, perpendicular to the floor. If the line joining the sacral promontory and the top of the symphysis pubis were to be extended, it would form an angle of 60° with the horizontal floor. Similarly, if a line

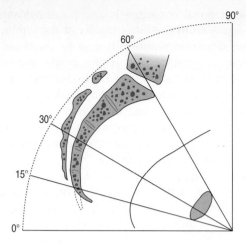

Figure 8.13 Median section of the pelvis showing the inclination of the planes and the axis of the pelvic canal.

joining the centre of the sacrum and the centre of the symphysis pubis were to be extended, the resultant angle with the floor would be 30°. The angle of inclination of the outlet is 15° (Fig. 8.13). When in the recumbent position, the same angles are made as in the vertical position; this fact should be kept in mind when carrying out an abdominal examination.

Pelvic planes

Pelvic planes are imaginary flat surfaces at the brim, cavity and outlet of the pelvic canal at the levels of the lines described above (Fig. 8.14).

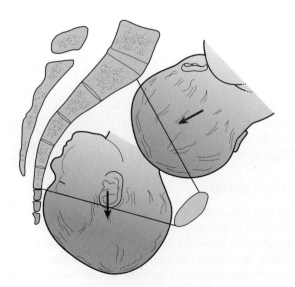

Figure 8.14 Fetal head entering plane of pelvic brim and leaving plane of pelvic outlet.

Axis of the pelvic canal

A line drawn exactly half-way between the anterior wall and the posterior wall of the pelvic canal would trace a curve known as the curve of Carus. The midwife needs to become familiar with this concept in order to make accurate observations on vaginal examination and to facilitate the birth of the baby.

The pelvic floor

The pelvic floor is formed by the soft tissues that fill the outlet of the pelvis. The most important of these is the strong diaphragm of muscle slung like a hammock from the walls of the pelvis. Through it pass the urethra, the vagina and the anal canal.

Functions

The pelvic floor is important in providing support for the pelvic organs and in the maintenance of continence as part of the urinary and anal sphincters. It also plays an important part in sexual intercourse.

During childbirth, the pelvic floor influences the passive movements of the fetus through the birth canal and relaxes to allow the exit of the fetus from the pelvis.

Muscle layers

The muscles of the pelvic floor are arranged into two layers, the superficial muscle layer and the deep muscle layer.

The superficial muscle layer

This layer is composed of five muscles (Fig. 8.15):

- the external anal sphincter, which encircles the anus, is attached posteriorly by a few fibres to the coccyx
- the transverse perineal muscles pass from the ischial tuberosities to the centre of the perineum
- the bulbocavernosus muscles pass from the perineum forwards around the vagina to the corpora cavernosa of the clitoris just under the pubic arch
- the ischiocavernosus muscles pass from the ischial tuberosities along the pubic arch to the corpora cavernosa

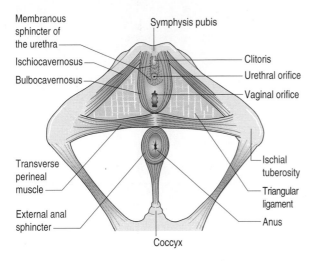

Figure 8.15   Superficial muscle layer of the pelvic floor.

- the membranous sphincter of the urethra is composed of muscle fibres passing above and below the urethra and attached to the pubic bones. It is not a true sphincter since it is not circular, but it acts to close the urethra.

The deep muscle layer

This layer consists of four main pairs of muscles (Fig. 8.16):

- the pubococcygeus and the puborectalis originate on the posterior inferior pubic rami and continue posteriorly becoming interlaced to a point of becoming inseparable. The pubococcygeus passes around the rectum and continues to its insertion on the coccyx

and the lower sacrum whereas the puborectalis fibres pass posteriorly encircling the rectum becoming part of the anorectal ring

- the iliococcygeus, which originates from the fascial covering of the obturator internus muscle, is directed posteriorly and medially. It converges with the pubococcygeus where it inserts into the coccyx and lower sacrum. The iliococcygeus forms a horizontal sheet that spans the opening in the posterior region of the pelvis providing a 'shelf' for the pelvic organs to rest on

- the ischiococcygeus originates from the ischial spine and adjacent sacroiliac fascia. It attaches to the coccyx, the lower sacrum and the median portion of the sacrotuberous ligament.

The pubococcygeus, the puborectalis, and the iliococcygeus, known collectively as the levatores ani, fix the pelvic structures and give support against which increased abdominal pressure may be exerted in the acts of lifting, coughing, defecation, urination and coitus. The ischiococcygeus and levatores ani combined form the pelvic diaphragm.

Between the muscle layers, and also above and below them are layers of pelvic fascia. This loose areolar tissue is used like packing material in the spaces. The tissue that fills the triangular space between the bulbocavernosus, the ischiocavernosus and the transverse perineal muscles is known as the triangular ligament.

The perineal body

The perineal body, a pyramid of muscle and fibrous tissue located between the vaginal introitus and anus, measures 4 cm in each direction. The apex, which is the deepest part, is formed from the fibres of the pubococcygeus muscle that cross over at this point. The base is formed from the transverse perineal muscles that meet in the perineum, together with the bulbocavernosus in front and the external anal sphincter behind.

Through its attachment to the cardinal and uterosacral ligaments, the rectovaginal septum stabilizes the perineal body, which is essentially suspended from the sacrum. The perineal body is further stabilized through the lateral attachments of the perineal membrane to the ischiopubic rami. Between the lateral and superior support, the downward mobility of the perineal body is limited. However, if this

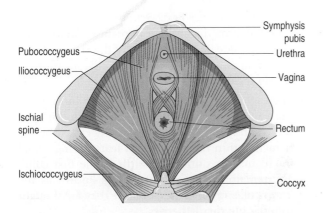

Figure 8.16   Deep muscle layer of the pelvic floor.

attachment is separated, as can occur during child-birth, the perineal body can become more mobile, leading to rectocele and perineal descent.

Blood supply

The internal pudendal artery is the primary blood supply to the pelvic floor.

Lymphatic drainage

Lymphatic drainage is through the common iliac nodes and the internal iliac nodes.

Nerve supply

The levatores ani is supplied by a branch from the fourth sacral nerve and by a branch of the pudendal nerve, which is sometimes derived from the perineal nerve and sometimes from the inferior haemorrhoidal nerve. The ischiococcygeus is supplied by a branch from the 4th and 5th sacral nerves.

The female reproductive system

The female reproductive system consists of the external genitalia, known collectively as the vulva and the internal reproductive organs: the vagina, the uterus, two uterine tubes and two ovaries. In the non-pregnant state, the internal reproductive organs are situated within the true pelvis.

The vulva

The vulva includes the mons pubis, labia majora, labia minora, clitoris and the perineum (Fig. 8.17).

- The mons pubis is a pad of fat lying over the symphysis pubis. It is covered with pubic hair from the time of puberty.
- The labia majora ('greater lips') are two folds of fat and areolar tissue covered with skin and pubic hair on the outer surface. They arise in the mons veneris and merge into the perineum behind.
- The labia minora ('lesser lips') are two thin folds of skin lying between the labia majora. Anteriorly they divide to enclose the clitoris; the frenum is formed by the two medial parts; posteriorly they fuse, forming the fourchette.

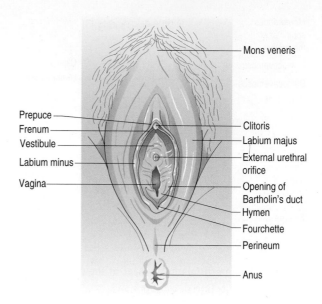

Figure 8.17   External female genital organs or vulva.

- The clitoris is a small rudimentary sexual organ corresponding to the male penis; the visible knob-like portion is located near the anterior junction of the labia minora, above the opening of the urethra and vagina. The prepuce a retractable piece of skin surrounds and protects the clitoris. Unlike the penis, the clitoris does not contain the distal portion of the urethra and functions solely to induce the orgasm of sexual intercourse.
- The vestibule is the area enclosed by the labia minora in which the openings of the urethra and the vagina are situated.
- The urethral orifice lies 2.5 cm posterior to the clitoris and immediately in front of the vaginal orifice. On either side lie the openings of the Skene's ducts, two small blind-ended tubules 0.5 cm long running within the urethral wall.
- The vaginal orifice, also known as the introitus of the vagina, occupies the posterior two-thirds of the vestibule. The orifice is partially closed by the hymen, a thin membrane that tears during sexual intercourse or during the birth of the first child. The remaining tags of hymen are known as the 'carunculae myrtiformes' because they are thought to resemble myrtle berries.

- Bartholin's glands are two small glands that open on either side of the vaginal orifice and lie in the posterior part of the labia majora. They secrete mucus, which lubricates the vaginal opening.

Blood supply

The blood supply comes from the internal and the external pudendal arteries. The blood drains through corresponding veins.

Lymphatic drainage

Lymphatic drainage is mainly via the inguinal glands.

Nerve supply

The nerve supply is derived from branches of the pudendal nerve. The vaginal nerves supply the erectile tissue of the vestibular bulbs and clitoris and their parasympathetic fibres have a vasodilator effect.

The vagina

The vagina is a hollow distensible fibromuscular tube that extends from the vaginal orifice in the vestibule to the cervix. It is approximately 10cm in length and 2.5cm in diameter (although there is wide anatomical variation). When a woman gives birth and during sexual intercourse, the vagina temporarily widens and lengthens.

The vaginal canal passes upwards and backwards into the pelvis along a line approximately parallel to the plane of the pelvic brim. When the woman stands upright, the vaginal canal points in an upward-backward direction and forms an angle of slightly more than 45° with the uterus.

Function

The vagina allows the escape of the menstrual fluids; receives the penis and the ejected sperm during sexual intercourse and provides an exit for the fetus during birth.

Relations

Knowledge of the relations of the vagina to other pelvic organs is essential for the accurate examination of the pregnant woman and the safe birth of the baby (Figs 8.18, 8.19).

- **Anterior** to the vagina lie the bladder and the urethra, which are closely connected to the anterior vaginal wall.

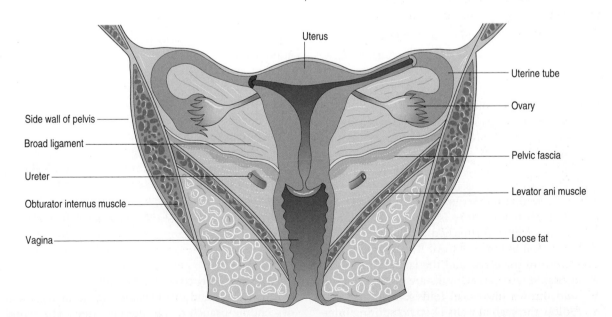

Figure 8.18 Coronal section through the pelvis.

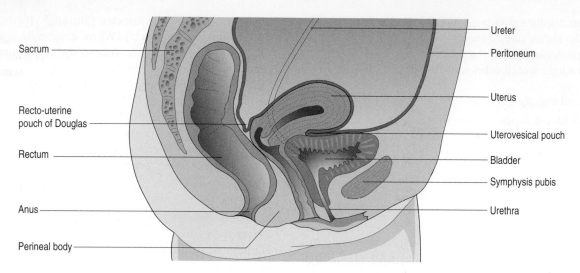

Figure 8.19 Sagittal section of the female pelvis.

- **Posterior** to the vagina lie the pouch of Douglas, the rectum and the perineal body; each occupying approximately one-third of the posterior vaginal wall.
- **Laterally** on the upper two-thirds are the pelvic fascia and the ureters, which pass beside the cervix; on either side of the lower third are the muscles of the pelvic floor.
- **Superior** to the vagina lies the uterus.
- **Inferior** to the vagina lie the external genitalia.

Structure

The posterior wall of the vagina is 10 cm long whereas the anterior wall is only 7.5 cm in length; this is because the cervix projects into its upper part at a right angle.

The upper end of the vagina is known as the vault. Where the cervix projects into it, the vault forms a circular recess that is described as four arches or fornices. The posterior fornix is the largest of these because the vagina is attached to the uterus at a higher level behind than in front. The anterior fornix lies in front of the cervix and the lateral fornices lie on either side. The vaginal walls are pink in appearance and thrown into small folds known as rugae. These allow the vaginal walls to stretch during intercourse and childbirth.

Layers

The vaginal wall is composed of three layers: mucosa, muscle and fascia. The mucosa is the most superficial layer and consists of squamous epithelium. Beneath the epithelium lies a layer of vascular connective tissue. The muscle layer is divided into a weak inner coat of circular fibres and a stronger outer coat of longitudinal fibres. Pelvic fascia surrounds the vagina and adjacent pelvic organs and allows for their independent expansion and contraction.

There are no glands in the vagina; however, it is moistened by mucus from the cervix and a transudate that seeps out from the blood vessels of the vaginal wall.

In spite of the alkaline mucus, the vaginal fluid is strongly acid (pH 4.5) owing to the presence of lactic acid formed by the action of Döderlein's bacilli on glycogen found in the squamous epithelium of the lining. These lactobacilli are normal inhabitants of the vagina. The acid deters the growth of pathogenic bacteria.

Blood supply

The blood supply comes from branches of the internal iliac artery and includes the vaginal artery and a descending branch of the uterine artery. The blood drains through corresponding veins.

Lymphatic drainage

Lymphatic drainage is via the inguinal, the internal iliac and the sacral glands.

Nerve supply

The nerve supply is derived from the pelvic plexus. The vaginal nerves follow the vaginal arteries to supply the vaginal walls and the erectile tissue of the vulva.

The uterus

The uterus is a hollow pear-shaped muscular organ located in the true pelvis between the bladder and the rectum. The position of the uterus within the true pelvis is one of anteversion and anteflexion. Anteversion means that the uterus leans forward and anteflexion means that it bends forwards upon itself. When the woman is standing, the uterus is in an almost horizontal position with the fundus resting on the bladder (Fig. 8.19).

Function

The main function of the uterus is to nourish the developing fetus prior to birth. It prepares for pregnancy each month and following pregnancy expels the products of conception.

Relations

Knowledge of the relations of the uterus to other pelvic organs (Figs. 8.18, 8.19) is desirable particularly when giving women advice about bladder and bowel care during pregnancy and childbirth.

- **Anterior** to the uterus lie the uterovesical pouch and the bladder.
- **Posterior** to the uterus are the recto-uterine pouch of Douglas and the rectum.
- **Lateral** to the uterus are the broad ligaments, the uterine tubes and the ovaries.
- **Superior** to the uterus lie the intestines.
- **Inferior** to the uterus is the vagina.

Supports

The uterus is supported by the pelvic floor and maintained in position by several ligaments, of which those at the level of the cervix (Fig. 8.20) are the most important.

- The transverse cervical ligaments fan out from the sides of the cervix to the side walls of the pelvis. They are sometimes known as the 'cardinal ligaments' or 'Mackenrodt's ligaments'.
- The uterosacral ligaments pass backwards from the cervix to the sacrum.

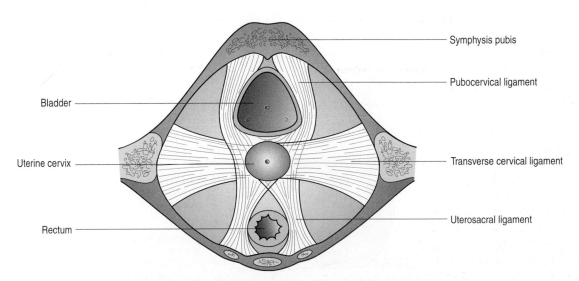

Figure 8.20 Supports of the uterus, at the level of the cervix.

- The pubocervical ligaments pass forwards from the cervix, under the bladder, to the pubic bones.
- The broad ligaments are formed from the folds of peritoneum, which are draped over the uterine tubes. They hang down like a curtain and spread from the sides of the uterus to the side walls of the pelvis.
- The round ligaments have little value as a support but tend to maintain the anteverted position of the uterus; they arise from the cornua of the uterus, in front of and below the insertion of each uterine tube, and pass between the folds of the broad ligament, through the inguinal canal, to be inserted into each labium majus.
- The ovarian ligaments also begin at the cornua of the uterus but behind the uterine tubes and pass down between the folds of the broad ligament to the ovaries.

It is helpful to note that the round ligament, the uterine tube and the ovarian ligament are very similar in appearance and arise from the same area of the uterus. This makes careful identification important when tubal surgery is undertaken.

Structure

The non-pregnant uterus is 7.5 cm long, 5 cm wide and 2.5 cm in depth, each wall being 1.25 cm thick (Fig. 8.21). The cervix forms the lower third of the uterus and measures 2.5 cm in each direction.

The uterus consists of the following parts:

- The cornua are the upper outer angles of the uterus where the uterine tubes join.
- The fundus is the domed upper wall between the insertions of the uterine tubes.
- The body or corpus makes up the upper two-thirds of the uterus and is the greater part.
- The cavity is a potential space between the anterior and posterior walls. It is triangular in shape, the base of the triangle being uppermost.
- The isthmus is a narrow area between the cavity and the cervix, which is 7 mm long. It enlarges during pregnancy to form the lower uterine segment.
- The cervix or neck protrudes into the vagina. The upper half, being above the vagina, is known as the supravaginal portion while the lower half is the infravaginal portion.

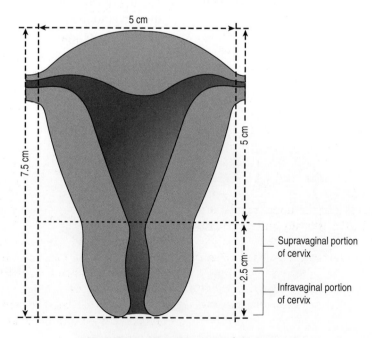

Figure 8.21 Measurements of the uterus.

- the internal os (mouth) is the narrow opening between the isthmus and the cervix.
- the external os is a small round opening at the lower end of the cervix. After childbirth, it becomes a transverse slit.
- the cervical canal lies between these two ora and is a continuation of the uterine cavity. This canal is shaped like a spindle, narrow at each end and wider in the middle.

Layers

The uterus has three layers: the endometrium, the myometrium and the perimetrium, of which the myometrium, the middle muscle layer, is by far the thickest.

The endometrium forms a lining of ciliated epithelium (mucous membrane) on a base of connective tissue or stroma. In the uterine cavity, this endometrium is constantly changing in thickness throughout the menstrual cycle (see Ch. 10). The basal layer does not alter, but provides the foundation from which the upper layers regenerate. The epithelial cells are cubical in shape and dip down to form glands that secrete an alkaline mucus.

The cervical endometrium does not respond to the hormonal stimuli of the menstrual cycle to the same extent. Here the epithelial cells are tall and columnar in shape and the mucus-secreting glands are branching racemose glands. The cervical endometrium is thinner than that of the body and is folded into a pattern known as the 'arbor vitae' (tree of life). This is thought to assist the passage of the sperm. The portion of the cervix that protrudes into the vagina is covered with squamous epithelium similar to that lining the vagina. The point where the epithelium changes, at the external os, is termed the squamo-columnar junction.

The myometrium is thick in the upper part of the uterus and is sparser in the isthmus and cervix. Its fibres run in all directions and interlace to surround the blood vessels and lymphatics that pass to and from the endometrium. The outer layer is formed of longitudinal fibres that are continuous with those of the uterine tube, the uterine ligaments and the vagina.

In the cervix, the muscle fibres are embedded in collagen fibres, which enable it to stretch in labour.

The perimetrium is a double serous membrane, an extension of the peritoneum, which is draped over the fundus and the anterior surface of the uterus to the level of the internal os. It is then reflected onto the bladder forming a small pouch between the uterus and the bladder called the uterovesical pouch. The posterior surface is covered to where the cervix protrudes into the vagina and is then reflected onto the rectum forming the recto-uterine pouch. Laterally the perimetrium extends over the uterine tubes forming a double fold, the broad ligament, leaving the lateral borders of the body uncovered.

Blood supply

The uterine artery arrives at the level of the cervix and is a branch of the internal iliac artery. It sends a small branch to the upper vagina, and then runs upwards in a twisted fashion to meet the ovarian artery and form an anastomosis with it near the cornu. The ovarian artery is a branch of the abdominal aorta, leaving near the renal artery. It supplies the ovary and uterine tube before joining the uterine artery. The blood drains through corresponding veins (Fig. 8.22).

Lymphatic drainage

Lymph is drained from the uterine body to the internal iliac glands and from the cervical area to many other pelvic lymph glands. This provides an effective defence against uterine infection.

Nerve supply

The nerve supply is mainly from the autonomic nervous system, sympathetic and parasympathetic, via the inferior hypogastric or pelvic plexus.

Uterine malformations

For pregnancy and labour to be achieved with minimal difficulty, a woman must have normal reproductive anatomy. When structural abnormality of the pelvic organs exists, problems arise that can place an extra burden on mother and fetus. The possible effects of such abnormalities are explained in Box 8.3.

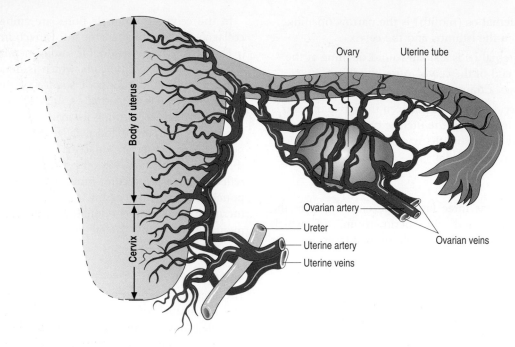

Figure 8.22   Blood supply of the uterus, uterine tubes and ovaries.

Box 8.3 Uterine malformations

Embryological development of the uterus

The female genital tract is formed in early embryonic life when a pair of ducts develops. These paramesonephric or Müllerian ducts come together in the midline and fuse into a Y-shaped canal. The open upper ends of this structure lead into the peritoneal cavity and the unfused portions become the uterine tubes. The fused lower portion forms the uterovaginal area, which further develops into the uterus and vagina.

Types of uterine malformation

Various types of structural abnormality can result from failure of fusion of the Müllerian ducts. Three of these abnormalities can be seen in Figure 8.23. A double uterus with an associated double vagina will develop where there has been complete failure of fusion. Partial fusion results in various degrees of duplication. A single vagina with a double uterus is the result of fusion at the lower end of the ducts only. A bicornuate uterus (one with two horns) is the result of incomplete fusion at the upper portion of the uterovaginal area. In rare cases, one Müllerian duct regresses and the result is a uterus with one horn – termed a unicornuate uterus.

Effect of abnormality on pregnancy

The outcome depends on the ability of the uterus to accommodate the growing fetus. A problem exists only if the tissue is insufficient to allow the uterus to enlarge for a full-term fetus lying longitudinally.

  If there is insufficient hypertrophy, the possible difficulties are miscarriage, premature labour and abnormal lie of the fetus. In labour, poor uterine function may be experienced.

  Minor defects of structure cause little problem and might pass unnoticed with the woman having a normal outcome to her pregnancy. Occasionally problems arise when a fetus is accommodated in one horn of a double uterus and the empty horn has filled the pelvic cavity. In this situation, the empty horn has grown owing to the hormonal influences of the pregnancy, and its size and position will cause obstruction during labour. Caesarean section would be the method of delivery.

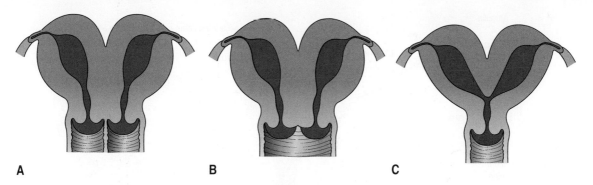

Figure 8.23 Uterine malformations: (A) Double uterus with duplication of body of uterus, cervix and vagina. (B) Duplication of uterus and cervix with single vagina. (C) Duplication of uterus with single cervix and vagina.

The uterine tubes

The uterine tubes, also known as fallopian tubes, oviducts and salpinges, are two very fine tubes leading from the ovaries into the uterus.

Function

The uterine tube propels the ovum towards the uterus, receives the spermatozoa as they travel upwards and provides a site for fertilization. It supplies the fertilized ovum with nutrition during its continued journey to the uterus.

Position

The uterine tubes extend laterally from the cornua of the uterus towards the side walls of the pelvis. They arch over the ovaries, the fringed ends hovering near the ovaries in order to receive the ovum.

Relations

- **Anterior**, posterior and superior to the uterine tubes are the peritoneal cavity and the intestines.
- **Lateral** to the uterine tubes are the side walls of the pelvis.
- **Inferior** to the uterine tubes lie the broad ligaments and the ovaries.
- **Medial** to the two uterine tubes lies the uterus.

Supports

The uterine tubes are held in place by their attachment to the uterus. The peritoneum folds over them, draping down below as the broad ligaments and extending at the sides to form the infundibulopelvic ligaments.

Structure

Each tube is 10 cm long. The lumen of the tube provides an open pathway from the outside to the peritoneal cavity. The uterine tube has four portions (Fig. 8.24):

The interstitial portion is 1.25 cm long and lies within the wall of the uterus. Its lumen is 1 mm wide.

The isthmus is another narrow part that extends for 2.5 cm from the uterus.

The ampulla is the wider portion where fertilization usually occurs. It is 5 cm long.

The infundibulum is the funnel-shaped fringed end that is composed of many processes known as fimbriae. One fimbria is elongated to form the ovarian fimbria, which is attached to the ovary.

Layers (Fig. 8.25)

The lining of the uterine tubes is a mucous membrane of ciliated cubical epithelium that is thrown into complicated folds known as plicae. These folds

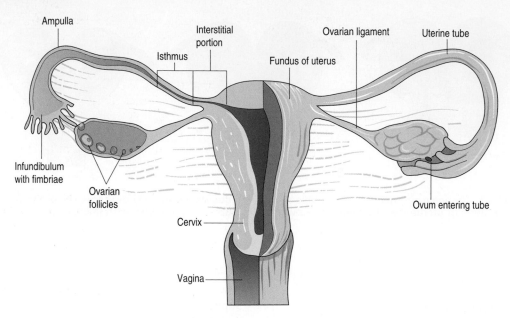

Figure 8.24   The uterine tubes in section. Note the ovum entering the fimbriated end of one.

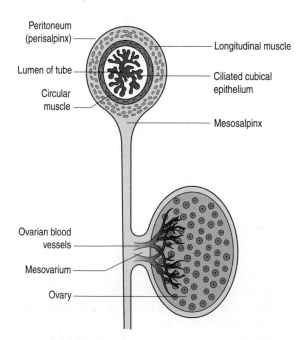

Figure 8.25   Cross-section of a uterine tube and ovary.

slow the ovum down on its way to the uterus. In this lining are goblet cells that produce a secretion containing glycogen to nourish the oocyte.

Beneath the lining is a layer of vascular connective tissue.

The muscle coat consists of two layers, an inner circular layer and an outer longitudinal layer, both of smooth muscle. The peristaltic movement of the uterine tube is due to the action of these muscles.

The tube is covered with peritoneum but the infundibulum passes through it to open into the peritoneal cavity.

Blood supply

The blood supply is via the uterine and ovarian arteries, returning by the corresponding veins.

Lymphatic drainage

Lymph is drained to the lumbar glands.

Nerve supply

The nerve supply is from the ovarian plexus.

The ovaries

The ovaries are components of the female reproductive system and the endocrine system.

Function

The ovaries produce oocytes and the hormones oestrogen and progesterone.

Position

The ovaries are attached to the back of the broad ligaments within the peritoneal cavity.

Relations

- **Anterior** to the ovaries are the broad ligaments.
- **Posterior** to the ovaries are the intestines.
- **Lateral** to the ovaries are the infundibulopelvic ligaments and the side walls of the pelvis.
- **Superior** to the ovaries lie the uterine tubes.
- **Medial** to the ovaries lie the ovarian ligaments and the uterus.

Supports

The ovary is attached to the broad ligament but is supported from above by the ovarian ligament medially and the infundibulopelvic ligament laterally.

Structure

The ovary is composed of a medulla and cortex, covered with germinal epithelium.

The medulla is the supporting framework, which is made of fibrous tissue; the ovarian blood vessels, lymphatics and nerves travel through it. The hilum where these vessels enter lies just where the ovary is attached to the broad ligament and this area is called the mesovarium (Fig. 8.25).

The cortex is the functioning part of the ovary. It contains the ovarian follicles in different stages of development, surrounded by stroma. The outer layer is formed of fibrous tissue known as the tunica albuginea. Over this lies the germinal epithelium, which is a modification of the peritoneum.

The cycle of the ovary is described in Chapter 10.

Blood supply

Blood is supplied to the ovaries from the ovarian arteries and drains via the ovarian veins. The right ovarian vein joins the inferior vena cava, but the left returns its blood to the left renal vein.

Lymphatic drainage

Lymphatic drainage is to the lumbar glands.

Nerve supply

The nerve supply is from the ovarian plexus.

The male reproductive system

The male reproductive system (Fig. 8.26) is a series of organs that are partly visible and partly hidden within the body. The visible parts are the scrotum

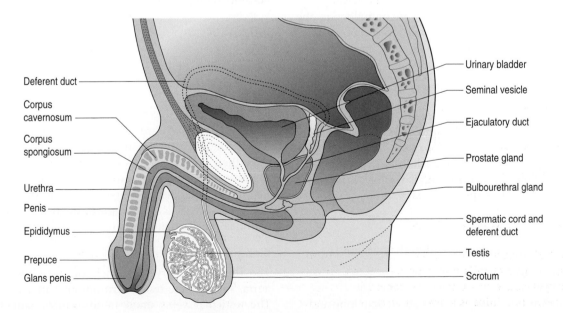

Figure 8.26 Male reproductive system.

and the penis. Inside the body are the prostate gland and tubes which link the system together. The male organs produce and transfer sperm to the female for fertilization.

The scrotum

The scrotum is part of the external genitalia. Also called the scrotal sac, the scrotum is a thin-walled, soft, muscular pouch located below the symphysis pubis, between the upper parts of the thighs behind the penis.

Function

The scrotum forms a pouch in which the testes are suspended outside the body keeping them at a temperature slightly lower than that of the rest of the body. A temperature around 34.4°C enables the production of viable sperm whereas a temperature of 36.7°C can be damaging to sperm count.

Structure

The scrotum is formed of pigmented skin and has two compartments, one for each testis.

The testes

Like the ovaries, to which they are homologous, the testes (also known as testicles) are components of both the reproductive system and the endocrine system. Each testis weighs about 25 g.

Function

The testes produce and store spermatozoa, and are the body's main source of the male hormone testosterone. Testosterone is responsible for the development of secondary sex characteristics. Together with follicle-stimulating hormone (FSH), it also promotes the production of spermatozoa.

Position

The testes are contained within the scrotum.

Structure

Each testis is an oval structure about 5 cm long and 3 cm in diameter.

Layers

There are three layers to the testis:

The **tunica vasculosa** is an inner layer of connective tissue containing a fine network of capillaries.

The **tunica albuginea** is a fibrous covering, ingrowths of which divide the testis into 200–300 lobules.

The **tunica vaginalis** is the outer layer, which is made of peritoneum brought down with the descending testis when it migrated from the lumbar region in fetal life.

The duct system within the testes is highly intricate:

The **seminiferous** ('seed-carrying') tubules are where spermatogenesis, or production of sperm, takes place. There are up to three of them in each lobule. Between the tubules are interstitial cells that secrete testosterone. The tubules join to form a system of channels that lead to the epididymis.

The **epididymis** is a comma-shaped, coiled tube that lies on the superior surface and travels down the posterior aspect to the lower pole of the testis, where it leads into the deferent duct or vas deferens.

The spermatic cord

The spermatic cord is the name given to the cord-like structure consisting of the vas deferens and its accompanying arteries, veins, nerves, and lymphatic vessels.

Function

The function of the deferent duct is to carry the sperm to the ejaculatory duct.

Position

The cord passes upwards through the inguinal canal, where the different structures diverge. The deferent duct then continues upwards over the symphysis pubis and arches backwards beside the bladder. Behind the bladder, it merges with the duct from the seminal vesicle and passes through the prostate gland as the ejaculatory duct to join the urethra.

Blood supply

The testicular artery, a branch of the abdominal aorta, supplies the testes, scrotum and attachments. The testicular veins drain in the same manner as the ovarian veins.

Lymphatic drainage

Lymphatic drainage is to the lymph nodes round the aorta.

Nerve supply

The nerve supply to the spermatic cord is from the 10th and 11th thoracic nerves.

The seminal vesicles

The seminal vesicles are a pair of simple tubular glands.

Function

The function of the seminal vesicles is production of a viscous secretion to keep the sperm alive and motile. This secretion ultimately becomes semen.

Position

The seminal vesicles are situated posterior to the bladder and superior to the prostate gland.

Structure

The seminal vesicles are 5 cm long and pyramid-shaped. They are composed of columnar epithelium, muscle tissue and fibrous tissue.

The ejaculatory ducts

These small muscular ducts carry the spermatozoa and the seminal fluid to the urethra.

The prostate gland

The prostate is an exocrine gland of the male reproductive system.

Function

The prostate gland produces a thin lubricating fluid that enters the urethra through ducts.

Position

The prostate gland surrounds the urethra at the base of the bladder, lying between the rectum and the symphysis pubis.

Structure

The prostate gland measures $4 \times 3 \times 2$ cm. It is composed of columnar epithelium, a muscle layer and an outer fibrous layer.

The bulbourethral glands

The bulbourethral glands are two very small glands, which produce yet another lubricating fluid that passes into the urethra just below the prostate gland.

The penis

The penis is the male reproductive organ and additionally serves as the external male organ of urination.

Functions

The penis carries the urethra, which is a passage for both urine and semen. During sexual excitement it stiffens (an erection) in order to be able to penetrate the vagina and deposit the semen near the woman's cervix.

Position

The root of the penis lies in the perineum, from where it passes forward below the symphysis pubis. The lower two-thirds are outside the body in front of the scrotum.

Structure

The penis has three columns of erectile tissue:

The **corpora cavernosa** are two lateral columns that lie one on either side in front of the urethra.

The **corpus spongiosum** is the posterior column that contains the urethra. The tip is expanded to form the glans penis.

The lower two-thirds of the penis are covered in skin. At the end, the skin is folded back on itself above the glans penis to form the prepuce or foreskin, which is a movable double fold. The penis is extremely vascular and during an erection the blood spaces fill and become distended.

The male hormones

The control of the male gonads is similar to that in the female, but it is not cyclical. The hypothalamus produces gonadotrophin-releasing factors. These stimulate the anterior pituitary gland to produce FSH and luteinizing hormone (LH). FSH acts on the seminiferous tubules to bring about the production of sperm, whereas LH acts on the interstitial cells that produce testosterone.

Testosterone is responsible for the secondary sex characteristics: deepening of the voice, growth of the genitalia and growth of hair on the chest, pubis, axilla and face.

Formation of the spermatozoa

Production of sperm begins at puberty and continues throughout adult life. Spermatogenesis takes place in the seminiferous tubules under the influence of FSH and testosterone. The process of maturation is a lengthy one and takes some weeks. The mature sperm are stored in the epididymis and the deferent duct until ejaculation. If this does not happen, they degenerate and are reabsorbed. At each ejaculation, 2–4 mL of semen is deposited in the vagina. The seminal fluid contains about 100 million sperm/mL, of which 20–25% are likely to be abnormal. The remainder move at a speed of 2–3 mm/min. The individual spermatozoon has a head, a body and a long, mobile tail that lashes to propel the sperm along (Fig. 8.27). The tip of the head is covered by an acrosome; this contains enzymes to dissolve the covering of the oocyte in order to penetrate it.

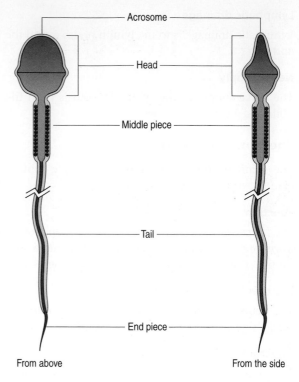

Figure 8.27   Spermatozoon.

FURTHER READING

Coad J with Dunstall M 2005 Anatomy and physiology for midwives, 2nd edn. Churchill Livingstone, Edinburgh

This comprehensive text provides a thorough review of anatomy and physiology applicable to midwifery from first principles through to current research, utilizing case studies for reflection.

Drake R, Vogl W, Mitchell A, 2005 Gray's anatomy for students. Churchill Livingstone, Edinburgh

This new edition of Gray's anatomy, which has been written for anatomy students, presents the essentials of clinical anatomy in clear terminology and explanatory diagrams. Chapter 5, which relates to the Pelvis and Perineum, is of particular relevance here.

Johnson M, Everitt B 2000 Essential reproduction, 5th edn. Blackwell Science, Oxford

In all respects, this text provides an unsurpassed source of information on the physiology of reproduction from a multidisciplinary perspective.

Stables D, Rankin J 2004 Physiology in childbearing with anatomy and related biosciences, 2nd edn. Baillière Tindall, Edinburgh

This textbook presents a, comprehensive and clear account of anatomy and physiology and related biosciences at all stages of pregnancy and childbirth.

Standring S, Healy J, Johnson D, et al 2004 Gray's anatomy: the anatomical basis of clinical practice, 39th edn. Churchill Livingstone, New York

This large volume, with detailed information about the anatomy of every part of the human body, provides the reader with much more insight into the structure and function of the reproductive organs. This edition includes specialist revision of topics such as the anatomy of the pelvic floor.

9 The female urinary tract

Mary E. Vance

The principal function of the urinary system, together with other body systems, is to maintain homeostasis. One aspect of this function is to rid the body of waste products that accumulate because of cellular metabolism. The urinary tract begins with the kidneys, and continues as a passage for urine in the ureters, the bladder and the urethra.

The kidneys

The kidneys are a pair of bean-shaped excretory glands that have both endocrine and exocrine functions. They are about 10 cm long, 6.5 cm wide and 3 cm thick and weigh around 120 g. Although similar in shape, the left kidney is a longer and more slender organ than the right kidney. Congenital absence of one or both kidneys, known as unilateral or bilateral renal agenesis, can occur.

Functions

The kidneys extract soluble wastes from the blood and excrete excess water and minerals. They also prevent substances that are needed by the body from being lost and have a part to play in red cell production and the maintenance of blood pressure.

The kidney functions can be summarized as the:

- elimination of wastes, particularly the breakdown products of protein, e.g. urea, urates, uric acid, creatinine, ammonia and sulphates
- elimination of toxins
- regulation of the water content of the blood and indirectly of the tissues
- regulation of the pH of the blood
- regulation of the osmotic pressure of the blood
- secretion of the hormones renin and erythropoietin.

Position and relations

The kidneys are in the posterior of the abdominal cavity, one on either side of the spine. They extend approximately from vertebra T12 superiorly to L3 inferiorly and however, because of the contents of the abdominal cavity the right kidney is located slightly lower than the left kidney. The anterior and posterior surfaces of the kidneys are related to numerous structures some of which come into direct contact with the kidneys whereas others are separated by a layer of peritoneum (Drake et al 2005). An adrenal gland sits on top of each kidney.

Supports

The kidneys are maintained in position by a generous packing of perinephric fat and by the closeness of neighbouring organs, particularly parts of the gastrointestinal tract in front and the musculature of the posterior abdominal wall behind.

Structure

Each kidney has a smooth surface covered by a tough fibrous capsule. There is a concave side facing medially; on this medial aspect is an opening called the hilum from which the renal artery, renal vein, nerves, and lymphatics enter and leave the kidney (Fig. 9.1). Internally the hilum is continuous with the renal sinus.

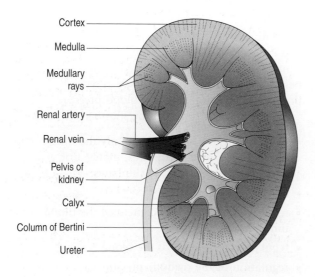

Cortex
Medulla
Medullary rays
Renal artery
Renal vein
Pelvis of kidney
Calyx
Column of Bertini
Ureter

Figure 9.1 Longitudinal section of the kidney.

Each kidney consists of an outer cortex and an inner medulla. The cortex sits directly beneath the kidney's fibrous capsule. Below the cortex lies the medulla which is divided into pyramids. There are approximately 12 pyramids and they contain bundles of tubules leading from the cortex. The tubules create a lined appearance known as the medullary rays. The base of each pyramid is curved and the cortex arches over it projecting downwards between them forming columns of tissue known as the columns of Bertini. Each pyramid together with the associated overlying cortex forms a renal lobe. The tip of each pyramid, known as a papilla, empties into a calyx, and the calices empty into the renal pelvis. Urine is transmitted from the renal pelvis to the urinary bladder via the ureter.

The nephrons

When the tissue of a normal adult kidney is examined under the microscope the basic functional unit, the nephron, of which there are more than 1 million, can be seen.

Each nephron starts at a knot of capillaries called a glomerulus (Fig. 9.2). It is fed by a branch of the renal artery, the afferent arteriole, and the blood is collected up again into the efferent arteriole. This is the only place in the body where an artery collects blood from capillaries. The pressure within the glomerulus is raised because the afferent arteriole has a wider bore than the efferent arteriole and this factor forces the filtrate out of the capillaries into the capsule. At this stage, any substance with a small molecular size will be filtered out.

Surrounding the glomerulus is a cup known as the glomerular capsule, into which fluid and solutes are exuded from the blood. The glomerulus and capsule together are known as the glomerular body (Fig. 9.2).

The cup of the capsule is attached to a tubule. The tubule initially winds and twists, then forms a straight loop that dips into the medulla, rising up into the cortex again to wind and turn before joining the straight collecting tubule, which receives urine from several nephrons. The first twisting portion of the nephron is the proximal convoluted tubule, the loop is termed the loop of Henle and the second twisting portion is the distal convoluted tubule. The

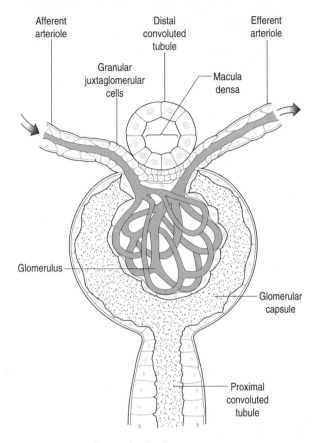

Afferent arteriole

Granular juxtaglomerular cells

Distal convoluted tubule

Macula densa

Efferent arteriole

Glomerulus

Glomerular capsule

Proximal convoluted tubule

Figure 9.2 A glomerular body.

whole nephron is about 3 cm in length (Fig. 9.3). The straight collecting tubule runs from the cortex to a medullary pyramid; it forms a medullary ray and receives urine from over 4000 nephrons along its length.

The distal convoluted tubule returns to pass alongside granular cells of the afferent arteriole and this part of the tubule is called the macula densa (Fig. 9.2). The two are known as the juxtaglomerular apparatus. The granular cells secrete renin whereas the macula densa cells monitor the sodium chloride concentration of fluid passing through.

Blood supply

The renal arteries are early branches of the descending abdominal aorta and divert about a quarter of the cardiac output into the kidneys. The artery enters at the renal hilum, sends numerous branches into the cortex and forms a glomerulus for each nephron. Blood is collected up and returned via the renal vein.

Lymphatic drainage

A rich supply of lymph vessels lies under the cortex and around the urine-bearing tubules. Lymph drains into large lymphatic ducts that emerge from the hilum and lead to the aortic lymph glands.

Nerve supply

The nerves of the kidney enter by the renal hilum and provide a sympathetic and parasympathetic nerve supply. Although small, there are about 15 in number.

Endocrine activity

The kidney secretes two hormones renin and erythropoietin. Renin is produced in the afferent arteriole and is secreted when the blood supply to the kidneys is reduced and in response to lowered sodium levels. It acts on angiotensinogen, which is present in the blood, to form angiotensin, which raises blood pressure and encourages sodium reabsorption. Erythropoietin stimulates the production of red blood cells.

Urine

The colour of urine ranges from a pale straw colour when very dilute to a dark brown colour when very concentrated. It should never be cloudy. In the newborn baby, it is almost clear. It has a recognizable smell, which in health is not unpleasant when freshly passed. An adult passes between one and 2 L of urine daily, depending on fluid intake.

The specific gravity of urine is 1.010–1.030. It is composed of 96% water, 2% urea and 2% other solutes. Urine is usually acid and contains no glucose or ketones, nor should it carry blood cells or bacteria. Women are susceptible to urinary tract infection but this is usually an ascending infection acquired via the urethra. A low bacterial count less than 100 000/mL is insignificant.

The production of urine

The production of urine takes place in three stages: filtration, reabsorption and secretion.

Filtration

Filtration is the simple process of water and the substances dissolved in it being passed from the glomerulus into the glomerular capsule because of the raised intracapillary pressure. Blood components such

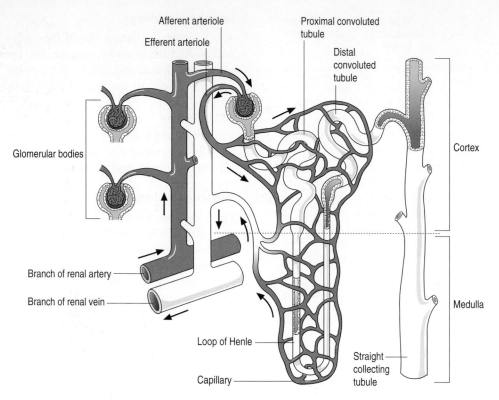

Afferent arteriole

Efferent arteriole

Proximal convoluted tubule

Distal convoluted tubule

Glomerular bodies

Cortex

Branch of renal artery

Branch of renal vein

Medulla

Loop of Henle

Straight collecting tubule

Capillary

Figure 9.3   A nephron.

as corpuscles and platelets as well as plasma proteins, which are large molecules, are kept in the blood vessel; water, salts and glucose escape through the filter as the filtrate (Fig. 9.4). A vast amount of fluid passes out in this way, about 2 mL per second or 120 mL per minute: 99% of this must be recovered, or the body would be totally drained of fluid within hours.

Reabsorption

The body selects from the filtrate the substances that it needs: water, salts and glucose. The posterior pituitary gland controls the reabsorption of water by producing antidiuretic hormone (ADH). If the body has lost fluid such as in sweating or if fluid intake has been low, more water is conserved and less urine passed, the urine appearing more concentrated. In the opposite circumstances, when the individual has consumed a lot of fluid and is sweating little, the urine is more copious and dilute. However, this is not always the case, for instance following the consumption of alcohol, urine flow increases because alcohol causes the acute inhibition of the

release of ADH. The absence of ADH causes segments of the kidney's tubule system to become impermeable to water, thus preventing it from being reabsorbed into the body (Epstein 1997). Newborn

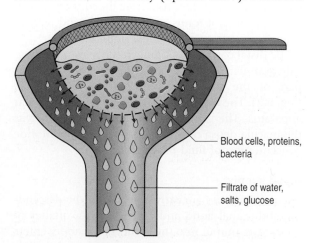

Blood cells, proteins, bacteria

Filtrate of water, salts, glucose

Figure 9.4   Filtration: larger molecules stay in the sieve (glomerulus) and smaller molecules filter out (into the glomerular capsule).

babies' ability to concentrate and dilute their urine is poor and preterm infants even more so. For this reason they are unable to tolerate wide variations in their fluid intake.

Minerals are selected according to the body's needs. The reabsorption of sodium is controlled by aldosterone, which is produced in the cortex of the suprarenal gland. The interaction of aldosterone and ADH maintains water and sodium balance. The pH of the blood must be controlled and if it is tending towards acidity then acids will be excreted. However, if the opposite pertains, alkaline urine will be produced. Often this is the result of an intake of an alkaline substance.

Secretion

Certain substances, such as creatinine and toxins, are added directly to the urine in the ascending arm of the loop of Henle.

The ureters

The ureters are hollow muscular tubes; the upper end is funnel-shaped and merges into the pelvis of the kidney where urine is received from the renal tubules.

Function

The ureters transport urine from the kidneys to the bladder by waves of peristalsis.

Structure

Each tube is about 3 mm in diameter and 25–30 cm long, running from the renal hilum to the posterior wall of the bladder (Fig. 9.5). They descend on the medial aspect of the psoas major muscle. At the pelvic brim, they descend along the side walls of the pelvis to the level of the ischial spines and then turn forwards to pass beside the uterine cervix and enter the bladder from behind passing through the bladder wall at an angle (Fig. 9.6).

Layers

The ureters are composed of three layers: a lining, a muscle layer and an outer coat. The lining is formed of transitional epithelium arranged in longitudinal folds. This type of epithelium consists of several layers of pear-shaped cells and makes an elastic and waterproof inner coat.

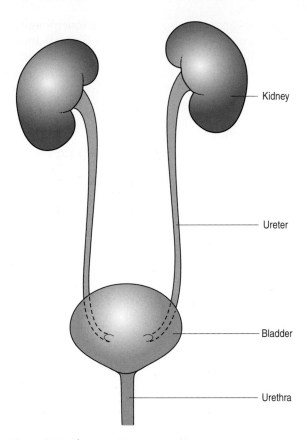

Figure 9.5   The ureters.

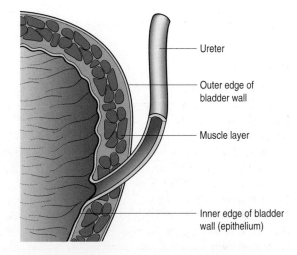

Figure 9.6   Diagram to show the entry of the ureter into the posterior wall of the bladder.

The muscular layer is arranged as an inner longitudinal layer, a middle circular layer and an outer longitudinal layer.

The outer coat is of fibrous connective tissue, which is continuous with the fibrous capsule of the kidney.

Blood supply

The upper part of the ureter is supplied similarly to the kidney. In its pelvic portion, it derives blood from the common iliac and internal iliac arteries and from the uterine and vesical arteries, according to its proximity to the different organs. Venous return is along corresponding veins.

Lymphatic drainage

Lymph drains into the internal, external and common iliac nodes.

Nerve supply

The nerve supply is from the renal, aortic, superior and inferior hypogastric plexuses.

The bladder

The bladder is a hollow, muscular, distensible pelvic organ which acts as a reservoir for the storage of urine until it is convenient for it to be voided.

Midwives need to be familiar with the anatomy and physiology of the bladder as pregnancy and childbirth can affect bladder control.

Position, shape and size

The empty bladder lies in the pelvic cavity with its base resting on the upper half of the vagina with its apex directed towards the symphysis pubis. However, as it fills with urine it rises up out of the pelvic cavity becoming an abdominal organ. It can be palpated above the symphysis pubis when full. During labour, the bladder is an abdominal organ as it is displaced by the descent of the fetus into the pelvic cavity.

When empty the bladder is described as being pyramidal, with its base being triangular. When it is full, it becomes more globular in shape as its walls are distended.

The empty bladder is of similar size to the uterus but when full of urine it becomes much larger. Its capacity is around 600 mL but it is capable of holding more, particularly under the influence of pregnancy hormones.

Relations (Fig. 9.7)

- **Anterior** to the bladder is the symphysis pubis, which is separated from it by a space filled with fatty tissue called the cave of Retzius.

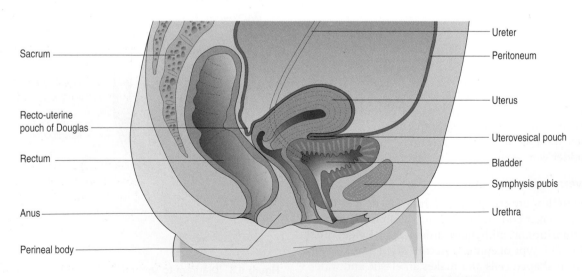

Figure 9.7   Sagittal section of the pelvis showing the relations of the bladder.

- **Posterior** to the bladder is the cervix and ureters.
- **Laterally** are the lateral ligaments of the bladder and the side walls of the pelvis.
- **Superiorly** lie the intestines and peritoneal cavity; in the non-pregnant female the anteverted, anteflexed uterus lies partially over the bladder.
- **Inferior** to the bladder is the urethra and the muscular diaphragm of the pelvic floor, which forms its main support, and on which its function partly depends.

Supports

There are five ligaments attached to the bladder. Two lateral ligaments extend from the bladder to the side walls of the pelvis. Two pubovesical ligaments extend from the bladder neck anteriorly to the symphysis pubis with the bladder neck resting on the pubococcygeus muscle. A fibrous band called the urachus extends from the apex of the bladder to the umbilicus.

Structure

The base of the bladder is termed the trigone. It is situated at the back of the bladder, resting against the vagina. Its three angles are the exit of the urethra below and the two slit-like openings of the ureters above. The apex of the trigone is thus at its lowest point, which is also termed the neck (Fig. 9.8).

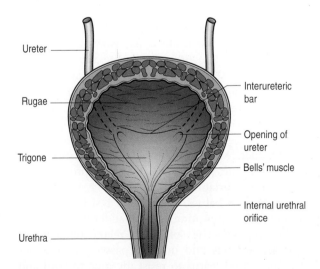

Figure 9.8 Section through the bladder.

The anterior part of the bladder lies close to the symphysis pubis and is termed the apex of the bladder. From it, the urachus runs up the anterior abdominal wall to the umbilicus. In fetal life, this is the remains of the yolk sac but in the adult is simply a fibrous band.

Layers

The lining of the bladder, like that of the ureter, is formed of transitional epithelium, which helps to allow the distension of the bladder without losing its water-holding effect. The lining, except over the trigone, is thrown into rugae, which flatten out as the bladder expands and fills. The mucous membrane lining lies on a submucous layer of areolar tissue that carries blood and lymph vessels and nerves.

The epithelium over the trigone is smooth and firmly attached to the underlying muscle.

The musculature of the bladder consists chiefly of the large detrusor muscle whose function is to expel urine. This muscle has an inner longitudinal, a middle circular and an outer longitudinal layer. Around the neck of the bladder, the circular muscle is thickened to form the internal urethral sphincter. The general elasticity of the numerous muscle fibres around the bladder neck tend to keep the urethra closed (Standring et al 2004). In the trigone, the muscles are somewhat differently arranged. A band of muscle between the ureteric apertures forms the interureteric bar. The urethral dilator muscle lies in the ventral part of the bladder neck and the walls of the urethra; it is thought to be of significance in overcoming urethral resistance to micturition (Standring et al 2004).

The outer layer of the bladder is formed of visceral pelvic fascia, except on its superior surface, which is covered with peritoneum (Fig. 9.7).

Blood supply

The vesical arteries are the main suppliers of blood. A few small branches from the uterine and vaginal arteries also bring blood to the bladder. Venous return is through corresponding veins.

Lymphatic drainage

Lymph drains into the internal iliac and the obturator glands.

Nerve supply

The nerve supply is parasympathetic and sympathetic and comes via the Lee-Frankenhäuser pelvic plexus in the pouch of Douglas. The stimulation of sympathetic nerves causes the internal urethral sphincter to contract and the detrusor muscle to relax, whereas the parasympathetic nerve fibres cause the sphincter to relax and the bladder to empty.

The urethra

The final passage in the urinary tract is the urethra, which is 4 cm long in the female and consists of a narrow tube buried in the outer layers of the anterior vaginal wall. It runs from the neck of the bladder and opens into the vestibule of the vulva as the urethral meatus. During labour, the urethra becomes elongated as the bladder is drawn up into the abdomen; becoming as much as several centimetres longer.

Structure

The urethra forms the junction between the urinary tract and the external genitalia. The epithelium of its lining reflects this. The upper half is lined with transitional epithelium whereas the lower half is lined with squamous epithelium. The lumen is normally closed unless urine is passing down it or a catheter is in situ. When closed, it has small longitudinal folds. Small blind ducts called urethral crypts open into the urethra, of which the two largest are Skene's ducts, which open just beside the urethral meatus. There is the possibility of them becoming infected with an organism such as the gonococcus.

The submucous coat of the urethra is composed of epithelium, which lies on a bed of vascular connective tissue.

The musculature is arranged as an inner longitudinal layer, continuous with the inner muscle fibres of the bladder, and an external circular layer. The inner muscle fibres help to open the internal urethral sphincter during micturition.

The outer layer of the urethra is continuous with the outer layer of the vagina and is formed of connective tissue.

At the lower end of the urethra, voluntary, striated muscle fibres form the so-called membranous sphincter of the urethra. This is not a true sphincter but it gives some voluntary control to the woman when she desires to resist the urge to urinate. The powerful levator ani muscles, which pass on either side of the uterus, also assist in controlling continence of urine.

Blood supply

The blood to the urethra is circulated by the inferior vesical and pudendal arteries and veins.

Lymphatic drainage

Lymph drains through the internal iliac glands.

Nerve supply

The internal urethral sphincter is supplied by sympathetic and parasympathetic nerves but the membranous sphincter is supplied by the pudendal nerve and is under voluntary control.

Micturition

The bladder fills and then contracts as a reflex response. The internal sphincter opens by the action of Bell's muscles (Fig. 9.8). If the urge is not resisted, the external sphincter relaxes and the bladder empties. This action, known as micturition, may be speeded by raising intra-abdominal pressure either to initiate the process or throughout voiding.

The urge to pass urine is felt when the bladder contains about 200–300 mL of urine, but also when psychological stimuli operate such as waking after sleep, arriving or leaving home, and from external stimuli such as the sound and feel of water and the feel of the toilet seat. Helpless laughter or paroxysmal coughing may also trigger a desire to empty the bladder. Micturition can be temporarily postponed but the full bladder becomes progressively more uncomfortable.

In newborn babies, there is no resistance to the spontaneous prompting of the bladder that it wishes to be emptied. The sphincters relax, the detrusor muscle contracts and urine is passed. After about 2 years a child learns to resist the urge to void and by adulthood it is taken for granted. Many women, particularly pregnant and parous women, have trouble in maintaining continence under the stress of coughing, laughing, sneezing and other factors that raise intra-abdominal pressure. Regular muscular exercise such as walking, swimming, running and pelvic floor exercises help to raise the tone of the voluntary muscles.

Changes to the urinary tract in pregnancy

In pregnancy, the enlarging uterus affects all the parts of the urinary tract (see Ch. 14) at various times with the hormones of pregnancy having an even greater influence than the mechanical effects. For instance, progesterone relaxes the walls of the ureters and allows dilatation and kinking (Fig. 9.9). In some women, this is quite marked and it tends to result in a slowing down or stasis of urinary flow, making infection a greater possibility. In addition, large amounts of urine are produced because in pregnancy, glomerular filtration is increased as it helps to eliminate the additional wastes created by maternal and fetal metabolism. In the first post-partum days, there is a rapid and sustained loss of sodium and a major diuresis occurs. A midwife will commonly observe a woman who has recently given birth voiding upwards of 1 L on a single occasion.

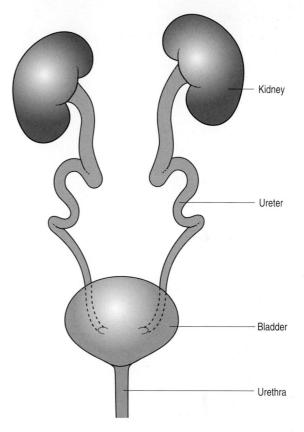

Kidney

Ureter

Bladder

Urethra

Figure 9.9 Dilated, kinked ureters in pregnancy.

REFERENCES

Drake R L, Wayne V, Mitchell A D M 2005 Gray's anatomy for students. Churchill Livingstone, Edinburgh, p 320–327

Epstein M 1997 Alcohol's impact on kidney function. Alcohol Health & Research World 21(1):84–93. Online. Available:

http://pubs.niaaa.nih.gov/publications/arh21-1/84.pdf 22nd April 2007

Standring S, Healy J, Johnson D et al 2004 Gray's anatomy: the anatomical basis of clinical practice, 39th edn. Churchill Livingstone, New York

---

FURTHER READING

Beischer N A, Mackay E V 1997 Obstetrics and the newborn, 3rd edn. W B Saunders, London

Chapter 38 in this book offers an account of changes in pregnancy with radiological/ultrasound illustrations, as well as addressing urinary tract problems associated with childbearing.

Coad J, with Dunstall M 2005 Anatomy and physiology for midwives, 2nd edn. Churchill Livingstone, Edinburgh

Chapter 2 of this book gives a very accessible account of the urinary system and a number of examples of clinical applications. A stylized diagram of urine production may help the individual who learns best from visual representation.

Stables D, Rankin J 2004 Physiology in childbearing with anatomy and related biosciences, 2nd edn. Baillière Tindall, Edinburgh

This text offers a fuller account of the urinary system, including changes in pregnancy and a short account of the postnatal period.

10 Hormonal cycles: fertilization and early development

Iolanda G. J. Serci

CHAPTER CONTENTS

Monthly physiological changes take place in the ovaries and the uterus, regulated by hormones produced by the hypothalamus, pituitary gland and ovaries. These cycles commence at puberty and occur simultaneously and together are known as the female reproductive cycle. The functions of the cycle are to prepare the *egg* often referred to as the *gamete* or *oocyte* for fertilization by the *spermatozoon* (sperm), and to prepare the uterus to receive and nourish the fertilized egg. If fertilization has not taken place the inner lining of the uterus or endometrium and the egg are shed and bleeding occurs per vagina, and the cyclic events begin again.

The first-ever occurrence of cyclic events is termed *menarche*, meaning the first menstrual bleeding. The average age of menarche is 12 years, although between the ages 8 and 16 is considered normal. Factors such as heredity, diet and overall health can accelerate or delay menarche. Interference with the hormonal-organ relationship during the reproductive years is likely to cause menstrual cycle dysfunction which may result in failure to ovulate. The cessation of cyclic events is referred to as the *menopause*, and signifies the end of reproductive life. Each woman has an individual reproductive cycle that varies in length, although the average cycle is normally 28 days long, and recurs regularly from puberty to the menopause except when pregnancy intervenes (Fig. 10.1).

The ovarian cycle

The ovarian cycle (Fig. 10.2) is the name given to the physiological changes that occur in the ovaries essential for the preparation and release of an oocyte.

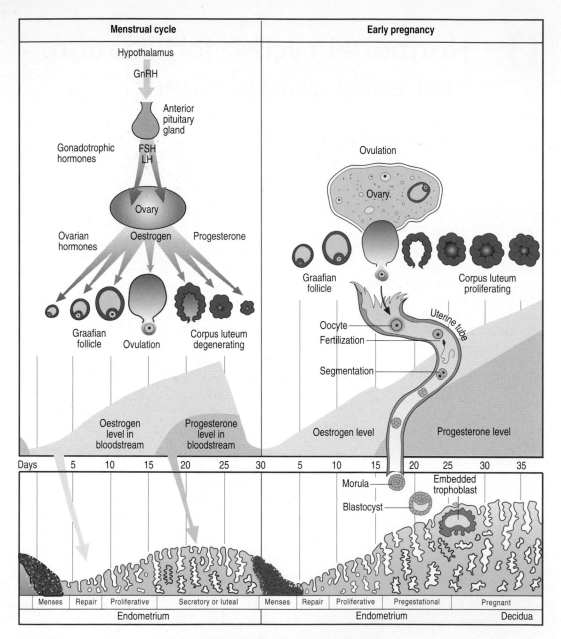

Figure 10.1   The female reproductive cycle.

The ovarian cycle consists of three phases, all of which are under the control of hormones.

The follicular phase

Throughout the year small *primordial follicles* containing primary oocytes, have been developing into large *preovulatory or Graafian follicles* containing secondary oocytes (Fig. 10.3), in a process known as *folliculo-genesis* (oocytes undergo *mitosis* (cell division) prior to birth and until puberty in a process known as *oogenesis*).

Low levels of oestrogen and progesterone stimulate the hypothalamus to produce gonadotrophin releasing hormone (GnRH). This releasing hormone

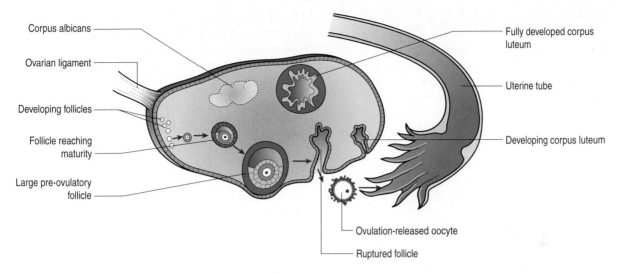

Figure 10.2   The cycle of a Graafian follicle in the ovary.

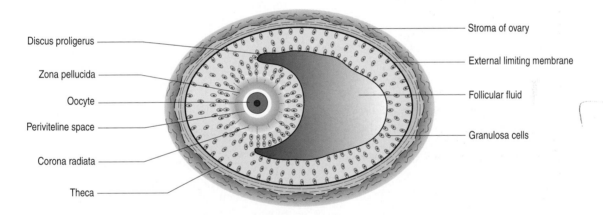

Figure 10.3   A ripe Graafian follicle.

causes the production of follicle stimulating hormone (FSH) and luteinizing hormone (LH) by the anterior pituitary gland. FSH controls the growth and maturity of the Graafian follicles. The Graafian follicles begin to secrete oestrogen, which comprises oestradiol, oestrone and oestriol. Rising levels of oestradiol cause a surge in LH. When oestradiol reaches a certain peak, the secretion of FSH is inhibited. The reduced FSH secretion causes a slowing in follicle growth and eventually leads to follicle death, known as *atresia*. The largest and dominant follicle secretes *inhibin*, which further suppresses FSH. This dominant follicle prevails and forms a bulge near

the surface of the ovary, and soon becomes competent to ovulate. The time from the growth and maturity of the Graafian follicles to ovulation is normally around 1 week, day 5–14 of a 28-day cycle of events. Occasionally the follicular phase may take longer if the dominant follicle does not ovulate and the phase will begin again.

Ovulation

Ovulation is the process whereby the dominant follicle ruptures and discharges the secondary oocyte into the uterine tube where it awaits fertilization. Ovulation is stimulated by a sudden surge in LH which matures the oocyte and weakens the wall of the follicle. This LH surge occurs around day 12–13 of a 28-day cycle and lasts 48hrs. Stringy clear mucus appears in the cervix, ready to accept the sperm from intercourse. During ovulation some women experience varying degrees of abdominal pain known as *mittelschmerz*, which can last several hours. There may be some light bleeding caused by the hormonal changes taking place. Following ovulation the fertilized or unfertilized oocyte travels to the uterus.

The luteal phase

The *luteal phase* is the process whereby the cells of the residual ruptured follicle proliferate and form a yellow irregular structure known as the *corpus luteum*. The corpus luteum produces oestrogen and progesterone for approximately 2 weeks, to develop the endometrium of the uterus, which awaits the fertilized oocyte. The corpus luteum continues its role until the placenta is adequately developed to take over. In the absence of fertilization the corpus luteum degenerates and becomes the corpus albicans (white body), and progesterone and oestrogen, and inhibin levels decrease. In response to low levels of oestrogen and progesterone the hypothalamus produces GnRH. The rising levels of GnRH stimulate the anterior pituitary gland to produce FSH and the ovarian cycle commences again (Stables and Rankin 2004).

The menstrual or endometrial cycle

The *menstrual cycle* is the name given to the physiological changes that occur in the uterus, and which are essential to receive the fertilized oocyte. The menstrual cycle consists of three phases.

The menstrual phase

This phase is often referred to as *menstruation, bleeding, menses,* or a *period*. Physiologically this is the terminal phase of the reproductive cycle of events and is simultaneous with the beginning of the follicular phase of the ovarian cycle. The spiral arteries of the endometrium go into spasm withdrawing the blood supply to it, and the endometrium dies, referred to as *necrosis*. The endometrium is shed down to the basal layer along with blood from the capillaries and the unfertilized oocyte. Failure to menstruate is an indication that a woman may have become pregnant. The term *eumenorrhea* denotes normal, regular menstruation that lasts for typically 3–5 days, although 2–7 days is considered normal. The average blood loss during menstruation is 50–150mL. The blood is inhibited from clotting due to the enzyme plasmin contained in the endometrium. The term *menorrhagia* denotes heavy bleeding.

Some women experience uterine cramps caused by muscular contractions to expel the tissue. Severe uterine cramps are known as *dysmenorrhea*.

The proliferative phase

This phase follows menstruation, is simultaneous with the follicular phase and lasts until ovulation. There is the formation of a new layer of endometrium in the uterus, referred to as the proliferative endometrium. This phase is under the control of oestradiol and other oestrogens secreted by the Graafian follicle and consist of the re-growth and thickening of the endometrium in the uterus. During the first few days of this phase the endometrium is re-forming, described as in the *regenerative phase*. At the completion of this phase the endometrium consists of three layers. The *basal layer* lies immediately above the myometrium and is approximately 1mm thick. It contains all the necessary rudimentary structures for building new endometrium. The *functional layer*, which contains tubular glands, is approximately 2.5mm thick, and lies on top of the basal layer. It changes constantly according to the hormonal influences of the ovary. The *layer of cuboidal ciliated epithelium* covers the functional layer. It dips down to line the tubular glands of the functional layer. If fertilization occurs, the fertilized oocyte implants itself within the endometrium.

The secretory phase

This phase follows the proliferative phase and is simultaneous with ovulation. It is under the influence of progesterone and oestrogen secreted by the corpus luteum. The functional layer of the endometrium thickens to approximately 3.5mm and becomes spongy in appearance because the glands are more tortuous. The blood supply to the area is increased and the glands produce nutritive secretions such as glycogen. These conditions last for approximately 7 days, awaiting the fertilized oocyte.

Fertilization

Human fertilization, known as conception, is the fusion of the sperm with the secondary oocyte, to form the zygote (Fig. 10.4). The process takes approximately 24 hrs and normally occurs in the ampulla of the uterine tube. Following ovulation, the oocyte, which is about 0.15 mm in diameter, passes into the uterine tube. The oocyte, having no power of loco-motion, is wafted along by the cilia and by the peristaltic muscular contraction of the uterine tube. At the same time the cervix which is under the influence of oestrogen, secretes a flow of alkaline mucus that attracts the spermatozoa. In the fertile male at intercourse approximately 300 million sperm are deposited in the posterior fornix of the vagina. Those that reach the loose cervical mucus survive and propel themselves towards the uterine tubes while the rest are destroyed by the acid medium of the vagina. Once inside the uterine tubes the sperm undergo a process known as *capacitation*. Influenced by

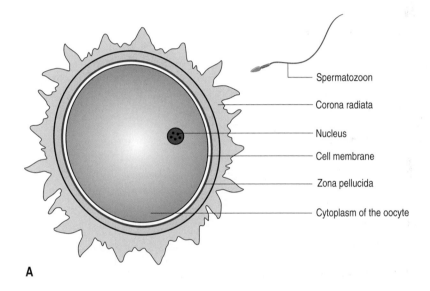

- Spermatozoon
- Corona radiata
- Nucleus
- Cell membrane
- Zona pellucida
- Cytoplasm of the oocyte

A

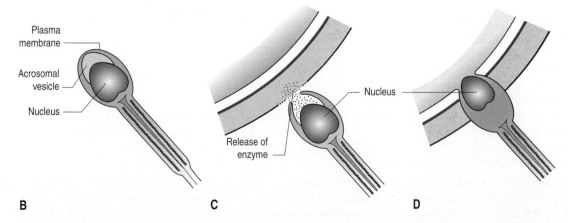

Plasma membrane

Acrosomal vesicle

Nucleus

Release of enzyme

Nucleus

B　　　　**C**　　　　**D**

Figure 10.4　Fertilization. Diagrammatic representation of the fusion of the oocyte and the spermatozoon. (Note that B, C and D are more greatly magnified than A.)

secretions from the uterine tube the sperm undergo changes to the plasma membrane, resulting in the removal of the glycoprotein coat. The acrosomal layer of the sperm becomes reactive and releases the enzyme hyaluronidase known as the *acrosome reaction*, which disperses the corona radiata (the outermost layer of the oocyte) allowing access to the zona pellucida (Fig. 10.4C). The first sperm that reaches the zona pellucida penetrates it (Fig. 10.4D). Penetration of the zona pellucida occurs with the aid of several enzymes processed by the sperm which break down the proteins of the zona layer. Upon penetration a chemical reaction known as the *cortical reaction* occurs. The cortical reaction alters the zona pellucida making it impermeable to other sperm. The plasma membranes of the sperm and oocyte fuse. The oocyte at this stage completes its second meiotic division, and becomes mature. The pronucleus now has 23 chromosomes, referred to as *haploid*. The tail and mitochondria of the sperm degenerate as the sperm penetrates the oocyte, and there is the formation of the male pronucleus. The male and female pronuclei fuse to form a new nucleus that is a combination of the genetic material from both the sperm and oocyte, referred to as a *diploid* cell. The male and the female gametes each contribute half the complement of chromosomes to make a total of 46 (Box 10.1). This new cell is called a *zygote*.

Development of the zygote

The development of the zygote can be divided into three periods. The first 2 weeks after fertilization referred to as the *pre-embryonic period* includes the implantation of the zygote into the endometrium; weeks 2–8 are known as the *embryonic period*; and weeks 8 to birth, are known as the *fetal period*.

The pre-embryonic period

During the first week the zygote travels along the uterine tube towards the uterus. At this stage a strong membrane of glycoproteins called the zona pellucida surrounds the zygote. The zygote receives nourishment, mainly glycogen, from the goblet cells of the uterine tubes and later the secretory cells of the uterus. During the travel the zygote undergoes mitotic cellular replication and division referred to as *cleavage*, resulting in the formation of smaller cells known as *blastomeres*. The zygote divides into two cells at 1 day, then four at 2 days, eight by 2.5 days, 16 by 3 days, now known as the *morula*. The cells bind tightly together in a process known as *compactation*. Next *cavitation* occurs whereby the outermost cells secrete fluid into the morula and a fluid-filled cavity or *blastocele* appears in the morula. This results in the formation of the blastula or *blastocyst*, comprising 58 cells. The process from the development

---

Box 10.1 Chromosomes

Each human cell has a complement of 46 chromosomes arranged in 23 pairs, of which two are sex chromosomes. The remainder are known as autosomes. During the process of maturation, both gametes shed half their chromosomes, one of each pair, during a reduction division called *meiosis*. Genetic material is exchanged between the chromosomes before they split up. In the male, meiosis starts at puberty and both halves redivide to form four sperm in all. In the female, meiosis commences during fetal life but the first division is not completed until many years later at ovulation. The division is unequal; the larger part will eventually go on to form the oocyte while the remainder forms the first polar body. At fertilization the second division takes place and results in one large cell, which is now mature, and a much smaller one, the second polar body. At the same time, division of the first polar body creates a third polar body.

When the gametes combine at fertilization to form the zygote, the full complement of chromosomes is restored. Subsequent division occurs by mitosis where the chromosomes divide to give each new cell a full set.

Sex determination

Females carry two similar sex chromosomes, XX; males carry two dissimilar sex chromosomes, XY. Each sperm will carry either an X or a Y chromosome, whereas the oocyte always carries an X chromosome. If the oocyte is fertilized by an X-carrying sperm a female is conceived, if by a Y-carrying one, a male.

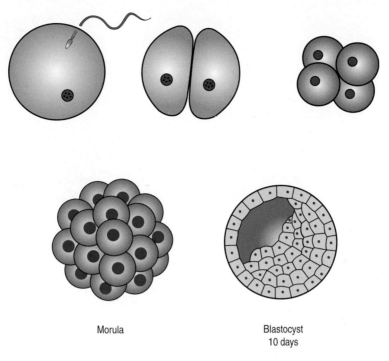

Morula

Blastocyst
10 days

Figure 10.5   Diagrammatic representation of the development of the zygote.

of the morula to the development of the blastocyst is referred to as *blastulation* and has occurred by around day 4 (Fig. 10.5). The surrounding zona pellucida begins to disintegrate and the volume of fluid increases. Around days 3–5 the blastocyst enters the uterus. The blastocyst possesses an *inner cell mass* or *embryoblast*, and an *outer cell mass* or *trophoblast*. The trophoblast becomes the placenta and chorion, while the embryoblast becomes the embryo, amnion and umbilical cord (Carlson 2004).

During week 2, the trophoblast proliferates and differentiates into 2 layers: the outer *syncytio-trophoblast* or *syncytium* and the inner *cytotrophoblast* (cuboidal dividing cells) (Fig. 10.6). Implantation of the trophoblast layer into the endometrium now known as the *decidua* begins (see Ch. 11). Implanta-tion is usually to the upper posterior wall. At the implantation stage the zona pellucida will have totally disappeared. The syncytiotrophoblast layer invades the decidua by forming finger-like projec-tions called *villi* that make their way into the decidua and spaces called *lacunae* that fill up with the mother's blood. The villi begin to branch, and con-tain blood vessels of the developing embryo, thus allowing gaseous exchange between the mother and embryo. Implantation is assisted by hydrolytic enzymes secreted by the syncytiotrophoblast cells that erode the decidua and assist with the nutrition of the embryo. The syncytiotrophoblast cells also produce human chorionic gonadotrophin (hCG), a hormone that prevents menstruation and maintains pregnancy by sustaining the function of the corpus luteum.

Simultaneously to implantation, the embryo is developing from the embryoblast. The cells of the embryoblast differentiate into two types of cells: the *epiblast* (closest to the trophoblast) and the *hypo-blast* (closest to the blastocyst cavity). The epiblast cells give rise to cells of the embryo. Each layer of epiblast cells, of which there are three, will form par-ticular parts of the embryo. The first appearance of these layers, collectively known as the *primitive streak*, is around day 15.

- The **ectoderm** is the start of tissue that covers most surfaces of the body: the epidermis layer of the skin, hair and nails. Additionally it forms the nervous system.

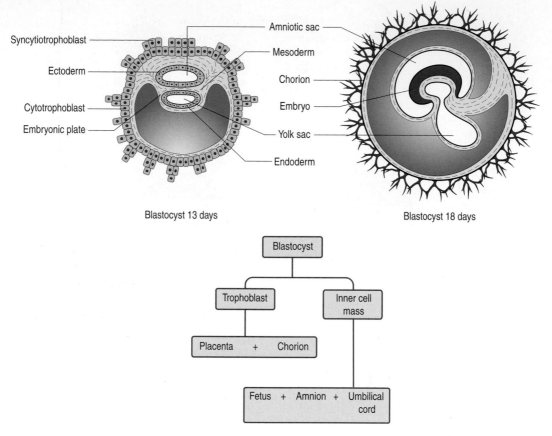

Blastocyst 13 days

Blastocyst 18 days

Figure 10.6 The development of the blastocyst.

- The **mesoderm** forms the muscle, skeleton, dermis of skin, connective tissue, the urogenital glands, blood vessels and blood and lymph cells.

- The **endoderm** forms the epithelia lining of the digestive, respiratory and urinary systems, and glandular cells of organs such as the liver and pancreas.

The epiblast separates from the trophoblast and forms a cavity, known as the *amniotic cavity*. The amniotic cavity derives from the ectoderm layer. The cavity is filled with fluid, and gradually enlarges and folds around the developing structures of the embryo to enclose it. The amnion forms from the lining of the cavity. It swells out into the *chorionic cavity* and eventually obliterates it when the amniotic and chorionic membranes come into contact.

The hypoblast layer of the embryoblast gives rise to extra-embryonic structures only, such as, the yolk sac. Hypoblast cells migrate along the inner cytotrophoblast lining of the blastocele secreting extracellular tissue which becomes the yolk sac. The yolk sac is lined with extraembryonic endoderm, which in turn is lined with extraembryonic mesoderm. The yolk sac serves as a primary nutritive function, carrying nutrients and oxygen to the embryo. The endoderm and mesoderm cells contribute to the formation of some organs, such as the primitive gut arising out of the endoderm cells; blood islands which later go on to develop blood cells arise from the mesodermal layer; the remainder resembles a balloon floating in front of the embryo until it atrophies by the end of the 6th week when blood forming activity transfers to embryonic sites. After birth, all that remains of the yolk sac is a vestigial structure in the base of the umbilical cord, known as the *vitelline duct*.

The pre-embryonic period is crucial in terms of initiation and maintenance of the pregnancy and early embryonic development. Inability to implant properly results in miscarriage. Additionally chromosomal defects and abnormalities in structure and organs can occur during this time (Moore & Persaud 2003).

REFERENCES

Carlson B M 2004 Human embryology and developmental biology, 3d edn. Mosby, Philadelphia

Moore K L, Persaud T V N 2003 Before we are born, essentials of embryology and birth defects, 6th edn. Saunders, London

Stables D, Rankin J 2004 Physiology in childbearing, 2nd edn. Elsevier, London

FURTHER READING

Coad J, with Dunstall M 2001 Anatomy and physiology for midwives. Mosby, Edinburgh

A very full and clear explanation of endocrine activity is given in Chapter 3. Chapter 4 addresses the reproductive cycles in similar detail with clear diagrams to assist the reader.

Johnson M H, Everitt B J 2000 Essential reproduction, 5th edn. Blackwell Science, Oxford

This authoritative volume provides the interested reader with a much greater depth of information than is possible in the present book and is recommended for those who wish to study the hormonal patterns of reproduction in detail.

11 The placenta

Mary E. Vance

The placenta is a complex organ, which originates from the trophoblastic layer of the fertilized ovum. When fully developed it serves as the interface between the mother and the developing fetus carrying out functions that the fetus is unable to perform for itself during intrauterine life. The survival of the fetus depends upon the placenta's integrity and efficiency.

Early development

Within a few days of fertilization, the zygote (see Ch. 10) develops into a blastocyst, a spherical structure composed of two distinct cell types, the inner cell mass, which will develop into the fetus and an outer ring of trophoblast cells, which will develop into the placenta and membranes. By 8 days, the trophoblasts begin to make human chorionic gonadotrophin (hCG), a hormone that ensures that the endometrium will be receptive to the implanting embryo.

Implantation

Once the blastocyst makes contact with the endometrium, the trophoblast layer adheres to the endometrial surface and the process of placentation begins (Fig. 11.1). By 10 days, the blastocyst is completely buried in the endometrium, which is now called the decidua.

The trophoblasts have a potent invasive capacity, which if left unchecked would spread throughout the uterus. This potential is moderated by the decidua, which secretes cytokines and protease inhibitors that modulate trophoblast invasion.

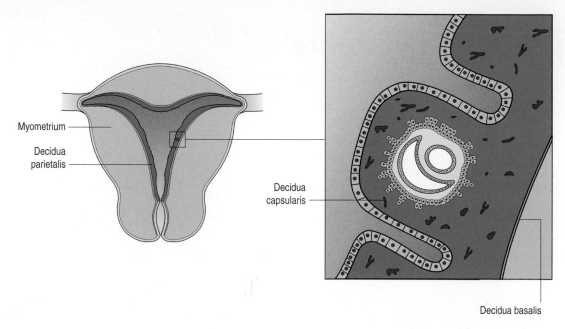

Figure 11.1   Early implantation of the blastocyst.

Chorionic villi

Initially the blastocyst appears to be covered by fine, downy hair, which consists of the projections from the trophoblastic layer. These proliferate and branch from about 3 weeks after fertilization, forming the *chorionic villi*. The villi become most profuse in the area where the blood supply is richest, the *decidua basalis*. This part of the trophoblast, which is known as the *chorion frondosum*, eventually develops into the placenta. The portion of decidua surrounding the blastocyst, where it projects into the uterine cavity, is known as the *decidua capsularis*. The villi under the decidua capsularis gradually degenerate forming the *chorion laeve*, which is the origin of the chorionic membrane (Fig. 11.2). The remaining decidua is known as the *decidua parietalis*. As the fetus enlarges and grows to fill the uterus the decidua capsularis thins and disappears and the chorion meets the decidua parietalis on the opposite wall of the uterus.

The villi erode the walls of maternal blood vessels as they penetrate the decidua, opening them up to form a lake of maternal blood in which they float. The opened blood vessels are known as sinuses, and the areas surrounding the villi as blood spaces. The maternal blood circulates slowly, enabling the villi to absorb food and oxygen and excrete waste. These are

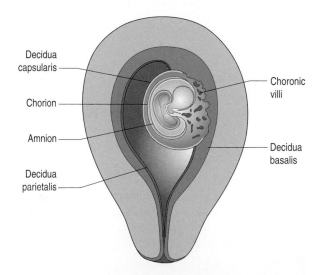

Figure 11.2   Implantation site at 3 weeks.

known as the *nutritive* villi. A few villi are more deeply attached to the decidua and are called *anchoring* villi.

Each chorionic villus is a branching structure arising from one stem. Its centre consists of mesoderm and fetal blood vessels, and branches of the umbilical artery and vein. These are covered by a single

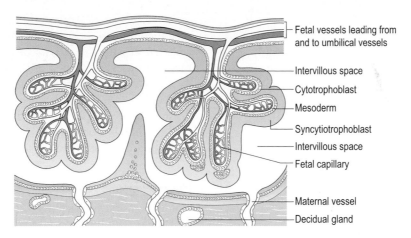

Fetal vessels leading from
and to umbilical vessels

Intervillous space

Cytotrophoblast

Mesoderm

Syncytiotrophoblast

Intervillous space

Fetal capillary

Maternal vessel

Decidual gland

Figure 11.3   Chorionic villi.

layer of *cytotrophoblast* cells and the external layer of the villus is the *syncytiotrophoblast* (Fig. 11.3). This means that four layers of tissue separate the maternal blood from the fetal blood making it impossible for the two circulations to mix unless any villi are damaged.

The mature placenta

The placenta is completely formed and functioning 10 weeks after fertilization. Between 12 and 20 weeks' gestation, the placenta weighs more than the fetus because the fetal organs are insufficiently developed to cope with the metabolic processes of nutrition. Later in pregnancy, some of the fetal organs, such as the liver, begin to function, so the cytotrophoblast and the syncytiotrophoblast gradually degenerate and this allows easier exchange of oxygen and carbon dioxide.

Functions

The placenta performs a variety of functions for the developing fetus.

Respiration

During intrauterine life, no pulmonary exchange of gases can take place so the fetus must obtain oxygen and excrete carbon dioxide through the placenta. Oxygen from the mother's haemoglobin passes into the fetal blood by simple diffusion; similarly, the fetus gives off carbon dioxide into the maternal blood.

Nutrition

The fetus needs nutrients for growth and development. For instance, amino acids are required for body building, large quantities of glucose for energy and growth, calcium and phosphorus for bones and teeth, and iron and other minerals for blood formation. These nutrients are actively transferred from the maternal to the fetal blood through the walls of the villi. The placenta is able to select those substances required by the fetus, even depleting the mother's own supply in some instances.

Water, vitamins and minerals also pass to the fetus. Fats and fat-soluble vitamins (A, D and E) cross the placenta only with difficulty and mainly in the later stages of pregnancy. Some substances, including amino acids, are found at higher levels in the fetal blood than in the maternal blood.

Storage

The placenta metabolizes glucose, stores it in the form of glycogen and reconverts it to glucose as required. It can also store iron and the fat-soluble vitamins.

Excretion

The main substance excreted from the fetus is carbon dioxide. Bilirubin will also be excreted as red blood cells are replaced relatively frequently. There is very little tissue breakdown apart from this and the amounts of urea and uric acid excreted are very small.

Protection

The placenta provides a limited barrier to infection. Few bacteria can penetrate with the exception of the treponema of syphilis and the tubercle bacillus. However, substances including alcohol, some chemicals associated with smoking cigarettes and several types of viruses, such as human cytomegalovirus and rubella are not filtered out. These substances can cross the placental barrier freely and may cause congenital abnormalities.

Although some drugs will cross the placental barrier to the fetus, many will be harmless and others, such as antibiotics administered to a pregnant woman with syphilis, are positively beneficial. However, there are exceptions (see Ch. 49).

Towards the end of pregnancy, antibodies in the form of immunoglobulin G (IgG) are transferred across the placental barrier to the fetus conferring passive immunity on the baby for the first 3 months of extrauterine life. However, it is important to realize that only those antibodies that the mother herself possesses can be passed on.

Endocrine

Human chorionic gonadotrophin (hCG) is produced by the cytotrophoblastic layer of the chorionic villi. Initially it is present in very large quantities, peak levels being achieved between the 7th and 10th week, but these gradually reduce as the pregnancy advances. hCG forms the basis of the many pregnancy tests available, as it is excreted in the mother's urine. Its function is to stimulate the growth and activity of the corpus luteum.

Oestrogens are growth stimulating hormones, which are secreted in large amounts throughout pregnancy. They are produced by the placenta as the activity of the corpus luteum declines, the fetus providing the placenta with the vital precursors for their production. The amount of oestrogen produced (measured as urinary or serum oestriol) is an index of fetoplacental well-being.

Progesterone is made in the syncytial layer of the placenta in increasing quantities until immediately before the onset of labour when its level falls. It may be measured in the urine as pregnanediol. The main function of progesterone is to act on tissues that have already been receptive to oestrogen.

Human placental lactogen (hPL) has a role in glucose metabolism in pregnancy. It appears to have a connection with the activity of human growth hormone, although it does not itself promote growth. As the level of hCG falls, so the level of hPL rises and continues to do so throughout pregnancy. Monitoring the level of hPL with the intention of assessing placental function has been disappointing in predicting fetal outcome.

Placental circulation

Maternal blood is discharged in a pulsatile fashion into the intervillous space by 80–100 spiral arteries in the decidua basalis. It spurts toward the chorionic plate and flows slowly around the villi, eventually returning to the endometrial veins and the maternal circulation. There are about 150 mL of maternal blood in the intervillous spaces, which is exchanged 3 or 4 times/min.

Fetal blood, low in oxygen, is pumped by the fetal heart towards the placenta along the umbilical arteries and transported along their branches to the capillaries of the chorionic villi where exchange of nutrients takes place between the mother and fetus. Having yielded up carbon dioxide and waste products and absorbed oxygen and nutrients, the blood is returned to the fetus via the umbilical vein (Fig. 11.4).

The membranes

There are two membranes, an outer membrane, the *chorion*, and an inner membrane, the *amnion*. As long as the membranes remain intact, they protect the fetus against ascending bacterial infection.

The chorion is a thick opaque friable membrane derived from the trophoblast. It is continuous with the chorionic plate, which forms the base of the placenta and adheres closely to the uterine wall.

The amnion is a smooth tough translucent membrane derived from the inner cell mass. It lines the chorion and the surface of the placenta continuing over the outer surface of the umbilical cord. When first formed the amnion is in contact with the embryo, but 4–5 weeks after conception the amniotic fluid begins to accumulate within it.

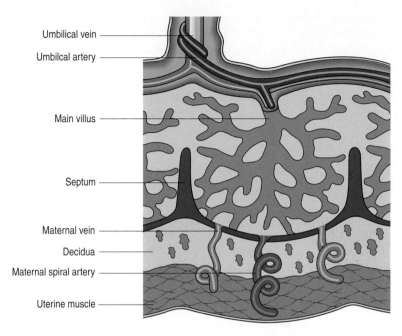

Umbilical vein

Umbilcal artery

Main villus

Septum

Maternal vein

Decidua

Maternal spiral artery

Uterine muscle

Figure 11.4 Blood flow around chorionic villi.

Amniotic fluid

Amniotic fluid is a clear alkaline and slightly yellowish liquid contained within the amniotic sac.

Functions

Amniotic fluid distends the amniotic sac allowing for the growth and free movement of the fetus and permitting symmetrical musculoskeletal development. It equalizes pressure and protects the fetus from jarring and injury. The fluid maintains a constant intrauterine temperature, protecting the fetus from heat loss and providing small quantities of nutrients to the fetus. In labour, as long as the membranes remain intact it protects the placenta and umbilical cord from the pressure of uterine contractions. It also aids effacement of the cervix and dilatation of the uterine os, particularly where the presenting part is poorly applied.

Origin

The source of amniotic fluid is thought to be both fetal and maternal. Some fluid is exuded from maternal vessels in the decidua and some from fetal vessels in the placenta. It is secreted by the amnion, especially the part covering the placenta and umbilical cord. Fetal urine also contributes to the volume from the 10th week of gestation onwards. The water in amniotic fluid is exchanged approximately 3-hourly.

Constituents

Amniotic fluid consists of 99% water with the remaining 1% being dissolved solid matter including food substances and waste products. In addition, the fetus sheds skin cells, *vernix caseosa* and *lanugo* into the fluid. Abnormal constituents of the liquor, such as *meconium* in the case of fetal compromise, may give valuable diagnostic information about the condition of the fetus. Aspiration of amniotic fluid for examination is termed *amniocentesis*.

Research has found that amniotic fluid is a plentiful source of non-embryonic stem cells (De Coppi et al 2007). These cells have demonstrated the ability to differentiate into a number of different cell-types, including brain, liver and bone.

Volume

During pregnancy, amniotic fluid increases in volume as the fetus grows. The volume is greatest at approximately 38 weeks' gestation, when there is about 1 L. It then diminishes slightly until term, when approximately 800 mL remains.

There are very wide variations in the amount, however if the total amount of fluid exceeds 1500 mL, the condition is known as *polyhydramnios* and if less than 300 mL, *oligohydramnios*. Such abnormalities are often associated with congenital malformations of the fetus (see Ch. 46).

The umbilical cord

The umbilical cord, which extends from the fetal surface of the placenta to the umbilical area of the fetus, is formed by the 5th week of pregnancy. It originates from the duct that forms between the amniotic sac and the yolk sac and transmits the umbilical blood vessels.

Functions

The umbilical cord transports oxygen and nutrients to the developing fetus, and removes waste products.

Structure

The umbilical cord contains two arteries and one vein (Fig. 11.5), which are continuous with the blood vessels in the chorionic villi of the placenta. The blood vessels are enclosed and protected by *Wharton's jelly*, a gelatinous substance formed from mesoderm. The whole cord is covered in a layer of amnion that is continuous with that covering the placenta. There are no nerves in the umbilical cord, so cutting it following the birth of the baby is not painful.

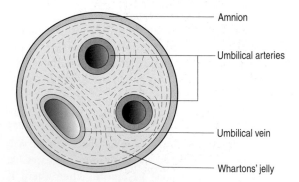

Figure 11.5 Cross-section through the umbilical cord.

The presence of only two vessels in the cord is sometimes related to abnormalities in the fetus, but may occur without accompanying abnormalities.

Measurements

The cord is approximately 1–2 cm in diameter and 40–50 cm in length. This length is sufficient to allow for the birth of the baby without applying any traction to the placenta.

A cord is considered short when it measures <40 cm. There is no specific agreed length for describing a cord as too long, but the disadvantages of a very long cord are that it may become wrapped round the neck or body of the fetus or become knotted. Either event could result in occlusion of the blood vessels, especially during labour.

Compromise of the fetal blood flow through the umbilical cord vessels can have serious deleterious effects on the health of the fetus and newborn. True knots should always be noted on examination of the cord, but they must be distinguished from false knots, which are lumps of Wharton's jelly on the side of the cord and are not significant.

The placenta at term

At term, the placenta is a round flat mass about 20 cm in diameter and 2.5 cm thick at its centre. It weighs approximately one-sixth of the baby's weight, although this proportion may be affected by the time at which the cord is clamped owing to the varying amounts of fetal blood retained in the vessels.

The maternal surface of the placenta is dark red in colour due to maternal blood and because part of the basal decidua will have been separated with it (Fig. 11.6A). The surface is arranged in about 20 cotyledons (lobes), which are separated by *sulci* (furrows), into which the decidua dips down to form *septa* (walls). The cotyledons are made up of lobules, each of which contains a single villus with its branches. Sometimes deposits of lime salts may be present on the surface, making it slightly gritty. This has no clinical significance.

The fetal surface of the placenta has a shiny appearance due to the amnion covering it (Fig. 11.6B). Branches of the umbilical vein and arteries are visible, spreading out from the insertion of the umbilical cord, which is normally in the centre. The amnion

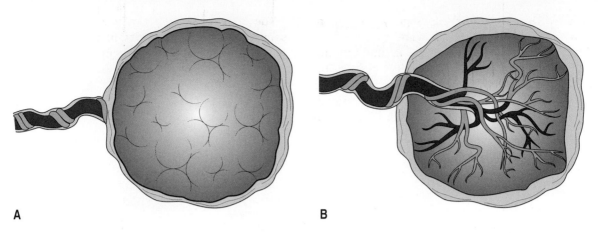

Figure 11.6 The placenta at term. (A) Maternal surface. (B) Fetal surface.

A

B

can be peeled off the surface of the chorion as far back as the umbilical cord, whereas the chorion, being derived from the same trophoblastic layer as the placenta, is continuous with the chorionic plate and cannot be separated from it.

Anatomical variations of the placenta and cord

A *succenturiate lobe* of placenta is the most significant of the variations in conformation of the placenta. A small extra lobe is present, separate from the main placenta, and joined to it by blood vessels that run through the membranes to reach it (Fig. 11.7). The danger is that this small lobe may be retained *in utero* after the placenta is delivered, and if it is not removed, it may lead to infection and haemorrhage. Every placenta must be examined for evidence of a retained succenturiate lobe, which can be identified by a hole in the membranes with vessels running to it.

In *circumvallate* placenta, an opaque ring is seen on the fetal surface of the placenta. It is formed by a doubling back of the chorion and amnion and may result in the membranes leaving the placenta nearer the centre instead of at the edge as usual (Fig. 11.8). This placental variation is associated with prematurity, prenatal bleeding, abruption, multiparity and early fluid loss.

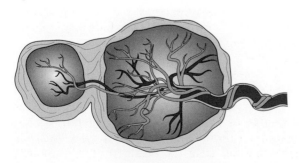

Figure 11.7 Succenturiate lobe of placenta.

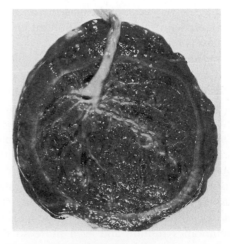

Figure 11.8 Circumvallate placenta.

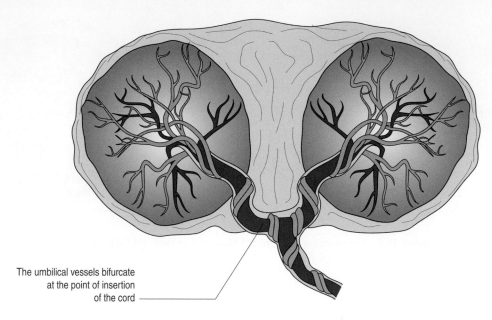

The umbilical vessels bifurcate at the point of insertion of the cord

Figure 11.9   Bipartite placenta.

In *bipartite placenta*, two complete and separate parts are present, each with a cord leaving from it. The bipartite cord joins a short distance from the two parts of the placenta (Fig. 11.9). This is different from the two placentas in a twin pregnancy, where there are also two separate umbilical cords. A *tripartite placenta* is similar to a bipartite placenta but it has three distinct parts.

In *battledore* insertion of the cord, the cord is attached at the very edge of the placenta in the manner of a table tennis bat. It is unimportant unless the attachment is fragile (Fig. 11.10).

A *velamentous* insertion of the cord, occurs when the cord is inserted into the membranes some distance from the edge of the placenta. The umbilical vessels run through the membranes from the cord to the placenta (Fig. 11.11). If the placenta is normally situated, no harm will result to the fetus, but the cord is likely to become detached upon applying traction during active management of the third stage of labour. However if the placenta is low-lying, the vessels may pass across the uterine os (*vasa praevia*). In this case, there is great danger to the fetus when the membranes rupture and even more so during artificial rupture, as the vessels may be torn, leading to rapid exsanguination of the fetus. If the onset of haemorrhage coincides with rupture of the membranes, fetal haemorrhage should be assumed and the birth expedited. It is possible to distinguish fetal blood from maternal blood by Singer's alkali-denaturation test, although, in practice, time is so short that it may not be possible to save the life of the baby. If the baby survives, haemoglobin levels should be estimated after birth.

Apart from the dangers noted above, these varieties of conformation have no clinical significance.

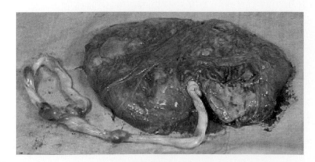

Figure 11.10   Battledore insertion of the cord.

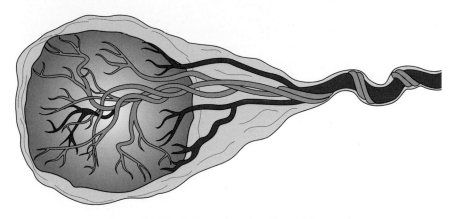

Figure 11.11 Velamentous insertion of the cord.

REFERENCES

De Coppi P, Bartsch G Jr, Siddiqui M M, et al 2007 Isolation of amniotic stem cell lines with potential for therapy. Nature Biotechnology 25(1):100–105.

FURTHER READING

Coad J, with Dunstall M 2005 Anatomy and physiology for midwives, 2nd edn. Churchill Livingstone, Edinburgh

Chapter 8 of this comprehensive text provides a detailed account of the placenta.

Johnson M H, Everitt B J 2000 Essential reproduction, 5th edn. Blackwell Science, Oxford

Chapter 10 of this volume provides detail about the development of the placenta and helps the reader to a fuller understanding of its function and the interdependence of maternal and fetal systems.

Oats J K, Abraham S 2005 Llewellyn-Jones fundamentals of obstetrics and gynaecology, 8th edn. Mosby, London

This book has a section on the placenta (Ch. 3) that the reader may find useful.

Stables D, Rankin J 2004 Physiology in childbearing with anatomy and related biosciences, 2nd edition. Baillière Tindall, Edinburgh

The placental hormones are explained in detail in Section 2a and a diagram (12.2) gives a clear visual representation of different forms of placental transfer.

Standring S, Healy J, Johnson D, et al 2004 Gray's anatomy: The anatomical basis of clinical practice, 39th edn. Churchill Livingstone, New York

Section 7 of this authoritative and comprehensive volume provides descriptions of the placenta and its functioning for the interested student.

12 The fetus

Iolanda G.J. Serci

CHAPTER CONTENTS

The midwife's role in embryological and fetal development is focused on health education for maternal and fetal well-being. This involves providing parents with information about the effects of maternal lifestyle, such as diet, smoking, alcohol, drugs and exercise, on fetal growth and development (see Ch. 13). Additionally, an understanding of fetal development is of value when a baby is born before term.

Time scale of development

Embryological development is complex and occurs from weeks 2–8; and includes the development of the zygote in the first 2–3 weeks after fertilization. Fetal development occurs from week 8 until birth. The interval from the beginning of the last menstrual period (LMP) until fertilization is not part of pregnancy. However, this period is important for the calculation of the expected date of birth. Figure 12.1 illustrates the comparative lengths of these prenatal events.

A summary of embryological and fetal development categorized into 4-week periods is provided in Box. 12.1. This should be used to complement the text below.

Fetal growth and maturation

From the 9th week, fetal growth is rapid. Tissues grow by cell proliferation, cell enlargement and accretion of extracellular material. An adequate supply of nutrients and oxygen from the placenta to the fetus is crucial for growth. In developed countries the

Box 12.1 Summary of embryological and fetal development

0–4 weeks

- Primitive streak appears
- Some body systems laid down in primitive form
- Primitive central nervous system forms
- Heart develops and begins to beat
- Covered with a layer of skin
- Limb buds form
- Gender determined.

4–8 weeks

- Very rapid cell division
- More body systems laid down in primitive form
- Blood is pumped around the vessels
- Lower respiratory system begins
- Head and facial features develop
- Early movements
- Visible on ultrasound from 6 weeks.

8–12 weeks

- Rapid weight gain
- Eyelids fuse
- Urine passed
- Swallowing begins
- External genitalia present but gender not distinguishable
- Fingernails develop
- Lanugo appears
- Some primitive reflexes present.

12–16 weeks

- Rapid skeletal development – visible on X-ray
- Meconium present in gut
- Nasal septum and palate fuse
- Gender distinguishable.

16–20 weeks

- Constant weight gain

- 'Quickening' – mother feels fetal movements
- Fetal heart heard on auscultation
- Vernix caseosa appears
- Skin cells begin to be renewed.

20–24 weeks

- Most organs functioning well
- Eyes complete
- Periods of sleep and activity
- Ear apparatus developing
- Responds to sound
- Skin red and wrinkled.

24–28 weeks

- Legally viable and survival may be expected if born
- Eyelids open
- Respiratory movements.

28–32 weeks

- Begins to store fat and iron
- Testes descend into scrotum
- Lanugo disappears from face
- Skin becomes paler and less wrinkled.

32–36 weeks

- Weight gain 25 g/day
- Increased fat makes the body more rounded
- Lanugo disappears from body
- Head hair lengthens
- Nails reach tips of fingers
- Ear cartilage soft
- Plantar creases visible.

36 weeks–Birth

- Birth is expected
- Shape rounded
- Skull formed but soft and pliable.

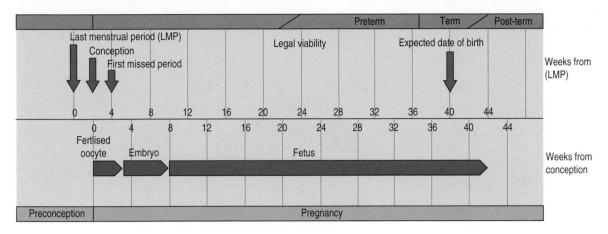

Figure 12.1 Timescales of prenatal events.

average birth weight is around 3400g and half of this is reached by 30 weeks' gestation. The fetus gains approximately 25g/day between weeks 32 and 40. A visual representation of growth in terms of height is provided in Figure 12.2.

As fetal growth is an indicator of fetal health and well-being, monitoring of growth is crucial. This is done by visual observation of the uterus for size, fundal height measurements and ultrasonography.

The cardiovascular system

The early development of the cardiovascular system in the 3rd week coincides with the lack of yolk sac, and the urgent need to supply the growing embryo with oxygen and nutrients from the maternal blood through the placenta.

The cardiovascular system is the first to function in the embryo. The heart and vascular system commences development in the 3rd week, and by the 4th week a primitive heart is visible and is beginning to function, beating at around 22 days. Blood is pumped around the vessels from the 4th week. The first signs of the heart are the appearance of paired endothelial strands in the cardiogenic mesoderm, which canalize to become heart tubes and then fuse to become a tubular heart.

By the 4th week, three paired veins drain into the heart. The vitelline veins return poorly oxygenated blood from the yolk sac. The hepatic veins and the portal vein develop from the vitelline veins and their networks. The umbilical vein carries oxygenated blood from the placenta to the embryo. A structure called the *ductus venosus* develops to connect the umbilical vein to the inferior vena cava. The common cardinal veins return poorly oxygenated blood from the embryo. These veins constitute the main venous drainage system of the embryo, draining the cranial and caudal parts of the embryo, respectively.

There are three phases of red blood cell formation: the *yolk sac* period from weeks 3–13; the *hepatic/liver* period from weeks 5–36; and the *bone marrow* period from weeks 12 throughout life. Red blood cells known as *erythrocytes* produced by the yolk sac and liver contain fetal haemoglobin. Fetal haemoglobin (HbF) has a much greater affinity for oxygen and is found in greater concentrations (18–20g/dL at term) than adult haemoglobin (HbA), thus enhancing the transfer of oxygen across the placental site. Fetal erythrocytes have a life span of 90 days, shorter than adult erythrocytes, which is around 120 days. The short life span of fetal erythrocytes contributes to neonatal physiological jaundice (see Ch. 47). Genes

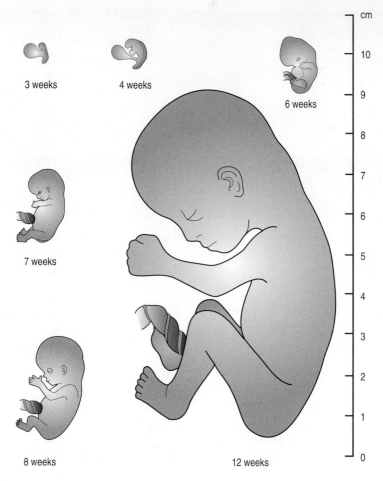

3 weeks

4 weeks

6 weeks

7 weeks

8 weeks

12 weeks

cm

10

9

8

7

6

5

4

3

2

1

0

Figure 12.2 Sizes of embryos and fetus between 3 and 12 weeks' gestation.

passed from both parents determine the fetal blood group and Rhesus factor.

The respiratory system

The development of the respiratory system begins in the 4th week. The lower respiratory tract and lungs develop simultaneously. The lungs originate from a bud growing out of the pharynx, which sub-divides again and again to form the branching structure of the bronchial tree. Lung development occurs on several levels and continues after birth until about 8 years of age when the full number of bronchioles and alveoli will have developed. The development of type II

alveolar cells commences around 20 weeks. These cells are necessary for the production of *surfactant*, a lipoprotein that reduces the surface tension in the alveoli and assists gaseous exchange. The amount of surfactant increases until the lungs are mature at 30–34 weeks.

There is some movement of the thorax from the 3rd month of fetal life and more definite diaphragmatic movements from the 6th month. This does not constitute breathing as gaseous exchange is via the placenta.

At term, the lungs contain about 100 mL of lung fluid. About one-third of this is expelled during birth and the rest is absorbed and carried away by the lymphatics and blood vessels as air takes its place.

Babies born before 24 weeks' gestation have a reduced chance of survival owing to the immaturity of the capillary system in the lungs and the lack of surfactant (see Ch. 44).

The urogenital system

The urogenital system is divided functionally into the *urinary/renal* system and the *genital/reproductive* system. Both systems develop from the intermediate mesoderm.

The kidneys develop from the 4th week and produce small amounts of urine from the 9th week. They become more functional around the 15th week when more urine is produced. The urine does not constitute a route for excretion as elimination of waste products is via the placenta. The urine forms much of the amniotic fluid and production increases with maturity.

The superior vesical arteries arise from the first few centimetres of the hypogastric arteries, which lead to the umbilical arteries. A single umbilical artery at birth is suggestive of abnormalities of the renal tract (see Ch. 46).

The sex of the embryo is determined at fertilization. The gonads develop in the 5th week from intermediate mesoderm. In the two sexes, genital development is similar and is referred to as the *indifferent state of sexual development*. Differentiation occurs from the 7th week, but female gonad development occurs slowly and the ovaries may not be identifiable until the 10th week. External genitalia in both sexes develops in the 9th week, but males and females are not distinguishable until about the 12th week.

The endocrine system

The adrenal glands develop from mesoderm and neural crest cells from the 6th week, and grow to 10–20 times larger than the adult adrenals. Their size regresses during the first year of life. They produce the precursors for placental formation of oestriols. They influence maturation of the lungs, liver and epithelium of the digestive tract. Also, it is thought that they play a part in the initiation of labour; the exact mechanism is not fully understood (Johnson & Everitt 2000).

The digestive system

The primitive gut develops from the endodermal layer of the yolk sac in the 4th week. It starts as a straight tube, and proceeds on several levels: foregut; midgut and hindgut. By the 5th week, the foregut (oesophagus, stomach and duodenum) is visible. The liver, gallbladder and pancreas bud form the gut tube around the 4th–5th week. The liver grows rapidly and from the 5th–10th week fills much of the abdominal cavity. It is responsible for about 10% of fetal weight by the 9th week. Towards the end of pregnancy, iron stores are laid down in the liver. The liver cells produce bile from the 12th week. The midgut (small intestine, caecum and vermiform appendix, ascending colon and transverse colon) undertakes much of its development in the 6th week, while the hindgut (rectum and anal canal) completes its development in the 7th week.

Around 12 weeks, the digestive tract is well formed and the lumen is patent. Most digestive juices are present before birth and act on the swallowed substances to form *meconium*. Bile enters the duodenum from the bile duct during the 13th week, giving the intestinal contents a dark green colour. Meconium is *normally* retained in the gut until after birth when it is passed as the first stool of the newborn.

Insulin is secreted from 10 weeks and glucagon from 15 weeks; both increase steadily with increasing fetal age.

The nervous system

The brain begins to develop from around day 19 and three structures are visible: forebrain, midbrain and hindbrain. By the 5th week the major regions, the thalamus and the hypothalamus are differentiated.

The neural tube is derived from the ectoderm. The ectoderm folds inwards by a complicated process to form the neural tube, which is then covered over by skin. Closure of the neural tube is essential and takes place by 26 days. This process is occasionally incomplete, leading to open neural tube defects (see Ch. 46).

The development of the sense organs, including the transmission of sensory input to the brain and output from the brain occurs under complex processes. The eyes and ears are associated with the development of the head and neck, which begin early and continues until the cessation of growth in the late teens. Although the eyes develop from around 22 days, for normal vision to occur many complex structures within the eye must properly relate to neighbouring structures. The eye is complete by 20 weeks but the eyelids are fused until around the 6th month. The developing eyes are sensitive to light.

The inner ear, which contains the structures for hearing and balance, commences early but is not complete until around 25 weeks.

Motor output controlled by the basal ganglia in the form of movement begins around 8 weeks. These movements are not usually felt by the mother until around 16 weeks, and are referred to as *quickening*. As the nervous system matures fetal behaviour becomes more complex and more defined. The fetus develops behavioral patterns: sleep with no eye or body movements; sleep with periodic eye and body movements known as *REM* sleep; wakefulness with subtle eye and limb movements; active phase with vigorous eye and limb movements.

Integumentary, skeletal and muscular systems

The epidermis develops from a single layer of ectoderm to which other layers are added. By the end of the 1st month, a thin outer layer of flattened cells covers the embryo. Further development continues until the 6th month. From 18 weeks, the fetus is covered with a white, creamy substance called *vernix caseosa*. This protects the skin from the amniotic fluid and from any friction against itself. Hair begins to develop during the 9th–12th week. At 20 weeks, the fetus is covered with a fine downy hair called *lanugo*; at the same time the head, hair and eyebrows begin to form. Lanugo is shed from 36 weeks and by term, there is little left. Fingernails develop from about 10 weeks but the toenails do not form until about 18 weeks. By term, the nails usually extend beyond the fingertips.

All skeletal tissue arises from the mesodermal and neural crest cells but skeletal tissue in different parts of the body are diverse in morphology and tissue architecture. The skeleton first appears as cartilage and at specific periods the cartilage is replaced by true bone through a process of ossification. However, the skull and facial bones develop from direct ossification with no intermediate cartilage stage. Skeletal, cardiac and smooth muscle is formed and continues into childhood (Carlson 2004, Moore & Persaud 2003).

The fetal circulation

The placenta is the source of oxygenation, nutrition and elimination of waste for the fetus. There are several temporary structures in addition to the placenta and the umbilical cord that enable the fetal circulation (Fig. 12.3) to occur. These are:

- The *ductus venosus* which connects the umbilical vein to the inferior vena cava
- The *foramen ovale* which is an opening between the right and left atria
- The *ductus arteriosus* which leads from the bifurcation of the pulmonary artery to the descending aorta
- The *hypogastric arteries* which branch off from the internal iliac arteries and become the umbilical arteries when they enter the umbilical cord.

The fetal circulation takes the following course:

Oxygenated blood from the placenta travels to the fetus in the umbilical vein. The umbilical veins divide into two branches; one that supplies the portal vein in the liver, the other the ductus venosus joining the inferior vena cava. Most of the oxygenated blood that enters the right atrium passes across the foramen ovale to the left atrium and from here into the left ventricle, and then the aorta. The head and upper extremities receive approximately 50% of this blood via the coronary and carotid arteries, and the subclavian arteries respectively. The rest of the blood travels down the descending aorta, mixing with deoxygenated blood from the right ventricle.

Deoxygenated blood collected from the upper parts of the body returns to the right atrium in the superior vena cava. Blood that has entered the right atrium from the superior vena cava and inferior vena cava passes into the right ventricle. A little blood travels to the lungs in the pulmonary artery, for their development. Most blood passes through the ductus arteriosus into the descending aorta. This blood, although low in oxygen and nutrients is sufficient to supply the lower body. It is also by this means that deoxygenated blood travels back to the placenta via the internal iliac arteries, which lead into the hypogastric arteries, which lead into the umbilical arteries.

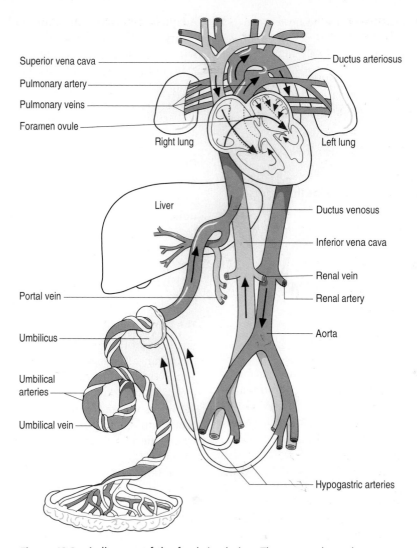

Figure 12.3   A diagram of the fetal circulation. The arrows show the course taken by the blood. The temporary structures are labelled in colour.

Adaptation to extrauterine life

At birth, there is a dramatic alteration to the fetal circulation and an almost immediate change occurs. The cessation of umbilical blood flow causes a cessation of flow in the ductus venosus, a fall in pressure in the right atrium and closure of the foramen ovale. As the baby takes the first breath, the lungs inflate, and there is a rapid fall in pulmonary vascular resistance. The ductus arteriosus constricts due to bradykinin released from the lungs on initial inflation. The effect of bradykinin is dependant on the increase in arterial oxygen. In the term baby, the ductus arteriosus closes within the first few days of birth.

These structural changes become permanent and become as follows:

- The umbilical vein becomes the *ligamentum teres*
- The ductus venosus becomes the *ligamentum venosum*

- The ductus arteriosus becomes the *ligamentum arteriosum*
- The foramen ovale becomes the *fossa ovalis*
- The hypogastric arteries are known as the *obliterated hypogastric arteries* except for the first few centimetres, which remain open as the superior vesical arteries.

Adaptation to extrauterine life also involves (Stables & Rankin 2004):

- Maintenance of a nutritional state through the establishment of breastfeeding
- Elimination of waste via the kidneys and gastro-intestinal system
- Temperature control
- Communication developed through parent–child interactions.

The fetal skull

The fetal head is large in relation to the fetal body compared with the adult (Fig. 12.4). Additionally, it is large in comparison with the maternal pelvis and is the largest part of the fetal body to be born.

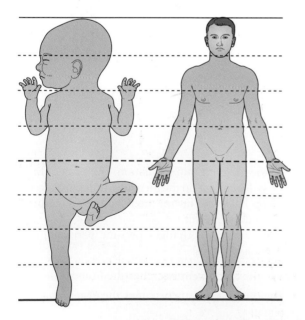

Figure 12.4 Comparison of a baby's proportions to those of an adult. The baby's head is wider than the shoulders and one-quarter of the total length.

Adaptation between the skull and the pelvis is necessary to allow the head to pass through the pelvis without complications. The bones of the vault are thin and pliable and if subjected to great pressure damage to the underlying delicate brain may occur. Important intracranial membranes, venous sinuses and structures can be seen in Figures 12.5 and 12.6.

Divisions of the fetal skull

The skull is divided into the *vault,* the *base* and the *face* (Fig. 12.7). The base comprises bones that are firmly united to protect the vital centres in the medulla. The face is composed of 14 small bones which are also firmly united and non-compressible. The vault is the large, dome-shaped part above an imaginary line drawn between the orbital ridges and the nape of the neck.

The bones of the vault

The bones of the vault (Fig. 12.8) are laid down in membrane. They ossify from the centre outwards in a process known as *ossification*. Ossification is incomplete at birth, leaving small gaps between the bones, known as the *sutures* and *fontanelles*. The ossification centre on each bone appears as a *protuberance*. Ossification of the skull is not complete until early adulthood.

The bones of the vault:

- The *occipital bone* lies at the back of the head. Part of it contributes to the base of the skull as it contains the foramen magnum, which protects the spinal cord as it leaves the skull. The ossification centre is the *occipital protuberance*.
- The two *parietal bones* lie on either side of the skull. The ossification centre of each is called the *parietal eminence*.
- The two *frontal bones* form the forehead or sinciput. The ossification centre of each is the *frontal eminence*. The frontal bones fuse into a single bone by 8 years of age.
- The upper part of the *temporal bone* on both sides of the head forms part of the vault.

Sutures and fontanelles

The *sutures* are the cranial joints formed where two bones meet. Where two or more sutures meet, a

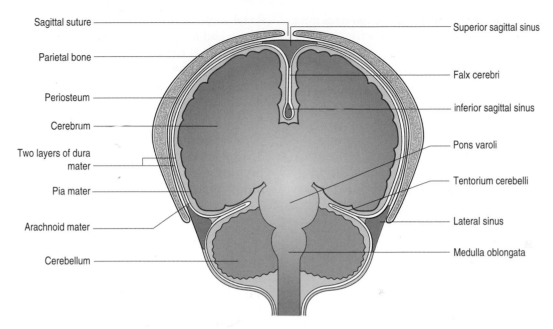

Figure 12.5 Coronal section through the fetal head to show intracranial membranes and venous sinuses.

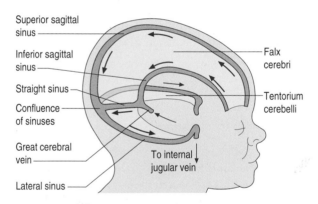

Figure 12.6 Diagram showing intracranial membranes and venous sinuses. Arrows show direction of blood flow.

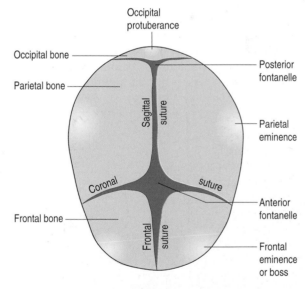

Figure 12.8 View of fetal head from above (head partly flexed), showing bones, sutures and fontanelles.

fontanelle is formed (Fig. 12.8). The sutures and fontanelles described below permit a degree of overlapping of the skull bones during labour.

- The *lambdoidal suture* separates the occipital bone from the two parietal bones.
- The *sagittal suture* lies between the two parietal bones.

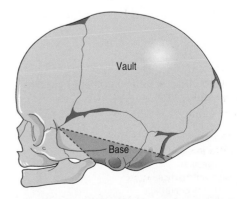

Figure 12.7 Divisions of the skull showing the large, compressible vault and the non-compressible face and base.

- The *coronal suture* separates the frontal bones from the parietal bones, passing from one temple to the other.
- The *frontal suture* runs between the two halves of the frontal bone. Whereas the frontal suture becomes obliterated in time, the other sutures eventually become fixed joints.
- The *posterior fontanelle* or lambda (shaped like the Greek letter lambda, λ) is situated at the junction of the lambdoidal and sagittal sutures. It is small, triangular in shape and can be recognized vaginally because a suture leaves from each of the three angles. It normally closes by 6 weeks of age.
- The *anterior fontanelle* or *bregma* is found at the junction of the sagittal, coronal and frontal sutures. It is broad, kite-shaped and recognizable vaginally because a suture leaves from each of the four corners. It measures 3–4 cm long and 1.5–2 cm wide and normally closes by 18 months of age. Pulsations of cerebral vessels can be felt through it.

Regions and landmarks of the fetal skull

The skull is further separated into regions and within these, there are important landmarks (Fig. 12.9). The midwife feels for the landmarks on vaginal examination as they help ascertain the position of the fetal head.

- The *occiput region* lies between the foramen magnum and the posterior fontanelle. The part below the *occipital protuberance* (landmark) is known as the *sub-occipital region*.
- The *vertex region* is bounded by the posterior fontanelle, the two parietal eminences and the anterior fontanelle.
- The *forehead/sinciput region* extends from the anterior fontanelle and the coronal suture to the orbital ridges.
- The face extends from the orbital ridges and the root of the nose to the junction of the *chin* or *mentum* (landmark) and the neck. The point between the eyebrows is known as the glabella.

Diameters of the fetal skull

Knowledge of the diameters of the skull alongside the diameters of the pelvis allows the midwife to determine the relationship between the fetal head and the mother's pelvis.

There are six longitudinal diameters (Fig. 12.10) and two transverse diameters (Fig. 12.11).

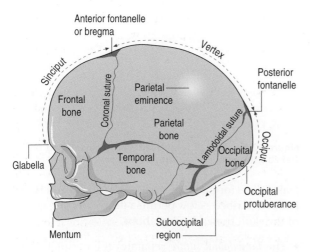

Figure 12.9 Fetal skull showing regions and landmarks of clinical importance.

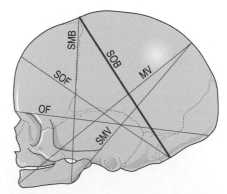

Figure 12.10 Diagram showing the longitudinal diameters of the fetal skull.

Diameter	Length (cm)
SOB, sub-occipitobregmatic	9.5
SOF, sub-occipitofrontal	10.0
OF, occipitofrontal	11.5
MV, mentovertical	13.5
SMV, sub-mentovertical	11.5
SMB, sub-mentobregmatic	9.5

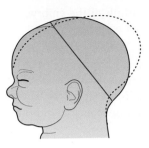

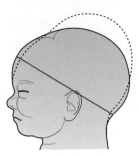

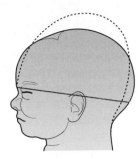

Figure 12.15 Vertex presentation, head well flexed.

Figure 12.16 Vertex presentation, head partially flexed.

Figure 12.17 Vertex presentation, head deflexed.

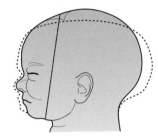

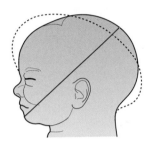

Figure 12.18 Face presentation.

Figure 12.19 Brow presentation.

Figures 12.15–12.19 Series of diagrams showing moulding when the head presents. Moulding is shown by the dotted line.

is softer and has wider sutures than that of the term baby, and hence may mould excessively.

Venous sinuses are closely associated with the intracranial membranes (Fig. 12.6) and if membranes are torn due to excessive moulding, there is danger of bleeding. A tear of the tentorium cerebelli may result in bleeding from the great cerebral vein.

REFERENCES

Carlson B M 2004 Human embryology and developmental biology, 3rd edn. Mosby, Philadelphia

Johnson M H, Everitt B J 2000 Essential reproduction, 5th edn. Blackwell Science, Oxford

Moore K L, Persaud T V N 2003 Before we are born, essentials of embryology and birth defects, 6th edn. Saunders, London

Stables D, Rankin J 2004 Physiology in childbearing, 2nd edn. Elsevier, London

FURTHER READING

Coad J, with Dunstall M 2001 Anatomy and physiology for midwives, Mosby, Edinburgh

A detailed discussion of embryonic and fetal development appears in Ch. 9. The fetal circulation and adaptation to neonatal life are addressed in Ch. 15 along with other adaptations at birth.

England M A 1983 A colour atlas of life before birth, Wolfe Medical Publications, Netherlands

This text serves to illustrate embryological and fetal development in photographic form. For the student who requires a detailed understanding of prenatal events and in particular the hormonal influences, this book

is unsurpassed. It is important to be aware that it addresses reproduction in various species and discusses how much our knowledge of the physiology of sheep or goats can inform us of events in the human. Useful statements at the head of each small section give the principles that are relevant.

Wolpert L 1991 The triumph of the embryo. Oxford University Press, Oxford

Originating in a series of Christmas lectures at the Royal Institution, this text explores the unifying principles that may account for the way embryos develop. Written for the non-specialist, it invites the reader to think broadly and aims to inspire as well as instruct.

3

Section 3
Pregnancy

SECTION CONTENTS

13

Preparing for pregnancy

Diane Barrowclough

Actively preparing for pregnancy is a constructive step towards achieving a positive pregnancy outcome and provides prospective parents with the opportunity to make conscious decisions about their health and lifestyle, options that may not be available once a pregnancy is confirmed. The challenge to health professionals is that pregnancies are often unplanned or women seek care too late for any effective interventions. As part of a primary care team the midwife is in a position to promote and be involved in this aspect of preventive medicine and aid a couple to be physically, psychologically and socially prepared for conception and parenthood.

The chapter aims to:

- discuss the aims of preconception care and describe the methods of preconception screening
- review the general health, medical and environmental factors that affect pregnancy outcome
- provide an overview of genetic principles and counselling
- give an overview of infertility management and describe the assisted conception techniques available
- draw attention to some of the complications of assisted conception techniques
- highlight the psychosocial, psychological, psychosexual and ethical issues associated with the management of infertility.

Preconception care

There has been increasing recognition that a woman's health status, lifestyle and history prior to conception strongly influence the achievement of a healthy pregnancy outcome. Once a pregnancy is confirmed interventions which could have influenced pregnancy outcome are either lost or ineffectual. Preconception care can be defined as 'a set of interventions that identify and modify biomedical, behavioural and social risks to a woman's health and future pregnancies' which are aimed at both partners achieving optimum health prior to conception (Centers for Disease Control and Prevention 2006, Korenbrot et al 2002).

Preconception advice is readily available in the mass media and the internet. However, the provision of preconception care is still not universal with the majority of services being provided by primary care practitioners most of them opportunistic (Wallace & Hurwitz 1998). Heyes et al (2004) in a study of preconception services found that while agreement of the importance of preconception care was evident, factors that hindered the delivery of such provision were lack of training, resources and practice policies. The Department of Health recognize that half of all pregnancies are unplanned but have made recommendations regarding the availability of pre-conception information for parents including what becoming a parent might be like (National Service Framework, [NSF] 2004).

The preconception period refers to a time span of anything from 3 months to 1 year before conception (Bussell 2000) but ideally should include the time when both the oocyte and sperm mature, which is approximately 100 days before conception (Bradley & Bennett 1995).

A preconception programme takes time to complete; therefore adequate time needs to be allowed for the initial consultation and the subsequent follow-ups where results, advice and treatment may be given. Box 13.1 outlines the information and investigations that may be included.

General health factors

Body weight

Assessment of body type is done by the Quetelet or body mass index (BMI) and is calculated by dividing the weight in kg by the height in m^2. It is a reflection of weight for height and therefore a high BMI identifies those people who are relatively overweight irrespective of their height.

Example: For someone who weighs 60 kg and is 1.65 m tall, the BMI is calculated as follows:

$$\frac{\text{(weight in kg)}}{\text{(height in m}^2)} = \frac{60}{1.65 \times 1.65} = 22.06$$

BMI charts and calculators are readily available. The desirable or healthy range is between 18.5 and 24.9. The underweight, overweight and obese categories can lead to long-term health hazards (Table 13.1).

Box 13.1 Information and investigations in a preconception programme

History

- Family history
- Medical history
- Menstrual history
- Obstetric history
- Method of contraception
- Medication
- Occupation
- Diet
- Smoking
- Alcohol

Observation–investigations

- Height and weight
- Blood pressure
- Urinalysis
- Stool sample
- Blood tests – haemoglobin
- Folic acid and vitamin levels
- Rubella immunity
- VDRL (venereal diseases research laboratory)
- Haemoglobinopathies
- Lead and trace elements
- Hair analysis (controversial)
- Male – semen analysis
- Female – cervical smear, high vaginal swab (HVS).

Table 13.1 Classification of body mass index (BMI)

BMI (kg/m²)	NICE classification	BMI classification
Under 18.5	–	Underweight
18.5–24.9	Healthy weight	Normal
25.0–29.9	Overweight	Overweight
30.0–34.9	Obesity I	Obese
35.0–39.9	Obesity II	–
≥40	Obesity III	Morbidly obese

Source: Lewis 2007.

By the time a pregnancy is confirmed, much of the cell organization, differentiation and organogenesis has already taken place. Suboptimal conditions at this time can result in fetal damage and stunted growth. An optimum BMI for maximum fertility and for producing a healthy baby of normal birth weight appears to be around 23 (Wynn & Wynn 1983, 1990). Low maternal weight before conception is associated with an increased risk in low birth weight babies and symmetrical growth restriction (Bussell 2000).

The prevalence of obesity has developed into one of the most serious public health challenges in Europe. The last two decades has seen a three-fold rate increase and overweight and obesity are known to shorten life expectancy and increase health risks (WHO 2006). Kanagalingham et al (2005) observed over a decade an increase in the proportion of obese women and the mean booking body mass index (BMI) in a UK maternity hospital. The risk of pregnancy complications and adverse pregnancy outcomes in overweight and obese women are increased. Even moderate overweight is a risk factor for gestational diabetes and hypertensive disorders of pregnancy, whereas overt obesity also includes a higher incidence of caesarean delivery (Bergholt et al 2007). It is most likely that midwives will encounter women who are either overweight or obese prior to and during pregnancy and that obesity related complications will continue to increase. It is now recommended that BMI should be calculated at the beginning of pregnancy (NICE 2003, 2008). The aim of preconception care is to help such women achieve an appropriate BMI prior to conception to enhance pregnancy outcome.

Principles of a healthy diet

Information and advice about a healthy diet is easily obtained from the Food Standards Agency (FSA) website http://www.eatwell.gov.uk/healthydiet. The principles of a healthy diet are to eat more starchy foods such as cereals, bread and wholegrain, at least five portions of fruit and vegetables daily, less fat, salt and sugar and some protein foods such as meat, fish, eggs and pulses. It is important to eat a variety of foods to ensure sufficient vitamins and minerals are included. According to the National Diet and Nutrition Survey (2004) intakes of salt, saturated fat and sugar were above the daily recommended values although total fat was lower. Mean intakes of some vitamins and minerals were low and adults living in households in receipt of benefits also had lower average intakes of energy and some nutrients compared with adults in non benefit households. A large proportion of men and women exceeded recommendations for alcohol consumption. From this brief synopsis it becomes apparent that dietary advice should be offered at every opportunity in an effort to enhance nutritional status. The challenge is to try and alter people's nutritional attitudes and eating habits.

Folate, folic acid and neural tube defects

Folic acid is a water-soluble vitamin belonging to the B complex. The term 'folates' is used to describe the folic acid derivatives that are found naturally in food and the term 'folic acid' is used to refer to the synthetic form used in vitamin supplements and fortification of foods. The main sources of folate in the UK diet are dark green vegetables, potatoes, fruit and fruit juices, beans and yeast extract. Folates are vulnerable to heat and readily dissolve in water; therefore considerable losses can occur as a result of cooking or prolonged storage. Folic acid is more stable and better absorbed than folate and is added to many brands of bread and breakfast cereals. All women are recommended to increase their daily folate and folic acid intake by an additional 400µg prior to conception and during the first 12 weeks of pregnancy to reduce the risk of first occurrence of neural tube defects (NTD) (DH 1992).This can be achieved by:

- eating more folate-rich foods
- eating more fortified foods such as bread and breakfast cereals
- taking a daily folic acid supplement of 400µg

Women with a history of a previous child with NTD should be prescribed 5mg of folic acid daily to reduce the risk of recurrence.

It is acknowledged that approximately half of all pregnancies are unplanned and that compliance with the recommendations is difficult. An increasing number of countries have introduced mandatory fortification such as the USA, Canada and South Africa where significant reductions in NTD-affected pregnancies have been reported (Bille et al 2007). Mandatory fortification does have its concerns particularly in relation to older people with vitamin B12 deficiency and the possibility of adverse neurological function, however mandatory fortification has been recommended along with a requirement to reduce folic acid intakes from voluntarily fortified foods and to monitor the effects of long-term exposure above the set limits. Even if mandatory fortification becomes a reality the recommendations of a 400µg/5mg supplement are still applicable (Scientific Advisory Committee on Nutrition (SACN) 2006).

Vitamin A

Vitamin A is essential for embryogenesis, growth and epithelial differentiation, but a high intake of the retinol form of vitamin A is known to be teratogenic. Rothman et al (1995) found a high dietary intake of vitamin A produced an increased frequency of craniofacial and heart defects among the babies born to women who had consumed high levels of vitamin A before the 7th week of pregnancy.

Vitamin A comes in two forms – retinol from animal sources and plant carotenoids which are vitamin A precursors. It is the preformed retinol which is of concern. In livestock production the diet is supplemented with retinol and concentrations reflected in animal products with levels being the highest in calf liver and lowest in chicken liver at 25200 and 10500µg/100mg. There is evidence to suggest that the retinol content of liver has decreased over time. However, women who are pregnant or planning a pregnancy are still advised to avoid eating liver, liver products or supplements including fish liver oils containing retinol. The lowest supplemental dose associated with teratogenic risk is 3000µg/day (DHSS 1990, SACN 2005).

Mercury

High levels of mercury are found in fish such as shark, swordfish and marlin which can be harmful to the neurological development of the fetus. Women should be advised to avoid eating these kinds of fish and to restrict the consumption of tuna to no more than two fresh tuna steaks or four medium-size cans a week (FSA 2007).

Listeria

Listeria monocytogenes is a bacterium that can cause spontaneous abortion, pre-term labour or stillbirth. Although the incidence during pregnancy is rare, pregnant women or women planning a pregnancy should be advised to avoid eating mould-ripened cheeses such as Brie or Camembert, blue veined cheeses or pate and to ensure that meat or reheated foods are thoroughly cooked (FSA 2007).

Pre-existing medical conditions and drugs

Diabetes

Diabetes mellitus is the most common pre-existing medical condition in pregnancy and the prevalence of both type 1 and type 2 diabetes is increasing. Infants of insulin-dependent diabetics are at an increased risk of congenital abnormalities and perinatal morbidity and mortality (Macintosh et al 2006).

Preconception care is associated with a significantly lower risk of major and minor congenital abnormalities yet many women neither plan their pregnancies nor achieve adequate glycaemic control before conception (Ray et al 2001). In England, Wales and Northern Ireland in 2002–2003, less than half of pregnant women with pre-existing diabetes had preconception counselling, testing for glycaemic control or folic acid supplementation. The most important aim of preconception care is to achieve the best possible glycaemic control before pregnancy as the teratogenic effects of hyperglycaemia occur during organogenesis. Diabetic complications such as retinopathy and nephropathy may worsen during pregnancy. Tight control however is associated with asymptomatic hypoglycaemia and women need to be specifically counselled about prevention and management strategies (Taylor & Davison 2007). Varughese et al (2007) found that diabetic women of childbearing age attending general diabetic clinics were not provided with appropriate counselling regarding the reproductive issues associated with their condition and that some patients were on potentially teratogenic medications. The standards of preconception and pregnancy care need to be improved (CEMACH 2007). The Diabetes NSF recommends that service provision should include all members of the multidisciplinary team (NSF 2001).

Epilepsy

Women with epilepsy need accurate information and counselling throughout the life stages, including conception in order to make informed choices. It is not known whether pregnancy increases the risk of sudden death in epilepsy (SUDEP), however six out of the 11 deaths in the confidential enquiry into maternal deaths met the criteria (Lewis 2007). The aim of preconception care is to help the woman plan her pregnancies carefully and to keep her seizure free on the lowest possible dose of anti-epileptic drugs (AEDs). Folic acid supplements of 5 mg/day should be offered. The risks and benefits of treatment with individual drugs need to be discussed in relation to major malformations as well as longer term neurological and cognitive outcomes (Adab et al 2004). Such assessment is difficult in relation to the newer AEDs as clinical data are limited (NICE 2004a). In a systematic review Adab et al (2004) acknowledged the difficulties highlighted above and cautiously concluded that the consensus of clinical advice was to continue medication during pregnancy using monotherapy at the lowest dose required to achieve seizure control and to avoid polytherapy.

Phenylketonuria

Phenylketonuria (PKU) is an inborn error of metabolism resulting from a deficiency of phenylalanine hydroxylase and characterized by mental retardation (see Ch.48). It is treatable by a low phenylalanine diet although some women with PKU discontinue treatment during childhood. Unless careful dietary control is resumed pre or peri-conception, the toxic effect of phenylalanine (Phe) on the developing embryo/fetus results in a high incidence of microcephaly, mental retardation and congenital heart defects (Rouse et al 2000). An international collaborative study has demonstrated that careful monitoring and controlled dietary phenylalanine restriction during pregnancy decreases the incidence of these morbidities. Optimum fetal outcomes occurred when maternal blood Phe levels of 120–360 µmol/L were achieved by 8–10 weeks of gestation and maintained throughout pregnancy (Koch et al 2003). Maternal dietary control and compliance with therapy is not easy for some women therefore they need help and support (Clarke 2003). Lee et al (2003) argue that this preventable situation is as a result of a lack of appropriate resources for these high risk women. The cognitive and behavioural development of the offspring of these women is also of concern and needs further research (Waisbren & Azen 2003).

Oral contraception

Oral contraception should be stopped at least 3 months and preferably 6 months prior to planning a pregnancy to allow for the resumption of natural hormone regulation and ovulation. The oral contraceptive pill is associated with vitamin and mineral imbalances that may need correcting. Copper levels are raised while zinc levels are reduced and can result in a deficiency of the latter mineral. Vitamin metabolism is also affected, which may lead to deficiencies of folate, B complex and vitamin C and an increase in vitamin A (Bradley & Bennett 1995). Other forms of contraception such as barrier methods will need to be advised during this time.

Drug abuse

The prevalence of taking drugs has decreased slightly in England in the 16–24 age groups with cannabis being the most frequently reported drug used. This was followed by ecstasy, cocaine and amphetamines (DH 2004). Disruption of the menstrual cycle is common among women using drugs like ecstasy, amphetamines, opiates and anabolic steroids, and heavy drug use during pregnancy is associated with miscarriage, preterm labour, low birth weight, stillbirth and abnormalities. Drug users are unlikely to present for preconception care as a high proportion of these women conceal their drug use (Illman 2001).

Environmental factors

Smoking

Smoking can affect women's sexual and reproductive health as well as the longer-term health status of themselves and their children. Studies suggest that women who smoke may suffer menstrual problems and an early menopause. In terms of fertility, women who smoke are twice as likely to be infertile or take longer to conceive than non-smokers. In men, smoking affects sperm morphology and can cause lower sperm counts. Couples who smoke are also known to have a poorer response to fertility treatments. The adverse effects of smoking during pregnancy are well known with increased risks of ectopic pregnancy, spontaneous abortion, low birth weight, fetal malformations and pre-term labour. Passive smoking is also associated with low birth weight and preterm labour. Other health risks include an increased risk of heart disease and stroke in women who use the oral contraceptive pill and malignant cancer of the cervix. Stopping smoking can reduce or reverse these risks. It is known that smoking is associated with social disadvantage and is more prevalent in the lower social classes and younger age groups. Women whose partners smoke are less likely to succeed in stopping smoking during pregnancy and are more likely to return to smoking after the baby is born (British Medical Association 2004). Lumley et al (2002) in a review of interventions for promoting smoking cessation during pregnancy programmes found that smoking cessation rates were increased and the incidence of low birth weight babies and pre-term labour reduced. Stanton et al (2004) also demonstrated that targeting men for smoking cessation at the time that their partners were pregnant appeared to be an effective strategy. Women should be offered smoking cessation interventions as part of antenatal care (NICE 2008).

Alcohol

Consuming large quantities of alcohol can reduce appetite and affect nutritional status (Goldberg 2000). High alcohol intakes in women have been associated with menstrual disorders and decreased fertility (Jensen et al 1998). Alcohol is a teratogen and fetal alcohol syndrome (FAS) is used to describe the congenital malformations associated with maternal alcohol intake during pregnancy. Fetal alcohol spectrum disorder (FASD) is used to describe the condition associated with alcohol exposure during pregnancy but where the full characteristics of FAS are not fully manifested (see Ch. 46). In view of the fact that the exact dose of alcohol that is safe in pregnancy is as

> **Box 13.2** Units of alcohol
>
> 1 unit of alcohol = ½ pint of ordinary strength beer, lager or cider
>
> = ¼ pint of strong beer or lager
>
> = 1 small glass wine
>
> = 1 single measure of spirit
>
> = 1 small glass sherry

yet inconclusive the safest approach is to abstain from drinking alcohol while trying to conceive and during pregnancy. For those women who wish to continue drinking alcohol the advice is to drink small amounts of no more than two units not more than once or twice a week as this has not been shown to be harmful (Mukherjee et al 2005, RCOG 2006).

Counting units of alcohol is an effective way of calculating alcohol consumption although consideration should be given to the amount and type of alcohol consumed as home measures tend to be larger (Box 13.2). Women who have difficulty in reducing their alcohol intake should be referred to local counselling or support services.

Exercise

Moderate exercise is known to be beneficial for health and the benefits of regular exercise for the healthy pregnant woman appear to outweigh the risks (see Ch.16). Clapp (2006) advises that healthy women who exercised regularly in the preconception period should be encouraged to continue either at an equivalent level or at least half of that level and sedentary women should be encouraged to increase their recreational activity. A randomized comparative trial of the efficacy and safety of exercise during pregnancy is currently being conducted for women at risk of gestational hypertension or preeclampsia (Yeo 2006). The outcomes of this study will be of interest to midwives and obstetricians.

Workplace hazards and noxious substances

Humans are exposed to many environmental agents that may be hazardous to their reproductive capacity and much of this exposure may occur in the workplace.

Some occupational exposure to hazards can reduce male or female fertility (RCOG 2004) although the Health and Safety Executive (2006) require employers to ensure that exposure to substances that can cause occupational asthma, cancer, or damage to genes that can be passed from one generation to another, is reduced as low as is reasonably practicable. Reports of miscarriages or birth defects among workers using visual display units (VDUs) have not been borne out.

Genetic counselling

Any couple who has a family history of genetic disorders or who has had a previous baby affected with a congenital abnormality will inevitably want to discuss the reasons why it happened or the implications of such conditions for any future offspring they may have. Turnpenny & Ellard (2005) describe genetic counselling as a process of communication and education where the overarching principles are to:

- adopt a non-directive approach
- diagnose the problem and its implications in relation to prognosis and possible treatment
- determine the mode of inheritance and the risk of developing or transmitting the disorder
- discuss available choices or options
- support the people involved so that they can reach their own fully informed decisions.

The concept of risk is not always easy to understand for some people and risk figures are often quoted as either odds or percentages (see Ch. 18). It is important therefore that a consistent and clear approach is adopted to avoid any confusion and the couple's perspective of the problem ascertained so that they are able to decide for themselves what constitutes a 'high' or 'low' risk (Turnpenny & Ellard 2005).

Chromosome abnormalities

Chromosome aberrations include the trisomies, such as trisomy 21 (Down syndrome) and the rarer trisomy 13 and 18. Age factors are significant particularly in Down syndrome, for which the risk is 1% for a woman around 40 years of age. Monosomies are usually lethal and non-viable autosomal trisomies are extremely common in spontaneous abortions. Sex chromosome abnormalities, such as Turner's syndrome (XO) and Klinefelter's syndrome (XXY) have a rare recurrence rate in families. Translocation is where genetic material is transferred from one chromosome to another and is regarded as reciprocal where there is exchange of chromosome material but no change in chromosome number. The incidence of reciprocal translocations is approximately 1 in 500 in the general population (Turnpenny & Ellard 2005).

Mendelian inheritance

Genetic disorders can occur as a result of Mendelian inheritance and are either dominant or recessive. An autosomal dominant disorder manifests when the condition is present in the heterozygous state (i.e. only one gene of a pair of chromosomes need be affected). The risks associated with this inheritance pattern are relatively straightforward – there is a 1 in 2, or 50%, risk in a couple where one of them is affected with the condition. An autosomal recessive disorder manifests only in the homozygous state (i.e. both chromosomes of a pair must be affected), which means that any offspring of an affected individual are obligatory carriers given that the other partner is unaffected.

Consanguinity is an important consideration in relation to autosomal recessive disorders. The incidence of congenital malformations in the children of first cousins is approximately twice that seen in the children of unrelated parents. Rates of consanguinity vary from <1% in Northern Europe to >50% in some Arab states (Turnpenny & Ellard 2005).

Multifactorial inheritance

The commoner congenital malformations, such as cleft lip and congenital heart disease do not follow any recognized pattern of Mendelian inheritance. These conditions arise as a result of a combination or interaction of environmental and genetic factors and are referred to as showing multifactorial inheritance even though they show a definite familial tendency and an increased incidence in close relatives (Turnpenny & Ellard 2005).

Prenatal diagnosis

Prenatal diagnosis is an option for couples who are at high risk of having a child with a serious genetic condition. For some couples such an option inevitably includes the difficult decision of whether to terminate the pregnancy or not. Ideally, for a couple to truly benefit from this option they should be identified and assessed before a pregnancy is planned so that they can be counselled and given the time to consider the risk and come to a decision based on the options available to them. Preimplantation genetic diagnosis is also an option particularly for couples undergoing assisted conception (Turnpenny & Ellard 2005).

Infertility/subfertility

The National Institute for Clinical Excellence (NICE 2004b, p 10) define infertility as 'failure to conceive after regular unprotected sexual intercourse for two years in the absence of known reproductive pathology'. Approximately one in seven couples in the UK has difficulty conceiving. It is further estimated that of 100 couples trying to conceive naturally, 85 will conceive within 1 year and 95 within 2 years (Human Fertilization and Embryology Authority (HFEA) 2007). Couples who have been unable to achieve a conception after 1 year are referred to as being subfertile. Infertility is categorized as primary if there has been no prior conception and secondary if there has been a previous conception. There have been no major changes in the prevalence of fertility problems although more people now seek help than did so previously. The trend is for women to have fewer children and to delay childbearing until a later age when there is an associated decline in fertility (RCOG 2004). Natural human fertility is low compared with other species and the chance in the most fertile of couples conceiving within one menstrual cycle is no higher than 33% therefore to expect a higher chance of pregnancy than this from any fertility treatment is unrealistic (Cahill & Wardle 2002).

The factors responsible for infertility are many and varied, with an incidence in men up to 30% (Box 13.3) and in women up to 40% (Box 13.4). Of these, approximately 39% of cases of infertility involve problems with both partners. In 30% of couples the causes of infertility remain unexplained (RCOG 2004).

Box 13.3 Causes of male infertility

Defective spermatogenesis

- Endocrine disorders
  - Dysfunction – hypothalamus, pituitary, adrenals, thyroid
  - Systemic disease – diabetes mellitus, coeliac disease, renal failure
- Testicular disorders
  - Trauma
  - Environmental – congenital, occupational, acquired
  - Cancer treatment

Defective transport

- Obstruction or absence of seminal ducts
- Impaired secretions from prostate or seminal vesicles

Ineffective delivery

- Psychosexual problems (impotence)
- Drug-induced (ejaculatory dysfunction)
- Physical disability or anomalies.

Box 13.4 Causes of female infertility

Defective ovulation

- Endocrine disorders
  - Dysfunction – hypothalamus, pituitary, adrenals, thyroid
  - Systemic disease – diabetes mellitus, coeliac disease, renal failure
- Physical disorders
  - Obesity, low BMI
- Ovarian disorders
  - Hormonal, polycystic ovarian disease, ovarian endometriosis

Defective transport

- Oocyte
  - Tubal obstruction – previous surgery, fimbrial adhesions, endometriosis, infection
- Sperm
  - Hostile mucus
  - Antisperm antibodies in mucus
  - Psychosexual problems (vaginismus)

Defective implantation

- Hormonal imbalance, congenital anomalies, fibroids or infection.

Initial management of the infertile couple

Much of the initial management of the infertile couple is via primary care, therefore the preliminary investigation of both partners and subsequent referral to specialist care will be through the general practitioner. Early referral is indicated where the female partner is over 38 years, has a history of infertility of more than 3 years, has indicative tubal disorder, ovulation disorder or where the male partner has an abnormal semen analysis. The investigative process is aimed at achieving an accurate diagnosis and definition of any cause, an accurate estimation of the chance of conceiving with and without treatment and a full appraisal of treatment options. Providing information, counselling and support are also an integral part of the management to help the couple cope with the stress of treatment and the possibility of failure (Cahill & Wardle, 2002).

It is important that both partners are involved in the management of their infertility and that full explanations are given to the couple at each stage in the investigation and treatment. This should be backed up with written information including a list of addresses of relevant organizations and fertility support groups. Rubella status should be confirmed and folic acid supplementation commenced for the female partner. A detailed drug history should be taken from both partners including any history of drug abuse and any occupational factors. General advice regarding lifestyle factors such smoking and alcohol should be given to both partners and weight control advice for the female partner if appropriate. The couple should be advised that sexual intercourse every 2–3 days optimizes the chance of pregnancy. The male partner should have semen analysis undertaken as part of the initial assessment (Box 13.5). Women with regular menstrual cycles are likely to be ovulating but women

> **Box 13.5** Semen analysis
>
> WHO Normal semen analysis values (WHO 1999):
>
> - semen volume >2–5 mL
> - sperm concentration >20 million/mL
> - motility >50% progressive motility
> - morphology >30% normal forms
> - white blood cells <1 million/mL.

with regular cycles and a history of more than 2 years infertility should have measurement of serum progesterone levels to confirm ovulation. Women with irregular or prolonged irregular cycles should have serum progesterone and serum gonadotrophin levels measured (RCOG 2004). Most investigations are relatively simple but more specialized investigations need to be undertaken in a dedicated, infertility clinic where there is access to a specialist team as this is likely to improve effectiveness, efficiency and patient satisfaction. The most important predictors of a successful conception in infertile couples undergoing investigation and treatment are the female partner's age, the duration of infertility, previous pregnancy history and the quality of the sperm. The success rate for *in vitro* fertilization treatment declines with increasing age and previous IVF failure (RCOG 2004).

Regulation

Any centre that provides techniques that involves fertilization outside the body has to be regulated by the Human Fertilization and Embryology Authority (HFEA), a statutory body that was created in 1991 following the passing of the Human Fertilization and Embryology Act in 1990. Its primary responsibility is to license and monitor clinics in the UK that offer *in vitro* fertilization (IVF) and donor insemination (DI) treatments, human embryo research and to regulate the storage of eggs, sperm and embryos. The HFEA Code of Practice (2003) imposes obligations upon centres to take account of the welfare of the relevant children, to give and record information and to provide counselling.

Assisted conception techniques

The aim of all assisted conception techniques is to promote the chances of fertilization and subsequent pregnancy by bringing the sperm and egg close to each other. A range of assisted reproduction techniques is available to treat the infertile couple and it is important that the appropriate treatment option is offered (Rowell & Braude 2003).

Ovulation induction

The principles of management of ovulation disorders include diagnosis and treatment of underlying causes and once an adequate sperm count and tubal patency have been confirmed ovulation induction can be commenced.

The World Health Organization classifies ovulation disorder into three groups:

Group I – hypothalamic pituitary failure (hypothalamic amenorrhoea or hypogonadotrophic hypogonadism)

Group II – hypothalamic pituitary dysfunction (predominately polycystic ovary syndrome)

Group III – ovarian failure.

Clomifene citrate and tamoxifen are referred to as anti-oestrogens and are a first-line treatment for Group II ovulation disorders. Clomifene citrate works by blocking oestrogen receptors in the hypothalamus inducing negative feedback, gonadotrophin secretion and follicular growth stimulation. Adverse effects of such therapy include multiple pregnancy, ovarian hyperstimulation, abdominal discomfort and hot flushes. Treatment should be for up to 12 months and women should be informed of the risks of treatment and offered ultrasound monitoring at least during the first cycle of treatment (RCOG 2004).

Women with clomifene-resistant polycystic ovarian syndrome can be treated with gonadotrophins, either human menopausal gonadotrophin, urinary follicle-stimulating hormone or recombinant follicle-stimulating hormone. Ultrasound monitoring is undertaken throughout the treatment to measure follicular size and number to reduce the risks of multiple pregnancy and ovarian hyperstimulation syndrome (RCOG 2004).

Dopamine agonists such as bromocriptine and cabergoline are safe and effective treatments for women with ovulatory disorders due to hyperprolactinaemia (Cahill & Wardle 2002).

Intrauterine insemination (IUI)

IUI is indicated as a first-line management where there are problems such as hostile cervical mucus, antisperm antibodies or male fertility problems such as a low sperm count or premature ejaculation although tubal patency of the female partner must be assured. It is also useful for cases of unexplained infertility. In order to increase the chances of success, ovulation is monitored and often induced and the sperm prepared to maximize its fertilizing ability before being inserted high into the uterus. If the sperm used for the procedure is freshly produced from the male partner then a license is not required. If the sperm from the male partner has been previously frozen or if donor sperm is used then the clinic carrying out the procedure must be licensed by the HFEA for the storage of sperm. The probability of a successful conception with IUI is greater in the first four attempts with the likelihood of success being reduced thereafter (Jenkins et al 2003).

In vitro fertilization/embryo transfer (IVF/ET)

In vitro fertilization describes the laboratory technique where fertilization occurs outside the body and is one of the main types of assisted conception techniques used. IVF is indicated in cases where the female partner has uterine tube occlusion, endometriosis or cervical mucus problems, or where male factors are the main problem. It may be appropriate for cases of unexplained infertility or when less invasive methods have been unsuccessful. It also provides an opportunity to detect specific sperm abnormalities and the fertilizing ability of the sperm. Stimulation of the ovaries to produce more than one egg is required and treatment starts with pituitary desensitization followed by gonadotrophin injections. The use of gonadotrophin releasing hormone (GnRH) agonists and more recently GnRH antagonists facilitates better control of cycles by preventing the physiological surge of luteinizing hormone and oocyte release. Transvaginal ultrasound monitoring of the ovaries is recommended and an injection of HCG is given 34–38 hrs before egg collection. Transvaginal follicle aspiration is now the method of choice for oocytes retrieval and is conducted under mild sedation. The oocytes are examined for maturity and if suitable are then placed with the prepared sperm from the male partner or donor and incubated. Embryo transfer is usually performed on the 2nd or 3rd day after insemination at the four- or eight-cell stage (Balen & Jacobs 2003). No more than two embryos can be transferred to women aged <40 years and no more than three in women aged over 40 years in any one cycle regardless of the procedure used. Any remaining embryos may be frozen for later use if the clinic is able to offer this facility (HFEA 2003).

Intracytoplasmic sperm injection

Developed in 1992, intracytoplasmic sperm injection (ICSI) is a highly specialized variant of IVF treatment that involves the injection of a single sperm into the cytoplasm of an egg with a fine glass needle. It is a useful technique when sperm quality is poor and in azoospermic men sperm can be obtained surgically from the epididymis or extracted from the testis itself (Braude & Rowell 2003a). Ovulation stimulation is required as in IVF and only mature oocytes that have extruded the first polar body are suitable for use.

Gamete intrafallopian transfer and zygote intrafallopian transfer

Both gamete intrafallopian transfer (GIFT) and zygote intrafallopian transfer (ZIFT) are laparoscopic techniques that offer little clinical advantage over *in vitro* fertilization and are no longer recommended (NICE 2004b).

Complications of assisted conception techniques

Ovarian hyperstimulation syndrome

One of the most serious iatrogenic problems associated with superovulation is ovarian hyperstimulation syndrome (OHSS), which can be a potentially life-threatening event. Incidence is between 0.6 and 10% of IVF cycles and 0.5% and 2% in its severe form. Associated risk factors include polycystic ovarian syndrome, young age, lean physique, HCG administration and multiple-pregnancy. Management and treatment is dependent upon the severity but should be in a specialist hospital and should include monitoring and multidisciplinary team involvement (Braude & Rowell 2003b).

Ectopic pregnancy

Ectopic pregnancy occurs in approximately 0.5–1% of all pregnancies but can rise to around 4–5% following assisted conception therapies. It is associated with significant mortality but is often detected early due to ultrasound monitoring (Balen & Jacobs 2003).

Multiple-pregnancy

Multiple-pregnancy, especially higher order multiples are associated with more complications during pregnancy and significant morbidity and mortality mainly due to the increased risk of preterm birth. The rate of triplet and other higher order births has been linked to the advent of assisted conception techniques. Ovulation induction requires careful monitoring and may result in cancelled cycles to reduce the risk. Only two embryos may be transferred in an IVF treatment cycle except in special circumstances (HFEA 2003).

Intracytoplasmic sperm injection and *in vitro* fertilization

There are concerns regarding the risk of major birth defects after intracytoplasmic sperm injection (ICSI) and *in vitro* fertilization (IVF). According to Hansen et al (2002), infants conceived with the use of such techniques have twice as high a risk of a major birth defect as that of infants conceived naturally. Devroey & Van Steirteghem (2004) also state that ICSI is associated with a significant increase in de novo chromosomal aberrations. The use of ICSI has transformed the treatment of severe male infertility and has resulted in a substantial number of couples being able to have their own genetic child instead of artificial insemination with donor sperm. It is argued that the increased risk may be due to factors associated with infertility and the need for ICSI or IVF in the first place. The likelihood of chromosomal abnormalities increases as sperm counts decrease therefore males may pass on to their sons the same aberration that would render them sterile also. According to Devroey & Van Steirteghem (2004) follow-up studies in infertile couples obtaining spontaneous

pregnancies and pregnancies after reduction of ovulation and after mild ovarian stimulation are needed in order to judge the congenital malformation rate after IVF or ICSI. In view of these risks couples undergoing such procedures should be offered appropriate genetic counselling and testing (RCOG 2004).

Sperm and egg donation

Any person considering donation of either sperm or eggs must undergo an assessment and screening process before any gametes are provided, and be aged over 18 and under 35 years for women and under 45 years for men. A medical and family history is taken including details of any donations that have been made elsewhere. Only 10 live birth events defined as the birth of a child or children, i.e. twins and triplets, are permissible from donors of gametes or embryos under the HFEA (2003) regulations. The screening process aims to prevent the transmission of serious genetic disorders and includes screening for human immunodeficiency virus (HIV), cytomegalovirus (CMV) and hepatitis B antibodies.

Donors are encouraged to provide as much non-identifying biographical information as possible that can be made available to prospective parents and to a donor-conceived person when they reach the age of 18. This information usually includes a physical description, ethnic group and whether the donor has any children, and now includes the donor's parents' ethnic group, whether the donor was adopted, the donor's marital status and where applicable, the gender of any children. Since April 2005, a donor-conceived person can ask for the donor's name now and name at birth if different, the date and place of the donor's birth and their last known address or the address that was recorded at the time of registration. Donors who made donations prior to April 2005 can remain anonymous if they wish but can decide to re-register as an identifiable donor and consent for identifying information to be given to donor-conceived people created using their donation once they reach the age of 18. Although the donor will be the genetic parent, in law they have no legal relationship, legal rights or obligations to any child created from their donations.

The HFEA's role as the UK's Fertility Regulator is to ensure that the fertility services people receive are safe, appropriate and sensitive to their needs. The last 5 years have seen a 2.5-fold increase in the number of single women having IVF and a four-fold increase in lesbian couples having IVF (HFEA 2006).

Surrogacy

Legal arrangements for surrogacy require the commissioning couple to both be over the age of 18, married to each other and the child genetically related to at least one of them. Civil ceremonies are not recognized and neither is any contractual arrangement legally binding (Surrogacy UK 2007). This means that either a fertile woman can be artificially inseminated with the sperm of the husband of the commissioning couple or the commissioning couple can undergo an IVF procedure and produce an embryo. The surrogate mother then acts as a host as the embryo is placed in her uterus. The commissioning couple can then apply for a parental order within 6 months of the birth as long as the child is living with them. The surrogate mother must still register the birth, as consent to the parental order cannot be given until 6 weeks after the birth of the child and no money other than reasonable expenses must have been paid. When a court has granted the parental order, the Registrar General will make an entry in a separate Parental Order Register re-registering the child. Adults who are the subject of parental orders are able to gain access to their original birth certificates after being offered counselling.

Psychosocial and psychological aspects of infertility

The inability to conceive children is a stressful situation for couples and individuals alike and can have deleterious social and psychological consequences. Commonly reported feelings are of guilt, anger, depression, anxiety, inadequacy, grief, loss of control and low self-esteem (Read 2004). Many of these symptoms persist over extended periods of time. The psychological distress appears to be more common in the partner with the fertility problem and infertile women are reported to have significantly higher levels of depressive symptoms relative to fertile women although men can also experience considerable distress. Most infertility patients, especially women consider the evaluation and treatment of infertility to be the most upsetting experience of their lives and the negative psychological impact of infertility by many health providers and mental health clinicians is underestimated. Women often have to undergo the bulk of the invasive procedures and are responsible for the daily monitoring activities required of treatment regimes and its subsequent disruption of their lives. Even when the reproductive impairment lies with the partner, women tend to carry the psychological burden although men appear to negotiate the transition to a childless lifestyle more easily than their wives (Cousineau & Domar 2007). However, infertility can also have positive effects with couples feeling closer by improved communication, having increased sensitivity to partner's feelings and a sense of closeness (Leiblum 1997).

Fertility clinics should aim to address the psychosocial and emotional needs of their patients, as well as their medical needs. The availability of appropriately trained counsellors is essential in the management of the infertile couple, as there are fundamental differences in their requirements from those of other disease-oriented consultations. The first is that the central focus is the couple's inability to fulfil their desire to have children. The second issue is that the interests of the child that may be conceived must be considered. Third, the treatment process often involves repeated therapies that if unsuccessful, create further stress and disappointment, and finally the couple are obliged to share intimate details of their sexual behaviour (Boivin et al 2001). In a systematic review, Boivin (2003) found that psychosocial interventions in infertility were more effective in reducing negative effects than in changing interpersonal functioning and although pregnancy rates were unlikely to be affected by such interventions, group interventions such as relaxation training were more effective across a range of outcomes than counselling interventions. Both men and women were found to benefit equally from such interventions.

One of the most difficult aspects of infertility treatment for a couple is deciding when to stop. Integral to the process is a realistic appraisal of the couple's problems before they start and an honest view of the cumulative chance of conception and live birth after a certain number of cycles. Most couples find stopping treatment extremely traumatic and they need help with preparing for this decision. After unsuccessful treatment cycles the number of further treatment cycles need to be discussed and then treatment terminated after that agreed limit (Balen & Jacobs 2003). The couple must then decide whether to remain childless or consider adoption.

Psychosexual aspects of infertility

The stress of infertility and its treatments may cause or exacerbate sexual difficulties for both men and women. For men, this may include erectile or ejaculatory failure, particularly when repeated semen samples are required and for women, the distress or anxiety may lead to arousal difficulties. Couples may also begin to avoid intercourse so as not to remind one or other partner of the fertility problem and feelings of only being wanted, when there is a chance of conception can lead to psychological issues of power and control. Such stresses conspire to alienate couples from the recreational aspects of sexual relations, resulting in an obsessive focus on the procreative aspects instead. Infertility examinations should include an evaluation of a couple's sexual behaviour including overt and clear questioning about their sexual activity with special reference to frequency and timing of intercourse and whether penetrative sex is actually occurring (Read 2004).

Ethical issues associated with infertility

The advancing reproductive technologies, while achieving the goal for many infertile couples are fraught with ethical dilemmas for all concerned. Resourcing and financial issues result in decisions being made as to who can be treated and who cannot. Issues arise relating to the welfare of the child, the ages of the prospective parents, the loss of anonymity of donors, the child's rights to know about its genetic origins, surrogacy and the creation of surplus embryos are to name but a few. Although these issues cannot be discussed in this chapter, everyone involved with infertility treatments and assisted conception techniques must be aware of them.

The role of the midwife

The psychological and psychosocial distresses associated with fertility treatments are not only complex and individual to the couples concerned but their effects can be persistent, leaving both partners with feelings of anxiety and low self-esteem. It is important that the midwife is aware of the types and implications of fertility treatments that are currently available and is able to provide care which is empathetic and sensitive to their needs not only throughout the pregnancy but also into the postnatal period as couples who have experienced infertility can also experience difficulties adjusting to parenthood (Balen & Jacobs 2003).

REFERENCES

Adab N, Smith C, Vinten J et al 2004 Common antiepileptic drugs in pregnancy in women with epilepsy (Review). The Cochrane Library Issue 3

Balen A H, Jacobs H S 2003 Infertility in practice. Churchill Livingstone, Edinburgh

Bergholt T, Lim L K, Jorgensend J S et al 2007 Maternal body mass index in the first trimester and risk of cesarean delivery in nulliparous women in spontaneous labor. American Journal of Obstetrics and Gynecology 196:163.e1–163.e5

Bille C, Murray J C, Olsen S F 2007 Folic acid and birth malformations. British Medical Journal 334: 433–434

Boivin J 2003 A review of psychological interventions in infertility. Social Science and Medicine 57: 2325–2341

Boivin J, Appleton T C, Baetons P et al 2001 Guidelines for counseling in infertility. Human Reproduction 16(6):1301–1304

Bradley S G, Bennett N 1995 Preparation for pregnancy. Glendaruel, Argyll, p 23–32

Braude P, Rowell P (2003a) Assisted conception II – In vitro fertilization and intracytoplasmic sperm injection. British Medical Journal 327:852–855

Braude P, Rowell P (2003b) Assisted conception III – Problems with assisted conception. British Medical Journal 327:920–923

British Medical Association 2004 Smoking and reproductive health. Online. Available: http://www.bma.org.uk/ap.nsf/Content/SmokingReproductiveLife 26 May 2007

Bussell G 2000 The dietary beliefs and attitudes of women who have had a low-birth weight baby: a retrospective pre-conception study. Journal of Human Nutrition and Dietetics 13(1):29–39

Cahill D J, Wardle P G 2002 Management of infertility. British Medical Journal 325: 28–32

Centers for Disease Control and Prevention (CDC) 2006 Preconception health and care. Online. Available: http://www.cdc.gov/ncbddd/preconception/documents/At-a-glance-4–11-06.pdf 24/05/07

CEMACH (Confidential Enquiry into Maternal and Child Health) 2007 Diabetes in pregnancy: Are we providing the best care? Findings of a National Enquiry: England, Wales and Northern Ireland. CEMACH, London

Clapp J F 2006 Influence of endurance exercise on diet and human placental development and fetal growth. Placenta 27:527–534.

Clarke J T R 2003 The maternal phenylketonuria project: A summary of progress and challenges for the future. Pediatrics 112(6):1584–1587

Cousineau T M, Domar A D 2007 Psychological impact of infertility. Best Practice & Research Clinical Obstetrics and Gynaecology 21(2):293–308

Devroey P, Van Steirteghem A 2004 A review of ten years experience of ICSI. Human Reproduction Update 10(1):19–28

DH (Department of Health) 2004 Statistics on young people and drug misuse: England 2003. Statistical Bulletin 2004/13

DH (Department of Health) 1992 Folic acid and the prevention of neural tube defects: report from an expert advisory group. DH Publication Unit, Heywood

DHSS (Department of Health and Social Security) 1990 Vitamin A and pregnancy. PL/CMO (90) 11, PL/CNO (90). HMSO, London

FSA (Food Standards Agency) 2007 Trying for a baby. Online. Available: http://www.eatwell.gov.uk/agesandstages/pregnancy/trybaby 24 May 2007)

Goldberg G R 2000 Nutrition in pregnancy. Advisa Medica London 1(2):1–3

Hansen M, Kurinczuk J J, Bower C et al 2002 The risk of major birth defects after intracytoplasmic sperm injection and in vitro fertilization. The New England Journal of Medicine 346(10):725–730

Heyes T, Long S, Mathers N 2004 Preconception care: Practice and beliefs of primary care workers. Family Practice 21:22–27

Health and Safety Executive 2006. Online. Available: http://www.hse.gov.uk 27 May 2007)

HFEA (Human Fertilization and Embryology Authority) Facts and figures. Online. Available: http://www.hfea.gov.uk/en/1215.html 21 April 2007)

HFEA (Human Fertilization and Embryology Authority) 2006 Single women and lesbian couples urged to speak out on the fertility services they receive. Press Release, October. HFEA, London

HFEA (Human Fertilization and Embryology Authority) 2003 Code of practice, 6th edn. HFEA, London

Illman L 2001 Promoting a health lifestyle. In: Andrews G (ed.) Women's sexual health. Baillière Tindall, Edinburgh, p 38–41

Jenkins J, Corrigan L, Chamber R 2003 Infertility matters in health care. Radcliffe Medical Press, Oxon, p 1–72

Jensen T K, Hjollund N H I, Henriksen T B et al 1998 Does moderate alcohol consumption affect fertility? Follow up study among couples planning first pregnancy. British Medical Journal 317(7157):505–510

Kanagalingham M G, Forouhi N G, Greer I A et al 2005 Changes in booking body mass index over a decade: retrospective analysis from a Glasgow Maternity Hospital. British Journal of Obstetrics and Gynaecology 112:1431–1433

Koch R, Hanley W, Levy H et al 2003 The maternal phenylketonuria international study: 1984–2002. Pediatrics 112 (6):1523–1529

Korenbrot C C, Steinburg A, Bender C et al 2002 Preconception care: A systematic review. Maternal and Child Health Journal 6(2):75–88

Lee P, Lilburn M, Baudin J 2003 Maternal phenylketonuria: Experiences from the United Kingdom. Pediatrics 112 (6):1553–1556

Leiblum S R 1997 Love, sex and infertility: the impact of infertility on couples. Infertility: psychological issues and counselling strategies. John Wiley, Chichester, p 149–166

Lewis, G (ed.) (2007) The Confidential Enquiry into Maternal and Child Health (CEMACH). Saving mothers' lives: reviewing maternal deaths to make motherhood safer 2003–2005. The seventh report on Confidential Enquiries into Maternal Deaths in the United Kingdom. CEMACH, London

Lumley J, Oliver S, Waters E 2002 Interventions for promoting smoking cessation during pregnancy (Review). The Cochrane Library Issue 3

Macintosh M C M, Fleming K M, Bailey J A et al 2006 Perinatal mortality and congenital anomalies in babies of women with type 1 or type 2 diabetes in England Wales and Northern Ireland: population based study. British Medical Journal 333 (7560):177

Mukherjee R A S, Hollins S, Abou-Saleh M T et al 2005 Low level alcohol consumption and the fetus. British Medical Journal 330:375–376

National Diet & Nutrition Survey: adults aged 19–64 years 2004 Summary Report, Vol 5. The Stationery Office, London

NICE (National Institute for Clinical Excellence) 2003. Antenatal care: routine care for the healthy pregnant woman. Clinical Guidelines. RCOG Press, London

NICE (National Institute for Clinical Excellence) 2004a The epilepsies: The diagnosis and management of the epilepsies in adults and children in primary and secondary care. Clinical Guideline 20. NICE, London

NICE (National Institute for Clinical Excellence) 2004b Fertility: assessment and treatment for people with fertility problems. Clinical Guideline 11. NICE, London

NICE (National Institute for Clinical Excellence) 2008 Antenatal care: routine care for the healthy pregnant woman. Clinical Guideline 62. NICE, London.

NSF (National Service Framework) for children, young people and maternity services 2004. DH, London

NSF (National Service Framework) for diabetes (England) standards 2001. Department of Health: The Stationery Office, London

Ray J G, O'Brien T E, Chan W S 2001 Preconception care and the risk of congenital anomalies in the offspring of women with diabetes mellitus: a meta-analysis. Quarterly Journal of Medicine 94:435–444

RCOG (Royal College of Obstetricians and Gynaecologists) 2006 Alcohol and pregnancy: information for you. RCOG, London

RCOG (Royal College of Obstetricians and Gynaecologists) 2004 Fertility: assessment and treatment for people with fertility problems. RCOG, London

Read J 2004 Sexual problems associated with infertility pregnancy and ageing. British Medical Journal 329 (7465):559–561

Rothman K J, Moore L L, Singer M R et al 1995 Teratogenicity of high vitamin A intake. New England Journal of Medicine 333(21):1369–1373

Rouse B, Matalon R, Koch R et al 2000 Maternal phenylketonuria syndrome: congenital heart defects microcephaly and developmental outcomes. Journal of Pediatrics 136(1):57–61

Rowell P, Braude P 2003 Assisted conception I – General principles. British Medical Journal 327:799–801

SACN (Scientific Advisory Committee on Nutrition) 2006 Folate and disease prevention. The Stationery Office, London

SACN (Scientific Advisory Committee on Nutrition) 2005 Review of dietary advice on vitamin A. The Stationery Office, London

Stanton W R, Lowe J B, Moffat J et al 2004 Randomised control trial of smoking cessation intervention directed at men whose partners are pregnant. Preventive Medicine 38:6–9

Surrogacy UK 2007 Online. Available: http://www.surroga-cyuk.org/FAQ.htm 21 April 2007)

Taylor R, Davison J M 2007 Type 1 diabetes and pregnancy. British Medical Journal 334:742–745

Turnpenny P, Ellard S 2005 Emery's elements of medical genetics. Churchill Livingstone, Edinburgh

Varughese G I, Chowdhury S R, Warner D P et al 2007 Pre-conception care of women attending adult general diabetes clinics – Are we doing enough? Diabetes Research and Clinical Practice 76:142–145

Waisbren S E, Azen C 2003 Cognitive and behavioural development in maternal phenylketonuria offspring. Pediatrics 112(6):1544–1547

Wallace M, Hurwitz B 1998 Preconception care: who needs it, who wants it, and how should it be provided? British Journal of General Practice 48:963–966

WHO (World Health Organization) 2006 European Ministerial Conference on Counteracting Obesity

WHO (World Health Organization) 1999 Laboratory manual for the examination of human semen and sperm-cervical mucus interaction, 4th edn. Cambridge University Press, Cambridge

Wynn M, Wynn A 1990 The need for nutritional assessment in the treatment of the infertile couple. Journal of Nutritional Medicine 1:315–324

Wynn M, Wynn A 1983 The prevention of handicap of early pregnancy origin. Some evidence of good health before conception. Foundation for Education and Research in Childbearing, London

Yeo S 2006 A randomised comparative trial of the efficacy and safety of exercise during pregnancy: Design and methods. Contemporary Clinical Trials 27:531–540

FURTHER READING

Andrews G (ed.) 2001 Women's sexual health. Baillière Tindall, Edinburgh.

This is an excellent text that covers all aspects of women's health.

USEFUL WEBSITES

Action on Smoking and Health (ASH):
http://www.ash.org.uk

British Agencies for Adoption and Fostering (BAAF):
http://www.baaf.org.uk/index.shtml

British Epilepsy Association:
http://www.epilepsy.org.uk

British Infertility Counselling Association (BICA):
http://74.220.203.213/bica/index.php

British Pregnancy Advisory Service (BPAS):
http://www.bpas.org

Diabetes UK:
http://www.diabetes.org.uk

Endometriosis UK:
http://www.endo.org.uk

Foresight:
http://www.foresight-preconception.org.uk

Human Fertilization and Embryology Authority:
http://www.hfea.gov.uk

Miscarriage Association:
http://www.miscarriageassociation.org.uk

NHS Pregnancy smoking helpline,
Tel: 0800 169 9169

Quit:
http://www.quit.org.uk

Resolve: The National Fertility Association:
http://www.resolve.org/site/PageServer

14 Change and adaptation in pregnancy

Irene Murray Jenny Hassall

The anatomical and physiological adaptations occurring throughout pregnancy affect virtually every body system. The timing and intensity of the changes vary between systems but all are designed to support fetal growth and development and prepare the mother for birth and motherhood. The midwife's appreciation of the normal adaptations to pregnancy and recognition of abnormal findings are fundamental in the management of normal as well as high risk pregnancies, enabling her to provide appropriate midwifery care to all women including those affected by pre-existing illness. A common feature of these changes is the dynamic and symbiotic partnership between the uteroplacental unit and the mother, which is influenced by physical, mechanical, genetic and hormonal factors. Many aspects of the physiology of pregnancy remain poorly understood and controversies continue to be researched.

The chapter aims to:

- provide an overview of the adaptation of each body system during pregnancy and the under-lying hormonal changes
- identify physiological changes that mimic or mask disease
- provide rationale for the common disorders in pregnancy enabling midwives to advise women appropriately
- review the diagnosis of pregnancy.

Changes in the woman's emotional state due to hormonal factors are discussed in Chapter 36, section A and changes in the breast are detailed in Chapter 41.

Physiological changes in the reproductive system

The uterus

The uterus plays an essential role in pregnancy by protecting and supporting the fetus, placenta and amniotic fluid (LaMar & Hamernik 2003). For most of the 40 weeks of pregnancy, it expands to accommodate the growing fetus and remains relatively quiescent, yet at the time of labour it is able to contract regularly and forcibly to expel the fetus due to its unique properties of contractility and elasticity. The uterine wall consists of three layers: an external serous epithelial layer or *perimetrium*, the middle muscle layer or *myometrium*, and the internal layer of *endometrium* (*decidua*) (Blackburn 2007).

The perimetrium

The perimetrium is a thin layer of peritoneum that protects the uterus (see Ch. 8). It provides a relatively inelastic base upon which the myometrium develops tension to increase intrauterine pressure. During pregnancy, the peritoneal sac is greatly distorted as the uterus enlarges and rises out of the pelvis, carrying the adjoining anatomical parts with them (Whitmore et al 2002). The increasing tension exerted on the broad ligaments causes them to become longer and wider and the anterior and posterior folds open out so they are no longer in apposition and can therefore accommodate the greatly enlarged uterine and ovarian arteries and veins (Cunningham et al 1997). The round ligaments undergo considerable hypertrophy and increase in both length and diameter (Cunningham et al 2005, p 24). Frequently, spasm of the round ligaments occurs with movement in pregnancy causing sharp groin pains – usually on the right side due to the dextrorotation of the uterus to the right (Gabbe et al 2004).

Myometrium

The myometrium is the main component in the enlargement of the uterus during pregnancy (Chard & Grudzinskas 1994) and is the distinct muscular layer of the uterine wall which is involved in contraction during labour. The lymphatics, immune cells and myometrial cells all increase in size and number, supported by the accumulating fibrous and elastic tissue which provides an expanding framework as the uterus distends (Rehman et al 2003). Despite historic descriptions of the myometrium having three layers of muscle fibres, it has recently been identified that these layers were observed in other species, such as rodents and lower mammals and that, contrary to traditional understanding, the human myometrium is not composed of well-defined circular and longitudinal layers (Young 2007).

The outer layer of the myometrium lying under the serosal perimetrium is a very thin sheet of smooth muscle, approximately $200\mu m$ thick, densely packed with myocytes and devoid of connective tissue (Young & Hession 1999). This structure is so thin in comparison with the remainder of the wall of the uterus that it is unlikely that it contributes significantly to the contractility of the uterus (Young 2007). However, the increase in elastin in this layer with resulting increase in elasticity allows the uterus to grow and stretch to accommodate the growing fetus (Blackburn 2007). Beneath this outer elastic layer lies another thin 'transitional' muscle layer approximately 0.5–1mm thick, containing bridging bundles of myocytes spanning from the outer to the inner layer (Young 2007).

The bulk of the uterine wall lies beneath these two thin layers and consists of a thick layer of myocytes organized into cylindrical, sheet-like and 'fibre' bundles or *fasciculata* with communicating bridges which merge and intertwine with each other to form an interlacing network and a contiguous pathway allowing coordinated contraction. The myocytes within each bundle all contract and relax in a longitudinal direction only (as with a spring).These fasciculi are well ordered, running transversely across the fundus of the uterus, obliquely down the anterior and posterior walls of the uterus and transversely across the lower uterine segment (Young & Hession 1999) (Fig. 14.1). Each fasciculata is 1–2mm in diameter and is surrounded and supported by fibrous tissue, collagen and elastin (Martin & Hutchon 2004).

In the first 12 weeks of pregnancy, uterine growth is due partly to *hyperplasia* (increased numbers of myocytes due to division) but mainly to hypertrophy (increased size of myocytes) under the influence

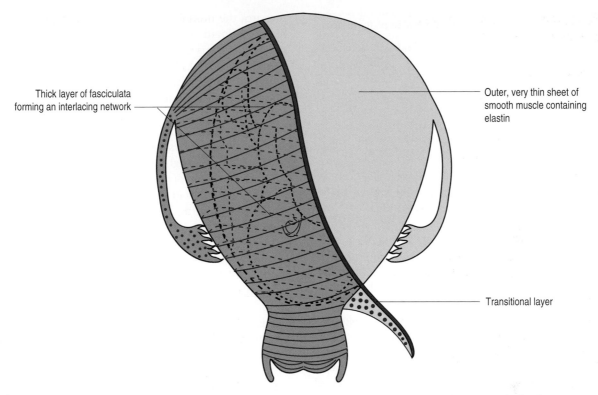

Thick layer of fasciculata
forming an interlacing network

Outer, very thin sheet of
smooth muscle containing
elastin

Transitional layer

Figure 14.1 Myometrium showing the very thin outer layer, the transitional layer and the inner bulk of myometrium with the arrangement of the fasciculata running transversely across the fundus between the fallopian tubes, obliquely down anterior and posterior walls and transversely around the lower uterine segment.

of high levels of oestradiol and progesterone (Cunningham et al 2005). The myometrial cells stretch in length by up to 15-fold (Baker 2006). Throughout the remainder of the pregnancy, uterine growth is predominantly due to fetal growth causing mechanical tension on the myometrium (Breuiller-Fouche & Germain 2006).

Although the walls of the corpus become considerably thicker during the first few months of pregnancy, as gestation advances they gradually thin so that by term they are only about 1.5 cm thick or even less and the uterus is changed into a muscular sac with thin, soft, readily indentable walls through which the fetus can easily be palpated (Cunningham et al 2005; Degani et al 1998). The walls become even thinner during active labour although significant thickening occurs at the implantation site after placental separation (Buhimschi et al 2003).

During pregnancy the uterus undergoes a 10-fold increase in weight (Symonds & Symonds 2004)

however, the dimensions vary considerably depending on the age and parity of the woman (Cunningham et al 2001). A study by Esmaelzadeh et al (2004) suggested that differences in dimensions may also be due to factors such as race, heredity, environment and diet (Table 14.1).

Although the primary function of the uterus is **not** to contract for the majority of the pregnancy in order to accommodate the developing fetus (Young 2007), the myometrium is never completely quiescent during pregnancy. By 7 weeks' gestation contractions are mild, irregular and non-synchronized, although not felt by the woman. As pregnancy progresses they are felt as 'tightenings', often appearing unpredictably and sporadically, particularly at night (Blackburn 2007). Late in pregnancy they become more rhythmic and may be as often as every 10–20 min, causing some discomfort and accounting for the so-called 'false labour' (Cunningham et al 2005) but not causing cervical dilatation. First observed by

Table 14.1 Increases in weight and size of the uterus during pregnancy

	Nulliparous	Parous	At term
Weight of uterus (g)	60–80	90–100	1100
Size of uterus (cm)	6–8 × 5 × 2.5	9–10	30 × 22.5 × 20

Cunningham et al 2001, Esmaelzadeh et al 2004.

Braxton Hicks in 1873, they are still known by his name today (Chard & Grudzinskas 1994).

Synchronous contractions of the uterus are dependent on the electrical coupling together of myometrial cells by gap junctions composed of connexin. Connexin 43 forms intercellular channels, which allow the transmission of electrical impulses, and perhaps metabolic communication, among the myometrial cells. Throughout most of pregnancy the number of these cell-to-cell channels is low, which results in poor electrical coupling. This favours myometrial quiescence and the maintenance of pregnancy. Several days prior to the onset of labour, the gap junctions markedly increase, leading to increased electrical conduction and coordination of myometrial cells and tissue necessary for effective contractions. The increase in gap junctions may be controlled by changing oestrogen and progesterone levels in the uterus (Garfield & Maner 2007).

The junctional zone is a separate and distinct functional unit within the uterus and lies between the myometrium and decidua. This area lacks a protective submucosal layer so that the endometrial glands lie in direct contact with the myometrium (Fusi et al 2006). Evidence has accumulated in recent years suggesting that this specialized zone plays a central role in the processes of sperm transport and implantation. Contractions arising in this area can facilitate or compromise the early survival of the embryo (Lesny & Killik 2004).

Decidua

The first signs of the re-modelling of endometrial stromal cells, matrix and blood vessels into the *decidua* (decidualization) (see Ch. 10) can be seen as early as day 23 of the normal menstrual cycle (Brosens & Gellersen 2006). Decidualization prepares the uterine lining for the invading trophoblasts (Kliman 2000). The decidua in the cervix and the isthmus are less well developed than in the corpus (Honda et al 2005), which prevents implantation in this region. Ultrasonography has identified that implantation usually occurs superiorly in the body of the uterus, and slightly more often on the posterior wall (Moore & Persaud 2003). Driven by rising levels of progesterone, decidualization spreads progressively throughout the endometrium during the first trimester of pregnancy (Jones et al 2006), but is most marked in the early weeks when the endometrial glands are best developed beneath the implantation site (Hempstock et al 2004). Over the first trimester, the decidua basalis gradually reduces from approximately 5 mm thick at 6 weeks to 1 mm thick at 14 weeks. The glands also gradually regress but still communicate with the intervillous space until at least 10 weeks (Hempstock et al 2004).

The glands within the decidua may provide an important source of nutrients, growth factors and cytokines for the fetoplacental unit (Hempstock et al 2004). Relaxin produced by the decidua plays a part in myometrial quiescence (Carvajal & Weiner 2003). The decidua also produces large amounts of prostaglandins, which either enhances uterine quiescence or initiates labour, depending on the specific receptor to which it is coupled (Blackburn 2007). The full significance of decidual cells is not understood but it has been postulated that they may protect maternal tissue against uncontrolled invasion by the syncytiotrophoblast (Moore & Persaud 2003).

Blood supply

Uterine blood flow in pregnancy supplies the myometrium, endometrium and placenta, with the latter receiving nearly 90% of the total uterine blood flow near term (Ross et al 2002) (see Chs 8 and 11). The diameters of the uterine arteries dilate to 1.5 times those seen in the non-pregnant state. The arcuate arteries that supply the placental bed become 10 times larger (Symonds & Symonds 2004). The highly coiled spiral arteries of the decidua and myometrium undergo marked physiological changes that disrupt their muscular and elastic elements and convert them from narrow spiral arteries into large calibre, uncoiled uteroplacental arteries which reach 30 times their pre-pregnancy diameter and permit expansion of the myometrial smooth muscle as it hypertrophies during pregnancy (Metaxa-Mariatou et al 2002). This re-modelling enhances their capacity to accommodate the increased blood volume needed within the intervillous spaces of the placenta leading to a large pool of blood within the uterus to maintain fetoplacental blood flow and oxygenation. The uterine veins also undergo significant adaptations to accommodate the massively increased uteroplacental blood flow (Blackburn 2007).

For the first 10–12 weeks blood supply into the intervillous spaces is limited due to the temporary occlusion of the tips of the spiral arteries by the invasive trophoblast (Blackburn 2007). Thereafter, the action of the invasive trophoblasts on the maternal spiral arteries leads to a very low resistance uteroplacental circulation which facilitates the marked increase in blood flow seen in these vessels at term (Kliman 2000). As a result of increase in maternal cardiac output and decline in uterine vascular resistance, as well as hormonal and chemical influences, the uterine blood flow progressively increases during gestation, from approximately 50mL/min at 10 weeks' gestation, increasing to 200mL/min by 28 weeks (Blackburn 2007), reaching as high as 750 mL/min at term, representing an almost 17-fold increase in uterine blood flow (Kliman 2000). Thus by term, the uterus is receiving between 10% and 20% of the maternal cardiac output (Blackburn 2007).

The passage of blood through the dilated uterine vessels produces a soft blowing sound synchronous with the maternal pulse known as the *uterine souffle*. It is heard most distinctly near the lower portion of the uterus. It should not be confused with the *placental souffle*, a muffled 'ocean-like' sound of blood coursing through the placenta which is synchronous with the fetal heart and found in the immediate vicinity of the placenta.

Changes in uterine size

Comparisons between the uterus and fruit has become a fairly reliable mental benchmark for uterine sizing in early pregnancy. At 5 weeks' gestation, the uterus feels like a small, unripe pear. By 8 weeks it feels like a large orange and by 12 weeks it is about the size of a grapefruit (Margulies & Miller 2001). The traditional method of assessing gestational age

is to relate the progressive increase in the height of the fundus at different gestations to abdominal landmarks throughout pregnancy (see Ch 17).

Changes in uterine shape

12th week of pregnancy

For the first few weeks of pregnancy, the increase in uterine size is limited principally to the anteroposterior diameter and the uterus maintains its original pear shape with the fundus being a flattened convexity between tubal insertions. As pregnancy advances, however, the corpus and fundus assume a more globular form becoming almost spherical by 12 weeks and too large to remain totally within the pelvis (Cunningham et al 2005). Physical movement of the uterus is normal in pregnancy, allowing the uterus to move relatively freely in all planes and thus to rise up out of its state of anteflexion (O'Grady & Pope 2006) (Fig. 14.2).

16th week of pregnancy

Between 12 and 16 weeks' gestation, the fundus becomes dome-shaped (Blackburn 2007). With the ascent of the uterus from the pelvis it usually undergoes dextrorotation to the right, possibly because of the rectosigmoid on the left side of the pelvis. The uterus now increases more rapidly in length than in width. From about 16 weeks, the internal os gradually relaxes and the lower uterine segment develops from the greatly expanded and thinned out muscular isthmus (Cunningham et al 2005).

20th week of pregnancy

As the uterus rises in the abdomen, it assumes an ovoid shape, the round ligaments appear to insert at the junction of the middle and upper thirds of the organ and the uterine tubes elongate (Cunningham et al 2005). By 20 weeks, the isthmus has fully developed into the lower uterine segment and the cervical canal expands from above downwards in a wedge-shaped fashion

30th week of pregnancy

As the uterus continues to enlarge it contacts the anterior abdominal wall, displacing intestines laterally and superiorly and continues to rise, ultimately

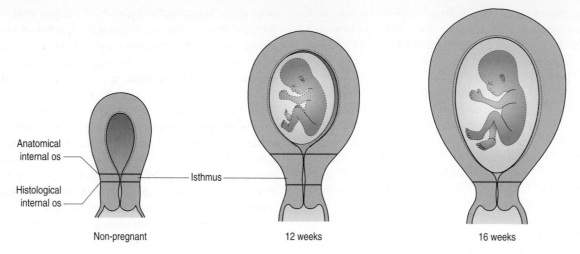

Figure 14.2   Changes in uterus from non-pregnant to 16 weeks' gestation. (From Hanretty 2003.)

reaching almost to the liver. The abdominal wall supports the uterus and unless it is quite relaxed, maintains this relation between the long axis of the uterus and the axis of the pelvic inlet. In the supine position the uterus falls back to rest on the vertebral column and the adjacent great vessels, in particular the inferior vena cava and aorta (Cunningham et al 2005).

36th week of pregnancy

By the end of the 36th week of pregnancy, the enlarged uterus almost fills the abdominal cavity. The fundus is at the tip of the xiphoid cartilage, which is pushed forward. The liver, transverse colon, stomach and spleen are crowded into the vault of the abdominal cavity. The small intestines are crowded above, behind, and to the sides of the uterus. The diaphragm is pressed upward, reducing the vertical diameter of the chest cavity by as much as 4 cm (Childbirth Connection 2007). By this stage, about half of the cervical canal is incorporated into the lower uterine segment.

38th week of pregnancy

By 38 weeks' gestation, the insertion of the uterine tubes and broad and round ligaments is located slightly above the middle of the uterus, exerting tension on the ligaments. The lower uterine segment is almost fully developed and the physiological retraction ring develops at the junction between lower and upper segments. The consistency of the lower uterine segment is much less firm. It is distended and much more passive while the upper uterine segment is quite hard, firm and contractile. Because the fasciculata run transversely across this area (Young 2007) and also because of its relative avascularity and quiescence in the puerperium this is the site of choice for the incision for a caesarean delivery.

Descent of the fetal head into the pelvic brim (*engagement*) leads to slight lowering of the fundus, known as *lightening* which causes a change in shape of the abdomen. Women describe this as 'the baby dropped'. When this occurs breathing becomes easier and heartburn occurs less frequently but the increased pressure on the bladder may lead to urinary frequency. As pressure increases in the pelvis constipation may occur and as the pelvic ligaments are stretched more, low backpain may be experienced. All the studies reviewed by Dietze (2001) suggested that engagement in nulliparous women is less common antenatally than is described in textbooks, ranging from 50% to 83%. Ambwani (2004) also commented on the extremely variable incidence, noting that in their study 21% of primigravidae had a floating head at term and calling for an attitude of watchful expectancy to avoid unnecessary intervention.

The cervix

Within 1 month of conception, the cervix becomes softer and cyanosed due to oedema and increased vascularity (Cunningham et al 2005). The collagen fibres become less dense with thinner and more loosely packed fibres. The arrangement of elastin and tightly wound, circumferential, collagen fibres, which are bonded together by a firm ground substance helps to form a rigid, tubular structure, which holds the canal closed and provides strength to retain the fetus in pregnancy (Gee 2004). The elastin:collagen ratio is greatest at the internal os where muscle content is lowest (Blackburn 2007). The glands of the cervix undergo such marked hypertrophy and hyperplasia that by the end of pregnancy they occupy half of the entire cervical mass as opposed to the small fraction in the nonpregnant state. They become everted so that the tissue tends to become red and velvety and bleeds even with minor trauma such as taking Pap smears. The basal cells near the squamocolumnar junction may be more prominent in shape and size due to oestrogen which renders the Pap smear less efficient (Cunningham et al 2005).

The endocervical mucosal cells produce copious amounts of a tenacious mucus resulting in the development of an antibacterial plug in the cervix. The consistency of the mucus changes during pregnancy under the influence of progesterone so that the typical *ferning* seen in very early pregnancy changes to a beaded pattern (Cunningham et al 2005).

In the last 6 weeks of pregnancy, the cervix undergoes many changes ('*ripening*') in preparation for expelling the fetus (Carbonne et al 2000). Cervical ripening involves inflammatory cells, but is likely dependent upon endogenously produced prostaglandins. Rearrangement and degradation of collagen fibres creates an increase in the space between them, shortens them and increases acidic solubility (Garfield et al 1998) along with reduced capacity to retain water (Chard & Grudzinskas 1994). The ground substance becomes fluid changing the cervix to a soft, distensible structure with reduced resistance to effacement and dilatation (Gee 2004). Cervical thinning, softening and effacement can be readily detected on vaginal examination.

The cervical canal shortens from above downwards from about 2 cm long to a mere circular orifice with almost paper-thin edges. The muscular fibres at the level of the internal cervical os are pulled upward or 'taken up' into the lower uterine segment while the external os remains unchanged. Effacement can be compared with a funneling process in which the whole length of a narrow cylinder is converted into a very obtuse, flaring funnel with a small circular orifice for an outlet. This process causes the expulsion of the mucus plug as a *bloody show* at the onset of labour. There are controversies around when cervical shortening occurs (Dijkstra et al 1999). Carvalho et al (2003) demonstrated a spontaneous shortening in the pregnant cervix from the first to the second trimester of pregnancy. Haram et al (2003) observed that the shorter the cervix, the greater the risk of pre-term labour.

Classically cervical effacement and dilatation has been thought to be due to fundal contractions causing a radial pulling of the cervix over the uterine contents. However, Young (2007) suggests effacement and dilatation is primarily the result of increased intrauterine pressure caused by contractions of the uterine wall. In this formulation the weakest point of the sphere – the thinner lower uterine segment and ripened cervix – bulges, thins, and dilates with each episode of increased pressure. In nulliparous women effacement usually takes place prior to the commencement of labour but in parous women effacement may take place simultaneously with cervical dilatation (Gee 2006). By term, assuming a well-fitting presenting part, only about the lower third of the cervical canal plus the external os remain to be dilated in the first stage of labour. Hormonal control of cervical ripening is a complex process that involves a cascade of changes in oestradiol, progesterone and relaxin (Blackburn 2007). Nitric oxide production increases in the cervix at the end of pregnancy (Garfield et al 1998) but its role in cervical ripening remains unclear (Blackburn 2007).

The vagina

During pregnancy, increased vascularity and hyperaemia develop in the skin and muscles of the perineum and vulva with softening of the underlying connective tissue. Increased vascularity affects the vagina and results in the violet colour characteristic of *Chadwick's sign*. In preparation for the distension that occurs in labour the vaginal walls undergo striking changes: the mucosa thickens, the connective tissue loosens and the smooth muscle cells hypertrophy. The increased volume of vaginal secretions due to high levels of oestrogen results in a thick, white discharge known as *leucorrhoea* (Cunningham et al 2005).

In pregnancy, larger amounts of glycogen are deposited in the vaginal epithelium due to high oestrogen availability (Boskey et al 2001). Glycogen is metabolized to lactic acid by the *Lactobacillus acidophilus*, ('Döderlein's bacillus'), a normal commensal of the vagina. This leads to increased vaginal acidity (pH varying from 3.5–6).

Changes in the cardiovascular system

Pregnancy is associated with profound but predominantly reversible changes in maternal haemodynamics and cardiac function. These complex adaptations are necessary to:

- meet evolving maternal changes in physiological function
- to promote the growth and development of the uteroplacental-fetal unit
- to compensate for blood loss at the end of labour.

All components of the system undergo a degree of adaptation in pregnancy (Table 14.2). The key physiological changes that occur are; an increase in blood

Table 14.2 A summary of the key components and functions of the cardiovascular system including changes in pregnancy

Component	Key change in pregnancy
The heart	Increases in size Shifted upwards and to left
Arteries	Dramatic systemic and pulmonary vasodilation to increase blood flow
Capillaries	Increased permeability
Veins	Vasodilation and impeded venous return in lower extremities
Blood	Haemodilution Increased capacity for clot formation

Adapted from Torgersen & Curran 2006.

volume, cardiac output, stroke volume and heart rate together with a decrease in systemic vascular resistance, blood pressure, pulmonary vascular resistance and colloid osmotic pressure (Table 14.3). They are accompanied by widespread peripheral vasodilation resulting in the high flow, low resistance haemodynamic state with marked haemodilution, characteristic of a healthy pregnancy.

It is critical to achieve a balance between fetal requirements and maternal tolerance. In most women, these demands are accommodated by physiological adaptations without compromising the mother.

Blood volume

The increase in total blood volume (TBV) is essential to:

- protect the mother (and fetus) against the harmful effects of impaired venous return
- meet the demands of the enlarged uterus with a significantly hypertrophied vascular system and provide extra blood flow for placental perfusion
- supply the extra metabolic needs of the fetus
- provide extra perfusion of kidneys and other organs
- counterbalance the effects of increased arterial and venous capacity
- safeguard the mother against adverse effects of excessive blood loss at birth.

The first step in the circulatory changes in pregnancy is extreme vasodilation mediated by rising pregnancy hormone levels (particularly progesterone) and circulating nitric oxide (Van Mook & Peeters 2005).

Vasodilation causes an 'underfilling' of the maternal circulation which subsequently initiates fluid and electrolyte retention, expansion of the plasma and extra cellular fluid volumes and a concurrent increase in cardiac output. This occurs prior to full placentation and is accompanied by a parallel increase in renal blood flow and glomerular filtration rate. These changes may be mediated by a systemic and renal vasodilator unique to pregnancy (Varga et al 2000).

The mechanisms for maintaining homeostasis are modified to accommodate and maintain these changes (Weissgerber & Wolfe 2006). Renin and aldosterone activity are increased by oestrogens, progesterone and prostaglandins, leading to increased

Table 14.3   Key physiological changes in cardiovascular system in pregnancy

Parameter	Adaptation	Magnitude	Non-pregnant (average value)	Timing of peak; average peak value
Plasma volume	Increase	50%	2600 mL	32 weeks; 3850 mL
Red cell mass	Increase	–	1400 mL	30 weeks; 1550 mL
Total blood volume	Increase	30–45%	4000 mL	32 weeks; 4600 mL
Cardiac output	Increase	35–50%	4.9 L/min	28 weeks; 7 L/min
Stroke volume	Increase			20 weeks
Heart rate	Increase	10–15 bpm	75 b.p.m.	Trimester 1; 90 b.p.m.
Systemic vascular resistance	Decrease	21%	–	Trimester 2
Pulmonary vascular resistance	Decrease	35%	–	34 weeks
Diastolic blood pressure	Decrease, returning to normal by term	10–15 mmHg	–	24 weeks
Systolic blood pressure	Minimal, no decrease	5–10 mmHg	–	24 weeks
Serum colloid osmotic pressure	Decrease	10–15%	–	14 weeks

Data from Blackburn 2007 and Nelson-Piercy 2006.

fluid and electrolyte retention. Oestrogen reduces the transcapillary escape rate of albumin, which promotes intravascular protein retention and shifts extra cellular fluid volume distribution while lowering the osmotic threshold for ADH (anti-diuretic hormone) release. Despite the progressive increase in blood volume as pregnancy progresses the secretion of ANP (atrial natriuretic peptide) is not increased because the ANP-volume relationship is reset during pregnancy (Weissgerber & Wolfe 2006). While ANP levels are slightly reduced, plasma renin activity tends to be increased. This supports the theory that the increase in plasma volume represents 'underfilling' due to systemic vasodilatation and the consequent rise in vascular capacity, rather than true blood volume expansion (Varga et al 2000).

Cardiac output

Cardiac output increase allows blood flow to the brain and coronary arteries to remain unchanged, while distribution to other organs is modified as pregnancy advances. The increased cardiac output is due to increases in both stroke volume and heart rate; the relative contributions of these factors to cardiac output vary with gestational age. Most of the increase in heart rate occurs during the first trimester thus contributing to early changes in cardiac output.

Increases in stroke volume facilitate second trimester increases in cardiac output augmented by plasma volume expansion. The stroke volume increases by 10% during the first half of pregnancy, and reaches a peak at 20 weeks' gestation that is maintained until term (Girling 2001) (Fig. 14.3).

Cardiac output in pregnancy is extremely sensitive to changes in body position. This sensitivity increases with lengthening gestation, because the uterus impinges upon the inferior vena cava, thereby decreasing blood return to the heart. Large variations in cardiac output, pulse rate, blood pressure and regional blood flow may follow trivial changes of posture, activity or anxiety.

Blood pressure and vascular resistance

While cardiac output is raised, arterial blood pressure is reduced by 10%, therefore resistance to flow must be decreased (de Sweit 1998a). This can be accounted for by the decrease in systemic vascular resistance, particularly in the peripheral vessels. The decrease begins at 5 weeks' gestation, reaches a nadir in the second trimester (a 21% reduction) and then gradually rises as term approaches. Numerous modifications occur in the mechanisms controlling vascular activity; agents responsible for peripheral vasodilation include; prostacyclin, nitric oxide and

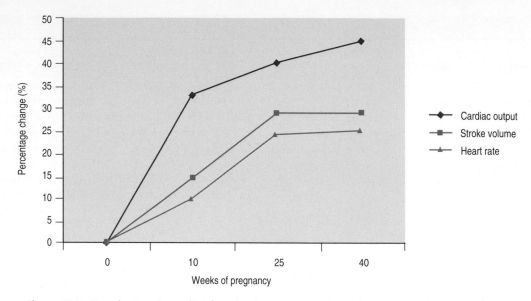

Figure 14.3 Key changes in cardiac function in pregnancy. (Data from Cunningham et al 2005.)

progesterone and vasoactive prostaglandins. The changes are not limited to the uteroplacental circulation but are apparent throughout the body in a healthy pregnancy. Increased heat production in pregnancy further contributes to the reduced resistance by stimulating vasodilation particularly in heat loss areas such as hands and feet (Blackburn 2007).

Early pregnancy is associated with a marked decrease in diastolic blood pressure but minimal reduction in systolic pressure. With reduced peripheral vascular resistance the systolic blood pressure falls an average of 5–10mmHg below baseline levels and the diastolic pressure falls 10–15mmHg by 24 weeks' gestation. Thereafter, blood pressure gradually rises, returning to the pre-pregnant levels at term. Despite the increased blood volume, systemic venous pressures do not rise significantly in pregnancy; the exception to this is in the lower limbs.

Postural changes that affect cardiac output also have a major effect on blood pressure. The enlarging uterus compresses both the inferior vena cava and the lower aorta when the woman lies supine. This reduces venous return to the heart with a consequential fall in pre-load and cardiac output of 30–40%. Most women are capable of compensating for the resultant decrease in stroke volume by increasing systemic vascular resistance and heart rate. Blood from the lower limbs may also return collateral conduits, however if these are not well developed or adequately perfused, the pregnant woman may suffer from *supine hypotensive syndrome*. This consists of hypotension, bradycardia, dizziness, light-headedness, nausea and even syncope, if she remains in the supine position too long and occurs in approximately 10% of pregnant women. The fall in blood pressure may be severe enough for the mother to lose consciousness due to reduced cerebral blood flow. By rolling the woman on to her left side, the cardiac output can be instantly restored (Burnett 2001). Compression of the aorta may lead to reduced uteroplacental and renal blood flow and fetal compromise.

The heart

In pregnancy, the heart is enlarged by both chamber dilation and myocardial hypertrophy. Myocardial hypertrophy in early pregnancy leads to a 10–15% increase in ventricular wall muscle. Blood volume expansion in the second and third trimesters results in increased diastolic filling (particularly in the left ventricle), and progressive distension of the heart chambers. Despite cardiac enlargement, efficiency is maintained by lengthening of muscle fibres and reduction in after load, facilitated by marked peripheral vasodilation.

The growing uterus elevates the diaphragm, the great vessels are unfolded and the heart is correspondingly displaced upward and to the left to produce a slight anterior rotation of the heart on its long axis. This can give an exaggerated impression of cardiac enlargement (de Sweit 1998a), and accounts for variations in parameters used for cardiac assessment including ECG and radiographic assessments. Atrial or ventricular extrasystoles are frequent and there is increased susceptibility to supraventricular tachycardia (de Sweit 1998a). While these symptoms are relatively common in normal pregnancies it is imperative that signs of severe disease are not overlooked.

Regional blood flow

As blood volume increases with gestation, a substantial proportion (10–20%), is distributed to the uteroplacental unit.

Renal vasodilation early in pregnancy results in increased renal blood flow and glomerular filtration rate accommodating the increased cardiac output before blood flow significantly increases to the uteroplacental unit (Varga et al 2000). Renal blood flow increases by as much as 70–80% by the 16th week of pregnancy which helps to enhance excretion.

Blood flow to the brain, coronary arteries and liver is not significantly changed in pregnancy. Pulmonary blood flow increases secondary to the increase in cardiac output and is facilitated by reduced pulmonary vascular resistance. Blood flow in the lower limbs is slowed in late pregnancy by compression of the iliac veins and inferior vena cava by the enlarging uterus and the hydrodynamic effects of increased venous return from the uterus (Broughton-Pipkin 2001). Reduced venous return and increased venous pressure in the legs contributes to the increased distensibility and pressure in the veins of the legs, vulva, rectum and pelvis, leading to dependent oedema, varicose veins of legs and vulva and haemorrhoids. These changes are more pronounced in the left leg due to compression of the left iliac vein by the overlying right iliac artery and the ovarian artery. This anatomical variation accounts for the fact that 85% of venous thrombosis in pregnancy occur in the left leg (Nelson-Piercy 2006) (Box 14.1).

Blood flow is increased to the capillaries of the mucous membranes and skin, particularly in hands and feet. This helps to eliminate the excess heat produced by the increased metabolism of the maternal-

---

Box 14.1 Varicosities

Varicosities develop in approximately 40% of women, and are usually seen in the veins of the legs, but may also occur in the vulva and as haemorrhoids in the anal area. The effects of progesterone and relaxin on the smooth muscles of the vein walls, and the increased weight of the growing uterus all contribute to the increased risk of valvular incompetence. A family tendency is also a factor (Blackburn 2007). Some suggestions for alleviating them include: spraying the legs with hot and cold water, resting with the legs elevated and wearing supportive stockings.

---

fetal mass and cardiorespiratory work of pregnancy. The associated peripheral vasodilation explains why pregnant women 'feel the heat', sweat profusely at times, have clammy hands and often suffer from nasal congestion (Broughton-Pipkin 2001).

Haematological changes

In parallel with the 30–45% increase in maternal blood volume, plasma volume increases by 50% (1250–1600 mL) over the course of the pregnancy (Burnett 2001), followed by a relatively smaller increase in red blood cell volume (Table 14.4). These changes are responsible for the hypervolaemia of pregnancy leading to numerous modifications to parameters commonly assessed in blood tests (Table 14.5).

Table 14.4 Key haematological changes in pregnancy

		Weeks of pregnancy		
	Non-pregnant	20	30	40
Plasma volume (mL)	2600	3150	3750	3850
Red cell mass (mL)	1400	1450	1550	1650
Total blood volume (mL)	4000	4600	5300	5500
Haematocrit (PCV) (%)	35.0	32.0	29.0	30.0
Haemoglobin (g/dL)	13.3	11.0	10.5	11.0

After Llewellyn-Jones 1999 p 34.

Table 14.5 Normal values in pregnant/non-pregnant women

Test	Non-pregnant (typical range)	Pregnant (typical range)	Comments
Biochemistry			
Alanine transaminase (ALT) (U/L)	6–40	No change	Raised levels indicate liver damage
Alkaline phosphatase (IU/L)	40–120	Doubled by late pregnancy	Usually elevated in third trimester due to placental production of enzyme
Bile acids (total) (µmol/L)	<9		Values of total bile acids ≥14 µmol/L are viewed as abnormal, indicating cholestasis
Bilirubin (µmol/L)	<17		Little change in non-pregnant range
Creatinine (µmol/L)	50–100	75 approx is upper limit of normal	Lower in mid-pregnancy but rises towards term
Potassium (mmol/L)	3.5–5.3	Unchanged	Unchanged in pregnancy
Albumin (g/L)	30–48	25–35	Total protein and albumin are both lower in pregnancy
Urea (mmol/L)	2–6.5	Usually ≤4.5	Lower in pregnancy
Uric acid (µmol/L)	150–350	Lowest values in second trimester, 10 × gestational age in weeks is approx upper limit of normal	Increases with gestation, although lower levels than non-pregnant
Haematology[a]			
Clotting time (min)	12	8	Observe whether blood is clotting or oozing from venepuncture sites in high-risk groups
Fibrin degradation products (µg/mL)	Mean 1.04	High values in third trimester and especially around time of birth	
Fibrinogen (g/L)	1.7–4.1	By term 2.9–6.2	Marked increase in pregnancy especially in third trimester and around time of birth
Haemotocrit (L/L)	0.35–0.47	0.31–0.35	Lower in pregnancy
Haemoglobin (g/dL)	11.5–16.5	10.0–12.0 should be ≥10 in third trimester	Good iron stores needed to maintain pregnancy levels. Fall in first trimester whether or not iron and folate taken
Platelets (× 10^9 L)	150–400	Slight decrease in normal pregnancy lower limit of 'normal' = 120	No functional significance
White cell count (× 10^9 L)	4.0–11.0	9.0–15.0; Higher values up to 25.0 around time of birth	Normal increase in pregnancy. Rise in infections

[a]Note: Pregnancy is a hypercoagulable state and prothrombin, partial thromboplastin and thrombin times are slightly faster than controls.
From Fraser & Cooper 2008, p 646–647, adapted from Ramsay 2000.

The changes begin at 6–8 weeks of pregnancy. Plasma volume, placental mass and birth weight positively correlate in a healthy pregnancy (Duffy 2004). Excessive increases in plasma volume have been associated with multiple pregnancy, prolonged pregnancy, maternal obesity, and infants large for gestational age while inadequate increases have been associated with pre-eclampsia.

Red cell mass, which represents the total volume of red cells in circulation, increases during pregnancy by approx 18% in response to increased levels of erythropoietin. This is stimulated by maternal hormones (prolactin, progesterone, human placental lactogen and oestrogen) and the extra oxygen requirements of maternal and placental tissue (Cunningham et al 1997). This homeostatic mechanism is discrete from that which controls fluid balance and increased plasma volumes. Therefore in spite of the increased production of red blood cells, the marked increase in plasma volume causes dilution of many circulating factors. As a result the red cell count, haematocrit and haemoglobin concentration all decrease (Letsky 1998), resulting in 'apparent anaemia', characteristic of a healthy pregnancy (Fig. 14.4). The disproportionate increase in plasma volume is clearly advantageous. By reducing blood viscosity, resistance to blood flow is reduced leading to improved placental perfusion and reduced maternal cardiac effort (Cunningham et al 1997).

Red blood cells become more spherical with increased diameter due to the drop in plasma colloid pressure encouraging more water to cross the erythrocyte cell membrane. Mean cell volume also increases due to the higher proportion of young larger red blood cells (reticulocytes). There is still disagreement as to the exact increase in red cell mass and measurements have been influenced by iron medication.

While **total** haemoglobin increases from 85–150g, the **mean** haemoglobin concentration falls. In healthy women with adequate iron stores this drops by about 2g/dL from an average of 13.3g/dL in the non-pregnant state to 11.0g/dL in early pregnancy. It is at its lowest at around 32 weeks' gestation when plasma volume expansion is maximal, and after this time rises by approximately 0.5g/dL, returning to 11g/dL around the 36th week of pregnancy. A haemoglobin level below 10.5g/100mL at 28 weeks should be investigated (NICE 2008a Ch. 21).

Iron metabolism

A fall in haemoglobin is a physiological adjustment to pregnancy, whereas a high haemoglobin level can be a sign of pathology (McFadyen 1995). The total iron requirements of pregnancy average about 1000mg. About 500mg are required to increase the red blood cell mass, and about 300mg are transported to the fetus, mainly in the last 12 weeks of pregnancy. The remaining 200mg are needed to compensate for insensible loss in skin, stool and urine. Practically all of the increased iron requirements occur in the last half of the pregnancy, averaging 6–7mg/day. Since this amount is not available from body stores in most women, the red cell volume and haemoglobin level fall with the rising plasma volume. In spite of this, even if the mother has severe iron deficiency anaemia, the placenta is still able to provide the needed iron from maternal serum for the fetal production of haemoglobin. However, if the woman enters pregnancy with depleted iron stores, in spite of the moderate increase in iron absorption from the gut the amount of iron absorbed from the diet plus that mobilized from stores may be insufficient to meet the demands imposed by pregnancy. The purpose of iron supplementation, therefore, is to maintain iron stores in

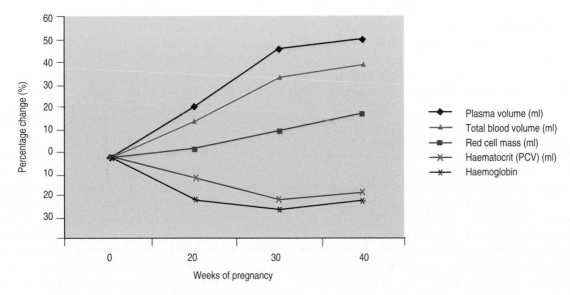

Figure 14.4 Key haematological changes in pregnancy. (Data from Cunningham et al 2005.)

order to prevent the development of true anaemia, rather than to raise the haemoglobin level (see Ch. 21) (Letsky 1998). Iron supplementation, however, should not be offered routinely to all pregnant women as it is of no benefit to mother or baby and has unpleasant maternal side-effects (NICE 2008a).

Plasma protein

Haemodilution leads to a fall in total serum protein content within the first trimester which remains reduced throughout pregnancy. Despite oestrogen reducing the transcapillary escape rate of albumin, albumin concentration falls abruptly in early pregnancy and then more slowly until late pregnancy (Table 14.5). Albumin plays an important role, not only as a carrier protein for some hormones, drugs, free fatty acids and unconjugated bilirubin, but also because of its influence in decreasing colloid osmotic pressure. A 10–15% fall in colloid osmotic pressure (Nelson-Piercy 2006) allows water to move from the plasma into the cells or out of vessels, and plays a part in the increased fragility of red blood cells and oedema of the lower limbs. It is now accepted that peripheral oedema in the lower limbs in late pregnancy is a feature of normal, uncomplicated pregnancy (Girling 2001).

Clotting factors

Changes in the coagulation system lead to the characteristic hypercoagulable state of normal pregnancy. The increased tendency to clot is caused by increases in clotting factors and fibrinogen accompanied by reduced plasma fibrinolytic activity and an increase in circulating fibrin degradation products in the plasma.

From 12 weeks' gestation there is a 50% increase in synthesis of plasma fibrinogen concentration (factor I). This may be necessary for the body to deal with the frequent disruptions in the integrity of the vascular tree in the placental bed (Coustan 1995). It is also critical in the prevention of haemorrhage at the time of placental separation. The development of a fibrin mesh to cover the placental site to control the bleeding requires 5–10% of all the circulating fibrinogen. When this process is impaired, as for example in inadequate uterine action or incomplete placental separation, there is rapid depletion of fibrinogen reserves, which can lead to exsanguination and death (Campbell & Lees 2000).

Coagulation factors VII, VIII and X increase in pregnancy (Burnett 2001), while factors II (prothrombin) and V remain constant or show a slight fall. Both the prothrombin time (normal 10–14s) and the partial thromboplastin time (normal 35–45s) are shortened slightly as pregnancy advances. The clotting times of whole blood, however, are not significantly different in normal pregnancy. The platelet count declines slightly as pregnancy advances, which is explained partially by haemodilution. However, there is a substantial increase in platelet volume, which may be due to the hyper-destruction of platelets in pregnancy, and as young platelets are larger than old ones the balance is pushed towards an overall increase in size (Steinfeld & Wax 2001).

A decrease in some endogenous anticoagulants (antithrombin, protein S and activated protein C resistance) occur in pregnancy and are intended to reduce the risk of haemorrhage at the time of birth; however, along with the physiological vasodilation of pregnancy, this contributes to a six-fold increase in the risk of thromboembolism in pregnancy (Girling 2001).

White blood cells (leucocytes) and immune function

Pregnancy presents a paradox for the mother's immune system as the mechanisms which are essential to protect her from infection have the potential to destroy the genetically disparate conceptus.

The total white cell count rises from 8 weeks' gestation and reaches a peak at 30 weeks. This is mainly because of the increase in numbers of neutrophil polymorphonuclear leucocytes, monocytes and granulocytes, the latter two producing a far more active and efficient phagocytosis function, which enhances the blood's phagocytic and bactericidal properties. Numbers of eosinophils, basophils, monocytes, lymphocytes and circulating T cells and B cells remain relatively constant. Lymphocyte function is depressed, and natural killer cytokine activity is down regulated by progesterone particularly in latter stages of pregnancy. Chemotaxis is suppressed resulting in a delayed response to some infections. There is decreased resistance to viral infections such as herpes, influenza, rubella, hepatitis, poliomyelitis and malaria. The metabolic activity of granulocytes increases during pregnancy, possibly resulting from the stimulation of oestrogen (Steinfeld & Wax 2001).

It is clear that the immunological relationship between the mother and the fetus involves a two-way communication involving fetal antigen presentation and maternal recognition of and reaction to these antigens by the immune system. There is evidence that immunological recognition of pregnancy is important for the maintenance of gestation and inadequate recognition of fetal antigens might result in failed pregnancy (Szekeres-Bartho 2001).

Maternal immune response is biased toward an enhancement of innate (humoral) immunity and away from cell-mediated response that could be harmful to the fetus. The stimulus for these changes is predominantly hormonal involving progesterone, HPL, prostaglandins, corticosteroids, human chorionic gonadotrophin (hCG), prolactin and serum proteins.

Despite the placental barrier, small trophoblastic fragments have been shown to enter the maternal circulation stimulating the maternal inflammatory response. This is modified in specific areas such as uteroplacental interface by pregnancy zone protein. This has been shown to increase in pregnancy by 100–200% (Blackburn 2007).

Changes in the respiratory system

Pregnancy is associated with marked changes in respiratory physiology mediated by biochemical and mechanical factors. These accommodate the progressive increase in oxygen consumption and the physical impact of the enlarging uterus. Normal oxygen consumption is 250 mL/min at rest and increases by 20% in pregnancy in order to meet the 15% increase in the maternal metabolic rate (Nelson-Piercy 2006). Changes in pregnancy result in an overcompensation to this respiratory demand. The resulting hyperventilation causes the arterial oxygen tension to increase and arterial carbon dioxide tension to fall, accompanied by a compensatory fall in serum bicarbonate. A mild respiratory alkalosis is therefore normal in pregnancy (Table 14.6).

Table 14.6 Summary of changes in respiratory function

Parameter	Adaptation	Magnitude (%)	Non-pregnant (average value)	Timing of peak; average peak value
Oxygen consumption	Increase	18	250 mL/min	300 mL/min
Metabolic rate	Increase	15	–	Peaks at term with increases up to 8 fold reported (Blackburn 2007)
Minute volume: amount of air/minute moved into and out of the lungs	Increase	40	7.5 L/min	Peaks at term; 10.5 L/min
Tidal volume: amount of air inspired and expired with normal breath	Increase	40	500 mL	700 mL
Vital capacity: maximum amount of air that can be forcibly expired after maximum inspiration	No change	–	3200 mL	3200 mL
Functional residual capacity: amount of air in lungs at resting expiratory level	Decrease	20	1700 mL	1350 mL
Blood gas analysis				
Arterial oxygen tension (PaO_2)	Increase		95–100 mmHg	Peak end trimester 1; 106–108 mmHg
Arterial carbon dioxide tension ($PaCO_2$)	Decrease		35–40 mmHg	27–32 mmHg
Serum bicarbonate	Decrease			18–22 mmol/L
Arterial pH	Small increase			7.44 (A mild respiratory alkalosis)

de Swiet 2002, Nelson Piercy 2002.

The driving force for change is the stimulatory effect of progesterone on the respiratory centre, which lowers the threshold and increases sensitivity to carbon dioxide (Jensen et al 2005). Up to 75% of pregnant women with no underlying pre-existing respiratory disease experience some dyspnoea possibly due to an increased awareness of the physiological hyperventilation (Nelson-Piercy 2006). Hyperventilation can be extremely uncomfortable and may lead to dyspnoea and dizziness. Although it is not usually associated with pathological processes, care must be taken not to dismiss it lightly and miss a warning sign of cardiac or pulmonary disease (Steinfeld & Wax 2001) (Box 14.2).

From early pregnancy onwards, the overall shape of the chest alters; the lower ribs flare outwards prior to any mechanical pressure from the growing uterus. This progressively increases the subcostal angle, from 68° in early pregnancy to 103° at term (Fig 14.5). The shape of the chest changes as the anteroposterior and transverse diameters increase, by about 2 cm, resulting in a 5–7 cm expansion of the chest circumference. The flaring of the lower ribs, causes the diaphragm to rise by up to 4 cm, its contribution to the respiratory effort increasing with no evidence of being impeded by the uterus. These changes are thought to be mediated by the effect of progesterone, which together with relaxin, increases ribcage elasticity by relaxing ligaments. Progesterone also mediates

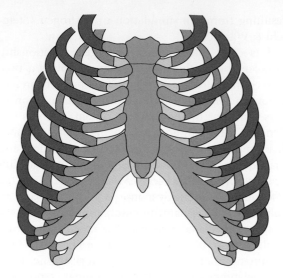

Figure 14.5 Displacement of the ribcage in pregnancy (dark) and the non-pregnancy state (light) showing elevated diaphragm, the increased transverse diameter and circumference, flaring out of ribs and the increased subcostal angle (de Sweit, 1998b, p 115, with permission from Wiley-Blackwell Publishing Ltd).

Box 14.2 Breathlessness

Breathlessness during pregnancy occurs in approximately 60% of women with exertion and under 20% at rest. This physiological dyspnoea often occurs early in pregnancy and does not interfere with daily activities and usually diminishes as term approaches. Although mechanical impediment by the uterus is often blamed, hyperventilation is due to altered sensitivity to CO_2. Distinguishing this physiological dyspnoea from breathlessness caused by disorders complicating pregnancy or diseases that might coexist with pregnancy is essential. It can be alleviated by maintaining an upright posture and holding hands above the head while taking deep breaths. Avoiding excessive exertion is advisable.

---

bronchial and tracheal smooth muscle relaxation thereby reducing airway resistance. This improves air flow along the bronchial tree, and explains why women with respiratory problems in pregnancy rarely deteriorate as much as women suffering from other chronic disorders (Campbell & Lees 2000).

Expansion of the rib cage causes *tidal volume* to increase by 30–40%. It rises early in pregnancy continuing to rise until term. Although the respiratory rate is little changed in pregnancy from the normal 14 or 15 breaths/min, breathing is deeper even at rest. The *minute volume* that facilitates gas exchange is increased by 30–40%, from 7.5–10.5 L/min, and minute oxygen uptake increases appreciably as pregnancy advances (Cunningham et al 1997). The enhanced tidal volume contributes to an increase in *inspiratory capacity* while *vital capacity* is unchanged. As a result the *functional residual capacity* is decreased by 20%. This reduces the amount of used gas mixing with each new inspiration thereby enhancing alveolar gas exchange by 50–70%.

Blood volume expansion and vasodilation of pregnancy result in hyperaemia and oedema of the upper respiratory mucosa, which predispose the pregnant woman to nasal congestion, epistaxis and even changes in voice. The changes to the upper respiratory tract may lead to upper airway obstruction and bleeding making both mask anaesthesia and tracheal intubation more difficult. These can be further exacerbated by fluid overload or oedema associated with pregnancy-induced hypertension or pre-eclampsia.

Blood gases

Despite overcompensation of the respiratory system to maternal oxygen requirements, alveolar oxygen partial pressure and the arterial oxygen partial pressure (PaO_2) are only slightly increased from non-pregnant values (98–100 mmHg) to pregnant values of (101–104 mmHg). This is accounted for by the increased oxygen consumption and oxygen carrying capacity of the blood (Broughton-Pipkin 2001). The 'hyperventilation of pregnancy' causes a 15–20% decrease in maternal arterial carbon dioxide partial pressure ($PaCO_2$) from an average of 35–40 mmHg in the non-pregnant woman to 30 mmHg or lower in late pregnancy (Girling 2004). Because fetal $PaCO_2$ is 44 mmHg, the carbon dioxide gradient from fetus to mother is increased, which facilitates the transfer of CO_2 from the fetus to the mother and causes carbon dioxide to be washed out of the lungs (Campbell & Lees 2000). Clinical implications of these changes are that maternal blood gases should never be performed in the supine position which may give a false impression of hypoxia.

The body has a considerable capacity for storing carbon dioxide in blood, largely as bicarbonate. To compensate, renal excretion of bicarbonate is significantly increased which may limit the buffering capacity in pregnancy. The fall in $PaCO_2$ is therefore matched by an equivalent fall in plasma bicarbonate concentration from the non-pregnant values of 24–30 mEq/L to the pregnant values of 18–21 mEq/L. Although maternal arterial pH changes very little, the resulting mild alkalaemia (arterial pH 7.40–7.45) further facilitates oxygen release to the fetus (Steinfeld & Wax 2001).

Central nervous system

Research suggests that the dramatic hormonal fluctuations occurring throughout childbearing may remodel the female brain, increasing the size of neurons in some regions and producing structural changes in others (Russell et al 2001). The pituitary gland increases in size by 30–50% in pregnancy (Carlson 2002). Prolactin and β endorphin production increase progressively as pregnancy advances accounting for much of the increased pituitary activity. The opioid active form of β endorphin produced by the pituitary is thought to play a major role in raising the maternal threshold for pain and discomfort in the latter stages of pregnancy.

The adaptations in neural circuitry in the mother's brain are initiated by pregnancy hormones. Oestrogen and progesterone readily enter the brain acting on a multitude of nerve cells changing the balance between inhibition and stimulation. Other pregnancy hormones, such as relaxin and lactogen also act on the brain. The stage of pregnancy is signalled to the brain by the pattern of secretion of these hormones.

Oxytocin is imperative for labour stimulating expulsive uterine contractions and plays a significant role in the bonding process (Ginesi & Niescierowicz 1998). While oxytocin production is increased in pregnancy, release is inhibited and levels build up in the posterior pituitary. Oxytocin neurons are inhibited from releasing the stored oxytocin prematurely through several hormonal mechanisms involving progesterone, oestrogen and opioid peptides. At term, progesterone secretion falls and the inhibitory mechanism modified to allow gradual release of oxytocin in labour followed by a surge at the time of birth.

Box 14.3 Sleep disturbances

Sleep disturbances are a common complaint of pregnancy. Various hormonal and mechanical influences promote insomnia leading to disturbed sleep during pregnancy in most women (Santiago et al 2001). This worsens toward the end of pregnancy and continues to some extent for 3 months postpartum (Hedman et al 2002).

Interventions include establishing sleep – wake habits, avoiding caffeine, relaxation techniques, massage, heat and support for lower back pain, modifying sleep environment, limiting fluids in the evening and avoiding passive smoking. Sleep medications should be avoided. Some studies have shown that sleep loss in the last few weeks of pregnancy are associated with increased labour length and LSCS rates (Lee & Gay 2004).

Pregnant women's sleep patterns are affected by both mechanical and hormonal influences. These include nocturia, dyspnoea, nasal congestion, stress and anxiety as well as muscular aches and pains, leg cramps and fetal activity (Box 14.3).

Changes in the urinary system

Kidneys and ureters

The changes to renal physiology in healthy pregnancy can both hide and mimic renal disease. Due to the increase in total blood volume renal blood flow increases. This causes a swelling of the kidneys so that they appear larger on ultrasonography. The renal pelvis, calyces, and ureters dilate and can appear obstructed (Williams 2004). The overall dimensions of the kidney increase by approximately 1 cm and renal volume increases by as much as 30%. Dilatation of the collecting system occurs in 80% of women by mid-pregnancy leading to a physiological hydronephrosis and hydroureter which can persist for several weeks postpartum (Jeyabalan & Lain 2007). The dilated collecting system can hold up to 300 mL of urine, serving as an excellent reservoir for bacteria. After the uterus rises out of the pelvis it rests on the ureters laterally displacing and compressing them at the pelvic brim. During the last half of pregnancy, the upper portion of the ureters above the pelvic brim elongate and become more tortuous, being thrown into single or double curves of varying sizes (Cunningham et al 2005). Dilatation of the ureters, which is rarely present below the pelvic brim, is possibly due to mechanical compression by the enlarging uterus and ovarian plexus. However, the early onset of ureteral dilatation suggests that smooth muscle relaxation caused by progesterone possibly plays an additional role (Gabbe et al 2004). The dilatation is more marked on the right side than on the left, because of the cushioning effect of the sigmoid colon on the left and also the uterine tendency to dextrorotation (Girling 2004).

Significant anatomical changes occur in the bladder from 12 weeks. Due to the increased size of the uterus, the hyperaemia affecting all pelvic organs, and the hyperplasia of the muscle and connective tissues, the bladder trigone is elevated and its posterior margin is thickened. As pregnancy continues, the trigone becomes increasingly deep and wide. The bladder mucosa becomes more oedematous and the blood vessels increase in size and become more tortuous (Cunningham et al 2005). Decreased bladder tone leading to incompetence of the vesicoureteral valve and reflux of urine is seen in up to 3.5% of pregnant women especially in the third trimester (Blackburn 2007). Although decreased bladder tone may lead to increased capacity, the enlarging uterus displaces the bladder superiorly and anteriorly and flattens it. The normal convex surface is converted into a concavity. On cystoscopy an indentation of the bladder dome by the enlarged uterus is visible and the ureteric orifices are visualized in a higher position than in the non-pregnant state. This doubles the intravesical pressure and may therefore decrease capacity. To compensate for reduced bladder capacity urethral length increases, and to preserve continence intraurethral pressure increases. In spite of this, most women experience a degree of urinary incontinence during pregnancy (Box 14.4). Pressure of the presenting part impairs drainage of blood and lymph from the base of the bladder which may cause the area to become oedematous, easily traumatized and more susceptible to infection (Cunningham et al 2005). Progesterone may be involved in the relaxation of bladder smooth muscle, and in extreme cases, detrusor inactivity and retention of urine (Fitzgerald & Graziano 2007). All of the above factors can lead to urinary stasis and an increased risk of urinary tract infection in pregnancy (Fig. 14.6) (see Ch. 21). Glycosuria provides substrates for bacterial growth and is therefore another cause of asymptomatic bacteriuria (Blackburn 2007) (Box 14.5).

Box 14.4 Urinary incontinence

Urinary incontinence can begin early in pregnancy and the incidence increases as pregnancy progresses. Stress incontinence appears to be more common than urge incontinence although mixed symptoms are frequent. Women's descriptions of their incontinence range from mild to 'terrible'. There is some evidence that pelvic floor strengthening can prevent incontinence during pregnancy and in the postpartum period. Normal function usually returns for most women soon after the birth of the baby (Fitzgerald & Graziano 2007).

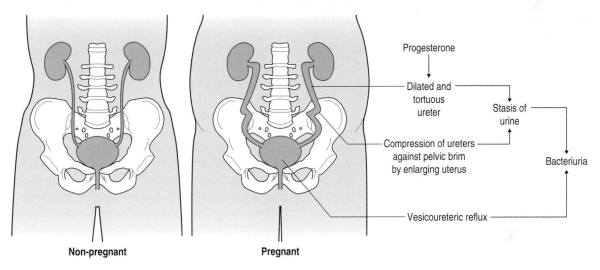

Figure 14.6 Changes in urinary tract in pregnancy and the factors predisposing women to urinary tract infection in pregnancy.

> **Box 14.5** Asymptomatic bacteriuria
>
> Asymptomatic bacteriuria, the presence of a positive urine culture in an asymptomatic person, occurs in 2–7% of pregnancies, often developing in the first month (Hooton & Stamm 2007). This diagnosis has traditionally been identified with greater than 100 000 colony-forming units (CFU)/mL on two consecutive first-void clean-catch urine specimens. More recently, isolation of >20 000 CFU/mL of a single bacterium has been considered to represent infection and has been associated with subsequent development of pyelonephritis (Wing 2002).

Alterations in renal haemodynamics are among the earliest and most dramatic maternal adaptations to pregnancy (Jeyabalan & Conrad 2007). Due to reduced resistance in the afferent and efferent arterioles of the kidney, and mediated by relaxin, renal plasma flow (RPF) increases most dramatically in the first trimester, from about 1.2 L/min in the non-pregnant state to at least 1.5 L/min. A 60–70% increase in RPF is reached by the beginning of the third trimester, with a subsequent decline towards term (Jeyabalan & Lain 2007), but is very dependent on posture. The GFR rises 25% by week 4 and 50% by the beginning of the second trimester (Williams 2004), remaining elevated until term even although renal plasma flow decreases during late pregnancy (Cunningham et al 2005). Because they are freely filtered at the level of the glomerulus there is a significant decrease in serum urea, creatinine, blood urea nitrogen (BUN) and uric acid levels during normal pregnancy (Blackburn 2007).

Serum urea levels may be only 63% of non-pregnant values by the third trimester (Blackburn 2007), falling from around 4.3–3.1 mmol/L. Serum creatinine also falls. By the end of the first and second trimesters the upper limit for serum creatinine is 80 μmol/L and 65 μmol/L, respectively (Nelson-Piercy 2004; de Swiet et al 2002), thus levels which are normal in the non-pregnant woman could represent quite severe renal disease in the pregnant woman (de Swiet et al 2002). It is important that appropriate pregnancy-specific normal ranges are used when managing both normal pregnancies and those of women with renal diseases (Baker 2006).

When measured by 24 h creatinine clearance test the GFR increases from 100 to around 150 mL/min by the beginning of the second trimester (Williams 2004). While the dilated collecting system can interfere with the accuracy of 24-h urine collections (Blackburn 2007), creatinine clearance is a useful test to estimate renal function in pregnancy.

As a consequence of increased GFR and/or reduced proximal tubular reabsorption, serum uric acid concentrations fall by 25% from non-pregnant values by 8 weeks' gestation, and by 35% throughout most of normal pregnancy. The rise toward non-pregnant levels near term may be due to a progressively increasing renal tubular reabsorption (Jeyabalan & Conrad 2007). The increased GFR increases concentration of solutes and volume of fluid within the tubules by 50–100%. Tubular reabsorption increases in order to prevent rapid depletion of sodium, chloride, glucose, potassium and water from the body. However, tubular reabsorption is not always able to cope with the increased filtered load, resulting in an increase in the excretion of substances such as glucose, amino acids, protein, electrolytes and vitamins (Blackburn 2007).

Glycosuria is common in pregnancy and can vary from day-to-day and within any 24-h period. Urinary glucose values may be 10–100-fold greater than the non-pregnant values, particularly in the third trimester (Blackburn 2007). Gestational glycosuria usually reflects reduced tubular glucose reabsorption rather than abnormal carbohydrate metabolism (Williams 2004). Glucose reabsorption occurs secondarily to the absorption of sodium and therefore other factors contributing to volume homeostasis and sodium retention may be involved in the physiological glycosuria of pregnancy (Baker 2006). Because of these changes in renal handling of glucose and the normal appearance of glucose in the urine, the use of glycosuria as a screen for pregnancy-related glucose intolerance is not particularly helpful (Jeyabalan & Lain 2007) and is not recommended (NICE 2008b).

Excretion of amino acids, urea and protein is markedly increased in pregnancy. Protein excretion rises from <100 mg/24 h up to 300 mg/24 h, with marked day-to-day variations. Proteinuria occurs more frequently during pregnancy due to the capacity of tubular reabsorption being exceeded. Values of 1+ protein on dipsticks are common and do not necessarily indicate glomerular pathology or pre-eclampsia. Potassium excretion is decreased with retention of an additional 300–350 mEq due to increased proximal tubular reabsorption. Serum potassium levels do not rise as the extra potassium is used for maternal tissues and by the fetus. Urinary calcium excretion is increased, possibly due to the increased GFR, and serum calcium and phosphorus levels decrease. This is balanced by increased intestinal absorption of calcium from the diet (Blackburn 2007).

The amount of water filtered by the kidneys increases by 50% due to the increased GFR (Blackburn 2007), but in pregnancy the woman must retain additional fluid and electrolytes to meet her own needs and the needs of the fetus. On average she gains 6–8 kg of fluid: 1.2 L is intravascular. Plasma volume expansion is positively correlated with fetal size (Williams 2004). Interstitial fluid volume increases gradually with the greatest accumulation in the second half of pregnancy. Accumulation of more than 1.5 L of interstitial fluid is associated with oedema (Blackburn 2007). During the day, pregnant women tend to accumulate water in the form of dependent oedema and at night while recumbent, they mobilize this fluid and excrete it via the kidneys (Cunningham et al 2005).

Urinary frequency (>7 daytime voidings), urgency, incontinence (Box 14.4) and nocturia may be experienced. It is primarily due to the effects of hormonal changes, hypervolaemia, increased renal blood flow and glomerular filtration rate (Blackburn 2007) although the increased fluid intake during pregnancy may also play a part (Fitzgerald & Graziano 2007). Later in pregnancy it is likely to be caused by the enlarged uterus, or descent of the presenting part.

Due to the increased GFR, the filtered load of sodium increases by up to 50%, however adaptation of the renal tubule results in 99% being reabsorbed in the tubules. Sodium retention occurs gradually with an increase in late pregnancy. It is used by the fetus and placenta and the rest is distributed in maternal blood and extracellular fluid. In spite of these alterations the woman responds normally to changes in water and sodium balance in pregnancy. Water excretion is enhanced by the lateral recumbent position although this position interferes with the ability of the woman to concentrate urine. Sodium excretion may be decreased in the supine and sitting positions.

Sodium retention is associated with weight gain and ankle oedema that comes and goes rapidly according to the woman's activities. During the day, water and sodium are trapped in the lower extremities because of venous stasis and pressure of the uterus on the iliac vein and inferior vena cava. This pressure is reduced at night when the woman is lying down resulting in increased venous return, cardiac output, renal blood flow and glomerular filtration rate with subsequent increase in urinary output. Nocturia may also be due to the large amounts of sodium (and therefore water), which are excreted at night as opposed to daytime (Blackburn 2007).

The kidney also acts as an endocrine organ that produces erythropoietin, vitamin D and renin. The production of these hormones increases during healthy pregnancy, but their effects are masked by other changes, e.g. lowered blood pressure, physiological anaemia and halving of parathyroid hormone levels (Williams 2004).

Renin leads to a cascade of events. The renin-angiotensin-aldosterone system is important in fluid and electrolyte homeostasis and maintaining arterial blood pressure (Fig. 14.7). This system must be altered in pregnancy to react appropriately to the new equilibrium. Renin peaks at levels two to three times higher than normal during the first trimester and remains elevated, then reaches a plateau at about 32 weeks' gestation. Renin release is stimulated by oestrogens, lower blood pressure, increased levels of plasma and urinary prostaglandin and progesterone. There is a 60% decrease in sensitivity to the hypertensive effect of angiotensin II so that rather than the blood pressure rising, it decreases along with the peripheral vascular resistance. Angiotensinogen levels also peak at 30–32 weeks. Aldosterone reaches levels 8–10 times

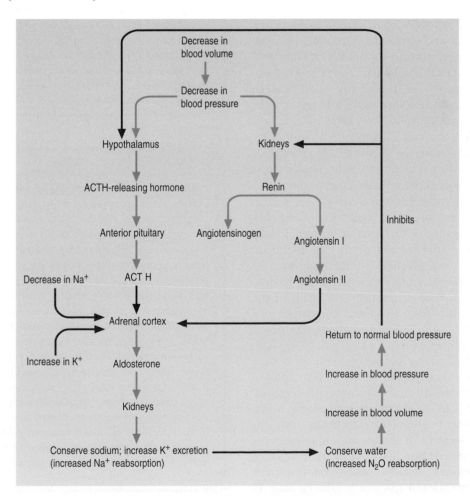

Figure 14.7   The renin-angiotensin system. (From Wallace 2005 p. 232, with permission of Elsevier.)

higher than those in nonpregnant women by 36 weeks. This opposes the sodium-losing effects of progesterone and allows a progressive accumulation of sodium in maternal and fetal tissues. It may also be necessary to maintain the expanded extracellular volume (Blackburn 2007). Although various hormones have been implicated in the gestational renal haemodynamic alterations, their effects are unclear and researchers offer conflicting opinions (Jeyabalan & Conrad 2007).

Changes in the gastrointestinal system

Anatomical and physiological changes take place in each organ of the gastrointestinal system. Influenced by oestrogen the gums become highly vascularized and oedematous. Associated with this is dental plaque, calculus and debris deposits which increase during pregnancy. Advanced gingivitis can lead to a specific angiogranuloma known as *epulis*. This is a purplish red mass, 2cm in diameter, often between the upper anterior maxillary teeth. It is very friable, bleeds easily and often interferes with chewing. It is usually painless but may ulcerate and become painful. It normally regresses spontaneously after birth but may recur in the same location in subsequent pregnancies. Occasionally these growths require to be excised (Blackburn 2007).

Pregnancy does not cause tooth decay. Fetal calcium requirements are drawn from maternal body stores, not from the teeth. Due to gingival alterations, however, the pregnant woman may become more aware of pre-existing or newly developed dental caries which may deteriorate as a result of the more acidic saliva (Box 14.6) and the nausea and vomiting of pregnancy. There may also be a transient increase in tooth mobility.

Nausea and vomiting is experienced by more than half of all pregnant women (Box 14.7). In spite of this, an increase in appetite is common in pregnancy and may be due to the effects of progesterone, which acts as an appetite stimulant (Blackburn 2007) or due to the movement of glucose and other nutrients to the fetus (Williamson 2006) or to the alterations in taste threshold. Food consumption has been reported to increase up to 20%, beginning early in

pregnancy, peaking at mid-gestation and decreasing near term (Chamberlain & Steer 2001).

Reduced physical activity as well as changes in metabolism lead to more efficient utilization and absorption of nutrients during pregnancy, which means that for many nutrients an increase in dietary intake over and above that which is normally required is not necessary (Williamson 2006).

Taste often changes early in pregnancy. Even before the first missed period, there may be a loss

---

Box 14.6 Ptyalism

Ptyalism (excessive salivation) is rare in pregnancy. It begins early in pregnancy and ceases with the birth of the baby. It may be associated with gastro-oesophageal reflux (Blackburn 2007) or due to stimulation of the salivary glands by the ingestion of starch. Much more common is the perception of an increased saliva production rather than an actual increase in saliva volume, due to difficulty in swallowing saliva during the period of nausea and vomiting in early pregnancy.

Box 14.7 Nausea and vomiting

Nausea and vomiting (popularly known as 'morning sickness') is experienced by more than half of all pregnant women and may occur at any time of day or night. Symptoms usually begin between 4 and 7 weeks and usually resolve by 16–20 weeks. Women need to know that it is not usually associated with a poor pregnancy outcome and should be advised that ginger, P6 (wrist) acupressure and antihistamines appear to be effective in reducing symptoms (NICE 2008a). Most women do not require treatment but it can have profound effects on the life of the woman and her family. If the condition persists and is severe it can progress to hyperemesis gravidarum (see Ch. 19) (Festin 2006). The exact cause and function is unknown. Many theories have been proposed but none are sufficiently supported by evidence (Blackburn 2007). Nausea is frequently triggered by hypoglycaemia, hence its occurrence on wakening in the morning. If severe it may be accompanied by food cravings and aversions.

of taste for something usually enjoyed (Chamberlain & Steer 2001). The development of cravings or aversions to food is also often reported. The most common cravings are for dairy products and sweet foods. Common aversions include tea and coffee, alcohol, fried foods and eggs and later in pregnancy, sweet foods (Williamson 2006). *Pica*, the persistent craving and compulsive consumption of non-food substances is poorly understood (Box 14.8). The increase in thirst in pregnancy noticed by many women may be due to a resetting of the central osmostat controlling thirst and vasopressin secretion as a result of the actions of relaxin on the brain (McKinley & Johnson 2004).

Gastrointestinal tone and the resting pressure of the lower gastro-oesophageal sphincter is decreased in pregnancy due to increased circulating levels of progesterone, oestrogen and motilin resulting in prolonged intestinal transit time (Suresh & Radfar 2004). The abdominal distension, which ensues can cause the woman to feel 'bloated' (Box 14.9). Progesterone is also responsible for the common problems of constipation and haemorrhoids (Box 14.10). By 20 weeks' gestation the gravid uterus exerts pressure on the stomach causing its upward displacement and rotation which alters the angle of the gastro-oesophageal junction and increases intragastric pressure (Rudra 2005). The altered position of the

---

Box 14.8 Pica

Pica is the persistent craving and compulsive consumption of substances such as ice, clay, soap, coal or starch. Several theories have been proposed to explain the condition, such as nutritional deficiencies of zinc or iron, or the sensory enjoyment of the taste, texture or smell of the substance. Some pica practices have cultural roots and some believe it is a behavioural response to stress, a habit or disorder or a manifestation of an oral fixation (Mills 2007). Pica can cause a number of medical problems, such as nutritional deficiencies, constipation, electrolyte imbalance, gastrointestinal and metabolic disturbances, lead poisoning, dental complications and weight gain (Mills 2007). Some cravings are potentially dangerous, such as eating mothballs, which can cause fetal haemolytic anaemia (Cunningham et al 2005). Patel et al (2004) noted that the prevalence of anaemia was 15% in women with pica compared with 6% in those without it, and the rate of pre-term birth at <35 weeks was noted to be twice as high in women with pica. The incidence of pica within the UK appears to have declined in recent years (Williamson 2006), however it may be commoner than generally believed, since it is known to be underreported by women due to embarrassment and guilt. When diagnosed it is important that a non-judgemental understanding and culturally sensitive approach to care is taken. Treatment will depend on the cause but may include iron supplementation, homeopathic remedies and counselling (Mills 2007).

Box 14.9 Abdominal distension

Abdominal distension and a 'bloated' feeling occur when nutrients and fluids remain in the intestinal tract for longer, particularly in the third trimester due to the prolonged transit time. Increased flatulence may also occur due to decreased motility and pressure of the uterus on the bowel (Blackburn 2007).

Box 14.10 Constipation and haemorrhoids

Constipation occurs because progesterone enhances absorption of sodium and water in the colon resulting in smaller stools with lower water content. Iron supplements may also aggravate constipation. Pregnant women are advised to consider changing the type of iron supplement (if used), to increase their intake of bran or wheat fibre and fluids and to take gentle exercise to alleviate this problem. Dietary bulking agents may also be helpful (Williamson 2006).

Haemorrhoids are also fairly common in pregnancy due to both constipation and pressure in veins below the level of the enlarging uterus (Cunningham et al 2005). Poor support for haemorrhoidal veins in the anorectal area and lack of valves in these vessels can lead to reversal in the direction of blood flow and stasis of blood (Blackburn 2007). Women should be offered dietary advice and if symptoms remain troublesome should consider standard haemorrhoid creams (NICE 2008a).

stomach, increased intragastric pressure due to the enlarging fetus, and decreased pressure of the lower gastro-oesophageal sphincter contribute to the common problem of heartburn (Cunningham et al 2005) (Box 14.11). While some confusion remains about how pregnancy affects gastric contents, recent evidence suggests that gastric emptying of fluids is not altered during pregnancy (O'Sullivan & Scrutton 2003) and gastric emptying of solids does not appear to be delayed during at least the first half of pregnancy (Rayner & Micell 2005). Following an extensive review of research studies for the development of fasting guidelines, the American Society of Anesthesiologists support the view that gastric emptying is normal in all three trimesters of pregnancy (Maltby 2000).

Although gastric acidity is reduced due to the influence of oestrogen during the first and second trimesters it is increased in the third trimester (Blackburn 2007). The comparative study by Hong et al (2005) confirms that women fasting prior to elective caesarean delivery at term had much greater and more acidic gastric contents than the non-pregnant patients preoperatively, however, it is recognized that this may be influenced by preoperative anxiety (Blackburn 2007).

Box 14.11 Heartburn

Heartburn or acid reflux into the lower oesophagus during pregnancy occurs in 30–80% of women, particularly during the third trimester (Rayner & Micell 2005). Frequent or more severe heartburn can interfere with sleep and deter the woman from eating adequately. Lifestyle modifications may be necessary, for example elevating the head of the bed 6 inches, stopping smoking, sleeping on the left side, avoiding reclining for 2–3 hrs after a meal. Dietary modifications which may be helpful include eating less fat and more protein, avoiding chocolate and certain drinks such as coffee, citrus juices, tomato products, and alcoholic or fizzy drinks (Charan & Katz 2001). Antacids such as Gaviscon or ranitidine may provide relief, however, it should be remembered that long-term therapy affecting gastric acidity can impair iron absorption (Rayner & Micell 2005).

The enlarging uterus causes the intestines to extend upwards and laterally (Cunningham et al. 2005) leading to a gradual displacement and lateral rotation of the caecum and appendix. In the first trimester the appendix remains within the right iliac fossa, moving to the pelvic brim during the second trimester and to lower right upper quadrant in the third trimester (Chawla et al 2003). Recent MRI studies have suggested that in spite of these anatomical changes the most common presenting symptom of appendicitis in pregnancy is pain in the right lower quadrant of the abdomen regardless of gestational age rather than the upper quadrant as previously believed (Oto et al 2006).

Gall bladder volume is increased and emptying rate is decreased, especially during the second and third trimesters due to its reduced muscle tone and motility under the influence of progesterone. The residual gall bladder volume after fasting is nearly twice that of the non- pregnant woman. As a result bile is more dilute with a decreased ability to make cholesterol soluble. The sequestered cholesterol precipitates formation of crystals and stones which increases the tendency to gall stones. Reduced gall bladder tone leads also to the tendency to retain bile salts which can lead to pruritus (Blackburn 2007).

Although the size of the liver remains the same during pregnancy it is displaced superiorly, posteriorly and anteriorly by the enlarging uterus. Hepatic blood flow is reduced by 35% in spite of the increased cardiac output, due to diversion to the uteroplacental circulation. Liver production of plasma proteins, bilirubin, serum enzymes and serum lipids is altered due to effects of oestrogen and haemodilution (see Table 14.5).

Changes in metabolism

The major changes in the utilization of carbohydrate, fat and protein during pregnancy are closely linked with the functions of the various endocrine glands. The placenta is already secreting hormones that affect metabolism within a few weeks of conception (see Ch. 11). Metabolic changes are essential for the continuous supply of glucose and amino acids for fetal growth as well as for meeting the increased physiological demands of the woman during pregnancy, labour and lactation. Food intake and appetite are increased, activity is decreased, approximately 3.5 kg of fat is deposited, energy reserves of approximately 30 000 kcal are established and 900 g of new protein is synthesized by the mother, fetus and placenta.

The products of conception, uterus and maternal blood are relatively rich in protein. In the first half of pregnancy, maternal storage of protein increases. Most of it is transported to the fetus but some is retained in maternal tissues. During the second half of pregnancy more protein is conserved with decreased urinary nitrogen excretion (Blackburn 2007). This increasing nitrogen balance suggests more efficient use of dietary protein as pregnancy progresses (Cunningham et al 2005).

Changes in lipid metabolism promote the accumulation of maternal fat stores in early and mid-pregnancy and enhance fat mobilization in late pregnancy (Butte 2000). Later in pregnancy, as fetal nutritional demands increase, maternal fat storage decreases. Leptin, a peptide hormone, is secreted by both placenta and adipose tissue and plays a key role in the regulation of body fat and energy expenditure. Serum leptin levels progressively increase, peaking during the second trimester and rising to a plateau at term in concentrations three to four times higher than the non-pregnant woman. Fats are used by the woman as an alternative energy substrate allowing her to conserve glucose for the fetus and her central nervous system during the second half of pregnancy. After a meal maternal fat stores are replenished by increased glucose uptake, incorporation of glucose to glycerol and taking up of fatty acids by adipocytes (Blackburn 2007).

Carbohydrate metabolism, however, demonstrates the most dramatic changes. During the first two trimesters in response to fetal and maternal needs, glucose secretion increases by 15–30% with increased peripheral glucose use without increases in insulin resistance. Maternal glucose levels are generally 10–20% lower than in non-pregnant women. From 20 weeks' gestation until term, insulin secretion increases three-fold and resistance increases with decreased glucose uptake by muscle and adipose tissue. Increasing insulin resistance promotes the flow of nutrients from the mother to the fetus and promotion of adipose tissue accumulation. Insulin resistance is mediated by the increasing levels of oestrogen, progesterone, hPL, cortisol and prolactin. In late pregnancy, although basal insulin levels are elevated, maternal blood glucose levels are similar to non-pregnant levels and do not drop as rapidly as usual even with higher circulating levels of insulin. This diabetogenic state protects the fetus even if the mother is fasting by keeping glucose in the blood and thus available for placental transfer (Blackburn 2007).

After a meal however, the pregnant woman's levels of glucose and insulin are higher than those of non-pregnant woman and glycogen is suppressed, resulting in hyperinsulinaemia, hyperglycaemia and insulin resistance. These changes increase glucose availability for transport to the fetus. Maternal blood glucose levels may rise transiently to 7.2–7.8 mmol/L and insulin resistance is increased by 60–70%. The hyperinsulinaemic response is most marked during the third trimester because of hypertrophy and hyperplasia of islet β cells, which become more responsive to alterations in blood glucose and amino acid levels. The increased insulin levels after eating overcome the insulin resistance to allow glucose uptake by muscles for storage as glycogen. Even with increased production of insulin however, overall glucose levels are maintained although at a relatively lower level than in the non-pregnant woman because of the counterbalancing effects of oestrogen, progesterone and hPL (Blackburn 2007).

The hyperglycaemic state after meals changes rapidly to a fasting state characterized by decreased levels of plasma glucose and amino acids. During fasting plasma concentrations of fatty acids, triglycerides and cholesterol are higher. This pregnancy-induced switch in fuels from glucose to lipids is known as *accelerated starvation* and ketonaemia rapidly appears (Cunningham et al 2005). During the overnight fast, plasma glucose levels decline more dramatically in the pregnant woman due to the continuous transfer of glucose and amino acids to the fetus (the *fetal siphon*). The woman compensates by using fat stores to meet her energy needs with breakdown of glycerol to glucose. As early as 15 weeks' gestation, maternal glucose levels after a 12–14 h fast are 0.8–1.1 mmol/L lower than levels in non-pregnant women. This becomes more noticeable during the second and third trimesters when the switch to fat oxidation takes place after 2–3h in comparison with 14–18h in the non-pregnant woman. Hypoglycaemia and lower insulin levels between meals and overnight lead to more rapid development of ketosis. This may contribute to the increased maternal appetite and sometimes a feeling of faintness during pregnancy. Optimal blood glucose levels in the pregnant woman range between 4.4 and 5.5mmol/L.

There is a two-fold increase in intestinal absorption of calcium during pregnancy to meet the calcium needs for fetal bone mineralization and breastmilk production. In spite of this maternal bone loss may occur in the last months of pregnancy when the fetal skeleton is rapidly mineralizing. The average daily transfer of calcium in the first trimester is 2–3mg/day, whereas the rate at 35–36 weeks' gestation is estimated to be 250mg/day. This places the woman at an increased risk of osteoporosis later in life. Maternal diet has little effect on the amount of mineral transferred (Kalwarf & Specker 2002). Serum albumin is required for binding calcium, however since albumin levels are decreased due to the greatly expanded intravascular fluid volume, maternal plasma calcium concentration falls (Cunningham et al 2005).

Low calcium levels are no longer believed to be associated with leg cramp and the most effective intervention for cramp remains unclear (Blackburn 2007). Calcium supplements are not generally thought to be necessary, however, women at risk of vitamin D deficiency are advised to take 10µg of vitamin D per day (NICE 2008a).

Maternal weight

Most of the weight gain during pregnancy is attributable to the uterus and its contents, the breasts, increases in blood volume and extracellular fluid (see Table 14.7). A smaller fraction of the increased weight is the result of metabolic alterations known as *maternal reserves* (Cunningham et al 2005). Approximately 62% of weight gain consists of water, which is retained in all systems of the body.

While initial maternal weight and the weight gained during pregnancy are highly associated with birth weight, it remains unclear what role maternal

Table 14.7 Distribution of average increase in weight

	Weight gain (kg)	Percentage of total weight
Maternal		
Uterus	0.9	
Breasts	0.4	
Fat	4.0	64
Blood	1.2	
Extracellular fluid	1.2	
Total	7.7	
Fetal		
Fetus	3.3	25
Placenta	0.7	11
Amniotic fluid	0.8	
Total	4.8	
Grand total	12.5	

fat or water have in fetal growth. Studies in well-nourished women at term suggest that maternal body water rather than fat contributes more significantly to infant birth weight (Cunningham et al 2005). The recommended pattern for normal weight gain is approximately 3kg in the first trimester followed by about 0.4kg/week for the remainder of the pregnancy. This pattern results in approximately 3kg of fat stores accumulating in the first half of pregnancy, while weight gained in the second half goes toward the growth of the fetus and maternal supportive tissues. Fetal growth is slow in the first 2 months during organogenesis but then accelerates rapidly. Maximum growth rate is achieved between the 4th and 8th month when the fetus grows at the rate of 5–9% per week. Until 15–16 weeks the placenta is larger than the fetus but by term the fetus is five to six times heavier than the placenta. Amniotic fluid increases from 7mL at 8 weeks, 30mL by 10 weeks, 190mL by 16 weeks, to a mean of about 800mL by 35 weeks after which it decreases to about 400mL by 42 weeks. The increase in the weight of the uterus is more rapid in the first 20 weeks (Blackburn 2007). The weight of breasts, blood volume and total body water increases steadily throughout pregnancy. The pitting oedema of ankles and legs, which is seen in most pregnant women, especially at the end of the day may amount to over 1L (Cunningham et al 2005).

There are currently no official recommendations for weight gain during pregnancy in the UK. Weight gain averages between 11 and 16 kg but variations are large. A birth weight of 3.1–3.6 kg has been associated with optimal maternal and fetal outcomes. Maternal nutritional status at the time of conception is very important for fetal growth and development. It is important to attain a healthy body weight prior to conception (see Ch. 13)

Skeletal changes

Mechanical and hormonal influences result in progressive modifications of posture, gait and joint mobility throughout pregnancy. The evolutionary derived curvature and reinforcement of the lumbar vertebrae enable women to compensate for the bipedal obstetric load (Whitcome et al 2007). Posture alters to compensate for the enlarging uterus, and a progressive lordosis shifts the woman's centre of gravity back over her legs. There is increased mobility of the sacroiliac and sacrococcygeal joints, which may contribute to the alteration in maternal posture leading to the characteristic 'waddling' gait of pregnancy and low back pain (Box 14.12). The muscles of the abdominal wall may stretch and lose some tone further aggravating back pain (Lowdermilk & Perry 2004).

Relaxation of the pelvic joints is predominantly due to hormonal influences. Oestrogen modifies the connective tissue making it more pliable. This causes the joint capsules to relax, making the pelvic joints mobile. Progesterone has the effect of relaxing or weakening the pelvic ligaments. Relaxin plays a major role in the changes, remodelling collagen fibres and softening pelvic joints and ligaments in preparation for birth (Marnach et al 2003). This allows some expansion of the pelvic cavity during descent of the fetal head in labour but further predisposes the woman to pelvic girdle instability.

Skin changes

Changes in the skin, hair, nails, sebaceous and sweat glands are predominantly modulated by hormonal, immunologic, and metabolic factors (Box 14.13). Certain changes have been shown to have a genetic predisposition, particularly striae gravidarum and pigmentation changes (Muallem & Rubeiz 2006).

Almost all women note some degree of skin darkening as one of the earliest signs of pregnancy. While the exact pathogenesis remains unclear, it is generally attributed to an increase in melanocyte stimulating

---

Box 14.12 Back pain

Back pain occurs in approximately 70% of pregnant women. The weight of the pregnant uterus and altered posture (compensatory lordosis) increase susceptibility which is exacerbated by progesterone and relaxin causing softening and relaxation of the ligaments of the pelvis. Simple measures to reduce pain include limiting physical activity, alteration of posture, wearing low-heeled shoes and adequate rest. Supportive pillows beneath the knees and abdomen and local application of heat may relieve pain. A physiotherapist may teach the woman back and abdominal muscle exercises to strengthen these muscles, or apply a sacroiliac or trochanteric support (see Ch. 16). Research suggests that exercises and acupuncture can reduce back pain (Pennick & Young 2007). While not substantiated by research, reports suggest a range of alternatives may be beneficial including massage, yoga, relaxation therapy, water exercises and osteopathy (Wang et al 2005).

Box 14.13 Hair growth

Hair growth has been shown to follow a common pattern in pregnancy. Women commonly report a thickening and increased volume of scalp hair. Stimulated by oestrogen, the growing period for hairs is increased in pregnancy so the woman reaches the end of pregnancy with many overaged hairs. This ratio is reversed after birth so that sometimes alarming amounts of hair are shed during brushing or washing. Normal hair growth is usually restored by 6–12 months. Mild hirsutism is common during pregnancy, particularly on the face (Muallem & Rubeiz 2006). Actions that may help include reducing damage to the hair by not combing when it is wet, and avoiding hairstyles that pull and stress hair, using shampoos and conditioners that contain biotin and silica. Diet that is high in fruits and vegetables containing flavonoids and antioxidants may provide protection for the hair follicles and encourage growth.

hormone, progesterone and oestrogen serum levels. Hyperpigmentation is more marked in dark-skinned women and is more pronounced in areas that are normally pigmented, e.g. areola, genitalia and umbilicus, in areas prone to friction, such as the axillae and inner thighs (Muallem & Rubeiz 2006) and in recent scars.

The linea alba is a line that lies over the midline of the rectus muscles from the umbilicus to the symphysis pubis. Hyperpigmentation causes it to darken resulting in the linea nigra. Pigmentation of the face affects up to 75% of pregnant women (Muallem & Rubeiz 2006). Known as chloasma or melasma, or 'mask of pregnancy' it is caused by melanin deposition into epidermal or dermal macrophages, further exacerbated by sun exposure. The chloasma usually regresses postpartum but may persist in approx 10% of women. Oral contraceptives may aggravate melasma and should be avoided in susceptible women (Cunningham et al 1997). If chloasma persists postpartum it can be treated with a variety of topical agents, including hydroquinone, tretinoin, kojic acid and vitamin C (Katsambas & Stratigos 2001).

As maternal size increases, stretching occurs in the collagen layer of the skin, particularly over the breasts, abdomen and thighs. In some women, this results in striae gravidarum (stretch marks) caused by thin tears occurring in the dermal collagen. These appear as red stripes changing to glistening, silvery white lines approximately 6 months after birth. The aetiology of striae has yet to be defined but may be compounded by hormones adrenocorticoids, oestrogens and relaxin which modify collagen and possibly elastic tissue.

Pruritus in pregnancy (not due to liver disease) can be distressing. In the absence of a rash, aspirin is recommended. If there is a rash chlorphenindione (chlorpheniramine) may be more effective (Young & Jewell 2002).

A rise in temperature by 0.2–0.4°C occurs as a result of the effects of progesterone and the increased basal metabolic rate (BMR). As a result, pregnant women 'feel the heat' and often sweat profusely, particularly in hot, humid climates. Peripheral vasodilation and acceleration of sweat gland activity help to dissipate the excess heat produced by maternal, placental and fetal metabolism (Lowdermilk & Perry 2004).

Table 14.8 Breast changes in chronological order

Time	Changes
3–4 weeks	Prickling, tingling sensation due to increased blood supply particularly around nipple
6–8 weeks	Increase in size, painful, tense and nodular due to hypertrophy of the alveoli. Delicate, bluish surface veins become visible just beneath the skin
8–12 weeks	Montgomery's tubercles become more prominent on the areola. These hypertrophic sebaceous glands secrete sebum, which keeps the nipple soft and supple. The pigmented area around the nipple (the primary areola) darkens and may enlarge and become more erectile
16 weeks	Colostrum can be expressed. The secondary areola develops with further extension of the pigmented area that is often mottled in appearance
Late pregnancy	Colostrum may leak from the breasts; progesterone causes the nipple to become more prominent and mobile

Angiomas or vascular spiders (minute red elevations on the skin of the face, neck, arms and chest) and palmar erythema (reddening of the palms) frequently occur, possibly as a result of high oestrogen levels. They are of no clinical significance, and disappear after pregnancy (Cunningham et al 1997). Most conditions have a tendency to resolve spontaneously within a few months postpartum. Nevertheless, changes may mask more serious conditions such as malignant neoplasms as well as herpes gestationis, and intrahepatic cholestasis of pregnancy. It is therefore imperative to assess for specific dermatoses of pregnancy which may be associated with maternal systemic symptoms and fetal mortality and morbidity if severe and untreated.

Changes in the breasts are summarized in Table 14.8.

Changes in the endocrine system

Successful physiological adaptation to pregnancy is due to the alterations in steroid and protein hormone production by the maternal endocrine system and the trophoblast (Cunningham et al 2005). Early effects of placental hormones are described in Chapter 10. Later physiological effects caused by hormones are now summarized.

Placental hormones

hCG levels increase rapidly in early pregnancy, doubling every 2 days, with maximal levels being attained at about 8–10 weeks' gestation. Thereafter levels begin to decline and a nadir is reached by around 20 weeks, after which this lower level is maintained for the remainder of pregnancy (Fig. 14.8). The detection of hCG in blood or urine is almost always indicative of pregnancy. Since hCG is also synthesized in the fetal kidneys it is also found in fetal blood and amniotic fluid (Cunningham et al 2005). Besides stimulating the maternal thyroid gland, the main function of hCG is to maintain the corpus luteum in order to ensure secretion of progesterone (and to a lesser extent relaxin) until placental production is adequate after 10–11 weeks, after which concentrations of hCG gradually decrease until it has completely disappeared 2 weeks after birth (Blackburn 2007).

The steady rise in maternal hPL plasma level, until it peaks around 34–36 weeks' gestation, is linked mainly to placental mass (Cunningham et al 2005). The primary role of hPL is to regulate glucose availability for the fetus. hPL is an insulin antagonist that increases maternal metabolism and use of fat for energy and reduces glucose uptake and use by maternal cells. As a result more glucose is available for transport to the fetus. When there is less glucose in the blood there is increased hPL secretion. By thus altering maternal protein, carbohydrate and fat metabolism, hPL promotes fetal growth (Blackburn 2007). While prolonged maternal starvation in the first half of pregnancy leads to an increase in the plasma concentration of hPL, short-term changes in plasma glucose or insulin have little effect on plasma levels of hPL (Cunningham et al 2005).

The placenta secretes over 20 different oestrogens into the maternal circulation but the major ones are oestradiol, oestrone, oestriol, the latter being the largest fraction. Oestradiol and oestrone are directly synthesized by the syncytiotrophoblast. Urinary and plasma oestriol levels increase progressively throughout pregnancy until 38 weeks' gestation (Symonds & Symonds 2004). The production of oestrogens is dependent on interaction of the maternal-fetal-

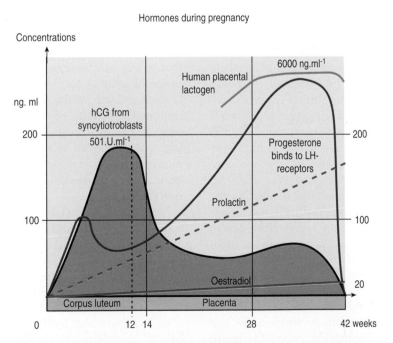

Figure 14.8 Variations in plasma hormone concentrations during a normal pregnancy. (From Paulev P 1999, with permission of Copenhagen Medical Publishers. Online. Available: http://www.mfi.ku.dk/ppaulev/chapter29/kap29.htm)

placental unit. Approximately 90% of the precursors for oestriol are derived from the fetal adrenal glands and the liver (Cunningham et al 2005). Oestrogen levels are low in the first trimester, then increase markedly in the second trimester and remain steadily elevated until labour (Ticconi et al 2006). During the last few weeks of pregnancy, huge amounts of oestrogens, in particular oestradiol, are produced each day by the syncytiotrophoblast, the majority of which are released into maternal circulation and eventually excreted in maternal urine (Cunningham et al 2005).

High oestrogen levels of pregnancy stimulate production of thyroxine-binding proteins and induce an increase in cortisol binding globulin (CBG) which in turn increases corticotrophin releasing hormone (CRH), adrenocorticotrophin hormone (ACTH), and total cortisol levels to maintain an adequate free cortisol concentration (Utz 2005). Oestrogens act to increase the number of glandular ducts of the breast, enhance myometrial activity, promote myometrial vasodilation, increase sensitivity of the maternal respiratory centre to carbon dioxide, soften fibres in the cervical collagen tissue, increase pituitary secretion of prolactin, increase serum binding proteins and fibrinogen, decrease plasma proteins and increase the sensitivity of the uterus to progesterone in late pregnancy (Blackburn 2007).

Progesterone is the principal pro-pregnancy factor. Placental production of progesterone increases steadily throughout pregnancy until it reaches maximal levels around 38 weeks. It is produced initially by the corpus luteum under the influence of hCG during the first 6–8 weeks after conception. Thereafter it is synthesized primarily by the syncytiotrophoblast. Some 90% is secreted into maternal circulation and the remaining 10% is used by the fetal adrenals to produce glucocorticoids and mineralocorticoids. During pregnancy progesterone acts to maintain myometrial quiescence, constrict myometrial vessels, inhibit prolactin secretion, help suppress maternal immunological responses to fetal antigens and therefore prevent rejection of the fetus, relax smooth muscle in the gastrointestinal and urinary systems, increase basal body temperature and increase sodium and chloride excretion (Blackburn 2007). It also stimulates the appetite, fat storage and the respiratory centres (de Sweit et al 2002).

Pituitary gland and its hormones

The anterior pituitary gland develops a more convex, dome-shaped surface and increases in size and weight during pregnancy by 30–50% from an average of 660 mg in the non-pregnant woman to 760 mg during pregnancy. The weight increase is due largely to an oestrogen induced hypertrophy and hyperplasia of the prolactin-secreting cells (Blackburn 2007). Pituitary FSH secretion is inhibited by the negative feedback of progesterone and oestrogen and also by *inhibin* (a glycoprotein hormone produced in the corpus luteum and placenta) and thus ovulation is prevented during pregnancy (Cunningham et al 2005) (see Ch. 10). Levels of FSH and LH are low by 6–7 weeks and are undetectable by mid-pregnancy (Blackburn 2007).

Thyroid-stimulating hormone (TSH) falls during the first trimester as a result of the mild thyrotrophic effect of hCG (British Thyroid Association 2006). It then rises rapidly by 20 weeks and plateaus until term. TSH increases both the synthesis and release of thyroxine (T4) and triiodothyronine (T3) (Shennan 2004). ACTH secretion and plasma levels increase progressively in the second and third trimesters to a peak during labour, thus stimulating release of cortisol by the adrenal gland (Blackburn 2007).

Prolactin concentrations in pregnancy reach levels that would be considered pathological in the non-pregnant woman (Baker 2006), increasing 10-fold to peak at birth. Although the anterior pituitary is responsible for most of the increase, prolactin is also produced by the breasts, the decidua and is found in high concentrations in amniotic fluid. Prolactin has many effects, the most important of which is to promote mammary development and stimulate lactation (see Ch. 41).

The posterior pituitary gland produces two hormones: vasopressin and oxytocin. Vasopressin levels are within normal ranges in pregnancy, however, the threshold at which it is secreted is reset with a decline in plasma osmolality. It also modulates blood pressure, electrolyte balance and ACTH release (Blackburn 2007). Oxytocin is produced not only by the posterior maternal and fetal pituitary glands but also by the myometrium, decidua, placenta and fetal membranes. Under the influence of oestrogen, the uterus becomes increasingly sensitive to oxytocin throughout pregnancy as oxytocin receptors in the myometrium increase 100-fold by 32 weeks and up to 300-fold by term. In spite of this, oxytocin concentration in the maternal circulation does not begin to rise until the expulsive stage of labour begins (Heffner & Schust 2006), when it stimulates contractions in the myometrium, and after the baby is born, causes contraction of myoepithelial cells of the breast, resulting in milk ejection (see Ch. 41).

Thyroid function

There is moderate enlargement of the thyroid gland in pregnancy due to a relative iodide deficiency as a result of the siphoning of maternal iodide by the fetus and also as a result of the increased glomerular filtration rate which increases renal clearance and excretion (Symonds & Symonds 2004). Enlargement can also be attributed to increased thyroid volume and blood flow in the intra-thyroid vessels (Fister et al 2006). However, enlargement should not be pathological and any goitre requires to be investigated (Cunningham et al 2005). While many studies have reported an increase of up to 50% in thyroid size in iodine-deficient areas, enlargement up to 15% has also been reported in areas with adequate iodine intake.

Thyroid function *per se* does not change during pregnancy (Blackburn 2007). In response to high oestrogen levels and the elevated hCG, there is a marked increase in levels of thyroid-binding globulin (TBG) by the liver which reach a peak around 20 weeks and then stabilize for the remainder of the pregnancy (Fig. 14.9). This leads to an increase in the bound forms of serum thyroxine (T4) and triiodothyronine (T3), which rise to a peak at 10–15 weeks' gestation and then plateau at levels 40–100% higher than non-pregnant values (Cunningham et al 2005). This suppresses thyroid stimulating hormone (TSH) secretion which decreases transiently from 8–14 weeks' gestation at the time of the hCG peak, returning to non-pregnant levels by the second trimester (Blackburn 2007). The circulating concentrations of unbound/free (and therefore active) forms of T3 and T4 decrease in the second and third trimesters and may fall below the reference range derived from non-pregnant women. The changes in maternal thyroid hormones are essential for the normal

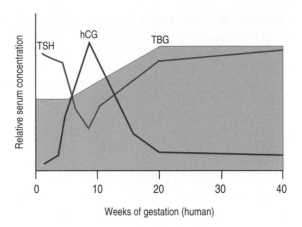

Figure 14.9 Relative levels of thyroid-stimulating hormone (TSH), thyroid-binding globulin (TBG) and human chorionic gonadotrophin (hCG) in pregnancy (From Bowen 1999, with permission.)

development of the fetal brain (British Thyroid Association 2006) and for supporting the altered carbohydrate, protein and lipid metabolism of pregnancy and changes in basal metabolic rate. However, as these changes mimic hyperthyroidism by causing palpitations, sweating and heat intolerance they can cause diagnostic confusion (Becks & Burrow 2000).

Adrenal glands

The adrenal gland increases only slightly in size during pregnancy due to hypertrophy and widening in the glucocorticoid area which suggests increased secretion of these hormones. Regulated by corticotrophin releasing hormone (CRH) and adrenocortocotrophin (ACTH), glucocorticoids control metabolism and blood glucose and suppress immune functions (Blackburn 2007). Because CRH is also produced by the trophoblast cells, maternal CRH levels increase dramatically and have a role in regulating the activity of the fetal adrenal glands and the myometrium and possibly the maternal adrenal gland (Baker 2006).

During pregnancy, the adrenal gland is more responsive to ACTH (Blackburn 2007). Although levels of ACTH are reduced strikingly in early pregnancy (Symonds & Symonds 2004), they increase approximately two-fold after the first trimester which stimulates a parallel increase in cortisol. Most of the cortisol circulates bound either to globulin or albumin (total cortisol), and only 10% is free (measured by 24h urinary free cortisol) with the result that the free cortisol fraction remains within the normal range (Garner 2002). Consequently, although total plasma cortisol increases from 3 months and peaks at term at levels 3–8 times higher, the pregnant woman does not show signs of hypercortisolism. Urinary cortisol increases up to three-fold by term and the diurnal secretion is blunted but maintained (Blackburn 2007).

Aldosterone, an anti-natriuretic hormone is the other major circulating mineralocorticoid produced by the adrenal gland. It regulates fluid and electrolyte imbalance by controlling sodium reabsorption and potassium and bicarbonate excretion in the distal renal tubule. Aldosterone levels in pregnancy increase four-fold by 8 weeks and continue to increase reaching a 10-fold increase by term (Garner 2002). Rising levels of progesterone with its natriuretic properties possibly influence the production of aldosterone (Baker 2006). The function of the adrenal medulla remains unchanged so that levels of catecholamine remain as in the non-pregnant state. However, during labour there are often massive increases in both adrenaline and noradrenaline as a result of stress and muscle activity (Symonds & Symonds 2004).

Diagnosis of pregnancy

The signs and symptoms of pregnancy are often enough to cause a woman to suspect pregnancy (Table 14.9) (Baker 2006). Diagnosis of pregnancy usually begins when a woman presents with such symptoms and possibly a positive home pregnancy test (Cunningham et al 2005).

Traditionally diagnosis has been based on history and physical examination. Important aspects of the menstrual history must be obtained. Items that may confuse the diagnosis of early pregnancy are an atypical last menstrual period, contraceptive use and a history of irregular periods. As many as 25% of women bleed during their first trimester, which may further complicate the assessment (Likes & Rittenhouse 2004). The signs of pregnancy described below are mainly of historic significance and although it is possible that they may still be of value in some parts of the world, they have generally been rendered obsolete in the developed world by more modern and sophisticated methods.

Hegar's (or Goodell's) sign

On bimanual examination, a firm cervix is felt in contrast with the softer body and compressible, softer isthmus at about 6–8 weeks menstrual age (Cunningham et al 2005).

Chadwick's sign

This is the dark purplish red discoloration and congestion of the vulva and vaginal mucous membranes (Cunningham et al 2005). First detected between the 4th and 8th weeks of pregnancy it reaches its maximum intensity at the 16th week and then persists throughout pregnancy (Mudaliar et al 1990).

Osiander's sign

This is the stronger and harder vaginal pulsations caused by the greatly increased blood supply and the enlarged uterine artery. This may also occur in the non-pregnant woman due to fibroids and pelvic inflammation.

Quickening

The first fluttering movements of the fetus are felt around 20 weeks in a first pregnancy and 18 weeks in subsequent pregnancies, however many women experience fetal movements earlier than these times. The woman's report should be recorded. Fetal movements can begin to be detected by the examiner around 20 weeks (see Table 14.9).

Most women use a home pregnancy test (HPT), which is private and easy to use. Measurement of hCG produced by the trophoblast from the day of implantation forms the basis for the standard modern pregnancy test using maternal urine although progesterone and early pregnancy factor (EPF) can also be measured (Likes & Rittenhouse 2004). hCG can be detected in maternal serum and urine 7–8 days after ovulation or around the time of implantation and can give a positive indication of pregnancy by 3 weeks after conception. Concentrations of hCG in maternal serum double every 2–3 days until peak values are reached 60–90 days after conception (Blackburn 2007). Women should be made aware that accuracy is variable and is

Table 14.9 Signs of pregnancy

Sign	Time of occurrence	Differential diagnosis
Possible (presumptive) signs		
Early breast changes (unreliable in multigravida)	3–4 weeks +	Contraceptive pill
Amenorrhoea	4 weeks +	Hormonal imbalance Emotional stress Illness
Morning sickness	4–14 weeks	Gastrointestinal disorders Pyrexial illness Cerebral irritation, etc.
Bladder irritability	6–12 weeks	Urinary tract infection Pelvic tumour
Quickening	16–20 weeks +	Intestinal movement, 'wind'
Probable signs		
Presence of human chorionic gonadotrophin (hCG) in:		
Blood	9–10 days	Hydatidiform mole
Urine	14 days	Choriocarcinoma
Softened isthmus (Hegar's sign)	6–12 weeks	
Blueing of vagina (Chadwick's sign)	8 weeks +	
Pulsation of fornices (Osiander's sign)	8 weeks +	Pelvic congestion Tumours
Changes in skin pigmentation	8 weeks +	
Uterine souffle	12–16 weeks	Increased blood flow to uterus as in large uterine myomas or ovarian tumours
Braxton Hicks contractions	16 weeks	
Ballottement of fetus	16–28 weeks	
Positive signs		
Visualization of gestational sac by		
Transvaginal ultrasound	4.5 weeks	
Transabdominal ultrasound	5.5 weeks	
Visualization of heart pulsation by		
Transvaginal ultrasound	5 weeks	
Transabdominal ultrasound	6 weeks	
Fetal heart sounds by		
Doppler	11–12 weeks	
Fetal stethoscope	20 weeks +	No alternative diagnosis
Fetal movements		
Palpable	22 weeks +	
Visible	Late pregnancy	
Fetal parts palpated	24 weeks +	
Visualization of fetus by X-ray	16 weeks +	

dependent on how, when and by whom the test is used and on the brand of the test. By waiting 2 weeks after the missed period, pregnancy will be confirmed accurately in 97% of women (Symonds & Symonds 2004). Early pregnancy detection allows for the commencement of prenatal care, potential medication changes and lifestyle changes to promote a healthy pregnancy (Likes & Rittenhouse 2004).

Common disorders arising from adaptations to pregnancy

Throughout this chapter, reference has been made to the multitude of symptoms the physiological changes may produce within a woman's body. While deemed physiological, women may experience these as unpleasant, and even distressing or debilitating. Due to their common, natural and non-pathological nature and the fact that they generally resolve spontaneously, caregivers are often guilty of a dismissive or trivializing approach towards them. Since these changes are expressions of the normal physiology of pregnancy it is both difficult and possibly ill-advised to take measures to prevent them.

The two key issues for midwives to build into their practice are:

1. Ensure that their assessment of women's symptoms is accurate, differentiating clearly between physiological and potentially pathological symptoms.

2. Develop a sympathetic approach to women experiencing these discomforts and ensure they offer appropriate advice to help women ameliorate or better tolerate the symptoms of pregnancy.

REFERENCES

Ambwani B 2004 Primigravidas with floating head at term or onset of labour. Internet Journal of Gynecology and Obstetrics 3(1). Online. Available:http://www.ispub.com/ostia/index.php?xmlFilePath=journals/ijgo/vol3n1/float.xml

Baker P (ed.) 2006 Obstetrics by ten teachers, 18th edn. Edward Arnold, London

Becks G, Burrow G 2000 Thyroid disorders and pregnancy. Thyroid foundation of Canada. Online. Available: http://www.thyroid.ca/Articles/ENGe11a.HTML January 2008

Blackburn S 2007 Maternal, fetal and neonatal physiology, 2nd edn. W B Saunders, Philadelphia

British Thyroid Association, Association of Clinical Biochemistry, British Thyroid Foundation 2006 UK guidelines for the use of thyroid function tests. Online. Available: http://acb.org.uk/docs/tftguidelinefinal.pdf April 2008

Broughton-Pipkin F 2001 Clinical physiology in obstetrics. Blackwell Science, Oxford, p 114–115

Boskey E, Cone R, Whaley K et al 2001 Origins of vaginal acidity: high D/L lactate ratio is consistent with bacteria being the primary source. Human Reproduction 16 (9):1809–1813

Bowen R 1999 Thyroid and parathyroid glands. In: Pathophysiology of the endocrine system. Online. Available: http://www.vivo.colostate.edu/hbooks/pathphys/endocrine/thyroid/thyroid_preg.html January 2008

Breuiller-Fouche M, Germain G 2006 Gene and protein expression in the myometrium in pregnancy and labor. Reproduction 131:837–850

Brosens J, Gellersen B 2006 Death or survival – progesterone-dependent cell fate decisions in the human endometrial stroma. Journal of Molecular Endocrinology 36:389–398

Buhimschi C, Buhimshci I, Malinow A et al 2003 Myometrial thickness during human labour and immediately post partum. American Journal of Obstetrics and Gynecology 188(2):553–559

Burnett A 2001 Clinical obstetrics and gynaecology. Blackwell Science, Oxford.

Butte N 2000 Carbohydrate and lipid metabolism in pregnancy: normal compared with gestational diabetes mellitus. American Journal of Clinical Nutrition 71(5):1256s–1261s

Campbell S, Lees C (eds) 2000 Obstetrics by ten teachers. Oxford University Press, New York

Carbonne B, Dallot E, Haddad B et al 2000 Effects of progesterone on prostaglandin E2-induced changes in glycosaminoglycan synthesis by human cervical fibroblasts in culture. Molecular Human Reproduction 6(7):661–664

Carlson H 2002 The pituitary gland in pregnancy and the puerperium. In: Melmed S (ed.) The pituitary. Blackwell Science, Oxford

Carvajal J, Weiner C 2003 Mechanisms underlying myometrial quiescence during pregnancy. Fetal and Maternal Medicine Review 14(3):209–237

Carvalho M, Bittar R, Brizot M et al. 2003 Cervical length at 11–14 weeks' and 22–24 weeks' gestation evaluated by transvaginal sonography, and gestational age at delivery. Ultrasound in Obstetrics and Gynaecology 21(2):135–139

Chamberlain G, Steer P 2001 Turnbull's obstetrics, 3rd edn. Churchill Livingstone, Edinburgh

Charan M, Katz P 2001 Gastrooesophageal reflux disease in pregnancy. Current Treatment Options in Gastroenterology 4:73–81

Chard T, Grudzinskas J 1994 The uterus. Cambridge University Press, Cambridge

Chawla S, Vardhan S, Jog S 2003 Appendicitis during pregnancy. Medical Journal of the Armed Forces India 59(3):212–215

Childbirth Connection 2007 Online. Available: http://www.childbirthconnection.org/article.asp?ck=10242 January 2008

Coustan D 1995 Maternal physiology. In: Coustan D, Haning R, Singer D (eds) Human reproduction – growth and development. Little, Brown, London

Cunningham F, MacDonald P, Gant N et al 1997 William's obstetrics, 20th edn. Prentice Hall, London.

Cunningham F, Gant N, Leveno K et al. 2001 William's obstetrics, 21st edn. McGraw-Hill, New York.

Cunningham F, Leveno K, Bloom S et al. 2005 William's obstetrics, 22nd edn. McGraw-Hill, New York.

Degani S, Leibovitz Z, Shapiro I et al. 1998 Myometrial thickness in pregnancy: longitudinal sonographic study. Journal of Ultrasound in Medicine 17:661–665

de Sweit M 1998a The cardiovascular system. In: Chamberlain G, Broughton Pipkin F (eds) Clinical physiology in obstetrics, 3rd edn. Blackwell Science, Oxford.

de Sweit M 1998b The respiratory system. In: Chamberlain G, Broughton Pipkin F (eds) Clinical physiology in obstetrics, 3rd edn. Blackwell Science, Oxford de Sweit M 2002 Medical disorders in obstetric practice, 4th edn. Blackwell, Oxford.

de Swiet M, Chamberlain G, Bennett P (eds) 2002 Basic science in obstetrics and gynaecology, 3rd edn. Churchill Livingstone, Edinburgh

Dietze M 2001 A Re-evaluation of the mechanism of labour for contemporary midwifery practice. Midwifery Matters 88:3–8. Online. Available:http://www.radmid.demon.co.uk/physiology.htm July 2007

Dijkstra K, Janssen H, Kuczynski E, Lockwood C 1999 Cervical length in uncomplicated pregnancy: A study of sociodemographic predictors of cervical changes across gestation. American Journal of Obstetrics and Gynecology 180(3):639–644

Duffy T 2004 Haematologic aspects of pregnancy. In: Burrows G N, Duffey T P, Copel J A (eds) Medical complications in pregnancy, 6th edn. Saunders, Philadelphia

Esmaelzadeh S, Rezael N HajiAhmadi M 2004 Normal uterine size in women of reproductive age in northern Islamic Republic of Iran. Eastern Mediterranean Health Journal 10 (3):437–441

Festin M 2006 Nausea and vomiting in early pregnancy. British Medical Journal Clinical Evidence. Online. Available: www.clinicalevidence.com

Fister P, Gaberscek S, Zaletel K et al 2006 Thyroid volume and intrathyroidal blood flow increase during pregnancy. Clinical Endocrinology 65:828–829

Fitzgerald M, Graziano S 2007 Anatomic and functional changes of the lower urinary tract during pregnancy. Urologic Clinics of North America 34:7–12

Fraser D M, Cooper M A 2008 Survival Guide to Midwifery, Churchill Livingstone Elsevier, Edinburgh

Fusi L Cloke B, Brosens J 2006 The uterine junctional zone. Best Practice and Research Clinical Obstetrics and Gynaecology 20(4):479–491

Gabbe S, Niebyl J, Simpson J et al (eds) 2004 Obstetrics: normal and problem pregnancies, 4th edn. Churchill Livingstone, Edinburgh

Garfield R, Saade G, Buhimschi C et al 1998 Control and assessment of the uterus and cervix during pregnancy and labour. Human Reproduction Update 4(5):673–695

Garfield R, Maner W 2007 Physiology and electrical activity of uterine contractions. Seminars in Cell and Developmental Biology 18:289–295

Garner P 2002 Adrenal disorders of pregnancy, Ch. 2B. Online. Available: http://www.endotext.com/pregnancy/pregnancy2/pregnancy2b.htm January 2008

Gee H 2004 Routine intrapartum care: an overview. In: Luesley D, Baker P (eds) Obstetrics and gynaecology – an evidence-based text for MRCOG. Arnold, London.

Gee H 2006 Poor progress in labour. In: James D, Steer P, Weiner C et al (eds) High risk pregnancy. Elsevier, Philadelphia

Ginesi L, Niescierowicz R 1998; Neuroendocrinology and birth 1: stress. British Journal of Midwifery 6(10):659–663

Girling J 2001 Physiology of pregnancy. Obstetrics, anaesthesia and intensive care medicine. Medicine Publishing Company, Abingdon, p 167–170. Online. Available:www.medicinepublishing.com/girl_ 1–4

Girling J 2004 Physiology of pregnancy. Anaesthesia and Intensive Care Medicine 5(7):215–218.

Hanretty K 2003 Obstetrics illustrated, 6th edn. Churchill Livingstone, Edinburgh

Haram K, Mortensen J, Wollen A 2003 Preterm delivery: an overview. Acta Obstetricia et Gynecologica Scandinavica 82:687–704

Hedman C, Pohjasvaara T, Tolonen U et al. 2002 Effects of pregnancy on mothers' sleep. Sleep Medicine (1):37–42

Heffner L, Schust D 2006 The reproductive system at a glance, 2nd edn. Blackwell, Oxford.

Hempstock J, Cindrova-Davies T, Jauniaux E et al. 2004 Endometrial glands as a source of nutrients, growth factors and cytokines during the first trimester of human pregnancy: A morphological and immunohistochemical study. Reproductive Biology and Endocrinology 2:58

Honda T, Hasegawa M, Nakahori T et al 2005 Perinatal management of cervicoisthmic pregnancy. Journal of Obstetrics and Gynaecology Research 31(4):332–336

Hong J, Park J, Jong I 2005 Comparison of preoperative gastric contents and serum gastrin concentrations in pregnant and nonpregnant women. Journal of Clinical Anesthesia 17(6):451–455

Hooton T, Stamm W 2007 Urinary tract infections and asymptomatic bacteriuria. UpToDate. Online. Available: http://patients.uptodate.com/print.asp?print=true&file=u-ti_infe/7516 January 2008

Jensen D, Wolfe L, Slatkovska L et al 2005 Effects of human pregnancy on the ventilatory chemoreflex response to carbon dioxide. American Journal of Physiology. Regulatory, Integrative and Comparative Physiology 288:R1369–R1375

Jeyabalan A, Conrad K 2007 Renal function during normal pregnancy and preeclampsia. Frontiers in Bioscience 12:2425–2437

Jeyabalan A, Lain K 2007 Anatomic and functional changes of the upper urinary tract during pregnancy. Urologic Clinics of North America 34:1–6

Jones R, Findlay J, Salamonsen L 2006 The role of activins during decidualization of human endometrium. Australian and New Zealand Journal of Obstetrics and Gynaecology 46:245–249

Kalwarf H, Specker B 2002 Bone mineral changes during pregnancy and lactation. Endocrine 17 (1):49–53

Katsambas A D, Stratigos A J. 2001 Depigmenting and bleaching agents: coping with hyperpigmentation. Clinical Dermatology 19:483–488

Kliman H 2000 Uteroplacental blood flow. The story of decidualization, menstruation and trophoblast invasion. American Journal of Pathology 157(6):1759–1768

LaMar K, Hamernik C 2003 Life inside the womb: implications for newborn and infant nurses. Newborn & Infant Nursing Reviews 3(4):136–142

Lee K A, Gay G 2004 Sleep in late pregnancy predicts length of labor and type of delivery. American Journal of Obstetrics and Gynecology 191(6):2041–2046

Lesny P, Killik S 2004 The junctional zone of the uterus and its contractions. British Journal of Obsetrics and Gynaecology 111:1182–1189

Letsky E 1998 The haematological system. In: Chamberlain G, Broughton Pipkin F (eds) Clinical physiology in obstetrics. Blackwell Science, Oxford

Likes R, Rittenhouse E 2004 Pregnancy diagnosis. Online. Available: http://www.emedicine.com/med/topic3277.htm January 2008

Llewellyn-Jones D 1999 Fundamentals of obstetrics and gynaecology, 7th edn. Mosby, London

Lowdermilk D, Perry S 2004 Maternity and Women's Health Care, 8th edn Mosby, Missouri

Maltby J 2000 Pre-operative fasting guidelines. Issue 12, article 2, p 2. Online. Available: www.nda.ox.ac.uk/wfsa/html/u12/u1202_02.htm#dela January 2008

Margulies R, Miller L 2001 Fruit size as a model for teaching first trimester uterine sizing in bimanual examination. American Journal of Obstetricians and Gynecologists 98(2):341–344

Marnach M L, Ramin K D, Ramsey P S, et al 2003 Characterization of the relationship between joint laxity and maternal hormones in pregnancy. Obstetrics and Gynecology 101(2):331–335

Martin W, Hutchon S 2004 Mechanism and management of normal labour. Current Obstetrics and Gynaecology 14:301–308

Metaxa-Mariatou V, McGavigan C, Robertson K et al 2002 Elastin distribution in the myometrial and vascular and smooth muscle of the human uterus. Molecular Human Reproduction 8(6):559–565

McFadyen I 1995 Maternal physiology in pregnancy. In: Chamberlain G (ed.) Turnbull's obstetrics, 2nd edn. Churchill Livingstone, Edinburgh, Ch. 7

McKinley M, Johnson A 2004 The physiological regulation of thirst and fluid intake. News in Physiological Sciences 19:1–6

Mills M 2007 Craving more than food – the implications of pica in pregnancy. Nursing for Women's Health 11(3):267–273

Moore K, Persaud T 2003 The developing human, 7th edn. Saunders, Philadelphia, p 47, 120

Muallem M, Rubeiz N 2006 Physiological and biological skin changes in pregnancy. Clinics in Dermatology 24(2):80–83

Mudaliar A, Menon M, Palaniappan B 1990 Mudaliar and Menon's clinical obstetrics, 9th edn. Orient Longman, Anna Salai, Madras, India, p 49. Online. Available:http://books.google.com/books?id=Iipd0GIpw4cC&pg=PA49&lpg=PA49&dq=osiander's+sign&source=web&ots=KDgr7YVxpw&sig=W6wSqWMecKTtltudd1TADSnocwA January 2008

Nelson-Piercy C 2004 Renal disease. In: Luesley D, Baker P (eds) Obstetrics and gynaecology – an evidence-based text for MRCOG. Arnold, London

Nelson-Piercy C 2006 Handbook of obstetric medicine. Taylor and Francis, Oxford

NICE 2008a Antenatal care: routine care for the healthy pregnant woman. RCOG Press, London

NICE 2008b Diabetes in pregnancy: management of diabetes and its complications from preconception to the postnatal period. Clinical guideline 63. RCOG Press, London

O'Grady J, Pope C 2006 Malposition of the uterus. Online. Available: http://emedicine.com/med/topic3473.htm January 2008

O'Sullivan G, Scrutton M 2003 NPO during labour. Is there any scientific validation? Anesthesiology clinics of North America 21(1):87–98

Oto A, Srinivasan P, Ernst R et al (2006) Revisiting MRI for appendix location during pregnancy. AJR Women's Imaging 186:883–887

Patel M, Nuthalapaty F, Ramsey P et al 2004 A neglected risk factor for preterm birth. Obstetrics and Gynecology 103:68S

Paulev P 1999 Essentials and clinical problems, Section vii: Sexual Satisfaction, Reproduction and Disorders. Endocrine glands in humans. In: Paulev P (ed.) Textbook in medical physiology and pathophysiology, Ch. 29. Copenhagen Medical Publishers, Copenhagen. Online. Available: http://www.mfi.ku.dk/ppaulev/chapter29/kap29.htm January 2008

Pennick V E, Young G 2007 Interventions for preventing and treating pelvic and back pain in pregnancy (Cochrane Review). The Cochrane Database of Systematic Reviews, Issue 2

Rayner C, Micell G 2005 Dealing with gastro-oesophageal reflux disease during pregnancy. European gastroenterology review 2005. Online. Available: http://www.touchgastroenterology.com/dealing-with-gastro-oesophageal-a1351–1.html January 2008

Rehman K, Yin S, Mayhew B et al 2003 Human myometrial adaptation to pregnancy: cDNA microarray gene expression profiling of myometrium from non-pregnant and pregnant women. Molecular Human Reproduction 9(11):681–700

Ross M, Ervin M, Novak D 2002 Placental and fetal physiology. In: Gabbe S, Neibyl J, Simpson J (eds) Obstetric – normal and problem pregnancies, 4th edn. Churchill Livingstone, Edinburgh

Rudra A 2005 Airway management in obstetrics. Indian Journal of Anaesthesia 49(4):328–335

Russell J, Douglas A, Windle R 2001 The maternal brain: neurobiological and neuroendocrine adaptation and disorders in pregnancy & post partum. Elsevier Science, Edinburgh

Santiago J, Nolledo M, Kinzler, W et al 2001 Sleep and sleep disorders in pregnancy. Annals of Internal Medicine 134(5):396.

Shennan A 2004 Thyroid disease In: Luesley D, Baker P (eds) Obstetrics and Gynaecology – An evidence-based text for MRCOG. Arnold, London, p 59

Steinfeld J, Wax J 2001 Maternal physiologic adaptations to pregnancy. In: Seifer D, Samuels P, Kniss D (eds) The physiologic basis of gynecology and obstetrics. Lippincott, Williams and Wilkins, London

Suresh L, Radfar L 2004 Medical management update – pregnancy and lactation. Oral Surgery, Oral Medicine, Oral Pathology 97(6):672–668

Symonds E, Symonds I 2004 Essential obstetrics and gynaecology, 4th edn. Churchill Livingstone, Edinburgh

Szekeres-Bartho J 2001 Progesterone dependent immunomodulation. Chemical Immunology and Allergy 89:118

Torgersen K L, Curran CA 2006. A systematic approach to the physiological adaptations of pregnancy. Critical Care Nursing Quarterly 29:2–19

Ticconi C, Belmonte A, Piccione E et al. 2006 Feto-placental communication system with the myometrium in pregnancy and parturition: The role of hormones, neurohormones, inflammatory mediators, and locally active factors. Journal of Maternal-Fetal and Neonatal Medicine 19(3):125–133

Utz A 2005 Physiologic cortisol dynamics and Cushing's syndrome in pregnancy. The Neuroendocrine Clinical Center Bulletin 11(2)

Van Mook W, Peeters L 2005 Severe cardiac disease in pregnancy, Part II: impact of congenital and acquired cardiac diseases during pregnancy. Current Opinion in Critical Care 11(5):435–448

Varga I, Rigó, J Somos P et al 2000 Analysis of maternal circulation and renal function in physiologic pregnancies: Parallel examinations of the changes in the cardiac output and the glomerular filtration rate. Journal of Maternal Fetal Medicine 9(2):97–104

Wallace W 2005 Endocrine Function In: Montague S, Watson R, Hubert R (eds) Physiology for Nursing Practice, 3rd edn. Elsevier

Wang S M, De Zinno P, Fermo L 2005 Complementary and alternative medicine for low-back pain in pregnancy: a cross-sectional survey. Journal of Alternative and Complementary Medicine 11(3):459–464

Weissgerber T, Wolfe L 2006 Physiological adaptation in early human pregnancy: adaptation to balance maternal-fetal demands Applied Physiology, Nutrition and Metabolism 31:1–11

Whitcome K, Shapiro L, Lieberman D 2007 Fetal load and the evolution of lumbar lordosis in bipedal hominis. Nature 450:1075–1078

Whitmore I, Willan P, Gosling J et al 2002 Human anatomy: colour atlas and text, 4th edn. Mosby, Edinburgh

Williams D 2004 Renal disease in pregnancy. Current Obstetrics and Gynaecology 14:166–174

Williamson C 2006 Nutrition in pregnancy. Briefing Paper. British Nutrition Foundation Nutrition Bulletin 31:28–59

Wing D 2002 Urinary tract infection in pregnancy: from asymptomatic bacteriuria to pyelonephritis. In: Mishell D, Goodwin T, Brenner P eds. Management of common problems in obstetrics and gynecology, 4th edn. Blackwell, Oxford

Young R, Hession R 1999 Three-dimensional structure of the smooth muscle in the term-pregnant human uterus. Obstetrics and Gynecology 93(1):94–99

Young G, Jewell D 2002 Antihistamines versus aspirin for itching in late pregnancy (Cochrane review). In: The Cochrane Library, Issue 1. Update Software Oxford. Online. Available: www.update-software.com accessed 23 October 2007

Young R 2007 Myocytes, myometrium, and uterine contractions. Annals of New York Academy of Sciences 1101:72–84

15 Antenatal education: principles and practice

Nina Smith   Mary L. Nolan

Pregnancy is a time when women and their partners are especially open to reflecting on their lifestyles and healthcare options. For health professionals, it provides an opportunity to help women learn how to use healthcare services effectively, and to acquire information and skills that will enable them to have the best possible experience of birth and early parenting.

The chapter aims to:

- examine the nature and purpose of antenatal education
- discuss the elements of antenatal education
- suggest effective teaching activities responsive to a variety of learning styles
- consider appropriate antenatal education for very young women, women from minority ethnic groups, same sex couples and fathers
- discuss collaborative working in the provision of antenatal education services.

Political and social context

There has perhaps been a tendency to see antenatal education as part of a different enterprise from that of *Education*. Since the inception of the health service, the education of pregnant women has been the province of midwives and health visitors whose primary training is as clinicians rather than as educators. The mind-set of the clinician, particularly of clinicians working in areas closely allied to medicine, has traditionally been that of the *expert*, the person who *has knowledge*, who *decides* and who *takes responsibility for* the *patient*. This is a very different mind-set from that of the educator.

In recent years, this clinical mind-set has started to change as a result of pressure from central government, aiming to mould the NHS into a more patient-sensitive service. The 'new deal' was heralded by the publication in 1997 of the *NHS Plan* which recognized the expertise of patients in relation to their own health and ill health, and their democratic right to be consulted about a service for which they were paying increasingly heavily in their taxes. One policy document after another (DH 1993, 1997, 2003, 2004a, 2007) stressed that health professionals must *engage* with patients and assist them to achieve health and well-being by taking into account their individual life circumstances.

While such policies have at least started to find their way into practice when care is being delivered to powerful patient populations such as the ethnic majority, the articulate, the affluent and the socially confident, it continues to be the case that the disenfranchised are likely to be subjected to an authoritarian model of care in which their voice is not heard. As consumers of healthcare, the childbearing woman is disenfranchised by reason of her exceptional vulnerability which is dependent, in part, on increasing social hysteria regarding the 'dangers' of pregnancy and birth.

Education for challenge or conformity?

Within the current policy context, and given negative social perceptions of childbirth, antenatal education might be considered to have a major part to play. Yet it has become a 'Cinderella' service, under-funded for years and increasingly marginalized to the point where some Trusts have withdrawn provision altogether and many others have reduced it to a single session in late pregnancy. Has it been marginalized because midwives and other key players in maternity care services have become increasingly confused about whether antenatal education should be educating women to challenge the medical model of childbearing or to conform to it?

It is strange that midwives have generally failed to see the potential of antenatal education to empower not only those they serve but also themselves. It provides a golden opportunity to help women to believe in the ability of their bodies to give birth, and in the 'rightness' and safety of midwifery care for themselves and their babies. Who better to sell this message than those most immediately interested in having a strong midwifery profession?

Education for liberation

For 40 years at least, education has been explicitly linked to liberation (and implicitly so, of course, since Plato). In South America, the great liberation theologian and educator, Paulo Freire (1921–1997), wrote about the power of education to liberate the people from the ignorance and superstition which made them helpless in the face of exploitation by the educated and powerful. Education bestows political, social and personal power because it enables people to be self-directing. Being self-directing leads to greater self-esteem, and is, Knowles (1984) suggests, both the mark of adulthood and its ongoing goal.

Worldwide, the majority of women and men choose to become parents. Parents are the first teachers of the new citizens of the global community. As *becoming*-parents, pregnant women and their partners need exposure to a model of education that respects and enhances their autonomy and decision-making skills at the start of a long period in their lives which will be characterized by making decisions on behalf of vulnerable others, namely their children.

The goal of antenatal education is therefore to help pregnant women and their supporters to make, and take responsibility for, their own choices. This puts it firmly into the political arena in which government policy aims to create a public that is astute about healthcare, understands its limits, appreciates that people must match care provided by professionals with care they provide for themselves, and that there are no guaranteed outcomes. In order for pregnant and new parents to become part of this critical mass of healthcare consumers, they need:

- *information*: that they have *applied* to their unique personal and social situations
- *increased awareness of their own feelings*: gained from thinking through and discussing with others key issues around the birth and start of their children's lives
- *skills*: to enable them to be independent in caring for their children.

Information

Information is about facts but facts, although apparently objective, do not mean the same thing to everyone who has access to them. Couples who receive the information that unexplained stillbirth increases from 3/1000 babies to 6/1000 after 42 weeks of pregnancy will, should the woman go post-dates, use that information to make very different decisions (if invited to make a decision). A woman may know that smoking during pregnancy is bad for her baby and herself, but not *know* it within the context of her own life where smoking helps her relax and where best friends who smoke have given birth to apparently healthy babies. A terrified woman may be given the information that an epidural will help her relax, but *know* from bitter experience of abuse that lying passively on her back is not relaxing. Education cannot escape grappling with ontological dilemmas – what we know, how we know it, how we experience it – the nature of knowing itself. Therefore it cannot direct the learner, but only walk alongside her.

Self-awareness

Education extends people's knowledge of themselves. Becoming-parents may make decisions based on influences of which they are not fully aware. Education aims to increase *self-awareness* by exposing learners to different ways of thinking. Women who have been offered only a consultant unit in which to have their baby may find their feelings about birth transformed when taken to visit the local midwife-led unit and given the chance to situate their ideas about birth within a different birthing context. Antenatal education enables becoming-parents to exchange views, understand how facts are coloured by individual concepts of risk, and reach their own decisions.

Skills

Finally, in order to be self-directing in our lives, we need certain *skills* or competencies. These cannot be learned by observing others or from books. They have to be learned by *doing*. Nobody becomes confident in bathing a baby by watching someone else bathe a baby. Few people are confident in communicating with a person in authority without practising being assertive. Children are far more open to learning skills than adults – perhaps because nearly all their learning is, in their early years, around skills. Adults have generally become fearful of skills-learning because 'failure' is much more evident when practising a skill than when receiving information or participating in a discussion (Daines et al 2002). Yet parents-to-be crave competence in, for example, baby-care skills (Nolan 1997; Singh & Newburn 2000), and educators must become confident facilitators of practical learning activities.

Aims and outcomes

In summary: antenatal education aims to:

- enable *becoming-parents* to achieve a richer adulthood by enhancing their ability to make well-informed decisions appropriate to their individual circumstances
- increase their self-esteem so they can make a confident transition to parenthood through labour, birth and the early months of their children's lives
- nurture a critical mass of healthcare consumers able to act on an individual and political level to improve services.

The measurable outcomes of effective antenatal education will be:

- knowledgeable parents in possession of a range of evidence-based information which they can assess within the context of their personal circumstances
- self-aware parents who know why they are choosing to do things in certain ways and why others may choose to do things differently
- skilled parents who are able to carry out the day-to-day care of their children, and who can stand up for themselves.

Introductions and ice-breakers

Recent studies of the structure and functioning of the learning brain are of considerable assistance to educators in creating effective learning opportunities for becoming-parents. This new understanding can be applied whether working with parents-to-be on a one-to-one basis or in small groups. Neurophysiology tells us that there is a 'toggle switch' in the brain, the Reticular Activating System (RAS), which acts to switch off cognitive learning when the emotional centre of the brain – the amygdala – is highly stimulated (Hannaford 2005). Put simply: we cannot learn if we are feeling very emotional, anxious or self-conscious. Many parents-to-be meeting their midwife for the first time, or joining an antenatal class, will feel nervous about how they will be perceived by the midwife/educator and other parents in the group. Expectant parents who are receiving difficult or different news – perhaps that their baby has been diagnosed with Down Syndrome, or that they are having twins – are highly aroused emotionally and the cerebral cortex where learning takes place is consequently deactivated. They are not able to take in information, as anyone who has been with people in such situations or experienced them personally, will know very well.

In an antenatal class, parents must be at ease before they are able to engage with the teacher and each other in learning activities. Helping people relax when they are in a group means helping them to learn each other's names and start to get to know each other by identifying common ground. The importance of opening activities either in an individual interview or in a small group situation cannot be over-estimated.

There are many ice-breaker activities available, but the key features of all are that:

- they are non-threatening
- they encourage the group members to talk
- the group leader does very little talking
- people are helped to learn each other's names
- they find out about each other
- they have a laugh!

The introduction to the first class (and the first 10 min of *any* class) is therefore for *social* learning (Box 15.1). Parents will learn that this is *their* group; that their participation and what they have to say are valued, and that this class will be an enjoyable experience.

Being able to help people relax requires the group leader to be relaxed herself, not rushing into the

---

Box 15.1 Introduction by the group leader (session for mothers and partners)

These classes are going to focus on what *you* want to learn about. They're also a wonderful opportunity to make friends. So can I ask you to spend a few moments now talking to someone you don't know and finding out a little about them. You could start by asking them when their baby is due and what their pregnancy has been like. You could talk about which football team you support or what kinds of things you like to do in your spare time. Whether you've lived in this area a long time or are new to it … anything at all! I'm not going to ask you to introduce the person you've been talking to, so don't worry about remembering everything they tell you.

---

session at the last minute. Adult learners are fiercely pragmatic; their time is precious; they come to antenatal classes with expectations that they will acquire something which justifies the time (and perhaps the money) they are putting into them. Resentment and unease are instantly created if it appears that the group leader is not well prepared. Educators need to be available to learners, to be 'with' them in the same way that midwives are accustomed to understanding their role as being 'with' women during labour.

Agenda setting

Given that adult learners, whatever their background, like to feel that their individual needs are being addressed, allowing expectant parents to set their own agenda is important. Agenda setting in a group allows individual and collective uncertainties, worries or simply the need to know more, to be expressed in a safe way. It is often a good idea to split class participants into small groups to think about their agenda, perhaps basing the groups on gender, thus allowing the men to express their unique angle. Whatever the approach, it is beneficial to allow everyone to feel they can be as general or particular as they like in what they choose to include on the agenda, and also that they are not being forced to reveal more than they wish. Generally, an issue which one person is too shy or hesitant to articulate will be voiced by somebody else.

Once an agenda has been agreed, it is good practice to have it on display in each session so that everyone, including you, can keep an eye on it. When giving a 'trailer' for the following session, look at the agenda and relate what you plan to cover in the items stated there. This reassures people that you are mindful of their needs and therefore encourages future attendance.

Agendas should enable a course to be opened up, not closed down. Yet some educators will allow themselves to be restrained by an agenda and omit things from classes because 'they have not been asked for'. Careful use of an agenda can allow subjects which you know will be useful to be aired, yet which have not been specifically asked for. Many women and men coming to classes would say they are not sure what they need to know, because they do not know what it is they don't know! Some of the issues which are very real for them are hard to put into words. So agenda setting is just one of many ways of finding out what is on everyone's mind. It also puts the expectant parents centre stage which in itself helps to build confidence.

The two agendas in Box 15.2 are from real classes and are used as examples. The variety of agendas set by parents is infinite, as infinite as the personalities and backgrounds of the people you come across. Agenda 1 was put together by a group of women and Agenda 2 by a mixed gender group, but the men particularly asked for the first two and the last items.

There are a number of things to note:

- Both agendas give the facilitator a wide remit – they allow scope for exploration and will encourage class attenders to think broadly as well as specifically.

- Although from two different antenatal courses, it is interesting to note that some subjects came up on both agendas, as well as some different ones.

- Interestingly, Agenda 1 makes no mention of anything postnatal – although there are some obvious openings for introducing postnatal issues.

- Agenda 2 gives plenty of scope for sessions on care of the baby, mothers' postnatal physical and emotional health and fathers' emotional health, but there is nothing about physical skills for labour – although again there are some obvious openings.

- The brevity of Agenda 1 came as a surprise to the educator, and may not be typical of a women-only group; however, brief agendas do not have to be constraining.

So how can these agendas be extended and used?

Agenda 1

Postnatal issues for mother and baby can be drawn out of 'How maternity care works'. 'Partner's role in labour' can be extended into life beyond birth – as Agenda 2 already allows. 'What to take to hospital' can be used to look at maternal physical and emotional health. If physical skills had not been mentioned, pain relief options would have been the obvious trigger for including them.

Box 15.2 Example agendas

Agenda 1

- How maternity care works
- When to go to hospital
- Physical skills for labour
- Pain relief options
- Signs of labour
- Partner's role in labour
- What to take to hospital

Agenda 2

- Making the baby thing real
- 'B-Day' – what to expect
- Birth plans
- What happens at hospital
- Role of the father in labour and afterwards
- When to go to hospital
- What happens post-birth
- Anything to give confidence

Agenda 2

'B-Day' – what to expect' gives permission for developing physical skills as does 'the role of the father in labour' and 'anything to give confidence'. 'Making the baby thing real' is also a gift to the facilitator who can encompass so much under this heading.

The key is to value agendas and not to judge them. Agendas are as important for what they *do not* say as for what they do. If you are surprised that certain subjects have not been included, you can mention this and help the group consider aspects of the transition to parenting that they may not have thought about. The key is for you yourself to think broadly and imaginatively.

Teaching physical skills

The only way to acquire a practical skill is by *practising*.

> *I hear . . . I forget*
> *I see . . . and I remember*
> *I do . . . and I understand* (Ancient Chinese Proverb)

Ancient wisdom, many people's preference for kinaesthetic learning, and what everyone knows from experience – all confirm the need for practice. Yet many antenatal classes focus solely on information sharing and discussion and exclude skills work, thereby sending out a subliminal message to parents that labour is a cerebral event which can be talked through, rather than a profoundly physical event taking place principally in the pelvis!

Childbirth educators are often fearful of attempting practical work. They are nervous that parents will refuse to participate. Acquiring confidence in this area of antenatal education requires you to be clear in your own mind about why you are going to spend time practising physical skills for labour. Define your aims:

- To empower women to give birth to their babies using their own resources
- To minimize the use of potentially harmful interventions
- To increase partners' confidence as birth companions.

If your aims for antenatal classes are similar to these, you will already be convinced of the importance of practical skills work.

Prepare yourself:

- You need to be at ease with your body. Before you do any teaching, try demonstrating different positions for labour while looking at yourself in a full length mirror. Listen to yourself trying out the different noises you know women make during labour. Can you imitate them?
- Collect pictures of women labouring in different positions. Mount and laminate them to use as prompts for when you invite parents to practise.
- Be prepared to introduce a physical skills session with a vigorous rationale for why acquiring these skills will help women when they are in labour.

The vast majority of parents attending antenatal classes will respond positively if you yourself demonstrate what you want them to do, if you are confident when you invite them to participate (*'Can you all stand up now and try out the positions in the pictures I'm handing out'*), and if you give them lots of positive, humorous feedback while they are practising.

It is often said that *Practice makes perfect*. Practice *may* make perfect, but the only thing it is guaranteed to do is to make *permanent*. Therefore, the childbirth educator has to take responsibility for ensuring that parents practise physical skills safely and that they acquire effective rather than ineffective skills.

- For example: a tall man leaning over to comfort a woman as she kneels on all fours will put his back under great strain. He needs to position himself so that he can be close to his partner without putting himself at risk.
- Massage isn't effective if the person massaging the woman is tense with hunched shoulders and rigid hands. She or he needs to practise relaxing while giving massage.

All physical skills work for labour needs to be set in a realistic context. Ideally, the antenatal session will be held in a birthing room so that skills can be developed in the place where they will be put into practice (a marvellous idea – see Foster 2005). Otherwise, the educator needs to discuss with parents how they can use the furniture and equipment at the local consultant unit or birth centre to best effect. This can be done by taking photos of the birthing rooms and bringing them to classes so that parents can consider how the skills they are practising can be applied in the labour suite.

Physical skills work in antenatal classes is not all about preparing for labour; equally importantly, it is about preparing for parenting. The essential point remains the same – *clients only learn by having a go*. Demonstrating how to bath a baby does not improve your clients' manual dexterity, and seeing just how competent *you* are may tend to undermine their confidence.

While it is easy to scorn working with dolls and condemn it as silly and unrealistic, in our experience, clients *love* undressing an attractive baby doll, bathing it and then re-dressing it! *Doing* something stimulates them to think of the questions that are important to them and to reflect on what caring for their babies will be like. In the course of undertaking practical work, all sorts of discussions will arise, enabling parents to share information about such things as baby equipment and exchange ideas about styles of parenting. The job of the facilitator is merely to direct these conversations so that they are as fruitful as possible in helping parents prepare for what lies ahead.

Group work and discussions

Often, midwives do not know from session to session exactly how large or small the antenatal group will be (Box 15.3). This can make it hard to plan how you will manage discussions – will there be a lot of discussion in the whole group? Will small group work feature more? How small is a small group? If you only have four couples, is it still worth breaking up into smaller units? And so on. Much depends on your feel for the group – are they lively or quiet? Are there some dominant individuals? Are there some who will not take things seriously and disturb the others? Are there some who are very quiet? Are there some who seem totally disengaged? All group members will have a personal angle on the sessions and it is important to try and work *with* their personalities, not against them, for optimum learning.

Box 15.3 Benefits of small group work

- Small groups allow people to get to know each other better
- Quieter people are more inclined to participate
- Dominant people have a smaller stage and are more easily contained by the others
- Those who have not contributed in the large group can be given responsibility as note-takers and a role in feeding back
- In single gender groups, subjects can be aired which may seem embarrassing in a large, mixed group
- Single gender groups allow both women and men to feel their ideas are valued – this is especially important for the men
- When there is a lot of material to cover, small groups can focus on different aspects of a topic and existing knowledge is drawn out more easily
- People have to move to go into their groups; this prevents a class from becoming static
- When small groups feed back, class members take the lead and the focus shifts from the facilitator to themselves.

Splitting the large group randomly can be very productive, e.g. numbering off; a 'birthday line' – with groups chosen according to people's birthdays; by the babies' due dates; by where people live or where they were born. Alternatively, you may have particular reasons for arranging groups in certain ways – to get a good mix of personalities; to ensure that everyone has a chance to work with different class members; to bring those who might be having a similar experience together (e.g. couples/mothers expecting twins or anticipating an elective caesarean).

There are some key points to remember:

- Make clear when feedback from the small group is required and when it is not.
- Use and value feedback when it is given – don't ask for feedback and then ignore it.
- Address issues which arise as soon as possible – or make a note to return to them later.

- Visit each group early in the exercise to check that everyone knows what the task is.

- Be aware of what is happening in the groups but keep a discreet distance so that people do not feel you are eavesdropping on their discussions.

- Be on hand if a difficult issue arises which requires your presence in a group – and if it is something the whole class should hear, make sure that you mention it, or encourage it to be brought up by one of the parents when everyone is together again.

- Be clear about time-keeping – let everyone know at the outset how long their group discussion will be, and then give a few minutes warning before bringing it to a close.

Avoiding information overload

Sadly, the vast majority of information given in any class will have been forgotten by the next (Hughes 2000). This situation is particularly acute with adult learners who tend to operate a ruthless filtering system with regard to information, dumping whatever they do not perceive as immediately relevant, and storing in long-term memory only a very few items which appeal to their prejudices, they find exciting, or they feel they can use.

Among the antenatal teacher trainees whom the authors tutor, there is a tendency for students to lie awake in the early hours of the morning, worrying because they did *not* tell the parents who attended last evening's class something the student considers essential. Lying awake worrying about having given *too much* information would generally be more appropriate!

So how can the midwife/educator decide how much information is sufficient and what that information should be? She does not want to ration information or act as a censor, making a unilateral decision about how much this particular group needs to know. Adult educators recognize that much of what learners wish to learn they already know – if not individually, then as a group. To enable group members to learn from each other, topics can be introduced with an invitation to share existing knowledge and first or second-hand experiences:

- Do you know anyone who's had their labour induced? Why did they need an induction?

- What have your friends said about the first few months with a new baby?

- Do you know anyone who has suffered from post-natal depression? What helped them to recover?

Such questions enable parents to take the lead. They will express themselves in words that are accessible to the other group members, rather than in the medical language which health professionals tend to use. The midwife/educator learns what the people in the group know *rightly* and what they know *wrongly* and something about the group's attitudes towards the issue under discussion. If wrong information is shared, it is very usual for another parent to challenge what has been said, or to ask you for clarification, enabling the information to be corrected without any loss of face on the part of the person from whom it came.

Let's imagine how information about pethidine can be gathered from the group and how you can identify what further information people need to have:

Group Leader: Has anyone ever had pethidine or a strong painkiller?
Father: Yes, I had it when I broke my leg.
Group Leader: How did it make you feel?
Father: Brilliant! I didn't know where I was or what time of day it was. I was just floating!
Group Leader: So it really helped with the pain?
Father: Well – the pain was still there but it wasn't connected to me any more.
Mother: My sister had it with her first baby and it made her sick. She hated it. She said it didn't touch the pain at all.
Group Leader: Any other experiences?
Father: I think I had it when I had an injury at rugby. To be honest, I can't remember much about it, but I think it was OK.
Group Leader: Well, what you've said gives a perfect picture of pethidine. Some women find it really helps in labour; some find it useless and quite a few feel out of control after they've had it.
Father: So if it's only so-so for the mother, does it have any effect on the baby?

You can then reply to the question that has been asked, which will almost certainly generate more. The amount of information finally shared will depend on:

- what the group already knows
- what aspects of the topic they are interested in
- what the group leader feels are vital pieces of information that must be shared (such as that pethidine can make breastfeeding more difficult)
- and perhaps, if time is short, whether the group can easily find more information from resources to which you can point them.

Studies into how humans learn have shown that *emotional tagging*, which means ensuring that learners are helped to apply information within the context of their individual lives, increases retention (Pert 1997). At the end of any information-rich topic, you can invite people to discuss with their partner or their support person how they feel about what they have just learned. This encourages class participants to tag information with their own feelings, retaining what they judge to be relevant and helpful.

Environment of classes

You may, or may not, have choice in the location of your sessions for parent education. If you can choose, then opting for venues that are well-suited to the size of the group is important (participants don't like to feel either cramped or lost in a space that is too big). You need room to move about; seating that is comfortable both for the pregnant and the non-pregnant, and more than one type of seating to cater for different needs; easily accessible refreshments; the capacity to regulate the room temperature; privacy for work in small groups; somewhere to display visual aids easily, and lighting that is not too harsh but not too dim either.

This is the ideal – and often not available. So the issue for the facilitator is how to manage the environment she is in. A rather unpromising room can still be used very productively (Box 15.4).

Body language is important, and not being in one position as a facilitator reinforces what you are saying about active labour. Give permission early in the first session to change position during the class. Make links between the comfort of the room – or the lack of it – and managing the environment for comfort in labour (Box 15.5).

Box 15.4 Seating

Hard, uncomfortable chairs?
- Ask class attenders to bring along a couple of pillows or cushions – some will respond
- Encourage women to sit in different positions and relate these to labour, e.g. sitting astride the chair facing the back
- Suggest sitting on the floor
- Encourage women to stand occasionally and lean against the wall – this can help an individual who is losing concentration because of discomfort re-engage with the session (and is a great position for labour)
- Use surfaces in the room, e.g. tables, window sills, worktops as places for individuals to lean onto – more useful learning for labour
- Use birthing balls as seats

Soft chairs?
- Encourage movement to prevent anyone getting too comfortable – or for some, too uncomfortable.

You will need a seat too, but remember to keep moving around. Sometimes stand, sometimes sit – that will allow others to do the same.

A sense of *privacy* is important. Pregnancy is a time when people can feel that their privacy has been invaded and they have suddenly become 'public property'. One reason why some are reluctant to attend antenatal groups is that they fear that they will have to talk about subjects which could embarrass them in front of strangers. When dividing into small groups, try to ensure that the groups cannot overhear each other; use break-out rooms if available. During physical skills work for labour, dim the lights and encourage individuals/couples to move so that they are not alongside others (Box 15.6). Anything that inhibits people will undermine the effectiveness of teaching physical skills so good use of space is vital.

The warmth of the welcome you give is the most important thing. Less than ideal surroundings can be tolerated if the facilitator shows that she cares about individuals, is interested in them and is pleased to see them.

Box 15.5 Making use of the space

- Arranging seating in a horse-shoe shape keeps you closer to participants and allows movement more easily

- Encouraging the whole room to be used for physical skills, adapting the fixed and movable furniture to suit different labour positions, assists learning about the environment for labour

- If you are doing small group work, encourage the groups to spread to all parts of the room and create their own space

- If you are fortunate to have a break-out room, use it as much as you can for small groups

- Use wall space, notice boards, flip chart stands etc for displaying visual aids. You may have favourite illustrations and diagrams that you wish to have on show all the time

- Display any lists, diagrams, charts referred to or drawn up by the parents during the session. Over the course of the classes, there should be a gradual build up of displayed material, not only as a memory-jogger but also to value what the course members have contributed.

Box 15.6 Lighting and visual aids

- If there is a dimmer switch, make good use of it

- If overhead lighting is harsh, try using only half the lights

- Always check that the lights you do use are bright enough for everyone to see visual aids

- Ensure that everyone is well-positioned to see visual aids – get people to move if their view is obstructed or awkward.

Meeting shared and different needs

As a midwife, you probably already regard education as an integral part of your work when giving antenatal and postnatal care to mothers, with or without their partners. Many of your opportunities for parent education occur outside group situations, when you are caring on a one-to-one or a one-to-two basis. The fundamental skills required for delivering parent education in groups apply just as much to other encounters with parents (Box 15.7).

Box 15.7 Essential skills

Essential skills for parent education, wherever or however it is given, and whoever it is given to:

Listening – listen actively, with body language which is open and encouraging – don't sit back with your arms folded, for example, but sit forward and move the speaker on with nods and occasional words of encouragement; avoid fiddling with pens etc; reflect back what people are saying to ensure that you have understood.

Communication – this includes:

Use of language – appropriate, no technical jargon. Try to use terms and expressions which have meaning for the particular parent. Some will require detailed medical explanations because they feel 'fobbed off' if they do not receive such information. For others, anything too complicated will simply be ignored, forgotten or misunderstood creating fear and worry rather than relieving them. Only you can work out what the right pitch is, having first listened carefully to the woman or couple to discover what their needs are.

Tone – whatever you say, the tone in which you say it counts for a huge amount. *How* you say things is as important as *what* you say. Listening and observing will help you see how your approach is being received. If you get engagement and more questions, with no defensiveness, you can feel confident you are using the right tone.

Being non-judgmental – fundamental to all parent education, in any setting. Adults do not learn if they feel they are being judged, either as people or as parents. They will feel negative towards you if you appear to feel negative towards them. It is easy to stereotype and so important not to fall into that trap.

Being inclusive – achieved by careful use of language, and also by an open and welcoming attitude to all.

Young parents

People who may be considered to be members of particularly vulnerable groups still have many needs that are the same as those of any expectant parent. Caregivers need to demonstrate listening skills and a non-judgemental attitude just as they do for all parents. This does not mean that specialized skills are not also important. Standifird (2005) considers that caring for very young parents requires knowledge of the behavioural development of teenagers and understanding of the way that teenagers think. An in-depth appreciation of the issues surrounding teen-parenting leads to better focused parent education because educators can take into account the social context in which young people are bringing up their children (Cater & Coleman 2006).

Tips for working with teens

1. Be clear about what age group your classes are for. It is likely that 13-year-olds will be intimidated by 17-year-olds, and 18-year-olds will consider themselves in a very different phase in their lives from 15-year-olds. When you have decided the age range, do not make exceptions.

2. At the booking visit, ask young Mums for their consent to text them with useful information. Text the times and dates of classes. This has been found to be very effective in promoting attendance. Produce high quality flyers to advertise classes – young people live in a world of sophisticated advertising.

3. Make the class a social as well as an educational event; provide lunch or at least, interesting snacks. Focus on the young Mums as much as on their babies (Cheema 2002). Consider incentives such as a baby goody-bag to be handed out following attendance at all the classes.

4. Be relaxed about people arriving after the class has begun and leaving before it ends. Any attendance is better than none.

5. Tailor classes to fit the group's agenda as closely as possible. The young Mums themselves know what information they need. Financial worries, relationship difficulties and finding accommodation are important issues as is establishing a support network.

6. Encourage the Mums to come with a companion of their choice – sister, mum, boyfriend, best friend, etc.

7. Invite young Mums who have just had their babies to visit the classes and tell their pregnant peers 'what labour's really like'.

Women from minority ethnic groups

Singh and Newburn (2000) and Singh et al (2002) found that all the pregnant women in their survey had some unmet information needs but young women, women from lower socioeconomic and minority ethnic groups felt most in need of more information. This is echoed in Soltani and Dickinson's (2005) research, which showed that over half of a sub-group of non-professional women in their survey did not understand all of the written information given to them.

Caregivers benefit from a good understanding of the cultural norms and religious practices surrounding birth in a particular community. It is important to find out what are the barriers that prevent women from coming to classes. These have been identified by Byrom and Harding (2005) as the lack of an easily accessible venue, cultural issues and looking after older children. Women from minority ethnic groups are hungry for information to help them understand the local context of maternity care and make 'the system' work for them. Many have a need to de-brief previous experiences of birth and parenting. Most welcome the opportunity to meet others from the same background who are going through the same experiences. Ideally, educators who come from the cultural and religious background of the pregnant women will lead the classes and where this is not possible, thought should be given to training such people. In the experience of the authors, women are often delighted to be approached and offered training which will help them grow personally and professionally and enable them to be of service to members of their own community.

Fathers

Expectant fathers and mothers often have identical issues which need to be addressed both in antenatal classes and through individual contact. For both, worries about coping as parents are high (Matthey et al 2002, Singh & Newburn 2000), but inevitably, the two genders may have varying standpoints on a number of issues, and the background and the type of community fathers come from will also play a part in determining their particular learning agenda. According to McElligott (2001) men want to attend antenatal classes, but are often disappointed that there is little effort made to target their particular needs. Childbirth educators direct their attention at women participants, using language that excludes the fathers. Yet men have an exciting and varied learning agenda in pregnancy. While they are concerned about the birth, they are perhaps even more interested in thinking ahead to the postnatal period and exploring how life will change when the new baby arrives. Information about babies':

- sleeping/waking patterns
- signs of illness
- crying
- milestones
- day-to-day care
- and equipment needed and not needed

will be very warmly received.

Even more gratefully received will be the chance to *practise* babycare skills. Men are increasingly keen to be involved fathers rather than distant breadwinners, but are nervous about their ability to handle babies as confidently and competently as their partners. Helping men to acquire practical babycare skills is best done in single-sex small groups as women have a tendency to decry the efforts of fathers-to-be. In addition, inviting new fathers to classes to talk about their experiences at the birth and in the first few weeks of their babies' lives is an effective way of increasing men's understanding and making them feel special. Following a class which had been attended by three new Dads, one of the 'pregnant' fathers commented:

> It was great to hear it from a real Dad. It's always the mother's worries that the hospital's concerned about. Never mine. For the first time, I could ask exactly the questions I wanted answering without being considered selfish.

The idea of co-facilitation, with a female childbirth educator and a father worker leading the antenatal class together, is not new. Smith (2002) and Symon (2003) suggest that this is an effective way of meeting different gender needs. Friedewald et al (2005) also discuss projects for all-male groups. However, it may not be feasible to run fathers-only groups in your area; this does not mean that the benefits for men of sharing ideas with other men cannot be realized. The earlier section in this chapter looking at small group work provides ideas about how to use single gender groups to enable men to discuss the issues that are important to them, and to help them form a support network with other fathers whose babies will be of a similar age.

When visiting homes postnatally, you can target your approach to meet the particular practical, emotional and learning needs of both the mother and the father. Some men never attend classes and this might be the only time they have dedicated input from someone who is informed, and more particularly, seems to care about them. Remembering to address the needs of a father if he is present at a postnatal visit is important. Ignoring him will not only do him a disservice, it could be detrimental to the well-being of the mother and the baby as research suggests that women who have an understanding, well-informed partner are less at risk of postnatal depression (Barclay & Lupton 1999). Educating and supporting fathers is therefore an important area to think about (Smith 2002).o

Lesbian couples

It takes courage for lesbian parents to attend antenatal classes. Stewart's research (2002) reveals that same-sex couples are anxious about how they will be received by maternity services and society in general, as they approach becoming a family. Lesbian and homosexual parents remain a curiosity, and may be the subject of bigotry and hatred.

Members of 'minority' groups are looking for acceptance, respect and support, just as are any other parents. Stewart (2002) notes that lesbian parents *did not want a politically correct response, but wanted to be truly accepted on their own terms* (p 417). Schott and Priest (2002, p 214) ask childbirth educators who feel uneasy at the prospect of having a lesbian couple in their classes to ask themselves why:

On what do you base your views – verifiable fact, experience, media portrayals or hearsay?

While it is always important to choose your language carefully whenever you are teaching parents, it is especially so when the group includes a lesbian couple. Instead of 'Fathers' or 'Dads', you can refer to 'partners' or 'birth partners'. Single sex small group work needs consideration and probably discussion with the couple beforehand. It would also be useful to establish in advance of the first class, whether and how the couple wishes to discuss their situation with other class members.

Accepting the couple's relationship means avoiding becoming hyper-aware of everything that you say. It can be easy to make the couple feel different simply by your determined efforts not to do so.

> *It was annoying having someone struggle to be okay about it ... It was watching this person trying not to put their foot in it ... being careful ... an effort.*
>
> (Stewart 2002, p 417)

While it is important not to make any assumptions about the 'kind of people' a lesbian couple are, it is likely that their need for a support system is at least as great, and probably greater, than that of heterosexual couples attending classes. If through her respect, warmth and teaching skills, the childbirth educator can help the couple find a support network within the antenatal group, she is contributing to their having a successful and joyful parenting experience.

The future of parent education

The world of parent education is changing. The general direction of government policy is to strengthen support to women and families and thereby improve health outcomes for all. The *Child Health Promotion Programme* (DH 2004b) and plans for a *National Academy of Parenting Practitioners* (2007) could have far reaching effects on all who work with parents at whatever stage they first meet them. At the same time as antenatal classes are becoming less available within the NHS, the social networking and support gained from these groups have perhaps never been so important. The recent report from the National Perinatal Epidemiology Unit, *Recorded*

Delivery: a national survey of women's experience of maternity care 2006 (NPEU 2007) emphasized how lost some of the women who participated in the survey felt in the postnatal period, especially if they had not had the chance to make friends at antenatal classes:

> *I was appalled by the lack of antenatal classes available to me ... Antenatal classes were something I'd looked forward to about being pregnant. I have no friends with babies/pregnant and I would have benefited from meeting other women in my situation. (p 40)*

Mothers need support from others to validate their relationship with their babies (Hawthorne 2007). Brazelton (2007) talks of the urgent need for support in 'our stressful new world' where families are reorganized around the pursuit of employment and its demands, isolated from extended family, friends and traditional institutions of succour. There is no time for family rituals and the transmission of family traditions, including with regard to child-rearing. A great opportunity for support could be lost to parents if they do not have opportunities to learn in antenatal groups.

Today, there are many parents – asylum seekers, families who speak little or no English, travellers, women with learning difficulties, women in prison – whose educational needs require specialist knowledge and support as well as the universal skills needed for the education of all parents. At the end of this chapter is a list of useful contacts to help you help them. The sheer diversity and extent of need clearly suggest that the way forward in parent education is through collaboration and partnership between midwives and specific voluntary organizations so that knowledge, expertise and resources can be shared to the benefit of all parents. In Box 15.8 are the thoughts of a group of National Childbirth Trust teachers who are running antenatal classes at a large teaching hospital serving a rich multicultural community, having been invited to do so by the Director of Midwifery Services. There are also comments from an antenatal teacher working for *YWEB* (*Young Women Expecting Babies*) to which local midwives refer teenage parents. Collaboration certainly brings challenges, but as these examples show, there is mostly gain –particularly for the expectant parents.

Box 15.8 Collaboration in antenatal education and support for women

NHS Women's Healthcare Trust and the National Childbirth Trust

- The collaboration developed out of a long period of contact, both formal and informal between the hospital and the teachers; good relationships and trust make a solid foundation for collaboration
- The Director of Midwifery Services wanted the NCT teachers to encourage the women to challenge the hospital, to try to empower the women and their partners to get the kind of birth experience they would like
- The NCT teachers feel that their teaching has benefited from the collaboration with the hospital
- The challenge for the teachers is to maintain their independent voice.

NHS Community Services Trust and Young Women Expecting Babies (YWEB)

- Contact with local midwives ensures publicity for the antenatal classes. Young parents build up a good relationship with their teenage pregnancy midwife and will usually act on her recommendation. Midwives have a large caseload, so welcome sharing the work with the antenatal teacher who has time to explore issues with the girls.

REFERENCES

Barclay L, Lupton D 1999 The experience of new fatherhood: a socio-cultural analysis. Journal of Advanced Nursing 29(4):1013–1020

Brazelton T B 2007 Touchpoints: vulnerabilities and opportunities for early development. Keynote speech at the Conference, 'Learning from the baby: new ways of working with parents', Cambridge University, Cambridge, 27 March

Byrom S, Harding C 2005 Improving services for women of South Asian heritage. In: Nolan M, Foster J (eds) Birth and parenting skills: new directions in antenatal education. Edinburgh: Churchill Livingstone, p 103–106

Cater S, Coleman L 2006 'Planned' teenage pregnancy: Perspectives of young parents from disadvantaged backgrounds. The Policy Press, Bristol

Cheema K 2002 Supporting pregnant teenagers. MIDIRS 12(1):26–29

Daines J, Daines C, Graham B 2002 Adult learning, adult teaching, 3rd edn. Welsh Academic Press, Cardiff

Department of Health 1993 Changing childbirth. The Stationery Office, London

Department of Health 1997 The NHS Plan. The Stationery Office, London

Department of Health 2003 Building on the best: Choice, responsiveness and equity in the NHS. The Stationery Office, London

Department of Health 2004a National Service Framework for children, young people and maternity services. The Stationery Office, London

Department of Health 2004b The National Service Framework for Young People and Maternity Services: for parents. Appendix 1 – Overview of the Child Health Promotion Programme. The Stationery Office, London

Department of Health 2007 Maternity matters: choice, access and continuity of care in a safe service. The Stationery Office, London

Foster J 2005 Innovative practice in birth education: Birmingham Women's Hospital Birth Ideas Workshops. In: Nolan M, Foster J (eds.) Birth and parenting skills: new directions in antenatal education. Churchill Livingstone, Edinburgh, p 85–101

Friedewald M, Fletcher R, Fairbairn H 2005 All-male discussion forums for expectant fathers: evaluation of a model. Journal of Perinatal Education 14(2):8–18 (Commentary by Sally Marchant in MIDIRS Midwifery Digest 15(4):534)

Hannaford C 2005 Smart moves: why learning is not all in your head. Great Ocean Publishers, Arlington

Hawthorne J 2007 Introduction to the NBAS, speech at the Conference, 'Learning from the baby: new ways of working with parents', Cambridge University, Cambridge, 27 March

Hughes M 2000 Closing the learning gap. Network Educational Press, Stafford

Knowles M 1984 Introduction to andragogy in action. Jossey-Bass, London

Matthey S, Morgan M, Healey L 2002 Postpartum issues for expectant mothers and fathers. Journal of Obstetric Gynecological and Neonatal Nursing 31(4):428–435

McElligott M 2001 Antenatal information wanted by first time fathers. British Journal of Midwifery 9(9):556–558

National Academy of Parenting Practitioners 2007 Online. Available: www.everychildmatters.gov.uk/napp/ 2 August 2007

National Perinatal Epidemiology Unit 2007 Recorded delivery: a national survey of women's experience of maternity care 2006. NPEU, Oxford

Nolan M 1997 Antenatal education: failing to educate for parenthood. British Journal of Midwifery 5(1):21–26

Pert C 1997 The molecules of emotion. Touchstone Books, New York

Schott J, Priest J 2002 Leading antenatal classes: a practical guide. Books for Midwives, Oxford

Singh D, Newburn M 2000 Becoming a father: men's access to information and support about pregnancy, birth and life with a new baby. The National Childbirth Trust and Fathers Direct, London

Singh D, Newburn M, Smith N 2002 The information needs of first-time pregnant mothers. British Journal of Midwifery 10(1):54–58

Smith N 2002 Parenting education for men. In Nolan M (ed.) Education and support for parenting: a guide for health professionals. Bailliere Tindall, London, Ch. 6

Soltani H, Dickinson F M 2005 Exploring women's views on information provided during pregnancy. British Journal of Midwifery 13(10):633–636

Standifird K 2005 What expectant teens need from their caregivers. International Journal of Childbirth Education 20(2):15–18

Stewart M 2002 'We just want to be ordinary': lesbian parents talk about their birth experiences. MIDIRS, Bristol

Symon A 2003 Including men in antenatal education: evaluating innovative practice. Evidence Based Midwifery 1(1):12–19

USEFUL WEBSITES

The following is a list of websites where you can find specific information and expertise when running classes for different groups of parents.

All parents: www.nct.org.uk (The National Childbirth Trust)

Cultural identity: www.parentlineplus.org.uk/index.php?id=702

Fathers: http://www.fathersdirect.com www.sowingseeds.co.uk (Sowing Seeds works with ethnic minority families, and especially fathers, in African Caribbean and African communities)

Parents with Disabilities: www.disabledparentsnetwork.org.uk

Mothers and babies in prison: www.sheilakitzinger.com/Prisons.htm;www.birthcompanions.org.uk

One-Parent Families: http://www.oneparentfamilies.org.uk/

Teenage Parents: http://www.everychildmatters.gov.uk/health/teenagepregnancy http://www.dfes.gov.uk/teenagepregnancy/dsp_Content.cfm?PageID=85 http://www.connexions-direct.com/; www.tsa.uk.com/ (Trust for the Study of Adolescence)

Travellers: www.amicus-cphva.org/default.aspx?page=75 (CPHVA Community Practitioners and Health Visitors Association)

Teaching aids:

The National Childbirth Trust Sales (0870 112 1120) produces a catalogue *Resources for Health Professionals* which includes books and teaching aids, plus a teenage pregnancy toolkit suitable for use by professionals running parent education classes for young parents.

16 Special exercises for pregnancy and the puerperium

Judith Lee   Ros Thomas

The information in this chapter is relevant for group practice, or for use on a one-to-one basis, and includes advice for the whole of the childbearing year. For this purpose, the childbearing year is defined as the 12-month period between conception and 12 weeks postpartum.

The chapter aims to:

- give midwives an insight into the teaching of physical skills
- provide practical information about exercise during the childbearing year
- promote trouble free pregnancy through exercise
- provide practical information about relaxation and breathing for pregnancy, labour and the puerperium
- promote continence
- promote back-care in pregnancy and postpartum
- advise on when to refer to other health professionals.

The role of the women's health physiotherapist

The women's health physiotherapist is part of the multidisciplinary team caring for women in pregnancy, labour and the puerperium. Working together with midwives, both are ideally placed to promote good health and fitness during a woman's childbearing year and to prevent, identify and treat problems. This physiotherapist is specially trained to work with women at any stage of their lives in the specific areas of obstetrics, including pregnancy-related pelvic girdle pain, gynaecology and urology/continence, with both in- and outpatients.

A combined approach from the women's health physiotherapist, midwives, health visitors and other health professionals can provide an opportunity for education, discussion and health promotion in a group setting. They should aim to create a learning environment with a relaxed atmosphere, where parents-to-be can enjoy developing the confidence to cope with pregnancy, labour, birth and the early postnatal days. The physiotherapist is the ideal choice to teach the physical skills required for parenthood. However, where no physiotherapist is available, midwives may find themselves responsible for physical preparation as well as parent education in antenatal classes or on a one-to-one basis.

Anatomy, anatomical and physiological changes

Four pairs of abdominal muscles combine to form the anterior and lateral abdominal wall, and may be termed the abdominal corset. The deepest of the group is the transversus abdominis (TrA) which lies deep to the internal abdominal oblique (IO) and external abdominal oblique (EO) with the rectus abdominis (RA) central, anterior and superficial.

The deep muscles of the abdomen together with the pelvic floor muscles, multifidus (a deep muscle of the back) and the diaphragm, can be considered as a complete unit and may be termed the lumbo-pelvic cylinder (Fig. 16.1). When advising on exercise

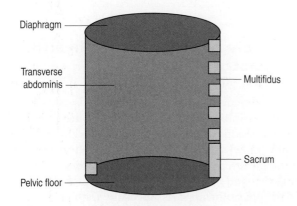

Figure 16.1 The lumbopelvic cylinder.

programmes relating to back-care and continence it is appropriate to consider the muscles of the cylinder as a working unit.

The coordinated actions of these muscles increase intra-abdominal pressure. At a high level, this facilitates expulsive actions of defaecation, micturition and parturition if in conjunction with a relaxed pelvic floor; and coughing, sneezing or vomiting if the diaphragm is relaxed. At a lower level, muscle activity exerts a force on the thoracolumbar fascia and a rise in intra-abdominal pressure that contributes to lumbar spine stability, crucial to pain-free resting posture and normal function.

The motor control of the muscles of the lumbo-pelvic cylinder is also significant in maintaining continence, controlling respiration and supporting the abdominal organs.

Optimal function of these muscles depends on timing of their recruitment, endurance, strength and coordination. This can be adversely affected by pain, postural malalignment, deficient nerve supply or fascial attachment.

The abdominal corset

The characteristics of the muscle fibres within the abdominal corset are variable.

The deepest TrA muscle is mainly slow twitch muscle fibres that are designed for endurance and postural control. The middle IO and EO muscles are a mix of slow and fast twitch fibres. This combination controls motion throughout movement, and may work eccentrically to decelerate movement, especially rotation. The most superficial RA has a bigger proportion of fast twitch muscle fibres that can produce and accelerate movement and act as shock absorbers of high loads.

The coordinated actions of all these muscles facilitate the maintenance of sustained postures and normal, pain-free movement of the lumbar spine.

The RA (Fig. 16.2) is a pair of two parallel long flat muscles, which extend vertically on each side of the midline along the front of the abdomen, being broader and thinner above the umbilicus than below and separated by a band of connective tissue called the linea alba (white line). Contained within the rectus sheath, it extends inferiorly from the pubic symphysis to the xiphisternum and lower costal

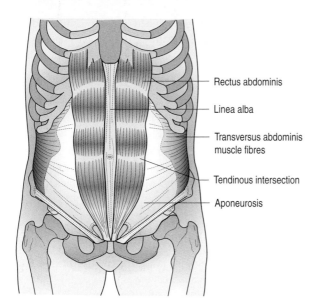

Figure 16.2 Rectus abdominis. (Reproduced from Brayshaw & Wright 1994, by kind permission.)

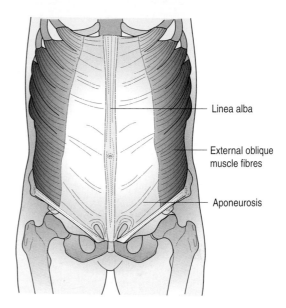

Figure 16.3 External oblique. (Reproduced from Brayshaw & Wright 1994, by kind permission.)

cartilages superiorly. The RA is a key postural muscle controlling pelvic girdle tilt and flexing the lumbar spine, as when doing a 'sit-up'. RA is assisted by EO and IO and works with the abdominal muscles to raise intra-abdominal pressure. By its attachment to the pubic symphysis it contributes to stability of this joint.

If the RA is bilaterally weak, posterior pelvic tilt will be much more difficult to control and perform, as will head and shoulder raising in the supine position. The difficulty in controlling pelvic tilt may increase the lumbar lordosis with possible associated low back pain.

As the baby grows during pregnancy, the two parallel rectus muscles within the rectus sheath elongate and move apart and may overstretch the linea alba. This is termed diastasis rectus abdominis muscle (DRAM).

The EO muscles (Fig. 16.3) are the largest and the most superficial of the flat muscles and are situated on the anterolateral aspect of each side of the abdomen. Each is broad, thin and irregularly quadrilateral; its muscular portion occupies the side of the abdomen and its aponeurosis (a flat tendon composed of layers of collagen fibres), the anterior wall.

The main muscle fibres run obliquely downwards and medially from the outer borders and costal cartilages of the lower ribs and insert by the aponeurosis into the linea alba forming the anterior part of the rectus sheath. The most lateral fibres pass from the lower four ribs almost vertically down to insert as the inguinal ligament.

The EO compresses the abdominal cavity, which increases the intra-abdominal pressure. It also participates in both flexion and side flexion and produces and controls rotation of the vertebral column.

The IO muscles (Fig. 16.4) form the middle layer of the flat abdominal muscles, lying just underneath the EO and just superficial to TrA. The fibres arise from the inguinal ligament, iliac crest and thoracolumbar fascia. Fibres insert into the crest of the pubis, pectineal line and upwards and medially at right angles to those of external oblique, by an aponeurosis, into the linea alba forming the posterior part of the rectus sheath as it passes behind RA. The most posterior fibres run vertically upwards to insert in the lower ribs.

The lower anterior fibres of the IO muscles work with TrA to compress and support the lower abdominal viscera. The upper anterior fibres of both IOs contract to flex the spine, support and compress the abdominal viscera, depress the thorax and assist in respiration. Contracting unilaterally, the upper anterior fibres of IO work with the anterior fibres

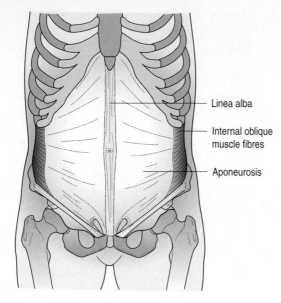

Figure 16.4 Internal oblique. (Reproduced from Brayshaw & Wright 1994, by kind permission.)

of the EO of the opposite side to produce and control rotation of the vertebral column. The lateral fibres of the IO on one side work with the lateral fibres of the EO on the same side to flex the trunk sideways.

TrA (Fig. 16.5) is a pair of muscles which are the deepest of the abdominal muscle sheets with fibres

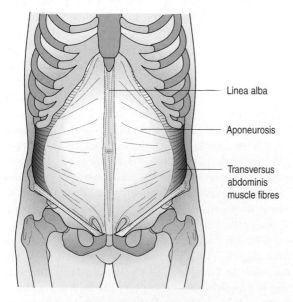

Figure 16.5 Transversus abdominis. (Reproduced from Brayshaw & Wright 1994, by kind permission.)

running transversely from the lateral one third of the inguinal ligament, the anterior two thirds of the inner lip of the iliac crest, the thoracolumbar fascia and the inner surfaces of the costal cartilages of the lower six ribs. Fibres run transversely to form and combine with the broad aponeurosis of the obliques and form the rectus sheath which encases RA and inserts into the linea alba.

The TrA muscles compress the abdominal viscera, giving support similar to a girdle and stabilize the lumbar spine by attachment to the thoracolumbar fascia.

The lumbopelvic cylinder

This consists of the TrA, diaphragm, multifidus and the pelvic floor muscles.

The *multifidus* consists of a number of fleshy and tendinous fasciculi, the fibres of which pass upwards and medially and fill up the groove on either side of the spinous processes of the vertebrae. These fasciculi vary in length: the most superficial, the longest, pass from one vertebra to the third or fourth above; those next in order run from one vertebra to the second or third above; while the deepest connect two contiguous vertebrae. Multifidus contributes to spinal segmental stability.

The *diaphragm* is a shelf of muscle extending across the bottom of the ribcage. It separates the thoracic from the abdominopelvic cavity. In its relaxed state, the diaphragm is shaped like a dome. Its convex upper surface forms the floor of the thoracic cavity, and its concave under surface, the roof of the abdominal cavity. Its peripheral part consists of muscular fibres, which take origin from the circumference of the thoracic outlet and converge to be inserted into a central tendon.

The diaphragm is pierced by a series of apertures to permit the passage of structures between the thorax and abdomen, most importantly the *aortic, oesophageal* and the *vena caval* openings. It is critically important in respiration. In order to draw air into the lungs, the diaphragm contracts, moving downwards, working with the EI thus enlarging the thoracic cavity and reducing intrathoracic pressure. When the diaphragm relaxes, air is exhaled by elastic recoil of the lung and the tissues lining the thoracic cavity.

It also helps to expel vomit, faeces and urine from the body by increasing intra-abdominal pressure.

The *pelvic floor* is a fascial and muscular sheet forming the inferior boundary of the abdomino-pelvic cavity. The main muscular components are the puborectalis, pubococcygeus, iliococcygeus and ischiococcygeus, collectively termed the levator ani (see Ch. 8). It is attached to the inner surface of the side of the lesser pelvis, and unites with its opposite fellow forming the greater part of the floor of the pelvic cavity. It supports the viscera and surrounds the structures, which pass through the cavity.

The coordinated action of levator ani, in the presence of intact fascia, generates a rise in intra-abdominal pressure to maintain organ support and urinary and faecal continence.

Influence of pregnancy on lumbopelvic stability and control of continence

During pregnancy, relaxin and progesterone affect the collagen fibres in fascia, tendons, aponeuroses and linea alba, causing these tissues to become more elastic and less supportive (Ostgaard 1997).

Anatomical and physiological changes

Lumbopelvic stability is the control of neutral position, which allows pain-free movement and effective load transfer through the spine and pelvis. According to Panjabi (1992a,b), this is achieved when the passive, active and neural systems work together. The passive structures are the bones, joints and joint ligaments; the active are the muscles of the abdominal corset and cylinder and the neural are the nerves supplying them. Instability and consequent pain may develop if any of these systems are dysfunctional.

Continence is maintained by a control mechanism of urethral sphincteric control and urethral support. The structures which provide support for the urethra include the passive system of the fascia which is anchored to the inside of the pelvic bones, the active system of the pelvic floor muscles and the neural system of nerves, which control the timing, endurance and strength of the muscle contraction. Stress urinary incontinence can result when there are problems with any of these systems (DeLancey 1994).

There is much evidence that pregnancy and childbirth can disrupt these systems (DeLancey et al 2003).

Ashton-Miller et al (2001) demonstrated that over-stretch and damage of the ventral and medial parts of pubococcygeus is evident in parous women and not in nulliparae.

Allen et al (1990) showed that vaginal birth causes partial denervation of the pelvic floor in most women having their first baby. This is sometimes severe and associated with urinary or faecal incontinence. Damage is increased during an active second stage longer than 83 min and birthweight over 3.14 kg.

Also, Tetzschner et al (1996) showed that vaginal birth could cause damage and delayed conduction of the pudendal nerve and subsequent decrease in urethral closure pressure. However, for the majority, vaginal birth is the safest and least problematic. Caesarean section should not be considered solely to protect the pelvic floor, as MacLennan et al (2000) showed there is no significant reduction in long-term pelvic floor morbidity associated with caesarean section versus spontaneous vaginal birth.

Safe exercise in the childbearing year

The exercise needs of the disabled woman during the childbearing year should be assessed individually, so that specific advice and information can be given (see *Fit and Safe* leaflet at: www.acpwh.org.uk).

Exercising during the childbearing year is not harmful to either mother or baby (Artal et al. 2003, Brown 2002, RCOG 2006) if the pregnancy is normal and the mother healthy (Arena and Maffulli 2002, Avery et al 1999, Goodwin et al 2000, Hefferman 2000, Riemann et al. 2000) and can be positively beneficial if at a mild to moderate level. *The aims of exercising in pregnancy should be to maintain, or slightly improve, the woman's level of fitness.*

Provided there are no specific obstetric or medical contraindications, fit women can safely *maintain* the same level of fitness during pregnancy. Pregnant women should not undertake new, vigorous exercise, which could make them too warm, tired or breathless and regular exercisers should reduce the intensity and duration of their training as the pregnancy progresses.

The American College of Obstetricians and Gynecologists (ACOG 2002) states that 'in the absence

Table 16.1 Borg Scale of Perceived Exertion and Talk Test guidelines

Borg scale	Level of exertion	Talk test guidelines
0	Nothing at all	Can easily carry on a conversation
1	Very easy	
2	Easy	
3	Moderate	You should be able to carry on a conversation
4	Somewhat hard	
5	Hard	
6		Can't talk continuously
7	Very hard	
8		Can't talk at all
9		
10	Maximal	

of either medical or obstetric complications, 30 min or more of moderate exercise a day on most, if not all, days of the week is recommended for pregnant women'.

All women should be encouraged to exercise at a moderate level to derive the associated health benefits (RCOG 2006). A moderate level is that intensity which can be maintained while able to carry on a conversation. The Borg Scale of Perceived Exertion (Noble et al. 1983), or the Talk Test can be used, preferably at level 3–5 (Table 16.1). This should be used in preference to a heart rate monitor, which is less reliable due to the pregnancy-induced increase in heart rate.

There are benefits to exercising in the childbearing year. The benefits according to the ACPWH may include:

- maintenance of cardiovascular fitness, respiratory and musculoskeletal status (Kramer 2000)
- maintenance of healthy weight range for mother
- improvement of body awareness, balance, co-ordination and posture
- improvement in circulation and lowered diastolic pressure
- an increase in both endurance and stamina
- increased feelings of social and emotional well-being, when exercise is combined with social interaction (Goodwin et al 2000, Horns et al 1996)

- a possible reduction in problems during labour and delivery. Labour may also be shorter and there may be fewer interventions (forceps, caesarean section) (Bungum 2000)
- evidence of neurological benefits to the baby and developing child (Friedman 1999)
- a reduction in common disorders of pregnancy
- suggestion of a more rapid postnatal recovery as the woman is likely to be fitter
- better glucose utilization by increasing insulin sensitivity (ACOG 2002, Hartmann et al 1999, Marquez-Sterling et al 2000)
- suggested improved placental growth, increased fetal growth.

However, further research on the benefits of exercise in pregnancy is needed and health professionals should remain up to date with current literature.

Most women will fall into one of the following four types of exerciser. Using the Borg Scale of Perceived Exertion is appropriate for all women, whatever their level of fitness or ability.

The non-exerciser These women will dislike exercise and not easily be persuaded of its benefits, especially during pregnancy. They may respond to encouragement to try some basic exercise.

The occasional exerciser These women may recognize the benefit of exercising when pregnant and may wish to increase the level of intensity, duration and regularity. They should be advised to avoid starting a new exercise programme until after the first trimester and should begin simply and gradually, preferably with the supervision of an adequately trained professional to oversee their progress.

The regular exerciser Guidelines for exercise in pregnancy (ACOG 2002) suggest that the woman who exercises regularly should:

- discuss her exercise programme with the obstetrician, GP, physiotherapist or midwife before continuing
- exercise at least three times per week for 20–30 min to improve aerobic capacity but discontinue contact or dangerous sports
- self-regulate both the level of intensity and duration of exercise as the pregnancy progresses. This will help to keep core temperature below 38°C

- always aim for low impact activity to reduce musculoskeletal stresses and wear supportive footwear
- prevent dehydration by maintaining an adequate fluid intake and should avoid exercising during hot and humid weather or with pyrexia
- ensure that they warm up and cool down for at least 5 minutes
- not overstretch because of the hormonal effects on the ligaments
- consult the relevant professional for advice on specific exercises, e.g. for the pelvic floor and abdominal muscles
- avoid certain movements like low squats, cross-over steps, rapid changes of direction and ballistic exercise
- avoid aortocaval compression by not exercising in the supine position (supine hypotension syndrome, Artal et al 2003)
- not restrict their calorific intake but aim to eat to appetite
- aim to pursue a variety of exercise activities in order to avoid overtraining
- not exercise to the point of fatigue nor become breathless.

The athlete These women are often the most difficult to advise as they are often highly motivated and competitive. They should follow the advice of regular exercisers. A safe level of aerobic exercise for the athlete will depend on the chosen sport and degree of fitness attained (Warren and Shantha 2000). The athlete will inevitably need to lower the intensity and length of her training sessions and they should be aware that the same warnings and contra-indications apply as for the regular exerciser.

Advisors of pregnant women athletes regarding safe exercise should remember that research into strenuous activity during pregnancy is limited, so should endeavour to keep updated of new information.

Antenatal exercise

It is best to continue with familiar activities rather than begin new types of exercise and the woman should listen to her body when exercising and stop if she feels uncomfortable, fatigued or unwell.

Basic exercise

Brisk walking during which the Borg Scale/Talk Test is correctly observed is an easy and accessible method of exercising for all.

Common exercise activities

Swimming is excellent exercise if aerobic changes are induced. Pelvic girdle pain can be avoided or reduced by using an alternative leg action during breaststroke so that forced adduction against resistance of the water is prevented. The lumbar spine should remain in the neutral position. The buoyancy of the water offsets the effects of gravity on the body and so tiredness is less likely though muscle strength and flexibility can be maintained or improved. Another effect of immersion in water is that of diuresis. It is sensible to avoid diving during pregnancy.

Exercising in water also raises the plasma beta endorphin levels significantly (McMurray et al 1990) and has a beneficial effect on the respiratory, cardiovascular and musculoskeletal systems and Hartmann and Bung (1999) state that water-based exercise can be highly recommended because of its beneficial effects provided potential dangers and contraindications are observed. Some women find aquanatal classes can fulfil both a social and physical need in a most enjoyable way. The classes should be led by a properly qualified professional following set guidelines (see ACPWH leaflets) and may be found in hospitals or community.

Cycling is a popular form of exercise which allows for good mobility of the lower limbs with the body-weight supported. It is an easy way to travel, although short distances are preferable and steep hills should be avoided.

Low impact aerobics is an adequate means of maintaining fitness levels. The intensity and duration of exercising may be increased initially to compensate for the high impact aerobic movements but as pregnancy progresses will need to be moderated.

Modified Pilates is a scheme of specially adapted non-aerobic exercises for pregnancy which offer both mental and physical training, targeting the deep postural muscles necessary to develop core stability and postural alignment and working to develop balance, posture, abdominal and back strength. The concentration on TrA and pelvic floor muscle strengthening makes it an ideal preparation for labour and postnatal recovery. A Pilates for Pregnancy video (Jackson 2001) will assist women who cannot get to classes to exercise in their own homes. Many women enjoy Pilates and Yoga but should check the instructor is qualified to teach pregnant women.

Back-care classes give an opportunity to educate and teach good back-care technique for life and can be adapted successfully for the pregnant woman.

Gym-based exercise is also very popular and many women wish to continue their training regimes. Equipment to encourage aerobic activity includes the static bicycle, treadmill or cross-trainer. Good technique is essential when strength training. Pregnant women should use lighter weights than they normally do and use sub-maximal lifts. Varying the exercise and using both upper and lower body muscle groups is good practice. Weights, sets and repetitions should be decreased further as pregnancy progresses (Avery et al 1999). Resistance should be varied according to ability.

Circuit training may be included but rest periods between activities may need to be longer and the intensity of the activity lowered and closely monitored.

Caution should be exercised before trying new types of classes that are introduced from time to time and where possible, seek recommendation of suitability from a physiotherapist.

Energetic and competitive sports activities which include jogging, hiking, rowing, cycling, dancing, skating, cross-country skiing, running and tennis can continue (ACOG 2002, SMA 2002).

Contact sports such as hockey, football or basketball pose a potential threat to the safety of the mother and fetus and should be avoided as should horse riding, skiing, and some racquet sports as they increase the risk of falling.

Special sports such as scuba diving and exertion at altitudes over 6000′ are dangerous.

Contraindications, precautions and warnings

Absolute contraindications to exercise in pregnancy

- serious cardiovascular, respiratory, renal or thyroid disease
- poorly controlled type 1 diabetes

- risk of, or current, premature labour
- cervical incompetence
- history or risk of IUGR and premature labour – reduce activity after 12 weeks
- hypertension – should be discussed with the woman's doctor
- placenta praevia after 26 weeks' gestation – should be discussed with the woman's doctor
- sudden swelling of ankles, hands or face
- acute infectious disease
- severe rhesus isoimmunization.

Precautions to exercise in pregnancy

The following conditions may require some caution and it is advisable to seek medical advice before commencing any exercise:

- asthma
- diabetes type 1. If insulin regimes are well controlled and exercise is moderate (Arena and Maffulli 2002), discuss with diabetic consultant, GP or specialist nurse
- history of miscarriage
- pre-pregnancy hypertension
- placenta praevia
- vaginal bleeding
- reduced fetal movement
- anaemia
- breech presentation
- extreme obesity
- extreme underweight BMI<12
- heavy smoking
- thyroid disease.

Warnings

All women should stop exercising immediately and seek advice from a midwife or doctor if they experience:

- abdominal pain
- leakage of amniotic fluid
- pelvic girdle pain
- pelvic girdle pain which may lead to difficulty in walking

- vaginal bleeding
- shortness of breath, dizziness, faintness, palpitations or tachycardia
- persistent severe headache
- calf pain
- absence of or reduced fetal movements.

Postnatal exercise

The aim of exercising after the baby is born is gradually to regain and then improve the former level of fitness. Once the baby is born, women should return to exercising as soon as they feel able but this should be a gradual process. Postnatal depression is less likely in women who return to exercising relatively soon after birth but only if the exercise sessions are positive rather than negative experiences (Koltyn & Schultes 1997).

High impact exercise should be avoided for a few months after birth to allow musculoskeletal changes of pregnancy to normalize. In women who experienced pregnancy-related pelvic girdle pain, there may be residual associated pelvic muscle imbalance. Increased caution and possible physiotherapy referral is necessary for these women. Athletes may be able to return to their sport more quickly. Pregnancy necessitates a reduction in maximal training but should not have a significant adverse impact on postnatal training regimes (Beilock et al 2001).

Coping skills for labour

Relaxation, breathing techniques, massage and encouragement to move and adopt an upright, or forward leaning, posture during labour will help the woman to cope with the discomfort and pain of contractions.

Relaxation

If feeling threatened, anxious, fearful or in pain, muscle tension increases and the body may unconsciously adopt an extreme posture. This is known as the fight or flight response, preparing the body for action. However, if the cause is not an enemy that can be fought with, or escaped from, the tension persists, becomes exhausting and causes physical changes in heart, lungs and other body systems. Relaxation is concerned with reducing body tension to a minimum and once learned can be used whenever increased tension is a problem. It can be particularly useful during pregnancy and labour and the early postnatal days. The most widely used relaxation technique used in pregnancy and labour is the Mitchell method of physical relaxation.

This technique (Box 16.1) involves a series of instructions and movements, which help the body to move away from the posture, caused by tension and so achieve a position of comfort, ease and relaxation. By following each individual instruction and movement, tension in that part of body will disappear.

Positions for labour

Early first stage of labour

Research shows that women who use upright positions during the first stage of labour:

- have more efficient contractions
- have shorter labours
- are less likely to use pethidine or an epidural for pain relief
- are less likely to have their labour accelerated artificially than women who were lying down (Enkin et al 2000).

A woman in labour should be encouraged to keep mobile and active. If there are no complications, she should try alternative positions of ease as change of position leads to productive uterine contractions (Roberts et al 1983). When discomfort increases, the woman should be encouraged to stay relaxed and concentrate on rhythmical easy breathing during contractions.

Coping with early first stage of labour

The following positions of ease may help during the early stages of labour and can be discussed and practised in the antenatal period:

- sitting against a table and relaxing forwards so that shoulders, arms and head are supported
- standing, leaning backwards against the wall of the room

Box 16.1 Physiological relaxation technique

For each part of the body where tension manifests itself there is a three-fold instruction:

1. An order to the reciprocal muscle group to work strongly
2. A command to that muscle group to stop working
3. A direction to the brain to recognize the new position of ease and to remember it.

Lie down comfortably on your side or sit in a chair with back and head supported.

Breathing. To begin the relaxation session take a deep breath in, expanding above the waist and lower ribs, then sigh out easily and continue to breathe gently, keeping the movement fairly low down in the chest.

The shoulders, arms and hands are usually the first areas to respond to stress so begin with these parts.

- *Shoulders.* Pull your shoulders towards your feet – stop pulling – concentrate on this new position of ease – your shoulders are relaxed and down

- *Arms.* Push your elbows slightly out from your body as though straightening the elbows – stop pushing, think about this position – your arms are relaxed and comfortably supported

- *Hands.* Let them rest on your tummy or thighs or the supporting surface – Open out the fingers and thumbs, keeping the wrists on the support. Stretch the fingers and thumbs – stop moving – feel the new position – comfortable, supported and relaxed.

The teacher moves on to the remainder of the body; the hips, knees, head and face, giving clear, precise instructions which can be found in full in the ACPWH leaflet.

Your body should end up in a position of ease and as relaxed as possible. Breathing is at your normal resting rate.

Relaxation can be adapted as labour progresses by adopting the most comfortable position for you, with easy breathing in the lower part of the chest.

- kneeling on all fours
- kneeling on the floor and leaning forwards onto a chair
- leaning forward against a partner
- sitting astride an armless chair with arms supported on the chair back and body relaxing forwards
- the birthing room may have additional aids, e.g. rocking chair, large ball and mat.

Pelvic rocking in any of these positions may be helpful.

Deep massage of the lower back or gentle stroking of the abdomen soothes many women and can be taught to the partner at couples' classes.

Later first stage of labour

As labour progresses, it becomes more difficult to find a comfortable position and frequent changes may be necessary. Many women however, are content to sit back against pillows on the bed at this stage and concentrate on relaxation and breathing. As each contraction builds up, the speed and depth of breathing sometimes alter but mothers must be encouraged to keep it as natural and easy as possible. They may find that 'sighing out slowly' (SOS) helps to avoid panic breathing and also relaxes physical tension, especially in the shoulders.

The emotional aspects of the end of the first stage of labour will be explained to couples antenatally and coping strategies need to be discussed. With a premature urge to push, an interrupted outward breath can be introduced (that is, two shorter breaths out followed by a longer breath out). This is often known as 'pant, pant, blow' or 'puff, puff, blow' breathing and it prevents the diaphragm from fixing with a subsequent increase in intra-abdominal pressure. A change in position will take away some of the urge to push, for example side-lying or prone kneeling with the forehead resting on the hands.

Second stage of labour

A review of research assessing the use of different positions during the second stage of labour showed that women who remained upright or lay on their sides to give birth, were more likely to have a shorter second stage and less likely to have an assisted birth (Gupta & Nikodem 2001).

Midwives can actively encourage women to choose the most comfortable position and to change position as and when they wish. They should acknowledge a preference for being upright in labour and discourage women from lying on their backs (MIDIRS 2003).

Coping with second stage of labour

Positions for second stage will depend on individual choice, method of pain relief and obstetric factors (see Ch. 27).

If there is pain in the pelvic girdle, particularly over the symphysis pubis or sacroiliac joints then undue abduction of the hips (by parting the knees beyond the woman's pain free range) should be avoided during labour, vaginal examinations and birth. The symphysis pubis joint may be protected from further disruption by limiting hip abduction and maintaining symmetry of hip positions. Prone kneeling or side-lying are the optimum positions for birth (ACPWH PGP leaflet, Fry 1997).

As the contraction starts, the mother is reminded to breathe in and out gently. Only when the urge to push becomes overwhelming should she bear down with the contraction, keeping the pelvic floor relaxed. Breath-holding longer than a few seconds should not be encouraged because of the danger of fetal hypoxia in an already compromised baby (Caldeyro-Barcia 1979).

To prevent pushing while the head is being born, deep panting may be useful.

Breathing control

Respiration is affected by stress and adapted breathing is one of the easiest ways of assisting relaxation. Breathing can be used to increase the depth of relaxation by varying its speed; slower breathing leads to deeper relaxation. Natural rhythmic breathing must not be confused with specific unnatural rates of breathing, which research has proved to be harmful to both mother and fetus (Bush 1992, Caldeyro-Barcia 1979). Women in labour frequently breathe very rapidly at the peak of a contraction but should be encouraged not to do so. Persistent rapid breathing or breath-holding is usually a sign of panic.

Very slow deep breathing can cause hyperventilation, which produces tingling in the fingers and may proceed to carpopedal spasm and even tetany.

Rapid shallow breathing or panting is only tracheal and can lead to hypoventilation with subsequent oxygen deprivation. During pregnancy, labour and birth, emphasis should be placed on easy, rhythmic breathing and on avoiding very deep breathing, shallow panting or long periods of breath-holding.

Antenatal and postnatal exercises and advice

Preventing and alleviating the early physical stresses of pregnancy and childbirth, should be taught as a priority. Common consequences of pregnancy and childbirth are the physical problems of pelvic girdle and low back pain or incontinence. The main aim in the postnatal period is to address healthcare needs and give advice and exercises to reduce the risk of future pelvic floor dysfunction or the possibility of long-term back problems, so that the woman may recover normal function free of both pain and symptoms.

Women whose pain or continence problems do not resolve with simple advice and exercises should be referred to a women's health physiotherapist.

Pain

Some 45% of all pregnant women suffer pregnancy-related pelvic girdle pain (PGP) and/or pregnancy-related low back pain (PLBP). Serious pain occurs in 25% of pregnant women and severe disability in 8% of pregnant women (Wu et al 2004).

Pelvic floor dysfunction (PFD) occurs in 52% of all pregnancy-related PGP/PLBP (Pool-Goudzwaard et al 2005).

Pelvic floor dysfunction

Pelvic floor disorders are very common and strongly associated with the female gender, ageing, pregnancy, parity and instrumental birth (MacLennan 2000).

- 31–47% report antenatal stress incontinence
- up to 34% report postnatal incontinence (Reilly et al 2002)
- 11.5% report faecal incontinence after a 3rd degree tear
- 25% report faecal incontinence after a 4th degree tear (Sangalli et al 2001).

For best compliance with the following advice and exercises, explain, demonstrate, supervise and practice at every opportunity.

Antenatal

Postural awareness and care of the back

Women should be advised that the weight of her baby, her altered centre of gravity and tiredness may alter her posture and place strain on her body, putting her at risk of low back and pelvic girdle pain. Her sustained posture when standing, sitting or lying plus repetitive movements may influence that risk and correction may prevent or reduce pain. Back-care advice should be developed relating to comfortable positions in sitting, standing, lying, general mobility and correct lifting.

Standing

For good standing posture, the centre of the head, shoulders and hips should fall in a line when viewed from the side. Standing tall, with shoulders relaxed, tummy gently drawn in and bottom tucked under, knees straight but not locked, and weight evenly distributed on both feet is advised (Fig. 16.6).

Sitting

The pregnant woman should choose a comfortable chair, which supports both her back and thighs (Fig. 16.7). She should sit well back and if necessary place a small cushion or folded towel behind the lumbar spine for additional comfort. Equal weight should be placed on each of her buttocks to prevent strain on the pelvic ligaments. The seat height should allow the feet to rest on the floor, or a small footstool or cushion may be placed under the feet to raise them slightly. Her workstation should be at the correct height such that she does not need to bend forwards. If relaxing in an easy chair, the head can be supported and the legs elevated slightly on a stool. Legs should not be crossed.

Lying

Sleep is a very valuable commodity during pregnancy and health professionals can advise and help women to find a comfortable position. Lying flat

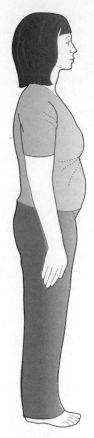

Figure 16.6 Posture in pregnancy.

on the back should be discouraged because of the risk of supine hypotension due to pressure from the gravid uterus on the inferior vena cava. However, if she wakes having been lying on her back she should be advised to lie on her side for a few moments before rising slowly. Most women will choose to lie on their side to sleep. Side-lying with pillows under the top forearm and knee is usually a comfortable position, and a small pillow under her waist supporting the increasing weight of her abdomen will help to maintain lumbar spine and pelvic girdle symmetry (Fig. 16.8).

Getting up from lying or rolling over in bed is easiest if she bends her knees, draws in the low abdominal and pelvic floor muscles, then uses her arms to push to roll over or to sit on to the edge of the bed.

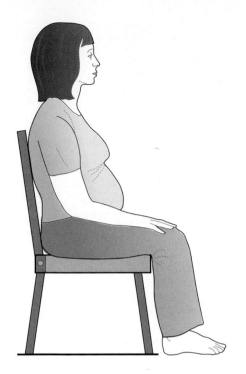

Figure 16.7   Good sitting posture.

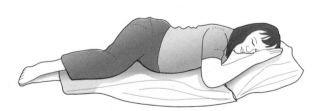

Figure 16.8   Side-lying supported with pillows.

Work activities

Women should be encouraged to make sure their seating and workstation is suitable, particularly if sitting for any length of time. Regular changes of task and alteration of positions is beneficial. If the woman's work involves constant standing she should ensure she sits at regular break times and be very careful if her work involves lifting or great physical effort. Many workplaces offer pregnancy risk assessments to employees.

Lifting and carrying

Lifting heavy or awkward objects should be avoided during pregnancy if at all possible. Twisting or bending while lifting is a particularly high-risk activity. If lifting is unavoidable, the thigh muscles, not those of the back, should take the strain. The abdominal and pelvic floor muscles should be drawn in for support and protection of the back and pelvis before bending the knees, holding the object or toddler close to the body, then lifting with the back straight (Fig. 16.9).

Toddlers should not be carried on one hip, or, at least, advise to alternate the hip. A rucksack carried on the back is much better for the back than a heavy shopping bag.

Pelvic floor exercises

There is evidence that pelvic floor muscle training used during a first pregnancy reduces the prevalence

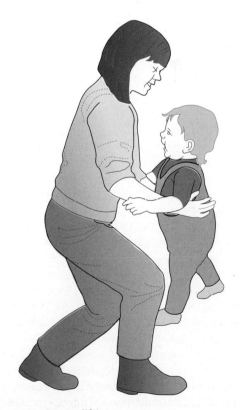

Figure 16.9   Correct lifting.

of urinary incontinence at 3 months following birth (Mason et al 2001).

The recommendation for preventive use of physical therapies is that pelvic floor muscle training should be offered to women in their first pregnancy as a preventive strategy for urinary incontinence. However, further studies need to be undertaken to evaluate the role and effectiveness of physical and behavioural therapies and lifestyle modifications in the prevention of urinary incontinence and long-term problems (NICE 2006).

Norwegian studies have shown that antenatal instruction in pelvic floor muscle exercises does reduce the likelihood of incontinence during and after pregnancy. The women in these studies had individual instruction in pelvic floor anatomy and how to contract the pelvic floor muscle correctly. Then they attended a 12-week intensive pelvic floor exercise programme supervised by a physiotherapist and were given a home exercise programme. The pelvic floor muscle strength, measured at 3 months postnatally had improved significantly (Morkved & Bø 2003).

It is impossible to provide this type of intensive women's health physiotherapy-led programme for all women during their pregnancy in the UK, but it is feasible that the multidisciplinary obstetric team could facilitate a satisfactory level of input to teach the exercises and encourage compliance. Women are regularly seen by their GP, hospital/community midwife or obstetrician and all women should have access to, and an opportunity to attend antenatal classes and receive written information about antenatal care (NICE 2008).

It is the recommendation of the Royal College of Obstetricians and Gynaecologists that every antenatal patient who is booked in should be asked about urinary and faecal incontinence and be given relevant advice or referral to continence services if symptomatic (RCOG 2006).

There are many opportunities for pelvic floor exercises to be encouraged and for trigger questions relating to urinary symptoms to be asked. The anatomy and function of the pelvic floor muscles should be taught (a model pelvis may help) and the risks of pelvic floor dysfunction explained, especially urinary incontinence in pregnancy and after childbirth (Box 16.2).

Box 16.2 Instructions for teaching the pelvic floor muscle exercise

- Sit, stand or lie down on your side. Imagine that you are trying to stop yourself passing wind and at the same time trying to stop the flow of urine
- The feeling should be of squeeze and lift, closing and drawing up the back and front passages
- Hold for as long as possible, up to 10 s, breathing normally, and then relax
- Repeat up to 10 times
- It is important to do this without tightening the buttocks or squeezing legs together and without holding your breath
- You should feel that your low tummy support muscle is working at the same time; this is good
- Try to practice this set of up to 10, 10-s squeezes at least 3 times a day This regime will help to build up, or maintain the endurance in the pelvic floor muscle during pregnancy
- The muscles should also be able to react to and maintain continence during sudden rises in intra-abdominal pressure as during a sneeze, cough or laugh; practising a few short, fast squeezes will help maintain this control
- Try to draw up the pelvic floor muscle gently when lifting.

Abdominal exercises

The deepest layer of muscles within the abdominal corset, TrA is important in postural control, controlling the neutral spine position and giving support to the weight of the growing baby. By its attachment to the aponeurosis, rectus sheath and linea alba, it may help to limit DRAM.

The mother should adopt a pain-free position, with good postural alignment. Sitting, standing, side-lying or four-point kneeling are good positions but she should avoid lying on her back after 16 weeks of pregnancy, because of the risk of supine hypotension. Figure 16.10 illustrates the transversus exercise, and Boxes 16.3 and 16.4 provide instructions for pelvic tilting and the TrA exercise.

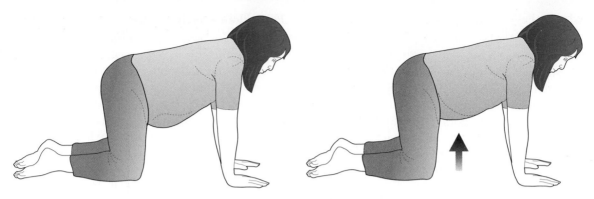

Figure 16.10 Transversus exercise.

Box 16.3 Instruction in pelvic tilting

- Place your hands on your abdomen
- Gently tighten your tummy muscles and buttocks and allow the back of your waist to slump backwards. Your pubic bone rocks up towards you. Breathe normally and hold the tilt for 5–10 s
- Relax and allow your back to hollow
- Repeat a few times. This is pelvic tilting
- The mid-way position is the neutral spine position and is safest for your back
- Practising the abdominal exercise is best done in the neutral spine position.

Box 16.4 Instructions for the TrA exercise

- Place your hands on lower part of abdomen
- Take a gentle breath
- As you breathe out, gently draw in and lift the lower tummy away from your hand, this time not allowing your back to move
- Keeping the tummy in, continue to breathe normally a few times
- Feel the muscle working under your hand as it supports the weight of your baby
- Relax
- Repeat up to 10 times, trying to hold each lift for 10 s, but don't hold your breath
- Repeat this set 6–8 times a day
- Try in different positions, and try to use this muscle during activity requiring effort.

Coping with common problems in pregnancy
(see also Ch. 14)

Leg cramps

Leg cramps are common and it can disturb sleep. Inadequate fluid intake, inactivity, prolonged sitting or wearing high heeled shoes may make the symptoms worse.

Advice: take a gentle walk, do foot and ankle circling, and gently stretch out the calf muscles. Have a warm bath before going to bed, and drink plenty of liquid.

Swollen ankles and varicose veins

Varicose veins are swollen, twisted, painful veins that have filled with an abnormal collection of blood. Prolonged standing and increased pressure within the abdomen may increase susceptibility to the development of varicose veins or aggravate the condition. Painless swelling of the feet and ankles is also a common problem.

Advice: rest with feet in elevation, take gentle exercise, avoid standing for long periods and consider wearing support tights.

Carpal tunnel syndrome

Fluid retention causing pressure on the median nerve within the carpal tunnel at the wrist may cause swelling, numbness, tingling or pain in the hands and fingers.

Advice: avoid repetitive movements, keep the hands cool and, if not resolving, refer to a women's health physiotherapist.

Postnatal

Rest

Adequate rest for the new mother is essential immediately after birth. The health professional may be able to suggest positions of ease in side-lying, with pillows under the abdomen and between the knees, or lying on the back with a soft pillow under the knees. If the new mother has learned a relaxation technique, she should use it to help her rest.

Getting in and out of bed

Rolling over and getting out of bed is easiest if she bends her knees, one at a time, supports her abdomen with a hand, especially if she has had a caesarean section draws in the low tummy muscles and rolls knees, hips and shoulders all over as one onto the side.

To get out of bed, push the body up by pressing down onto the mattress and allowing the feet to drop down to the floor. Sit for a few moments before standing by pushing up with both hands and standing tall.

Reverse the above instructions to get back into bed.

Sitting and feeding

Posture when feeding is important to protect the back. Aim for a pain-free, neutral spine posture and if sitting, use adequate pillows to lift baby to the breast or bottle, so that the mother's back is supported and shoulders relaxed.

Pelvic floor exercises and pelvic floor care

The pelvic floor muscles have been under strain during pregnancy and stretched during birth and it may be both difficult and painful to contract these muscles postnatally. Mothers should be encouraged to try the exercise as often as possible in order to regain full bladder control, prevent incontinence and prolapse and ensure normal sexual satisfaction for both partners in the future.

Studies have shown that women who had instruction by the physiotherapist on the postnatal ward and had been compliant with the exercises had reduced incidence of stress incontinence up to 1 year postnatally (Morkved & Bo 2003).

Pelvic floor exercise advice

Start exercises as soon after birth as possible, but if a urinary catheter is in place, wait until it is removed.

Try drawing in the muscles in varying positions; if the area is painful, side-lying is probably the most comfortable. If the area is painful and swollen, gentle rhythmical tightening and relaxing of the muscles will ease discomfort and promote healing.

Once the mother is more comfortable she should exercise the muscles as in the antenatal section, aiming to continue with a regular exercise regime for several months.

Other advice

Women should inform the midwife if they have not passed urine within 6 hrs of birth. It is the responsibility of the midwife to ensure local post-birth voiding protocols are adhered to and perinatal continence risk assessments completed, action taken as indicated and that any urinary incontinence is noted.

Empty the bladder regularly in first day or two after birth, but do not get into the habit of going to the toilet 'just in case'. Do not stop then start the flow of urine. Drink plenty of water for a healthy bladder, especially if breastfeeding.

When having a bowel movement, it may help to support the perineum with a pad or a hand on the abdomen if a caesarean section has been performed.

3rd and 4th degree tears

Faecal incontinence affects approximately 10% of female adults, with anal sphincter laceration during childbirth being the major risk factor, and accountable for 45% of incidence of postnatal faecal incontinence.

Following 3rd or 4th degree tears, 13% of primiparae and 23% of multiparae have on-going symptoms of urgency and/or faecal incontinence 3 months after birth (Sultan 1993).

All 3rd and 4th degree tears should be documented and a local care plan put in place to manage and review these women. A multidisciplinary team approach for these women is essential as pain management, advice regarding hygiene and care should be given postnatally and women should be advised about diet and position of defaecation to protect the anal sphincter. Compliance with the pelvic floor exercise programme is essential.

Faecal incontinence may also be caused by damage to the pelvic and pudendal nerves during vaginal birth and subsequent weakness of the pelvic floor and anal sphincter (Allen et al 1990).

It is a distressing and disabling condition, especially for new mothers but MacArthur et al (1997) found that only 14% of women with new faecal incontinence after childbirth had consulted a doctor and those doing so were unlikely to report incontinence voluntarily as one of their symptoms.

All postnatal women should be encouraged to exercise the pelvic floor and be asked about bladder and bowel function.

Abdominal exercises

The abdominal muscles become stretched and weakened by pregnancy. It is advisable to begin abdominal exercises to regain tone as soon as possible after birth in order that they recover to support the spine, prevent and relieve back pain and help the mother regain her 'former figure'.

Pelvic tilting as described in the antenatal section helps to locate the neutral spine position and also assists the relief of wind and nausea following caesarean section.

The TrA exercise

It is important to begin by exercising the deepest layer of muscles, the TrA, as described in the antenatal section.

The woman may now practise this exercise lying down with knees bent up and feet comfortably flat on the bed, with just one pillow beneath her head and arms by her side and in neutral spine position. This position is termed crook-lying. She should be advised to progress to exercising the muscle when sitting and standing, aiming for 10, 10 secs holds, three times a day and also to draw in the lower tummy when lifting, or bending forward to dress and change baby. This can be progressed further by trying the above exercise in four-point kneeling if comfortable. Women who have had a caesarean section should wait until this position is comfortable.

Progressing further

If, when trying the following exercise, abdominal doming occurs, the woman should revert to just the TrA exercise. If the doming persists after a few

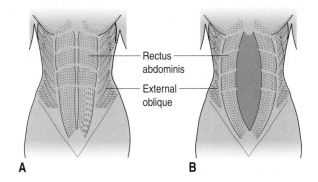

Figure 16.11 (A) Rectus muscles before pregnancy. (B) Diastasis of rectus muscles after pregnancy.

days, this may indicate that the rectus muscle has separated and the linea alba overstretched as in DRAM (Fig. 16.11). Contact should be made with the women's health physiotherapist who will advise on safe abdominal exercises and back-care.

Knee bends

In crook-lying, draw in the lower tummy, keeping the back still and bend one hip and knee up as far as is comfortable. Hold for 10 secs and slowly lower. Breathe easily throughout. Repeat, with the other leg. If able, repeat another three times for each side. This is a more challenging exercise for the abdominal corset and requires control by the oblique muscles to prevent trunk rotation.

Knee rolling

In crook-lying with lower tummy drawn in, gently lower both knees to the right as far as is comfortable, bring them back to the middle and relax, breathing easily throughout. Draw in the lower tummy and repeat to the other side. Repeat three times to each side.

Head lifts

This is not advisable for anyone who has neck pain.

In crook-lying, take a gentle breath in, then after the breath out, draw in the lower tummy and the pelvic floor muscles and lift head from the pillow, hold for 3 secs, lower and relax. Repeat up to 10 times. Progress by lifting the head and shoulders simultaneously.

Women should be advised to aim to practise abdominal exercises three times a day for at least 3 months after childbirth.

Care of the back after the birth

It may take up to 6 months before the ligaments completely resume their normal functions (Polden & Mantle 1992), so it is vital that new mothers receive advice on back-care in relation to everyday activities.

The mother should sit well supported to feed the baby. To prevent the mother from slouching forward, the baby should rest raised up on pillows. Nappy changing and bathing are best carried out on a surface at waist level or with the mother kneeling at a surface of coffee-table height.

Lifting anything heavier than the baby for the first 6 weeks should be avoided if at all possible but if unavoidable, good advice is:

- always try to bend the knees
- draw in the low tummy and pelvic floor muscles
- breathe out as you lift
- carry the toddler or object close to the body.

Baby chairs are heavy and are best carried by holding underneath and close to the body instead of by the carrying handle which puts a strain on one side of the body. Whenever possible, the chair should be carried empty and placed in the position required before the baby is put in it.

Baby slings should be comfortable and not cause an arched back. The weight should be well supported and the mother should use her TrA and pelvic floor muscles to ensure a good posture and prevent backache.

If back or pelvic girdle pain persists postnatally then referral to the women's health physiotherapist is indicated.

When/what to refer to the physiotherapist

Physiotherapists can advise on, or treat, the following conditions.

Antenatal problems may include:

- pregnancy-related pelvic girdle pain (PGP), which includes symphysis pubis dysfunction (SPD) and lower back pain
- divarication of RA
- coccydynia
- incontinence (see Haslam & Laycock 2008)
- carpal tunnel syndrome (CTS)
- co-existing disability with pregnancy.

Postnatal problems may include:

- pregnancy-related pelvic girdle pain (PGP) and lower back pain
- divarication of RA
- incontinence
- CTS
- co-existing disability
- 3rd/4th degree tears following birth
- coccydynia
- perineal pain including dyspareunia and scarring.

Promoting health and fitness

Opportunities for liaising with and sharing good practice with other health professionals to develop both specific and general health care measures should never be missed. Physiotherapists, midwives and health visitors have a duty of care to promote health and fitness to women and this may be possible in a variety of settings.

During pregnancy, labour and the puerperium, midwives and other healthcare professionals have many opportunities to influence parents-to-be, incorporating a sensible approach to exercise within the broader sphere of healthy routines for all family members. Walking, cycling, swimming and other forms of exercise should be encouraged as part of a general lifestyle as well as learning relaxation techniques as appropriate. Specific exercises for strengthening the pelvic floor and abdominal muscles, especially TrA, will have relevance far beyond the months of child bearing. Parents-to-be are an extremely receptive audience so opportunities to develop and promote specific and general healthcare measures should be optimized. Health professionals are well placed to encourage all women and their families to continue exercising for life.

REFERENCES

ACOG 2002 Exercise during pregnancy and the post partum period: Committee Opinion. Obstetrics and Gynecology 99:171–173

Allen R E, Hosker G L, Smith A R B, et al 1990 Pelvic floor damage and childbirth: a neurophysiological study. British Journal of Obstetrics and Gynaecology 97:770–779

Arena B, Maffulli N 2002 Exercise in pregnancy: how safe is it? Sports Medicine and Arthroscopy Review 10(1):15–22

Artal R, O'Toole M, White S 2003 Guidelines of the American College of Obstetricians and Gynaecologists for exercises during pregnancy and the postpartum period. British Journal of Sports Medicine 37:6–12

Ashton-Miller J A, Howard D, Delancey J O L 2001 The functional anatomy of the female pelvic floor and stress continence control system. Scandinavian Journal of Urology and Nephrology 207:S1–S7, S106–S125

Avery N D, Stocking K D, Tranmer J E et al 1999 Fetal responses to maternal strength conditioning exercises in late gestation. Canadian Journal of Applied Physiology 24(4):362–376

Beilock S L, Feltz D L, Pivarnik J M 2001 Training patterns of athletes during pregnancy and postpartum. Research Quarterly for Exercise and Sport 17(1):39–46

Brown W 2002 The benefits of physical activity during pregnancy. Journal of Science and Medicine in Sport 5(1):37–45

Bungum T J, Peaslee D L, Jackson A W et al 2000 Exercise during pregnancy and type of birth in nulliparae. Journal of Obstetric, Gynecologic and Neonatal Nursing 29(3):258–264

Bush A 1992 Cardiopulmonary effects of pregnancy and labour. Journal of the Association of Chartered Physiotherapists in Obstetrics and Gynaecology 71:3–4

Caldeyro-Barcia R 1979 The influence of maternal bearing-down efforts during second stage on fetal well-being. Birth and Family Journal 6:17–22

DeLancey J O L 1994 Structural support of the urethra as it relates to stress urinary incontinence: the hammock hypothesis. American Journal of Obstetrics and Gynecology 170(6):1713

DeLancey J O L, Kearney R, Chou Q et al 2003 The appearance of levator ani muscle abnormalities in magnetic resonance images after vaginal birth. Obstetrics and Gynecology 101:46–53

Enkin M, Keirse M J N C, Neilson J et al 2000 A guide to effective care in pregnancy and childbirth, 3rd edn. Oxford University Press, Oxford

Friedman E H 1999 Neurobiology of infants born to women who exercise regularly throughout pregnancy. American Journal of Obstetrics and Gynecology 181(4):1038–1039

Fry D 1997 Symphysis pubis dysfunction guidelines ACPWH. Physiotherapy 83(1):41–42

Goodwin A, Astbury J, McMeeken J 2000 Body image and psychological well being in pregnancy. A comparison of exercisers and non-exercisers. Australian and New Zealand Journal of Obstetrics and Gynaecology 40(4):442–447

Gupta J K, Nikodem C 2001 Maternal posture in labour. European Journal of Obstetrics, Gynecology and Reproductive Biology 92(2):273–277

Hartmann S, Bung P 1999 Physical exercise during pregnancy – physiological considerations and recommendations (review). Journal of Perinatal Medicine 27(3):204–215

Haslam J, Laycock J 2008 Therapeutic management of incontinence and pelvic pain, 2nd edn. Springer, London

Hefferman A E 2000 Exercise and pregnancy in primary care. Nurse Practitioner 25(3):42, 49, 53–56

Horns P N, Ratcliffe L P, Leggett J C et al 1996 Pregnancy outcomes among active and sedentary primiparous women. Journal of Obstetrics, Gynecology and Neonatal Nursing 25(1):49–54

Jackson 2001. Pilates in pregnancy DVD, with Lindsey Jackson. Enhance Wellbeing. Online. Available: lj.enhance@btinternet.com

Koltyn K F, Schultes S S 1997 Psychological effects of an aerobic exercise session and a rest session following pregnancy. Journal of Sports Medicine and Physical Fitness 37:287–291

Kramer M S 2000 Regular aerobic exercise during pregnancy Cochrane Database of Systematic Reviews, Issue 2: CD000180

Mason L, Glenn S, Walton I 2001 The relationship between antenatal pelvic floor muscle exercises and post partum stress incontinence. Physiotherapy 87(12):651–661

MacArthur C, Bick D, Keighly M R 1997 Faecal incontinence after childbirth. British Journal of Obstetrics and Gynaecology 104:46–50

Marquez-Sterling S, Perry A C, Kaplan T A et al 2000 Physical and psychological changes with vigorous exercise in sedentary primigravidae. Medicine and Science in Sports and Exercise 32(1):58–62

McMurray R G, Berry M J, Katz V L 1990 The beta-endorphin responses of pregnant women during aerobic exercise in water. Medicine and Science in Sports and Exercise 22(3):298–303

MacLennan A H, Taylor A W, Wison D H et al 2000 The prevalence of pelvic floor disorders and their relationship to gender, age, parity and mode of birth. British Journal of Obstetrics and Gynaecology 107(12):1460–1470

MIDIRS 2003 Positions in labour and birth. Informed Choice for Professionals, Leaflet 5

Morkved S, Bø K 2003 Pelvic floor muscle training during pregnancy to prevent urinary incontinence: a single-blind randomised controlled trial. Obstetrics and Gynaecology 101(2):313–319

NICE 2008 NICE Guidelines: antenatal care – routine care for the healthy pregnant woman, CG62. National Institute for Health and Clinical Excellence, London

NICE 2006 NICE Guidelines: urinary incontinence, CG40. National Institute for Health and Clinical Excellence, London

Noble B J, Borg G A, Jacobs I et al 1983 A category-ratio perceived exertion scale: Relationships to blood and muscle lactates and heart rate. Medicine and Science in Sports and Exercise 15(6):523–528

Ostgaard H C 1997 Lumbar back and posterior pelvic pain in pregnancy. In: Vleeming A, Mooney V, Dorman T et al (eds) Movement, stability and low back pain. Churchill Livingstone, Edinburgh, p 411–420

Panjabi M 1992a The stabilizing system of the spine. Part I: function, dysfunction, adaptation, and enhancement. Journal of Spinal Disorders 5(4):383

Panjabi M 1992b the stabilizing system of the spine. Part II. Neutral zone and instability hypothesis. Journal of Spinal Disorders 5(4):390

Polden M, Mantle J 1992 Physiotherapy in obstetrics and gynaecology. Butterworth and Heinemann, Oxford

Pool-Goudzwaard A L, Slieker Ten Hove M C P, Vierhout M E et al 2005 Relations between pregnancy related low back pain, pelvic floor activity and pelvic floor dysfunction. International Journal of Urogynecology 16(6):468–474

RCOG 2006 Royal College of Obstetricians and Gynaecologists setting standards to improve women's health. Standard No. 4, January 2006

Reilly E T C, Freeman R M, Waterfield M R et al 2002 Prevention of postpartum stress incontinence in primigravidae with increased bladder neck mobility: a randomised controlled trial of antenatal pelvic floor exercises. British Journal of Obstetrics and Gynaecology 109(1):68–76

Riemann M K, Kanstrup Hansen I L 2000 Effects on the fetus of exercise in pregnancy. Scandinavian Journal of Medicine and Science in Sports 10(1):12–19

Roberts J E, Mendez-Bauer C, Wodell D A 1983 The effects of maternal position on uterine contractility and efficiency. Birth 10:243–249

Sangalli M R, Curtin F, Morabia A et al 2001 Prevalence of anal incontinence and other anorectal symptoms in women. International Urogynaecology Journal 12(2):117–121

SMA 2002 Sports Medicine Australia Statement: the benefits and risks of exercise during pregnancy. Journal of Science and Medicine in Sports 5:11–19

Sultan A H 1993 Anal sphincter disruption during vaginal birth. New England Journal of Medicine 329:1905–1911

Tetzschner T, Sørensen M, Lose G et al 1996 Pudendal nerve recovery after a non-instrumented vaginal delivery. International Urogynecology Journal and Pelvic Floor Dysfunction 7(2):102–104

Warren M P, Shantha S 2000 The female athlete. Best Practice and Research in Clinical Endocrinology and Metabolism 14(1):37–53

Wu W H, Meijer O G, Uegaki K, et al 2004 Pregnancy-related pelvic girdle pain. Terminology and prevalence. European Spine Journal 13(7):575–589

FURTHER READING

Leaflets produced by the Association of Chartered Physiotherapists in Women's Health (ACPWH) (www.acpwh.org.uk):

- Aquanatal Guidelines

- Fit for Pregnancy leaflets

- Fit for Birth leaflets

- Fit for Motherhood (postnatal leaflet)

- Fit and Safe

- Pregnancy-related Pelvic Girdle Pain (information leaflets for either the health professional or guidance for mothers to be and new mothers)

- Exercises and advice after the stillbirth or death of your baby

- Pilates in Women's Health Physiotherapy

- The Mitchell Method of Simple Relaxation.

17 Antenatal care

Anne Viccars

Antenatal care refers to care given to a pregnant woman from the time conception is confirmed until the beginning of labour. The midwife should provide a woman-centred approach to the care of the woman and her family by sharing information with the woman to help her make informed choices about her care.

This chapter aims to:

- explore the role of the midwife in providing woman-centred care, addressing her physical, psychological and sociological needs. Emphasize the contribution of skilled communication to provide effective antenatal care
- discuss the initial assessment visit, define its objectives and consider the significance of the different components of the woman's history taken by the midwife
- describe the physical examination and psychological support of the woman at the initial assessment and during subsequent visits
- explore the midwife's role in carrying out an abdominal examination.

Introduction

Antenatal care was first offered in the late 1920s (Ministry of Health 1929). The model of antenatal care followed a traditional regime of monthly visits until 28 weeks' gestation, then fortnightly visits until 36 weeks, then weekly visits until the birth of the baby. This model was challenged in the 1980s by Hall et al (1980) whose retrospective analysis demonstrated that health professionals' expectations of antenatal care might not be met by this provision of care. They found that conditions requiring hospitalization, including pre-eclampsia, were neither prevented nor detected by antenatal care; and intrauterine growth restriction was over-diagnosed.

A more flexible approach to the timing of visits and place of consultation was incorporated into midwifery practice (Clement et al 1996, Jewell et al 2000, Sikorski et al 1996). This was in an attempt to improve maternal satisfaction by the provision of holistic, individualized care and organizational change in the pattern of care (DH 2004, 1993). Sikorski et al (1996) conducted a randomized controlled trial, with low risk pregnant women, to compare the acceptability and effectiveness of a reduced antenatal visit schedule of six to seven routine visits with the traditional 13 routine visits. No differences in clinical outcome between the two groups were found, but twice as many women in the reduced-visit group were dissatisfied with the frequency of attendance, compared with women who received the full range of visits. A substantial number of women in both groups felt that the gaps in their care were too long, with women in the reduced-visit group feeling less remembered from one visit to the next.

A report for The National Institute for Health and Clinical Excellence (NICE 2003) indicated that women may be less satisfied with a reduced pattern of antenatal visits, however, low risk women can be cared for with this reduced pattern without detrimental maternal or fetal effects. It is important to note, however, that the most recent study referred to by NICE (2003) was a large randomized controlled trial conducted in Saudi Arabia, Thailand, Cuba and Argentina, where less than 20% of women were cared for antenatally by a midwife as their main provider (Villar et al 2001). Comparing five visits with eight visits had minimal impact on maternal and perinatal outcomes (Villar et al 2001). The need to provide a more individualized, flexible approach to care, with increased psychosocial support for those pregnant women who needed it, was one of the main conclusions of this study. Clement et al (1996) and NICE (2003) agree that women who had a midwife willing to spend time with them and facilitate them to ask questions were more likely to be satisfied with reduced visits than those whose midwife did not offer this.

Traditional visiting versus flexible visiting, by a midwife, was studied in 11 primary care centres with 609 women (Jewell et al 2000). Comparing the two groups, no difference was found either in attitudes to pregnancy and motherhood or in women urgently reporting antenatal problems. However, women in the flexible care group would like to have been seen more often, although they liked the choices associated with the individualized approach to planning visits (Jewell et al 2000). Rates of obstetric complications did not differ between groups (Jewell et al 2000). Villar & Khan-Neelofur (2001), who reviewed randomized controlled trials involving 25 000 women, support this finding. Evidence supports the view that perinatal outcomes are not adversely affected by a reduction in visits, nor by midwife-led models of care when a woman's pregnancy is uncomplicated (Jewell et al 2000, Villar & Khan-Neelofur 2001). In 2008 NICE partially updated and replaced their 2003 antenatal guidelines, see Box 17.1 for the revised recommended visiting pattern.

Oakley et al (1990) explored a bespoke approach to antenatal care and showed that an individual approach best supported women's needs. A randomized controlled trial examined the effect of providing social support to women who had previously had one or more babies with a birth weight less than 2500 g. Women who had an increased

---

Box 17.1 Antenatal visiting pattern as advocated by NICE (2008)

- Booking appointment(s) with midwife by 10 weeks if possible
- 10–14 weeks: ultrasound scan for gestational age
- 16 weeks: midwife
- 18–20 weeks: ultrasound scan for fetal anomalies
- 25 weeks: midwife (nulliparous women)
- 28 weeks: midwife
- 31 weeks: midwife (nulliparous women)
- 34 weeks: midwife
- 36, 38 weeks: midwife
- 40 weeks: midwife (nulliparous women)
- 41 weeks: midwife (discuss options).

likelihood of being socially disadvantaged in pregnancy were identified and a research midwife gave additional support to them. The midwife visited this group of women a minimum of three times during their pregnancy. She could be contacted by telephone 24 hrs a day, gave practical advice and information, made referrals to other healthcare professionals as necessary but did not give any clinical care. Women and babies in this group experienced improved outcomes, fewer hospital admissions in pregnancy, fewer very low birth weight babies, reduced need for neonatal intensive care and women reporting healthier babies in the first few weeks of life, compared with the control group.

A year later, women felt less anxious about their babies and more positive about motherhood. Six years later, the psychological and health benefits in the intervention group had continued, compared with women in the control group (Oakley et al 1996). Government-led initiatives, such as Sure Start, support the findings of Oakley's work and have been developed throughout the UK; positive results for the health and well-being of under-5s in disadvantaged areas are clearly found (Barnes et al 2006). Extending the boundaries of midwifery care to offer social support demonstrates the positive effect of an holistic approach to care of women and their families with positive outcomes in terms of lifestyle, employment and the growth and development of children (Leamon & Viccars 2007).

The aim of antenatal care

The aim of antenatal care is to monitor the progress of pregnancy to optimize maternal and fetal health. It is essential that the midwife critically evaluates the physical, psychological and sociological effects of pregnancy on the woman and her family. The midwife achieves this by:

- developing a partnership with the woman
- providing a holistic approach to the woman's care that meets her individual needs
- promoting an awareness of the public health issues for the woman and her family
- exchanging information with the woman and her family, enabling them to make informed choices about pregnancy and birth

- being an advocate for the woman and her family during her pregnancy, supporting her right to choose care appropriate for her own needs and those of her family
- recognizing complications of pregnancy and appropriately referring women to the obstetric team or relevant health professionals or other organizations
- facilitating the woman and her family in preparing to meet the demands of birth, and making a birth plan
- facilitating the woman to make an informed choice about methods of infant feeding and giving appropriate and sensitive advice to support her decision
- offering parenthood education within a planned programme or on an individual basis.

Women will attend antenatal care if it offers them information and choice about childbirth. It needs to meet their expectations and support them to be in control of their childbirth experience. Women may have to meet demands of work, family and children, which can be stressors affecting the pregnancy. Education from health professionals, schools, the media, television and lay childbirth organizations give contrasting views about the normality of pregnancy and childbirth which can make decision-making during pregnancy challenging.

Midwives should be approachable, flexible and adapt to meet women's individual needs. Midwives provide the infrastructure for antenatal care within an environment of trust and safety and should offer evidence-based information for informed choices (see Ch. 4). Five steps to help to sensitivity and evidence for practice are (Page 2006, p 360):

1. Finding out what is important to the woman and her family.
2. Using information from the clinical examination.
3. Seeking and assessing evidence to inform decisions.
4. Talking it through.
5. Reflecting on outcomes, feelings and consequences.

This method, incorporating individual needs, with sources of credible evidence will facilitate optimum antenatal care. The midwife has roles as counsellor and mediator and may need to utilize skills to deal with conflict or communication difficulties. The midwife has a responsibility to refer the family to appropriate professional or lay organizations when provision of care extends beyond her role (NMC 2004).

A birth plan can be instrumental in assisting the woman towards having the birth experience of her choice or at least to consider what she might like to do during labour and what is important to her. Lundgren et al (2003) suggest that birth plans do not enhance the childbirth experience for all but some women felt that aspects of pain, fear and concern for their baby were alleviated by having a birth plan. Most satisfaction with childbirth in this study was related to the relationship women developed with their midwife in labour, irrespective of whether or not they had prepared a birth plan (Lundgren et al 2003). Thus, birth plans are likely to be most effective if they are written with the midwife sharing information to enable the woman to make plans that reflect current practice and care.

When women carry their own maternity records, it was found to enhance their satisfaction with antenatal care and communication with health professionals (NICE 2008, Webster et al 1996) and their feeling of control during pregnancy (Elbourne et al 1987, Homer et al 1999, NICE 2008).

The initial assessment (booking visit)

The purpose of this visit is to introduce the woman to the maternity service. Information is shared between the woman and midwife in order to discuss, plan and implement care for the duration of the pregnancy, the birth and postnatal period. General conversation about the woman's experiences can be a more useful way of sharing information between woman and midwife compared with asking a list of questions or filling in computer data (McCourt 2006).

Questions need to be open and facilitate a discussion to collect salient information. McCourt (2006) found that information shared did not differ between hospital and home. The way in which midwives communicated with women differed between those case holding where a partnership approach was used and a conventional model of care where a more 'professional/didactic' guiding technique was used (McCourt 2006).

Early contact with the midwife, ideally by 10 weeks, is important so that appropriate and valuable advice relating to nutrition and care of the developing fetal organs, which are almost completely formed by 12 weeks' gestation, may be given. Medical conditions, infections and lifestyle may all have a profound and detrimental effect on the fetus during this time.

Early stages of pregnancy may leave the mother feeling exhausted, nauseous and overwhelmed with the changes occurring in her body. Women are encouraged to access their midwife through their local health centre on confirmation or suspicion of a positive pregnancy test and should be facilitated to do this. They do not require referral from a GP, but the midwife may refer when known medical or psychological problems could impact on the pregnancy or the condition. It is important for the midwife to maintain continuity with the woman even if she is not providing total care during the pregnancy; she can act as an advocate for the woman to enhance care given (e.g. by accompanying her to consultant appointments). It is also important for the midwife to comprehend and promote normality within the context of high risk care.

Models of midwifery care

Women can choose from a variety of midwifery care options. However, there may be restrictions resulting from resource allocation to accessing some of these, dependent on where the woman lives and what services are offered locally. Options for place of birth include the home, a birth centre or a tertiary hospital. Midwives have been shown to exert the most influence over decisions about place of birth compared with other health professionals and lay personnel (Barber et al 2007, 2006a,b).

The majority of women receive antenatal care in the community, either in their own home or at a local clinic. Hospital or community based clinics are available for women who receive care from an obstetrician or physician in addition to their midwife. Women who have identified risk factors or develop complications during pregnancy will usually plan for a hospital birth. The Government is keen to promote birth at home as an option for all women with low risk pregnancies, but fundamental to this is women's choice (Redshaw et al 2006).

Introduction to the midwifery service

The woman's first introduction to midwifery care is crucial in forming her initial impressions of the maternity service. A friendly, professional approach will enable the development of a positive partnership between the woman and the midwife. The initial visit focuses on the exchange of information (Box 17.2). This helps the midwife and the woman to get to know each other. The midwife may meet other members of the family and in this way gain a more informed view of the woman's needs. The midwife will also recognize that there are occasions when the woman may need to spend time alone with her to facilitate discussion, which she may not feel able to have in the presence of family members. For example, it is important for the midwife to recognize her own attitudes to culture and religion and to accept individual differences

that may conflict with these (Schott & Henley 1996). Receiving antenatal care from a midwife in an unknown or unfamiliar environment may be the first time some women have experiences outside their own community.

Communication

The midwife requires many skills to achieve optimal antenatal care, fundamentally the ability to communicate effectively and sensitively. McCourt (2006) suggests that 'knowledge and confidence' in the woman will develop as her relationship with the midwife progresses. The National Service Framework for children, young people and the maternity service supports earlier policy in its emphasis on basic principles of care as a means of achieving satisfaction for women in pregnancy and childbirth (DH 2004, 1993).

Listening skills involve attending to or focusing on what the woman is saying, considering the words, phrases and general content of what is said (Morrison & Burnard 1997). The fluency, timing, volume and pitch of the woman's voice all impact on how the midwife listens to her. In addition, non-verbal responses, including facial expression, body position, eye contact, proximity to the midwife and touch, will affect the flow of information between woman and midwife.

The midwife can promote communication with the woman during discussion by gentle questioning, open-ended statements and reflecting back keywords from what is said, to encourage and facilitate exploration of what is meant (Stein-Parbury 1993). Communication encompasses writing accurate, comprehensive and contemporaneous records of information given and received and the plan of care that has been agreed (NMC 2006). This is essential when there is shared care within the multidisciplinary team, as well as to ensure that the woman understands the records she holds (NMC 2004).

First impressions

A midwife can gain much from the initial observation and assessment of a woman at the start of their first meeting. Previous experiences of the health or maternity services can impact on how the woman will respond to meeting her midwife and her emotional response to this may depend on the empathic

---

Box 17.2 Objectives for the initial assessment

- To assess levels of health by taking a detailed history and to offer appropriate screening tests

- To ascertain baseline recordings of blood pressure, urinalysis, blood values, uterine growth and fetal development to be used as a standard for comparison as the pregnancy progresses

- To identify risk factors by taking accurate details of past and present midwifery, obstetric, medical, family and personal history

- To provide an opportunity for the woman and her family to express and discuss any concerns they might have about the current pregnancy and previous pregnancy loss, labour, birth or puerperium

- To give public health advice and that pertaining to pregnancy in order to maintain the health of the mother and fetus

- To build the foundation for a trusting relationship in which the woman and midwife are partners in care.

and caring response she is met with on their first meeting. The assessment should be carried out sensitively, enabling the woman to express her concerns about this or previous experiences of pregnancy or birth. While it is important for the midwife to be welcoming and enthusiastic towards the woman, it must not be assumed that in all cases the pregnancy is wanted. Observation of physical characteristics is also important. Poor posture and gait can indicate back problems or previous trauma to the pelvis. The woman may be lethargic, which could be an indication of extreme tiredness, anaemia, malnutrition or depression.

Social history

It is useful to assess the response of the whole family to the pregnancy. Some families may experience overcrowding, and need support from the midwife to find out about re-housing. Some women may be overwhelmed by having to care for a new baby and other children; some children may find it difficult to accept the prospect of a new baby into the family. The woman may be a teenager, still under her parents' care and there may be issues of how much support they can offer their daughter during pregnancy and following the birth. Additional support from a range of lay and professionals will support the teenager through pregnancy in terms of accommodation and schooling for example (Ch. 3).

The Government is committed to improving health and reducing health inequalities in pregnant women and their young children (see Chs 3 and 51). The midwife may, in partnership with the woman, advocate referral to a social worker who has a role in alleviating some of these difficulties or to other multiprofessional agencies where assistance can be obtained.

Domestic violence is an ongoing problem and it is important for the midwife to explore sensitively this issue when possible with the woman during her antenatal care. Midwives should be trained to ask all women if they experience abuse during or prior to pregnancy (Lewis 2007). Support can then be offered with the multiprofessional team working together. Bacchus et al (2004) found that 23% of women had life experience of domestic violence. The woman may only disclose information if she is alone; the midwife must be vigilant during pregnancy for signs or symptoms of domestic violence (NICE 2003). The risk of domestic violence may be more significant in single or women separated from their partners or in those not cohabiting (Bacchus et al 2004, Mezey et al 2005).

General health

General health should be discussed and good habits reinforced, giving further advice when required. All women should be provided with information about healthy eating, and vitamin D supplementation will be recommended for women at risk of deficiency (NICE 2008).

Exercise

Usual aerobic or strength conditioning exercise should be continued (RCOG 2006). Not only will this enhance general well-being, but also reduce stress and anxiety and prepare the body for the challenge of labour. Any activity which can cause trauma or physical injury to the woman or fetus should be avoided (RCOG 2006) (see Ch. 16). Sexual intercourse during pregnancy may continue and has been found to reduce the likelihood of premature labour between 29 and 36 weeks (Sayle et al 2001).

Smoking

Evidence suggests that 33% of women smoke during pregnancy (DH 2005). Some women may be ready to cut down or give up smoking, while others may not want to change their smoking behaviour (Prochaska 1992). Motivating women to change their behaviour can be helpful; the midwife can be influential in setting goals to cut down or quit smoking (McLeod et al 2004, 2003, DH 2007a). Walker and Walker (2006) state that significant effects of smoking on the fetus occur in late pregnancy and therefore strategies to quit should be continued throughout pregnancy.

Babies born to women who smoke are frequently smaller by up to 458 g (Roquer et al 1995) (see Ch. 42), they frequently have respiratory problems at birth and in their first year; there are also higher rates of prematurity, stillbirth and low birthweight (Floyd et al 1993, Li & Windsor 1993). There is an increased risk of asthma and otitis media in these babies (Nafstad et al 1996). The midwife should offer referral to local organizations and the NHS Quit Smoking line (DH 2007a). Nicotine replacement therapy should be discussed with women having difficulty quitting smoking (NICE 2008).

The woman, her partner and other family members should be informed about the direct and passive effects of smoking on the baby. Smoking in pregnancy increases the risk of babies dying from sudden infant death syndrome (SIDS) (Blair et al 1996). Babies of women who smoke 15 cigarettes a day have a 15 times greater risk of dying from SIDS than babies of a non-smoker (Mitchell et al 1997).

Alcohol

The effects of alcohol on the fetus are marked, particularly in the 1st trimester when fetal alcohol syndrome can develop. This syndrome consists of restricted growth, facial abnormalities, central nervous system problems, behavioural and learning difficulties (CDC 2007, DH 2007b, NOFAS-UK 2007). It is recommended that pregnant women abstain from alcohol during pregnancy (DH 2007b) (see Ch. 48).

Menstrual history and expected date of delivery

An accurate menstrual history helps determine the expected date of delivery (EDD), enables the midwife to predict a birth date and subsequently calculate gestational age at any point in the pregnancy. However, midwives are often inaccurate in the way in which they do this (Stenhouse et al 2003). Midwives may wish to consider giving women a 'baby born by' date instead of an EDD which is the date at which they would be 42 weeks' pregnant. This may help to reduce the anxiety felt by women and their families once they reach term. The midwife has a role in helping the woman to understand that an EDD is 1 day between 37 and 42 weeks' gestation during which her baby is term, and may be born.

The EDD is calculated by adding 9 calendar months and 7 days to the date of the first day of the woman's last menstrual period (known as Naegele's Rule). This method assumes that:

- the woman takes regular note of regularity and length of time between periods
- conception occurred 14 days after the first day of the last period; this is true only if the woman has a regular 28-day cycle

- the last period of bleeding was true menstruation; implantation of the ovum may cause slight bleeding
- breakthrough bleeding and anovulation can be affected by the contraceptive pill thus impacting on the accuracy of a LMP.

The duration of pregnancy based on Naegele's rule suggests that the duration of a pregnancy is 280 days. However, it is useful to consider that if the woman has a 35 day cycle then 7 days should be added to the EDD owing to the long second menstrual phase; if her cycle is less than 28 days then the appropriate number of days is subtracted (see Ch. 10).

Controversy exists over the suitability of applying Naegele's rule to determine EDD. Predicted dates of delivery were studied in over 14 000 women with a reliable date of LMP, average length of pregnancy of 280 or 282 days (Nguyen et al 1999). They found the average discrepancies between dates of delivery predicted from the bi-parietal diameter, or BPD (on ultrasound in the second trimester) were 7.96 and 8.63 days, respectively. The error of the LMP method alone was reduced significantly by adding 282 days to the LMP instead of 280 days. This method would reduce the incidence of postterm pregnancy; however, the authors concluded that use of BPD alone is superior to the use of LMP, but if LMP is the only predictor available then 282 days should be added to the LMP.

These data support that of Tunon et al (1996) who found that if LMP and ultrasound differed by less than 8 days, then neither method could more accurately predict EDD. However, as the difference in gestational age between the two methods increases, ultrasound becomes the more accurate method for predicting the EDD. These findings do depend on the availability of and accessibility to an experienced ultrasonographer and the woman's consent to have an ultrasound scan. Kalish & Chervenak (2005) suggest that head circumference is the best measure for determination of gestational age. NICE (2008) now recommend crown–rump measurement between 10 weeks 0 days and 13 weeks 6 days and if above 84 mm, then measure head circumference. Nuchal translucency can be identified between 11 and 14 weeks as part of the 'combined test' for Down syndrome screening and the 18–20 week scan for structural abnormality screening (NICE 2008) (see Ch. 18). For women who book after 14 weeks, the triple or quadruple serum screening test can be offered between 15 and 20 weeks. Information about ultrasound will be offered by the midwife and peer reviewed leaflets can support this process (MIDIRS 2008a).

Obstetric history

Previous childbearing experiences have an important part to play in possible outcome prediction of the current pregnancy. In order to give a summary of a woman's childbearing history, the descriptive terms *gravida* and *para* are used. 'Gravid' means 'pregnant', gravida means 'a pregnant woman', and a subsequent number indicates the number of times she has been pregnant regardless of outcome. 'Para' means 'having given birth'; a woman's parity refers to the number of times that she has given birth to a child, live or stillborn, excluding abortions. A *grande multigravida* is a woman who has been pregnant five times or more, irrespective of outcome. A *grande multipara* is a woman who has given birth five times or more.

A sympathetic non-judgemental approach is required to elicit information and encourage the woman to talk freely about her experiences of previous births, miscarriages or terminations. The booking visit may be the first opportunity a woman has to discuss her last experience of labour and birth in detail. A pregnancy loss may have affected the way in which the woman accepted it at the time, perhaps grieving the loss of hopes and expectations of a pregnancy (Raphael-Leff 2005). This may lead to suppression of feelings, which could interfere with emotional adjustment to the present pregnancy. Any form of miscarriage/abortion occurring in a Rhesus negative woman requires prophylactic administration of anti-D immunoglobulin to reduce the risk of Rhesus incompatibility in a subsequent pregnancy (see Ch. 47).

Confidential information may be recorded in a clinic-held summary of the pregnancy and not in the woman's handheld record if she requests this. Repeated spontaneous fetal loss may indicate such conditions as genetic abnormality, hormonal imbalance or incompetent cervix (see Ch. 19). The woman may be more anxious about the pregnancy and will usually be relieved when it progresses past the date of previous fetal loss. Minor disturbances in pregnancy may be exacerbated and preoccupation with

the pregnancy may lead to other psychological, social or physical problems. The woman may be reassured if she hears the fetal heart or sees the image of her unborn baby on an ultrasound scan.

For completeness of the history, reference to old case notes should be made to elicit all the relevant information. A risk assessment should be carried out based on the woman's obstetric, medical and social history and current pregnancy. This will enable the midwife and woman to discuss the progress of her pregnancy and identify other health professionals who may need to be involved. If risk factors such as those listed in Box 17.3 are identified, they can help to determine the frequency of antenatal visits and alert staff to appropriate screening techniques. This should follow an individualized approach, using Page's five steps (Page 2006). The location of antenatal care will be determined by the availability of support services, senior obstetric staff and experienced midwives. Place of birth will also be influenced by the risk assessment but in all cases the ultimate decision is taken by the woman who should make an informed choice (MIDIRS 2008b).

Medical history

During pregnancy both the mother and the fetus may be affected by a medical condition, or a medical condition may be altered by the pregnancy; if untreated there may be serious consequences for the woman's health (Lewis 2007).

- Urinary stasis and reflux occur during pregnancy therefore a predisposition to urinary tract infections is important to note in pregnancy. A urinary tract infection (UTI) can easily develop into pyelonephritis, in 12–30% of women, which, untreated, may lead to kidney damage and cause preterm labour (Nowicki 2000, cited by Williams 2006).

- Women with a history of thrombosis are at greater risk of recurrence during pregnancy, more when over 30 years; have a BMI over 25; have prolonged bed rest; a family history of venous thromboembolism; have a caesarean delivery or travel by air (Farquharson & Greaves 2006). Thromboembolism remains the leading direct cause of maternal death in the UK (Lewis 2007).

- Hypertensive disorders encompass gestational hypertension (pre-eclampsia and eclampsia) and

Box 17.3 Factors that may require additional antenatal support or referral to an obstetrician/physician/other health professional

Initial assessment

- Age less than 18 years or 40 years and over
- Grande multiparity (more than six previous births)
- Vaginal bleeding at any time during pregnancy
- Unknown or uncertain expected date of birth
- Late booking.

Past obstetric history

- Stillbirth or neonatal death
- Baby small or large for gestational age
- Congenital abnormality
- Rhesus isoimmunization
- Pregnancy-induced hypertension
- Two or more terminations of pregnancy
- Three or more spontaneous miscarriages
- Previous pre-term labour
- Cervical cerclage in past or present pregnancy
- Previous caesarean section or uterine surgery
- Ante- or postpartum haemorrhage

- Precipitate labour
- Multiple pregnancy.

Maternal health

- Previous history of deep vein thrombosis or pulmonary embolism
- Chronic illness, e.g. epilepsy, severe asthma, hepatic or renal disease, cystic fibrosis
- Hypertension, cardiac disease
- History of infertility
- Uterine anomalies
- Family history of diabetes or genetic disorders
- Type I or Type II diabetes
- Substance abuse (drugs, alcohol or smoking)
- Psychological or psychiatric disorders.

Examination at the initial assessment

- Blood pressure 140/90 mmHg or above
- Maternal obesity or underweight according to BMI
- Blood disorders.

chronic/essential hypertension. Essential hypertension is the underlying factor in 90% of chronic cases (Walfish & Hallak 2006).

- Other conditions including asthma, epilepsy, infections and psychiatric disorders may require drug treatment, which may adversely affect fetal development (see Ch. 49). Suicide is a leading cause of maternal death, (Lewis 2007) therefore any psychiatric illness prior to the pregnancy must be fully explored so that the most appropriate multidisciplinary care can be offered (NICE 2007). Major medical complications such as diabetes and cardiac conditions require the involvement and support of a medical specialist (see Ch. 21).

Family history

Certain conditions are genetic in origin, others are familial or related to ethnicity, and some are associated with the physical or social environment in which the family lives. There is a higher mortality rate in babies born to mothers of Pakistan or Caribbean origin (DH 1999). Lewis (2007) demonstrated that women from minority ethnic groups were three times more likely to die than Caucasian women and the mortality rate was seven times higher in black African and asylum seekers than white women. There is also evidence of a high rate of consanguinity within Pakistani families which can adversely affect outcomes (Bundey & Alan 1991). Genetic disease in the baby is much more likely to occur if his biological parents are close relatives such as first cousins (Stoltenberg et al 1998).

Diabetes, although not inherited, leads to a predisposition in other family members, particularly if they become pregnant or obese. Hypertension also has a familial component and multiple pregnancy has a higher incidence in certain families. Some conditions such as sickle cell anaemia and thalassaemia are more common in black Caribbean, African-Caribbean, African, Pakistani, Cypriots, Bangladeshis and those of Chinese ethnicity (NICE 2008) (see Ch. 21). Screening for gestational diabetes is now recommended using a risk factor approach.

Physical examination

Prior to conducting the physical examination of a pregnant woman, her consent and comfort are primary considerations. Sophisticated biochemical assessments and ultrasound investigations can enhance clinical observations.

It is therefore important to look holistically at the woman and her family and assess fetal growth and development by recognized markers in conjunction with this knowledge.

Weight

Normal weight gain in pregnancy ranges from 7–18 kg for a 3–4 kg baby. Normal body mass index (BMI) should be calculated at booking, based on pre-pregnancy weight. Referral to an obstetrician should be made if it is <18 kg/m^2 or ≥30 kg/m^2 (NICE 2008) (see Ch. 13). Women with a BMI in the obese range are more at risk of complications of pregnancy. These may include gestational diabetes, PIH and shoulder dystocia. There may also be difficulty in palpating the fetal parts and defining presentation, position or engagement of the fetus. Overweight or underweight women should be carefully monitored, have additional care from an obstetrician, and be offered appropriate support including nutritional counselling within the multiprofessional team.

Blood pressure

Blood pressure is taken in order to ascertain normality and provide a baseline reading for comparison throughout pregnancy. Systolic blood pressure does not alter significantly in pregnancy, but diastolic falls in mid pregnancy and rises to near non-pregnant levels at term. The systolic recording may be falsely elevated if a woman is nervous or anxious; long waiting times can cause additional stress; white coat hypertension whereby the BP is higher than normal by 30 mmHg can occur during the procedure or in a doctor's surgery (Beevers et al 2001a). If the midwife

is aware of this she can arrange to see the woman at home so she is relaxed beforehand. A full bladder can also cause an increase in blood pressure. Blood pressure should be checked with the woman relaxed. The woman should be comfortably seated or resting in a lateral position on the couch for the measurement. Brachial artery pressure is highest when sitting and lower when in the recumbent position.

Current opinion is that Korotkoff V should be used (Beevers et al 2001a, Walfish & Hallak 2006). An elevation of more than 30 mmHg systolic or 15 mmHg diastolic on at least two occasions 6 hrs apart warrants investigation (Walfish & Hallak 2006). It has been recommended by NICE (2008, para 1.9.2.5) that if there is a 'single diastolic blood pressure of 110 mmHg or two consecutive readings of 90 mmHg at least 4 hrs apart and/or significant proteinuria (1+)', there should be an increase in surveillance. Steps that can be taken to increase accuracy of blood pressure measurement and recording are listed in Box 17.4.

Urinalysis

Urinalysis is performed at every visit to exclude proteinuria (NICE 2008, Way 2000). The woman can be shown how to test her own urine and encouraged to test it at subsequent visits. At the first visit a midstream

---

Box 17.4 Factors that increase accuracy of blood pressure measurement and recording (Beevers et al 2001a, b)

- The correct width of cuff should be chosen for the woman
- The arm should be horizontal and at the level of the heart
- The radial pulse should be estimated and the cuff pumped up 30 mmHg above this level before auscultating the brachial pulse
- Measurements should be recorded to the nearest mmHg
- The woman should be sitting, relaxed and comfortable
- Use a regularly serviced sphygmomanometer (conventional mercury sphygmomanometer is the most reliable, see Lewis & Drife 2001, p 76).

specimen may be sent to the laboratory for culture to exclude asymptomatic bacteruria. This condition exists when a culture is grown of a specific bacterium that exceeds 10^6 organisms/mL of urine. As it is asymptomatic the woman is unaware of disease and treatment will reduce the risk of preterm labour.

Other possible findings during subsequent routine urinalysis include:

- ketones due to fat breakdown caused by unmet fetal demands that may be due to vomiting, hyperemesis, starvation or excessive exercise
- glucose caused by higher circulating blood levels, reduced renal threshold or disease. NICE (2008) do not currently recommend routine testing for glycosuria
- protein due to contamination by vaginal leucorrhoea, or hypertensive disorders of pregnancy.

(See Chs 20 and 21 for further information.)

Blood tests in pregnancy

The midwife should explain why blood tests are carried out at the booking visit (NMC 2004). Women should be facilitated by the midwife to make an informed choice about the tests that are available. The midwife should be fully aware of the difference between screening and diagnostic tests, and their accuracy, and discuss these options with women. Blood tests taken at the initial assessment include the following:

ABO blood group and Rhesus (Rh) factor

It is important to identify the blood group, RhD status and red cell antibodies in pregnant women, so haemolytic disease of the newborn (HDN) can be prevented and to prepare for blood transfusion if it becomes necessary. Blood will be taken at booking and again at 28 weeks to determine if antibodies are present (NICE 2008). All Rh negative women will be offered anti-D at 28 and 34 weeks' gestation (NICE 2002). If the woman's partner is also Rh negative then anti-D prophylaxis will not be required (NICE 2002). Threatened miscarriage, amniocentesis or any other uterine trauma are indications for the administration of anti-D gammaglobulin within a few days of the event in pregnancy in addition to

that given at 28 and 34 weeks (NICE 2002). If the titration demonstrates a rising antibody response then more frequent assessment will be made in order to plan management by a specialist in Rhesus disease (see Ch. 47).

Full blood count

This is taken to observe the woman's general blood condition, and includes: *Haemoglobin (Hb) estimations* (see Ch. 14 for normal values). If the mean cell volume (MCV) is found to be low on the full blood count result, serum ferritin levels are also taken in order to assess the adequacy of iron stores. Haemoglobin below 11 g/L at booking is investigated at the 16-week check and iron supplementation considered. Further investigation of an Hb of 10.5 g/L or less will be carried out at 28 weeks when the physiological effects of haemodilution are becoming more apparent. Iron supplementation is not considered necessary in women who are taking adequate dietary iron and who have a normal Hb and MCV at the initial assessment.

The decision to use supplements should be made on an individual basis and include clear information about dietary iron sources. Maximum absorption of iron in meat or green leafy vegetables will be achieved by consuming vitamin C at the same time and avoiding caffeine. The intestinal mucosa has a limited ability to absorb iron and when this is exceeded extra iron is excreted in the stools. Folic acid (400 µg/day) should be taken prior to conception and for the first 12 weeks of pregnancy to reduce the risk of spina bifida (NICE 2008).

Venereal disease research laboratory (VDRL) test

This is performed for syphilis. Not all positive results indicate active syphilis; early testing will allow a woman to be treated in order to prevent infection of the fetus (see Ch. 23).

HIV antibodies

Routine screening to detect HIV infection should be offered in pregnancy (Ades et al 1999, NICE 2008) as treatment in pregnancy is beneficial in reducing vertical transmission to the fetus. There are many views as to the ethical issues involved in screening. It is important to gain informed consent for any blood tests undertaken and offer appropriate counselling before and after the screening is carried out.

Rubella immune status

This is determined by measuring the rubella antibody titre. Women who are not immune must be advised to avoid contact with anyone suffering from the disease and may wish to discuss termination of pregnancy if they have been exposed. The live vaccination is offered during the puerperium, and subsequent pregnancy must be avoided for at least 3 months.

Investigations for other blood disorders

All women should be offered screening for sickle cell disease or thalassaemias early in pregnancy. Some ethnic groups have a higher incidence than others and the type of screening will depend on the prevalence (NICE 2008). If a woman either has or is a carrier of one of these diseases her partner's blood should also be tested. The couple will be offered genetic counselling and management during pregnancy will be explained.

Hepatitis B

Screening is offered in pregnancy so that postnatal intervention can be planned to decrease the risk of mother-to-baby transmission (NICE 2003).

Hepatitis C and chlamydia

This is currently not recommended as a routine screening test in pregnancy because the effect and cost effectiveness have not yet been evaluated (NICE 2008).

Cytomegalovirus and toxoplasmosis

These are not routinely done in pregnancy because tests do not currently determine which pregnancies may result in an infected fetus (NICE 2008). Toxoplasmosis screening is not recommended because the risks of screening may outweigh the benefits; however, women need to be informed of how to avoid contracting the infection (NICE 2008) (See Ch. 47).

The midwife's examination

The midwife's examination of the woman, with consent, is performed by exchange of information between the woman and midwife and observation rather than physical examination. Communication has been shown to be most effective if the woman is sitting in a comfortable position making eye contact with the midwife.

The midwife's general examination of the woman should be holistic and should encompass her physical, social and psychological well-being. The usual social contact gives the midwife an opportunity to look at the woman's face and assess her health and general well-being. Sleeping patterns can be disrupted in pregnancy. Women frequently continue to work throughout pregnancy, therefore they are unlikely to be able to rest during the day and many need to go to bed earlier to alleviate the tiredness. If at any time the midwife notices any sign of ill health she should discuss this with the woman, and advocate referral to the most appropriate health professional.

The midwife should facilitate discussion about infant-feeding. Breastfeeding should be promoted in a sensitive manner, and information given about the benefits to both mother and baby (see Ch. 41, UNICEF 2007). Most women will not require an examination of their breasts. Current evidence does not support the benefits of nipple preparation (Alexander et al 1992). The midwife may also discuss the woman's experiences of breast changes so far in her pregnancy, and expected changes as pregnancy progresses.

Some women will appreciate information about the body changes taking place during pregnancy. Increasing abdominal size may be an acceptable body change but breast changes may not have been anticipated. For some women, breast size and appearance are an important part of their body image. Partners may also be affected by the changes. The midwife can be influential in discussions with women who had not realized the extent to which pregnancy would change their body. Open and honest discussion between the woman and her partner may help to resolve anxieties. A good relationship in which the couple feels able to share anxieties and fears may minimize some of the difficulties in making the transition to motherhood.

Bladder and bowel function may be discussed; dietary advice may be necessary at this visit or later in the pregnancy with reference to how hormonal changes may alter normal bowel and kidney function. Early referral within the multidisciplinary team will be necessary if treatment is required or problems identified. Vaginal discharge (leucorrhoea) increases in pregnancy; the woman may discuss any increase or changes with the midwife. If the discharge is itchy, causes soreness, is any colour other than creamy-white or has an offensive odour then infection is likely, and should be investigated further. Later in pregnancy the woman may report a change from leucorrhoea to a heavier mucous discharge.

The obstetrician will investigate vaginal bleeding during pregnancy; however, in early pregnancy spotting may occur at the time when menstruation would have been due. Early bleeding is not uncommon; the midwife should advise the woman to rest at this time and avoid sexual intercourse until the pregnancy is more stable. Ultrasound will usually confirm a diagnosis.

Abdominal examination

In the past midwives have palpated the uterus once it has entered the abdomen, from about 12 weeks' gestation, however current guidelines suggest that because of sophisticated scanning techniques there is no benefit in palpating the uterus prior to 25 weeks' gestation, at which time uterine growth can be measured (NICE 2008).

Oedema

This should not be evident during the initial assessment but may occur as the pregnancy progresses. Physiological oedema occurs after rising in the morning and worsens during the day; it is often associated with daily activities or hot weather. At visits later in pregnancy the midwife should observe for oedema and ask the woman about symptoms. Often the woman may notice that her rings feel tighter and her ankles are swollen. Pitting oedema in the lower limbs can be identified by applying gentle fingertip pressure over the tibial bone: a depression will remain when the finger is removed. If oedema reaches the knees, affects the face or is increasing in the fingers it may be indicative of hypertension of pregnancy if other markers are also present.

Varicosities

These are more likely to occur during pregnancy and are a predisposing cause of deep vein thrombosis. The woman should be asked if she has any pain in her legs. Reddened areas on the calf may be due to varicosities, phlebitis or deep vein thrombosis. Areas that appear white as if deprived of blood could be caused by deep vein thrombosis. The woman should be asked to report any tenderness that she feels either during the examination or at any time during the pregnancy. Referral should be made to medical colleagues as appropriate (NMC 2004). Support stockings will help alleviate symptoms although not prevent varicose veins occurring (NICE 2008).

Abdominal examination

Abdominal examination is carried out from 25 weeks' gestation to establish and affirm that fetal growth is consistent with gestational age during the pregnancy.

The specific aims are to:

- observe the signs of pregnancy
- assess fetal size and growth
- auscultate the fetal heart when indicated
- locate fetal parts
- detect any deviation from normal.

Preparation

Abdominal examination will be most effective if the woman is consistently in the same position at each antenatal check (Engstrom et al 1993). A study comparing supine, trunk elevation, knee flexion and trunk elevation with knee flexion found there were significant differences between each in estimating fundal height measurements (Engstrom et al 1993). A full bladder will make the examination uncomfortable; this can also make the measurement of fundal height less accurate. It is important that the midwife exposes only that area of the abdomen she needs to palpate, and covers the remainder of the woman to enhance privacy. The woman should be lying comfortably with her arms by her sides to relax the abdominal muscles. The midwife should discuss her findings throughout the abdominal examination with the woman.

Inspection

The size of the uterus is assessed approximately by visual observation. A full bladder, distended colon or obesity may give a false impression of fetal size, however.

The shape of the uterus is longer than it is broad when the lie of the fetus is longitudinal, as occurs in the majority of cases. If the lie of the fetus is transverse, the uterus is low and broad.

The multiparous uterus may lack the snug ovoid shape of the primigravid uterus. Often it is possible to see the shape of the fetal back or limbs. If the fetus is in an occipitoposterior position a saucer-like depression may be seen at or below the umbilicus. The midwife may observe fetal movements, or they may be felt by the mother; this can help the midwife determine the position of the fetus. The woman's umbilicus becomes less dimpled as pregnancy advances and may protrude slightly in later weeks.

Lax abdominal muscles in the parous woman may cause the uterus to sag forwards; this is known as *pendulous abdomen* or anterior obliquity of the uterus. In the primigravida it is a significant sign as it may be due to pelvic contraction.

Skin changes

Stretch marks from previous pregnancies appear silvery and recent ones appear pink. A *linea nigra* may be seen; this is a normal dark line of pigmentation running longitudinally in the centre of the abdomen below and sometimes above the umbilicus. Scars may indicate previous obstetric or abdominal surgery.

Palpation

The midwife's hands should be clean and warm; cold hands do not have the necessary acute sense of touch, they tend to induce contraction of the abdominal and uterine muscles and the woman may find palpation uncomfortable. Arms and hands should be relaxed and the pads, not the tips, of the fingers used with delicate precision. The hands are moved smoothly over the abdomen to avoid causing contractions.

In order to determine the height of the fundus the midwife places her hand just below the xiphisternum. Pressing gently, she moves her hand down the abdomen until she feels the curved upper border of the fundus, noting the number of fingerbreadths that can be accommodated between the two (Fig. 17.1). The distance between the fundus and the symphysis pubis can be determined with a tape measure which is consistent with current practice; the height of the fundus in centimetres should correspond with weeks of

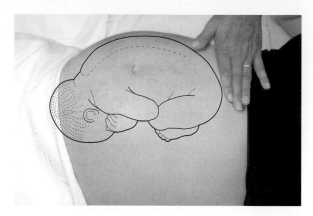

Figure 17.1 Assessing the fundal height in finger-breadths below the xiphisternum.

gestation to the nearest 3 cm (Neilson 2001). Measurements should be recorded in the pregnancy record or plotted on a chart that gives average findings for gestational age: a symphysis–fundal height chart (Gardosi & Francis 1999, NICE 2008).

Clinically assessing the uterine size to compare it with gestation does not always produce an accurate result but Figure 17.2 is a guide to fundal height at

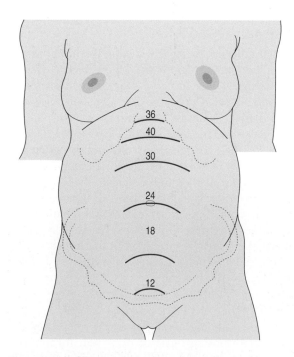

Figure 17.2 Growth of the uterus, showing the fundal heights at various weeks of pregnancy.

various weeks of pregnancy. If the uterus is unduly big the fetus may be large or it may indicate multiple pregnancy or polyhydramnios. When the uterus is smaller than expected the LMP date may be incorrect, or the fetus may be small for gestational age. Further investigation is warranted and an ultrasound scan will usually be required alongside medical referral (NMC 2004).

Fundal palpation

This determines the presence of the breech or the head. This information will help to diagnose the lie and presentation of the fetus. Talking through the palpation with the woman, making eye contact with her during the procedure, the midwife lays both hands on the sides of the fundus, fingers held close together and curving round the upper border of the uterus. Gentle yet deliberate pressure is applied using the palmar surfaces of the fingers to determine the soft consistency and indefinite outline that denotes the breech. Sometimes the buttocks feel rather firm but they are not as hard, smooth or well defined as the head. With a gliding movement the fingertips are separated slightly in order to grasp the fetal mass, which may be in the centre or deflected to one side, to assess its size and mobility. The breech cannot be moved independently of the body but the head can (Fig. 17.3). The head is much more distinctive in outline than the breech, being hard and round; it can be balloted (moved from one hand to the other) between the fingertips of the two hands because of the free movement of the neck.

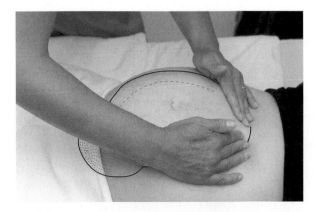

Figure 17.3 Fundal palpation. Palms of hands on either side of the fundus, fingers held close together palpate the upper pole of the uterus.

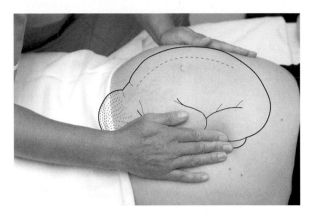

Figure 17.4 Lateral palpation. Hands placed at umbilical level on either side of the uterus. Pressure is applied alternately with each hand.

Lateral palpation

This is used to locate the fetal back in order to determine position. The hands are placed on either side of the uterus at the level of the umbilicus (Fig. 17.4). Gentle pressure is applied with alternate hands in order to detect which side of the uterus offers the greater resistance. More detailed information is obtained by feeling along the length of each side with the fingers. This can be done by sliding the hands down the abdomen while feeling the sides of the uterus alternately. Some midwives prefer to steady the uterus with one hand and, using a rotary movement of the opposite hand, to map out the back as a continuous smooth resistant mass from the breech down to the neck; on the other side the same movement reveals the limbs as small parts that slip about under the examining fingers.

'Walking' the fingertips of both hands over the abdomen from one side to the other is an excellent method of locating the back (Fig. 17.5). The fingers should be dipped into the abdominal wall deeply. Palpating from the neck upwards and inwards can locate the anterior shoulder.

Pelvic palpation

Pelvic palpation can cause contractions of the uterus therefore it is often carried out before fundal and lateral palpation to make the findings easier to determine. However, some would argue that it should be carried out last. Pelvic palpation will identify the pole

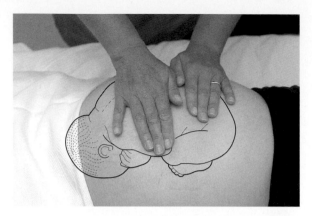

Figure 17.5 'Walking' the fingertips across the abdomen to locate the position of the fetal back.

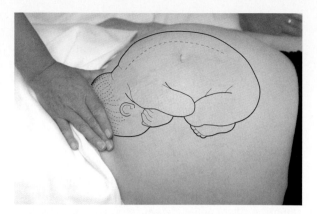

Figure 17.7 Pawlik's manoeuvre. The lower pole of the uterus is grasped with the right hand, the midwife facing the woman's head.

of the fetus in the pelvis; it should not cause discomfort to the woman. NICE (2008) recommend this is only done from 36 weeks onwards.

The midwife should ask the woman to bend her knees slightly in order to relax the abdominal muscles and also suggest that she breathe steadily; relaxation may be helped if she sighs out slowly. The sides of the uterus just below umbilical level are grasped snugly between the palms of the hands with the fingers held close together, and pointing downwards and inwards (Fig. 17.6).

If the head is presenting (towards the lower part of the uterus), a hard mass with a distinctive round, smooth surface will be felt. The midwife should also estimate how much of the fetal head is palpable above the pelvic brim to determine engagement. The two-handed technique appears to be the most comfortable for the woman and gives the most information.

Pawlik's manoeuvre, where the midwife grasps the lower pole of the uterus between her fingers and thumb, which should be spread wide enough apart to accommodate the fetal head (Fig. 17.7), is sometimes used to judge the size, flexion and mobility of the head, but undue pressure must not be applied. It should be used only if absolutely necessary: There is no research evidence to support one method over the other.

Engagement

Engagement is said to have occurred when the widest presenting transverse diameter has passed through the brim of the pelvis. In cephalic presentations this is the biparietal diameter and in breech presentations the bitrochanteric diameter. Engagement demonstrates that the maternal pelvis is likely to be adequate for the size of the fetus and that the baby will birth vaginally.

In a primigravid woman, the head normally engages at any time from about 36 weeks' pregnancy, but in a multipara this may not occur until after the onset of labour. Engagement of the fetal head is usually measured in fifths palpable above the pelvic brim. When the vertex presents and the head is engaged the following will be evident on clinical examination:

- only two- to three-fifths of the fetal head is palpable above the pelvic brim (Fig. 17.8)
- the head will not be mobile.

On rare occasions, the head is not palpable abdominally because it has descended deeply into the pelvis. If the head is not engaged, the findings are as follows:

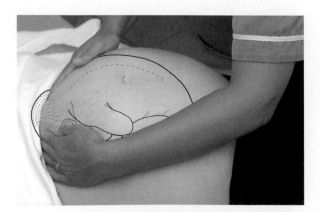

Figure 17.6 Pelvic palpation. The fingers are directed inwards and downwards.

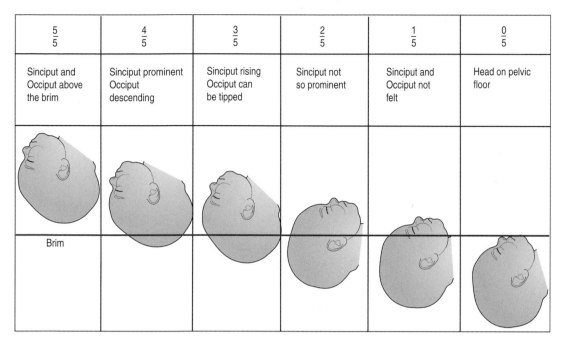

$\frac{5}{5}$	$\frac{4}{5}$	$\frac{3}{5}$	$\frac{2}{5}$	$\frac{1}{5}$	$\frac{0}{5}$
Sinciput and Occiput above the brim	Sinciput prominent Occiput descending	Sinciput rising Occiput can be tipped	Sinciput not so prominent	Sinciput and Occiput not felt	Head on pelvic floor

Figure 17.8 Descent of the fetal head estimated in fifths palpable above the pelvic brim.

- more than half of the head is palpable above the brim
- the head may be high and freely movable (ballotable) or partly settled in the pelvic brim and consequently immobile.

If the head does not engage in a primigravid woman at term, there is a possibility of a malposition or cephalopelvic disproportion. However, Roshanfekr et al (1999) found that 86% of nulliparous women with a non-engaged head at the onset of active labour proceeded to have a vaginal birth. Therefore, until labour commences, the midwife should assess the woman as usual and monitor the progress of her pregnancy. The force of labour contractions encourages flexion and moulding of the fetal head and the relaxed ligaments of the pelvis allow the joints to give. This may be sufficient to allow engagement and descent. Other causes of a non-engaged head at term include:

- occipitoposterior position
- full bladder
- wrongly calculated gestational age
- polyhydramnios
- placenta praevia or other space-occupying lesion
- multiple pregnancy
- pelvic abnormalities
- fetal abnormality

Presentation

Presentation refers to the part of the fetus that lies at the pelvic brim or in the lower pole of the uterus. Presentations can be *vertex*, *breech*, *shoulder*, *face* or *brow* (Figs 17.9–17.14). Vertex, face and brow are all head or cephalic presentations. When the head is flexed the vertex presents; when it is fully extended the face presents and when partially extended the brow presents (Figs 17.15–17.18). It is more common for the head to present because the bulky breech finds more space in the fundus, which is the widest diameter of the uterus, and the head lies in the narrower lower pole. The muscle tone of the fetus also plays a part in maintaining its flexion and consequently its vertex presentation.

Auscultation

Listening to the fetal heart has historically been an important part of the process. However, NICE (2008) do not recommend routine listening other than at maternal request because there is no clinical

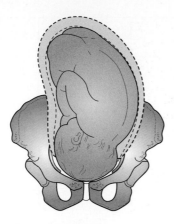

Figure 17.9   Vertex.

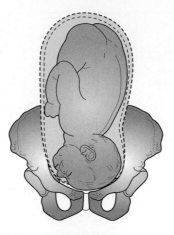

Figure 17.10   Brow.

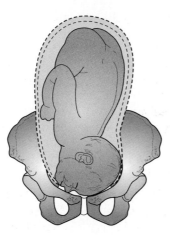

Figure 17.11   Face.

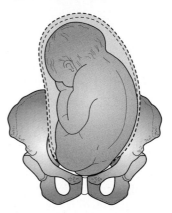

Figure 17.12   Breech.

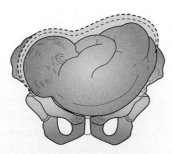

Figure 17.13   Shoulder, dorsoanterior.

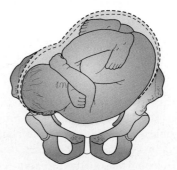

Figure 17.14   Shoulder, dorsoposterior.

Figures 17.9–17.14   The five presentations.

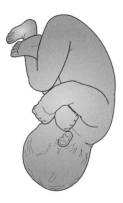

Figure 17.15 Vertex (well-flexed head).

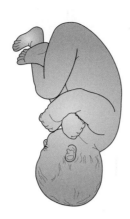

Figure 17.16 Vertex (deflexed head).

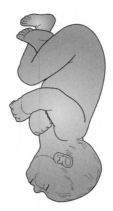

Figure 17.17 Brow.

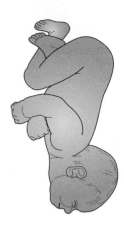

Figure 17.18 Face.

Figures 17.15–17.18 Varieties of cephalic or head presentation.

benefit. A Pinard's fetal stethoscope will enable the midwife to hear the fetal heart directly and determine that it is fetal and not maternal. The stethoscope is placed on the mother's abdomen, at right angles to it over the fetal back (Fig. 17.19). The ear must be in close, firm contact with the stethoscope but the hand should not touch it while listening because then extraneous sounds are produced. The stethoscope should be moved about until the point of maximum intensity is located where the fetal heart is heard most clearly. The midwife should count the beats per minute, which should be in the range of 110–160. The midwife should take the woman's pulse at the same time as listening to the fetal heart to enable her to distinguish between the two. In addition, ultrasound equipment (e.g. a sonicaid or Doppler) can be used for this purpose so that the woman may also hear the fetal heartbeat. However, use of a Pinard's stethoscope will enable the midwife to hear the actual heartbeat and not the reflected sound waves produced from the ultrasound equipment.

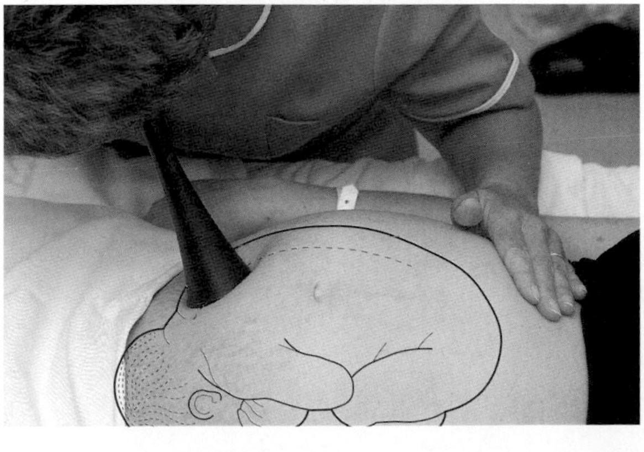

Findings

The findings from the abdominal palpation should be considered part of the holistic picture of the pregnant woman. The midwife assesses all the information she has gathered from inspection, palpation and auscultation and critically evaluates the well-being of the woman and her fetus. Deviation from the expected growth and development should be discussed with the woman and referral to an obstetrician can be arranged if required. Concerns about this screening process may also be discussed within the interprofessional team.

Lie

The lie of the fetus is the relationship between the long axis of the fetus and the long axis of the uterus (Figs 17.20–17.24). In the majority of cases the lie is *longitudinal* owing to the ovoid shape of the uterus; the remainder are oblique or transverse. *Oblique lie*, when the fetus lies diagonally across the long axis of the uterus, must be distinguished from *obliquity of the uterus*, when the whole uterus is tilted to one side (usually the right) and the fetus lies longitudinally within it. When the lie is *transverse* the fetus lies at right angles

Figure 17.19 Auscultation of the fetal heart. Vertex right occipitoanterior.

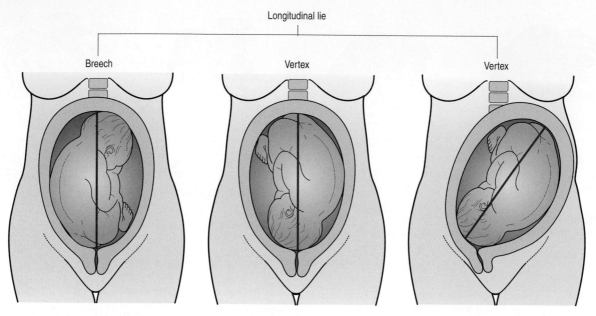

Longitudinal lie

Breech   Vertex   Vertex

Figures 17.20–17.22   Depict the longitudinal lie. Confusion sometimes exists regarding Figure 17.22, which gives the impression of an oblique lie, but the fetus is longitudinal in relation to the uterus and merely moving the uterus abdominally rectifies the presumed obliquity.

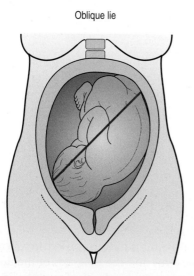

Oblique lie

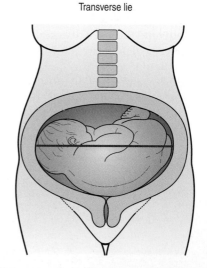

Transverse lie

Figure 17.23   Shows an oblique lie because the long axis of the fetus is oblique in relation to the uterus.

Figure 17.24   Shows a transverse lie with shoulder presentation.

Figures 17.20–17.24   The lie of the fetus.

across the long axis of the uterus. This is often visible on inspection of the abdomen.

Attitude

Attitude is the relationship of the fetal head and limbs to its trunk. The attitude should be one of flexion. The fetus is curled up with chin on chest, arms and legs flexed, forming a snug, compact mass, which utilizes the space in the uterine cavity most effectively. If the fetal head is flexed the smallest diameters will present and, with efficient uterine action, labour will be most effective.

Denominator

'Denominate' means 'to give a name to'; the denominator is the name of the part of the presentation, which is used when referring to fetal position. Each presentation has a different denominator and these are as follows:

- in the vertex presentation it is the occiput
- in the breech presentation it is the sacrum
- in the face presentation it is the mentum.

Although the shoulder presentation is said to have the acromion process as its denominator, in practice the dorsum is used to describe the position. In the brow presentation no denominator is used.

Position

The position is the relationship between the denominator of the presentation and six points on the pelvic brim (Fig. 17.25). In addition, the denominator may be found in the midline either anteriorly or posteriorly, especially late in labour. This position is often transient and is described as *direct anterior* or *direct posterior*.

Anterior positions are more favourable than posterior positions because when the fetal back is at the front of the uterus it conforms to the concavity of the mother's abdominal wall and the fetus can flex more easily. When the back is flexed the head also tends to flex and a smaller diameter presents to the pelvic brim. There is also more room in the anterior part of the pelvic brim for the broad biparietal diameter of the head. The positions in a vertex presentation are summarized in Box 17.5 (also see Figs 17.26–17.31)

Box 17.5 Positions in a vertex presentation

- **Left occipitoanterior (LOA)** The occiput points to the left iliopectineal eminence; the sagittal suture is in the right oblique diameter of the pelvis (Fig. 17.26).

- **Right occipitoanterior (ROA)** The occiput points to the right iliopectineal eminence; the sagittal suture is in the left oblique diameter of the pelvis (Fig. 17.27).

- **Left occipitolateral (LOL)** The occiput points to the left iliopectineal line midway between the iliopectineal eminence and the sacroiliac joint; the sagittal suture is in the transverse diameter of the pelvis (Fig. 17.28).

- **Right occipitolateral (ROL)** The occiput points to the right iliopectineal line midway between the iliopectineal eminence and the sacroiliac joint; the sagittal suture is in the transverse diameter of the pelvis (Fig. 17.29).

- **Left occipitoposterior (LOP)** The occiput points to the left sacroiliac joint; the sagittal suture is in the left oblique diameter of the pelvis (Fig. 17.30).

- **Right occipitoposterior (ROP)** The occiput points to the right sacroiliac joint; the sagittal suture is in the right oblique diameter of the pelvis (Fig. 17.31).

- **Direct occipitoanterior (DOA)** The occiput points to the symphysis pubis; the sagittal suture is in the anteroposterior diameter of the pelvis.

- **Direct occipitoposterior (DOP)** The occiput points to the sacrum; the sagittal suture is in the anteroposterior diameter of the pelvis.

In breech and face presentations the positions are described in a similar way using the appropriate denominator.

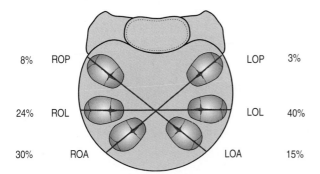

8% ROP LOP 3%

24% ROL LOL 40%

30% ROA LOA 15%

Figure 17.25 Diagrammatic representation of the six vertex positions and their relative frequency: LOA, left occipitoanterior; LOL, left occipitolateral; LOP, left occipitoposterior; ROA, right occipitoanterior; ROL, right occipitolateral; ROP, right occipitoposterior.

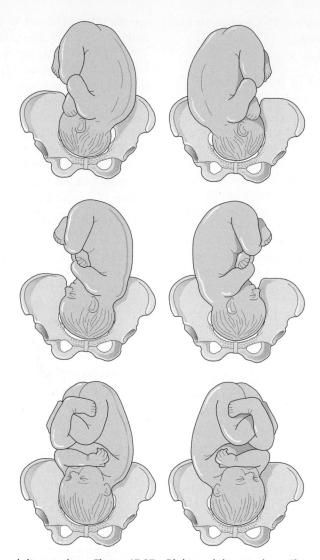

Figure 17.26   Left occipitoanterior.   **Figure 17.27**   Right occipitoanterior.   **Figure 17.28**   Left occipitolateral.
Figure 17.29   Right occipitolateral.   **Figure 17.30**   Left occipitoposterior.   **Figure 17.31**   Right occipitoposterior.

Figures 17.26–17.31   Six positions in vertex presentation.

Assessment of pelvic capacity

According to NICE (2008), routine antenatal pelvic examination is an inaccurate measurement of gestational age, and the likelihood of preterm birth or cephalopelvic disproportion, therefore it is not recommended.

Ongoing antenatal care

The information gathered during the antenatal visits will enable the midwife and pregnant woman to determine the appropriate pattern of antenatal care (NICE 2008). The timing and number of visits will vary according to individual need and changes should be made as circumstances dictate (e.g. as demonstrated in Box 17.6).

Indicators of fetal well-being

These include:

- increasing uterine size compatible with the gestational age of the fetus
- fetal movements that follow a regular pattern from the time when they are first felt
- fetal heart rate that is regular and variable with a rate between 110 and 160 beats/minute.

Eliciting information about recent fetal movement will reassure the mother. Patterns of fetal movements are a reliable sign of fetal well-being; evidence of usual fetal movements for the woman can be considered normal. However, NICE (2008) supported by Mangesi & Hofmeyr (2007) suggest that fetal movement counting does not prevent fetal morbidity or mortality and therefore is a poor indicator of fetal well-being.

Preparation for labour

During the latter weeks of pregnancy, plans for labour and birth will be a focus of discussion. Most hospitals provide a list of items that they require women to bring

Box 17.6 Risk factors that may arise during pregnancy

- Any chronic or acute illness or disease in the woman
- Hb lower than 10.5 g/dL
- Proteinuria
- BP: single diastolic of 110 mgHg or two of 90 mmHg at least 4 hrs apart; two systolic of above 160 mmHg at least 4 hrs apart
- Uterus large or small for gestational age
- Excess or decreased liquor
- Malpresentation
- Fetal movement pattern significantly reduced or changed
- Any vaginal, cervical or uterine bleeding
- Premature labour
- Infection
- Sociological or psychological factors

with them into hospital for themselves and their baby. If the woman has planned a home birth, she is visited by her midwife to make final arrangements for the birth. In both cases it is important to ensure that women know whom to contact if they need advice about the commencement of labour or have other concerns.

The focus on the positive progress of labour and birth, centering on normality, is a priority but if there is a need to change plans during labour then women and their families should be facilitated by the midwife to make an informed choice. Flexibility and adaptability should be built into the labour and birth plans to ensure an individual approach is adopted and the woman's needs are met. Parents' wishes should be recorded in the pregnancy labour notes in addition to discussions about care, which take place between the woman, her family, the midwife and other health professionals who are involved antenatally.

REFERENCES

Ades A, Sculpher M, Gibb D et al 1999 Cost effectiveness analysis of antenatal HIV screening in United Kingdom. British Medical Journal 319(7219): 1230–1234

Alexander J M, Grant A M, Campbell M J 1992 Randomised controlled trial of breast shells and Hoffman's exercises for inverted and non-protractile nipples. British Medical Journal 304(6833):1030–1032

Bacchus L, Mezey G, Bewley S 2004. Domestic violence: prevalence in pregnant women and associations with physical and psychological health. European Journal of Obstetrics, Gynecology, and Reproductive Biology 113(1):6–11

Barber T, Rogers J, Marsh S 2006a The birth place choices project: phase one. British Journal of Midwifery 14 (10):609–613

Barber T, Rogers J, Marsh S 2006b The birth place choices project: phase two initiative. British Journal of Midwifery 14(11):671–675

Barber T, Rogers J, Marsh S 2007 Increasing out of hospital births: what needs to change? British Journal of Midwifery 15(1):16–20

Barnes J, Cheng H, Howden B et al 2006 Changes in the characteristics of SSLP areas between 2000/1 and 2003/4. Online. Available: dfes/www.surestart.gov.uk

Beevers G, Lipe G, O'Brien E 2001a ABC of hypertension: blood pressure measurement. British Medical Journal 332:981–985

Beevers G, Lipe G, O'Brien E 2001b ABC of hypertension: blood pressure measurement Part II. British Medical Journal 322:1043–1047

Blair P, Bensley D, Smith I, et al 1996 Smoking and the sudden infant death syndrome: results from 1993–5 case-control study for confidential enquiry into stillbirths and deaths in infancy. British Medical Journal 313:195–198

Bundey S, Alan H 1991 Why do UK born Pakistani babies have high perinatal and neonatal mortality rates? Paediatrica Perinatal Epidemiology 5(1):101–114

Clement S, Candy B, Sikorski J et al 1996 Does reducing the frequency of routine antenatal visits have long term effects? Follow up of participants in a randomised controlled trial. British Journal of Obstetrics and Gynaecology 106 (4):367–370

CDC (Center for Disease Control) 2007 Fetal alcohol spectrum disorders. Online. Available: http://www.cdc.gov/ncbddd/fas/fasask.htm (accessed 7 October 2007)

DH 2007a Smoking and pregnancy. Online. Available: http://www.gosmokefree.co.uk/whygosmokefree/smokingpregnancy/index.php (accessed 6 April 2007)

DH 2007b Alcohol and Pregnancy. Online. Available: http://www.dh.gov.uk/en/News/DH_074968 (accessed 7 October 2007)

DH 2005 Social Services and Public Safety, Infant Feeding Survey. DH, London

DH 2004 The National Service framework for children, young people and the maternity services. DH, London

DH (Department of Health) 1993 Changing childbirth: report of the expert maternity group. HMSO, London

DH (Department of Health) 1999 Our healthier nation: reducing health inequalities: an action report. DH, London

Elbourne D, Richardson M, Chalmers I et al 1987 The Newbury maternity care study: a randomised controlled trial to assess a policy of women holding their own obstetric records. British Journal of Obstetrics and Gynaecology 94(7): 612–619

Engstrom J, Piscioneri L, Low L 1993 Fundal height measurement part 3 – the effect of maternal position on fundal height measurements. Journal of Nurse-Midwifery 38(1): 23–27

Farquharson and Greaves 2006 Thromboembolic disease. In: James, D, Steer P, Weiner C et al (eds) High risk pregnancy, 3rd edn. Saunders, London, p 938–948

Floyd R, Rimer B et al 1993 A review of smoking in pregnancy: effects on pregnancy outcomes and cessation efforts. Annual Review of Public Health 14:379–411

Gardosi J, Francis A 1999 Controlled trial of fundal height measurement plotted on customised antenatal growth charts. British Journal of Obstetrics and Gynaecology 106(4): 309–317

Hall M H, Cheng P K, MacGillivray I 1980 Is routine antenatal care worth while? Lancet ii:78–80

Homer C, Davis G, Everitt L 1999 The introduction of a woman-held record into a hospital antenatal clinic: the bring your own records study. Australian and New Zealand Journal of Obstetrics and Gynaecology 39(1):54–57

Jewell D, Sharp D, Sanders J et al 2000 A randomised controlled trial of flexibility in routine antenatal care. British Journal of Obstetrics and Gynaecology 107(10): 1241–1247

Kalish R, Chervenak F 2005 Sonographic determination of gestational age. Ultrasound Review of Obstetrics and Gynecology 5(4):254–258

Leamon J, Viccars A 2007 West Howe midwifery evaluation: the with me study. Bournemouth University, Bournemouth

Lewis G (ed.) 2007 Confidential Enquiry into Maternal and Child Health (CEMACH) Saving Mothers' Lives: reviewing maternal deaths to make motherhood safer 2003–2005. The 7th report on Confidential Enquiries into Maternal Deaths in the United Kingdom. CEMACH, London

Lewis G & Drife J 2001 Why Mothers Die 1997–1999. The fifth report of the confidential enquiries into maternal deaths in the United Kingdom. RCOG Press, London

Li C, Windsor R 1993 The impact on infant birthweight and gestational age of cotinine-validated smoking reduction in pregnancy. Journal of the American Medical Association 269:1519–1524

Lundgren I, Berg M Lindmark G 2003 Is the childbirth experience improved by a birth plan? Journal of Midwifery and Women's Health 48(5):322–328

Mangesi L, Hofmeyr G 2007 Fetal movement counting for assessment of fetal well-being. Cochrane Database of Systematic Reviews 1:CD004909

McCourt C 2006 Supporting choice and control? Communication and interaction between midwives and women at the antenatal booking visit. Social Science and Medicine 62:1307–1218

Mcleod M, Benn C, Pullon S et al 2004 Midwifery Education for women who smoke: A randomised controlled trial. Midwifery 20(1):37–50

Mcleod M, Benn C, Pullon S et al 2003 The midwife's role in facilitating smoking behaviour during pregnancy. Midwifery 19(4):285–297

Mezey G, Bacchus L, Bewley et al 2005. Domestic violence lifetime trauma and psychological health of childbearing women. British Journal of Obstetrics and Gynaecology 112(2):197–204

MIDIRS 2008a Ultrasound scans-what you need to know. Informed choice leaflet (3) for women. MIDIRS, Bristol

MIDIRS 2008b where will you have your baby? Informed choice leaflet (10) for women. MIDIRS, Bristol

Ministry of Health, 1929 Maternal mortality in childbirth. Antenatal clinics: their conduct and scope. HMSO, London

Mitchell E A, Tuohy P G, Brunt J M et al 1997 Risk factors for sudden infant death syndrome following the prevention campaign in New Zealand: a prospective study. Pediatrics 100:835–840

Morrison P, Burnard P 1997 Caring and communicating. Macmillan Press, London

Nafstad P, Jaakkola J J, Hagen J A et al 1996 Breastfeeding, maternal smoking and lower respiratory tract infections. European Respiratory Journal 9(12):2623–2629

Neilson J P 2001 Symphysis-fundal height measurement in pregnancy. In: The Cochrane Library, issue 3. Update Software, Oxford

Nguyen T, Larsen T, Enghollm G et al 1999 Evaluation of ultrasound-estimated date of delivery in 17 450 spontaneous singleton births: do we need to modify Naegele's rule? Ultrasound in Obstetrics and Gynecology 14(1):223–228

NICE 2008 Antenatal care: Routine care for the healthy pregnant woman. CG62 NICE, London

NICE 2007 Antenatal and postnatal mental health. NICE, London

NICE 2003 Antenatal Care: Routine care for the pregnant woman. NICE, London

NICE 2002 Guidance on the use of routine antenatal Anti D prophylaxis for RhD negative women. Appraisal Guidance No 41. NICE, London

NOFAS-UK National Organisation on Fetal Alcohol Syndrome UK 2007. Online Available: http://www.nofas-uk.org/index.asp (accessed 7 October 2007)

Nursing and Midwifery Council 2004. Midwives Rules and Standards. London: NMC

Nursing and Midwifery Council 2006. A–Z Advice Sheet: Records and record keeping. NMC, London

Oakley A, Rajan L, Grant A 1990 Social support and pregnancy outcome. British Journal of Obstetrics and Gynaecology 97:155–162

Oakley A, Hickey D, Rajan L 1996 Social support in pregnancy: does it have long term effects? Journal of Reproductive and Infant Psychology 14:7–22

Page L 2006 Being with Jane in childbirth: putting science and sensitivity into practice in: L. Page and R. McCandlish (eds) 2006 The new midwifery science and sensitivity in practice, 2nd edn. Churchill Livingstone, London

Prochaska J 1992 What causes people to change from unhealthy to health enhancing behaviour? In: Heller T, Bailey L, Patison S (eds) Preventing cancers. Open University Press, Buckingham, p 147–153

Raphael-Leff J 2005 Psychological processes of childbearing, 4th edn. Chapman & Hall, Anna Freud Centre, London

Redshaw M, Rowe R, Hockley C et al 2006 Recorded delivery: a national survey of women's experience of maternity care. Oxford: National Perinatal Epidemiology Unit

RCOG (Royal College of Obstetricians and Gynaecologists) 2006 Recreational exercise and pregnancy. Online. Available: http://www.rcog.org.uk/resources/public/pdf/recreational_exercise_pi.pdf (accessed 7 April 2007)

Roquer J, Figueras J, Botet F et al 1995 Influence on fetal growth of exposure to tobacco smoking during pregnancy. Acta Paediatrica 84:118–121

Roshanfekr D, Blakemore K J, Lee J et al 1999 Station at onset of active labor in nulliparous patients and risk of cesarean delivery. Obstetrics and Gynecology 93(3):329–331

Sayle A, Savitz D, Thorp J et al 2001 Sexual activity during late pregnancy and risk of pre-term delivery. Obstetrics and Gynecology 97:283–9

Schott J, Henley A 1996 Culture, religion and childbearing in a multiracial society. Butterworth Heinemann, London

Sikorski J, Wilson J, Clement S et al 1996 A randomised controlled trial comparing two schedules of antenatal visits: the antenatal care project. British Medical Journal 312:546–553

Stenhouse E, Wright D, Hattersley A et al 2003. How well do midwives estimate the date of delivery? Midwifery 19:125–131

Stein-Parbury 1993 Patient and person developing interpersonal skills in nursing. Churchill Livingstone, Edinburgh

Stoltenberg C, Magnus P, Lie R T et al 1998 Influence of consanguinity and maternal education on risk of stillbirth and infant death in Norway, 1967–1993. American Journal of Epidemiology 148(5):452–459

Tunon K, Eik-Nes S, Grottum P 1996 A comparison between ultrasound and a reliable last menstrual period as predictors of the day of delivery in 15 000 examinations. Ultrasound in Obstetrics and Gynaecology 8:178–185

UNICEF UK Baby Friendly Initiative 2007 The ten steps to successful breastfeeding. Online. Available: http://www.babyfriendly.org.uk/page.asp?page=60 (accessed 7 October 2007).

Villar J, Hassan B, Piaggio G et al 2001 WHO antenatal care randomized trial for the evaluation of a new model of routine antenatal care. The Lancet 357:1551–1564

Villar J, Khan-Neelofur D 2001 Patterns of routine antenatal care for low-risk pregnancy. In: The Cochrane Library, issue 3. Update Software, Oxford

Walfish A, Hallak M 2006 Hypertension. In: D. James P, Steer C, Weiner Bet al (eds) High risk pregnancy, 3rd edn. Elsevier, Philadelphia, p 772–797

Walker J, Walker A 2006. Substance abuse In: James D, Steer P, Weiner et al (eds) High risk pregnancy, 3rd edn. Elsevier, Philadelphia, p 721–741

Way S 2000 Core skills for caring and assessment. Books for Midwives, Manchester

Webster J, Forbes K, Foster S et al 1996 Sharing antenatal care: client satisfaction and use of the 'patient-held record'. Australian and New Zealand Journal of Obstetrics and Gynaecology 35(1):11–14

Williams, D 2006 Renal disorders In: James D, Steer P, Weiner et al (eds) High risk pregnancy, 3rd edn. Elsevier, Philadelphia, p 1098–1124

18 Specialized antenatal investigations

Amanda Sullivan   Beverley Kirk

CHAPTER CONTENTS

Antenatal assessment of the fetus is now a mainstream aspect of care for all pregnancies. In early to mid-pregnancy, a number of tests for fetal anomaly are offered to all mothers as part of the NHS Antenatal and Newborn Screening Programmes. Later in pregnancy, monitoring of fetal well-being may be required. Advances in technology mean that fetal assessments have become increasingly sophisticated and more widespread. For instance, ultrasound scan machines are now able to detect a number of abnormalities in the first trimester of pregnancy. Some centres already offer this facility. Inevitably, increased testing results in increased information for parents. Generally, test findings give a degree of reassurance, but they can also result in significant anxiety and devastating decisions about whether to end the pregnancy. Increased childbearing among older mothers (Langford 1992) has resulted in more age-related chromosomal abnormalities. Consequently, there are a number of factors that contribute to an ever-increasing emphasis on antenatal fetal assessments.

The chapter aims to explore:

- the psychological impact of fetal investigations
- the role of the midwife when caring for mothers considering or undergoing such tests
- effective information-giving techniques
- common screening and diagnostic procedures
- the use of new and emerging technologies.

Social and psychological impact of fetal investigations

Pregnancy is a profound and life-changing event. During this time, the mother has to adapt physically, socially and psychologically to the forthcoming birth of her child. Many women feel more emotional than usual (Raphael-Leff 1991) and may have heightened levels of anxiety (e.g. Dragonas & Christodoulou 1998, Tindall 1997). As Hawkey (1998) states, the increasing availability of fetal investigations has been shown to cause women even greater anxiety and stress. Any feelings of excitement and anticipation can quickly change when the mother is introduced to the idea that she is 'at risk' of having a baby with a particular problem (Fisher 2006).

There is evidence that mothers nearing the end of their reproductive years (with a higher risk of chromosomal abnormality) experience pregnancy in a way that is different to younger women. Older mothers are often more anxious and have fewer feelings of attachment to the fetus at 20 weeks of pregnancy (Berryman & Windridge 1995). Psychologists, sociologists and health professionals now generally accept the finding that high-risk women delay attachment to the fetus until they receive reassuring test results. Rothman (1986) classically termed this the 'tentative pregnancy', in a study of women undergoing amniocentesis.

Anxiety caused by consideration of possible fetal abnormality may be accompanied by moral or religious dilemmas. Tests that can diagnose chromosomal or genetic abnormalities also carry a risk of procedure-induced miscarriage. Many parents agonize about whether to subject a potentially normal fetus to this risk in order to obtain this information. Parents may then need to consider whether they wish to terminate or continue with an affected pregnancy. Some religious authorities only support prenatal testing so long as the integrity of the mother and fetus are maintained. There are also opposing views about the legitimacy of terminating a pregnancy, even when a serious disorder has been diagnosed. Such dilemmas are an unfortunate but inevitable cost of the choices associated with some fetal investigations.

Despite this, there are important advantages to the acquisition of knowledge about the fetus before birth. First, society greatly values the freedom of individuals to choose. People are encouraged to accept some responsibility when making decisions about treatment options, in partnership with healthcare professionals. A second advantage is that reproductive autonomy may be increased. Women can choose for themselves whether they wish to embark upon the lifelong care of a child with special needs. This may be viewed as empowering and as a means of preventing later suffering and hardship for child and family alike.

In summary, prenatal testing is a two-edged sword. It enables midwives and doctors to give people choices that were unheard of in previous generations and that may prevent much suffering. However, in some circumstances they actually increase the amount of anxiety and psychological trauma experienced in pregnancy. The long-term effects of such trauma on family dynamics are not currently understood.

The midwife's role and responsibilities

All midwives need to have a broad understanding of fetal investigations because they are responsible for offering, interpreting and communicating the results. The Midwives Rules and Standards (NMC 2004) state that midwives *'should enable the woman to make decisions about her care based on her individual needs, by discussing matters fully with her'* (p 16). Some midwives specialize in discussing complex testing issues with parents and become antenatal screening coordinators. The UK National Screening Committee (2004) recommends that dedicated screening coordinators oversee the running of screening programmes in every Trust. Screening coordinators also provide specialist advice and ensure that there is a line of referral for women whose needs are not met by routine services (Ferguson 2001).

When offering tests, it is necessary for the midwife to present and discuss the options, so that women can make a choice that best suits their circumstances and preferences. Midwives commonly recommend antenatal tests such as infectious disease screening, full blood count or cardiotocograph for reduced fetal movements. However, tests for fetal anomaly require a non-directive approach that enables the mother to make an informed choice (Clarke 1994). Consent must be obtained prior to all tests and this must be documented (National Institute for Clinical Excellence (NICE) 2003, UK National Screening Committee 2004). The information required to obtain consent is shown in Box 18.1 (DH 2001). It is noteworthy that obtaining consent is a process and not usually a one-off event. This means that tests should be discussed on more than one occasion and mothers should be given time to consider their options.

Midwives are required to discuss options for testing in a manner that enables shared decision making (Sullivan 2005). This means that the midwife and mother both share information and are jointly

---

Box 18.1 Information required to obtain informed consent

- purpose of the procedure
- all risks and benefits to be reasonably expected
- details of all possible future treatments that could arise as a consequence of testing
- disclosure of all available options (this may include tests that are offered by private providers where relevant)
- the option of refusing any tests
- the offer to answer any queries.

---

accountable for the decisions that are made. There may be mixed feelings about the final decision. Sometimes, it is helpful to consider what the mother's worst-case scenario would be, as that can help to decide the best way forward. Attention should be paid to documenting all discussions carefully for future reference and for continuity of care. The process for shared decision-making is shown in Figure 18.1.

Issues to consider when presenting information

When discussing tests, it is important to understand the motivations and thought processes of pregnant women. The motivation for testing is often different for mother and practitioner. Whereas the medical indication for testing is to identify fetal anomalies, mothers commonly accept these tests in order to gain reassurance that their fetus is normal (Farrant 1985). Mothers often think that fetal anomaly tests such as ultrasound scans are an integral or mandatory part of their antenatal care. They may also be unaware of the reasons for performing the test and this can compound the shock of finding problems or abnormalities (Health Technology Assessment 2000).

It is also evident that, when feeling anxious or under stress, people are less able to remember the information portrayed (Ingram & Malcarne 1995). Parents may feel vulnerable and less able to ask questions. This may lead to dissatisfaction with the quality of communications with healthcarers. Since an unborn

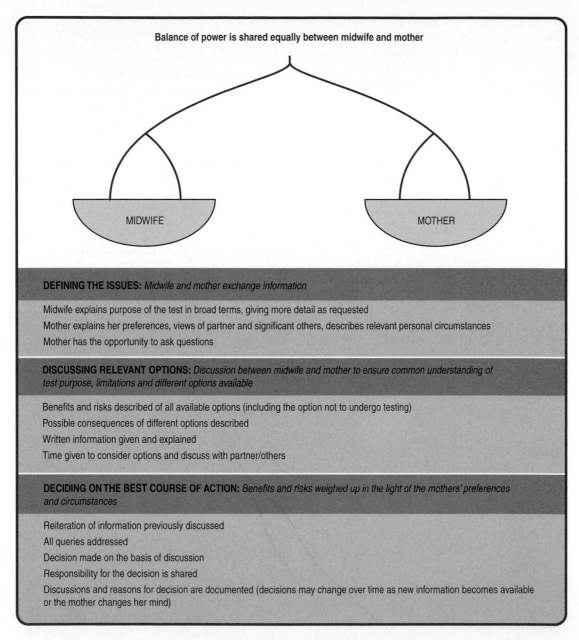

Balance of power is shared equally between midwife and mother

MIDWIFE

MOTHER

DEFINING THE ISSUES: *Midwife and mother exchange information*

Midwife explains purpose of the test in broad terms, giving more detail as requested

Mother explains her preferences, views of partner and significant others, describes relevant personal circumstances

Mother has the opportunity to ask questions

DISCUSSING RELEVANT OPTIONS: *Discussion between midwife and mother to ensure common understanding of test purpose, limitations and different options available*

Benefits and risks described of all available options (including the option not to undergo testing)

Possible consequences of different options described

Written information given and explained

Time given to consider options and discuss with partner/others

DECIDING ON THE BEST COURSE OF ACTION: *Benefits and risks weighed up in the light of the mothers' preferences and circumstances*

Reiteration of information previously discussed

All queries addressed

Decision made on the basis of discussion

Responsibility for the decision is shared

Discussions and reasons for decision are documented (decisions may change over time as new information becomes available or the mother changes her mind)

Figure 18.1 The shared decision-making process.

fetus is something of an enigma to parents, this may increase anxiety and sensitivity to real or imaginary cues. For example, professionals practising non-directive counselling may be perceived as evasive and as concealing bad news. One particular aspect of counselling that has been criticized by parents is the portrayal of risk estimates (Al-Jader et al 2000).

There is much evidence that people do not make consistent decisions about undertaking tests in pregnancy on the basis of the risk information received. For instance, a mother with a risk of Down syndrome of 1:200 may perceive herself to be at a very high risk and may request amniocentesis. However, others may view that same risk as very low. We do not fully understand the way in which parents interpret risk information, although it is clear that personal circumstances, preferences and beliefs are an integral part of this process. For this reason, it is vital that the midwife begins a consultation by investigating how mothers feel about testing and what they already know.

There are also common biases in the way people interpret risk information. The midwife should be aware of these in order to help parents choose the most appropriate course of action. For example, people tend to view an event as more likely if they can easily imagine or recall instances of it. This means that a mother whose friend or neighbour has a baby with Down syndrome may be sensitized to this possibility and overestimate the chances of it happening to her. In reality, her risk remains unchanged. Mothers who work with infirm people, or those with a disability, are most likely to seek prenatal diagnosis (Sjogren 1996). Perhaps these mothers are easily able to imagine the lifelong commitment of caring for a child with special needs. This common bias in risk perception is important because it means that some mothers may not easily be reassured by reiteration of the fact that the risk of abnormality may be comparatively rare.

Explaining risk

The way in which the midwife tells a mother about risk will also greatly influence how that risk is perceived. For example, a mother who is told that her risk of a particular condition is 1 in 10 may be more alarmed than if she had been informed that there was a 90% chance of normality. This is known as the *'framing'* effect (Kessler & Levine 1987).

People vary considerably in the ways that they consider and understand risk, so it is important that this information is presented in a variety of ways. As such, a midwife discussing a 1 in 100 risk of a disorder should also point out the fact that 99% or 99 out of 100 similar people will not experience that disorder. This may help people cope when considering tests or when anxiously awaiting results.

There are other general considerations to take into account when providing information (Hunter 1994):

1. Be clear. Explain everything in terms that are not medical jargon or complex terminology.

2. Be aware that people can remember only a limited amount of information at one time. Be simple, concise and to the point.

3. Give important information first. This will then be remembered best.

4. Group pieces of information into logical categories, such as treatment, prognosis and ways to cope.

5. Information may be recalled more easily if it has been presented in several forms. For example, leaflets can be helpful after a consultation.

6. Offer to answer any queries. Give contact numbers, in case people think of questions at a later date.

7. Do not make assumptions about information requirements on the basis of social class, age or ethnic group.

8. Repeat the information and ask people whether there is anything that remains unclear.

If a test is undertaken in pregnancy, it is good practice to ensure that parents are clear about how, when and from whom they will be able to obtain the result. If possible, there should be some options available.

Antenatal fetal tests

Broadly speaking, there are two types of test offered to pregnant women. They are known as screening or diagnostic tests.

Screening tests

Screening tests aim to identify individuals who are most likely to be affected by a named disorder. This makes it possible to target further investigations towards those with the greatest apparent need. Mothers who undergo screening tests will be classified as above or below an action limit for follow-up investigations. Traditionally, this classification has been known as 'screen positive' or 'screen negative'. However, this terminology has caused problems with interpretation. As such, many mothers given a 'screen positive' result have assumed that there is a positive certainty that they have an affected pregnancy. Likewise, a 'screen negative' result has been interpreted as the exclusion of a problem. In fact, positive or negative in this context simply means that the chances of a problem are higher or lower than specified by an action limit. For this reason, screening results are now referred to as 'high(er) risk' or 'low(er) risk'.

It is also important to note that the action limit (or the dividing point between high and low risk) is usually defined in line with the level of resources available for follow-up procedures. There is no agreed scientific means of calculating what defines high risk. Consequently, some mothers within the low-risk group will be sufficiently anxious to request follow-up, whereas some who are categorized as high risk will not wish to pursue subsequent investigations.

The performance of a screening test is defined in a number of ways:

- *Detection rate/sensitivity* – this is the proportion of affected pregnancies that would be identified as high risk.
- *False positive rate* – this is the proportion of unaffected pregnancies with a high risk classification. The higher the specificity, the fewer are the false positives.
- *False negative rate* – this is the proportion of affected pregnancies that would not be identified as high risk. The higher the sensitivity, the fewer are the false negatives.

National fetal screening programmes have been developed for a range of congenital abnormalities. These include fetal anomaly ultrasound screening, Down syndrome screening and haemoglobinopathy screening. These screening programmes should be offered to all pregnant women.

Diagnostic tests

Diagnostic tests are performed in order to confirm or disprove the presence of a particular abnormality. They may be offered as a consequence of screening test results. However, the diagnosis may not give certainty as to the severity of the disorder or the quality of life of a particular individual. Responses to a diagnosis will vary, according to cultural, social, moral and religious beliefs. Furthermore, we are not currently able to diagnose all fetal abnormalities and some will not be manifested until childhood or even adulthood. Examples of diagnostic tests include amniocentesis, chorionic villus sampling (CVS) and ultrasound scans (scans can be used to diagnose some structural anomalies such as spina bifida and they can also be used to screen for clue signs of disorders such as Down syndrome).

Fetal anomaly screening from maternal serum

Down syndrome screening

Down syndrome (also referred to as Down's syndrome) is the most common cause of severe learning difficulty in children. In the absence of antenatal screening, around 1 in 700 births would be affected (Kennard et al 1995). While some children with Down syndrome learn literacy skills and lead semi-independent lives, others remain completely dependent. Around one in three of these babies are born with a serious heart defect. The average life expectancy is about 60 years, although most people develop pathological changes in the brain (associated with Alzheimer's disease) after the age of 40 (Kingston 1994).

Maternal blood contains a number of hormones that can be used to assess the risk of Down syndrome. A growing number of hormones have been shown to have different average levels in Down syndrome compared with unaffected pregnancies and are therefore known as biochemical markers. These are shown in Table 18.1. One of the difficulties with using biochemical markers for screening is the fact that their levels fluctuate and are dependant on a number of factors, such as maternal weight. Consequently, a more accurate risk estimate can be obtained if several markers are used in combination. Levels of biochemical markers are never diagnostic for Down syndrome. The incidence of Down syndrome is also related to maternal age, so this is also factored into risk calculations. Older mothers are more likely to receive a higher risk result. The risk of Down syndrome by maternal age is shown in Table 18.2.

Biochemical markers, combined with maternal age, form part of the national Down syndrome screening programme. The UK National Screening Committee (2004) standards state that, whatever markers are used, tests should have a detection rate of >75% with a false positive rate of <3%. The cut-off point between higher and lower risk is 1:250. Some centres also add ultrasound markers (see Nuchal translucency measurement, p. 299) to maternal age and biochemical

Table 18.1 Biochemical markers used in Down syndrome screening

Marker	Derivation	Average levels in affected Down syndrome pregnancy	Most effective gestation for screening (weeks)
Pregnancy Associated Plasma Protein-A (PAPP-A)	Placental syncytiotrophoblasts	Lower	10–14
Human chorionic gonadotrophin (hCG) (free bhCG in both trimesters, intact bhCG in second trimester)	Embryo and later the trophoblast	Higher	10–22
Unconjugated oestriols (uE3)	Placenta and fetal adrenals	Lower	14–22
Alpha-fetoprotein (AFP)	Fetal liver and gastrointestinal tract	Lower	15–20
Inhibin A	Placenta	Higher	15–20

Table 18.2 Estimated risk of having a Down syndrome birth according to maternal age at birth (calculated using eight surveys)

Maternal age	Risk	Maternal age	Risk
15	1:1578	33	1:574
16	1:1572	34	1:474
17	1:1565	35	1:384
18	1:1556	36	1:307
19	1:1544	37	1:242
20	1:1528	38	1:189
21	1:1507	39	1:146
22	1:1481	40	1:112
23	1:1447	41	1:85
24	1:1404	42	1:65
25	1:1351	43	1:49
26	1:1286	44	1:37
27	1:1208	45	1:28
28	1:1119	46	1:21
29	1:1018	47	1:15
30	1:909	48	1:11
31	1:796	49	1:8
32	1:683	50	1:6

From Cuckle et al 1987.

screening tests. This greatly enhances the reliability and safety of Down syndrome screening. The aim is to maximize the detection rate, while minimizing the false positive results. This is very important because women with higher-risk results can only find out whether the baby is affected by undergoing invasive procedures such as amniocentesis or CVS. These tests carry a risk of causing a procedure-induced miscarriage. The types and safety levels of different screening tests are shown in Table 18.3, which shows increasing safety and effectiveness as more markers are added together.

It is noteworthy that the serum integrated and integrated tests are performed in two stages, with first and second trimester testing. Some clinicians find this concept problematic because it necessitates withholding test results until all phases of the testing process have been completed. Research is currently underway to explore the feasibility of this model in mainstream practice. One possible modification is known as contingency screening. A two-phase testing process occurs, but women above or below certain thresholds receive their results after the first phase. Higher risk mothers are offered diagnostic testing at this point and lower risk mothers are informed that their risk is low. Women in the middle range proceed to second trimester testing, since further information is advantageous in determining the risk classification.

When performing serum screening, it is essential that the gestation is accurately assessed. The scan dates should be used in preference to menstrual history, since scans give a more accurate indicator of the time of conception. Crown–rump length or biparietal diameter scan measurements should be used. Femur length is not a reliable indicator of gestational age. Serum screening is not indicated in multiple pregnancies because it is impossible to know how the levels relate to each fetus. Mothers with multiple pregnancies should be offered nuchal translucency scanning as an alternative. Serum levels also change with maternal weight (i.e. they are more concentrated in women with lower body mass and

Table 18.3 Types and safety of Down syndrome screening tests

Name of test	Markers used	Trimester for test	Number of women referred for diagnostic test	Number of unaffected pregnancies lost due to diagnostic test	Number of Down syndrome diagnosed per unaffected fetuses lost due to diagnostic test
Double (no longer recommended)	AFP, hCG	Second	6500	46	3.2
Triple	AFP, hCG, uE3	Second	4200	30	5.1
Quadruple	AFP, hCG, uE3, Inhibin A	Second	2500	18	8.5
Combined	PAPP-A, hCG, nuchal translucency	First	2300	17	9.0
Serum integrated	PAPP-A, Quadruple	PAPP-A in first, quadruple in second	800	6	25.4
Integrated	PAPP-A, nuchal translucency, Quadruple	PAPP-A and nuchal translucency in first, quadruple in second	300	2	76.3

Taken from the Department of Health (2003) Model of best practice for Down syndrome screening. Calculations derived from Wald et al (2003) Health Technology Assessment First and Second Trimester Antenatal Screening for Down Syndrome. Data based on modelled outcomes for 100 000 women screened, 152 diagnosed Down syndrome pregnancies with an 80% diagnostic test uptake and 0.9% procedure-related fetal loss rate.

circulating volume). It is therefore important to weigh the mother on the day of the test.

Neural tube defect screening and AFP

Traditionally, α-fetoprotein (AFP) has been used as a biochemical marker for neural tube defects such as spina bifida. This test has been superseded by the use of ultrasound to diagnose a range of neural tube defects. However, many centres still report high AFP levels at 15–20 weeks because this can be a prognostic indicator for other problems. Around 2% of mothers have a raised AFP level (Kennard et al 1995). Reasons include multiple pregnancy, incorrect gestation and threatened miscarriage. Raised AFP levels can be predictive of intrauterine growth restriction and pre-eclampsia. These pregnancies are therefore considered by some to be high risk and some centres offer increased fetal growth and fetal well-being monitoring in the third trimester.

Haemoglobinopathy screening

The NHS antenatal and newborn screening programmes include antenatal screening for fetal haemoglobinopathies. This should be linked with the newborn bloodspot screening programme, which tests for sickle cell disease. Haemoglobinopathies are inherited disorders of haemoglobin and are more prevalent in certain racial groups (NHS Sickle Cell and Thalassaemia Programme 2004; see Ch. 21).

Currently, antenatal screening is organized differently in different areas, based on population prevalence. High prevalence areas offer all pregnant women electrophoresis screening for haemoglobin variants and thalassaemia trait. Low prevalence areas use a family origins questionnaire to determine genetic ancestry for the last two generations (or more if possible). Women with genetic ancestry that includes high-risk racial groups are then offered electrophoresis testing. If the mother is found to be a haemoglobinopathy carrier, partner testing should be offered. Genetic ancestry is also important when interpreting screening results. It is also important to establish maternal iron levels when carrier status is suspected, since iron deficiency can give rise to similar red cell appearances. Haemoglobinopathies are recessively inherited, so the fetus would have a 1 in 4 chance of inheriting the disorder and a 1 in 2 chance of being a carrier. Diagnostic CVS or amniocentesis should be offered when both parents are carriers of a haemoglobinopathy.

Ultrasound scans for fetal testing

Pregnant women are offered two ultrasound scans in pregnancy. These include an early pregnancy scan and an 18–20-week fetal anomaly screening scan. Ultrasound scanning enables assessment and monitoring of many aspects of the pregnancy. It is used in order to screen for and to diagnose fetal abnormalities. Ultrasound works by transmitting sound at a very high pitch, via a probe, in a narrow beam. When the sound waves enter the body and encounter a structure, some of that sound is reflected back. The amount of sound reflected varies according to the type of tissue encountered. For example, fluid does not reflect sound and appears as a black image. Conversely, bone reflects a considerable amount of sound and appears as white or echogenic. Many structures appear as different shades of grey. Generally, pictures are transmitted in 'real time', which enables fetal movements to be seen.

Safety aspects of ultrasound

Ultrasound has been used as a diagnostic imaging tool since the 1950s, so we are now into the third generation of scanned babies. It seems reasonable to assume that any major adverse effects of this technology would have become apparent before now. However, modern machines have higher resolutions and indications for ultrasound scanning have greatly increased. This means that levels of exposure to ultrasound have increased in pregnancy and there is little research into the effects. Ultrasound should be used with respect and only when there is good indication.

Ultrasound waves have been shown to cause tissue heating, primarily within the first 40 s of exposure (Bosward et al 1993). There are also conflicting data regarding a possible association with low birth weight (Newnham et al 1993, Salvesen 1997), with dyslexia (Stark et al 1984) and with non-right-handedness (Salvesen et al 1993). Consequently, care should be taken to limit exposure time and the thermal indices should be controlled (European Committee of Medical Ultrasound Safety 2006). The use of ultrasound for entertainment or as a 'keep sake' is not recommended. Ultrasound is a diagnostic tool, but diagnosis can only be as reliable as the expertise of the operator and the quality of the machine. As Wood (2000) states, abnormalities may be missed or incorrectly diagnosed if the operator is inexperienced or inadequately trained.

Women's experiences of ultrasound

In general, women experience ultrasound as a pleasurable opportunity to have visual access to their unborn baby (Sandelowski 1994). Indeed, ultrasound scans have been shown to increase psychological attachment to the fetus (Sedgman et al 2006). Parents have a profound curiosity about their baby and a scan can turn something nebulous into something which seems much more real as a living individual (Furness 1990). This can be particularly important for a woman's partner and family, who do not have the immediate physical experience of the pregnancy. Women tend to regard their scan as providing a general view of fetal well-being: the fact that the fetus is alive, growing and developing. However, this reassurance is temporary and begins to wear off after a few weeks (Clement et al 1998). Mothers may then seek other forms of reassurance (e.g. monitoring fetal movements, auscultation of the fetal heartbeat). This initial reassurance may also create an enthusiasm for scans when there is no clinical indication.

However, scans may also cause considerable anxiety, particularly if there is a suspected or actual problem with the fetus. There is evidence to suggest that women who miscarry after visualization of the fetus on scan may feel a heightened sense of anguish because the fetus seemed more real. This may also be the case for parents considering termination of pregnancy on the grounds of fetal abnormality. However, others may view their scan as a treasured memory of the baby they lost (Black 1992).

The identification of fetal abnormality in the antenatal period has differing psychological effects for parents when the pregnancy is to continue. Some parents have reported feeling grateful that they were able to prepare for the birth of a child with a disability (Chitty et al 1996). However, others have reported feelings of wishing they had not known about their child's problems before birth because this created a powerful image of the fetus as a 'monster'. Some parents reported this to be far worse than the reality of caring for the baby after birth (Turner 1994). It is necessary for midwives to be mindful of the powerful psychological effects ultrasound scans have on pregnant women and their families, if sensitive and appropriate care is to be given at this potentially distressing time.

The midwife's role concerning ultrasound scans

As for all procedures, mothers should be fully informed about the purpose of the scan. Information should be given about which conditions are being checked for and which problems the scan would be unable to detect. Because of the pleasurable aspect of seeing the fetus, ultrasound scans have traditionally been tests that mothers undertake willingly, without prior discussion and consideration of potential consequences. It is advisable to remind mothers gently of the medical indications for scans, so that they can decide whether or not they wish to undergo a procedure that may bring unwelcome news. Women should be aware that ultrasound scans are optional and not an inevitable part of their care.

There is evidence that, although some mothers may find this information disturbing, most feel that this is outweighed by the positive aspects of seeing the baby and gaining reassurance (Oliver et al 1996). Indeed, extra information about the purpose of the scan has been shown to increase women's understanding and satisfaction with the amount of information received, while the proportion of women accepting a scan (99%) appears to remain unchanged (Thornton et al 1995).

The Royal College of Obstetricians and Gynaecologists recommends that, wherever scans are performed, a midwife or counsellor with a particular interest or expertise in the area should be available to discuss difficult news. Discussion about the implications of this should also take place with an obstetrician within one working day (RCOG 2000). Effective multidisciplinary team working and communication are therefore essential. It is also good practice for the midwife to liaise with the primary healthcare team, who would normally carry out the majority of antenatal care. With the increasing use of client-held records, mothers may have more opportunity to scrutinize the written results of their scan. Midwives may increasingly be called upon to explain and discuss these findings, both in hospital and in the community setting.

First trimester pregnancy scans

All women should be offered a first trimester scan. The purpose of this is to establish:

- that the pregnancy is viable and intrauterine (not ectopic)
- gestational age
- fetal number (and chorionicity or amnionicity in multiple pregnancies)
- detection of gross fetal abnormalities, such as anencephaly (absence of the cranial vault).

There is evidence to suggest that at least one scan is beneficial, mainly in reducing the need to induce labour for post-maturity (Neilson 1999). A gestation sac can usually be visualized from 5 weeks' gestation and a small embryo from 6 weeks. Until 13 weeks, gestational age can be accurately assessed by crown–rump length (CRL) measurement (the length of the fetus from the top of the head to the end of the sacrum). This is demonstrated in Figure 18.2. Care must be taken to ensure that the fetus is not flexed at the time

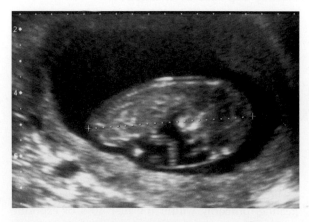

Figure 18.2 Crown–rump length.

of measurement. Mothers are asked to attend with a full bladder, since this aids visualization of the uterus at an early gestation.

Measurement of nuchal translucency at 10–14 weeks

Additional information about the fetus can be gained by measuring the nuchal translucency (NT) at 10–14 weeks' gestation. This is the thickness of the subcutaneous collection of fluid at the back of the neck, as shown in Figure 18.3. During the last decade, a series of studies have reported that increased NT is associated with chromosomal abnormalities, as well as other structural and genetic disorders (Nicolaides et al 1999). This information can be used in combination with maternal age and biochemical markers for Down syndrome.

The main advantage of this test is that it offers an early way of assessing the mother's risk for Down syndrome. In general, mothers greatly value the opportunity for early information about Down syndrome, so that they could consider the option of termination before they are visibly pregnant and can feel their baby's movements. Increased NT is also associated with other structural (mainly cardiac) and genetic syndromes, so increased pregnancy surveillance could be arranged. However, a disadvantage of this knowledge is that parents may suffer considerable anxiety until later scans offer some degree of reassurance.

Another potential disadvantage is that early identification of chromosomally abnormal pregnancies may mean that parents are faced with a decision about whether to terminate a pregnancy that may be destined to miscarry naturally. Approximately 40% of affected fetuses die between 12 weeks' gestation and term (Nicolaides et al 1999). Some parents may experience more feelings of guilt after a termination than they would have done had the pregnancy spontaneously miscarried.

Second trimester ultrasound scans

After 13 weeks of pregnancy, gestational age is primarily assessed using the biparietal diameter (BPD). This is the measurement between the two parietal eminences of the fetal skull. It is a very useful measurement during the second trimester, but becomes less accurate towards the end of pregnancy because the shape of the head may alter. Limbs are also measured, most notably the femur.

The detailed fetal anomaly screening scan

This scan is usually performed at 18–20 weeks of pregnancy, since visualization of fetal anatomy is more difficult before that time (Drife & Donnai 1991). The purpose of this scan is to reassure the mother that the fetus has no obvious structural anomalies that fall into the following categories:

- anomalies that are incompatible with life
- anomalies that are associated with significant morbidity and long-term disability
- anomalies which may benefit from intrauterine therapy
- anomalies which may require postnatal treatment or investigation.

Detection rates vary considerably, but it is thought that around 50% of significant abnormalities are identified at this time (Boyd et al 1998). This is influenced by the expertise of the sonographer and quality of the equipment. There may also be technical difficulties, such as fetal position, multiple pregnancy or maternal obesity.

Also, some structural problems do not have associated sonographic signs. An example of this would be tracheo-oesophageal fistula (an opening between the trachea and the lower oesophagus). Moreover, some fetal abnormalities, such as hydrocephalus and bowel obstructions, may not appear until later in pregnancy. Diagnosis may therefore be missed. Average detection rates for some abnormalities are

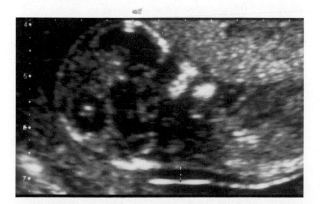

Figure 18.3 Nuchal translucency measurement.

Table 18.4 Detection rates of fetal abnormalities, if present, on detailed ultrasound scan

Problem	Chance of being seen (%)
Spina bifida	90
Anencephaly	99
Hydrocephalus	60
Major congenital heart problems	25
Diaphragmatic hernia	60
Exomphalos/gastroschisis	90
Major kidney problems	85
Major limb abnormalities	90
Cerebral palsy	Never seen
Autism	Never seen
Down syndrome	May be associated with heart or bowel problems in about 40%

RCOG (2000).

presented in Table 18.4. It is vital that mothers are fully aware of the precise purpose and limitations of the detailed scan. The comprehensive range of structures to be examined during the detailed scan are presented in Box 18.2. Examination of the four chambers of the fetal heart is shown in Fig. 18.4.

Box 18.2 Features examined on detailed fetal ultrasound scans

- Spine
- Head shape and internal structures (cavum pellucidum, cerebellum, ventricular size at atrium <10 mm)
- Abdominal shape and content – at level of the stomach
- Abdominal shape and content – at the level of kidneys and umbilicus
- Renal pelvis <5 mm
- Longitudinal axis, abdominal–thoracic appearance (diaphragm/bladder)
- Thorax – at level of four chamber cardiac view
- Arms – three bones and hand
- Legs – three bones and foot
- Face and lips
- Cardiac outflow tracts.

From RCOG 2000

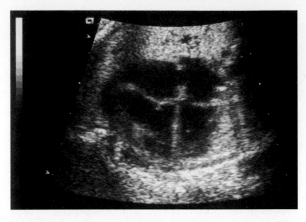

Figure 18.4 Four chamber view of the fetal heart. The opening between the atria (foramen ovale) can be seen.

Markers for chromosomal abnormality

Markers are minor sonographic clue signs, which may increase the chance that the fetus has a chromosomal abnormality (most are associated with Down syndrome). They are seen in many normal fetuses (at least 5%) and, when isolated, are of dubious value (Whittle 1997). Examples of such markers include the following:

Choroid plexus cyst This is a collection of cerebrospinal fluid within the choroids plexi, from where cerebrospinal fluid is derived.

Echogenic bowel This is a bright appearance of the bowel, equivalent to the brightness of bone. It is also associated with intra-amniotic bleeding and fetal swallowing of bloodstained liquor (Fig. 18.5).

Nuchal fold >5 mm at 20 weeks' gestation This is an increased thickness of fetal skin and fat at the back of the fetal neck. Subcutaneous fluid (NT) cannot usually be visualized after 14 weeks.

Echogenic foci in the heart These are bright echoes from calcium deposits in the fetal heart, often the left ventricle. They do not affect cardiac function.

Dilated renal pelvis >5 mm This may be due to slight backflow from the ureters and is more common in male fetuses.

Short femur This is a shorter than average thigh bone, when compared with other fetal measurements.

Sandal gap This is an exaggerated gap between the first and second toes.

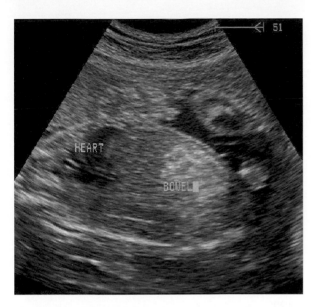

Figure 18.5 Echogenic bowel.

The strength of association between each individual marker and Down syndrome varies considerably. As such, an increased nuchal fold increases the chances of an affected pregnancy by 10 times the background risk. Conversely, echogenic foci in the heart increase the chances only by a marginal factor of 1.2 (Snijders & Nicolaides 1996). The UK National Screening Committee recommends that the Down syndrome screening risk should not be altered on the basis of a single ultrasound marker, unless it is at least as significant as an increased nuchal fold. It is also noteworthy that there is much debate about the validity of some of the above markers, particularly echogenic foci in the heart. It is possible that sonographers will not continue to report some of these markers in the future. Likewise, many new markers are emerging and may be incorporated into national screening programmes in the future. One example is the absence of nasal bone.

Advantages and disadvantages of fetal anomaly scans

Providing the sonographer has sufficient expertise, many lethal or severely disabling conditions can be detected during the 18–20 week scan. There is also an increase in first trimester diagnosis. Although this means that parents may be faced with difficult and unexpected decisions, it may be that later psychological trauma and physical suffering can be prevented. Furthermore, many parents are offered reassurance that no obvious abnormalities were seen. There is also evidence that, for neonates requiring early surgical or paediatric interventions, prior knowledge of the abnormality allows a plan of care to be evolved in advance of the birth. The mother can then give birth in a unit with appropriate facilities. This has been shown to reduce morbidity in the cases of gastroschisis (an abdominal wall defect, adjacent to the umbilicus, allowing the intestines and other abdominal organs to protrude outside the body), cardiac abnormalities and intestinal obstruction (Chang et al 1991, Romero et al 1989).

However, there is also the potential for false positive findings that are not confirmed postnatally. In particular, markers for chromosomal abnormalities may cause considerable anxiety without having any clinical significance for the baby. Indeed, they may be regarded as variants of normal, particularly if the fetal chromosomes are proven to be normal (see 'A testing time', Box 18.3).

There is also the problem of defining the prognosis for some recognizable abnormalities. In summary, the 18–20 week scan appears to confer psychological and health improvement benefits in some cases, but also has the capacity to cause great anxiety and distress. Care must be taken to ensure that parents are fully informed of the purpose, benefits and limitations of ultrasound scans before they consent to this procedure.

Third trimester pregnancy scans

In general, late pregnancy scans are performed in response to a specific clinical need and not as a screen of the low risk pregnant population. However, fetal abnormalities may come to light or be reassessed at this time. Many late scans are performed as a means of monitoring fetal well-being, growth and development.

Fetal growth

Many scans are performed in order to detect instances when growth deviates from the norm. Fetuses with excessive growth (*macrosomia*) have increased perinatal mortality and morbidity. There may be cephalopelvic disproportion or shoulder dystocia, with consequent birth asphyxia and trauma. In most cases, there is no apparent cause, but there is sometimes an association with maternal diabetes mellitus. Serial growth measurements are indicated in this latter group.

Fetuses may be small because they are preterm or because they are small for dates. Sometimes, these two problems overlap. In general, growth-restricted fetuses can be divided into two groups, symmetrical and asymmetrical growth restriction.

Symmetrical growth restriction

Most symmetrically small fetuses are entirely normal and may be genetically predetermined to be small. However, in some instances, this may be caused by chromosomal abnormalities, infection or environmental factors such as maternal substance misuse.

Asymmetrical growth restriction

These fetuses have a head size appropriate for gestational age, but thin bodies. This is generally caused by placental insufficiency, whereby the placenta is unable to provide sufficient nourishment for the fetus. Glycogen stores in the liver are reduced, so there are less energy reserves for the fetus during labour. Asymmetrically growth-restricted fetuses are therefore more likely to suffer antenatal or perinatal asphyxia, or both. Other potential problems include hypoglycaemia, hypothermia and premature birth.

In order to assess fetal growth, the gestational age must be accurately assessed on scan before 24 weeks. Women at high risk of having an abnormally grown fetus should have serial scans – often at 28, 32 and 36 weeks. Where there is a particular concern, growth may be measured every 2 weeks. The most important measurements are head circumference and abdominal circumference. In this way, trends in fetal growth can be assessed.

Biophysical profiling

Another measure of fetal well-being is the fetal biophysical profile. This is based on recognized fetal adaptations that occur as placental function declines. A score is calculated on the basis of five criteria (Manning et al 1980). These are listed as follows:

- *Fetal breathing movements* In the healthy fetus, breathing movements can be visualized in the third trimester of pregnancy. This helps develop respiratory muscles before birth. There should be at least 30 secs of sustained fetal breathing movements in 30 min of observation. Hiccoughs are considered breathing activity.
- *Fetal movements* Movement is often compromised in hypoxic fetuses. There should be three or more gross body movements in 30 min of observation. Simultaneous limb and trunk movements are counted as a single movement.
- *Fetal tone* There should be at least one episode of motion of a limb from a position of flexion to extension and rapid return to flexion. Absence of fetal movement is counted as absence of fetal tone.
- *Fetal reactivity* There should be two or more fetal heart accelerations of at least 15 b.p.m., within 40 min of observation. These should last at least 15 secs and be associated with fetal movement. This may best be recorded on a fetal CTG.
- *Qualitative amniotic fluid volume* There should be a pocket of amniotic fluid that measures at least 2 × 2 cm. Placental insufficiency often results in decreased renal perfusion in the fetus and reduced urinary output. Consequently, liquor volume can become reduced.

Doppler ultrasonography

Placental blood flow can be assessed using the Doppler shift (a change in the frequency of ultrasound wave reflection, according to the speed and direction of blood flow). Compromises in maternofetal circulation can be identified. Abnormalities in Doppler measurements may be detected before growth becomes impaired and can be used as a prognostic indicator. Doppler analysis of the umbilical artery is the only test that improves outcomes in high-risk pregnancies (Neilson & Alfirevic 2005). This is shown in Figure 18.6.

Findings from growth scans, biophysical profile scores and CTG recordings should be considered collectively, taking into account the full clinical picture and obstetric history.

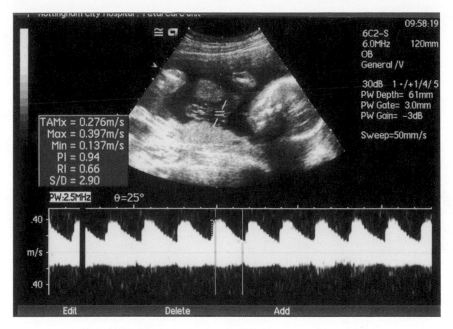

Figure 18.6 Measurement of umbilical artery Doppler flows.

Invasive diagnostic tests

If mothers are found to have an increased risk of chromosomal or genetic problems, they may wish to undergo a diagnostic procedure. The two most frequently used tests are chorionic villus sampling (CVS) and amniocentesis. They should be performed in specialist centres, by obstetricians with specific training and expertise. These tests provide the opportunity to examine the fetal karyotype (the number and structure of chromosomes, visible through a microscope during mitotic metaphase (see Fig. 18.7) or DNA analysis for particular gene mutations, or both.

Chorionic villus sampling

Chorionic villus sampling is the acquisition of chorionic villi (placental tissue) under continuous ultrasound guidance. Chorionic villi originate from the same cells as the fetus and therefore generally have the same genes and chromosomes. This may be performed at any stage after 10 weeks of pregnancy.

Access may be achieved transcervically (until 13 weeks' gestation) or via the transabdominal route.

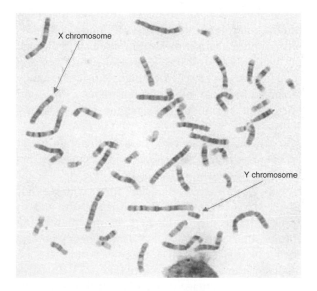

Figure 18.7 Normal male chromosomes.

When CVS is performed *transcervically*, a catheter is introduced through the cervix and is guided into the chorion frondosum. Suction is then applied to an attached syringe and 10–40 mg of tissue

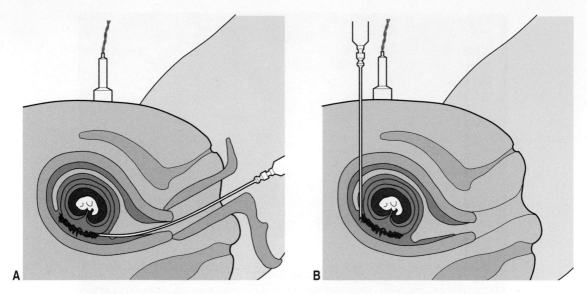

Figure 18.8 CVS procedures. (A) transcervical aspiration; (B) transabdominal puncture.

are aspirated. This procedure is represented in Figure 18.8.

The *transabdominal* approach involves the insertion of a needle into the maternal abdomen. Under ultrasound guidance, the needle is pushed through the uterine wall and into placental tissue. Tissue is aspirated via an attached syringe. Villi are carefully separated from maternal decidua under a dissection microscope, prior to cytogenetic (chromosome) analysis.

In general, there are two stages to the reporting of results. The initial result is issued after 24–48 hrs and counts specific chromosomes (e.g. to test for Down syndrome). Cells are then cultured for 14–21 days, to confirm the initial results and to allow more detailed cytogenetic examination of the chromosome structure. DNA (for genetic) or biochemical (for metabolic) diagnoses can also be obtained from chorionic villi tissue.

The main advantage of CVS is that this is the earliest way mothers can obtain definitive information about the chromosomal/genetic status of the fetus. Mothers who are known carriers of particular disorders often have high recurrence risks and so are anxious until their results are known. If the news is not

good and mothers wish to end their pregnancy, a surgical procedure can be performed. After 12–13 weeks, terminations are usually induced medically, in order to reduce the risk of causing cervical incompetence. This process of induction and vaginal birth can be very distressing. Decisions about termination of pregnancy may also become more difficult as the pregnancy progresses, since the mother begins to feel fetal movements and becomes visibly pregnant. Most women considering diagnostic procedures prefer to have an early test (Abramsky & Rodeck 1991). The main disadvantage with CVS is the procedure-induced risk of miscarriage. This is 0.5–2%, depending upon the experience of the operator (National Electronic Library for Health 2001) and occurs because of infection or bleeding. Also, ambiguous results are obtained in 1% of samplings (Holzgreve et al 1999).

Early CVS has been associated with limb reduction abnormalities. However, a large WHO international trial found the incidence of these abnormalities to be equal to the background rate (6/10 000), providing CVS was performed after 10 weeks. If CVS is performed prior to this gestation (i.e. during organogenesis), there is a higher chance that it may be harmful. Consequently, the WHO recommends 10 weeks as the earliest safe gestation for the procedure (Froster & Jackson 1996). In general, if an experienced operator with sufficient counselling support performs CVS, it is an effective and safe means of gaining early information about the fetus.

Amniocentesis

This is usually performed after 15 weeks' gestation, since early amniocentesis has a higher loss rate than early CVS (Nicolaides et al 1994). The procedure involves transabdominal insertion of a fine needle into the amniotic fluid cavity, under continuous ultrasound guidance; 15 mL of amniotic fluid are aspirated. Cytogenetic, molecular (DNA) and biochemical analyses are possible. Amniocytes are often examined. These comprise cells that have been shed from several fetal sites, including skin, lungs and renal tract. The risk of procedure-induced miscarriage is 1% (National Electronic Library for Health 2001), although 2–3% of mothers have some leakage of amniotic fluid (Simpson et al 1981). Miscarriage is usually caused by infection or spontaneous rupture of the membranes at the puncture site.

Amniocentesis has traditionally been performed more commonly than CVS, mainly because more obstetricians had the required training. However, recent clinical governance initiatives have resulted in a move towards performing invasive procedures only in specialist centres. This is important because procedure loss rates are so dependent on the operator. In the second trimester of pregnancy, CVS and amniocentesis have similar risks and benefits. The miscarriage risks are comparable and, in most cases, both tests provide the required information.

Recent advances in cytogenetic techniques mean that mothers can obtain an initial set of results (usually for Down syndrome) and then a full culture result after 2–3 weeks.

Fetal blood sampling

The use of this technique has declined in recent years because improved molecular and cytogenetic techniques allow more diagnoses to be made from chorionic villi or amniotic fluid. However, fetal blood may be advantageous when there are ambiguous findings from placental tissue. Also, when there is Rhesus isoimmunization, it may be necessary to determine the fetal haemoglobin. When this is low, an intrauterine transfusion may be performed. Blood can be sampled from the umbilical cord or intrahepatic umbilical vein. The latter is less risky, as there are no umbilical arteries in close proximity. The loss rate also depends upon the gestation and condition of the fetus. In uncomplicated procedures after 20 weeks, the loss rate is around 1% (Holzgreve et al 1999).

Rapid diagnostic techniques

Rapid diagnostic technologies are now available to women who undergo invasive testing. There are two main techniques in use today, FISH and QF-PCR.

Fluorescent *in situ* hybridization (FISH)

A specific probe 'paints' the chromosomes to be examined. For example, for Down syndrome, the probe appears fluorescent under a microscope when in contact with chromosome 21. Cells are examined to determine whether there are two or three signals for this chromosome. Two is the normal count, whereas three indicates Down syndrome. Since many mothers undergo testing because of a high risk serum screening result or identification of markers on scan, they are very anxious to obtain quick results. For this reason, the use of FISH has greatly enhanced service delivery. See Plate 1 for an example of this technique.

Quantitative fluorescence-polymerase chain reaction (QF-PCR, sometimes referred to as PCR)

This is a molecular technique for replicating DNA. Fetal DNA is extracted from the cells and is then multiplied. Fluorescent dyes are used to identify gene regions and to enable analysis. This technique is commonly used for 'genetic fingerprinting' and for paternity testing.

New and emerging technologies

Fetal imaging techniques

Ultrasound scans in pregnancy have been discussed at length in this chapter, since they are important fetal investigations. Women generally see two-dimensional (2D) images of their unborn baby. However, there is a growing market for three-dimensional ultrasound imaging (3D). As such, multiple images are stored digitally and then shaded to produce life-like pictures. This technique can assist the diagnosis of surface structural anomalies, such as cleft lip and spina bifida. However, there are a growing number of commercial enterprises that offer 3D or 4D (3D in real time) 'bonding' scans. This is a matter of concern, since such services have minimal regulation and vary considerably in their quality and marketing techniques. The level of pre- and post-test advice is also questionable in some cases.

Magnetic resonance imaging (MRI) has also been applied in the examination of the fetus over the last two decades. This technique has not been widely applied because ultrasound can give similar diagnostic information at a lower cost. However, MRI may have a contribution to make, particularly when examining the brain. There is evidence that this may provide additional information and change the counselling and management for a significant number of pregnancies where brain abnormalities are suspected (Levine et al 1997). A further possible application is that MRI could offer an alternative to postmortem following termination or perinatal death. This may offer information to parents who decline postmortem because of its invasive nature (Brookes & Hall-Craggs 1997). MRI may also be useful in providing serial brain images following asphyxia in the newborn. This may give us a better understanding of the evolution of brain injury (Maalouf et al 1998). More recently, MRI imaging has been used to refine the diagnosis of diaphragmatic hernias and sacrococcygeal teratomas (Kumar & O'Brien 2004).

Fetal cells in the maternal circulation

There has been extensive research into the use of fetal cells in maternal blood for genetic diagnosis. This would be helpful to mothers who want diagnostic information without the risk of procedure-induced miscarriage of a potentially normal fetus. Some progress has been made, such as fetal sexing and rhesus typing from maternal blood. However, this technology is not yet sufficiently well developed for wider application to general clinical care.

Fetal therapy

There are certain instances when therapeutic interventions may improve fetal prognoses. For instance, therapeutic amniocentesis may be performed to drain excess liquor. This may reduce the likelihood of preterm labour when the uterus is large-for-dates. Therapeutic amniocentesis is also sometimes performed in monochorionic twin pregnancies with twin-to-twin transfusion syndrome (discordant placental circulation and consequent discordant growth and liquor volume – if severe, this has a poor prognosis for both babies). Liquor is drained from the largest sac; this sometimes helps equal the pressures between the twins and allows both fetuses to grow satisfactorily.

Another treatment that is sometimes used is laser treatment to reduce pathological placental flow between the twins. Shunts can also be inserted into the fetus in order to drain pathological collections of fluid. These include ascites, renal obstruction and hydrocephalus. However, while there may be some improvement in outcome, much will depend on the underlying cause of the obstruction.

Conclusion

Fetal investigations are an integral aspect of antenatal care. Scientists and clinicians have developed a range of new diagnostic and imaging technologies. Some of these have been incorporated into national screening programmes and standards of care. The midwife must therefore ensure that women are informed about the benefits and risks associated with these technologies, so that they can make choices to suit their requirements. Undoubtedly, testing technologies profoundly influence women's experiences of pregnancy and their early attachment to their unborn child. Midwives therefore have a duty to prepare women for tests through sensitive and accurate communications and then to support parents in their assimilation of information and decision-making once the results are known.

Box 18.3 A testing time

I was called upon some time ago to outline my experiences of antenatal investigations to a midwives' research group, I did this and thought at the time that I was bearing my soul to 200 people that I had never met before. I can only guess at the readership of this textbook and so with great trepidation, I will attempt to give a taste of what antenatal investigations are like from the parents' side of the fence and hopefully 'bring alive' some of the traumas and dilemmas involved. The research, the facts, the paper evidence are there for all to see, whereas the emotions, considerations and 'angst' are less tangible; here is what it feels like to experience the process of diagnostic testing.

My husband and I knew early on in my pregnancy that I was expecting twins; having digested in some measure that awesome news, we nervously attended the hospital for my detailed scan. Everything seemed fine, the babies were assessed and all the checks made, except the position of the lower twin meant that the spine could not be seen clearly. We waited outside, I drank yet more water, though my bladder was bursting already, hoping that the baby would change position. We were euphoric, two baby girls on the way, how pleased our families would be, getting carried away, we even started to consider possible names: Amy, Alice, Emily, Lucy … (Fig. 18.9).

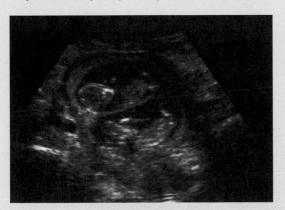

Figure 18.9 The scan of the twins.

We re-entered the room to continue the scan and among the, 'yes, that's fine, there's the other leg, etc.', we detected a different intonation in the radiographer's voice as she said, 'Ah, echogenic foci, there's a small marker near the baby's heart, a calcium deposit. It's probably nothing, but I'll tell you about it anyway even though some radiographers would not even mention it. An echogenic focus is a soft indicator of Down syndrome'. The words hit us like a hammer; there was nothing remotely 'soft' about what we had just heard. In literally a few minutes and the length of a hospital corridor the effect of that discovery was to have a devastating impact on us and our families.

We were ushered to the other end of the corridor where the facts were explained to us. We were told percentage risk factors for women of a certain age and Downrisk factors associated with amniocentesis; fact followed fact followed fact. That I was carrying twins complicated matters. Do we have both babies tested? How significantly does that increase the risk of miscarriage? What if one baby is fine and the other shows signs of abnormality? Would we be able to cope with a handicapped child? Can one baby be aborted? Question followed question followed question. We were given all the known evidence associated with our predicament and, while in our rational minds we understood the notion of professional ethics, we most desperately craved the one thing we could not have, a considered expert medical opinion. Fine, we knew about all the research, but how could we, with so little medical knowledge or familiarity with such situations, even begin to make such a monumental decision?

The journey home was a silent one; to say that we hardly knew how we got from A to B is not to overstate our sense of confusion and trauma. My parents were in the middle of a meal when we arrived. Having delivered the news about two grand-daughters there followed the giant, 10 feet tall letters of BUT … The effect was instantaneous; not another bite was eaten.

There followed 3 days of complete bewilderment as we tried to cope with the dilemma we faced and the monstrous decisions we had to make. We considered a million times the avenues available and canvassed everyone's opinion: family, friends, work colleagues, my local midwife, my health visitor, people we knew in the medical profession. Despite comforting and reassuring words, no respite came as we were forced to acknowledge any decisions were going to be exclusively ours; how desperately we needed advice!

We decided to have the amniocentesis on one baby and even now, the reasons as to why we chose this option are not clear, just as they were not at the time. Intuition, selfishness, whim, we really did not know if

Continued

Box 18.3 A testing time—cont'd

we were doing the right thing. In our minds, facts and research belong in textbooks; we were people craving guidance.

Funnily enough I did not find the actual test too awful. As we waited our turn, a member of the consultant's team shared with us similar cases she had dealt with where the results had been favourable and I will never forget her words when she said, 'I've got a good feeling about this, I'm sure everything will be fine'. This was the most human of comments from a professional that we had the pleasure to hear; it truly was like manna from heaven. Of course we knew that she could not possibly anticipate the results of the test, but her words at least made us feel there was some hope. Over the next 2 weeks we were to cling to those words time and time and time again. As we left the unit, we were told, 'give us a ring in a couple of weeks', and for what seemed like much longer than 2 weeks we were casually cast adrift to contemplate and imagine the results of the test.

Without wishing to jargonize or be drawn into using a cliché-ridden phrase, those 2 weeks were literally nightmarish. The comments people had made played over and over and over in our minds. 'I'll tell you this but it's probably nothing … echogenic-foci … soft indicator of Down … I've got a good feeling about

this …'. We merely functioned at work, nothing more; our lives were on hold and we were both emotionally and physically drained. We shrank from conversation with others and between ourselves on occasions; we considered innumerable times the possible outcomes. We slept fitfully; one night I sat on the stairs sobbing as I contemplated death, funerals and the fact that our babies may never exist in our world. My own midwife made a poignant and frighteningly accurate comment when she said that I was 'mourning' my babies – she was right. I was numb, we both were!

When the day for the result finally arrived there was absolutely no possibility that I could have made the call to the hospital. My husband was to phone up and then relay the news to me at work, but there were safety measures! Bad news, no call, no test results, no call, this gave me a get-out and ensured that hope could live on. To say I shook as I took my husband's phone call is a massive understatement and upon hearing the good news, I broke down, utterly and completely. The pent-up emotion of the previous 2 weeks poured out. That I hugged the headteacher, ignoring, forgetting or simply not caring about protocol, is an indication of the level of euphoria and relief I felt.

Our daughters were born on the 18 January 1999, weighing in at 5 lb 15 oz and 6 lb 11 oz (Fig. 18.10).

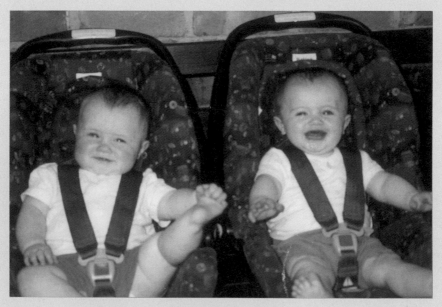

Figure 18.10 The twins.

Many, many issues were contemplated during this 'testing' experience – among them, can research be too advanced? A few years ago it is unlikely that such a marker would have been detected and a trouble-free pregnancy would have ensued! Most significantly, the role of counselling and support offered to women undergoing diagnostic tests must be considered as a vital component in the whole process.

I do not know if I am a better or different person as a result of my experience of diagnostic testing. I do know, however, that it is forever etched in my mind and heart; talking and writing about it even now feels incredibly emotional, vivid and raw.

(*Note*: the validity of 'echogenic focus' as a marker for Down syndrome has become increasingly debatable since this scan was performed. This makes the passage even more poignant. Also, rapid diagnostic technologies would mean that results would nowadays usually be available after 1–2 days. This greatly reduces the long period of uncertainty that women faced at that time.)

REFERENCES

Abramsky L, Rodeck C H 1991 Women's choices for fetal chromosome anomalies. Prenatal Diagnosis 11:23–28

Al-Jader L N, Parry Langdon N, Smith R J 2000 Survey of attitudes of pregnant women towards Down syndrome screening. Prenatal Diagnosis 20:23–29

Berryman J C, Windridge K C 1995 Motherhood after 35. A report of the Leicester motherhood project. Leicester University, Nestlé, Leicester

Black R B 1992 Seeing the baby: the impact of ultrasound technology. Journal of Genetic Counselling 1:45–54

Bosward K L, Barnett S B, Wood A K et al 1993 Heating of guinea pig fetal brain during exposure to pulsed ultrasound. Ultrasound in Medicine and Biology 19(5):415–424

Boyd P A, Chamberlain P, Hicks N R 1998 Six-year experience of prenatal diagnosis in an unselected population in Oxford. Lancet 352:1577–1581

Brookes J S, Hall-Craggs M A 1997 Postmortem perinatal examination: the role of magnetic resonance imaging. Ultrasound in Obstetrics and Gynaecology 9(3):145–147

Chang A C, Huhta J C, Yoon G Y 1991 Diagnosis, transport and outcome in fetuses with left ventricular outflow tract obstruction. Journal of Thoracic and Cardiovascular Surgery 102:841–848

Chitty L, Barnes C A, Berry C 1996 Continuing with the pregnancy after a diagnosis of lethal abnormality. British Medical Journal 313:701–702

Clarke A 1994 Genetic counselling. Practice and principles. Routledge, London

Clement S, Wilson J, Sikorski 1998 Women's experiences of antenatal ultrasound scans. In: Clement S (ed.) Psychological perspectives on pregnancy and childbirth. Churchill Livingstone, Edinburgh, p 117–132

Cuckle H S, Wald N J, Thompson S G 1987 Estimating a woman's risk of having a pregnancy associated with Down syndrome using her age and serum alpha feto-protein level. British Journal of Obstetrics and Gynaecology 94:387–402

Department of Health 2001 Good practice in consent implementation guide: consent to examination or treatment. Department of Health Publications (Crown Copyright), London. Online. Available: www.doh.gov.uk/consent

Department of Health 2003 Model of best practice. Down syndrome screening. Department of Health, London. Online. Available: www.screening.nhs.uk/downs/model_best practice.pdf

Dragonas T, Christodoulou G N 1998 Prenatal care. Clinical Psychology Review 18(2):127–142

Drife J O, Donnai D 1991 Antenatal diagnosis of fetal abnormalities. Springer-Verlag, London

European Committee of Medical Ultrasound Safety (ECMUS) 2006 Clinical safety statement for diagnostic ultrasound. Online. Available: www.efsumb.org

Farrant W 1985 Who's for amniocentesis? The politics of prenatal screening. In: Homans H (ed.) The sexual politics of prenatal screening. Gower Press, London

Ferguson P 2001 Skimming the surface: antenatal screening and testing. RCM Midwives Journal 4(8):262–264

Fisher J 2006 Pregnancy loss, breaking bad news and supporting parents. In: Sullivan A, Kean L, Cryer A (eds) Midwife's guide to antenatal investigations. Elsevier, London, p 31–42

Froster U G, Jackson L 1996 Limb defects after chorionic villus sampling: results from an international registry, 1992–1994. Lancet 347:489–494

Furness M E 1990 Fetal ultrasound for entertainment? Medical Journal of Australia 153(7):371

Hawkey M 1998 Psychological impacts on pregnancy: from hormones to genes. British Journal of Midwifery 6(5):310

Health Technology Assessment 2000 Ultrasound screening in pregnancy: a systematic review of the clinical effectiveness, cost-effectiveness and women's views. The National Coordinating Centre for HTA, Southampton

Holzgreve W, Tercanli S, Surbek D et al 1999 Invasive diagnostic methods. In: Rodeck C H, Whittle M J (eds) Fetal medicine: basic science and clinical practice. Churchill Livingstone, Edinburgh, p 417–434

Hunter M 1994 Counselling in obstetrics and gynaecology. British Psychological Society Books, Leicester

Ingram R, Malcarne V 1995 Cognition in depression and anxiety. Same, different or a little of both. In: Craig K, Dobson K (eds) Anxiety and depression in adults and children. Sage, London, p 37–56

Kennard A, Goodburn S, Golightly S et al 1995 Serum screening for Down syndrome. Royal College of Midwives Journal 108(1290):207–210

Kessler S, Levine E 1987 Psychological aspects of genetic counselling IV. The subjective assessment of probability. American Journal of Medical Genetics 28:361–370

Kingston H M 1994 ABC of clinical genetics. BMJ Publishing, London

Kumar S, O'Brien A 2004 Recent developments in fetal medicine. British Medical Journal 328(7446):1002–1006

Langford J 1992 Over 35 and at risk? New Generation 11 (4):4–5

Levine D, Barnes P D, Madsen J R et al 1997 Fetal central nervous system anomalies: MR imaging augments sonographic diagnosis. Radiology 204(3):635–642

Maalouf E F, Counsell S, Battin M et al 1998 Magnetic resonance imaging of the neonatal brain. Hospital Medicine 59:41–45

Manning F A, Platt L D, Sipros L 1980 Antepartum fetal evaluation: development of a fetal biophysical profile. American Journal of Obstetrics and Gynaecology 136:787–795

National Electronic Library for Health 2001 Down syndrome screening. Invasive diagnosis. Online. Available: www.nelh. nhs.uk/screening

Neilson J P 1999 Ultrasound for fetal assessment in early pregnancy. The Cochrane review. In: The Cochrane Library, Issue 3. Update Software, Oxford

Neilson J P, Alfirevic Z 2005 Doppler ultrasound for fetal assessment in high-risk pregnancies. The Cochrane Database of Systematic Reviews, Issue 1

Newnham J P, Evans S F, Mehael C A et al 1993 Effects of frequent ultrasound during pregnancy: a randomised controlled trial. Lancet 342:887–891

NHS Sickle Cell and Thalassaemia Screening Programme 2004. Online. Available: www.sickleandthal.org.uk

NICE (National Institute for Clinical Excellence) 2003 Antenatal care. Routine care for the healthy pregnant woman. National Collaborating Centre for Women's and Children's Health, RCOG Press, London. Online. Available: www.rcog.org.uk/resources/Public/pdf/ Antenatal_Care.pdf

Nicolaides K, de Lourdes B M, Patel F, et al 1994 Comparison of chorionic villus sampling and amniocentesis for fetal karyotyping at 10–13 weeks gestation. Lancet 344:435–439

Nicolaides K H, Souka A P, Noble P L 1999 Fetal nuchal translucency at 10–14 weeks of gestation. In: Rodeck C, Whittle M J (eds) Fetal medicine. Basic science and clinical practice. Churchill Livingstone, London, p 573–580

NMC (Nursing and Midwifery Council) 2004 Midwives rules and standards. NMC, London

Oliver S, Rajan L, Turner H et al 1996 A pilot study of 'informed choice' leaflets on positions in labour and routine ultrasound. NHS Centre for Reviews and Dissemination, York

Raphael-Leff J 1991 Psychological processes of childbearing. Chapman & Hall, London

RCOG (Royal College of Obstetricians and Gynaecologists) 2000 Routine ultrasound screening in pregnancy. Protocol, standards and training. Supplement to

ultrasound screening for fetal abnormalities report of the RCOG working party. RCOG, London. Online. Available: www.rcog.org.uk/index.asp? PageID=1185#20week

Romero R, Ghidini A, Costigan K et al 1989 Prenatal diagnosis of duodenal atresia: does it make any difference? Obstetrics and Gynaecology 71:739–741

Rothman B 1986 The tentative pregnancy. How amniocentesis changes the experience of motherhood. Norton Paperbacks, New York

Salvesen K A 1997 Epidemiology of diagnostic ultrasound exposure during human pregnancies. BMUS Bulletin November:32–34

Salvesen K A, Vatten L J, Eik-Nes S H et al 1993 Routine ultrasonography in utero and subsequent handedness and neurological development. British Medical Journal 307:159–164

Sandelowski M 1994 Channel of desire: fetal ultrasonography in two-use contexts. Qualitative Health Research 4:262–280

Sedgman B, McMahon C, Cairns D et al 2006 The impact of two-dimensional versus three dimensional ultrasound exposure on maternal-fetal attachment and maternal health behavior in pregnancy. Ultrasound in Obstetrics and Gynecology 27:245–251

Simpson J L, Socol M I, Aladam S 1981 Normal fetal growth despite persistent amniotic fluid leakage after genetic amniocentesis. Prenatal Diagnosis 1:277–279

Sjogren B 1996 Psychological indications for prenatal diagnosis. Prenatal Diagnosis 16:449–454

Snijders R, Nicolaides K 1996 Ultrasound markers for fetal chromosomal defects. Parthenon, London

Stark C, Orleans M, Haverkamp A et al 1984 Short and long-term risks after exposure to diagnostic ultrasound in utero. Obstetrics and Gynaecology 63:194–200

Sullivan A 2005 Skilled decision making: the blood supply of midwifery practice. In: Raynor M, Marshall J, Sullivan A (eds) Decision making in midwifery practice. Elsevier, London

Thornton J G, Hewison J, Lilford R J et al 1995 A randomised trial of three methods of giving information about prenatal testing. British Medical Journal 311:1127–1130

Tindall N 1997 Psychology of childbearing. Midwifery practice guides 6. Books for Midwives Press, Hale, Cheshire

Turner L 1994 Problems surrounding late prenatal diagnosis. In: Abramsky L, Chapple J (eds) Prenatal diagnosis. The human side. Chapman & Hall, London

UK National Screening Committee 2004 Antenatal screening working standards. National Down Syndrome Screening Programme for England. Online. Available: www.screening. nhs.uk/downs/working-standards.pdf

Wald N J, Rodeck C, Hackshaw A K et al 2003 First and second trimester antenatal screening for Down syndrome: the results of the Serum, Urine and Ultrasound Screening Study (SURUSS). Health Technology Assessment 7 (11):1–77

Whittle MJ 1997 Ultrasonographic 'soft markers' of fetal chromosomal defects. (Editorial.) British Medical Journal 314:918

Wood P 2000 Safe and (ultra)sound – some aspects of ultrasound safety. Royal College of Midwives Journal 3(2):48–50

FURTHER READING

Sullivan A, Kean L, Cryer A (eds) 2006 Midwifes' guide to antenatal investigations. Elsevier, London

A practical guide for midwives to use when discussing and interpreting antenatal test results. Covers maternal and fetal investigations.

USEFUL WEBSITES

Screening Choices: A learning resource for health professionals offering antenatal and newborn care. Prepared for UK National Screening Committee by Homerton School of Health Studies and Jill Rogers Associates, www.screening.nhs.uk/cpd/webfolder/web_nsc.html

Training resource covering genetics, understanding and communicating risk, informed choice, the parent perspective.

DIPEx – Patient experiences website, www.dipex. org/Experiences.aspx

Includes a range of pregnancy and screening experiences from the woman's perspective. Includes video clips of interviews with women who talk about their experiences

19 Abnormalities of early pregnancy

Ian M. Symonds

This chapter is concerned with conditions that occur during the first 20 weeks of pregnancy. These are a significant cause of maternal morbidity and even on occasion mortality. Midwives will often be the first point of contact by women seeking advice for these problems and be involved in care in both primary and secondary healthcare settings. Increased understanding of the abnormalities that can occur in early pregnancy will enhance the quality of midwifery care provided for these women.

The chapter aims to:

- consider the causes and diagnosis of the common presenting symptoms in early pregnancy of vaginal bleeding, abdominal pain and vomiting
- describe the main causes of pregnancy loss before 20 weeks
- emphasize the need for midwives to be able to offer support and care for mothers early in pregnancy.

Bleeding in early pregnancy

Vaginal bleeding occurs in up to 25% of pregnancies prior to 20 weeks. It is a major cause of anxiety for all women, especially those who have experienced previous pregnancy loss, and may be the presenting symptom of life-threatening conditions, such as ectopic pregnancy. Bleeding should always be considered as abnormal in pregnancy and investigated appropriately.

A small amount of bleeding may occur as the blastocyst implants in the endometrium 5–7 days after fertilization (implantation bleed). If this occurs at the time of expected menstruation it may be confused with a period and so affect calculations of gestational age based on the last menstrual period.

The common causes for bleeding in early pregnancy are miscarriage, ectopic pregnancy and benign lesions in the lower genital tract. Less commonly it may be the presenting symptom of hydatidiform mole or cervical malignancy.

Spontaneous miscarriage

The term miscarriage is normally used in preference to spontaneous abortion because of the association of the latter term with induced abortion. It is defined as the termination of pregnancy prior to 24 weeks' gestation or a fetal weight of <500 g. In practice, with fetal survival rates now of up to 50% at 23 weeks, the management of these babies can best be considered as part of the care of other extremely premature infants born before 26 weeks.

Incidence

A total of 15–20% of clinical pregnancies end in miscarriage. If all women who have had biochemical evidence of pregnancy (i.e. a positive serum hCG) are included, the pregnancy loss rate is as high as 30%. The majority of miscarriages occur prior to 13 weeks' gestation, although 1–2% occur between 13 and 24 weeks (Stirrat 1990).

The aetiology of miscarriage

In many cases no definite cause can be found for miscarriage. It is important to identify this group as the prognosis for future pregnancies is generally better than average (Regan & Rai 2000).

Genetic abnormalities

Up to 50% of sporadic miscarriages are associated with chromosomal abnormalities which result in failure of development of the embryo. The most common chromosomal defects are autosomal trisomies, which account for half the abnormalities, and polyploidy or monosomy X, which account for a further 20% each. Although chromosome abnormalities are common in sporadic miscarriage, parental chromosomal abnormalities are present in only 3–5% of partners presenting with recurrent pregnancy loss.

Endocrine factors

Progesterone is essential for the maintenance of a pregnancy, and early failure of the corpus luteum may lead to miscarriage. However, it is difficult to be certain whether falling plasma progesterone levels represent a primary cause of miscarriage or whether they are a result of a failing pregnancy. The prevalence of polycystic ovarian syndrome (PCOS) is significantly higher in women with recurrent miscarriage than in the general population. Women with poorly controlled diabetes and untreated thyroid disease are at higher risk of miscarriage and fetal malformation.

Maternal illness and infection

Infections such as syphilis, *listeria monocytogenes*, mycoplasma and *Toxoplasma gondii* and severe maternal febrile illnesses associated with infections, such as influenza, pyelitis and malaria predispose to miscarriage. The presence of bacterial vaginosis has been reported as a risk factor for preterm birth and second, but not first trimester, miscarriage (Hay et al 1994). Other severe illnesses involving the cardiovascular, hepatic and renal systems are also associated with increased rates of miscarriage.

Abnormalities of the uterus

Uterine anomalies, such as a bicornuate uterus or subseptate uterus, can be demonstrated in 15–30% of women experiencing recurrent miscarriages. There is an increased frequency of early pregnancy loss in the presence of submucosal fibroids (Benson et al 2001). Following damage to the endometrium and inner uterine walls, the surfaces may become adherent, thus partly obliterating the uterine cavity (Asherman syndrome). The presence of these synechiae may lead to recurrent miscarriage.

Cervical incompetence

Cervical incompetence results in painless dilatation of the cervix, spontaneous rupture of the membranes and miscarriage or early pre-term birth. The diagnosis has historically been made on the basis of the history of previous late pregnancy loss. However, ultrasound examination is being used increasingly to identify where there is an increased risk of premature cervical dilatation. The key feature is shortening of the cervical canal to <25 mm and funneling of the internal cervical os. Cervical incompetence may be associated with other congenital abnormalities of the genital tract but most commonly results from physical damage caused by mechanical dilatation of the cervix or by damage inflicted during childbirth.

Autoimmune factors and thrombophilic defects

The antiphospholipid antibodies lupus anticoagulant (LA) and anticardiolipin antibody (aCL) are present in 2% of women with normal reproductive histories but 15% of women with recurrent miscarriage. Without treatment the live birth rate in women with primary antiphospholipid syndrome may be as low as 10%. Defects in the natural inhibitors of coagulation – antithrombin III, protein C and protein S – are more common in women with recurrent miscarriage. The majority of cases of activated protein C deficiency are secondary to a mutation in the factor V (Leiden) gene.

Pregnancy loss in these conditions is thought to be due to thrombosis of the uteroplacental vasculature and impaired trophoblast function. In addition to miscarriage there is an increased risk of intrauterine growth restriction, pre-eclampsia and venous thrombosis.

Alloimmune factors

Research into the possibility of an immunological basis of recurrent miscarriage has generally explored the possibility of a failure to mount the normal protective immune response or if the expression of relatively non-immunogenic antigens by the cytotrophoblast may result in rejection of the fetal allograft. There is evidence that unexplained spontaneous miscarriage is associated with couples who share an abnormal number of HLA antigens of the A, B, C and DR loci (Beydoun & Saftlas 2005). Despite attempts to treat women with paternal lymphocytes, which initially appeared to reduce the incidence of recurrent miscarriage, subsequent studies have failed to confirm the initial findings.

Clinical presentation

Spontaneous miscarriage progresses through a number of stages with clinical symptoms of vaginal bleeding and lower abdominal pain.

Threatened miscarriage

The presence of bleeding from the uterus in an ongoing early pregnancy is described as a threatened miscarriage. Uterine size is normally consistent with the estimated gestation and the cervical os is closed. Lower abdominal pain is either minimal or absent. Some 80% of women presenting with a threatened miscarriage will continue with the pregnancy.

Inevitable/incomplete miscarriage

In inevitable miscarriage there is usually increasing abdominal pain associated with heavier vaginal bleeding. The cervix opens, and eventually products of conception are passed into the vagina. However, if some of the products of conception are retained, then the miscarriage remains incomplete.

Complete miscarriage

An incomplete miscarriage may proceed to completion spontaneously, when the pain will cease and vaginal bleeding will subside with involution of the uterus.

Miscarriage with infection

During the process of miscarriage – or after therapeutic termination of a pregnancy – infection may be introduced into the uterine cavity. The clinical findings are similar to those of incomplete miscarriage with the addition of uterine and adnexal tenderness. The vaginal loss may become purulent and the patient pyrexial. In cases of severe overwhelming sepsis, endotoxic shock may develop with profound and sometimes fatal hypotension. Other manifestations include renal failure, disseminated intravascular coagulopathy and multiple petechial haemorrhages. Organisms which commonly invade the uterine cavity are *Escherichia coli*, *Streptococcus faecalis*, *Staphylococcus albus* and *aureus*, *Klebsiella*, and *Clostridium welchii* and *C. perfringens*.

Missed or silent miscarriage

Early fetal demise occurs when a pregnancy is identified within the uterus on ultrasound, but despite a fetal pole being visible no fetal heartbeat is seen. In anembryonic pregnancy a gestational sac is seen on ultrasound but there is no evidence of a fetus or fetal parts (Fig. 19.1). There is usually some pain and bleeding and the uterus does not increase in size.

Recurrent miscarriage

Recurrent miscarriage is defined as three or more successive pregnancy losses prior to viability. The incidence of 1% is higher than would be expected by chance given that 15–20% of pregnancies miscarry suggesting that there are persistent factors operating in successive pregnancies to increase the risks of pregnancy loss. However, it is important to remember that after two consecutive miscarriages the likelihood of a successful third pregnancy is still

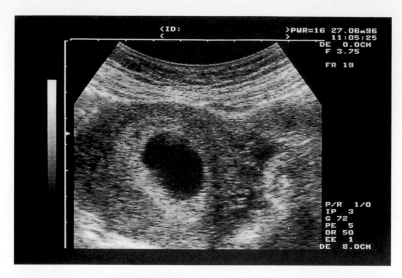

Figure 19.1 The empty gestation sac of a missed miscarriage. (From Symonds E M, Symonds I 2003 Essential Obstetrics and Gynaecology, 4th edn. Churchill Livingstone, Edinburgh.)

around 80%. Even after three consecutive miscarriages, there is still a 55–75% chance of success.

Diagnosis

An initial clinical assessment involves determining haemodynamic status and general condition for evidence of blood loss. Distension of the cervical canal by products of conception in an incomplete miscarriage can cause profound vagal response resulting in hypotension and bradycardia (cervical shock).

Where there is evidence of haemodynamic compromise the key differential diagnosis will be of ruptured ectopic pregnancy. Although there is often considerable lower abdominal pain associated with miscarriage there is not normally evidence of peritonism on abdominal examination.

A vaginal examination to assess whether the cervix is open and to look for the presence of products of conception will distinguish an inevitable or incomplete from a threatened miscarriage.

Transvaginal ultrasound will be required for the majority of women presenting with bleeding in early pregnancy and has a high predictive value for the confirmation of miscarriage. In approximately 10% of women with intrauterine pregnancies viability will be uncertain at the first assessment. This occurs when there is no evidence of a yolk sac or fetus and the gestation sac is <20 mm or there is a fetal pole of <6 mm with no evidence of fetal cardiac

activity. In these cases it will be necessary to repeat the scan a week later to confirm the diagnosis of viability or miscarriage (Fig. 19.1).

For most women presenting with bleeding, urine based human chorionic gonadotrophin (hCG) tests are sensitive enough to confirm pregnancy within 9–10 days of conception. The use of serial hCG measurements is mainly of value in distinguishing miscarriage from ectopic pregnancy. Serum hCG levels double approximately every 48 hrs in 85% of normal intrauterine pregnancies between 4 and 6 weeks' gestation.

Treatment options

For women with threatened miscarriage there is no specific treatment except reassurance that once viability has been confirmed the prognosis for ongoing pregnancy is usually good. There is no evidence that bed rest alters the risk of further bleeding. Where complete miscarriage has occurred no further treatment is indicated other than appropriate resuscitation and replacement of blood loss if indicated. Where there is evidence of retained products of tissue the options include expectant management, medical treatment or surgical uterine evacuation.

Surgical evacuation

Surgical uterine evacuation of retained products of conception (ERPOC) involves the removal of tissue by suction curettage of the uterine cavity under

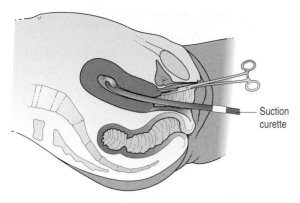

Figure 19.2 Surgical evacuation of retained products of conception. (From Symonds E M, Symonds I 2003 Essential Obstetrics and Gynaecology, 4th edn. Churchill Livingstone, Edinburgh.)

general or local anaesthetic (Fig. 19.2). Until recently, it was standard treatment for all women with miscarriage on the assumption that retained tissue increases the risk of infection and bleeding. In fact, if anything, infection rates are lower in women who are managed expectantly or medically (Demetroulis et al 2001). Despite this up to a third of women express a strong preference for surgical management once the diagnosis of miscarriage has been confirmed (Hindshaw 1997). Clinical indications for ERPOC include persistent excessive bleeding, haemodynamic instability, evidence of infected retained tissue and suspected gestational trophoblastic disease. Where infection is suspected antibiotic treatment should be given for 12–24 hrs before surgery. Preoperative treatment with prostaglandins makes it easier to dilate the cervix and reduces the risk of bleeding and cervical/uterine trauma.

Complications of surgery include uterine perforation, cervical tears, intra-abdominal trauma, intrauterine adhesions and bleeding. The overall incidence of serious morbidity is similar to that for surgical termination of pregnancy at 1–2%.

Women who have lower genital tract infections with chlamydia, gonorrhoea or bacterial vaginosis are at increased risk of pelvic inflammatory disease following surgical evacuation. Screening for chlamydia by urinary polymerase chain reaction (PCR) or endocervical swabs should be offered to women undergoing surgical management. The routine use of antibiotic prophylaxis prior to surgery has not been shown to reduce the incidence of postoperative pelvic inflammatory disease.

Expectant management

The natural history of most cases of miscarriage will be the spontaneous passage of products of conception. Waiting for this to happen is an effective and acceptable alternative to surgery for women where there is no infection or heavy bleeding. It is important that women who choose this option are aware that complete resolution may take several weeks, particularly where there is an intact gestation sac. Expectant management is more likely to be successful in incomplete miscarriage (94%; range 80–100%) than missed miscarriage (28%; range 14–47%) (Graziosi et al 2004).

Medical management

Various treatment regimes using prostaglandins with or without antiprogesterone have been described. Reported efficacy rates vary from 13–96%. Success rates for medical treatment vary according to the type of miscarriage, gestation, sac size (if present), total dose of prostaglandin and route of administration. Success rates for incomplete miscarriage are comparable to surgical treatment with equal patient satisfaction and lower rates of pelvic infection (Demetroulis et al 2001). Potential complicating factors are increased pain and blood loss and duration of bleeding.

Medical and expectant management can be undertaken on an outpatient basis. It is important that this is supported by access to 24 hrs telephone advice and emergency admission if required.

Anti-D immunoglobulin

Rhesus negative women who are non-sensitized should receive Anti-D immunoglobulin following any bleeding in pregnancy after 12 weeks' gestation including threatened miscarriage. In pregnancies <12 weeks anti-D should be given where the bleeding is heavy or associated with pain or after medical or surgical evacuation of the uterus. The discharge documentation should state whether anti-D was given (RCOG 2002).

Recurrent miscarriage

Recurrent miscarriage should be investigated by examining the karyotype of both parents and, if possible any fetal products. Maternal blood should be examined for lupus anticoagulant and anticardiolipin antibodies on at least two occasions, 6 weeks apart. An ultrasound scan should be arranged to assess ovarian morphology for polycystic ovarian syndrome (PCOS) and the uterine cavity (RCOG 2003). Women with persistent lupus anticoagulant and anticardiolipin antibodies can be treated with low-dose aspirin and heparin during subsequent pregnancies (Rai et al 1996). Those with karyotypic abnormalities should be referred to a clinical geneticist. Cervical cerclage carried out at 14–16 weeks in cases of cervical incompetence reduces the incidence of pre-term birth but has not been shown to improve fetal survival.

Organization of care

The efficiency of service and quality can be improved by the use of dedicated Early Pregnancy Assessment Units (EPAU). Admission to hospital can be avoided in 40% of cases and length of stay reduced in a further 20% (Bigrigg & Read 1991). Direct access should be available to GPs and selected patients such as those who have had a previous ectopic pregnancy or recurrent miscarriage. Facilities for transvaginal ultrasound scanning and rapid access to rhesus antibody testing and serum human chorionic gonadotrophin (hCG) estimation should be available. Except where bleeding is heavy or ectopic pregnancy suspected most women can be give an appointment to be assessed in the clinic during the day reducing the need for out-of-hours admission. These units function best when dedicated nursing staff use established diagnostic and therapeutic algorithms of care.

Psychological aspects of miscarriage

Miscarriage is often not regarded medically as 'serious' and is usually not investigated further when it occurs for the first time. As a result, many women do not receive an explanation of their loss. There is no evidence to associate miscarriage with an overall increased risk of psychiatric morbidity. However, feelings of anger, grief and guilt are common and almost half of all women are considerably distressed at 6 weeks following miscarriage.

Women who lose pregnancies in the second trimester face the same risks of postpartum 'mood disorder' as women in the normal puerperium. Grief reactions are usually more severe and may persist for up to 6 months following the loss of their pregnancy (see Ch. 38). (see Box 19.1 for key points)

Box 19.1 Summary of key points on miscarriage

1. Miscarriage is the spontaneous loss of pregnancy before 24 weeks.
2. The commonest causes are chromosome abnormalities in the fetus.
3. Most women can be offered medical or expectant management.
4. Grieving is an essential part of the recovery process following miscarriage.

Ectopic pregnancy

The term 'ectopic pregnancy' refers to any pregnancy occurring outside the uterine cavity (see Box 19.2). Ectopic pregnancy occurs in 1 in 100 pregnancies in the UK and accounted for 3% of pregnancy related deaths between 1994 and 1996. Between 1973 and 1996, the number of ectopic pregnancies per 1000 pregnancies increased from 4.9 to 11.5, while mortality fell from 16 to 4/10 000 cases (DoH 1998, Lewis & Drife 2001). The last 20 years have also seen major changes in both the diagnosis and treatment of the disease.

Pathology

The commonest site of extrauterine implantation is the uterine tube, usually in the ampullary region. Ectopic implantation may also occur on the ovary, in the abdominal cavity or in the cervical canal (Fig. 19.3). Abdominal pregnancy may result from direct implantation of the conceptus or it may result from extrusion of a tubal pregnancy with secondary implantation in the peritoneal cavity. As with normal pregnancy the conceptus produces hCG, which maintains the corpus luteum and the production of oestrogen and progesterone. This causes the uterus to enlarge and the endometrium to undergo decidual change.

Trophoblastic cells invade the wall of the tube and erode into blood vessels of the mesosalpinx. This process will continue until the pregnancy ruptures into the abdominal cavity or the broad ligament, or the embryo dies, thus resulting in a tubal mole. Under these circumstances, absorption or tubal miscarriage may occur. Expulsion of the embryo into the peritoneal cavity or partial miscarriage may also

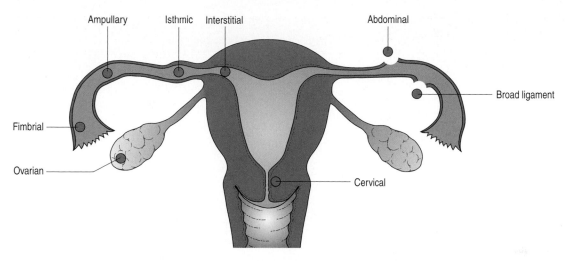

Figure 19.3 Sites of implantation of ectopic pregnancy. (From Symonds E M, Symonds I 2003 Essential Obstetrics and Gynaecology, 4th edn. Churchill Livingstone, Edinburgh.)

occur with continuing episodes of bleeding from the tube (Fig. 19.4). Vaginal bleeding occurs as a result of shedding of the decidual lining of the endometrium and progesterone levels fall with the failing pregnancy.

Predisposing factors

The majority of cases of ectopic pregnancy have no identifiable predisposing factor, but a previous history of ectopic pregnancy, sterilization, pelvic inflammatory disease and sub-fertility all increase the likelihood of an ectopic pregnancy. The increased risk for an intrauterine device (IUCD) applies only to pregnancies that occur despite the presence of the IUCD. Because of their effectiveness as contraceptives ectopic rates per year in IUCD users are lower than in women not using contraception (Table 19.1).

Clinical presentation

Acute presentation

The 'classical' pattern of symptoms includes amenorrhoea, lower abdominal pain and vaginal bleeding. The abdominal pain is typically of sudden onset starting on one side of the lower abdomen, but rapidly becomes generalized as blood loss extends into the peritoneal cavity. Sub-diaphragmatic irritation by blood produces referred shoulder tip pain and discomfort on breathing. There may be episodes of syncope.

The findings on clinical examination are hypotension, tachycardia and signs of peritonism including abdominal distension, guarding and rebound tenderness. On pelvic examination the cervix is closed and acutely tender when moved (cervical excitation) because of irritation of the pelvic peritoneum caused by the bleeding. This type of acute presentation occurs in no more than 25% of cases.

Subacute presentation

The majority of ectopic pregnancies present less acutely and some or all of the classic symptoms of pain, bleeding and amenorrhoea may be absent (Sperov et al 1994). Typically, there is a history of amenorrhoea or of an abnormally light last 'period' followed by irregular vaginal bleeding and abdominal pain. Any woman who develops lower abdominal pain following an interval of amenorrhoea should be assessed for a possible ectopic pregnancy. In its subacute phase, it may be possible to feel a mass in one fornix on vaginal examination although this should be undertaken with care because of the risk of provoking rupture of the ectopic pregnancy.

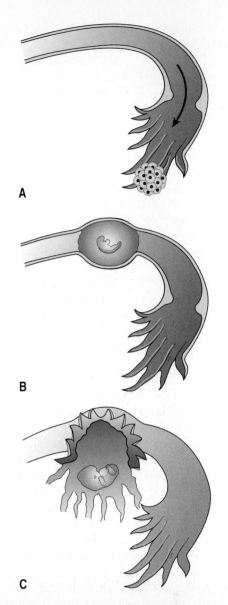

Figure 19.4 Possible outcomes of tubal pregnancy: (A) tubal abortion; (B) tubal mole; (C) tubal rupture.

Table 19.1 Risk factors and associated relative risk of ectopic pregnancy

Risk factor	Relative risk
Previous ectopic pregnancy	10
Failed IUCD	10
Failed sterilization	9
Previous tubal surgery	4.5
Previous pelvic inflammatory disease	4

Ling & Stovall 1994, Sperov et al 1994.

Diagnosis

While the diagnosis of the acute ectopic pregnancy rarely presents a problem, diagnosis in the subacute phase may be much more difficult. The commonest diagnosis to be made in error on clinical diagnosis is threatened or incomplete miscarriage. It may also be confused with complications of ovarian cysts or acute salpingitis. Because bleeding into the peritoneum can cause bowel irritation maternal deaths have been reported when the diagnosis has been delayed in patients presenting with symptoms of abdominal pain and diarrhoea (DoH 1998). The overall accuracy of clinical diagnosis is only 50% (Ling & Stovall 1994).

The high sensitivity of modern immunoassays for hCG (98% for urine and 100% for serum) (Sperov et al 1994) mean that a negative serum hCG will effectively exclude ectopic pregnancy. It should be possible to visualize a normal intrauterine pregnancy on transvaginal ultrasound when the serum level of hCG is >1500 IU/L (6000–6500 IU/L for transabdominal), although in multiple pregnancy this level may be higher. A rise of <66% in the serum hCG between two levels taken 48 hrs apart is associated with >80% of ectopic pregnancies (Kadar et al 1981) but is also seen in non-viable intrauterine pregnancies and in up to 15% of normal pregnancies (Sperov et al 1994).

The main value of ultrasound is to confirm intrauterine pregnancy. Confirmation of an intrauterine pregnancy does not exclude heterotopic pregnancy, which although rare in spontaneous conceptions (1/3000–4000), can be seen in up to 3% of pregnancies resulting from assisted reproduction. Ultrasound may also provide direct evidence of ectopic pregnancy (Table 19.2) with the commonest finding being an extraovarian solid tubal mass (Atri et al 1996) and free fluid in the peritoneal cavity. The combination of serial serum hCG measurement and transvaginal ultrasound has a sensitivity and specificity for the diagnosis of ectopic pregnancy that is comparable with laparoscopy (Sadek & Schiotz 1995).

Laparoscopy has been the mainstay of diagnosis for the last 30 years. False negatives occur in 3–4%

Table 19.2 Features of intrauterine and ectopic pregnancy on transvaginal ultrasound

Intrauterine pregnancy	Ectopic pregnancy
Intrauterine gestation sac (4–5 weeks)	Empty uterus
Yolk sac (5–6 weeks)	Poorly defined tubal ring with fluid in Pouch of Douglas
Double decidual sign (5 weeks)	Pseudosac in uterus
Fetal heartbeat (7 weeks)	Tubal ring with extrauterine heartbeat

Sadek & Schiotz 1995, Dodson 1991.

of cases and false positives in up to 5% (Ling & Stovall 1994), with interpretation being especially difficult in very early pregnancy and in the presence of previous pelvic pathology. Using algorithms incorporating quantitative hCG measurements, transvaginal ultrasound and clinical symptoms allows earlier diagnosis, results in fewer ruptured ectopics and reduces the need for diagnostic laparoscopy (especially those done out-of-hours) (Ling & Stovall 1994). Furthermore, the diagnostic accuracy of laparoscopy itself is improved when used together with the hCG and ultrasound results.

Surgical treatment

Laparotomy is indicated in the haemodynamically compromised patient and may be indicated in obese patients or those with extensive pelvic adhesions or haemoperitoneum depending on the experience and training of the operator in laparoscopic surgery.

The advantages of laparoscopic compared with open surgery include lower blood loss and reduced need for postoperative pain relief. Mean duration of hospital stay is 50% less than for open surgery (Vu et al 1996) and there are similar or greater reductions in the time to return to normal activity.

Whether the laparotomy or laparoscopy is used there are two main options for surgical removal of the ectopic: partial salpingectomy (removal of part of the tube) or salpingotomy (leaving the tube in place and removing the ectopic through an incision in the wall of the tube). Salpingotomy is associated with a higher rate of subsequent intrauterine pregnancy than salpingectomy but also results in a higher

rate of recurrent ectopic pregnancy. Of those women who attempt to conceive following salpingotomy for ectopic pregnancy, 61% achieve intrauterine pregnancy and 15% have further ectopic pregnancies (Yao & Tulandi 1997). It must be remembered that other factors influence subsequent fertility rates as much, if not more than the surgical treatment used. In particular, these are a previous history of infertility and the condition of the contralateral tube at the time of surgery (Pouly et al 1991, Yao & Tulandi 1997).

Where the tube is not removed, there is a risk that some gestational tissue may be left in place and continue to develop. Follow-up with weekly hCG measurements is therefore necessary after conservative surgery and it may take up to 10 weeks for these to return to normal.

Salpingectomy remains the treatment of choice where there is uncontrolled bleeding or a second ectopic pregnancy in the same tube. It should also be discussed where childbearing is complete or for a severely damaged tube.

Expectant management

A proportion of haemodynamically stable patients with falling hCG levels will show spontaneous resolution of ectopic pregnancy. The overall success rate of this approach is 69%, although higher rates have been reported where the initial hCG was <200 IU/L (Yao & Tulandi 1997). An hCG level of >2000 is an absolute contraindication to expectant management. Furthermore, tubal rupture has been reported even in low and falling levels of hCG. The efficacy and safety of systemic methotrexate make this a more attractive alternative to surgical management.

Medical management

Medical treatment has the advantage of avoiding the need for surgery with concomitant reductions in cost and surgical morbidity. The commonest drug used is methotrexate, an antimetabolite that interferes with the synthesis of DNA, given i.m. as a single dose of 1 mg/kg body weight or 50 mg/m^2. Multiple dose regimes have higher success rates but are associated with more side-effects. Weekly follow-up with serum hCG levels is required. Success rates of up to 92% have been reported but 5% of patients will require surgery for failed treatment. Subsequent intrauterine and ectopic pregnancy rates appear comparable with those reported for surgical treatment (54% and 8%, respectively) (Slaughter & Grimes 1995).

The success of medical treatment is related to the serum hCG level, size of the ectopic and the presence of fetal cardiac activity Although significant adverse effects are uncommon after systemic administration of methotrexate, up to 60% of patients experience increased abdominal pain 6–7 days after treatment (Yao & Tulandi 1997). Good patient compliance is essential for non-surgical treatment and selection of suitably reliable individuals is as important as the size of the ectopic itself.

Although promising, the clinical role for methotrexate, given the availability of highly effective and safe conservative surgical treatments, remains unproven. It can be considered as an alternative to surgical treatment where the serum hCG is <2000 IU/L and the ectopic <2 cm with no fetal cardiac activity seen (Shalev et al 1995).

Box 19.2 Summary of key points on ectopic pregnancy

1. Ectopic pregnancy is the commonest cause of direct maternal death in early pregnancy.

2. Ectopic pregnancy should be considered in any woman presenting with pain or bleeding in early pregnancy.

3. The use of diagnostic algorithms incorporating transvaginal ultrasound and serum hCG measurement allows most cases of ectopic pregnancy to be diagnosed without surgery.

4. Most cases of ectopic pregnancy can be treated laparoscopically.

5. Medical treatment with methotrexate is a suitable alternative to surgery in selected cases.

Trophoblastic disease

This is a group of disorders characterized by abnormal placental development. The chorionic villi are hydropic with vacuolation of the placenta and destruction of the normal stroma.

Incidence

Trophoblastic disorders affect 1.5 per 1000 pregnancies in the UK (Bagshawe et al 1986). There is considerable geographic variation in incidence, the highest being in countries of the Far East.

Pathology

Benign trophoblastic disease is usually either a complete hydatidiform mole, where there is no evidence of an embryo, or a partial hydatidiform mole which may be associated with an embryo (usually abnormal) (Szulman 1988). Other types of trophoblastic disease include invasive moles, placental site reactions, trophoblastic tumours and hydropic change.

Malignant trophoblastic disease (choriocarcinoma) complicates approximately 3% of complete moles although in 50% of cases of choriocarcinoma there is no history of immediately preceding trophoblastic disease. It may also occur following normal pregnancy. Blood-borne metastases may occur locally in the vagina but most commonly appear in the lungs.

Aetiology

Trophoblastic disease is thought to arise by fertilization of the oocyte by a single diploid spermatozoon or by two haploid sperm. If this occurs in the absence of any female nuclear material the resulting conceptus pregnancy is a complete mole with a diploid karyotype (46XX). A partial mole is thought to occur where fertilization occurs with the maternal chromosome and the conceptus is triploid (69XXX or 69XXY). Older women and those with a previous history of trophoblastic disease or an A type blood group are at increased risk (Lawler et al 1991).

Presentation

Molar pregnancy most commonly presents as bleeding in the first half of pregnancy, and is usually diagnosed initially as a threatened miscarriage. Occasionally, the passage of a 'grape-like' tissue raises a clinical suspicion but the diagnosis is normally made on ultrasound or after uterine evacuation. The uterus is larger than dates in about half the cases. Associated conditions include severe hyperemesis, pre-eclampsia and unexplained anaemia and ovarian cysts. The high circulating levels of hCG have a TSH like action and can cause clinical thyrotoxicosis. Choriocarcinomas may present with the symptoms of distant metastases (cerebral, pulmonary).

Diagnosis

A 'snowstorm' appearance with multiple highly reflective echoes and areas of vacuolation within the uterine cavity on ultrasound examination usually suggests molar disease. In a partial mole, a gestation sac with a fetus may also be present. Other imaging, such as chest X-rays, CT or MRI may be indicated to exclude pulmonary or cerebral metastases if choriocarcinoma is suspected. The diagnosis of trophoblastic disease is confirmed by histological examination of products of conception removed at the time of uterine evacuation.

Management

Once the diagnosis is established, the pregnancy is terminated by suction curettage. Occasionally, repeat evacuation may be required if there is persistent bleeding or a raised serum hCG but routine second evacuation is not helpful. All cases of molar pregnancy in the UK should be registered with one of the trophoblastic disease screening centres who will arrange follow-up.

The aim of follow-up is to detect persistent trophoblastic disease and choriocarcinoma. Because all trophoblastic tumours produce hCG patients can be monitored by measurement of urinary or serum hCG levels. Levels are checked fortnightly until the serum level is <2 IU/L, and then monthly for 6 months following this if the hCG is negative within 6 weeks of treatment. If the hCG takes longer than 6 weeks to become negative, follow-up is continued for a further 12 months (Newlands et al 2001, RCOG 2004). Patients should be counselled to avoid pregnancy until 6 months after the serum hCG levels fall to normal.

There is a 0.8–2.9% risk of recurrence in subsequent pregnancies after one mole, 15–28% after two moles and serum hCG levels should be checked 6 weeks after any subsequent pregnancy.

Chemotherapy with methotrexate (with folinic acid rescue) is indicated for a rising hCG level in the absence of a new pregnancy, an hCG persistently >20 000 IU/L by 4 weeks after treatment, persistent symptoms or evidence of metastatic disease. Subsequent fertility does not appear to be impaired by chemotherapy and there does not seem to be an increased incidence of other chromosomal abnormalities.

Other causes of bleeding in early pregnancy

Vaginal bleeding in pregnancy may occur from other lesions in the lower genital tract in the same way as in non-pregnant women of the same age. These may be normal physiological variants such as cervical ectropion, benign or malignant neoplastic lesions or infections.

Cervical ectropion (eversion)

This condition is commonly and erroneously known as cervical erosion. Following puberty and increasingly in pregnancy high levels of oestrogen cause proliferation of columnar epithelial cells, found in the cervical canal. As a result the area of columnar epithelium extends beyond the external cervical os onto the vaginal surface of cervix giving a dark red appearance (Fig. 19.5).

Hyperactivity of the endocervical cells increases the quantity of vaginal discharge. There is only a single layer of epithelial cells covering the underlying stroma and capillaries in columnar epithelium so this tends to be more friable and liable to bleed. This may cause intermittent bloodstained loss, or spontaneous bleeding, particularly following sexual intercourse. The ectropion will usually reduce in size during the puerperium and normally requires no treatment in pregnancy.

Cervical polyps

These are small, vascular pedunculated growths consisting of squamous or columnar epithelium covering a core of connective tissue and blood vessels. They are thought to arise by hyperplasia of the underlying epithelium and can arise from either the cervical canal or the ectocervix. They may be asymptomatic or cause bleeding during pregnancy. They can be visualized on speculum examination and no treatment is required during pregnancy, unless bleeding is profuse or a cervical smear suggests malignancy.

Carcinoma of the cervix

The incidence of cancer in pregnancy is 1 in 6000 live births (Lewis & Drife 2001). Carcinoma of the cervix is the most frequently diagnosed cancer in pregnancy. Some 80% of cases detected in pregnancy are diagnosed in the first or second trimester. The disease is

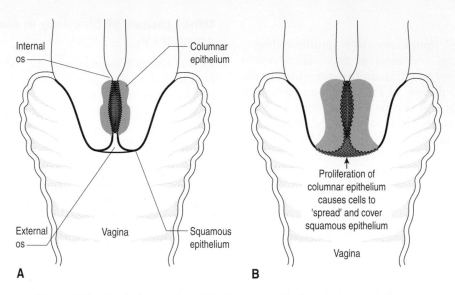

Figure 19.5 Cervical ectropion: (A) columnar epithelium becomes profuse in pregnancy; (B) cervical eversion caused by growth of columnar epithelial cells.

usually squamous cell carcinoma although up to 40% of cases now reported are adenocarcinomas.

Aetiology

Cervical neoplasia is strongly associated with infection with some serotypes of human papilloma virus (HPV). Two serotypes, 16 and 18, are found in >70% of cases of invasive disease. HPV infection is common (80% of women will have some evidence of exposure by the age of 50) and the reasons that some women develop neoplasia while others exposed to the virus do not is not clear, although it does appear related to how long the virus persists in the epithelium (NHSCSP 2005, Schlecht et al 2001).

Clinical presentation and diagnosis

The commonest presenting symptom is blood stained vaginal discharge. The diagnosis may be suspected on routine cervical screening or because of the appearance of the cervix on speculum examination. Confirmation of the diagnosis is made by colposcopy and cervical biopsy.

Treatment

Treatment depends on the stage of the disease and gestation.

Cone biopsy under general anaesthesia involves excision of cervical tissue and is both a diagnostic tool and a treatment for early stage disease. The cervix is highly vascular in pregnancy so that the risk of haemorrhage is high, and there is the possibility of causing the mother to miscarry.

If the changes to the cervix are advanced and diagnosis is made in the first or second trimester, the mother may have to make a choice as to whether to terminate the pregnancy in order to undergo treatment. If diagnosis is made later in pregnancy, a decision to deliver the fetus may be taken to allow the mother to commence treatment.

Cervical intraepithelial neoplasia

Cervical intraepithelial neoplasia (CIN) is the precursor to invasive cancer of the cervix and is normally diagnosed by colposcopy following referral for an abnormal Papanicolaou smear (Pap smear). The condition is asymptomatic and treatment can usually be deferred until after the pregnancy. For high-grade CIN, follow-up with colposcopy during the pregnancy is normally carried out to check for any signs of invasive disease.

Vaccination against HPV 16 and 18 became available in 2007 for women aged up to 26 and appears to be effective in preventing the development of CIN associated with these serotypes. The vaccines are not licensed for use during pregnancy. Vaccination will not obviate the need for cervical screening but should substantially reduce the risk of developing CIN/cervical cancer.

Midwives have a role in explaining the value of regular smear tests to mothers. National guidelines in the UK recommend that every woman between the ages of 25 and 49 has a cervical smear test every 3 years, and from 50–64 every 5 years. Where there is no evidence of a recent smear having been carried out, it may be appropriate for a smear to be taken during pregnancy. Simple explanations about the procedure can help overcome anxieties about the smear test. Cervical screening may be carried out at the 6-week postnatal examination. For women under the age of 26 this should now also be an opportunity to discuss the benefits of vaccination against HPV. Midwives acting as advocates for disadvantaged mothers should be aware that women who are at risk include those with learning disabilities, those from minority ethnic and those from indigenous populations. This group of women are vulnerable through sexual activity, sexual abuse and smoking and are less likely to access healthcare (NHSCSP 2000).

Lower genital tract infection

Inflammatory change in the cervix (cervicitis) or vagina can present with increased vaginal discharge or bleeding in pregnancy. Women in the reproductive age group, especially those aged 16–25 are at greatest risk of sexually transmitted infections such as *Chlamydia Trachomatis* and *Neisseria Gonorrhoea*. Non-STIs including candidiasis and bacterial vaginosis may also be associated with increased susceptibility of the vaginal mucosa to bleeding. Screening for chlamydia with urinary PCR should be included in the investigation of women presenting with lower genital tract bleeding (see also Ch. 23).

Nausea and vomiting in early pregnancy

Nausea and vomiting are common symptoms in early pregnancy usually starting between 4 and 10 weeks' gestation, and resolving before 20 weeks. *Hyperemesis gravidarum* is defined as persistent pregnancy-related vomiting associated with weight loss of >5% of body mass and ketosis. Affecting 0.3–3% of all pregnant women, this is associated with dehydration, electrolyte imbalance and thiamine deficiency. (see Box 19.3)

Aetiology

The aetiology of hyperemesis is uncertain, with multifactorial causes, such as endocrine, gastrointestinal and psychological factors proposed. Hyperemesis occurs more often in multiple pregnancy and hydatidiform mole, suggesting an association with the level of hCG. Although transient abnormalities of thyroid function are common this does not require treatment in the absence of other clinical features of hyperthyroidism. Infection with *Helicobacter pylori*, the organism implicated in gastric ulcers, may also contribute (Frigo et al 1998). Women with a previous history of hyperemesis are likely to experience it in subsequent pregnancies (Snell et al 1998).

Diagnosis

It is important to ask about the frequency of vomiting, trigger factors and whether any other members of the family have been affected. A history of vomiting in a previous pregnancy or outside pregnancy should be sought. Smoking and alcohol can both exacerbate symptoms, and should be enquired of. If this pregnancy resulted from fertility treatment, or there is a close family history of twins, a multiple pregnancy is more likely. Early pregnancy bleeding or a past history of trophoblastic disease may point to a hydatidiform mole.

The clinical features of dehydration include tachycardia, hypotension and loss of skin turgor. Causes of vomiting not due to pregnancy, such as thyroid problems, urinary tract infection or gastroenteritis, need to be excluded so the abdomen should be palpated for areas of tenderness, especially in the right upper quadrant, hypogastrium and renal angles. A dipstick analysis of the urine for ketones, blood or protein should be performed.

Routine investigations should include full blood count, electrolytes, liver and thyroid function tests. Elevated haematocrit, alterations in electrolyte levels and ketonuria are associated with dehydration. Urine should be sent for culture to exclude infection and an ultrasound arranged to look for multiple pregnancy or gestational trophoblastic disease.

Management

The impact of nausea and vomiting on the woman and her daily life should not be underestimated.

The midwife should enquire of all women attending for early antenatal care whether they are experiencing nausea or vomiting. If the vomiting is mild to moderate, and not causing signs of dehydration then usually, reassurance and advice will be all that is necessary.

Simple measures include:

- taking small, carbohydrate meals
- avoiding large volume drinks, especially milk and carbonated drinks
- raising the head of the bed if reflux is a problem.

A history of persistent, severe vomiting with evidence of dehydration requires admission to hospital for assessment and management of symptoms.

Hypovolaemia and electrolyte imbalance should be corrected by intravenous fluids. These should be balanced electrolyte solutions or normal saline as overly rapid rehydration with 5% dextrose can result in water intoxication.

Thromboprophylaxis with compression stockings and low molecular weight heparin should be considered. Most women will settle in 24–48 hrs with these supportive measures. Once the vomiting has ceased, small amounts of fluid, and eventually food can be re-introduced. It is worthwhile doing this gently. If rushed, many women relapse and require re-admission.

Antiemetic therapy is reserved for those women who do not settle on supportive measures, or who persistently relapse. The use of antiemetics in pregnancy received widespread publicity when links were found between thalidomide and severe malformations of children born to mothers who had taken the drug for morning sickness. Currently antihistamines are the recommended pharmacological first line treatment for nausea and vomiting, no antiemetic being approved for treatment. Metoclopramide and prochlorperazine have not been shown to be teratogenic in man (though metoclopramide is in animals).

Vitamin supplements including thiamine should be given, particularly where hyperemesis has been prolonged. If vomiting continues, and the history is suggestive of severe reflux or ulcer disease, endoscopy can be very valuable. It is a safe technique in pregnancy. If severe oesophagitis is confirmed then appropriate treatment with alginates and metoclopramide can be given. Ulcer disease will require H2 antagonist treatment (ranitidine) or if very severe, omeprazole, though there is limited experience of this in pregnancy.

Very occasionally, women do not settle with a combination of the above measures. Some of these women may improve with steroid therapy, though trials are still ongoing. Women in whom there is liver function derangement may benefit particularly. H2 antagonists must be given in conjunction with the steroid treatment. Parenteral nutrition is necessary for some that develop severe protein/calories malnutrition. Specialized nutrition units can be very helpful in this setting.

If hyperemesis is left untreated, the mother's condition worsens. Wernicke's encephalopathy is a complication associated with a lack of vitamin B_1 (thiamine). Coma and death have been reported because of hepatic and renal involvement. Termination of pregnancy may reverse the condition and has a place in preventing maternal mortality. Hyperemesis persisting into the third trimester should be further investigated as it may be symptomatic of serious illness such as acute fatty liver of pregnancy (Lewis & Drife 2001).

Box 19.3 Nausea and vomiting in pregnancy

- Hyperemesis gravidarum is severe persistent vomiting starting before 20 weeks in pregnancy and associated with ketosis and weight loss
- Prolonged vomiting can be associated with life-threatening complications including encephalopathy, renal and hepatic failure
- Hospital admission is indicated where there is evidence of dehydration or electrolyte imbalance
- Transient abnormalities of thyroid and liver function tests may occur in hyperemesis and do not require treatment.

Abdominal pain in early pregnancy

Abdominal pain is a common presenting symptom for miscarriage and ectopic pregnancy in early pregnancy. As in non-pregnant women, there is a long potential list of other differential diagnoses of causes and in some cases no definitive diagnosis will be reached and management will be symptomatic. This section concentrates on those causes that are specific to the reproductive tract other than miscarriage and ectopic pregnancy and some of the commoner non-gynaecological conditions that can present with pain in early pregnancy.

Retroversion of the uterus

Where the angle between the long axis of the uterus and the axis of the vagina is >180°, the uterus is said to be retroverted. In most cases this causes no problems during pregnancy and corrects spontaneously as the uterus rises out of the pelvis into the abdomen as pregnancy progresses.

Incarceration of the retroverted gravid uterus

If the retroverted uterus fails to rise out of the pelvic cavity by the 14th week, it is said to be incarcerated. The growing uterus is confined within the pelvis, beneath the sacral promontory. Pressure causes abdominal discomfort, and a feeling of pelvic fullness, low abdominal or back pain. Frequency of micturition, dysuria and paradoxical incontinence are the result of the urethra being elongated as the cervix is increasingly displaced. Compression of the bladder neck leads to urinary retention. Urinary stasis can result in infections developing, including pyelonephritis (Myers & Scotti 1995).

On examination, the bladder will be palpable abdominally. Demonstrating effective clinical practice the midwife should explain, and gain consent for catheterization to relieve the retention of urine. An indwelling catheter is used to keep the bladder empty, enabling the uterus to rise out of the pelvis.

Fibroids (leiomyomas)

These are firm, benign tumours of muscular and fibrous tissue, ranging in size from very small to very large. The incidence of detectable fibroids in pregnancy is 1%; the lowest risk being in Caucasian women, but risk increases in Afro-Caribbean women and women over 35-years-old (Lumsden & Wallace 1998).

Although ultrasound monitoring of fibroids has demonstrated that they do not significantly increase in size during pregnancy (Aharoni et al 1988, Davis et al 1990), they do become more vascular and oedematous. Red degeneration of a fibroid occurs when a rapidly growing fibroid occludes its own venous drainage. The central core necroses, and bleeding occurs into the middle. The mother experiences severe abdominal pain that is acute in nature (Katz et al 1989), the affected area is tender on palpation, and she may also have low-grade pyrexia.

Referral for ultrasound scan aids differential diagnosis of the pain, as the relationship between the placental site and the focus of pain can be established. The degeneration can be seen clearly on ultrasound. The pain is normally relieved by rest and analgesia; no other treatment is required (Lumsden & Wallace 1998).

Ovarian cysts

Incidence

Between 1 in 80 and 1 in 300 pregnancies are complicated by the presence of ovarian cysts (Singer 1989). The majority of these will be benign, the commonest being functional ovarian cysts (follicular cysts, corpus luteum). The commonest solid, benign ovarian cysts found in pregnancy are mature cystic teratomas (dermoid cysts). Most cystic neoplasms are epithelial (serous or mucinous cystadenomas). Between 2% and 5% of ovarian cysts in pregnancy will be malignant with an overall incidence of between 1 in 8000 and 1 in 20 000 pregnancies.

Diagnosis

Most lesions are asymptomatic and diagnosed following palpation of an abdominal or pelvic mass or on routine ultrasound scanning for fetal viability or abnormality. Symptoms usually arise as a result of complications, such as torsion or rupture of the cyst causing abdominal pain, nausea, vomiting and local tenderness. Torsion (but not haemorrhage and rupture) is more common in pregnancy and in the puerperium than at other times (complicates 10–15% of tumours). Ultrasound examination should be arranged to distinguish ovarian cysts from other types of pelvic mass. Definitive diagnosis can only be made by removal of the cyst at laparotomy.

Management

Asymptomatic cysts of <10 cm can be left and monitored by ultrasound. They will usually resolve without treatment after birth. It is important to remember that in the first trimester the continuation of the pregnancy is dependant on progesterone produced by the corpus luteum and if this is removed the pregnancy will miscarry unless progesterone supplements are given.

Laparotomy is indicated for cysts that are persistently >10 cm in diameter, are enlarging, or contain abnormal features on ultrasound scan (complex multilocular or solid areas). Unless indicated earlier because of an acute surgical complication of the cyst such as torsion, laparotomy is usually performed during the mid-trimester at 16 weeks (by which time the pregnancy is not dependant on the corpus luteum and miscarriage is less likely). Benign lesions are treated by unilateral cystectomy or salpingo-oophorectomy. Stage I ovarian carcinoma can be treated by unilateral salpingo-oophorectomy providing that there is no obvious invasion of the capsule or involvement of the contralateral ovary and no ascites. Where the diagnosis is made in the second trimester, a decision will need to be made on a case by case basis as to whether to delay treatment to allow the pregnancy to reach viability.

Other causes of abdominal pain in early pregnancy

Urinary tract infection

Lower urinary tract infection is common in pregnancy and should be treated because of the increased risk of ascending infection. Acute pyelonephritis occurs in 1–2% of pregnant women. The clinical features include fever, loin tenderness and urinary frequency. Treatment should be as an inpatient with intravenous antibiotics, fluids and adequate analgesia.

Urolithiasis

Renal colic occurs in 0.03–0.5% of pregnancies. Urinary calculi in pregnancy normally present with sudden onset abdominal pain, which is severe enough to warrant hospital admission, associated with urinary tract infection and haematuria. Ultrasound scan findings of unilateral hydronephrosis or a calcified area are suggestive of renal calculi. The management should be conservative with intravenous fluids, antibiotics and effective analgesia. If a calculus is large enough to cause obstruction then surgery may be required.

Appendicitis

Acute appendicitis complicates about 1/1000 of pregnancies. There is no increase in incidence during pregnancy but mortality is higher. During pregnancy the caecum and appendix are displaced upwards and to the right with advancing gestation. The pain is less well localized and tenderness, rebound and guarding less obvious. This leads to delay in diagnosis and treatment and an increased incidence of perforation (15–20% of cases), peritonitis and sepsis. When perforation occurs, maternal and fetal mortality reaches 17% and 43%, respectively. Early referral for surgical treatment is essential. In the first trimester this can be accomplished laparoscopically.

Cholecystitis

Acute cholecystitis complicates about 1 in 1000 pregnancies. Presentation is with sudden onset of right upper quadrant or epigastric colicky pain with associated nausea, vomiting and fever. Jaundice is uncommon. The diagnosis is made by the clinical features, biochemical tests and the presence of stones in the biliary tree on ultrasound scan. The treatment is by using the appropriate antibiotics, adequate analgesia and fluids. Surgery is indicated during pregnancy where there is associated pancreatitis or recurrent episodes but otherwise is deferred until after the puerperium.

Induced abortion (pregnancy termination)

In the UK, this is carried out in approved centres under the provision of the Abortion Act 1967. This Act requires that two doctors agree that continuation of the pregnancy would either involve greater risk to the physical or mental health of the mother or her other children than termination, or that the fetus is at risk of an abnormality likely to result in it being seriously handicapped. The most recent amendment to the Act (1990) sets a limit for termination under the first of these categories at 24 weeks, although in practice the majority of terminations are carried out prior to 20 weeks (see Box 19.4).

All women who are opting to terminate a pregnancy need adequate support and counselling, both before and after the procedure. Social, medical and psychological factors all contribute to the decision.

Box 19.4 Indications for termination of pregnancy under the Abortion Act 1967, as amended by Human Fertilization and Embryology Act 1990

A. The continuance of the pregnancy would involve risk to the life of the pregnant woman greater than if the pregnancy were terminated.

B. The termination is necessary to prevent grave permanent injury to the physical or mental health of the pregnant woman.

C. The pregnancy has not exceeded its 24th week and the continuance of the pregnancy would involve risk, greater than if the pregnancy were terminated, of injury to the physical or mental health of the pregnant woman.

D. The pregnancy has not exceeded its 24th week and the continuance of the pregnancy would involve risk, greater than if the pregnancy were terminated, of injury to the physical or mental health of the existing child(ren) of the family of the pregnant woman.

E. There is a substantial risk that if the child were born it would suffer from such physical or mental abnormalities as to be seriously handicapped.

Methods of termination of pregnancy

All women undergoing termination of pregnancy should be screened for sexually transmitted infection and/ or offered antibiotic prophylaxis. Following termination anti-D immunoglobulin should be given to all Rhesus negative women. All women should be offered follow-up appointment to check that there are no physical problems and contraceptive measures are in place.

Up to 12% of women requesting termination of pregnancy will have active infection with *C. trachomatis*. In these women, there is a 30% pelvic inflammatory disease if the appropriate antibiotic treatment is not given at the time of surgical termination.

Surgical termination of pregnancy

This is the method most commonly used in the first trimester. The cervix is distended using a series of graduated dilators and the conceptus removed using a suction curette. A variation involving piecemeal removal of the larger fetal parts with forceps (dilatation and evacuation) allows the method to be used for later second-trimester pregnancies. Although most procedures are carried out under general anaesthesia in the UK, the use of local anaesthetic for terminations under 10 weeks is widely used in many countries and reduces the time the patient needs to stay in the hospital or clinic.

Medical termination of pregnancy

This is the method most commonly used for pregnancies after 14 weeks and is increasingly being offered as an alternative to surgical termination in first trimester pregnancies (up to 9 weeks' gestation). The standard regimes for first trimester termination uses the progesterone antagonist mifepristone (RU 486) given orally followed 36–48 hrs later by prostaglandins administered either orally or as a vaginal pessary. There are several different regimes but all have a success rate of >95%. Second trimester terminations can be performed using vaginal prostaglandins given 3-hourly or as an extra-amniotic infusion through a balloon catheter passed through the cervix. Pretreatment with mifepristone significantly reduces the time from induction to abortion. After delivery of the fetus, an examination under general anaesthetic may be necessary to remove the placenta.

The mother needs to be cared for in a single room, her privacy being protected at all times. She should be offered information about the process so she is aware of what is happening. Adequate analgesia should be available and supportive staff identified to care for the mother and her family throughout the procedure (Kohner 1995). It may be appropriate for the named midwife to care for the mother during her termination.

Legal abortion should not result in a live birth and feticide may be carried out as part of or prior to the procedure. Amendments implemented in 1991 to the Abortion Act 1967 allowed for the reduction of multiple pregnancies where one or more of the fetuses, but not all, may be terminated (Paintain 1994).

Complications of termination

Early complications include bleeding, uterine perforation (with possible damage to other pelvic viscera), cervical laceration, retained products and sepsis. All the procedures also have a small failure rate (overall rate 0.7/1000). Late complications include infertility, cervical incompetence, isoimmunization and psychiatric morbidity. In the developing world, unsafe abortion is one of the five main causes of direct maternal death (WHO 1997). Septic abortion remains a major complication of an illegal abortion or one carried out in non-sterile conditions.

Psychological sequelae of termination

The majority of women who find themselves with an unwanted pregnancy are very distressed. Despite this, evidence shows that the majority of women do not experience medium- to long-term psychological sequelae following termination for psychosocial reasons. The available evidence is that the rate of psychiatric morbidity following termination of pregnancy decreases. The situation for women having a termination of pregnancy because of fetal abnormality is different. These are usually older women who have a much wanted pregnancy and whose problem has been diagnosed either because of a previous experience or as the

result of screening. The decision to terminate the pregnancy is usually reached only after much thought and anguish. The consequence of termination is, therefore, very much like the spontaneous loss of a more advanced pregnancy, that is to say, of a grief reaction. Most late terminations of pregnancy involve the induction of labour and a prolonged process of giving birth. This can be a distressing and traumatic experience, and psychological recovery will be improved by sensitive and compassionate handling by the doctor and midwifery or nursing staff. Their psychosocial recovery may be assisted by granting them the dignity of a naming and burial.

The role of the midwife

Midwives will primarily be caring for mothers for whom termination of pregnancy is an option they are considering as a result of the antenatal screening or diagnostic tests offered.

Within the terms of the Abortion Act 1967, if an individual has a conscientious objection then he or she is not required to assist with abortion. A midwife would normally be required to notify her manager of such an objection before any care was expected. The Act requires practitioners, however, to provide care to prevent harm to the pregnant woman so the exception to this would be in the event of an emergency when conscientious objection does not preclude the midwife from involvement. The midwife otherwise has a duty of care to mothers for whom she is the named midwife. Midwifery practice may involve assisting with blood tests or amniocentesis, the results of which could lead to a termination. The duty of care and exercise of professional accountability means that mothers should be given the necessary information and advice. Professional guidelines require the midwife to care for clients in a non-judgemental manner. This applies when caring for a mother terminating a current pregnancy or a mother who has undergone termination in a previous pregnancy.

REFERENCES

Abortion Act Abortion Act 1967 HMSO, London
Aharoni A, Reiter A, Golan D et al 1988 Patterns of growth of uterine leiomyomas during pregnancy. A prospective longitudinal study. British Journal of Obstetrics and Gynaecology 95:510–513

Atri M, Leduc C, Gillett P et al 1996 Role of endovaginal sonography in the diagnosis and management of ectopic pregnancy. Radiographics 16(4):755–774
Bagshawe K D, Dent J, Webb J 1986 Hydatidiform mole in England and Wales 1973–1983. Lancet ii:673–675

Benson C B, Chow J S, Chang-Lee W et al 2001 Outcome of pregnancies in women with uterine leiomyomas identified by sonography in the first trimester. Journal of Clinical Ultrasound 29(5):261–264

Beydoun H, Saftlas AF 2005 Association of human leucocyte antigen sharing with recurrent spontaneous abortions. Tissue Antigens 65(2):123–135

Bigrigg M A, Read M D 1991 Management of women referred to early pregnancy assessment unit: care and effectiveness. British Medical Journal 302:577–579

Davis J L, Ray-Mazumder S, Hobel C J et al 1990 Uterine leiomyomas in pregnancy: a prospective study. Obstetrics and Gynaecology 75(1):41–44

Demetroulis C, Saridogan E, Kunde D et al 2001 A prospective RCT comparing medical and surgical treatment for early pregnancy failure. Human Reproduction 16:365–369

Dodson M G 1991 Early ectopic pregnancy. In: Dodson M G (ed.) Transvaginal ultrasound. Churchill Livingstone, Edinburgh, p 165–214

DoH (Department of Health), Welsh Office, Scottish Home and Health Department, Department of Health and Social Services, Northern Ireland 1998. Why mothers die. Report on Confidential Enquiries into Maternal Deaths in the United Kingdom 1994–1996. Stationery Office, London

Frigo P, Lang C, Reisenberger K et al 1998 Hyperemesis gravidarum associated with *Helicobacter pylori* seropositivity. Obstetrics and Gynecology 91(4):615–617

Graziosi G C, Moi B W, Ankum W M et al 2004 Management of early pregnancy loss – a systematic review. International Journal of Gynaecology and Obstetrics 86:337–346

Hay P E, Lamont R F, Taylor-Robinson D et al 1994 Abnormal bacterial colonization of the genital tract and subsequent pre-term delivery and late miscarriage. British Medical Journal 308:295–298

Hindshaw H K S 1997 Medical management of miscarriage. In: Grudzinskas J G, O'Brien P M S (eds) Problems in early pregnancy: advances in diagnosis and management. RCOG press, London, p 284–298

Human Fertilization and Embryology Act 1990 HMSO, London

Kadar N, Caldwell B V, Romero R 1981 A method for screening for ectopic pregnancy and its indications. Obstetrics and Gynecology 58:162–165

Katz V L, Dotters D J, Droegemueller W 1989 Complications of uterine leiomyomas in pregnancy. Obstetrics and Gynecology 73(4):593–596

Kohner N 1995 Pregnancy loss and the death of a baby. Guidelines for professionals. SANDS, London

Lawler S D, Fisher R A, Dent J 1991 A prospective genetic study of complete and partial hydatidiform moles. American Journal of Obstetrics and Gynecology 164(5):1270–1277

Lewis G, Drife J (eds) 2001 Why mothers die. The fifth report of the Confidential Enquiries into Maternal Deaths in the UK 1997–1999. RCOG Press, London

Ling F W, Stovall T G 1994 Update on the diagnosis and management of ectopic pregnancy. In: Advances in Obstetrics and Gynecology. Mosby Year Book, Chicago, p 55–83

Lumsden M A, Wallace E M 1998 Clinical presentation of uterine fibroids. Baillière's Clinical Obstetrics and Gynaecology 12(2):177–195

Myers D L, Scotti R J 1995 Acute urinary retention and the incarcerated, retroverted, gravid uterus. A case report. Journal of Reproductive Medicine 40:487–490

Newlands E S, Seckl S J, Boultbee J E et al 2001 Gestational trophoblastic tumours. Information for medics. Hydatidiform mole and choriocarcinoma UK information and support service. Online. Available: http://www.hmole-chorio.org.uk 19 December 2001

NHSCSP (National Health Service Cancer Screening Programme) 2000 Good practice in breast and cervical screening for women with learning disabilities. NHSCSP, Sheffield

NHSCSP (National Health Service Cancer Screening Programme) 2005 The aetiology of cervical cancer. NHSCSP, Sheffield

Paintain D 1994 Induced abortion. In: Clements R V (ed.) Safe practice in obstetrics and gynaecology. A medico-legal handbook. Churchill Livingstone, Edinburgh, p 355

Pouly J L, Chapron C, Manhes H et al 1991 Multifactorial analysis of fertility after conservative laparoscopic treatment of ectopic pregnancy in a series of 223 patients. Fertility and Sterility 56:453–460

Rai R, Clifford K, Regan L 1996 The modern preventative treatment of recurrent miscarriage. British Journal of Obstetrics and Gynaecology 103:106–110

RCOG (Royal College of Obstetricians and Gynaecologists) 2002 Use of anti-d immunoglobulin for Rh prophylaxis (22). Online. Available: http://www.rcog.org.uk/index.asp?PageID=1972

RCOG (Royal College of Obstetricians and Gynaecologists) 2003 The investigation and treatment of couples with recurrent miscarriage (17). Online. Available: http://www.rcog.org.uk/resources/Public/pdf/Recurrent_Miscarriage_No17.pdf

RCOG (Royal College of Obstetricians and Gynaecologists) 2004 The management of gestational trophoblastic disease, evidence based guidelines. Online. Available: http://www.rcog.org.uk/index.asp?PageID=519

Regan L, Rai R 2000 Epidemiology and the medical causes of miscarriage. Best Practice and Research in Clinical Obstetrics and Gynaecology 14(5):839–854

Sadek A L, Schiotz H A 1995 Transvaginal sonography in the management of ectopic pregnancy Acta Obstetrica et Gynecologica Scandinavica 74:293–296

Schlecht N F, Kulaga S, Robitaille J et al 2001 Persistent human papillomavirus as a predictor of cervical intraepithelial neoplasia. Journal of the American Medical Association 286(24):3106–3114

Shalev E, Peleg D, Bustan M et al 1995 Limited role for intratubal methotrexate treatment of ectopic pregnancy. Fertility and Sterility 63:20–24

Singer A 1989 Malignancy and premalignancy of the genital tract in pregnancy In: Turnbull A, Chamberlain G (eds) Obstetrics. Churchill Livingstone, Edinburgh, p 657–672

Slaughter J L, Grimes D A 1995 Methotrexate therapy: non-surgical management of ectopic pregnancy. Western Journal of Medicine 162:225–228

Snell L H, Haughey B P, Buck G et al 1998 Metabolic crisis: hyperemesis gravidarum. Journal of Perinatal and Neonatal Nursing 12(2):26–37

Sperov L, Glass R H, Kase N G 1994 Ectopic pregnancy. In: Sperov L, Glass R H, Kase N G (eds) Clinical gynecologic endocrinology and infertility. Baltimore: Williams & Wilkins, p 947–964

Stirrat G M 1990 Recurrent miscarriage I: definition and epidemiology. Lancet 336:673–675

Szulman A E 1988 The biology of trophoblastic disease: complete and partial hydatidiform moles. In: Beard R W, Sharp F (eds) Early pregnancy loss, mechanisms and treatment. Springer-Verlag, London, p 309–316

Vu K, Gehlbach D L, Rosa C 1996 Operative laparoscopy for the treatment of ectopic pregnancy in a residency program. Journal of Reproductive Medicine 41(8):602–604

WHO 1997 Unsafe abortion: Global and regional estimates of incidence of mortality due to unsafe abortion with a history of available country data, 3rd edn. WHO, Geneva

Yao M, Tulandi T 1997 Current status of surgical and nonsurgical management of ectopic pregnancy. Fertility and Sterility 67:421–433

FURTHER READING

Kohner N, Henley A 2003 When a baby dies: the experience of late miscarriage, stillbirth and neonatal death. HarperCollins, London

RCOG (Royal College of Obstetricians and Gynaecologists) 2004 The care of women requesting termination; evidence based guideline No. 7. RCOG, London

RCOG (Royal College of Obstetricians and Gynaecologists) 2006 Management of early pregnancy loss; evidence based guidelines. Online. Available: http://www.rcog.org.uk/index.asp?PageID=515

20 Problems of pregnancy

Helen Crafter

Problems of pregnancy range from the mildly irritating to life-threatening conditions. Fortunately the life-threatening ones are rare because of improvements to the general health of the population, improved social circumstances and lower parity. However, as women delay childbearing (an increasing phenomenon in the developed world), they become more at risk of disorders associated with increasing age, such as malignancy, placenta praevia and problems associated with obesity. Regular antenatal checks beginning early in pregnancy are undoubtedly valuable. They help to prevent many complications and their ensuing problems, contribute to timely diagnosis and treatment, and enable women to form relationships with midwives, obstetricians and other health professionals who become involved with them in striving to achieve the best possible pregnancy outcomes.

The chapter aims to:

- provide an overview of problems of pregnancy
- describe the role of the midwife in relation to the identification, assessment and management of the more common disorders of pregnancy
- consider the needs of both parents for continuing support when a disorder has been diagnosed.

The midwife's role

The midwife's role in relation to the problems associated with pregnancy is clear. At initial and subsequent encounters with the pregnant woman, it is essential that an accurate health history is obtained. General and specific physical examinations must be carried out and the results meticulously recorded. The examination and recordings give direction towards future referral and management. Where the midwife detects a deviation from the norm which is outside her current sphere of practice, she must refer the woman to a suitable qualified health professional to assist her (NMC 2004, p 16). The midwife will continue to offer the woman care and support throughout her pregnancy and beyond. The woman who develops problems during her pregnancy is no less in need of the midwife's skilled attention; indeed, her condition and psychological state may be considerably improved by the midwife's continued presence and support. It is also the midwife's role in such a situation to ensure that the woman and her family understand the situation; are enabled to take part in decision-making; are protected from unnecessary fear and the midwife must ensure that all care from different health professionals is balanced and integrated – in short, the woman's needs remain paramount throughout.

Abdominal pain in pregnancy

Abdominal pain is a common complaint in pregnancy. It is probably suffered by all women at some stage, and therefore presents a problem for the midwife of how to distinguish between the physiologically normal (e.g. mild indigestion or muscle stretching), the pathological but not dangerous (e.g. degeneration of a fibroid) and the dangerously pathological requiring immediate referral to the appropriate medical practitioner for urgent treatment (e.g. ectopic pregnancy or appendicitis).

The midwife should take a detailed history and perform a physical examination in order to reach a decision about whether to refer the woman. Treatment will depend on the cause (Box 20.1) and the maternal and fetal conditions.

Many of the pregnancy-specific causes of abdominal pain in pregnancy listed in Box 20.1 are dealt with in this and other chapters. For most of these conditions, abdominal pain is one of many symptoms and not necessarily the overriding one. However, an observant midwife may be crucial in procuring a safe pregnancy outcome for a woman presenting with abdominal pain.

Uterine fibroid degeneration

The problems experienced in early pregnancy, as outlined in Ch. 19, may continue throughout the pregnancy as the muscle fibres continue to become hypertrophic and the fibroid (myoma) enlarges. Some women with fibroids will experience acute pain, and sometimes nausea, vomiting and mild pyrexia most commonly at 20–22 weeks' gestation (Mahomed 2006b) as fibroids situated within the myometrium may receive a diminished blood supply and, as the pregnancy progresses, there may be central core necrosis.

If the fibroid or fibroids were not diagnosed prior to pregnancy or in its early stages, diagnosis can be made at any stage by ultrasound, especially if a fibroid is seen where the pain is located. Often fibroids are easily palpable. The pain usually subsides within 4–7 days with adequate explanation to the woman, rest and analgesia. The pregnancy will usually progress to term. However, the pain is often recurrent, especially if more than one fibroid is present.

Occasionally, enlargement of the fibroid may impede the progress of labour. Rupture of the uterus at the affected site is a possibility that should always be considered when caring for the woman in labour.

Severe uterine torsion

As it grows during pregnancy, the uterus usually rotates to the right by no more than 40°. On rare occasions, the uterus rotates by more than 90° and this may cause abdominal pain in the latter half of pregnancy. There is almost always a predisposing factor in such cases of acute torsion, the most common being fibroid, congenital malformation of the uterus, adnexal mass or a history of pelvic surgery (Mahomed 2006a).

The condition is usually managed conservatively by bed-rest, altering the maternal position to correct the torsion spontaneously. Analgesia may be required and if administered then the well-being of both mother and fetus should be monitored, as in rare severe cases, the mother can become shocked and the fetus deprived of oxygen. In such cases, a laparotomy will need to be performed as it is difficult to make a clear diagnosis without surgical evidence. Sometimes

---

Box 20.1 Causes of abdominal pain in pregnancy

Pregnancy-specific causes

- Physiological
  - Heartburn, soreness from vomiting, constipation.
  - Braxton Hicks contractions
  - Pressure effects from growing/vigorous/malpresenting fetus
  - Round ligament pain
  - Severe uterine torsion (can become pathological).
- Pathological
  - Spontaneous miscarriage
  - Uterine leiomyoma
  - Ectopic pregnancy
  - Hyperemesis gravidarum (vomiting with straining)
  - Preterm labour
  - Chorioamnionitis
  - Ovarian pathology
  - Placental abruption
  - Spontaneous uterine rupture
  - Abdominal pregnancy
  - Trauma to abdomen (consider undisclosed domestic violence)

  - Severe pre-eclampsia
  - Acute fatty liver of pregnancy
- Incidental causes.

More common pathology

- Appendicitis
- Acute cholestasis/cholelithiasis
- Gastro-oesophageal reflux/peptic ulcer disease
- Acute pancreatitis
- Urinary tract pathology
- Inflammatory bowel disease
- Intestinal obstruction.

Miscellaneous

- Rectus haematoma
- Sickle cell crisis
- Porphyria
- Malaria
- Arteriovenous haematoma
- Tuberculosis
- Malignant disease
- Psychological causes.

Adapted from Mahomed 2006a.

---

the torsion can be corrected manually. Delivery by caesarean section may be performed, either preceded or followed by manipulation of the uterus.

Pelvic girdle pain/symphysis pubis dysfunction

Symphysis pubis dysfunction (SPD), or pelvic girdle pain (PGP) as it is increasingly being called, is characterized by abnormal relaxation of the ligaments supporting the pubic joint (see Ch. 16). This is brought about by high levels of pregnancy hormones (particularly relaxin), biomechanical and genetic factors, and affects about 1 in 300 women (Ambrose & Repke 2006). The result of the relaxation is increased mobility of the joint; the pubic bones move up and down alternately as the woman walks. Strain on the sacroiliac joints may also occur, particularly in grande multiparae. The woman will complain of pain in the pubic region, and also of backache, at any time from the 28th week of pregnancy. It may start in the early postnatal period. Pain may be experienced in the abdominal muscles owing to an attempt to stabilize the bones by muscular action. On examination, the mother will complain of tenderness over the symphysis pubis. She may be extremely debilitated by the condition.

The midwife should note whether there is any history of pelvic fractures that may be aggravated by the pregnancy. Otherwise the midwife should explain to the mother the cause of this condition and advise her that as much rest as possible will be beneficial, especially as the pregnancy advances and abdominal distension increases. The woman should also aim to reduce non-essential weight-bearing activities and avoid straddle movements, which abduct the hips, e.g. squatting (Fry et al 1997). A supportive panty girdle or 'tubigrip' and comfortable shoes may also help when the woman is up and mobile. There is an increased risk of deep vein thrombosis if the woman's mobility is reduced.

The midwife should notify the doctor if she suspects PGP and of the advice she has given. Advice and treatment from an obstetric physiotherapist will be of great help to the woman. In severe cases, bedrest may be necessary on a firm mattress.

The ligaments should slowly return to normal following birth. However, the woman should be informed during pregnancy that the pain and discomfort may last for some time afterwards, to give her the opportunity to make appropriate arrangements. Postnatal physiotherapy will aid the strengthening and stabilization of the joint.

The Association of Chartered Physiotherapists (www.acpwh.co.uk) has produced a National Clinical Guideline for the care for women with SPD/PGP and its website: www.pelvicpartnership.org.uk provides further detailed information.

Antepartum haemorrhage

Bleeding from the genital tract in late pregnancy, after the 24th week of gestation and before the onset of labour, is referred to as an antepartum haemorrhage (APH). This may place the life of the mother and fetus at risk.

Effect on the fetus

Fetal mortality and morbidity are increased as a result of severe vaginal bleeding in pregnancy. Stillbirth or neonatal death may occur. Premature placental separation and consequent hypoxia may result in severe neurological damage in the baby (Manolitsas et al 1994).

Effect on the mother

If bleeding is severe, it may be accompanied by shock and disseminated intravascular coagulation (DIC) (see blood coagulation failure). The mother may die or be left with permanent ill health.

Types of APH

If bleeding from local lesions of the genital tract (incidental causes) is excluded, vaginal bleeding in late pregnancy is due to placental separation from placenta praevia or placental abruption (Table 20.1).

Initial appraisal of a woman with APH

When a woman first loses blood from the vagina during pregnancy, she may call the midwife or present herself at hospital. She may fear that she is losing her baby; her partner may fear for the lives of both mother and child. The midwife's role at this stage is to be supportive and ascertain as much detail as possible of the history and the circumstances surrounding the blood loss. This will assist both in assessing the woman's condition and in making a diagnosis. However, the midwife will also be aware that APH is unpredictable and the woman's condition can deteriorate rapidly at any time; she must therefore make a rapid decision about the urgency of need of a medical or paramedic presence, or both, often at the same time as observing and talking to the woman and her partner.

Table 20.1 Causes of bleeding in late pregnancy	
Cause	**Incidence (%)**
Placenta praevia	31.0
Placental abruption	22.0
'Unclassified bleeding'	47.0
Marginal	60.0
Show	20.0
Cervicitis	8.0
Trauma	5.0
Vulvovaginal varicosities	2.0
Genital tumours	0.5
Genital infections	0.5
Haematuria	0.5
Vasa praevia	0.5
Other	0.5

Adapted from Konje & Taylor (2006). *Note*: Konje & Taylor do not explain the lost 2.5% of 'unclassified bleeding'.

Sometimes bleeding that the woman had presumed to be from the vagina will in fact be from haemorrhoids. The midwife should consider this differential diagnosis and confirm or exclude this as soon as possible by careful questioning and examination.

Assessment of physical condition

Maternal condition

The first priority is the well-being of the mother. The midwife should look for any pallor or breathlessness, which may indicate shock. She should also assess the woman's emotional state as she greets her and begins to ask for a history of events. She must generate the trust of both partners and remain calm.

Observation of pulse rate, respiratory rate, blood pressure and temperature will be made and recorded. The midwife must assess the amount of blood lost in order to ensure adequate fluid replacement. She will discuss with the couple how much has been lost earlier and should ask to see all soiled articles, retaining them for the doctor's inspection.

A gentle abdominal examination is made, observing for signs that the woman is going into labour. On no account must any vaginal or rectal examination be made nor may an enema or suppository be given to a woman suffering from an APH, as these procedures could exacerbate the bleeding.

Fetal condition

The mother should be asked if the baby has been moving as much as normal. The midwife must attempt to auscultate the fetal heart and may use ultrasound apparatus to obtain information.

Factors to aid differential diagnosis

The location of the placenta is perhaps the most critical piece of information that will be needed in order to make a correct diagnosis; initially the midwife will not usually have this fact at her disposal. However, if she is able to elicit the following information from her observations and talking to the woman and her partner, then this will help her to arrive at a provisional diagnosis:

Pain: Did the pain precede bleeding and is it continuous or intermittent?

Onset of bleeding: Was this associated with any event such as abdominal trauma or sex?

Amount of visible blood loss: Is there any reason to suspect that some blood has been retained *in utero*?

Colour of the blood: Is it bright red or darker in colour?

Degree of shock: Is this commensurate with the amount of blood visible or more severe?

Consistency of the abdomen: Is it soft or tense and board-like?

Tenderness of the abdomen: Does the mother recoil from abdominal palpation?

Lie, presentation and engagement: Are any of these abnormal when taking account of parity and gestation?

Audibility of the fetal heart: Is the fetal heart heard?

Ultrasound scan: Does a scan suggest that the placenta is in the lower uterine segment?

The relevance of the findings from these observations is further discussed in the context of the various causes of APH.

Supportive treatment

Alongside emotional support, the first need is for restoration of physical condition if this is being compromised. This will necessitate fluid replacement first with a plasma expander and subsequently with whole blood if necessary. If the mother is in severe pain, she should be offered strong analgesia to help counteract shock. If the midwife is in attendance at home she must decide how best to arrange transfer to hospital. She may summon the emergency obstetric unit where this exists, or alternatively the ambulance service. If she carries intravenous equipment, she can site an infusion. The obstetric registrar or paramedic will carry and infuse a plasma expander before transfer of the woman to hospital.

Subsequent management depends on the definite diagnosis.

Placenta praevia

In this condition the placenta is partially or wholly implanted in the lower uterine segment on either the anterior or posterior wall.

The lower uterine segment grows and stretches progressively after the 12th week of pregnancy. In later weeks this may cause the placenta to separate and severe bleeding can occur. Bleeding is caused by shearing stress between the placental trophoblast and maternal venous blood sinuses. In some instances bleeding may be precipitated by sex. A separating placenta praevia places the mother and fetus at high risk and it constitutes an obstetric emergency. Medical assistance is vital if the lives of the mother and fetus are to be saved. Women with suspected placenta praevia should be transferred to a consultant obstetric unit.

Degrees of placenta praevia

Type 1 placenta praevia

The majority of the placenta is in the upper uterine segment (Figs. 20.1 and 20.5). Vaginal birth is possible. Blood loss is usually mild and the mother and fetus remain in good condition.

Type 2 placenta praevia

The placenta is partially located in the lower segment near the internal cervical os (marginal placenta praevia) (Figs. 20.2 and 20.6). Vaginal birth is possible, particularly if the placenta is anterior. Blood loss is usually moderate, although the conditions of the mother and fetus can vary. Fetal hypoxia is more likely to be present than maternal shock.

Type 3 placenta praevia

The placenta is located over the internal cervical os but not centrally (Figs. 20.3 and 20.7). Bleeding is likely to be severe, particularly when the lower segment stretches and the cervix begins to efface and dilate in late pregnancy. Vaginal birth is inappropriate because the placenta precedes the fetus.

Type 4 placenta praevia

The placenta is located centrally over the internal cervical os (Figs. 20.4 and 20.8) and torrential haemorrhage is very likely. Caesarean section is essential in order to save the lives of the mother and baby.

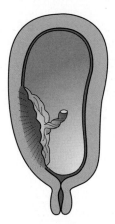 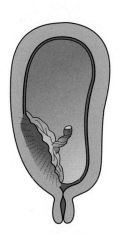 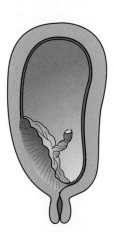 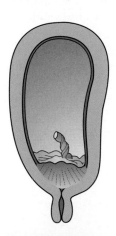

Figure 20.1 Type 1   **Figure 20.2** Type 2   **Figure 20.3** Type 3   **Figure 20.4** Type 4

Figures 20.1–20.4 Types of placenta praevia.

Figure 20.5 Type 1   **Figure 20.6** Type 2   **Figure 20.7** Type 3   **Figure 20.8** Type 4

Figures 20.5–20.4 Relation of placenta praevia to cervical os.

Indications of placenta praevia

Bleeding from the vagina is the only sign and it is painless. The uterus is not tender or tense. The presence of placenta praevia should be considered when the presenting part of the fetus is above the pelvis and/or the lie is unstable.

Localization of the placenta using ultrasonic scanning will confirm the existence of placenta praevia and establish its degree.

It is noteworthy that the degree of placenta praevia does not necessarily correspond to the amount of bleeding. A type 4 placenta praevia may never bleed before elective caesarean section in late pregnancy or the onset of spontaneous labour; conversely, some women with placenta praevia type 1 may experience relatively heavy bleeding from early in their pregnancy.

Assessing the mother's condition

The amount of vaginal bleeding is variable; some mothers may have a history of a small repeated blood loss at intervals throughout pregnancy whereas others may have a sudden single episode of vaginal bleeding after the 20th week. However, severe haemorrhage occurs most frequently after the 34th week of pregnancy.

The haemorrhage may be mild, moderate or severe, is often not associated with any particular type of activity and may occur at rest. The colour of the blood is bright red, denoting fresh bleeding. The low placental location allows all of the lost blood to escape unimpeded and a retroplacental clot is not formed. For this reason, pain is not a feature of placenta praevia.

General examination

If the haemorrhage is slight the woman's blood pressure, respiratory rate and pulse rate may be normal. In severe haemorrhage however, the blood pressure will be low and the pulse rate raised because of shock. The degree of shock correlates with the amount of blood lost from the vagina. Respirations are also rapid and the mother may have air hunger due to a reduction in the number of red blood cells in the circulation available for the uptake of oxygen. The mother's colour will be pale and her skin cold and moist. With severe bleeding she may lose consciousness.

Abdominal examination

The midwife may find that the lie of the fetus is oblique or transverse and the fetal head may be high in a primigravida near term. The uterine consistency is normal and pain is not experienced by the mother when her abdomen is palpated.

The midwife must not attempt to do a vaginal examination as this could precipitate a torrential haemorrhage and worsen the situation.

An attempt should be made to quantify the amount of blood lost and all blood-soaked material used by the mother should be saved. Although this will not provide an accurate estimation of the quantity, it may be a helpful clue in assessing fluid replacement.

Assessing the fetal condition

The mother should be asked whether fetal activity has been normal. She may be aware of diminution or cessation of fetal movements, which may occur if fetal hypoxia is severe. Excessive fetal movement is sometimes said by midwives to be an indicator of fetal hypoxia although no good quality research evidence exists to support this.

The midwife should assess the fetal condition using an ultrasound fetal monitor such as a cardiotocograph (CTG) or handheld device. A Pinard fetal stethoscope may be used if these are not available. Fetal oxygenation depends upon the proportion of the placenta remaining attached. Fetal hypoxia is an emergency and medical assistance should be called urgently.

Management of placenta praevia

The management of placenta praevia depends on:

- the amount of bleeding
- the condition of mother and fetus
- the location of the placenta
- the stage of the pregnancy.

Conservative management

This is appropriate if bleeding is slight and the mother and fetus are well. The woman will be kept in hospital at rest until bleeding has stopped. A speculum examination will have ruled out incidental causes. Further bleeding is almost inevitable if the placenta encroaches into the lower segment; therefore it is usual to require the woman to remain in, or close to hospital for the rest of the pregnancy. Placental function is monitored by means of fetal kick charts and antenatal CTG. Ultrasound scans are repeated at intervals in order to observe the position of the placenta in relation to the cervical os as the lower segment grows. Fetal growth is also monitored as placental perfusion across the lower segment is less efficient than that in a fundally situated placenta, and intrauterine growth restriction may result.

A woman who is asked to stay in hospital for many weeks will have particular psychological and social needs. If she has other children, she will be anxious to know that good arrangements have been made for their care and they must be allowed to visit her frequently. She should be offered parent education and sometimes it may be possible to continue with a group she has been attending. Occupational therapy may help to alleviate the boredom often felt during long-stay hospital admission. A visit to the Special Care Baby Unit, perhaps with her family, and answering any questions she has may also help to prepare her for the possibility of pre-term birth.

A decision will be made with the woman about how and when the birth will be managed. If the woman does not have further severe bleeding, she can give birth when the fetus reaches maturity, vaginally if the placental location allows. Vaginal ultrasound allows for a more accurate estimation of placental site, on which the decision about mode of birth will be based.

Vaginal birth is usual with type 1 placenta praevia and possible with type 2, unless the placenta is situated immediately above the sacral promontory where it is vulnerable to pressure from an advancing fetal head and may impede descent. The degrees of placenta praevia that are amenable to vaginal birth may be termed minor. Labour is likely to be induced from 37 weeks' gestation.

The midwife should be aware that, even if vaginal birth is achieved, there remains a danger of postpartum haemorrhage. This is because the placenta has been situated in the lower segment where there is paucity of oblique muscle fibres and therefore the living ligature action will be poor.

Active management

Severe vaginal bleeding will necessitate immediate delivery by caesarean section regardless of the location of the placenta. This should take place in a unit with facilities for the appropriate care of the new-born, especially if the baby will be pre-term.

Blood will be taken for a full blood count, cross-matching and clotting studies. An intravenous infusion will be in progress and several units of blood may need to be transfused quickly, with the woman's consent. In an emergency, it may be necessary to give group O blood, if possible of the same Rhesus group as the mother.

An anaesthetist will be involved in the woman's care, assessing her fluid requirements and output and helping her to make a decision about the use of regional or general anaesthesia (if she is able). During the assessment and preparation for theatre the mother will be extremely anxious and the midwife must comfort and encourage her, sharing information with her as much as possible. The partner will also need to be supported, whether he is in the operating theatre or waits outside.

Konje & Taylor (2006) describe the procedure of 'double set up' (p 1264), whereby a woman is examined in an operating theatre with full preparation to proceed to caesarean section if her condition worsens. This procedure can be useful where attempted placental localization by diagnostic ultrasound scanning proves inconclusive.

If the placenta is situated anteriorly in the uterus, this may complicate the surgical approach as it underlies the site of the normal incision. In major degrees of placenta praevia (types 3 and 4) caesarean section is required even if the fetus has died in utero. Such management aims to prevent torrential haemorrhage and possible maternal death.

Incidence

Placenta praevia occurring after 20 weeks' gestation complicates 3–6 of every 1000 pregnancies (Lockwood & Funai 1999). It is more common in multigravidae, with an incidence of 1 in 90 births. (Placenta praevia rates rise in women with increasing age and increasing parity.) In primigravidae the incidence is 1 in 250 births. Its aetiology is unknown, but a raised incidence is also seen in women who smoke and those who have had a previous caesarean section. The recurrence rate for women who have had a previous placenta praevia is in the order of 4–8%.

Complications include:

- maternal shock, resulting from blood loss and hypovolaemia
- anaesthetic and surgical complications, which are more common in women with major degrees of placenta praevia, and in those for whom preparation for surgery has been suboptimal (Lewis 2007)
- placenta accreta, in up to 15% of women with placenta praevia
- air embolism, an occasional occurrence when the sinuses in the placental bed have been broken
- postpartum haemorrhage: occasionally uncontrolled haemorrhage will continue, despite the administration of uterotonic drugs at delivery – even following the best efforts to control it, and a ligation of the internal iliac artery, a caesarean hysterectomy may be required to save the woman's life
- maternal death, a very rare outcome of this condition in the developed world (Lewis 2007)
- fetal hypoxia and its sequelae due to placental separation
- fetal death, depending on gestation and amount of blood loss.

Placental abruption

Premature separation of a normally situated placenta occurring after the 22nd week of pregnancy is referred to as placental abruption. The aetiology of this type of haemorrhage is not always clear, but it is often associated with severe pre-eclampsia, although not chronic hypertension (Ananth et al 1997). Abruption can follow a sudden reduction in uterine size, for instance when the membranes rupture or after the birth of a first twin, and rarely is a result of direct trauma to the abdomen, perhaps through a road traffic accident (Reis et al 2000), seat-belt injury (Eckford et al 1995) or deliberate violence. All of these may partially dislodge the placenta. Abu-Heija et al (1998) found in their large case–control study of 18256 women that high parity was a significant aetiological factor. Rasmussen et al (1999) found that caesarean section in the previous delivery increased the risk of placental abruption by 40%. There also appears to be a correlation between placental abruption and cigarette smoking (Andres 1996).

Interestingly, some researchers are starting to find links between pregnancy-induced hypertension, intrauterine growth restriction and preterm birth in that they may share a common early to mid-pregnancy aetiology of placental dysfunction, which may then manifest itself as placental abruption in the second half of pregnancy (Ananth & Wilcox 2001, Rasmussen et al 1999, 2000). This theory clearly needs to be tested in future research.

Placental abruption occurs in 0.49–1.8% of all pregnancies (Konje & Taylor 2006). Partial separation of the placenta causes bleeding from the maternal venous sinuses in the placental bed. Further bleeding continues to separate the placenta to a greater or lesser degree. If blood escapes from the placental site it separates the membranes from the uterine wall and drains through the vagina. Blood that is retained behind the placenta may be forced into the myometrium and it infiltrates between the muscle fibres of the uterus. This extravasation can cause marked damage and, if observed at operation, the uterus will appear bruised and oedematous. This is termed Couvelaire uterus or uterine apoplexy. There is no vaginal bleeding, but the mother will have all the signs and symptoms of hypovolaemic shock, caused by concealed bleeding into the muscle of the uterus. The concealed haemorrhage causes uterine enlargement and extreme pain. Concealed haemorrhage is said to account for 20–35% of abruptions (Konje & Taylor 2006).

A combination of these two situations where some of the blood drains via the vagina and some is retained behind the placenta is known as a mixed haemorrhage.

Types of placental abruption

The blood loss from a placental abruption may be defined as revealed, concealed or mixed haemorrhage, as described above. An alternative classification, based on the degree of separation and therefore related to the condition of the mother and baby, is of mild, moderate and severe haemorrhage. The midwife cannot rely on visible blood loss as a guide to the severity of the haemorrhage; on the contrary, the most severe haemorrhage is often that which is totally concealed.

Assessing the mother's condition

There may be a history of pre-eclampsia. A recent history of headaches, nausea, vomiting, epigastric pain and visual disturbances may be a feature. Physical domestic violence should be considered by the midwife, which the woman may be too frightened to reveal (Bewley & Gibbs 2001). Road traffic accidents are a cause of trauma to the abdomen. External cephalic version injudiciously performed may also result in placental separation. The midwife should be aware of the possibility of placental separation after the birth of a first twin or loss of copious amounts of amniotic fluid.

The mildest degrees of placental abruption are relatively pain free, although the mother may experience a slight localized pain. The blood loss is revealed. More severe degrees are associated with abdominal pain and the midwife should enquire about the time of onset and whether the bleeding began simultaneously or later.

General examination

The woman is likely to be anxious, experiencing abdominal pain, and her skin will be pale and moist if she is shocked. On clinical examination, the mother may have obvious oedema of the face, fingers and pretibial area of the lower limbs attributable to pre-eclampsia.

The blood pressure and pulse should be taken immediately. A low blood pressure and raised pulse rate are signs of shock; if the mother has pregnancy-induced hypertension then the blood pressure may be within normal limits, having been raised prior to the haemorrhage. The respirations may be normal or rapid, and reduced oxygenation may lead to air hunger. The temperature will usually be normal but, as placental abruption may be caused by severe infection, it should be taken.

The amount of any visible blood loss should be estimated and its colour noted. Freshly lost blood is bright red; blood that has been retained *in utero* for any length of time changes to a brown colour.

Abdominal examination

Concealed haemorrhage may lead to uterine enlargement in excess of gestation. The uterus has a hard consistency and there is guarding on palpation of the abdomen. Palpation may be difficult and should not be attempted if the uterus is rigid and excessively painful. Fetal parts may not be palpable. In less

severe cases palpation should be kept to a minimum in order to avoid further pain and damage. The nature and location of the pain should be established.

The fetal heart is unlikely to be heard with a fetal stethoscope if there has been any concealed haemorrhage; an ultrasound scanner, CTG or hand-held device should be used. If the haemorrhage is severe, fetal death is a common outcome.

Assessing the fetal condition

The woman may be aware of a cessation of fetal movements. A CTG recording will give more complete information about fetal condition, as will an ultrasound scan of the heart chambers. Failure to elicit heart sounds with a Pinard stethoscope is not confirmation of fetal death.

The midwife should take care how she conveys information about the fetus to the mother. If the heart is inaudible on first examination, she should explain that a fetal monitor is needed to establish the condition of her baby. It is rarely, if ever, appropriate to attempt to conceal fetal death from the mother.

Management

Any woman with a history suggestive of placental abruption needs urgent medical attention. She should be transferred speedily to a consultant obstetric unit, preferably by the emergency obstetric service. The midwife or a paramedic may site an intravenous cannula prior to transfer.

On arrival at the hospital the woman is admitted to the labour suite and the registrar or consultant obstetrician is informed. The midwife should offer the woman comfort and encouragement by attending to her physical and emotional needs, including her need for information.

Pain exacerbates shock and must be alleviated. As it may be extreme, a suitable analgesic would be morphine 15 mg or pethidine 100–150 mg. If the woman has had a narcotic drug prior to admission, the midwife must alert those in attendance to the fact that analgesia has been given.

The acute pain of concealed haemorrhage from placental abruption is due to the extravasation of blood between the muscle fibres of the uterus. This must be differentiated from the pain of uterine contraction due to the onset of labour and from subcapsular liver haemorrhage as a result of pre-eclampsia. The nature of the pain should be discussed because labour may supervene following placental abruption.

Shock may be due to hypovolaemia, to extravasation and consequent pain or to consumptive coagulopathy. The latter is due to tissue damage and the liberation of thromboplastins into the circulation with resulting disseminated intravascular coagulation (see below).

If blood is not available for immediate transfusion, hypovolaemia may be reduced by administering a suitable plasma expander. Letsky (1995) favours the use of Haemacel, which does not interfere with platelet function or subsequent blood grouping and cross-matching of blood. It also helps to improve renal function. However, this is only a temporary palliative and blood transfusion must follow as quickly as possible.

The woman should rest on her side in order to prevent vena caval occlusion and aortic compression by the gravid uterus. If shock becomes severe and medical assistance cannot be immediately obtained, or intravenous access secured, placing the woman flat with a wedge, or in a semirecumbent position with the legs only raised will help to sustain the circulation to her upper body for a short period. However, under no circumstances should the foot of the bed be elevated as this will cause pooling of blood in the vagina and is unlikely to reduce shock.

Observations

Once the maternal and fetal conditions have been assessed, decisions will be made about management. If resuscitation of the woman is required her condition should be stabilized before surgery is undertaken. Likewise, if the woman and fetus are not in imminent danger (or the fetus has died) some time will elapse before surgery is considered, and at this time it is crucial that the midwife maintains continual and accurate observations.

The mother's blood pressure, respirations and pulse rate should be taken at frequent intervals, which will depend on the severity of her condition. If a pyrexia is present, the temperature may be recorded every 1–2 hrs; if the woman is not feverish, a 4-hourly recording is adequate. A central venous line is usually inserted in order to monitor the central venous pressure every 2 hrs, or more frequently, as necessary (see Ch. 33). If the haemorrhage is not severe enough to warrant intravenous infusion, a cannula will be sited in case the haemorrhage suddenly worsens.

Urinary output is accurately assessed by the insertion of an indwelling catheter. Oliguria or anuria indicates suppression of renal function, which may persist until a postpartum diuresis occurs. The urine should be tested for the presence of protein, which may also be linked to pre-eclampsia. Fluid intake must also be recorded accurately and fluid balance assessed with the aid of the central venous pressure recordings.

Fundal height and abdominal girth may be measured at regular intervals. An increase indicates continued bleeding behind the placenta. If the fetus is alive, the fetal heart rate should be monitored continuously with the aid of a CTG.

Any deterioration in the maternal or fetal conditions must be reported immediately to the obstetrician.

Investigations

As soon as practicable following admission a full blood count, cross-match and clotting studies should be obtained. Blood samples may be needed at intervals in order to monitor the progress of the condition. If pre-eclampsia is suspected the relevant blood tests should also be ordered. If the woman is Rhesus negative she should be offered anti-D immunoglobulin. If the Kleihauer is positive more anti-D will be required (Konje & Taylor 2006).

Management of different degrees of placental abruption

In mild separation of the placenta, the placental separation and the haemorrhage are slight. Mother and fetus are in a stable condition. There is no indication of maternal shock and the fetus is alive with normal heart sounds. The consistency of the uterus is normal and there is no tenderness on abdominal palpation. It may be difficult to differentiate this condition from placenta praevia and from an incidental cause of vaginal bleeding.

An ultrasound scan can determine the placental location and identify any degree of concealed bleeding. Fetal condition should be continually assessed while bleeding persists by frequent, if not continuous, monitoring of the fetal heart rate. Subsequently CTG should be carried out once or twice daily because any degree of abruption by definition involves partial separation of the placenta.

If the woman is not in labour and the gestation is <37 weeks, she may be cared for in an antenatal ward for a few days. She may then go home if there is no further bleeding and the placenta has been found to be in the upper uterine segment. Women who have passed the 37th week of pregnancy may be offered induction of labour, especially if there has been more than one episode of mild bleeding. Further heavy bleeding or evidence of fetal compromise may indicate that a caesarean section is necessary.

It should also be noted that if the mother is already severely anaemic then even an apparently mild abruption should cause concern.

Moderate separation of the placenta describes placental separation of about one-quarter. Some or all of the blood may escape from the vagina; some or all may be retained behind the placenta as a retroplacental clot or an extravasation into the uterine muscle. The mother will be shocked, with a raised pulse rate and a lowered blood pressure. There will be a degree of uterine tenderness and abdominal guarding. The fetus may be alive although hypoxic; intrauterine death is also a possibility.

The immediate aims of care are to reduce shock and to replace blood loss. Fluid replacement should be monitored with the aid of a central venous pressure line. The fetal condition should be assessed with continuous CTG if the fetus is alive, in which case immediate caesarean section may be indicated once the woman's condition is stabilized.

If the fetus is in good condition or has already died, vaginal birth may be contemplated. Such management is advantageous because it enables the uterus to contract and control the bleeding. The spontaneous onset of labour frequently accompanies moderately severe placental abruption, but if it does not then amniotomy is usually sufficient to induce labour. Oxytocin may be used with great care if necessary. Birth is often quite sudden after a short labour. The use of drugs to attempt to stop labour is usually inappropriate.

Moderate separation of the placenta may on occasion deteriorate into a more serious degree of separation.

Severe separation of the placenta

This too is an acute obstetric emergency; at least two-thirds of the placenta has become detached and a life-threatening amount of blood is lost from the circulation. Most or all of the blood can be concealed behind the placenta. The woman will be severely shocked, perhaps to a degree far beyond what might be expected from the amount of visible blood loss. The blood pressure will be lowered; the reading may lie within the normal range owing to a preceding hypertension. The fetus will almost certainly be dead. The woman will have very severe abdominal pain with excruciating tenderness; the uterus has a board-like consistency.

Features associated with severe haemorrhage are coagulation defects, renal failure and pituitary failure. Treatment is the same as for moderate haemorrhage. Whole blood should be transfused rapidly and subsequent amounts calculated in accordance with the woman's central venous pressure. Labour may begin spontaneously in advance of amniotomy and the midwife should be alert for signs of uterine contraction causing periodic intensifying of the abdominal pain. However, if bleeding continues or a compromised fetal heart rate is present, caesarean section may be required as soon as the woman's condition has been adequately stabilized. The woman requires constant explanation and psychological support, despite the fact that, because of her shocked condition, she may not be fully conscious. Pain relief must also be considered. The woman's partner will also be very concerned, and should not be forgotten in the rush to stabilize the woman's condition.

Care of the baby

Preparation should be made for an asphyxiated baby. The paediatrician must be present at the birth to resuscitate the infant. The baby may require neonatal intensive care following birth and the staff of the neonatal unit will have been alerted. In addition to the insult of the haemorrhage, the baby may suffer from the effects of preterm birth and the stay in the neonatal unit may be prolonged. A baby who is born in good condition will of course require minimal resuscitation and will stay with the mother.

Psychological care

When a woman has a placental abruption she and her partner must be kept fully informed of what is happening at all times. The doctor should have a full and frank discussion with them about the events and the prognosis. The midwife should ensure that the partner is offered support and adequate explanation if the woman requires emergency surgery, or if her condition deteriorates suddenly. Whenever possible, he should continue to be present.

If the fetus is alive, a midwife or nurse from the neonatal unit should visit the couple in order to explain where the baby will be cared for after birth. The partner should be encouraged to visit the unit.

When the baby is born, if it is at all possible, the parents should be given a chance to see and handle their child before transfer to the neonatal unit. It is most helpful to have a photograph taken, which the mother can keep beside her, and the father should visit the baby at the earliest opportunity. Later the mother will be taken to see the baby, if necessary in her bed or in a wheelchair. As soon as she is able, she will be encouraged to participate in caring for her baby.

At a suitable time following her recovery, the mother must be invited to discuss the events and the prognosis for her baby. She may ask about the possibility of haemorrhage occurring in future pregnancies. There is some evidence that a previous abruption is a risk factor for abruption in the next pregnancy (Misra & Ananth 1999, Rasmussen et al 1997).

Complications

- DIC is a complication of moderate to severe placental abruption.

- Postpartum haemorrhage may occur as a result of the Couvelaire uterus and disseminated intravascular coagulation, or both. Intravenous ergometrine 0.5 mg is given at birth as a prophylactic measure.

- Renal failure may occur as a result of hypovolaemia and consequent poor perfusion of the kidneys.

- Pituitary necrosis is another possible consequence of prolonged and severe hypotension (also known as Sheehan's syndrome; see medical texts for details of this rare condition).

- The maternal mortality rate due to placental abruption is 1% (Konje & Taylor 2006).

Blood coagulation failure

Normal blood coagulation

Haemostasis refers to the arrest of bleeding, its function being to prevent loss of blood from the blood vessels. It depends on the mechanism of coagulation. This is counterbalanced by fibrinolysis which ensures that the blood vessels are reopened in order to maintain the patency of the circulation.

Blood clotting occurs in three main stages:

1. When tissues are damaged and platelets break down, thromboplastin is released.
2. In the presence of calcium ions, thromboplastin leads to the conversion of prothrombin into thrombin.
3. Thrombin is a proteolytic (protein-splitting) enzyme that converts fibrinogen into fibrin.

Fibrin forms a network of long, sticky strands that entrap blood cells to establish a clot. The coagulated material contracts and exudes serum, which is plasma depleted of its clotting factors. This is the final part of a complex cascade of coagulation involving a large number of different clotting factors. These factors have been assigned Roman numerals (for instance 'Factor IV') in order of their discovery.

It is equally important for a healthy person to maintain the blood as a fluid in order that it can circulate freely. The coagulation mechanism is normally held at bay by the presence of heparin, which is produced in the liver.

Fibrinolysis is the breakdown of fibrin and occurs as a response to the presence of clotted blood. Unless fibrinolysis takes place, coagulation will continue. It is achieved by the activation of a series of enzymes culminating in the proteolytic enzyme plasmin. This breaks down the fibrin in the clots and produces fibrin degradation products (FDPs).

Disseminated intravascular coagulation

DIC is a situation of inappropriate coagulation within the blood vessels, which leads to the consumption of clotting factors. As a result clotting fails to occur at the bleeding site. DIC is rare when the fetus is alive and it usually starts to resolve when the baby is born (Enkin et al 2000).

Aetiology

DIC is never a primary disease – it always occurs as a response to another disease process. Such an event triggers widespread clotting with the formation of microthrombi throughout the circulation. Clotting factors are used up. The DIC triggers fibrinolysis and the production of FDPs. FDPs reduce the efficiency of normal clotting. A paradoxical feedback system is therefore set up, in which clotting is the primary problem, but haemorrhage is the predominant clinical finding.

When DIC occurs during or after birth, the reduced level of clotting factors and the presence of FDPs prevent normal haemostasis at the placental site. FDPs inhibit myometrial action and prevent the uterine muscle from constricting the blood vessels in the normal way. Torrential haemorrhage may be the outcome. Visible blood loss may be observed to remain uncoagulated for several minutes and even when clotting does occur, the clot is unstable.

Microthrombi may cause circulatory obstruction in the small blood vessels. The effects of this vary from cyanosis of fingers and toes to cerebrovascular accidents and failure of organs such as the liver and kidneys.

Events that trigger DIC

There are a number of obstetric events that may precipitate DIC:

- placental abruption
- intrauterine fetal death including delayed miscarriage
- amniotic fluid embolism
- intrauterine infection including septic abortion
- pre-eclampsia and eclampsia.

Each of these conditions is dealt with in the appropriate chapter and only those aspects relating to DIC are discussed here.

Placental abruption

Owing to the damage of tissue at the placental site large quantities of thromboplastin are released into the circulation and may cause DIC. If the placenta is delivered as soon as possible after the abruption the risk of DIC is reduced. (However, vaginal birth where possible is often favoured over caesarean birth to reduce the risk of postpartum haemorrhage.)

Intrauterine fetal death

If a dead fetus is retained *in utero* for more than 3 or 4 weeks, then thromboplastins are released from the dead fetal tissues. These enter the maternal circulation and deplete clotting factors. If labour does not follow fetal death spontaneously, then it should be induced, with the woman's consent. If fetal death is known to have occurred some time previously, clotting studies should be performed prior to induction of labour; if DIC is diagnosed the appropriate medical action should be taken.

Amniotic fluid embolism

If death does not occur from maternal collapse, DIC may develop. Thromboplastin in the amniotic fluid is responsible for setting off the cascade of clotting.

Intrauterine infection

The causes of this include septic abortion, hydatidiform mole, placenta accreta and endometrial infection before or after birth. DIC is caused by endotoxins entering the circulation and damaging the blood vessels. Therefore, as well as treating the DIC, the infection itself must be aggressively treated with antibiotics. It should be noted that if the woman develops haemolytic septicaemia, any blood administered may be destroyed by the bacteria in the bloodstream. The baby may need treatment following birth if the infection was antepartum. In postpartum infection, any retained products must be evacuated from the uterus.

Pre-eclampsia and eclampsia

The occurrence of DIC with severe pre-eclampsia is fully dealt with in Ch. 22.

Management

The aims of the management of DIC are summarized in Box 20.2.

The midwife should be aware of the conditions that may cause DIC. She should be alert for signs that clotting is abnormal and the assessment of the nature of the clot should be part of her routine observation

Box 20.2 Aims of management of DIC

- To manage the underlying cause and remove the stimulus provoking DIC
- To ensure maintenance of the circulating blood volume
- To replace the 'used up' clotting factors and destroyed red blood cells.

(Anthony 2006)

during the third stage of labour. Oozing from a venepuncture site or bleeding from the mucous membrane of the mother's mouth and nose must be noted and reported. As well as a full blood count and blood grouping, the doctor will carry out clotting studies and also measure the levels of platelets, fibrinogen and FDPs.

Treatment involves the replacement of blood cells and clotting factors in order to restore equilibrium. This is usually done by the administration of fresh frozen plasma and platelet concentrates. Banked red cells will be transfused subsequently. The use of fresh whole blood is not now common, partly because the screening processes undertaken in the modern transfusion service can take up to 24 hrs and the components are best given separately. In situations where the transfusion service is not so sophisticated, whole blood will be used.

Management is carried out by a team of obstetricians, anaesthetists, haematologists, midwives and other health professionals who must strive to work together harmoniously and effectively to achieve the best possible clinical outcomes.

Care by the midwife

DIC causes a frightening situation that demands speed both of recognition and of action. The midwife has to maintain her own calmness and clarity of thinking as well as helping the couple to deal with the situation in which they find themselves. Frequent and accurate observations must be maintained in order to monitor the woman's condition. Blood pressure, respirations, pulse rate and temperature are recorded. The general condition is noted. Fluid balance is monitored with vigilance for any sign of renal failure.

The partner in particular is likely to be baffled by a sudden turn in events, when previously all seemed to be under control. The midwife must make sure that someone is giving him appropriate attention and he will need to be kept informed of what is happening and be excluded as little as possible. The carers need to be aware that he may find it impossible to absorb all that he is told and he may require repeated explanations. He may be the best person to help the woman to understand. The death of the mother is a real possibility.

Hepatic disorders and jaundice in pregnancy

Some liver disorders are specific to pregnant women, and some pre-existing or co-existing disorders may complicate the pregnancy (Box 20.3).

Causes of jaundice in pregnancy are listed in Box 20.4.

Intrahepatic cholestasis of pregnancy

ICP is an idiopathic condition that begins in pregnancy, usually in the third trimester but occasionally as early as the first trimester. It resolves spontaneously following birth, but has up to a 9% recurrence rate in subsequent pregnancies (Nelson-Piercy 2002). The prevalence rate is seven cases per 1000 pregnancies in low-risk populations, which include Caucasians, but it is seen most frequently in Scandinavia, Chile, Poland, Australia and China and in

Box 20.3 Hepatic disorders of pregnancy

Specific to pregnancy

- intrahepatic cholestasis of pregnancy
- acute fatty liver in pregnancy
- pre-eclampsia and eclampsia
- severe hyperemesis gravidarum.

Pre- or co-existing in pregnancy

- gall bladder disease
- hepatitis.

> **Box 20.4** Causes of jaundice in pregnancy
>
> **Not specific to pregnancy**
>
> - viral hepatitis – A, B, C, D and E are the most prevalent
> - hepatitis secondary to infection, usually cytomegalovirus, Epstein–Barr virus, toxoplasmosis or herpes simplex
> - gall stones
> - drug reactions
> - alcohol/drug abuse
> - Budd–Chiari syndrome.
>
> **Pregnancy-specific causes**
>
> - acute fatty liver
> - HELLP (haemolysis, elevated liver enzymes, low platelets) syndrome
> - intrahepatic cholestasis of pregnancy
> - hyperemesis gravidarum.
>
> *Note*: Jaundice is not an inevitable symptom of liver disease in pregnancy.

women of South-Asian origin (Williamson & Girling 2006). Its cause is unknown although genetic, geographical and environmental factors would appear to be at play. Almes (1995), Davidson (1998) and Gaudet et al (2000) put forward a group of theories that suggest the biochemistry of bile metabolism is altered; this is possibly due to a genetic inherited hypersensitivity to oestrogens. A subsequent increase in serum bile acid levels then negatively affects placental blood flow, putting the fetus at risk. Disturbances in fetal steroid metabolism may also be implicated. It is not a life-threatening condition for the mother, but she is at increased risk of pre-term labour, fetal compromise and meconium staining and her stillbirth risk is increased by 15% unless there is active management of her pregnancy.

Affected women will first start to notice pruritus at night, and may complain of fatigue and insomnia because of this. Two weeks later, 50% of women affected will develop mild jaundice, which will persist until the birth. Fever, abdominal discomfort and nausea and vomiting are not uncommon symptoms. Women may notice that their urine is darker and stools are paler than usual.

If this condition is suspected, blood will be tested for an increase in bile acids, serum alkaline phosphatase, bilirubin and transaminases. Hepatic viral studies, an ultrasound scan of the hepatobiliary tract and an autoantibody screen (for primary biliary cirrhosis) are also indicated as of value in excluding differential diagnoses. The woman will be prescribed local antipruritic agents, for instance antihistamines, and advised to keep any sores caused by scratching clean. Drugs, such as ursodeoxycholic acid (UDCA), dexamethasone and cholestyramine have disappointing results in controlling symptoms (Williamson & Girling 2006) and there has been little follow-up of the babies to date. The woman may be prescribed Vitamin K 10 mg orally daily as her absorption will be poor, leading to prothrombinaemia, which will predispose her to obstetric haemorrhage.

Because of concern about the implications of this condition for the fetus, the resultant jaundice and the severity of the itching, this woman will require sensitive psychological care. Fetal well-being should be monitored, possibly by Doppler analysis of the umbilical artery blood flow, and elective delivery considered when the fetus is mature (usually at 35–38 weeks' gestation) or earlier if the fetal condition appears to be compromised by the intrauterine environment.

The woman can be advised that her pruritus will resolve within 3–14 days after the birth. She should be carefully monitored if she uses oral contraception in the future. The pruritus is often so severe and distressing that many women who have suffered from this condition will avoid future pregnancy.

Further information and support is available at: www.ocsupport.org.uk

Acute fatty liver of pregnancy

AFLP is a rare condition of unknown aetiology (although fetal long-chain hydroxyacyl co-enzyme A dehydrogenase (LCHAD) deficiency has recently been implicated). It has an incidence in various studies of between 1 in 7000 and 1 in 13 000 pregnancies (Williamson & Girling 2006). It is frequently fatal for the mother and baby unless there is a speedy diagnosis and the correct treatment is given.

Typically, an obese woman will present with vomiting and a headache in her third trimester. She will quickly complain of malaise and severe abdominal pain, followed by jaundice and drowsiness. Fagan (2002) comments that over 50% of these women have symptoms of pre-eclampsia (hypertension and proteinuria), and so there is an inherent danger that the pre-eclampsia will mask the presentation of AFLP.

The condition is diagnosed by the clinical picture. The woman's liver is tender but not enlarged, and an ultrasound or computerized tomography (CT) scan of the liver demonstrates fatty infiltration. Liver biopsy is contraindicated owing to the risk of coagulopathy. The liver enzymes are moderately raised and the woman will also quickly show signs of renal failure and will become hypoglycaemic.

Management will first involve correcting any coagulopathy by measures such as infusing fresh frozen plasma. The woman must be delivered immediately. Caesarean section is said to have many advantages for the baby, but it is safest for the mother to birth vaginally if this is possible. Epidural analgesia is contraindicated in all but the mildest cases owing to the coagulopathy problems, unless these have been corrected first.

Convalescence is prolonged but usually complete. In the few cases where further pregnancy has been undertaken and recorded in the medical literature, recurrence has been low.

Gall bladder disease

Pregnancy appears to increase the likelihood of gallstone formation but not the risk of developing acute cholecystitis. Diagnosis of gall bladder disease is made by listening to the woman's previous history or an ultrasound scan of the hepatobiliary tract, or both. She will require symptomatic treatment of the biliary colic by analgesia, hydration, nasogastric suction and antibiotics. Surgery should be avoided if at all possible.

Viral hepatitis

Viral hepatitis is the most common cause of jaundice in pregnancy (Fagan 2002). Acute infection affects approximately 1 in 1000 pregnancies and has an incubation period of 1–6 months. Symptoms include nausea, vomiting, anorexia, pain over the liver, mild diarrhoea, jaundice lasting several weeks and malaise. Fever is rare and for many the disease is asymptomatic, or mimics mild influenza. Its main spread is by blood, blood products and sexual activity. The virus can also be transmitted across the placenta. Hepatitis B is more common in tropical and developing countries, especially where nutrition is poor and the use of barrier contraceptives is limited, but it is also a particular problem among injecting drug users who share needles in the Western world (Fagan 2002). The more common infections are known as hepatitis A, B and C (D and E strains also exist and have many clinical and epidemiological features which overlap; concise diagnosis is made by blood tests).

Hepatitis A (HAV) occurs as an acute infection spread predominantly by ingesting water contaminated with faecal matter. It is endemic worldwide. Mother to baby transmission is rare but can occur at birth. HAV is a self-limiting illness which invariably results in complete recovery in otherwise healthy individuals. Vaccination is available. Strict hygiene and hand washing in health care settings reduces the risk of cross infection.

Hepatitis B (HBV) is a more serious infection because 5–10% of those infected become chronic carriers, and 25–30% of these will die as a result years later (Silverman 2006). In the Western world 0.5–5% of the population are chronic HBV carriers (Fagan 2002), continuing to test positive for the HBV surface antigen (HBsAg). However, in healthy adults 90% of primary cases of HBV resolve completely within 1–3 months. In the remaining 5–10%, hepatitis B surface antigen (HBsAg) remains in the serum and the woman is considered to be a chronic carrier. Some of these will clear the antigen over the course of the next 6 months and the rest will develop chronic active hepatitis, and the symptoms described above will also continue. A few will develop hepatic failure, which can result in death unless liver transplantation is available (Box 20.5). If hepatitis B is transmitted from mother to fetus and immunization does not prevent infection in the baby, the child will be at increased risk of chronic liver disease, cirrhosis and primary liver cancer in later life, these childhood implications often being severely underestimated (Fagan 2002). In

Box 20.5 Pregnancy and liver transplantation

There have now been a number of pregnancies in women who have undergone liver transplantation before or during their pregnancy, many with successful outcomes. Although not desirable, liver transplantation in women of childbearing age is becoming increasingly common and such women now have the opportunity to consider having a family. However, the risks to pregnancy are great and these women require expert medical and midwifery care at a specialized centre equipped to deal with all of the complications, both of a physical and psychological nature, that such women may face.

pregnancy, the risk is considered to be greater to the fetus than the mother through transplacental passage of the virus and particularly through blood and body fluids at birth. Caesarean section does not prevent mother to fetus transmission. Diagnosis is made from the woman's history of her symptoms and lifestyle. Serological studies will be performed, but it can be difficult to distinguish hepatitis B from other forms of viral hepatitis during the acute presentation, before antibodies have formed. Treatment is of the symptoms as they arise. Infection control measures should be instituted where the woman is considered to be infectious, and information not only about the disease, but also nutrition and sexual advice, should be offered. Liver function will be monitored and fetal condition assessed. Household contacts should be offered immunization once their HBsAg seronegativity is established. Sexual partners should be traced and offered testing and vaccination. Postnatally the mother will be encouraged to accept vaccination for the baby. Breastfeeding is not contraindicated (Fagan 2002).

Hepatitis C virus (HCV) was first identified in 1989 (Silverman 2006). The usual risk factors for transmission are blood and blood products and the use of shared intravenous needles. At least 90% of post-blood transfusion hepatitis can be traced to HCV, commonly from a blood donor who had yet to sero-convert at the time of blood donation and testing. (This suggests that blood transfusion should always be carefully considered and never undertaken without good clinical need.) Acute HCV has an incubation period of 30–60 days but 75% of those infected will be asymptomatic. In the remaining 25% symptoms include transient nausea and jaundice; 50% of those infected will progress to chronic HCV which is associated with B cell lymphomas and chronic liver disease. In the USA, the HCV rate appears to be 2.3–4.5% in pregnant women and placental (vertical) transmission rate suggests the risk to the baby is <5% (Silverman 2006). Optimal route of birth and safety of breastfeeding have yet to be established. While more difficult to acquire than HBV, HCV carries a much higher long term risk of chronic liver disease. No vaccine is available yet and the long-term outcome for infected newborns appears to be unreported at present in large epidemiological studies.

Skin disorders

Many skin changes are noticed by pregnant women; most of these are so common as to be described as physiological.

Treatment of pre-existing skin disorders, such as eczema or psoriasis, should continue as required, bearing in mind that some topical agents should be used with caution in pregnancy (such as steroid creams and applications containing nut oil derivatives).

Many women suffer from physiological pruritus in pregnancy, especially over the abdomen. Often emotional support, and the application of calamine lotion over the affected area, will suffice. However, for some women, pruritus with or without a rash will be a symptom of a more serious condition. Generalized pruritus should always be referred to a medical practitioner, as it may be a symptom of conditions such as intrahepatic cholestasis, liver or thyroid disease, lymphoma or scabies.

Pemphigoid gestationis (herpes gestationis)

This is a disease specific to pregnancy that usually occurs in the mid-trimester and persists into the postnatal period, although sometimes it starts after the birth. It affects 1 in 10 000 to 1 in 50 000 pregnancies (Engineer et al 2000) and its aetiology is unknown; however, it is thought that the condition is initiated by a maternal autoimmune response to paternal antigens and persists under the influence of pregnancy hormones. Despite its name, this skin condition is not related to the herpes virus – the misnomer came about in the nineteenth century when 'herpes' referred to skin blisters, rather than the virus.

The woman will complain of generalized itching and a burning sensation, and an erythematous rash will appear (see Plate 2). This is initially over the abdomen, but spreads to involve the remainder of the trunk and limbs. Blisters develop that may become infected and purulent, especially if the woman scratches.

The midwife should refer the woman to a medical practitioner and be supportive to her throughout her care. A skin biopsy may be needed to confirm the diagnosis. Topical or oral steroids may be prescribed depending on the severity of the disease. The lesions should be kept clean and may be covered to prevent the woman scratching. A diet high in vitamins should be encouraged. The woman may have her labour induced at about the 37th week of pregnancy, as there is controversial evidence that there is a greater incidence of intrauterine growth restriction with this condition, which is suggestive of a link with placental insufficiency (Kroumpouzos & Cohen 2006). The baby may have a rash when born and will need paediatric examination for any skin lesions, although these are usually clinically mild.

Without excessive scratching or secondary infection, the woman's lesions will heal without scarring, although this may take some time and occasionally a few years. Once the condition has been activated by pregnancy, flare-ups may occur during menstruation, at ovulation or when the woman takes an oral contraceptive (Kroumpouzos & Cohen 2006). The condition may recur in subsequent pregnancies, especially with the same partner.

Disorders of the amniotic fluid

Normal amniotic fluid increases in amount throughout pregnancy from a few millilitres until 38 weeks, when there is about 1 L. After this, it diminishes to approximately 800 mL at term. Amniotic fluid is not static; the water of which it is largely composed changes every hour and the solutes change about every 3 hrs.

There are two chief abnormalities of amniotic fluid: hydramnios (or polyhydramnios) and oligohydramnios. These conditions are sometimes suspected on palpation and diagnosis is made ultrasonographically.

Hydramnios

The amount of liquor present in a pregnancy can be estimated by measuring 'pools' of liquor around the fetus with ultrasound scanning. The single deepest pool is measured to calculate the amniotic fluid volume (AFV). However, where possible a more accurate diagnosis may be gained by measuring the liquor in each of four quadrants around the fetus in order to establish an amniotic fluid index (AFI).

Hydramnios is said to be present when the deepest vertical pool of liquor (DP) exceeds 8 cm, or the calculated AFI is above the 95th centile for gestational age (Taylor & Fisk 2006). It is present in 0.2% of pregnancies, most commonly in a mild to moderate form.

Causes and predisposing factors

These include:

- oesophageal atresia
- open neural tube defect
- multiple pregnancy, especially in the case of monozygotic twins
- maternal diabetes mellitus
- rarely, an association with Rhesus isoimmunization
- chorioangioma, a rare tumour of the placenta
- anencephalic fetus.

However, in many cases the cause is unknown.

Types

Chronic hydramnios

This is gradual in onset, usually starting from about the 30th week of pregnancy. It is the most common type.

Acute hydramnios

This is very rare. It usually occurs at about 20 weeks and comes on very suddenly. The uterus reaches the xiphisternum in about 3 or 4 days. It is frequently associated with monozygotic twins or severe fetal abnormality.

Recognition

The mother may complain of breathlessness and discomfort. If the hydramnios is acute in onset, she may have severe abdominal pain. The condition may cause exacerbation of symptoms associated with pregnancy such as indigestion, heartburn and constipation. Oedema and varicosities of the vulva and lower limbs may be present.

Abdominal examination

On inspection, the uterus is larger than expected for the period of gestation and is globular in shape. The abdominal skin appears stretched and shiny with marked striae gravidarum and obvious superficial blood vessels.

On palpation, the uterus feels tense and it is difficult to feel the fetal parts, but the fetus may be balloted between the two hands. A fluid thrill may be elicited by placing a hand on one side of the abdomen and tapping the other side with the fingers. A wave of fluid will move across from the side that is tapped and this is felt by the opposite examining hand. It may be helpful to measure the abdominal girth (Fig. 20.9), particularly in cases of acute hydramnios, in order to observe the rate of increase.

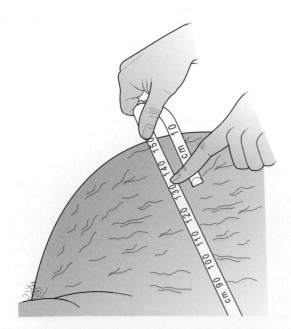

Figure 20.9 Measuring abdominal girth in a case of polyhydramnios.

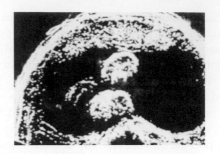

Figure 20.10 Polyhydramnios: ultrasonogram

Auscultation of the fetal heart can be difficult if the quantity of fluid allows the fetus to move away from the stethoscope.

Ultrasonic scanning is used to confirm the diagnosis of hydramnios (Fig. 20.10). As well as calculating the DP, AFV and AFI, and therefore the severity of the hydramnios, scanning may reveal a multiple pregnancy or fetal abnormality. X-ray examination is not often performed and the images are usually hazy where there is a large quantity of amniotic fluid.

Complications

These include:

- maternal ureteric obstruction
- increased fetal mobility leading to unstable lie and malpresentation
- cord presentation and prolapse
- pre-labour (and often preterm) rupture of the membranes
- placental abruption when the membranes rupture
- pre-term labour
- a higher incidence of pre-eclampsia
- increased incidence of caesarean section
- postpartum haemorrhage
- raised perinatal mortality rate.

Management

The aim of managing this condition is to relieve maternal symptoms and optimize the length of gestation, prolonging it if safe. The cause of the condition should be determined if possible and fetal karyotyping may be indicated. The woman may be admitted to a consultant obstetric unit. Subsequent care will depend on the condition of the woman and fetus, the cause and degree of the hydramnios and the stage of pregnancy. Diabetes mellitus will be managed as an entity; the hydramnios is managed much as in other cases. The presence of fetal abnormality will be taken into consideration in choosing the mode and timing of birth. If gross abnormality is present, labour may be induced; if the fetus is suffering from an operable condition such as oesophageal atresia, transfer will be arranged to a neonatal surgical unit.

Mild asymptomatic hydramnios is managed expectantly. The woman is not usually admitted to hospital, but should be advised that if she suspects that her membranes have ruptured immediate admission is recommended. She should be encouraged to get adequate rest, and if she is working it may be helpful to discuss commencing maternity leave, although the physical nature of her job and the stress that may be engendered by stopping work should be assessed with the woman before making recommendations. Panting-Kemp et al (1999) suggest that if the hydramnios is found to be idiopathic, as is more likely in mild asymptomatic cases, she can be reassured that fetal outcome is likely to be good.

Regular ultrasound scans will reveal whether or not the hydramnios is progressive. Many cases of idiopathic hydramnios resolve spontaneously as pregnancy progresses (Hendricks et al 1991).

For a woman with symptomatic hydramnios, an upright position will help to relieve any dyspnoea and she may be given antacids to relieve heartburn and nausea. If the discomfort from the swollen abdomen is severe, then therapeutic amniocentesis, or amnioreduction, may be considered. However, this is not without risk, as infection may be introduced or the onset of labour provoked. It is at best a temporary relief as the fluid will rapidly accumulate again and the procedure may need to be repeated. Acute hydramnios managed by amnioreduction has a poor prognosis for the baby. The usual course of events is that the fluid continues to increase at an alarming rate, the membranes rupture spontaneously and the fetus or fetuses are born, grossly premature, in a river of amniotic fluid.

Administration of drugs such as indomethacin and sulindac reduce fetal urine production and consequently amniotic fluid, but use of these drugs is still experimental until the risks have been more fully ascertained (Taylor & Fisk 2006).

The woman may need to have labour induced in late pregnancy if the symptoms become worse. The lie must be corrected if it is not longitudinal and the membranes will be ruptured cautiously, allowing the amniotic fluid to drain out slowly in order to avoid altering the lie and to prevent cord prolapse. Placental abruption is also a hazard if the uterus suddenly diminishes in size.

Labour is usually normal but the midwife should be prepared for the possibility of postpartum haemorrhage. The baby should be carefully examined for abnormalities and the patency of the oesophagus ascertained by passing a nasogastric tube.

Oligohydramnios

Oligohydramnios is an abnormally small amount of amniotic fluid. At term it may be 300–500 mL but amounts vary and it can be even less. When diagnosed in the first half of pregnancy it is often found to be associated with renal agenesis (absence of kidneys) or Potter's syndrome in which the baby also has pulmonary hypoplasia. When diagnosed at any time in pregnancy before 37 weeks, it may be due to fetal abnormality or to pre-term pre-labour rupture of the membranes where the amniotic fluid fails to re-accumulate. The lack of amniotic fluid reduces the intrauterine space and over time will cause compression deformities. The baby has a squashed-looking face, flattening of the nose, micrognathia (a deformity of the jaw) and talipes. The skin is dry and leathery in appearance.

Oligohydramnios sometimes occurs in the post-term pregnancy and is believed to be linked with the development of placental insufficiency. As placental function reduces, so too does perfusion to the fetal organ systems including the kidneys. The decrease in fetal urine formation leads to oligohydramnios, as the major component of amniotic fluid is fetal urine.

Recognition

On inspection, the uterus may appear smaller than expected for the period of gestation. The mother who has had a previous normal pregnancy may have noticed a reduction in fetal movements. When the abdomen is palpated the uterus is small and compact and fetal parts are easily felt. Breech presentation is possible. Auscultation is normal.

Ultrasonic scanning will enable differentiation of oligohydramnios from intrauterine growth restriction (although both may occur together where there is placental insufficiency). Renal abnormality may be visible on the scan. As with hydramnios, measurement of amniotic fluid and calculation of the AFI below the 5th centile will aid diagnosis.

Management

The aim in managing oligohydramnios is to establish its cause by investigating the aetiology and fetal effects. The woman may be admitted to hospital. If the ultrasound scan demonstrates renal agenesis the baby will not survive. Liquor volume will also be estimated from the ultrasound scan, and if renal agenesis is not present then further investigations will include careful questioning of the woman to check the possibility of pre-term rupture of the membranes. Placental function tests will also be performed.

Where fetal anomaly is not considered to be lethal, or the cause of the oligohydramnios is not known, prophylactic amnioinfusion with normal saline, Ringer's lactate or 5% glucose may be performed in order to prevent compression deformities and hypoplastic lung disease, and prolong the pregnancy. Little evidence is available to determine the benefits and hazards of this intervention in midpregnancy. However, Pitt et al (2000) in a metaanalysis of randomized controlled trials concluded that prophylactic intrapartum amnioinfusion in women with oligohydramnios resulted in lower caesarean section rates and improved neonatal outcome for structurally normal babies. Early indications are that this is a useful intervention.

In the case of term pregnancy, Grant (2006) reports that fetal surveillance by cardiotocography, amniotic fluid measurement by ultrasound and Doppler assessment of fetal and uteroplacental arteries is unlikely to predict the fetal outcome reliably. Furthermore, Grant et al (1989) demonstrated that maternal counting, recording and reporting of fetal movement was not effective in reducing stillbirths. Oligohydramnios in prolonged pregnancy in the absence of ruptured membranes remains a poorly understood phenomenon, and its management therefore remains highly controversial.

At any stage of pregnancy labour may intervene, or be induced where the fetus is viable because of the possibility of placental insufficiency. Epidural analgesia may be indicated because uterine contractions are often unusually painful with this condition. Impairment of placental circulation or cord compression may result in fetal hypoxia and therefore continuous fetal heart rate monitoring is desirable. In rare cases the membranes may adhere to the fetus. Also, if meconium is passed in utero it will be more concentrated and represent a greater danger to an asphyxiated baby during birth.

Pre-term pre-labour rupture of the membranes

PPROM occurs before 37 completed weeks' gestation, where rupture of the fetal membranes occurs without the onset of spontaneous uterine activity resulting in cervical dilatation. (Term pre-labour rupture of the membranes is discussed in Ch. 30.)

PPROM affects 2% of pregnancies. Placental abruption is evident in 4–7% of women who present with PPROM. The condition has a 17–34% recurrence rate in subsequent pregnancies of affected women (Svigos et al 2006). It may be associated with cervical incompetence (although it is likely that uterine contractions accompany the rupture of membranes with this condition). There is a strong association between PPROM and maternal vaginal colonization with potentially pathogenic micro-organisms, with the incidence of subclinical chorioamnionitis said to be around 30% (Svigos et al 2006). Infection may both precede (and cause) or follow PPROM.

Risks of PPROM

These include:

- labour, which may intervene at any time, resulting in a preterm birth
- chorioamnionitis, which may be followed by fetal and maternal systemic infection if not treated promptly
- oligohydramnios if prolonged PPROM occurs, with associated fetal problems including pulmonary hypoplasia

- psychosocial problems resulting from uncertain fetal and neonatal outcome and long term hospitalization
- cord prolapse
- malpresentation associated with prematurity
- primary antepartum haemorrhage.

Management

Because the pathophysiology of PPROM is still not fully understood, and trials into different management options have not been conclusive in their findings, contemporary management of the condition remains controversial.

Psychological consideration of the woman's, and her partner's, circumstances must always be considered with PPROM as it is known to be an extremely disturbing condition for parents, not least because causes and predictions of the outcome cannot be given. If PPROM is suspected, the woman will be admitted to the labour suite where a careful history is taken and rupture of the membranes confirmed by a sterile speculum examination of any pooling of liquor in the posterior fornix of the vagina. Very wet sanitary towels over a 6 hrs period will also offer a reasonably conclusive diagnosis if urine leakage has been excluded, but a positive Nitrazine test should not be considered conclusive when it is the only sign (Svigos et al 2006). Where diagnosis is in doubt, a fetal fibronectin immunoenzyme test is useful in confirming rupture of the membranes, and ultrasound scanning has some value.

Digital vaginal examination should be avoided to reduce the risk of introducing infection. Observations must also be made of the fetal condition from the fetal heart rate (an infected fetus may have a tachycardia) and maternal infection screen, temperature and pulse, uterine tenderness and any purulent or offensively smelling vaginal discharge. A decision on future management will then be made.

If the woman has a gestation of <32 weeks, the fetus appears to be uncompromised and APH and labour have been excluded, she will be managed expectantly. She is likely to be hospitalized and offered frequent ultrasound scans to check the growth of the fetus and the extent and complications of any oligohydramnios. She should be given corticosteroids as soon as PPROM is confirmed in case

the baby is born (Crowley 2001), and if labour intervenes then tocolytic drugs will be considered to prolong the pregnancy. Known vaginal infection should be treated with antibiotics and prophylactic antibiotics may also be offered to women without symptoms of infection as the present evidence suggests that antibiotic administration following preterm rupture of the membranes (PROM) is associated with a statistically significant reduction in major markers of neonatal morbidity (but not mortality) and the data support the routine use of antibiotics from PPROM. The choice of antibiotic however, remains less clear but erythromycin seems to be the drug of choice for most women (Kenyon et al 2007). Sometimes the leak will re-seal (especially if it is a hindwater leak) and the pregnancy may proceed with no further complications. However, 're-sealing' is said to occur in only 8% of cases of PPROM occurring in mid-trimester (Sciscione et al 2001). Serial amnioinfusion for otherwise normal pregnancies is an intervention that is gaining increasing interest; for instance Locatelli et al (2000) report improved perinatal outcomes where PPROM and oligohydramnios have occurred at <26 weeks' gestation, although Taylor & Fisk (2006) report that the fluid usually leaks out again. Research is ongoing looking at cervical occlusion with fibrin gel. If membranes rupture before 24 weeks of gestation the outlook is not good; the fetus is likely to succumb either to the problems caused by oligohydramnios or to those caused by pre-term birth. The mother in such cases may be offered, and may accept termination of the pregnancy.

If the woman is more than 32 weeks' pregnant, the fetus appears to be compromised and APH or intervening labour is suspected or confirmed, active management will ensue. The mode of birth will be decided and induction of labour or caesarean section performed.

Malignant disease in pregnancy

It is estimated that 1 in 1000–1500 pregnancies are complicated by cancer (Munkarah et al 2006). The most common malignancies associated with pregnancy are, in descending frequency: cervix, ovary, breast, melanoma, leukaemia, lymphoma and colorectum (Allen & Nisker 1986, quoted in Munkarah et al 2006). The incidence of cancer occurring along-side pregnancy increases as women delay childbearing (see Ch. 19 for Cervical carcinoma). Pregnancy may adversely affect the course of the disease, and cancer in the mother can metastasize to the placenta and fetus, melanoma being the most likely to do so.

If cancer is discovered before pregnancy is embarked upon, it should be treated and followed up before pregnancy is attempted. Once successfully treated, and as long as the reproductive organs are not damaged, pregnancy is rarely contraindicated for medical reasons. However, cancer discovered during pregnancy leads to a host of management dilemmas. The options involve balancing the effects of the treatment, the disease and birth on both the mother and her fetus.

If the woman is in early pregnancy, her first dilemma may be whether or not to continue with the pregnancy. If she continues, the next dilemma will be whether to treat the disease during the pregnancy or await birth, as both chemotherapy and radiation therapy may have toxic effects, particularly on the fetus. Surgery is the treatment least likely to affect the pregnancy adversely, particularly if it takes place in later pregnancy, but it may not be the treatment of first choice for the particular condition.

Elective pre-term birth is often favoured by medical practitioners involved in the woman's care and the woman herself, after which her condition can be assessed and more appropriate treatment of the disease administered.

Obesity and failure to gain weight in pregnancy

Although evidence exists to refute strongly the value of frequent routine weighing of all pregnant women in predicting various perinatal outcomes, surprisingly little is known about optimal weight gain and the effects of large and low weight gain in pregnancy. However, it is becoming increasingly clear that women who have a poor diet and their fetuses are at greater risk than well-nourished women (Dallison & Lobstein 1995).

Weight is no more than a very crude indicator of a woman's health status in pregnancy. However, the midwife's observation of a very obese woman, or a very thin one, should alert her to some of the risks such women may face during pregnancy and the longer term risks to both women and their children (see Ch. 13 for Quetelet index).

A woman who starts pregnancy while obese, or puts on an excessive amount of weight during pregnancy, appears to be at greater risk of hypertensive disturbances, including pregnancy-induced hypertension (see Ch. 22). She is also at greater risk of gestational diabetes (see Ch. 21) and both of these conditions make her more likely to be delivered by caesarean section. She is also at increased risk of urinary tract infection, uncertain fetal position, postpartum haemorrhage and thrombophlebitis. She is more likely to give birth to a large for gestational age infant, although if her pregnancy has been otherwise uncomplicated she is not statistically at greater risk of shoulder dystocia (Wildschut 2006). There is conflicting evidence of a relationship between maternal obesity and perinatal mortality. The woman is also more prone to wound infection following operative delivery. Obesity may also be associated with malnourishment from essential nutrient deficiency. However the Confidential Enquiries into Maternal Deaths in the United Kingdom (Lewis 2007) reports that over half of the women who died (2003–2005) were overweight or obese. Obesity is, therefore, an important risk factor for maternal death.

As well as excessive weight increase during pregnancy being a greater risk factor for the onset of hypertensive disorders, its sudden onset may signal occult oedema. If such weight gain is noted by the woman or the midwife it is prudent to take the woman's blood pressure and test her urine for protein.

Once oedema has been excluded, the midwife should make tactful attempts to discuss the woman's diet with her, when it becomes apparent that her weight may raise her risk of complications. Ideally all women should be given the opportunity to discuss diet, as well as other general lifestyle factors, from as early on in their pregnancy as possible, or even before, and at regular intervals thereafter. Midwives should discuss diet, nutrition, exercise and the reasons why excessive weight gain in pregnancy is undesirable. There is no advantage to dieting during pregnancy (and strict dieting may be dangerous), so sensible eating should be advocated. Referral to a dietician may be helpful.

Blood pressure measurements should always be taken accurately with a correctly sized cuff, and gestational diabetes and urinary tract infection screened for. Frequent routine weighing is rarely of any practical benefit, and may only reduce a woman's self-esteem and make her dread her antenatal appointments. The midwife should also bear in mind that obesity can be a symptom of another disease, such as hypothyroidism, polycystic ovarian syndrome or Cushing's disease, and in such cases diet will have only a minimal effect on weight.

Conversely, the midwife may observe that a woman appears to be thin during her pregnancy and not laying down healthy fat stores. Detailed discussion should attempt to elicit the quality and quantity of the woman's diet and her weight pattern over previous years. Some women are naturally very slim and remain so because of genetic factors and a high metabolic rate, going on to produce a healthily sized baby. Of the rest, a medical disorder such as a malabsorption condition may be present, or starvation, if the woman has been living until recently in a country struck by famine.

The midwife needs to be aware that pregnant women can be afflicted by anorexia nervosa or bulimia, or both, often chronic conditions that may have been previously undetected despite their obsessive nature, or labelled 'dieting'.

Where a woman is suffering from nutritional deprivation she is at greater risk of anaemia and intrauterine growth restriction and its sequelae, including birth asphyxia and perinatal death. Bulimia may be wrongly diagnosed as hyperemesis gravidarum.

The midwife's role in the care of such women will depend on the cause. She should always involve the medical practitioner because of the risk of intrauterine growth restriction, and in cases with a medical cause. Where an eating disorder such as anorexia nervosa or bulimia is suspected, or admitted to, the involvement of a clinical psychologist or psychiatrist may be of value but, of course, the woman must be amenable to this. (It should also be said that if a midwife cares for a woman who has resolved a former eating disorder it would be inappropriate to suggest that the woman requires psychiatric support

in her pregnancy because of her history.) Dietary discussion and advice, including the use of supplements such as multivitamins and referral to a dietician, should be discussed with the woman. Quality of nutrition is as important, if not more so, than quantity. Where a woman is known to be suffering from an eating disorder, the importance of non-judgemental support from all of her carers cannot be overestimated in maintaining her well-being. As with the obese woman, some of the problem may lie with lowered self-esteem.

Problems associated with pregnancy following assisted conception

The rate of assisted conceptions has risen dramatically in the last few years. Couples who achieve pregnancy following assisted conception may be at greater risk of complications during the pregnancy than those who conceive naturally, for a number of reasons.

The cause of the fertility problem may be a medical problem in itself that is aggravated by pregnancy, such as some forms of malignancy and their treatments. It is also known that with some forms of assisted conception there is an increased rate of multiple pregnancy, which will in turn increase the risk of pre-eclampsia, preterm labour and so on. Women who undergo assisted conception are likely to be an older age group, either having previously tried for some time to conceive a baby naturally or having fertility problems because of their increased age. Increased maternal age has slight associations with multiple pregnancy and pre-eclampsia, and the older a woman is the more lifetime she has lived to develop a medical problem such as essential hypertension or diabetes mellitus, or a gynaecological problem such as fibroids.

The desire of many couples to be parents can override potential risk to the woman and a couple may present a compelling case to the fertility clinic whose help they seek. Also, women who achieve pregnancy with medical assistance are more likely to be closely monitored, particularly with ultrasound scans and perhaps closer follow-up of otherwise mild symptoms. The couple themselves may feel greatly reassured to have their pregnancy the subject of such close medical scrutiny. However, the combination of the increased use of technology, and the stress engendered by searching for problems (which in today's open environment means explaining what each problem may entail) in a so-called 'precious pregnancy', can themselves invoke a perception of a more complicated pregnancy than may actually be the case.

REFERENCES

Abu-Heija A, Al-Chalabi H, El-Iloubani N 1998 Abruptio placentae: risk factors and perinatal outcome. Journal of Obstetrics and Gynaecology Research 24(2):141–144

Almes L T 1995 Intrahepatic cholestasis of pregnancy. Journal of the Society of Obstetricians and Gynaecologists of Canada 17(4):343–351

Ambrose A, Repke J 2006 Puerperal problems. In: James D K, Steer P J, Weiner C P and Gonik B (eds) High risk pregnancy management options. W B Saunders, Philadelphia, p 1579–1605

Ananth C V, Wilcox A J 2001 Placental abruption and perinatal mortality in the United States. American Journal of Epidemiology 153(4):332–337

Ananth C V, Savitz D A, Bowes W A et al 1997 Influence of hypertensive disorders and cigarette smoking on placental abruption and uterine bleeding during pregnancy. British Journal of Obstetrics and Gynaecology 104(5):572–578

Andres R L 1996 The association of cigarette smoking with placenta previa and abruptio placentae. Seminars in Perinatology 20(2):154–159

Anthony J 2006 Major obstetric haemorrhage and disseminated intravascular coagulation. In: James D K, Steer P J, Weiner C P and Gonik B (eds) High risk pregnancy management options. W B Saunders, Philadelphia, p 1606–1623

Beischer N A, Mackay E V, Colditz P B 1997 Obstetrics and the newborn, 3rd edn. W B Saunders, London

Bewley C, Gibbs A 2001 Domestic abuse and pregnancy. MIDIRS Midwifery Digest 11(2):183–187

Crowley P 2001 Prophylactic steroids for preterm birth. In: The Cochrane Database of Systematic Reviews. Update Software, Oxford, Issue 2

Dallison J, Lobstein T 1995 Poor expectations. NCH Action For Children, London

Davidson K M 1998 Intrahepatic cholestasis of pregnancy. Seminars in Perinatology 22(2):104–111

Eckford S D, Vyas S, Mills M S et al 1995 Delayed placental abruption after road traffic accident. Journal of Obstetrics and Gynaecology 15(3):186–187

Engineer L, Bhol K, Ahmed A R 2000 Pemphigoid gestationalis: A review. American Journal of Obstetrics and Gynaecology 183:483–491

Enkin M, Keirse M J N C, Neilson J et al 2000 A guide to effective care in pregnancy and labour. Oxford University Press, Oxford

Fagan E A 2002 Disorders of the liver, biliary system and pancreas. In: de Swiet M (ed.) Medical disorders in obstetric practice. Blackwell Science, Oxford, p 282–345

Fry D, Hay-Smith J, Hough J, et al 1997 National Clinical Guideline for the care of women with symphysis pubis dysfunction. Midwives 110(1314):172–173

Gaudet R, Merviel P, Berkane N et al 2000 Fetal impact of cholestasis of pregnancy: experience at Tenon Hospital and literature review. Fetal Diagnosis and Therapy 15(4):191–197

Grant A, Elbourne D, Velentin L et al 1989 Routine formal movement counting and risk of antepartum late death in normally formed singletons. Lancet ii:345–349

Grant J M 2006 Prolonged pregnancy. In: James D K, Steer P J, Weiner C P, Gonik B (eds) High risk pregnancy management options. W B Saunders, London, p 1376–1382

Hendricks S K, Conway L, Wang K et al 1991 Diagnosis of polyhydramnios in early gestation: Indication for prenatal diagnosis? Prenatal Diagnosis 11(8):649–654

Kenyon S, Boulvain M, Neilson J 2007 Antibiotics for preterm rupture of membranes. The Cochrane Database of Systematic Reviews, Issue 3

Konje J C, Taylor D J 2006 Bleeding in late pregnancy. In: James D K, Steer P J, Weiner C P et al (eds) High risk pregnancy management options. W B Saunders, London, p 1259–1275

Kroumpouzos G K, Cohen L M 2006 Skin disease. In: James D K, Steer P J, Weiner C P et al (eds) High risk pregnancy management options. W B Saunders, London, p 1138–1162

Letsky E A 1995 Coagulation defects. In: de Swiet M (ed.) Medical disorders in obstetric practice. Blackwell Science, Oxford, p 71–115

Lewis G (ed.) 2007 The Confidential Enquiry into Maternal and Child Health (CEMACH). Saving mothers' lives: reviewing maternal deaths to make motherhood safer – 2003–2005. The Seventh Report on Confidential Enquiries in the United Kingdom. CEMACH, London

Locatelli A, Vergani P, Di Pirro G et al 2000 The role of amnioinfusion in the management of premature rupture of membranes at less than 26 weeks' gestation. American Journal of Obstetrics and Gynecology 183(4):878–882

Lockwood C J, Funai E F 1999 Placenta previa and related disorders. In: Queenan J T (ed.) High-risk pregnancy. Blackwell Science, Massachusetts, p 466–474

Mahomed K 2006a Abdominal pain. In: James D K, Steer P J, Weiner C P et al (eds) High risk pregnancy management options. W B Saunders, Philadelphia, p 1231–1247

Mahomed K 2006b Non malignant gynaecology. In: James D K, Steer P J, Weiner C P et al (eds) High risk pregnancy management options. W B Saunders, Philadelphia, p 1248–1258.

Manolitsas T, Wein P, Beicher N A et al 1994 Value of cardiotocography in women with antepartum haemorrhage – is it too late for caesarean section when the cardiotocograph shows ominous features? Australian and New Zealand Journal of Obstetrics and Gynaecology 34(4):403–408

Misra P, Ananth C V 1999 Risk factor profiles of placental abruption in first and second pregnancies; heterogeneous etiologies. Journal of Clinical Epidemiology 52(5):453–461

Munkarah A R, Morris R T, Schimp V L 2006 Malignant disease. In: James D K, Steer P J, Weiner C P et al (eds) High risk pregnancy management options. W B Saunders, Philadelphia, p 1163–1173

Nelson-Piercy C 2002 Handbook of obstetric medicine. Martin Dunitz, London.

NMC (Nursing and Midwifery Council) 2004 Midwives Rules and Standards. NMC, London

Panting-Kemp A, Nguyen T, Chang E et al 1999 Idiopathic polyhydramnios and perinatal outcome. American Journal of Obstetrics and Gynecology 181(5):1079–1082

Pitt C, Sanchez-Ramos L, Kaunitz A M et al 2000 Prophylactic amnioinfusion for intrapartum oligohydramnios: a meta-analysis of randomized controlled trials. Obstetrics and Gynecology 96(5):861–866

Rasmussen S, Irgens L M, Dalaker K 1997 The effect of the likelihood of further pregnancy of placental abruption and the rate of its reoccurrence. British Journal of Obstetrics and Gynaecology 104(11):1292–1295

Rasmussen S, Irgens L M, Dalaker K 1999 A history of placental dysfunction and risk of placental abruption. Paediatric and Perinatal Epidemiology 13(1):9–21

Rasmussen S, Irgens L M, Dalaker K 2000 Outcome of pregnancies subsequent to placental abruption: a risk assessment. Acta Obstetrica et Gynecologica Scandinavica 79(6):495–501

Reis P M, Sander C M, Pearlman M D 2000 Abruptio placenta after auto accidents: a case-control study. Journal of Reproductive Medicine 45(1):6–10

Sciscione A C, Manley J S, Pollock M et al 2001 Intracervical fibrin sealants: a potential treatment for early preterm premature rupture of the membranes. American Journal of Obstetrics and Gynecology 184(3):368–373

Silverman N S 2006 Hepatitis virus infections. In: James D K, Steer P J, Weiner C P et al (eds) High risk pregnancy management options. W B Saunders, Philadelphia, p 606–619

Svigos J M, Robinson J S, Vigneswaran R 2006 Prelabour rupture of the membranes. In: James D K, Steer P J, Weiner C P et al (eds) High risk pregnancy management options. W B Saunders, Philadelphia, p 1321–1333

Taylor M J O, Fisk N M 2006 Hydramnios and oligohydramnos. In: James D K, Steer P J, Weiner C P et al (eds) High risk pregnancy management options. W B Saunders, Philadelphia, p 272–290

Wildschut H I J 2006 Prepregnancy antecedents of a high risk pregnancy. In: James D K, Steer P J, Weiner C P et al (eds) High risk pregnancy management options. W B Saunders, Philadelphia, p 3–41

Williamson C, Girling G 2006 Hepatic and gastrointestinal disease. In: James D K, Steer P J, Weiner C P et al (eds) High risk pregnancy management options. W B Saunders, Philadelphia, p 1032–1060.

21 Medical disorders associated with pregnancy

Carmel Lloyd

Pregnancy may be complicated by a variety of disorders and conditions that can profoundly affect the woman and her family. Care for women with pre-existing medical disorders (PEMD) should ideally take place before conception in multidisciplinary pre-pregnancy clinics. This process should begin during adolescence with discussions about family planning, contraception and pregnancy. A complete medical history and assessment of health at this time, including obtaining up-to-date investigations, enables a risk assessment for pregnancy to be made. These risks should be discussed with the woman and her family so that appropriate choices can be made.

The pathophysiology of these disorders may adversely affect the pregnancy. Similarly, the physiological changes occurring in pregnancy may modify the clinical course of these disorders and their management. Women with PEMD have high-risk pregnancies and a collaborative multidisciplinary approach is recommended to ensure careful monitoring of both the woman and her fetus.

The chapter aims to:

- outline the common medical disorders
- describe the effects of the different disorders on the woman and her fetus or neonate
- identify the treatment required and implications for midwifery care
- consider the midwifery care and support required by the woman and her family pre-pregnancy, during pregnancy, labour and the postnatal period.

Introduction

During pregnancy, women with PEMD require regular review by the multidisciplinary team hence total midwife-led care is inappropriate, however it is important that they have 'routine' midwifery input and support. The frequency of visits at hospital clinics will depend on the underlying condition and it must be decided early in pregnancy if all care is at the hospital or if shared with the community team. Women who miss appointments should be immediately contacted and followed up. Women should be counselled about potentially worrying symptoms and advised to attend hospital if such symptoms develop or if they feel unwell. Equally midwives and doctors need to be aware and recognize the clinical signs and symptoms of deteriorating maternal health (NICE 2007). Recognition of acute illness is often delayed and its subsequent management may be inappropriate leading to late referral to senior medical care, admission to a critical care unit and may lead to maternal death, particularly where the initial standard of care is suboptimal (Lewis 2007).

Labour and birth in women with PEMD can be a time of additional challenges. Timing and mode of birth should be carefully planned and should take place in a hospital with neonatal facilities. Promoting normality is key although invasive monitoring may be required in symptomatic women and those with severe disease. In general, vaginal birth is preferred and a caesarean section should only be undertaken if clinically indicated (Bridges et al 2003).

Where there is chronic illness this can have a profound effect on the physical, psychological, sexual and social aspects of women's lives. Involvement of the woman and her family in decisions regarding her care engenders feelings of autonomy and control over a condition that has the potential to result in the medicalization of childbirth. Midwives have a role in supporting women and their families, ensuring that their needs are met and that the pregnancy is treated as normal, so far as is possible (Harrison et al 2003).

Cardiac disease

In most pregnancies, heart disease is diagnosed before pregnancy. There is, however, a small but significant group of women who will present at an antenatal clinic with an undiagnosed heart condition. Although heart disease complicates <1% of maternities, it continues to contribute significantly to maternal morbidity and mortality and is the leading cause of maternal death overall in the UK (Lewis 2007). Heart disease can be broadly classified into 'congenital' and 'acquired'. Those more likely to be seen in pregnancy are described below.

Congenital heart disease

The most common congenital heart diseases (CHD) found in pregnancy are atrial septal defect (ASD), ventricular septal defect (VSD), patent ductus arteriosus (PDA), pulmonary stenosis, aortic stenosis and tetralogy of Fallot. The majority of these lesions will have been corrected surgically in childhood resulting in a growing population of women with CHD compatible with pregnancy. Uncorrected lesions may cause pulmonary hypertension, cyanosis and severe left ventricular failure and are therefore high risk for pregnancy. CHD is also associated with increased fetal complications linked with the maternal functional class and the degree of cyanosis. These include fetal loss, intrauterine growth restriction, pre-term birth and an increased risk of fetal CHD (Head & Thorne 2005).

Particularly high risk cardiac conditions for pregnancy include:

Eisenmenger's syndrome happens when a large left-right shunt of blood, usually through a VSD, ASD or PDA, is not corrected. This results in an increase in the pulmonary blood flow, which over time leads to fibrosis and the development of pulmonary hypertension and cyanosis (Raja & Basu 2005). When right heart pressures exceed left heart pressures, the shunt reverses, worsening cyanosis. Women with this condition are advised against pregnancy as maternal mortality lies in the region of 30–50%. The greatest risk to the fetus is prematurity which contributes to the high perinatal mortality rate (Siu & Colman 2001).

Marfan's syndrome is caused by an autosomal dominant defect on chromosome 15. It is a connective tissue disease that affects the musculoskeletal system, the cardiovascular system and the eyes. The cardiovascular abnormalities are the most life-threatening as the elastic fibres in the media of the blood vessels weaken. This results in dilatation of the ascending and descending aorta, which may be followed by dissection or rupture, or both. The mean age at which these events occur is 32 years and it often results in premature death. Pregnancy poses a significant risk because of the increased stress on the cardiovascular system and there is a 50% chance of a child inheriting Marfan's syndrome if one parent is affected. Women and their partners should be counselled carefully regarding these potential outcomes before embarking on a pregnancy (Lipscomb et al 1997). Women who have minimal cardiovascular involvement and normal aortic root dimensions have a better pregnancy outcome. Careful monitoring is required throughout pregnancy including the use of serial echocardiography to identify progressive aortic root dilatation. Prophylactic antihypertensive therapy using beta-blockers is recommended to reduce blood pressure and the rate of aortic dilatation (Siu & Colman 2001).

Acquired heart disease

Rheumatic heart disease

Rheumatic heart disease (RHD) has declined progressively in Europe and North America but worldwide it remains the most common cardiac problem. RHD causes inflammation and scarring of the heart valves and results in valve stenosis, plus or minus regurgitation. The mitral valve is most often affected with stenosis, occurring in two-thirds of cases. This condition is often diagnosed because of severe breathlessness and tiredness for the first time during pregnancy – particularly in immigrant or refugee women who have not had access to medical care. Most women with valvular heart disease can be managed medically which aims to reduce the work rate of the heart. During pregnancy, this involves bed rest, oxygen therapy and the use of cardiac drugs e.g. diuretics (reduce fluid load), digoxin (reduces and regulates the heart rate) and heparin (reduces risk of thromboembolic disease). Women with more severe symptomatic disease may require surgical intervention such as balloon valvoplasty or valve replacement, although both of these procedures carry a degree of maternal and fetal mortality. Antibiotic prophylaxis is recommended for all women with valvular lesions during labour (Gelsen et al 2007, Prasad & Ventura 2001).

Myocardial infarction and ischaemic heart disease

Myocardial infarction (MI) and ischaemic heart disease (IHD) are uncommon cardiac complications but are an increasing cause of maternal death in the UK. Identifiable risk factors include increasing maternal age, obesity, diabetes, pre-existing hypertension, smoking, family history and inequalities in health (BCS 2007, Lewis 2007). A myocardial infarction is most likely to occur in the third trimester and peripartum period when haemodynamic changes are having their maximum effect and there is a higher risk of thrombotic events due to the hypercoagulability induced by hormonal changes. In the immediate postpartum period, spontaneous coronary artery dissection is the most common cause of MI. Typically, women present with ischaemic chest pain in the presence of an abnormal ECG and elevated cardiac enzymes although these signs and symptoms may be masked during labour and birth (Ray et al 2004). Atypical features include abdominal or epigastric pain and vomiting. Primary percutaneous transluminal coronary angioplasty (PTCA) which improves the patency of blocked arteries is first line therapy for this condition (Baird & Kennedy 2006).

Aortic dissection (acute)

Aortic dissection (acute) may occur in pregnancy in association with severe hypertension (systolic >160 mmHg) due to pre-eclampsia, coarctation of the aorta or connective tissue disease such as Marfan's syndrome. The woman typically presents with severe chest or intrascapular pain. Early diagnosis using computed tomography chest scan or MRI or transoesophageal echocardiogram is critical as maternal mortality is high (Lewis 2007, Ray et al 2004).

Endocarditis

Endocarditis is an inflammation of the heart usually involving the heart valves. Although rare in pregnancy, it is one of the most serious complications of heart disease. Women with valvular heart disease, prosthetic valves, a previous history of endocarditis, periodontal disease and intravenous substance misusers are particularly vulnerable to this condition. Streptococcal organisms are the most common cause and give rise to the subacute form of the disease. Acute endocarditis is due to more virulent organisms such as *Staphylococcus aureus*, *Streptococcus pneumoniae* and *Neisseria gonorrhoeae*. Primary prevention includes recognition of risk factors and use of strategies to minimize bacteraemia, e.g. good dental hygiene, avoidance of drug misuse, early treatment of sepsis and administration of antibiotic prophylaxis to women with high risk cardiac conditions (Stuart 2006).

Peripartum cardiomyopathy

Peripartum cardiomyopathy is a relatively rare but potentially fatal disease; mortality rates range from 25% to 50% with a significant number of deaths occurring shortly after the onset of signs and symptoms. Diagnosis is made within a specific period of time, occurring between the last month of pregnancy and the first 5 months postpartum and commonly women have no previous history of heart disease. It is associated with older and multiparous women, hypertension, pre-eclampsia, obesity and diabetes. It has also been linked to myocarditis, viral infection, long-term oral tocolytic therapy and cocaine misuse. Inflammation and enlargement of the myocardium (cardiomegaly) give rise to left ventricular heart failure and thromboembolic complications. Treatment involves use of medication (oxygen, diuretics, vasodilators) to decrease pulmonary congestion and fluid overload, inotropic agents to improve myometrial contractility and anticoagulation therapy. As the cardiomegaly resolves there should be a corresponding improvement in the woman's condition but this process may take up to 6 months and there is a risk of recurrence in a subsequent pregnancy. In some women, left ventricular dysfunction persists and unless a heart transplant is performed mortality will be high (Palmer 2006, Pryn et al 2006).

Changes in cardiovascular dynamics during pregnancy

In normal pregnancy the haemodynamic profile alters in order to meet the increasing demands of the growing fetoplacental unit (see Ch. 14). Normal, healthy pregnant women are able to adjust to these physiological changes quite easily. In women with coexisting heart disease, however, the added workload can precipitate complications. The three peak periods of cardiovascular stress (28–32 weeks of pregnancy, during labour, 12–24hrs postpartum) are the most critical and life threatening for women with heart disease (Cox et al 2005).

Recognition of cardiac compromise

Many of the symptoms of normal pregnancy resemble those of heart disease. The symptoms and signs of cardiac compromise include: fatigue, shortness of breath (dyspnoea), difficulty in breathing unless upright (orthopnoea), palpitations, bounding/collapsing pulse, chest pain, development of peripheral oedema, distended jugular veins and progressive limitation of physical activity. Severity of cardiac disease may be classified by the degree of functional compromise (Table 21.1).

Diagnosis

Along with the signs and symptoms, physical assessment and laboratory tests can assist with the diagnosis of cardiac disease and determine the type of lesion together with an assessment of current functional capacity. These may include:

- full cardiovascular examination, history and assessment of lifestyle risk factors
- blood tests – full blood count, clotting studies and cardiac enzymes (Troponin)
- 12-lead electrocardiogram

Table 21.1 The New York Heart Association's functional classification of cardiac disease

Class	Definition
Class I	No limitation of physical activity. Ordinary activity does not cause undue fatigue, palpitations, dyspnoea or angina
Class II	Slight limitation of physical activity. Comfortable at rest. Ordinary physical activity results in fatigue, palpitations, dyspnoea or angina
Class III	Marked limitation of physical activity. Comfortable at rest. Less than ordinary physical activity results in fatigue, palpitations, dyspnoea or angina
Class IV	Inability to carry on any physical activity without discomfort. Symptoms of cardiac insufficiency or angina may be present even at rest, and are intensified by activity

Dobbenga – Rhodes & Pride 2006

- echocardiogram to look at cardiac chambers, valves and great vessels
- chest radiograph to assess cardiac size and outline, pulmonary vasculature and lung fields. Chest X-rays, with appropriate abdominal screening, should always be done when clinically indicated e.g. in women with chest pain (Lewis 2007, Lewis & Drife 2004)
- other imaging – CT chest scan or MRI.

Risks to mother and fetus

The majority of pregnancies complicated by maternal heart disease can be expected to have a favourable outcome for both mother and fetus. The risk for morbidity and mortality depends on: (1) the nature of the cardiac lesion, (2) its affect on the functional capacity of the heart and (3) the development of pregnancy-related complications such as hypertensive disorders of pregnancy, infection, thrombosis and haemorrhage. Congestive heart failure precipitated by the altered haemodynamic state is a serious complication that may result in maternal death and can occur at any time during pregnancy (Lewis & Drife 2004). Adverse fetal effects are the result of decreased uterine blood flow or decreased maternal oxygenation. This can lead to spontaneous abortion, intrauterine growth restriction, fetal hypoxia, preterm birth and intrauterine death. If either parent has a congenital heart defect this may be inherited by their offspring (Tan 1999).

Preconception care

Women with known heart disease should seek advice from a cardiologist and an obstetrician before becoming pregnant. Preconception and antenatal counselling offer women information regarding the risks of the pregnancy to themselves and their baby, enables assessment of their functional status and whether pregnancy should be avoided. The woman's condition should be optimized and general health advice given by the midwife.

Antenatal care

The symptoms of normal pregnancy can mimic the signs and symptoms of heart disease, e.g. dypsnoea on exertion, orthopnoea, palpitations, dizziness, fainting, a bounding pulse, tachycardia, peripheral oedema, distended jugular veins and alterations in heart sounds. Maternal investigations should be carried out prior to and at the onset of pregnancy to gain baseline referral points.

Management

Management requires a multidisciplinary approach involving midwives, obstetricians, cardiologists and anaesthetists (Badawy & El-Metwally 2001). During the antenatal period women with heart disease are monitored more frequently than healthy pregnant women. The aim is to maintain a steady haemodynamic state and prevent complications, as well as promote physical and psychological well-being. Visits to a joint clinic run by a cardiologist and obstetrician are usually every 2 weeks until 30 weeks' gestation and weekly thereafter until birth. At each visit the woman is asked about cardiac symptoms and whether there is any limitation on her activities. The severity of the heart lesion is assessed by clinical examination.

Evaluation of fetal well-being includes use of:

- ultrasound examination to confirm gestational age and congenital abnormality
- assessment of fetal growth and amniotic fluid volume both clinically and by ultrasound
- monitoring the fetal heart rate by CTG
- measurement of fetal and maternal placental blood flow indices by Doppler ultrasonography.

Physical and psychological care

The midwife can give advice with regard to modifying and adjusting physical activity during pregnancy. Some women will need to commence maternity leave earlier than anticipated. In late pregnancy, women may require admission to hospital for rest and close monitoring. Psychological support by the midwife is important. Where possible, care in the community is preferable, although the importance of adequate rest should be emphasized.

Dietary advice

Guidance should be given about what constitutes a well-balanced diet. Cholesterol, sodium-rich foods and salt should be restricted. Weight gain should be monitored in these women as excess weight gain will place additional strain on the heart. Compliance with taking iron and folic acid supplementation is important for preventing anaemia.

Prevention of infection

Infections often cause a pyrexia and tachycardia, which will put an added strain on the heart. In addition the infective organism can cause further damage in women with heart lesions by causing endocarditis. The midwife needs to advise the woman about how she may identify respiratory, urinary and vaginal infections and the necessity of seeking treatment as quickly as possible. An early dental examination is important to detect and treat caries and gum disease, which may precipitate endocarditis. Prophylactic antibiotic therapy is recommended for women who are at high risk of endocarditis (Endocarditis Working Party of the British Society of Antimicrobial Chemotherapy 1990). All invasive procedures should be carried out using a strict aseptic technique and the number of vaginal examinations in labour should be kept to a minimum.

Antithrombotic therapy

The hypercoagulable state in pregnancy increases the risk of thromboembolic disease in women who have arrhythmias, mitral valve stenosis or who have had mechanical cardiac valve replacements.

The treatment of women requiring antithrombotic therapy during pregnancy is difficult. Warfarin is commonly used in the non-pregnant state but is teratogenic in early pregnancy and is associated with a high fetal loss rate. It also predisposes the woman and her fetus to haemorrhage when used in the third trimester. Subcutaneous low molecular weight heparins, such as enoxaparin, are useful for thromboprophylaxis (Ellison 2000) but may not be suitable for women with mechanical heart valves. The advice of a haematologist should be sought. High thromboembolic support stockings should be worn if the woman is admitted for rest and assessment. They should also be worn during labour and in the immediate postnatal period.

Intrapartum care: the first stage of labour

A coordinated team approach with good communication between the midwife, obstetrician, cardiologist, neonatologist, anaesthetist, the woman and her family is essential. Women with heart disease may have uncomplicated labours. Vaginal birth is preferred unless there is an obstetric indication for caesarean section. The advantages of a vaginal birth are: less blood loss, greater haemodynamic stability, avoidance of surgical stress and less chance of postoperative infection and pulmonary complications (Ray et al 2004). Optimal management involves monitoring the maternal condition to include: temperature, pulse, respiration, blood pressure, fluid intake and urine output. Observation of the fetal condition is also required using electronic fetal monitoring. Continuous electrocardiography (ECG) is recommended in nearly all cases and pulse oximetry may be utilized to assess arterial haemoglobin saturation, which may be reduced in women with heart disease owing to disruption of normal gas exchange between the lungs and blood. If oxygen saturation levels fall below 92%, oxygen therapy will be required. The use of invasive haemodynamic studies via an arterial line may be required in women with moderate to severe heart disease. Blood and urine tests are undertaken during labour to determine the haematological and metabolic changes.

Fluid balance

Fluid management requires judicial use of intravenous fluids and fluid may need to be restricted. Overload will lead to an increase in the circulating blood volume and development of pulmonary oedema and congestive heart disease (Witcher & Harvey 2006).

Pain relief

The midwife should help the woman to use the techniques that she has learned for coping with stress. An epidural may be the analgesia of choice as it is an effective form of analgesia that decreases cardiac output and heart rate. It causes peripheral vasodilatation and decreases venous return, which alleviates pulmonary congestion. Nitrous oxide and oxygen and pethidine are usually considered safe, but it is important to consult a doctor before administering any form of pain-relieving drug to a woman with a heart condition (Durbridge et al 2006).

Positioning

Cardiac output is influenced by the position of the woman during labour. Women with heart disease are particularly sensitive to aortocaval compression by the gravid uterus in the supine position. It may be necessary to recommend an upright position or left lateral position for some women to adopt during labour and the birth, according to their individual condition.

Pre-term labour

Beta sympathomimetic drugs widely used for the treatment of preterm labour are contraindicated in women with heart disease, since they cause tachycardia and predispose to pulmonary oedema. Consideration may be given in individual cases if it is safe to use oxytocin antagonists.

Induction

The least stressful labour for a woman with cardiac disease will be spontaneous in onset. Prostaglandins should be used with caution as they are potent vasodilators and cause a marked increase in cardiac output. Oxytocin by intravenous infusion causes a degree of fluid retention and it is important for the midwife to keep a careful record of fluid balance if this is used.

The second stage of labour

This should be short without undue exertion on the part of the mother. Prolonged pushing with held breath (the Valsalva manoeuvre), may be dangerous for a woman with heart disease. It raises the intrathoracic pressure, pushes the blood out of the thorax and impedes venous return, with the result that cardiac output falls. The midwife should encourage the woman to breathe normally and follow her natural desire to push, giving several short pushes during each contraction. Forceps or ventouse may be used to shorten the second stage. Care should be taken when the woman is in the lithotomy position, where the lower part of the body is higher than trunk, as this produces a sudden increase in venous return to the heart, which may result in heart failure (Durbridge et al 2006). A wedge should be used to avoid aortocaval compression.

The third stage of labour

This is usually actively managed owing to the increased risk of postpartum haemorrhage (PPH). Oxytocin is the drug of choice but its use in the prevention of PPH must be balanced against the risk of oxytocin-induced hypotension and tachycardia in women with cardiovascular compromise (Lewis & Drife 2004). Administration should follow the guidance in the British National Formulary (BMA & RPS 2001) and when given as an intravenous bolus the drug should be given slowly in a dose that should not exceed 5IU. Ergot-containing preparations such as ergometrine are contraindicated in cardiac conditions which would be worsened by a rise in blood pressure.

Postnatal care

The first 48hrs following birth are critical for the woman with significant heart disease. The heart must be able to cope with the extra volume of blood (autotransfusion) from the uterine circulation as well as the increased venous return following relief of aortocaval compression of the uterus. Conversely, total blood volume may be diminished by loss at birth and during the postnatal period and the heart will need to compensate if blood flow is impaired due to postpartum haemorrhage. Close monitoring of haemodynamic changes is required at this time and the midwife should identify early signs of infection, thrombosis or pulmonary oedema (Ramsay 2006). Breastfeeding should be encouraged as cardiac output is not affected by lactation although drug therapy for specific heart conditions may need to be reviewed for safety during breastfeeding. The midwife provides support with breastfeeding as is usual (see Ch. 41), with emphasis placed on the need for adequate rest and a dietary intake with sufficient calories to support breastfeeding. Discharge planning is particularly important for women with heart disease. The midwife can evaluate the help and support that will be available in the home during the postnatal period. Relatives and friends often fulfill this need but community support services should be considered if necessary. The woman and her partner should discuss with the cardiologist and obstetrician the implications of a future pregnancy and be given appropriate contraceptive advice (Thorne et al 2006).

Respiratory disorders

Asthma

The prevalence of active asthma in the UK is 5.8% (Pinnock & Shah 2007) and affects 3–12% of pregnant women worldwide with 5.8% of women hospitalized for asthma during pregnancy (Murphy et al 2006). Prevalence is increasing mainly due to environmental factors such as: change in indoor environment, smoking, family size, pollution and diet (Rees 2005).

Effect of asthma on pregnancy

Pregnancy does not consistently affect asthmatic status; some women experience no change in symptoms whereas others have a distinct worsening of the disease. The mechanisms that contribute to the varying changes in asthma during pregnancy are not well understood, although increases in maternal circulating hormones (cortisol, oestradiol and progesterone), altered β_2-adrenoreceptor responsiveness and immune function or the presence of a female fetus may be involved (Murphy et al 2005). When asthma is well controlled maternal and fetal outcomes are similar to those in women without asthma. Women with severe disease and those who have poor control of asthma seem to have an increased incidence of adverse maternal and neonatal outcomes including preterm labour (Schatz et al 2006).

Diagnosis

The characteristic symptoms of asthma are: chest tightness, dyspnoea, wheezing and coughing. Measuring peak expiratory flow (PEF) using a PEF meter is a useful tool for making a diagnosis and determining how well a person's asthma is controlled (Booker 2007). PEF monitors the level of resistance in the airways caused by inflammation or bronchospasm, or both and values are lower than predicted in people with asthma. A range of normal values can be predicted for each person according to sex, height and age. Knowledge of the usual PEF and self-monitoring at home will enable a person with asthma to determine when to take or increase their medication and when to seek medical attention. Hospital admission is usually required if the PEF is <50% of the normal value and the person is too breathless to complete sentences.

Management

The BTS & SIGN (2005) guidelines recommend a stepwise approach to management of asthma. Therapy should be initiated to establish quick control of the asthma symptoms and then stepped down to the minimum medication necessary to maintain control. Treatment relies on inhaled bronchodilators and inhaled steroids with or without oral steroids. Nebulized drugs are given during acute attacks of asthma.

Antenatal care

Care should ideally be provided jointly between the midwife, GP, chest physician and obstetrician. At the booking interview the midwife should be able to discuss with the woman the frequency and severity of her asthma, family history, any known asthma triggers and current treatment. The main anxiety for women and those providing care relates to the use of asthma medication and its effect on the fetus. In general, the medications used in the treatment of asthma, including systemic steroids, are considered safe to use in pregnancy (BTS & SIGN 2005). It is crucial that therapy is maintained during pregnancy as a severe asthma attack may result in a deterioration in the maternal condition and a reduction in the oxygen supply to the fetus. Respiratory tract infections should be diagnosed and treated promptly in order to prevent an acute asthma attack. If during the pregnancy there are any difficulties in controlling the symptoms of asthma the woman should be admitted to hospital.

Intrapartum care

An increase in cortisone and adrenaline (epinephrine) from the adrenal glands during labour is thought to prevent attacks of asthma during labour (BTS & SIGN 2005). If an asthma attack does occur this should be treated in the usual way. Women should continue their usual asthma medications during labour and it is important that they remain well hydrated. Maternal and fetal condition should be monitored closely, namely: respiratory function, pulse oximetry, oxygen therapy and continuous fetal heart rate monitoring. All forms of pain relief may be used although regional anaesthesia reduces hyperventilation and the stress response to pain. It is also advocated for operative delivery as it avoids the potential complications of ventilating people with asthma

(Kuczkowski 2005). Certain aspects of labour management in women with asthma require special attention. These include: the use of β_2-adrenergic antagonists for the treatment of hypertension and the use of ergometrine or carboprost (prostaglandin F2a) for the management of postpartum haemorrhage. These drugs may cause bronchospasm and should be avoided or used with caution (Kuczkowski 2005). Oxytocin and prostaglandin E2 are safe to use for the induction of labour (BTS & SIGN 2005). Women who have received corticosteroids in pregnancy (>7.5 mg prednisolone/day for >2 weeks prior to the onset of labour) should receive parenteral hydrocortisone 100 mg 6–8-hourly during labour (BTS & SIGN 2005).

Postnatal care

Breastfeeding should be encouraged, particularly as it may protect infants from developing certain allergic conditions. None of the drugs used in the treatment of asthma is likely to be secreted in breastmilk in sufficient quantities to harm the baby.

Cystic fibrosis

Cystic fibrosis (CF) is an autosomal recessive multisystem disorder which significantly reduces life expectancy (Rowe et al 2005). People with CF develop chronic obstructive lung disease (poor peak flow, reduced forced expiratory volume (FEV1) and decreased oxygen saturation). Obstruction of the pancreatic ducts leads to a loss of acinar cells and replacement by fibrous tissue and fat. Loss of pancreatic function causes poor digestion, malnutrition and the development of type 1 diabetes. Many women with CF now live into their reproductive years in good health and although fertility may be slightly reduced, principally because of alteration in the chemical make-up of the cervical mucus, pregnancies are possible.

Pre-pregnancy care

One in 25 people carry the defective gene and therefore if the partner is a carrier there is a one in two chance that their children will have CF. Specific changes in respiratory, cardiac and pancreatic function as well as increased nutritional demands during pregnancy pose a serious health risk for many women with CF and should be assessed prior to pregnancy (McMullen et al 2006).

Antenatal care

Midwifery, obstetric, dietetic, medical, nursing and physiotherapy expertise are essential. Specific assessment includes pulmonary function tests, arterial blood gases, sputum culture, liver function tests, glucose tolerance test, chest radiogram, electrocardiogram, echocardiogram and monitoring of weight gain. Compliance with antibiotic therapy must be stressed as the potential risks to the fetus are outweighed by the risk of the mother developing a severe lung infection. In addition, it is important to pay attention to nutrition and CF-related diabetes, the risks of which increase with age and are more likely to be problematic in pregnancy (Bussey & Mittelstaedt 2003).

Intrapartum care

During labour close monitoring of cardiorespiratory function will be required and an anaesthetist should be involved at an early stage. Fluid and electrolyte management requires careful attention as women with CF may easily become hypovolaemic from the loss of large quantities of sodium in sweat. Epidural analgesia is the recommended form of pain relief in labour and general anaesthesia should be avoided because of the potential risks from respiratory complications (Cameron & Skinner 2005, Holdcroft & Thomas 2000).

Postnatal care

Women should be cared for in a high dependency unit as cardiorespiratory function often deteriorates following birth. Sodium concentration in breastmilk has been found to be similar to women without CF and therefore breastfeeding is not contraindicated. However, in order for breastfeeding to be successful women need to be well nourished and maintain an adequate calorie intake. As CF is the UK's most common life-threatening inherited disease, it is recommended that universal neonatal testing is undertaken as part of the UK newborn blood spot screening programme (UKNSPC 2005).

Pulmonary tuberculosis

Tuberculosis (TB) is an air-borne infectious disease caused by the tubercule bacillus, *Myobacterium tuberculosis*. It is transmitted through inhalation of infected air-borne droplets from a person with infectious TB. It may also be contracted from infected cattle through the consumption of milk and dairy products that have not been pasteurized. The lungs are the organ most commonly affected (pulmonary TB) although it may spread to other areas parts of the body typically bones, joints and the lymphatic, genitourinary and central nervous system (extrapulmonary TB). All forms of TB are notifiable under the Public Health (Control of Disease) Act 1984 and therefore primary healthcare workers including midwives are among the first to be involved in the prevention, screening and treatment of TB (NICE 2006, Royal College of Physicians 2006). Contributory factors leading to the increasing incidence of this disease include: (1) women and children who have immigrated to the UK from areas where TB is endemic, principally South-Asia and sub-Saharan African countries, (2) the development of drug-resistant organisms and (3) increases in adults and children who have become infected with HIV (HPA 2007). Most cases occur in inner city areas where additional social factors such as poverty, homelessness, substance misuse, poor nutrition and crowded living conditions contribute to the transmission of the disease (HPA 2007, Kothari et al 2006). TB is primarily a disease of poverty and almost all cases are preventable.

Diagnosis

The onset of primary TB is often insidious and the symptoms are non-specific: fatigue, malaise, loss of appetite, loss of weight, alteration in bowel habit and low grade fever. These can be interpreted as usual symptoms occurring in pregnancy leading to a delay in diagnosis (Kothari et al 2006). The classic symptoms of chronic cough, intermittent fever, night sweats, haemoptysis, dyspnoea and chest pain occur quite late in the disease process and are often absent when the TB is extrapulmonary.

Measures to increase awareness about TB in the immigrant population and in the community, and to provide access to medical care could reduce delays in diagnosis (DH 2007). The presence of risk factors requires assessment via the Mantoux tuberculin skin test and/or an interferon-γ (secreted by lymphocytes in the presence of antigens to TB) test. A thorough history and physical examination should also be undertaken. A positive tuberculin test should be further evaluated with a chest X-ray; abdominal shielding for this procedure keeps fetal exposure to a minimum. Microscopic examination and culture of sputum are also required to confirm active mycobacterial infection and identify drug sensitivity (HPA 2006, Ormerod 2001). Once active TB has been diagnosed, the need for contact tracing must be assessed and testing and treatment of asymptomatic household and other close contacts implemented in order to prevent spread of the disease (NICE 2006).

Management

All pregnant women with TB should be under the care of a specialist physician and a named key worker with full training in the disease who manage the clinical aspect of the woman's treatment (NICE 2006). It is important that they work collaboratively with the midwife, GP and obstetrician. The key to a successful outcome is to ensure that the woman is involved in treatment decisions and adheres to the prescribed treatment. Figueroa-Damian & Arredondo-Garcia (2001) found that maternal morbidity and mortality are significantly higher where active TB remains untreated and when treatment is started late in pregnancy. In addition, neonates of women with TB have a higher risk of prematurity and perinatal death and low birth weight.

Standard anti-tuberculous therapy is considered safe in pregnancy (HPA 2006). TB is treated in two phases. The first involves taking rifampicin, isoniazid, pyrazinamide and ethambutol daily for 2 months. In the second (continuation) phase, rifampicin and isoniazid are taken for a further 4 months (NICE 2006). Congenital deafness has been reported in infants with exposure to streptomycin *in utero* and therefore this anti-tuberculous drug is avoided in pregnancy. Part of the midwife's role during this time is to assist the named key worker to ensure that women are compliant with the drug therapy and understand the importance of adhering to the regimen in order to cure the disease and prevent the bacillus becoming resistant to the drugs. The majority of women will require minimum supervision and a monthly review will be sufficient to monitor progress (Kothari et al 2006). For those women at risk of non-adherence care is planned individually and thrice weekly directly observed therapy (DOTS) may be required (NICE 2006).

Attention should also be placed on rest, good nutrition and education with regard to preventing the spread of the disease. TB usually becomes non-infectious by 2 weeks of treatment. Where possible the treatment is undertaken in the woman's home to disrupt family life as little as possible. Some women may require admission to hospital because of the severity of the illness or adverse effects of drug therapy, for obstetric reasons such as the onset of labour, for social reasons or for further investigations. Risk assessment should be made in order to determine appropriate infection control measures.

Providing all TB bacteria are killed, the person with TB is cured. In a small number of people, the disease can return if not all bacteria have been killed. This is more likely to occur where there is poor/no compliance with drug treatment or where there is multi-drug resistant (MDR) TB.

Postnatal care

Following birth, babies born to mothers with infectious TB should be protected from the disease by the prophylactic use of isoniazid syrup (5 mg/kg per day) and pyridoxine (5–10 mg/day) for 6 weeks and then to be tuberculin tested. If negative, the neonatal Bacille Calmette–Guérin (BCG) vaccination should be given and drug therapy discontinued. If the tuberculin test is positive the baby should be assessed for congenital or perinatal infection and drug therapy continued if these are excluded (HPA 2006). The baby cannot be infected by the mother via the breastmilk unless she has tuberculous mastitis. Additionally the concentration of the anti-tuberculous drugs in breastmilk is insufficient to cause harm in the neonate, therefore in the majority of cases breastfeeding should be encouraged (HPA 2006).

Caring for a child at home makes great demands on the mother and extra help should be arranged if possible. Midwives should explain that poor nutrition, stress and overtiredness will encourage a recurrence of active disease. Family planning advice is an integral part of postnatal and preconception care and it is advisable for a woman with TB to avoid further pregnancies until she has been disease-free for at least 2 years. When choosing her method of family planning, the woman needs to be aware that rifampicin reduces the effectiveness of oral contraception (BMA & RPS 2001). Long-term medical and social follow-up is necessary.

The outcome for both mother and baby is improved by early diagnosis and effective treatment. Midwives are pivotal in ensuring compliance with drug therapy and providing general health education during pregnancy in order to reduce the incidence of TB in both the obstetric and the general population.

Renal disease

A knowledge of the changes in renal physiology and function in healthy pregnancy is crucial to the midwife's understanding of the impact of pregnancy on existing renal disease and the predisposition women have to develop urinary tract infections (see Ch. 14).

Urinary tract infection

Urinary tract infection (UTI) is the presence of significant bacteria in a clean-catch or catheter specimen of urine, most commonly described as a colony of at least 100 000 bacteria/mL of urine. Infection in the lower urinary tract may originate in the urethra (urethritis) or bladder (cystitis) and if untreated ascend into the upper urinary tract and affect the kidneys (pyelonephritis). Symptoms of a lower urinary tract infection include burning or pain on urination (dysuria), frequent passing of small amounts of urine (frequency), a change in the smell of the urine, the presence of blood in the urine (haematuria) and discomfort in the suprapubic area. The presence of fever (pyrexia >38°C), rigors, tachycardia, nausea and vomiting leading to dehydration, pain and tenderness over the kidney area is indicative of pyelonephritis.

Acute pyelonephritis occurs in 1–2 % of pregnant women (Norman et al 2001) and Sharma & Thapa (2007) found that it most commonly occurs: in nulliparous women; the younger age group (20–29 years) and at the end of the second/beginning of the third trimester and the puerperium. Examination of the urine shows it to be cloudy with the presence of white blood cells (leucocytes) and the infecting organism is often *Escherichia coli*.

UTIs in pregnancy need to be treated promptly to prevent the development of maternal morbidity (chronic renal insufficiency, transient renal failure, acute respiratory distress syndrome (ARDS), sepsis and shock) as well as fetal morbidity and mortality (pre-labour rupture of membranes, chorioamnionitis, preterm labour and birth) (Gilstrap & Ramin 2001, Vazquez & Villar 2003).

Management

The diagnosis of UTI/pyelonephritis is usually made on presenting symptoms and dipstick urinalysis using nitrite and leucocyte detectors (Bent et al 2002); this may be confirmed by urine microscopy and culture. Vaginal infections and sexually transmitted diseases such as *Chlamydia trachomatis* may mimic symptoms of UTI and should be excluded. Referral to a doctor is required and in cases of pyelonephritis admission to hospital is usual in order that intravenous antibiotics can be administered. During the early stages of the illness the woman will feel quite ill. Severe nausea and vomiting will lead to dehydration and intravenous fluids may be required. A record of fluid balance is maintained to assess renal function. The midwife should provide general nursing care; this will include regular observation of temperature, pulse, blood pressure and respiratory rate. The temperature should be reduced by tepid sponging and antipyretics. Uterine activity should be monitored to detect the onset of pre-term labour. The midwife should also take steps to prevent complications of immobility such as deep vein thrombosis. This requires use of antithrombotic stockings and the doctor may prescribe low dose heparin therapy.

Antibiotic therapy is effective in curing urinary tract infections although there is insufficient data to recommend any one specific treatment regime. Many different drugs may be used, given by oral or i.v. route with the course of treatment dependent on the drug used. Repeat cultures should be done 2 weeks after completion of the course of treatment and monthly until birth in order to ensure there is no recurrence. Women who develop recurrent UTI may require prophylactic antibiotic treatment throughout pregnancy. Follow-up examination of the renal system (excretion urography) is often undertaken 3 months postnatally as persistent or recurrent infection, with or without symptoms, may be associated with an abnormality of the renal tract.

Asymptomatic bacteriuria

All pregnant women should be screened for bacteriuria using a clean voided specimen of urine at their first antenatal visit. A diagnosis of asymptomatic bacteriuria (ASB) (significant bacteriuria without symptoms of UTI) is made when there are >100 000 bacteria/mL of urine. ASB occurs in 2–10% of pregnant women as a result of the physiological changes in the urinary tract during pregnancy. If ASB is not identified and treated, 20–30% of these women will develop a symptomatic urinary tract infection such as cystitis or pyelonephritis. Treatment with antibiotics is recommended to reduce the incidence of symptomatic kidney infection and pregnancy complications (Smaill & Vazquez 2007).

Chronic renal disease

When a woman has renal disease, most often the outcome of the pregnancy depends on the severity of rather than type of kidney disease. In order to determine the impact of pregnancy on a woman with chronic renal disease, the following factors need to be considered:

- general health status of the woman
- presence or absence of hypertension
- presence or absence of proteinuria
- type of kidney disease and current renal function
- pre-pregnancy drug therapy.

If the renal disease is under control maternal and fetal outcome is usually good. In some instances renal function may deteriorate and the chance of pregnancy complications subsequently rises. Renal disease combined with hypertension is associated with fetal growth restriction, pre-term birth and increased perinatal mortality. Pregnant women with mild renal insufficiency (serum creatinine [Scr] <125 μmol/L or 1.4 mg/dL) have relatively few complications of pregnancy. Moderate or severe renal insufficiency (Scr 125–250 μmol/L or 1.4–2.6 mg/dL) in pregnancy may accelerate the underlying disease and reduce fetal survival. Complications are frequent and include a rise in hypertension, high grade proteinuria (urinary excretion >3g in 24hrs) and loss of renal function, which may persist up to 1 year following birth. Around 10% of cases will progress to end-stage renal failure necessitating dialysis during or shortly after pregnancy; this is most likely to occur when the Scr is >250μmol/L or 2.8mg/dL at the beginning of pregnancy (Davison 2001).

Care and management

Assessment of renal function prior to conception is important in order to advise a couple appropriately on the risks of pregnancy. The aim of pregnancy care is to detect deterioration in renal function. This will necessitate more frequent attendance for antenatal care and close liaison between the midwife, obstetrician and nephrologist. Renal function can be assessed on a regular basis by measuring serum urate levels, serum electrolyte and urea, 24hrs creatinine clearance and serum creatinine. Urinalysis is undertaken for glycosuria, proteinuria and haematuria. Regular urine cultures will detect infection and advice should be given regarding the signs and symptoms so that women can seek treatment early. The emergence and severity of hypertension and pre-eclampsia are monitored by recording blood pressure, undertaking urinalysis and utilizing pre-eclampsia blood screening tests. A full blood count will detect anaemia as the production of erythropoietin is suppressed in chronic renal disease. Fetal surveillance includes fortnightly ultrasound scans from 24 weeks, Doppler blood flow studies and monitoring fetal activity. Admission to hospital is advised when there is evidence of fetal compromise, if renal function deteriorates and proteinuria increases or the blood pressure rises. If the maternal condition becomes life-threatening, the risks and benefits of continuing with the pregnancy need to be discussed with the woman and her family.

Women on haemodialysis/peritoneal dialysis

Women who develop end-stage renal failure prior to or during pregnancy may require dialysis. End-stage renal failure results in hypothalamic-gonadal dysfunction causing infertility; however, dialysis lessens the hormonal dysfunction and those who conceive and continue a pregnancy are at significant risk for adverse maternal and fetal outcomes. Pregnancy will increase the length and frequency of dialysis required in order to achieve a serum urea below 20mmol/L. Higher levels are associated with an increased risk of fetal demise (Norman et al 2001). During dialysis, it is important to prevent fluid overload and the development of hypertension, which will be influenced by other factors, such as electrolyte imbalance. The anaemia of chronic renal disease is exacerbated and this may require erythropoietin (Epo) therapy and blood transfusions to resolve. Hypertension and superimposed pre-eclampsia are common maternal complications. Many pregnancies in dialysed patients end in early spontaneous abortion, therapeutic abortion and pre-term birth with only 40–50% of pregnancies resulting in a successful outcome (Davison 2001).

Renal transplant

Renal transplantation reverses abnormal renal, endocrine and sexual functions and therefore women are more likely to become pregnant following a renal transplant. Preconception advice is particularly important as the woman must be in optimal health before embarking on a pregnancy. It is advisable for her to wait a minimum of 2 years before attempting pregnancy as this allows time for the success of the graft to be evaluated and pregnancy outcome is more likely to be successful (Davison 2001). During pregnancy women are monitored closely by the multidisciplinary team. Clinic visits are likely to be more frequent, during which time renal function including urinalysis, blood pressure, haemoglobin levels and the status of the graft are assessed. Close monitoring of the fetus is also required to detect fetal growth restriction. Immunosuppressive therapy is usually continued during pregnancy although the effect on the pregnancy and the fetus is unknown (Davison 2001). It is likely, however, to make the woman more vulnerable to infection. The newborn baby will also be more prone to infection as immunosuppressive therapy reduces the transmission of maternal antibodies to the fetus.

Kuvacic et al (2000) identified the following specific factors that appear to contribute to the higher rate of therapeutic and spontaneous abortion, pre-term birth and low birth weight infants in pregnancies following renal transplant:

- transplant–pregnancy interval <2 years
- maternal hypertension
- elevated serum creatinine levels
- asymptomatic bacteriuria.

The anaemias

Anaemia is a reduction in the oxygen-carrying capacity of the blood; this may be caused by a decrease in red blood cell (RBC) production, or reduction in haemoglobin (Hb) content of the blood, or a combination of these. It is often defined by a decrease in Hb levels to below the normal range of 13.5 g/dL (men), 11.5 g/dL (women) and 11.0 g/dL (children and pregnant women) (Higgins 2000). The effect on the individual will depend on the severity and speed of onset of the anaemia and the degree to which the oxygen-carrying capacity of the blood is diminished. Signs and symptoms include pallor of the mucous membranes, fatigue, dizziness and fainting, headache, exertional shortness of breath, tachycardia and palpitations. Severe anaemia is defined as Hb <7 g/dL and requires medical treatment. Very severe anaemia is defined as a Hb <4 g/dL; in pregnant women this is a medical emergency due to the risk of congestive heart failure and maternal death (WHO 2001). It is estimated that nearly half of the pregnant women in the world are considered to be anaemic; 52% in non-industrialized as compared with 23% in industrialized countries, and is a contributory factor to women developing health problems and dying during pregnancy and childbirth (WHO 2001).

Physiological anaemia of pregnancy

During pregnancy the maternal plasma volume gradually expands by 50%, or an increase of approximately 1200 mL by term. The total increase in RBCs is 25%, or approximately 300 mL. This relative haemodilution produces a fall in Hb concentration, which reaches its lowest level during the second trimester in pregnancy and then rises again in the third trimester. These changes are not pathological but are considered to represent a physiological alteration of pregnancy necessary for the development of the fetus. Fetal outcomes appear to mirror this U-shaped curve, with an increased incidence of low birthweight and pre-term birth in mothers who have either a very low or very high haemoglobin concentration (Rasmussen 2001). A low Hb level is likely to affect the ability of the maternal system to transfer sufficient oxygen and nutrients to the fetus. High Hb levels are considered to reflect poor plasma volume expansion as found in some pathological conditions such as pre-eclampsia (Yip 1996).

Iron deficiency anaemia in pregnancy

Iron deficiency anaemia (IDA) is the most common cause of anaemia in pregnant women worldwide. It is defined as a condition in which there are no mobilizable iron stores and compromised supply to body tissues. The more severe stages of iron deficiency are associated with anaemia but even mild-moderate iron deficiency will have adverse consequences. During pregnancy iron deficiency increases the risk of haemorrhage, sepsis, maternal mortality, perinatal mortality and low birthweight (WHO 2001). IDA in women is usually due to:

- reduced intake or absorption of iron; this includes dietary deficiency and gastrointestinal disturbances such as diarrhoea, hyperemesis, coeliac disease or inflammatory bowel disease
- excess demand such as frequent, numerous or multiple pregnancies
- chronic infection, particularly of the urinary tract
- acute or chronic blood loss, e.g. menorrhagia, bleeding haemorrhoids, or antepartum or postpartum haemorrhage.

In non-industrialized countries other common causes include hookworm infestation, infections such as amoebic dysentery, malaria due to *Plasmodium falciparum* and haemoglobinopathies.

Iron and pregnancy

When giving advice in early pregnancy regarding the dietary intake of iron, the midwife needs to take into consideration how the intake of iron may be affected by social, religious and cultural preferences. She also needs to explain how iron is absorbed and identify the optimal sources of iron (bioavailability). The absorption of iron is complex and tends to decrease during the first trimester and then rises throughout the remainder of the pregnancy and during the first months of the puerperium. Iron absorption is also influenced by the bioavailability of iron in the diet. Iron is most easily absorbed in the form found in red meat and wholegrain products such as wholemeal bread (haem iron). Where the diet is mainly vegetarian (non-haem), iron is of low bioavailability. Absorption of iron is inhibited by tea and coffee but enhanced by ascorbic acid, which is present in orange juice and fresh fruit (Bothwell 2000). It is estimated that a median amount of 840–1210mg of iron needs to be absorbed over the course of the pregnancy (Beard 2000). The demand for absorbed iron increases from 0.8mg/day in early pregnancy to 6mg/day in late pregnancy owing to the increase in maternal Hb, and in oxygen consumption by both mother and fetus, fetal growth and deposition of iron, placental circulation, the replacement of daily loss through stools, urine and skin, the replacement of blood lost at birth and in the postnatal period and lactation (Bothwell 2000). WHO (2001) data on the prevalence of anaemia in women suggest that the normal dietary intakes of iron are insufficient to meet these requirements for the majority of women and recommend that all pregnant women should be given iron and folic acid daily in pregnancy.

Assessing iron status in pregnancy

Assessing iron status in pregnancy can be difficult (see Ch 14). A low haemoglobin (Hb) concentration indicates anaemia is present but it does not reveal the cause. The mean cell volume (MCV = the average volume occupied by the red cell, normal value 80–95 fL) and the mean cell haemoglobin concentration (MCHC) indicating how well filled with Hb the cells are (normal value 32–36g/dL), are usually used to identify the cause of anaemia. Iron deficiency anaemia is microcytic (low MCV) and hypochromic (low MCHC). By the time the Hb falls, the iron stores will already be depleted. Relative total iron body stores can also be assessed by measuring serum ferritin (iron storage protein) levels (normal range 15–300µg/L). Serum ferritin levels fall in proportion to the decrease

in iron stores and will show changes before the Hb level falls (Higgins 2000) although in late pregnancy this test becomes unreliable as serum ferritin levels diminish even when bone marrow iron is present (WHO 2001).

Management

Decisions about whether to prescribe prophylactic iron supplements during pregnancy in order to maintain the Hb at 11g/dL remain controversial. A number of authors have contributed to the debate (e.g. Beard 2000, Beaton 2000, Bothwell 2000, Rasmussen 2001, Scholl & Reilly 2000, Strong 2006).

The first-line treatment for women with iron deficiency anaemia is oral iron preparations 120–240 mg/day in divided doses. Common iron preparations include ferrous sulphate, 200 mg tablets containing 60 mg of available iron, and ferrous gluconate, 300 mg tablets containing 35mg of available iron. There are gastrointestinal side-effects of oral iron therapy that women need to be aware of. These are largely dose related and include nausea, epigastric pain and constipation. These discomforts can be reduced by taking iron supplements after meals. Some women may find one form of iron salts more tolerable than another; slow release preparations, although more expensive, are relatively free from side-effects.

Iron can also be given intramuscularly or intravenously bypassing the gastrointestinal tract. This can be beneficial in women who are unable to take, tolerate or absorb oral preparations. Intramuscular iron is given in the form of iron sorbitol. The injection should be given using a 'Z technique' deep in to the muscle to prevent staining and irritation at the injection site. Injections should not be given in conjunction with oral iron as this enhances the toxic effects such as headache, dizziness, nausea and vomiting.

Iron dextran is given as total dose intravenous infusion. The dosage is calculated by taking account of bodyweight and the Hb concentration deficit. Side-effects include allergic reaction, which may take the form of severe anaphylactic shock. The infusion should therefore be administered slowly under close surveillance. Joint pain occurring within 24hrs of the infusion is not uncommon.

Oral, intramuscular and intravenous administrations of iron result in similar rates of increase in the Hb concentration. An increase of 0.8 g/dL per week is usual irrespective of the route of administration. Blood transfusion is rarely used to treat iron deficiency anaemia in pregnancy. It may be considered where there is an inadequate amount of time to treat severe anaemia prior to birth.

In women with iron deficiency anaemia, oral iron supplementation should continue postnatally particularly if they are breastfeeding. Blood tests should be repeated at the 6-week postnatal check and further investigation undertaken should iron deficiency anaemia remain.

Folic acid deficiency anaemia

Folic acid is needed for the increased cell growth of both mother and fetus but there is a physiological decrease in serum folate levels in pregnancy. Anaemia is more likely to be found towards the end of pregnancy when the fetus is growing rapidly. It is also more common during winter when folic acid is more difficult to obtain and in areas of social, economic and nutritional deprivation. The MRC Vitamin Study Research Group (1991) found a positive correlation between folate deficiency and the development of neural tube defects in the fetus.

The cause of folic acid deficiency anaemia is primarily a reduced dietary intake or reduced absorption, or a combination of these. In some instances, there may be excessive demand and loss of folic acid. In haemolytic anaemia, there is an increased demand for the production of new red cells and consequently for folic acid. Multiple pregnancy also results in an increased demand. Some drugs may interfere with the utilization of folic acid, e.g. anticonvulsants, sulphonamides and alcohol.

Investigation

The signs and symptoms are varied and may be mistaken as 'minor disorders of pregnancy', such as pallor, lassitude, weight loss, depression, nausea and vomiting, glossitis, gingivitis and diarrhoea. Examination of the red cell indices will reveal that the red cells are reduced in number but enlarged in size. This condition is termed *macrocytic* or *megaloblastic anaemia*. The MCV rises, the MCHC may remain the same but as there are fewer cells the Hb level falls.

Management

The risk of folic acid deficiency can be reduced by advising pregnant women on foods that are high in folic acid (see Ch. 13). Following the MRC trial in 1991, the DoH Expert Advisory Group recommended a folic acid supplement of 0.4 mg/day (DoH 1992). Some women require extra folate supplements from early pregnancy in order to prevent megaloblastic anaemia. The recommended daily supplement is 5–10 mg orally in the following circumstances:

- diagnosed folate deficiency
- malabsorption syndrome
- haemoglobinopathy
- epilepsy requiring anticonvulsant treatment
- multiparity
- multiple pregnancy
- adolescence.

Vitamin B_{12} deficiency anaemia

Deficiency of vitamin B_{12} also produces a megaloblastic anaemia. Vitamin B_{12} levels fall during pregnancy but anaemia is rare because the body draws on its stores. Deficiency is most likely in vegans, who eat no animal products at all, and should therefore take vitamin B_{12} supplements during pregnancy (Strong 2006).

Haemoglobinopathies

This term describes inherited conditions where the haemoglobin is abnormal. Haemoglobin consists of a group of four molecules, each of which has a haem unit made up of an iron porphyrin complex and a protein or globin chain. A total of 97% of adult Hb (HbA) has two α- and two β-chains; the remaining 3% is HbA_2 and is composed of two α- and two δ-chains. Fetal Hb (HbF) has two α- and two γ-chains; by 6 months of age this has been replaced by adult haemoglobin. The type of globin chain is genetically determined. Defective genes lead to the formation of abnormal haemoglobin; this may be as a result of impaired globin synthesis (thalassaemia syndromes) or from structural abnormality of globin (haemoglobin variants such as sickle cell anaemia). These conditions prevail in certain geographical areas because the heterozygous (trait) form of thalassaemia and sickle cell offers some protection against malaria. It is found mainly in people whose families come from Africa, the West Indies, the Middle East, the eastern Mediterranean and Asia (Higgins 2000). As these conditions are inherited, and in the homozygous form can be fatal, screening of the population at risk should be carried out. Blood is examined by electrophoresis, which detects the different types of haemoglobin. Prospective parents who are known to have (or carry genes for) abnormal haemoglobin need genetic counselling in order to help them make an informed decision regarding contraception, pregnancy and prenatal diagnostic techniques (NHS Sickle Cell and Thalassaemia Screening Programme Centre 2006).

Thalassaemia

This condition is most commonly found in people of Mediterranean, African, Middle and Far Eastern origin. The basic defect is a reduced rate of globin chain synthesis in adult haemoglobin. This leads to ineffective erythropoiesis and increased haemolysis with a resultant inadequate haemoglobin content. The red cell indices show a low Hb and MCHC level but raised serum iron level. Definitive diagnosis may require DNA analysis. The severity of the condition depends on the number of abnormal genes. There are also different types of thalassaemia (Box 21.1). The key issues should be: test everyone (as the gene pools are thoroughly mixed up); partner testing when the mother is positive; offer couples who are both positive

early prenatal diagnosis, as some combinations of haemoglobinopathies are fatal and others very serious, to enable termination choice to be made.

Alpha thalassaemia major

α-Thalassaemia major is incompatible with extra-uterine life.

Beta thalassaemia major

The defective genes present result in severe haemoglobin deficiency, which may result in cardiac failure and death in early childhood. In those that survive, the ineffective erythropoiesis and increased haemolysis cause hypersplenism. A splenectomy is often performed in order to increase RBC survival and reduce the need for frequent blood transfusions. Blood transfusions increase the possibility of survival to childbearing age. Until recently, the high mortality rate made pregnancy in transfusion-dependent thalassaemia rare. However, advances in paediatric and haematological management have resulted in good maternal and fetal outcomes in women with β-thalassaemia major.

Alpha and beta thalassaemia minor

α- and β-thalassaemia minor is the most common problem encountered among pregnant women. This heterozygous condition produces an anaemia that is similar to iron deficiency in that the Hb, the MCV and the MCH are all lowered. A definitive diagnosis needs DNA analysis. A deficiency in iron is not, however, usually a problem because RBCs are broken down more rapidly than normal and the iron is stored for future use. In pregnancy, oral iron and folate supplements are necessary in order to maintain the iron stores. Parenteral iron should never be given. Blood transfusions may be required if the haemoglobin is thought to be inadequate for the stress of labour and blood loss at birth (Strong 2006).

Sickle cell disorders

Sickle cell disorders are found most commonly in people of African or West Indian origin. Defective genes produce abnormal haemoglobin alpha or beta chains; the resulting Hb is called HbS. In sickle cell anaemia (HbSS, or SCA) abnormal genes have been inherited from both parents, whereas in sickle cell trait (HbAS) only one. abnormal gene has

---

Box 21.1 Types of thalassaemia and their inheritance

α-chains are formed by two genes from each parent.

β-chains are formed by one gene from each parent.

Therefore:

α-thalassaemia major	= four defective α genes
α-thalassaemia intermedia	= three defective α genes
α-thalassaemia minor	= two or one defective α genes
β-thalassaemia major	= two defective β genes
β-thalassaemia minor	= one defective β gene

been inherited (Khattab et al 2006a). The introduction of a national antenatal and neonatal screening programme for haemoglobinopathies in England will improve healthcare and reduce childhood morbidity and mortality significantly (NHS Sickle Cell and Thalassaemia Screening Programme Centre 2006).

Sickle cell anaemia

Sickle cells have an increased fragility and shortened life span of 17 days, which results in chronic haemolytic anaemia and causes episodes of ischaemia and pain, known as *attacks of pain* or *sickle cell crises*. Sickling crisis may occur whenever oxygen concentration is low. Precipitating factors that affect oxygen uptake include psychological stress, cold climate and extreme temperature changes, smoking-induced hypoxia, strenuous physical exertion and fatigue, respiratory disease, infection and pregnancy. When subjected to low oxygen tension, HbS contracts damaging the cell and causing it to assume a sickle shape. Sickle cells easily adhere to the vascular epithelium causing a reduced blood flow, vascular obstruction and hypoxia. This results in acute pain, particularly in the bones, joints and abdominal organs.

Painful episodes last for a few hours to a few days and are often poorly managed and undertreated by nursing, midwifery and medical staff in pregnancy. Effective management of sickle cell crisis can be achieved by:

- utilization of pain assessment tools to determine severity of the pain
- administration of effective analgesia within 30 min of admission to hospital starting with a non-opioid analgesia, e.g. paracetamol before moving to opioid analgesia for moderate/severe pain
- liaison with the acute pain management team to ensure adequate and continuing pain relief
- administration of oral and intravenous fluids to correct dehydration and electrolyte imbalance caused by pyrexia, vomiting or diarrhoea
- pulse oximetry to assess oxygen saturation and the administration of oxygen therapy if indicated
- antibiotic treatment if infection is suspected
- assessment of haematological indices and liaison with the haematology department

- keeping warm and promoting rest
- provision of social, psychological and physical support to alleviate symptoms associated with chronic pain.

Blood transfusion therapy is key to the management of sickle cell anaemia as it increases the oxygen carrying capacity of blood by increasing the haemoglobin concentration and decreasing the percentage of sickle haemoglobin. However, due to the risk of developing red cell antibodies and iron overload the indications for the use of blood transfusion therapy include: acute chest syndrome, heart failure, multiorgan failure, stroke, splenic sequestration and aplastic crisis. New therapies include the use of drugs such as hydroxyurea, which inhibits the development of sickle cells by increasing fetal haemoglobin production. Bone marrow and stem cell transplantation can cure SCA but is still in the early stages of development and not generally available (Claster & Vichinsky 2003, Khattab et al 2006b, National Institutes of Health 2002). Life expectancy for people with sickle cell anaemia has improved considerably over the last decade although overtime major organ damage results in a chronic illness requiring long term physical and psychosocial support (Okpala et al 2002, Thomas & Taylor 2002).

Maternal and fetal effects. There have been significant decreases in both maternal and perinatal mortality. Women with SCA are at an increased risk for medical complications during pregnancy. Maternal risks include antenatal and postnatal attacks of pain, infections, pulmonary complications, anaemia, pre-eclampsia and caesarean section. Fetal and neonatal complications include spontaneous abortion, pre-term birth, intrauterine growth restriction and perinatal death (Sergeant et al 2004, Sun et al 2001).

Preconception care. All women should be offered haemoglobin electrophoresis in early pregnancy and for any with positive results it is important to have their partner tested. Where both parents have abnormal results, counselling regarding prenatal diagnosis should be offered at a dedicated obstetric/haematology clinic. If both parents are carriers for HbS (i.e. heterozygous) there is a one in four chance that the fetus will inherit the more serious condition, sickle cell anaemia (Fig. 21.1) (Zack-Williams 2007).

Antenatal care. Antenatal care aims to minimize the maternal and fetal complications as 35–50% of

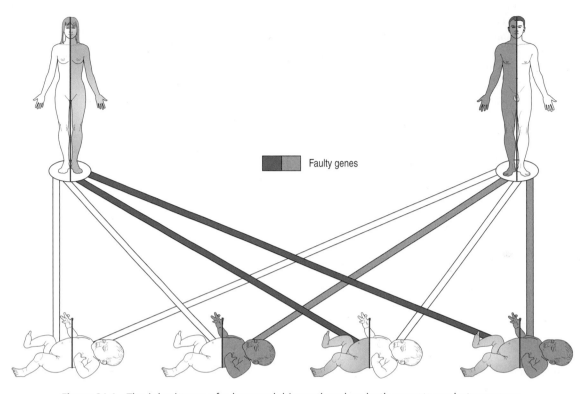

Faulty genes

Figure 21.1 The inheritance of a haemoglobinopathy when both parents are heterozygous.

women with SCA will experience sickle crises during pregnancy which requires hospital admission and treatment (Rahimy et al 2000, Sun et al 2001). Monitoring of pregnancy is performed at frequent intervals by a multidisciplinary team involving a midwife, obstetrician, haematologist, specialist nurse and physician, maintaining close liaison and discussion with the woman and her family. Midwives have an important role in providing information and education about SCA and how it affects pregnancy, particularly in emphasizing the factors that may precipitate sickle crisis. In addition to the tests routinely performed as part of antenatal care, initial blood tests should include screening for red cell antibodies, haemoglobin electrophoresis, serum iron, total iron-binding capacity, serum ferritin levels, liver function tests, blood urea nitrogen and serum creatinine. Regular monitoring of the haemoglobin concentration is required throughout pregnancy; this is usually in the range of 6–9g/dL. Fluid intake should be well maintained to prevent dehydration and it is important to detect bacterial infections, particularly genitourinary and respiratory infections, at an early stage. Good nutrition and folic acid supplements assist in maintaining a steady haematological state. The use of prophylactic blood transfusions to improve the outcome of pregnancy remains controversial. The potential benefits for the pregnancy have to be offset against the disadvantages of transfusions. Most authors recommend a policy of transfusing only when indicated, for example in symptomatic anaemia, severe anaemia with a haematocrit <18%, sickle crisis, cardiac failure or prior to caesarean section. Fetal assessment includes regular ultrasound scans to assess fetal growth. If growth restriction is identified, then more intensive monitoring will be required utilizing biophysical profiles and uterine Doppler blood flow studies (Dauphin-McKenzie et al 2006, Rahimy et al 2000).

Intrapartum care. Timing and mode of birth is gauged according to maternal and fetal health, induction of labour or caesarean section should be performed for obstetric reasons. Good pain relief and adequate hydration are essential to reduce the risk of a sickle crisis; an epidural is usually recommended.

Oxygen therapy via a nasal prong or mask is advised to maintain adequate oxygenation and improve cardiac function. Prophylactic antibiotics may be considered to prevent infection. Prolonged labour should be avoided and active management or a caesarean section may be advised on clinical grounds. CTG monitoring is recommended, especially where there is intrauterine growth restriction.

Postnatal care. Women with SCA are at a high risk of developing thromboembolic disorders therefore early ambulation and wearing antiembolic stockings should be encouraged. To prevent puerperal sepsis, antibiotic cover is continued throughout the postnatal period. Neonatal screening of babies must be undertaken by obtaining a sample of neonatal capillary or venous blood at birth. Those with positive results should be followed-up by a haematologist. In order to prevent the high incidence of infant mortality from sickle cell anaemia, early diagnosis combined with prophylaxis against infection, parental education and adequate follow-up are recommended (NHS Sickle Cell and Thalassaemia Screening Programme Centre 2006).

Sickle cell trait is usually asymptomatic. The blood appears normal, although the sickle screening test is positive. The woman may be mildly anaemic in pregnancy and folate 5 mg daily is recommended to help erythropoiesis.

Combinations of abnormal haemoglobins

Sickle cell disease can be combined with other disorders and therefore individual advice from a haematologist is necessary.

Other rare inherited disorders

Glucose-6-phosphate dehydrogenase

Glucose-6-phosphate dehydrogenase (G6PD) deficiency is an X-linked, hereditary genetic defect. G6PD is an enzyme necessary for the survival of the red cell; when it is deficient RBCs are destroyed in the presence of certain substances. These include fava beans, sulphonamides, vitamin K analogues, salicylates and camphor (found in products such as 'Vicks VapoRub'). To prevent haemolysis these substances should be avoided (Cappellini & Fiorelli 2008).

Spherocytosis

Spherocytosis is found in northern Europe. In this condition, the red cells are spherical instead of biconcave and are easily destroyed. In this disease the abnormal gene is dominant. Midwives need to be aware that women with this condition might have had a splenectomy.

Diabetes mellitus

Diabetes is a chronic and progressive disorder which has a significant impact on almost all aspects of life. Approximately 2–5% of pregnancies involve women with diabetes (NICE 2008). The St Vincent Declaration of the European Association for the Study of Diabetes and of the UK Task Force (SVD Working Party 1990) was an agreement to work towards achieving pregnancy outcome for women with diabetes equal to that of women without diabetes. Research by the Confidential Enquiry into Maternal and Child Health (CEMACH) found that babies of women with diabetes in England, Wales and Northern Ireland are five times more likely to be stillborn, three times more likely to die in their first months of life and twice as likely to have a major congenital abnormality. Additionally, the study showed that nearly one in three mothers with diabetes have type 2 diabetes and that the risk for poor outcome for these women is similar to those with type 1 diabetes (CEMACH 2005, Macintosh et al 2006). Critical to reducing the incidence of poor outcome is the need for good preconception care, near normal glycaemic control before and around conception and throughout pregnancy. Efforts to improve outcome should also focus on identifying at risk groups, particularly women who have difficulties accessing appropriate care either because of language difficulties or unfamiliarity with the healthcare system (CEMACH 2007). Midwives are increasingly the initial contact in early pregnancy and have a vital role, working collaboratively with the woman and the obstetric and diabetes team, to ensure that women with diabetes have a 'positive experience of pregnancy and childbirth and receive care that promotes their physical health and well-being and optimizes the health of their babies' (DH 2001, p 35).

The term *'diabetes mellitus'* (DM) describes a metabolic disorder that affects the normal metabolism of carbohydrates, fats and protein. It is characterized by hyperglycaemia and glycosuria resulting from defects in insulin secretion, or insulin action, or both. The classic signs and symptoms are excessive thirst (polydipsia), excessive urinary excretion (polyuria) and unexplained weight loss. The long-term effects of DM are reflected in the development of macrovascular and microvascular disease producing coronary heart disease, peripheral arterial disease, kidney disease (diabetic nephropathy), loss of vision (diabetic retinopathy) and nerve damage (diabetic neuropathy). It can also affect mental health and well-being.

A normal fasting blood glucose of <6.1 mmol/L is regulated by the pancreatic hormones insulin and glucagon. Following the ingestion of carbohydrates, the rising blood glucose stimulates the pancreas to secrete insulin, which reduces blood glucose. Falling blood glucose levels induce glucagon production, which prevents further glucose reduction. The combined action of these two hormones maintains the blood glucose within normal limits.

Hyperglycaemia is usually the result of insulin deficiency or when there is a high secretion of hormones antagonistic to insulin action; severe hyperglycaemia (blood glucose >25.0 mmol/L) may result in diabetic ketoacidosis, coma or death.

Hypoglycaemia is defined as a blood glucose <2.2 mmol/L. Symptoms of a falling blood glucose include tremor, sweating and tachycardia. Severe hypoglycaemia, particularly in neonates, can result in fits, coma and death. Repeated severe episodes of hypoglycaemia are associated with the risk of permanent brain damage (Higgins 2001).

Classification

Type 1 diabetes

This occurs when β cells in the islets of Langerhans in the pancreas are destroyed, stopping insulin production. Insulin therapy is required in order to prevent the development of ketoacidosis, coma and death. It presents more commonly in childhood, but can occur at any age and in some cases is attributable to an autoimmune process (WHO 1999).

Type 2 diabetes

This results from a defect in the action of insulin. Insulin therapy is not always needed. The risk of developing this type of diabetes increases with age, obesity and lack of physical activity. It occurs more frequently in women with prior gestational diabetes mellitus and in individuals with hypertension. Its frequency varies between different racial or ethnic groups and there is some suggestion of a genetic predisposition (WHO 1999).

Gestational diabetes mellitus

Gestational diabetes mellitus (GDM). This is defined as carbohydrate intolerance resulting in hyperglycaemia of variable severity, with its onset or first recognition during pregnancy (WHO 1999).

Impaired glucose regulation

This includes *impaired* glucose tolerance (IGT) and *impaired fasting glycaemia* (IFG), which are metabolic states intermediate between normal glucose homeostasis and diabetes. IGT is categorized as carbohydrate metabolism resulting in slightly raised post-meal blood glucose levels of >7.8 mmol/L. IFG refers to fasting glucose concentrations that are lower than those required to diagnose diabetes but higher than the 'normal' reference range (i.e. >6.1 mmol/L but <7.0 mmol/L). Individuals with impaired glucose regulation are at increased risk of developing diabetes and cardiovascular disease (WHO 1999).

The demographic pattern of diabetes is changing with increasing numbers of young people diagnosed as having type 1 diabetes and the number of people diagnosed as having type 2 diabetes increasing predominantly among people in Black, Asian or other minority ethnic groups (DH 2001, Hotu et al 2004). Among pregnancies complicated by diabetes, 25% of cases involve pre-existing type 1 diabetes, 10% involve pre-existing type 2 diabetes and, the remaining 65% involve gestational diabetes which may or may not resolve after pregnancy.

Diagnosis

WHO (1999) recommend the following criteria for diagnosing diabetes:

1. Diabetes symptoms of increased thirst, increased urine volume, unexplained weight loss, plus

2. – a random venous plasma glucose concentration >11.1 mmol/L or,
   – a fasting plasma concentration >7.0 mmol/L or,
   – a 2 hrs plasma concentration >11.1 mmol/L 2 hrs after 75 g anhydrous glucose in an oral glucose tolerance test (OGTT);

3. without symptoms, diagnosis should not be based on a single glucose determination but requires confirmatory plasma venous determination taken on another day;

4. the OGTT should always be used to diagnose gestational diabetes mellitus and impaired glucose regulation.

Monitoring diabetes

The main objective of diabetic therapy is to maintain blood glucose levels as near to normal as possible and to reduce the risk of long-term complications. People with diabetes are therefore encouraged to monitor their blood glucose concentration regularly by obtaining a finger-prick sample of capillary blood and using reagent test strips (e.g. BM test) with or without a reflectance glucose meter. Blood glucose can also be estimated by testing urine for glucose using reagent strips, although this is less accurate than the blood test and not recommended in pregnancy. Long-term blood glucose control can be determined by undertaking a laboratory test to measure glycosylated haemoglobin (HbA_{1c}). Around 5–8% of haemoglobin in the red blood cells carries a glucose molecule and is said to be glycosylated. The degree of haemoglobin glycosylation is dependent on the amount of glucose the red blood cells have been exposed to during their 120-day life. A random blood test measuring the percentage of haemoglobin that is glycosylated will reflect the average blood glucose during the preceding 1–2 months. The higher the HbA_{1c} the poorer is the blood sugar control. Good diabetic control is defined as an HbA_{1c} of <6.5% (Higgins 2001).

Carbohydrate metabolism in pregnancy

Pregnancy is characterized by several factors that produce a diabetogenic state so that insulin and carbohydrate metabolism is altered in order to make glucose more readily available to the fetus. Increasing levels of oestrogen, progesterone and prolactin produce progressive hyperplasia of the pancreatic β-cells resulting in the secretion of 50% more insulin (hyperinsulinaemia) by the third trimester. However, progesterone, human placental lactogen and cortisol are insulin antagonists and reduce the effectiveness of insulin. This is considered to be a 'glucose-sparing mechanism', which enables large quantities of glucose to be taken up by the maternal circulation and transferred to the fetus via the placenta by a process known as 'facilitated diffusion'. After the placenta is delivered, insulin resistance and requirements decrease rapidly and the pre-pregnancy sensitivity to insulin is restored. Gestational diabetes is most likely to emerge during the third trimester when the extra demands on the pancreatic beta cells precipitate glucose intolerance. Women with diabetes do not have the capacity to increase insulin secretion in response to the altered carbohydrate metabolism in pregnancy and therefore glucose accumulates in the maternal and fetal system leading to significant morbidity and mortality.

Pre-pregnancy care

The National Service Framework (NSF) for Diabetes: Standards (DH 2001) and the NICE guideline on diabetes in pregnancy (NICE 2008) set out standards and key interventions that will reduce the risks of adverse pregnancy outcomes. Women with diabetes who are planning to become pregnant should be informed that establishing good glycaemic control before conception and continuing throughout pregnancy will reduce but not eliminate the risk of miscarriage, congenital malformation (predominately cardiac anomalies, urogenital anomalies and neural tube defects [NTD]), stillbirth and neonatal death.

Pre-pregnancy care aims to achieve optimal glycaemic control in women with diabetes and provides an opportunity for genetic counselling, diabetes care, preconception care and family planning options (Hofmanova 2006). A comprehensive obstetric, gynaecological and diabetic history is essential and assessment is made of current diabetic control. Individualized targets for self-monitoring of blood glucose should be agreed with women with pre-existing diabetes taking into account the risk of hypoglycaemia. If safely achievable, women should aim for an HbA_{1c}

below 6.1% (NICE 2008). Women with type 1 diabetes will need their insulin dosage reviewed and an explanation given of the adjustments that will be required during pregnancy. Women with type 2 diabetes who have poor glycaemic control will require insulin during pregnancy and those taking oral hypoglycaemics will need to change to insulin to prevent the possibility of teratogenesis. Pregnancy may lead to a deterioration of diabetes and for this reason, the presence of renal, cardiovascular or retinal changes need to be assessed. Angiotensin-converting enzyme (ACE) inhibitors used to control hypertension in women with diabetes are contraindicated in pregnancy because of possible teratogenesis and therefore alternative antihypertensive therapy such as methyldopa or nifedipine is required. Nutritional and dietary advice should be given as weight gain will influence the insulin requirements and affect its absorption. Folic acid supplementation, 5 mg/day, is recommended when planning a pregnancy and should be continued until 12 weeks pregnant to reduce the risk of having a baby with a NTD. General health measures, including checking rubella status and smoking cessation, need to be discussed in addition to giving advice regarding the effect of diabetes on pregnancy and of pregnancy on diabetes (DH 2001, Diabetes UK 2005, NICE 2008, SIGN 2001).

Antenatal care

Antenatal care for women with diabetes should be provided by a multidisciplinary team in a joint diabetes and antenatal clinic (NICE 2008). The woman is seen as often as required in order to maintain good glycaemic control; this may entail 2–4 weekly visits until 28 weeks' gestation and then 1–2 weekly until term. Glycaemic control is particularly difficult to maintain in early pregnancy owing to the effects of pregnancy on diabetes and this may be exacerbated by other pregnancy disorders such as nausea and vomiting. Blood glucose levels should be monitored frequently (four times a day using a calibrated blood glucose meter correctly) and insulin levels adjusted to achieve a fasting blood glucose of between 3.5 and 5.9 mmol/L and 1 hr postprandial <7.8 mmol/L (NICE 2008). Additional estimations of blood glucose control such as HbA_{1c} (or fructosamine) measurements are also required. Intensive glycaemic control means that women with diabetes are also more likely to become severely hypoglycaemic, particularly at night-time and in gestational weeks 10–20. Loss of hypoglycaemic awareness and warning symptoms are also common (Temple 2007). Women and their relatives need to be warned of this and advice should be given regarding recognition, management and treatment of hypoglycaemia. Temple (2007) recommends the following treatments for hypoglycaemia: 3–5 glucose tablets, 250–300 mL isotonic Lucozade, 75–120 mL carbonated lemonade or 4–6 jelly babies repeated as necessary. This should be followed by one piece of fruit, one or two plain biscuits or a piece of bread. In addition, a glucagon kit should be supplied and the woman's partner and relatives instructed on how to use it.

Dietary advice and monitoring is continued throughout pregnancy as the need for carbohydrate increases as the fetus grows. A diet that is high in fibre is beneficial as carbohydrates are released slowly and therefore a more constant blood glucose level can be achieved. Glycosuria is common in pregnancy owing to the increased glomerular filtration rate (GFR) and decreased renal threshold. Women with diabetes have a predisposition to urinary and vaginal infections during pregnancy; these should be discussed with the midwife so women can recognize the signs and symptoms and seek treatment as soon as possible.

Pre-existing vascular disease will increase the risk of a woman with diabetes developing hypertensive disorders in pregnancy. It will also cause a deterioration of diabetic retinopathy; retinal assessment should therefore be undertaken in the first and third trimesters. Renal function should also be monitored and referral made to a nephrologist if the serum creatinine is 120 μmol/L or more or total protein excretion exceeds 2 g/day (NICE 2008).

In view of the increased risk of congenital malformations, a detailed anomaly ultrasound scan should be performed at 20 weeks' gestation. It is also recommended that fetal echocardiography is undertaken at 20 weeks to detect any cardiac abnormalities. Serum screening for Down syndrome is altered with maternal diabetes and care should be taken when interpreting the results.

Fetal growth must be observed carefully because of the risk of growth restriction due to maternal vascular disease, pre-eclampsia, or a combination of both. Poor glycaemic control will result in fetal macrosomia.

A dating ultrasound scan should be undertaken in the first trimester (8–10 weeks). Monitoring of fetal growth should be offered monthly from 28 weeks' gestation. Serial ultrasound should also assess fetal well-being in late pregnancy through monitoring of amniotic fluid volume.

As far as possible, the woman monitors her diabetes at home and diabetic care is provided on an outpatient basis. It is important that the midwife assesses the progress of the pregnancy in the normal way in order to detect any complications. Hospital admission may be required because of poor glycaemic control, a destabilizing illness or obstetric complications.

Intrapartum care

For women with uncomplicated diabetes the spontaneous onset of labour and normal birth is recommended but this should take place in a hospital with neonatal intensive care facilities (SIGN 2001). Routine induction of labour or planned caesarean section before 38 weeks' gestation is not recommended as it does not reduce the perinatal mortality rate, is more likely to result in neonatal respiratory morbidity and contributes to the high caesarean section rate for women with diabetes. However, Diabetes UK (2005) and NICE (2008) recommend that labour should commence after 38 completed weeks' gestation in order to minimize the risk of late fetal death. Poor glycaemic control or a deterioration in the maternal or fetal condition may necessitate earlier, planned birth. Induction of labour may also be considered where the fetus is judged to be macrosomic (birth weight >4000g). Fetal lungs mature more slowly when the mother is diabetic and it is important to take this into account if early induction of labour is planned. In addition, steroids such as dexamethasone, which may be used to aid lung maturation and surfactant production, will increase insulin requirements in women with diabetes.

The aim of intrapartum care is to maintain normoglycaemia in labour (i.e. 4.0–7.0mmol/L) by use of an insulin infusion titrated according to blood glucose levels. Maternal hyperglycaemia (>8mmol/L) leads to an increase in fetal insulin production, which will cause neonatal hypoglycaemia. Fetal compromise is more common as placental blood flow is reduced and glycosylated haemoglobin decreases oxygen carriage in women with diabetes. In addition, maternal ketoacidosis may result from dehydration and unstable diabetes. If the mother becomes acidotic, ketones will cross the placenta and affect the fetal acid–base status. CTG monitoring is recommended and fetal blood sampling should be utilized if acidosis is suspected.

Postpartum care

Immediately after the third stage of labour the insulin requirements will fall rapidly to pre-pregnancy levels. The insulin infusion rate should be reduced by at least 50%. Carbohydrate metabolism returns to normal very quickly and women can resume their pre-pregnancy insulin regimen as soon as they are able to eat. Women with type 2 diabetes who were previously on oral hypoglycaemics or dietary control need to be reviewed prior to recommencing therapy. Monitoring of blood glucose levels should continue during this interim period. Breastfeeding should be encouraged in all women with diabetes. An additional carbohydrate intake of 40–50g is recommended and insulin therapy may need to be adjusted accordingly. Operative birth, together with diabetes, predisposes these women to infection and delayed healing. The administration of antibiotics may be a useful preventative measure in this instance. All women should be offered contraceptive advice so that optimum glycaemic control is achieved prior to planning the next pregnancy. The issues governing choice of contraception for women with diabetes are similar to those for women without diabetes; all contraceptive methods are considered safe, acceptable and effective. Women with diabetes should be reviewed at 6 weeks, ideally at a combined diabetes/obstetric clinic especially if they are breastfeeding.

Neonatal care

All babies should remain with their mothers unless there is a specific medical indication for admission to a neonatal unit (CEMACH 2004, CEMACH 2007, DH 2001, Diabetes UK 2005, NICE 2008). The development of complications in the neonate is related to maternal hyperglycaemia during pregnancy leading to fetal hyperinsulinaemia. This will result in the following neonatal problems: macrosomia (see Chs 33 and 45 for birth difficulties); hypoglycaemia (see Ch. 48); polycythaemia (see Ch. 43); and respiratory distress syndrome (see Ch. 44).

Gestational diabetes

The incidence of gestational diabetes (GD) varies widely across different ethnic groups. In Caucasians, it is 1–2%, in Afro-Caribbeans 2–3% and in Asians 4–5% (Lowy 1997). An agreement as to what is considered a 'normal' blood glucose level in pregnancy and at what level maternal and fetal morbidity ensues remains elusive. Hence, the significance of GDM is difficult to determine (Mitchell 2001). The strongest evidence suggests that fetal macrosomia and caesarean section rates are increased. In the longer term, there appears to be an association between raised glucose levels *in utero* and the development of obesity and diabetes in later life. There is also evidence to suggest that women who develop GDM are at risk of developing type 2 diabetes (Virjee et al 2001). Davey & Hamblin (2001) identify that some women are at high risk of developing GDM and there may be some benefit in selective screening for GDM in women where the following risk factors are identified:

- previous baby weighing >4.5 kg
- diabetes affecting a first degree relative
- high risk racial heritage, e.g. Asian-Indian, Middle Eastern, black-Caribbean
- BMI >30 kg/m^2.

NICE (2008) guidance for screening and diagnosis of GDM includes:

- if the woman has had GDM before, to self-monitor blood glucose or a 2 hrs 75 g OGTT at 16–18 weeks and again at 28 weeks if normal
- if any other risk factors, do an OGTT at 24–28 weeks.

Treatment will depend on the blood glucose levels. The midwife should involve both the diabetic nurse (or midwife) specialist and dietician in dietary interventions to regulate carbohydrate intake and restrict fat and sugars. Advice regarding exercise in pregnancy will be of benefit and smoking cessation strategies where appropriate. Grossly abnormal results are likely to require insulin therapy. Blood glucose monitoring should continue on a regular basis throughout pregnancy in order to detect hyperglycaemia. Fetal macrosomia is the main complication and therefore fetal growth and well-being should be closely monitored for the remainder of the pregnancy. Decisions can then be made about the optimal mode and time of birth. Following birth the baby should be closely monitored for hypoglycaemia. If the woman is on insulin therapy, this is withdrawn immediately after the birth of the baby. It is recommended that a postnatal OGTT is performed at 6 weeks; if the results are abnormal then appropriate referral should be made. Those with normal glucose levels require advice regarding the implications for future pregnancies and the development of type 1 or type 2 diabetes. If the woman adopts a healthy lifestyle and avoids obesity this risk may be reduced.

Epilepsy

Epilepsy is a common serious chronic neurological disorder. MacDonald et al (2000) estimate that approximately 7 out of 1000 people have epilepsy. It can affect anyone at any age but the disorder commonly develops before 20 years of age, 30% of cases occurring in early childhood. Due to the wide variation of epileptic syndromes this results in significant difficulties in the diagnosis, management and treatment of the condition and morbidity mortality can be high (APPG 2007).

Between 2003–2005, 11 women died as a result of epilepsy (Lewis 2007). Key to a successful pregnancy includes ensuring that:

- women with epilepsy are receiving appropriate information and counselling about contraception, conception and pregnancy so that they can make informed decisions about their care (APPG 2007, Stoneman 2005)
- care is provided by a multidisciplinary team comprising a named midwife, obstetrician and neurologist in order to prevent significant morbidity/mortality in either the mother or fetus
- clinical guidelines, such as the National Institute for Health and Clinical Excellence (NICE 2004), the Scottish Intercollegiate Guidelines Network (SIGN 2003) and the National Service Framework for Long-term (Neurological) Conditions (DH 2005) are implemented.

Aetiology

An epileptic seizure results from abnormal electrical activity in the brain, which is manifest by brief disturbances of sensory, motor and autonomic function. These disturbances recur spontaneously and are classified according to the parts of the brain affected. Seizures may be described as *partial*, usually arising from the temporal or frontal lobe of the brain, or *generalized*, resulting from disturbances involving both halves of the brain. General seizures may be further classified as *absence seizures* (petit mal), *myoclonic seizures*, *tonic-clonic seizures* (grand mal), *atonic seizures* and *status* epilepticus (Taylor 2000).

The cause of epilepsy in most instances is unknown. There is some suggestion of a genetic component, which in certain circumstances predisposes an individual to epileptic seizures. In other cases, an underlying cause such as hypoglycaemia, encephalitis, meningitis, cerebral hypoxia, toxicity from alcohol or drugs, or structural damage or abnormality of the brain may result in epilepsy. A number of 'trigger' factors have been identified that may precipitate an attack in those who have been diagnosed with epilepsy; these include emotional stress, sleep deprivation/physical exhaustion, increased body temperature (fever, hot steamy environments), environmental factors (strobe lighting, noise), non-compliance with drug therapy. In women, the hormonal changes at the onset of menstruation may trigger epileptic seizures (Jackson 2006) and women with pre-existing epilepsy may find that seizures cluster peri-menstrually (Reddy 2007).

Diagnosis

Identification of the type and cause of epilepsy is important in the treatment of epilepsy, there are however approximately 30 different epileptic syndromes and over 38 different types of seizure. Diagnosis is therefore complex and involves a number of investigations: taking a clear history including eyewitness accounts is fundamental; blood tests to determine haematology, biochemistry and toxicology assays; neuroimaging such as magnetic resonance imaging (MRI) and computerized tomography (CT) to identify any structural abnormalities and neurological lesions; electroencephalogram (EEG) to classify seizure type by identifying the origin of the abnormal electrical discharge and telemetry which uses video and EEG to observe and identify the seizure type; neuropsychological assessment to evaluate any learning disability and cognitive dysfunction (NICE 2004).

Treatment

The aim of treatment is to identify the cause of the seizure and provide appropriate therapy to prevent recurrence. For the majority of people the control of seizures can be achieved through the use of one anti-epileptic drug (AED). In some individuals a combination of drugs (polytherapy) may be required and a few will require surgery. Most of the drugs have side-effects, which include drowsiness, sedation, nausea and skin rashes; these are most notable when the drug is first taken or if the dosage is too high. The ideal treatment therefore is a single AED prescribed at the lowest effective dose. AED therapy must be started under the guidance of a specialist physician and will need to be reviewed at regular intervals and at a minimum once a year. Women who take AEDs have a 4% chance of having a baby with a major congenital malformation and therefore the dosage and type of drug will need to be reviewed and adjusted in pregnancy in order to reduce this risk (NICE 2004).

Health education

The provision of appropriate advice in primary care and prompt referral to secondary care is vital for people with epilepsy. Midwives and other health professionals have an important role in the education of women and their families and for ensuring that they are provided with a range of information including:

- knowledge of epilepsy in general
- the significance of trigger factors which may precipitate a seizure
- a guide to AEDs, how they work, their side effects and the importance of compliance
- an explanation of what happens during a seizure, recognizing status epilepticus, what to do and when to get medical help (NSE 2007)
- implications for employment, education, sports activities, driving and maintaining independent living
- psychological and sociological issues
- effects of treatment on fertility and pregnancy and the risk of congenital abnormalities
- sudden death in epilepsy (SUDEP) (APPG 2007, Hanna et al 2002)

- knowledge of voluntary organizations that provide information and support, for example, Epilepsy Action (www.epilepsy.org.uk) and National Society for Epilepsy (www.epilepsynse.org.uk).

Effect of epilepsy on the fetus and neonate

In general, women whose epilepsy is well controlled have few problems in pregnancy and can expect a normal, uncomplicated pregnancy and birth. Some women may experience an increase in seizures and the risk of complications in pregnancy is increased when epilepsy is poorly controlled (EURAP Study Group 2006). This is often due to non-compliance with the drug regimen, sleep deprivation during pregnancy and the decline in plasma concentrations of the AED as the pregnancy progresses. Prolonged and/or serial seizures during pregnancy increase the risk of fetal morbidity and mortality caused by hypoxia or placental abruption. There is also an increased risk of maternal death. Particular emphasis should be placed on the first aid measures that should be adopted following an epileptic seizure in order to prevent aspiration, the dangers of hot baths inducing fainting and consequent drowning and the risk of SUDEP (Lewis 2007). The majority of women on antiepileptic drugs have physically normal babies, however evidence suggests there is a two–four-fold increased risk of major congenital malformations in babies of women with epilepsy which is directly related to the type and number of drugs the woman is taking (Morrow et al 2006).

Pre-pregnancy care

Preconception advice is essential for women with epilepsy and a review of AED therapy is crucial before women consider becoming pregnant (Lewis & Smith 2006). In some instances, the gradual withdrawal of AED therapy may be considered prior to pregnancy in order to reduce the risk of congenital malformation in the fetus. This may be possible where the woman (a) suffers from seizures that are unlikely to harm the fetus such as absence, partial or myoclonic or (b) has been seizure free for more than two years and a recurrence is unlikely (Tomson & Hiilesmaa 2007). Folic acid supplementation (5 mg/day) should be commenced before pregnancy and continued throughout pregnancy to prevent

congenital malformation and the development of anaemia (NICE 2004).

Antenatal care

Pregnancy has no effect on seizure control and most women with epilepsy will remain seizure free (EURAP Study Group 2006). Close monitoring of the maternal and fetal condition is required and antenatal care should be provided by a multidisciplinary team which includes a named midwife, obstetrician and a neurologist or physician with a specialist interest in epilepsy in pregnancy (Lewis 2007). Care should include a detailed anomaly scan at 18–22 weeks. Epilepsy is not an indication for early induction of labour or elective caesarean section.

Intrapartum care

The EURAP Study Group (2006) found that labour and birth carry an increased risk for tonic-clonic seizures with 2–5% of women with epilepsy having seizures at this time. Careful observation and monitoring of the maternal and fetal condition by the midwife is required through labour and the early postnatal period. AEDs should be administered as scheduled throughout labour and it is important to prevent the development of possible 'trigger' situations such as sleep deprivation, hypoglycaemia, stress, hyperventilation and anaemia, all of which may arise during the course of labour. Women with epilepsy should be offered the same choices for pain relief in labour as other women, including epidural analgesia.

Postnatal care

Following birth, women with epilepsy may be at an increased risk of seizures due to fluctuating hormone levels and sleep disturbance. Safety precautions in the home should be discussed with the woman and her partner. This will include giving advice about how to minimize risks when feeding, bathing, changing and transporting the baby.

AEDs cross the placenta freely and decrease production of Vitamin K leading to the risk of Vitamin K deficiency bleeding in the newborn (Ch. 45). This can be prevented by routine administration of oral vitamin K (20 mg/day) to the mother from 36 weeks' gestation and to the baby (1 mg i.m.) shortly after birth (NICE 2004). Breastfeeding is generally safe but specific information must be obtained for each agent. How much AED passes into breastmilk must be considered, as well as the rate of clearance by the neonate. Some AEDs have a sedative effect, causing drowsy babies less efficient at feeding and gaining weight more slowly. Advice should be sought from a neonatologist and some breastfeeds may need to substituted with formula feeds. The British National Formulary (JFC 2007) will indicate which AEDs are contraindicated when a women is breastfeeding.

AED therapy should be reviewed soon after birth by the neurology team and the dosage adjusted to pre-pregnancy levels if it has been increased. Future pregnancy plans should be discussed and appropriate contraceptive advice given. All methods of contraception are available to women with epilepsy, although oral contraceptives are less effective with some AEDs as they induce hepatic enzymes which metabolize oestrogen faster. Women taking these AEDs will require oral contraceptives with a higher dosage of oestrogen (i.e. >50mg oestrogen) in order to prevent the risk of an unplanned pregnancy due to contraceptive failure (Gilmour-White 2000, NICE 2004).

Autoimmune disease

Autoimmune disease arises from a disruption in the function of the immune system of the body, resulting in the production of antibodies against the body's own cells. Antigens normally present on the body's cells stimulate the development of autoantibodies, which, unable to distinguish the self antigens from non-self or foreign antigens, act against the body's cells to cause localized and systemic reactions. The cause of these conditions is unknown but it is thought to be multifactorial with genetic, environmental, hormonal and viral influences. Many autoimmune diseases are more prevalent in women, particularly between puberty and the menopause, which suggests that female hormonal factors may play a role. They broadly fall into two groups:

1. Multisystem disease such as systemic lupus erythematosus (SLE).
2. Tissue- or organ-specific disorders such as autoimmune thyroid disease.

These disorders are characterized by periods of remission interrupted by periods of crisis, which may require hospitalization. This cyclical variation appears to be related to some external factors, for example excessive emotional stress. Treatment is aimed at lessening the severity of the symptoms rather than effecting a cure. Mild cases usually respond to anti-inflammatory drugs; more severe illnesses may require steroids or immunosuppressant therapy.

Systemic lupus erythematosus

Systemic lupus erythematosus (SLE), or lupus, is an autoimmune, connective tissue disorder with a wide range of clinical manifestations. Connective tissue is found throughout the body; therefore SLE produces multisystem disorders affecting muscles, bone, skin, blood, eyes, nervous system, heart, lungs and kidneys. Ethnic groups, particularly those with African or Asian ancestry are at greatest risk of developing the disorder and one of the highest prevalence is seen in the UK Afro-Caribbean populations (D'Cruz et al 2007). Most people with SLE have a normal life expectancy and serious complications are rare. Infection is the major cause of mortality at all stages of SLE; early deaths are usually due to active SLE and late deaths are attributed to thromboembolic disorders (Ruiz-Irastorza et al 2001).

Diagnosis

The diagnosis of SLE is based on a collection of signs and symptoms particularly when joint pain, skin conditions and fatigue occur in combination or evolve over time. The initial manifestation of SLE is often arthritis accompanied by fever, fatigue, malaise, weight loss, photosensitivity and anaemia. A wide range of skin lesions are seen and an erythematous facial 'butterfly' rash is characteristic of the disorder. Depending on the organs involved, inflammatory conditions such as pruritus, pericarditis, glomerulonephritis, neuritis and gastritis may arise. Renal disease and neurological abnormalities are the most serious manifestations of the disease. Blood tests are used to confirm the diagnosis and comprise full blood count, erythrocyte sedimentation rate (ESR) and testing for antinuclear antibody (ANA). There is often normochromic normocytic anaemia, the ESR is elevated even when the disease is in remission and >95% of people with SLE will have ANA (D'Cruz et al 2007).

Antiphospholipid syndrome (Hughes syndrome)

Antiphospholipid syndrome (APS) is a prothrombotic disorder characterized by arterial and/or venous thrombosis, recurrent spontaneous miscarriage, neurological disease including stroke in the presence of circulating antiphospholipid antibodies (aPL). Approximately 30–40% of women with SLE have aPL antibodies and some will develop APS. A blood test will detect aPL and lupus anticoagulant. APS in conjunction with SLE increases the risk of these women developing thromboembolic disorders in pregnancy and is associated with a higher risk of pregnancy loss, intrauterine growth restriction, placental insufficiency, pre-eclampsia and pre-term birth. Reducing the risk of thrombosis through the use of antithrombolytic therapy during pregnancy significantly improves the chance of a successful pregnancy outcome (Khamashta 2006, Tincani et al 2006).

Effects of SLE on pregnancy

As SLE occurs primarily in women during their childbearing years it is likely to complicate pregnancy and it may arise for the first time in pregnancy. The effect of SLE on pregnancy is variable although lupus flares (worsening of SLE symptoms) are common. The frequency of the flares is lower in women with mild and well-controlled disease and providing the disease is in remission at the time of conception, it is less likely that it will become active during the course of the pregnancy. Exacerbation of SLE with major organ involvement (such as the kidneys and central nervous system) may occur in approximately 20% of cases (Classen et al 1998).

Overall pregnancies in SLE women have an increased incidence of adverse pregnancy outcome. Approximately one-third will result in fetal loss owing to spontaneous abortion, therapeutic abortion, intrauterine death or stillbirth. Maternal renal disease and the presence of aPL have been found to be significant predictors of fetal loss, development of pre-eclampsia and intrauterine growth restriction. The rate of preterm birth and intrauterine growth restriction is closely related to the incidence of pre-eclampsia and many women with SLE give birth before 37 weeks (Yasmeen et al 2001).

Neonatal lupus syndrome is rare but may occur as a result of the transplacental passage of maternal IgG autoantibodies. The neonate presents with a mild form of lupus that is transient and resolves when the antibodies are cleared in a few months following birth. A more severe form of the disease results in fetal anaemia, leucopenia and thrombocytopenia. When anti-Ro and/or anti-La antibodies have passed to the fetus, then there is a risk of developing congenital heart block (CHB), which is permanent and carries significant morbidity and mortality. Over 60% of affected children require lifelong pacemakers (Tincani et al 2006).

Preconception care

Women with SLE should be counselled about planning a pregnancy in order to allow time to optimize their health prior to pregnancy. The management of SLE should start before conception so that baseline assessments and alterations to drug therapy can be undertaken. It is recommended that the disease has been in remission for at least 6 months prior to conception. SLE in conjunction with pulmonary hypertension, renal nephritis or APS confers a high risk of maternal morbidity and mortality (Mackillop et al 2007).

Antenatal care

Women should be referred as soon as possible to a centre that specializes in the care of people with lupus disorders. Antenatal care should be provided by a multidisciplinary team in combined clinics. The frequency of antenatal visits is dependent on the severity of the disease, but women with SLE may have additional social and psychological needs requiring consistent midwifery care and support. A minimum of monthly visits until 28 weeks, fortnightly visits to 36 weeks and then weekly visits is recommended (Khamashta 2006). Baseline investigations include: full blood count; urea, creatinine and electrolytes; liver function tests; immunological blood tests to detect antibodies; blood pressure; urinalysis and 24 hrs urine collection for creatinine clearance and total protein to assess renal function is also recommended (Mackillop et al 2007).

An early first trimester scan is undertaken to confirm fetal viability and an anomaly scan is performed at 18–20 weeks. Women with SLE and APS are offered a fetal cardiac anomaly scan at 24 weeks' gestation and echocardiography to detect CHB at intervals in the second and third trimesters.

In view of the high incidence of intrauterine fetal death, careful monitoring of fetal growth and well-being should begin at 28–32 weeks. This should include serial ultrasound examinations for fetal growth, placental Doppler studies and amniotic fluid volume, as well as CTG. Doppler assessment of uterine artery blood flow studies at 20–24 weeks may also be undertaken to predict pre-eclampsia and intrauterine growth restriction (Khamashta 2006).

During pregnancy, the aim is to control disease activity and achieve clinical remission while keeping drug therapy to a minimum. Avoidance of emotional stress and the promotion of a healthy lifestyle may play a part in reducing the likelihood of flares or exacerbations of SLE arising during pregnancy. Alternative therapies and low impact exercise may be utilized by women to reduce the effects of pain, joint stiffness and fatigue. Simple analgesics such as paracetamol and codeine derivatives may be used for symptomatic relief. Women who have a mild form of the disease or are in remission require minimal to no medication. Mild flares with joint pain, skin lesions and fatigue respond well to low dose prednisolone (up to 10mg/day). Antimalarial drugs are effective as maintenance therapy in women with frequent flares and hydroxychloroquine is considered safe to use in pregnancy. Advanced renal disease and women with more severe SLE will require higher doses of prednisolone and immunosuppression. Women with SLE and APS have associated recurrent miscarriage, thrombosis and thrombocytopenia and it is recommended that treatment with anticoagulants such as low dose aspirin and/or heparin is commenced as soon as pregnancy is diagnosed (Mackillop et al 2007). Thromboprophylaxis promotes successful embryonic implantation in the early stages of pregnancy and protects against thrombosis of the uteroplacental vasculature after successful implantation.

Intrapartum care

Generally, intrapartum care falls into the high risk category and women with SLE should be cared for in hospital although a normal labour and vaginal birth should be the aim. Close liaison is required between all healthcare professionals involved: the midwife, obstetrician, rheumatologist, anaesthetist, paediatrician and haematologist. The woman and her family should continue to be involved in the development of the care pathway and the decision making process.

Women with SLE are particularly prone to infection, hypertension, thrombocytopenia and thromboembolic disorders. Careful hand-washing, strict aseptic techniques with invasive procedures and limiting the number of vaginal examinations will reduce the risk of infection. Close monitoring of the maternal condition is required by the midwife, obstetrician and anaesthetist to evaluate cardiac, pulmonary and renal function. Blood tests should be undertaken to screen for haematological conditions, which may lead to clotting disorders. Comfort measures, nursing interventions and the use of TED stockings can reduce the risk of pressure sores and the development of deep vein thrombosis. Women who have been on long-term and/or high doses of steroid therapy will require parenteral steroid cover during labour. SLE may compromise the uteroplacental circulation therefore continuous fetal monitoring in conjunction with fetal blood gas estimation is recommended (Classen et al 1998).

Postpartum care

During the immediate postpartum period, the midwife should observe closely for: signs of SLE flares that may occur as a result of the stress of labour, signs and symptoms of infection, pre-eclampsia, renal disease, thrombosis and neurological changes. Careful consideration needs to be given to breastfeeding as most of the drugs used to treat SLE are excreted in breastmilk: paracetamol is the drug of choice for postpartum analgesia; low dose steroids and hydroxychloroquine are considered safe; immunosuppressive therapy is contraindicated; large doses of aspirin should be avoided and non-steroidal antiinflammatory drugs (NSAIDs) are contraindicated when breastfeeding jaundiced neonates.

The midwife has a role in advising women with regard to her contraceptive options as the choice for a woman with SLE may be limited. Combined oral contraception increases the risk of hypertension, thrombosis and SLE flares. Low dose oestrogen combined pills may be considered in women with well-controlled SLE without a history of thromboembolic disease or APS. Intrauterine contraceptive devices are associated with an increased risk of infection in SLE women. Progestogens and barrier methods represent the safest options and may be suitable for those women where other methods are contraindicated (Mok & Wong 2001).

Thyroid disease

Thyroid disease is the second most common endocrine disorder affecting women of reproductive age. The thyroid gland comprises two lobes connected by the isthmus. Follicular cells within the lobes produce the thyroid hormones. *Thyroxine* (T_4) and *tri-iodothyronine* (T_3) are iodine-containing hormones, which are essential for normal body growth in infancy and childhood and affects the metabolic rate of the body. The thyroid gland also produces *calcitonin*, which is required for calcium metabolism. The production and release of T_3 and T_4, is regulated by *thyroid-stimulating hormone* (TSH), which is secreted through a negative feedback mechanism by the anterior pituitary gland. Production of the thyroid hormones depends on dietary consumption of iodine and calcium. After digestion and synthesis the thyroid hormones become bound to a transport protein called *thyroid-binding globulin* (TBG) and are stored within the thyroid. Stored thyroid hormone is capable of supplying the body with the required amount of hormone for 2–3 months. When released into the circulation 99% of T_4 and T_3 are bound to plasma proteins and serve as a reservoir or store of thyroid hormones in the body. Less than 1% remains as 'free' (unbound to protein) T_4 and T_3, which can be utilized metabolically and act as indicators of the thyroid level in the body, stimulating the release of TSH when T_4 and T_3 levels fall (Rashid & Rashid 2007). In pregnancy, hypothalamic and pituitary regulation maintain normal levels of TSH; however, thyroid function is affected by four factors that increase the basal metabolic rate by 20%:

1. Oestrogen stimulates the production of TBG, which binds more of the thyroid hormones resulting in a doubling of the total serum levels of T_4 and T_3.
2. Human chorionic gonadotrophin (HCG) secreted by the placenta appears to stimulate the thyroid gland directly as TSH levels fall in early pregnancy

and then increase in the second and third trimesters, with a corresponding rise and then fall in the level of HCG. This overstimulation of the thyroid in early pregnancy may partly explain the hyperemesis of pregnancy.

3. A rise in the glomerular filtration rate in pregnancy leads to increased renal clearance of iodine, resulting in an increase in dietary iodine requirement.
4. The fetal thyroid begins concentrating iodine at 10–12 weeks' gestation and is controlled by fetal pituitary TSH by approximately 20 weeks' gestation. Fetal levels will be dependent on maternal levels of iodine.

Clinical assessment of thyroid dysfunction is difficult as pregnancy-related symptoms are similar to hyperthyroidism and hypothyroidism. Thyroid function can be assessed by biochemical tests that measure, free thyroxine (FT_4), free T_3 (FT_3) and TSH (Higgins 2000).

Hyperthyroidism

Hyperthyroidism (also called thyrotoxicosis) occurs in 0.1–0.2% of pregnancies (Lao 2005). The most common cause of hyperthyroidism in pregnancy is *Graves' disease*. This is an autoimmune disorder that results in TSH receptor stimulating antibody (TSHRAb) activation of the thyroid gland. The gland becomes enlarged and secretes an increased amount of thyroid hormone. The metabolic processes of the body are accelerated resulting in sweating, tachycardia, dyspnoea, diarrhoea, mood lability and fatigue. Clinical diagnosis may be difficult as the physiological signs and symptoms that pregnant women normally exhibit may mask this condition. Maternal and fetal complications include miscarriage, placenta abruption, pre-term labour and birth, pre-eclampsia and intrauterine growth restriction (Rashid & Rashid 2007).

A serious complication of untreated or poorly controlled hyperthyroidism is *thyroid storm*. This may occur spontaneously or be precipitated by infection, surgery or stress such as labour and birth. It is characterized by signs and symptoms associated with an extreme hypermetabolic state: hyperthermia (>41°C) leading to dehydration, tachycardia, acute respiratory distress and cardiovascular collapse. This is a medical emergency requiring the administration of oxygen, use of antipyretics, cooling blanket, hydration, antibiotics and drug therapy to stop the production and reduce the effect of thyroid hormone. Thyroid storm is a rare occurrence in pregnancy but carries a high risk of maternal heart failure, fetal or neonatal hyperthyroidism and stillbirth hence intensive maternal and fetal monitoring will be required (Sheffield & Cunningham 2004).

Treatment

Treatment of hyperthyroidism is achieved through the use of antithyroid medication. Propylthiouracil (PTU), methimazole and carbimazole may be used in pregnancy. PTU is the drug of choice as less of it crosses the placenta and only small amounts are found in breastmilk. The aim of treatment is to use the lowest dose possible as these drugs may cause goitre and hypothyroidism in the fetus. During childbirth the midwife should be aware of factors that may precipitate thyroid storm, such as infection, the stress of labour and caesarean section. The woman should be seen monthly by the endocrinologist for clinical evaluation and monitoring of her thyroid levels. Fetal well-being should also be monitored closely (Rashid & Rashid 2007).

Hypothyroidism

Hypothyroidism occurs as the result of decreased activity of the thyroid gland and occurs in 2.5% of pregnancies and may lead to maternal and neonatal complications as well as being a cause of infertility. The most common cause of hypothyroidism in pregnancy is *autoimmune thyroiditis* (*Hashimoto's disease*). It may also be induced following treatment for Graves' disease. Slowing of the body's metabolic processes may occur giving rise to mental and physical lethargy, excessive weight gain, constipation, cold intolerance and dryness of the skin. However, the symptoms may be non-specific and the condition can be difficult to diagnose.

Thyroid hormone is essential for human brain development and the fetus obtains its hormone almost entirely from its mother; reduced availability for fetal requirements results in impaired neurological development in childhood (Haddow et al 1999, Pop et al 2003). In addition, untreated hypothyroidism in pregnancy is associated with increased risk of miscarriage, pre-eclampsia, fetal growth restriction, placental abruption, perinatal mortality and neonatal morbidity (Lao 2005). Women should be encouraged to increase their dietary iodine intake during pregnancy. A study undertaken by Kibirige et al (2004) in the north-east of England found that 40% of pregnant women had iodine deficiency.

It is important to identify and treat hypothyroidism with daily thyroxine as early as possible in order to improve pregnancy outcome. Following birth, thyroid status in the neonate should be checked to identify whether neonatal hypothyroidism is present. There is no contraindication to breastfeeding but the dose of thyroxine may need adjustment postpartum because of maternal weight loss following childbirth.

Postpartum thyroiditis

This is an autoimmune disorder and is a form of Hashimoto's thyroiditis. It occurs in 10% of women within 12 months following childbirth (Lazarus & Premawardhana 2005). It is a transient thyroid disorder, characterized by a period of mild hyperthyroidism 1–4 months after the birth of her baby, followed by a phase of hypothyroidism. In both phases the disorder presents with fatigue and a painless goitre; the condition may also mimic postpartum depression. Treatment is not required as recovery is usually spontaneous but the disorder tends to recur in subsequent pregnancies and may progress to permanent hypothyroidism (Muller et al 2001).

Screening for thyroid disorders

Due to the maternal obstetric complications and reduced neonatal and child neurological development, it is recommended by some authors that a screening programme for thyroid dysfunction should be undertaken in early pregnancy (Lazarus & Premawardhana 2005, Rashid & Rashid 2007). The evidence base for this is currently being assessed; interim measures to improve pregnancy outcome include: optimum iodine nutrition during pregnancy and identifying women with (a) known thyroid disease and (b) increased risk of thyroid disease, e.g. those with other autoimmune disorders. All babies in the UK are screened for congenital hypothyroidism as part of the newborn blood spot programme (UKNSPC 2005).

REFERENCES

APPG (All Party Parliamentary Group on Epilepsy) 2007 Wasted money, wasted lives. The human and economic cost of epilepsy in England. Joint Epilepsy Council of UK and Ireland, Leeds. Online. Available:www.jointepilepsycouncil.com

Badawy A M, El-Metwally A G 2001 Cardiac disease during pregnancy: who will manage? Journal of Obstetrics and Gynaecology 21(1):36–38

BCS (British Cardiovascular Society) 2007 British Cardiovascular Society working group report and recommendations for Women's Heart Health. BCS, London

Baird S, Kennedy B 2006 Myocardial infarction in pregnancy. Journal of Perinatal & Neonatal Nursing 20(4):311–321.

Beard J L 2000 Effectiveness and strategies of iron supplementation during pregnancy. American Journal of Clinical Nutrition 71:1288S–1294S

Beaton G H 2000 Iron needs during pregnancy: do we need to rethink out targets? American Journal of Clinical Nutrition 72:265S–271S

Bent S, Nallamothu B K, Simel D L et al 2002 Does this woman have an acute uncomplicated urinary tract infection? Journal of the American Medical Association 287 (20):2701–2710

BMA, RPS (British Medical Association, Royal Pharmaceutical Society of Great Britain) 2001 British National Formulary 42. BMJ Books, London

Booker R 2007 Peak expiratory flow measurement. Nursing Standard 21(39):42–43

Bothwell T H 2000 Iron requirements in pregnancy and strategies to meet them. American Journal of Clinical Nutrition 72(1):257S–264S

Bridges E J, Womble S, Wallace M et al 2003 Haemodynamic monitoring in high-risk obstetric patients, I – Expected haemodynamic changes in pregnancy. Critical Care Nurse 23(4):53–62

BTS (British Thoracic Society), SIGN (Scottish Intercollegiate Guidelines Network) 2005 British Guideline on the Management of Asthma – a national clinical guideline. BTS, SIGN, London. Online. Available www.brit-thoracic.org.uk and www.sign.ac.uk

Bussey C G, Mittelstaedt E A 2003 Pregnant with cystic fibrosis. AWHONN Lifelines 7(1):40–46

Cameron A J D, Skinner T A J 2005 Case report – Management of a parturient with respiratory failure secondary to cystic fibrosis. Anaesthesia 60:77–80

Cappellini M D, Fiorelli G 2008 Glucose-6-phosphate dehydrogenase deficiency. Lancet 371:64–74

CEMACH (Confidential Enquiry into Maternal and Child Health) 2004 Maternity services in 2002 for women with type 1 and type 2 diabetes. England, Wales and Northern Ireland. RCOG, London

CEMACH 2005 (Confidential Enquiry into Maternal and Child Health) Pregnancy in women with type 1 and type 2 diabetes in 2002–2003. England, Wales and Northern Ireland. RCOG, London

CEMACH (Confidential Enquiry into Maternal and Child Health) 2007 Diabetes in pregnancy: are we providing the best care? Findings from a National Enquiry: England, Wales and Northern Ireland. CEMACH, London

Classen S R, Paulson P R, Zacharias S R 1998 Systemic lupus erythematosus: perinatal and neonatal implications. Journal of Obstetric, Gynaecological and Neonatal Nursing Sept/ Oct:493–500

Claster S, Vichinsky E P 2003 Managing sickle cell disease. British Medical Journal 327:1151–1155

Cox P, Boris W, Gogarten W et al 2005 Maternal cardiac disease. Current Opinion in Anaesthesiology 18(3):257–262

Dauphin-McKenzie N, Gilles J M, Jacques E et al 2006 Sickle cell anaemia in the female patient. Obstetrical and Gynaecological Survey 61(5):343–352

Davey R X, Hamblin P S 2001 Selective versus universal screening for gestational diabetes mellitus: an evaluation of predictive risk factors. Medical Journal of Australia 174:118–121

Davison J M 2001 Renal disorders in pregnancy. Current Opinion in Obstetrics and Gynaecology 13:109–114

D'Cruz D P, Khamashta M A, Hughes G R V 2007 Systemic lupus erythematosus. Lancet 369:587–596

DH (Department of Health) 2001 The National Service Framework for Diabetes (England) Standards. The Stationery Office, London

DH (Department of Health) 2005 National Service Framework for Long-term Conditions. The Stationery Office, London

DH (Department of Health) 2007 Tuberculosis prevention and treatment: a toolkit for planning, commissioning and delivering high quality services in England. The Stationery Office, London

Diabetes UK 2005 Recommendations for the management of pregnant women with diabetes (including gestational diabetes). Diabetes UK, London. Online. Available: www.diabetes.org.uk

Dobbenga-Rhodes Y A, Pride A M 2006 Assessment and education of women with cardiac disease in pregnancy. Journal of Perinatal and Neonatal Nursing 20(4):295–302

DoH (Department of Health), Scottish Office Home and Health Department, Welsh Office, Department of Health & Social Services, Northern Ireland 1992 Folic acid and the prevention of neural tube defects. Report from an expert advisory group. Health Publications Unit, Lancashire

Durbridge J, Dresner M, Harding K R et al Pregnancy and cardiac disease – peripartum aspects. In: Steer P J, Gatzoulis M A, Baker P (eds) Heart disease in pregnancy 2006. RCOG Press, London

Ellison J, Walker I D, Greer I A 2000 Antenatal use of enoxaparin for prevention and treatment of thromboembolism in pregnancy. British Journal of Obstetrics and Gynaecology 107:1116–1121

Endocarditis Working Party of the British Society of Antimicrobial Chemotherapy 1990 Antibiotic prophylaxis of infective endocarditis. Recommendations. Lancet 335:88–90

EURAP Study Group 2006 Seizure control and treatment in pregnancy. Observations from the EURAP epilepsy pregnancy registry. Neurology 66:354–360

Figueroa-Damian R, Arredondo-Garcia J L 2001 Neonatal outcome of children born to women with tuberculosis. Archives of Medical Research 32(1):66–69

Gelsen E, Gatzooulis M, Johnson M 2007 Valvular heart disease. British Medical Journal 335:1042–1045

Gilmour-White S 2000 Epilepsy. In: Lee A, Inch S, Linnigan D (eds) Therapeutics in pregnancy and lactation. Radcliffe Medical, Oxford

Gilstrap L C, Ramin S M 2001 Urinary tract infections during pregnancy. Obstetric and Gynaecology Clinics of North America 28(3):581–591

Haddow J E, Palomaki G E, Allan W C et al 1999 Maternal thyroid deficiency during pregnancy and subsequent neuropsychological development of the child. New England Journal of Medicine 341(8):549–555

Hanna N J, Black M, Sander J W et al 2002 Related death: epilepsy – death in the shadows. The National Sentinel Clinical Audit of Epilepsy. The Stationery Office, London

Harrison M J, Kushner K E, Benzies K 2003 Women's satisfaction with their involvement in health care decisions during high-risk pregnancy. Birth 20(2):109–115

Head C E G, Thorne S A 2005 Congenital heart disease in pregnancy. Postgraduate Medical Journal 81:292–298

Higgins C 2000 Understanding laboratory investigations. A text for nurses and healthcare professionals. Blackwell Science, Oxford

Higgins C 2001 Diagnosing diabetes: blood glucose and the role of the laboratory. British Journal of Nursing 10 (4):230–236

Hofmanova I 2006 Pre-conception care and support for women with diabetes. British Journal of Nursing 15 (2):90–94

Holdcroft A, Thomas T A 2000 Principles and practice of obstetric anaesthesia and analgesia. Blackwell Science, Oxford

Hotu S, Carter B, Watson P D et al 2004 Increasing prevalence of type 2 diabetes in adolescents. Journal of Paediatric Child Health 40(4):201–204

HPA (Health Protection Agency) 2006 Pregnancy and tuberculosis. Guidance for Clinicians. HPA, London

HPA (Health Protection Agency) 2007 Tuberculosis in the UK. Annual report on TB surveillance and control in the UK 2007. HPA, London

Jackson M 2006 Epilepsy in women: a practical guide to management. Practical Neurology 6:166–179

JFC (Joint Formulary Committee) 2007 British National Formulary 53; Appendix 5. British Medical Journal and RPS Publishing, London

Khamashta M A 2006 Systemic lupus erythematosus and pregnancy. Best Practice and Research in Clinical Rheumatology 20(4):685–694

Khattab A D, Rawlings B, Ibitsam S A 2006a Care of patients with haemoglobin abnormalities: history and biology. British Journal of Nursing 15(18):994–998

Khattab A D, Rawlings B, Ibitsam S A 2006b Care of patients with haemoglobin abnormalities: nursing management. British Journal of Nursing 15(19):1057–1062

Kibirige M S, Hutchinson S, Owen C J et al 2004 Prevalence of maternal dietary iodine insufficiency in the north east of England: implications for the fetus. Archives of Disease in Childhood – Fetal and Neonatal edn 89:436–439

Kothari A, Mahadevan N, Girling J 2006 Tuberculosis and pregnancy – results of a study in a high prevalence area in London. European Journal of Obstetrics, Gynaecology and Reproductive Biology 126:48–55.

Kuczkowski K M 2005 Labor analgesia for the parturient with respiratory disease: what does the obstetrician need to know? Archives of Gynaecology and Obstetrics 272:160–166

Kuvacic I, Sprem M, Skrablin S et al 2000 Pregnancy outcome in renal transplant recipients. International Journal of Gynaecology and Obstetrics 70(3):313–317

Lao T T 2005 Thyroid disorders in pregnancy. Current Opinion in Obstetrics and Gynaecology 17:123–127.

Lazarus J H, Premawardhana L D 2005 Screening for thyroid disease in pregnancy. Journal of Clinical Pathology 58:449–452

Lewis G, Drife J (eds) 2004 Why mothers die 2000–2002. The Sixth Report of Confidential Enquiries into Maternal Deaths in the United Kingdom. RCOG Press, London

Lewis G (ed.) 2007 Saving mothers' lives: reviewing maternal deaths to make motherhood safer – 2003–2005. The Seventh Report of the Confidential Enquiries into Maternal Deaths in the United Kingdom. CEMACH, London

Lewis S, Smith D 2006 Counselling of women with epilepsy on anti-epileptic drugs: the value of nurse-led clinics. British Journal of Neuroscience Nursing 2(7):356–359

Lipscomb K J, Clayton Smith J, Clarke B et al 1997 Outcome of pregnancy in women with Marfan's syndrome. British Journal of Obstetrics and Gynaecology 104:201–206

Lowy C 1997 Diabetes and pregnancy. Medicine 25(7):57–58

MacDonald B K, Cockerell O C, Sander J W et al 2000 The incidence and lifetime prevalence of neurological disorders in a prospective community-based study in the UK. Brain 123:665–667

Macintosh M C M, Fleming K M, Bailey J A et al 2006 Perinatal mortality and congenital anomalies in babies of women with type 1 or type 2 diabetes in England, Wales and Northern Ireland: population based study. British Medical Journal 333:177–180

Mackillop L H, Germain S J, Nelson-Piercy C 2007 Systemic lupus erythematosus. British Medical Journal 335:933–936

McMullen A H, Pasta D J, Frederick P D 2006 Impact of pregnancy on women with cystic fibrosis. Chest 129:706–711

Mitchell M 2001 Gestational diabetes: a controversial concept. British Journal of Midwifery 91:26–34

Mok C C, Wong R W 2001 Pregnancy in systemic lupus erythematosus. Postgraduate Medical Journal 91:26–34

Morrow J, Russell A, Guthrie E et al 2006 Malformation risk of antiepileptic drugs in pregnancy: a prospective study from the UK Epilepsy and Pregnancy Register. Journal of Neurology, Neurosurgery and Psychiatry 77:193–198

MRC (Medical Research Council) Vitamin Study Research Group 1991 Prevention of neural tube defects: results of the Medical Research Council Vitamin Study. Lancet 338:131–137

Muller A F, Drexhage H A, Berghout A 2001 Postpartum thyroiditis and autoimmune thyroiditis in women of childbearing age; recent insights and consequences for antenatal and postnatal care. Endocrinology Review 22:605–630.

Murphy V E, Gibson P G, Smith R, Clifton V L 2005 Asthma during pregnancy: mechanisms and treatment implications. European Respiratory Journal 25:731–750

Murphy V E, Clifton V L, Gibson P G 2006 Asthma exacerbations during pregnancy: incidence and association with adverse pregnancy outcomes. Thorax 61:169–176

National Institutes of Health (National Heart, Lung and Blood Institute) 2002 The management of sickle cell disease. NIH, Bethesda. Online. Available: www.nhlbi.nih.gov

NHS Sickle Cell and Thalassaemia Screening Programme Centre 2006 NHS Sickle Cell and Thalassaemia Screening Programme. Standards for the linked antenatal and new-born screening programme. NHS Sickle Cell and Thalassaemia Screening Programme Centre, Kings College, London

NICE (National Institute for Health and Clinical Excellence) 2004 The epilepsies. The diagnosis and management of the epilepsies in adults and children in primary and secondary care. Clinical Guideline No. 20. NICE, London

NICE (National Institute for Health and Clinical Excellence) 2006 Tuberculosis. Clinical diagnosis and management of tuberculosis, and measures for its prevention and control. Clinical Guideline No. 33. NICE, London

NICE (National Institute for Health and Clinical Excellence) 2007 Acutely ill patients in hospital. Clinical Guideline No. 50. NICE, London

NICE (National Institute for Health and Clinical Excellence) 2008 Diabetes in pregnancy: management of diabetes and its complications from preconception to the postnatal period. Clinical Guideline No. 63. RCOG Press, London

Norman J C, Davison J M, Lindheimer M D 2001 Renal disorders in pregnancy. Contemporary Clinical Gynaecology and Obstetrics 1:59–67

NSE (National Society for Epilepsy) 2007 Information on epilepsy: first aid for epilepsy. Online. Available: www.epilepsy.nse.org

Okpala I, Thomas V, Westerdale N et al 2002 The comprehensive care of sickle cell disease. European Journal of Haematology 68:157–162

Ormerod P 2001 Tuberculosis in pregnancy and the puerperium. Thorax 56:494–499

Palmer D G 2006 Peripartum cardiomyopathy. Journal of Perinatal & Neonatal Nursing 20(4):324–332

Pinnock H, Shah R 2007 Asthma – BMJ Masterclass for GPs. British Medical Journal 334:847–850

Pop V J, Brouwers E P, Vader H L et al 2003 Maternal hypothyroxinaemia during early pregnancy and subsequent child development: a 3 year follow-up study. Clinics in Endocrinology 59:282–288

Prasad A K, Ventura H O 2001 Valvular heart disease and pregnancy. Postgraduate Medicine 110(2):69–88

Pryn A, Bryden F, Reeve W et al 2006 Cardiomyopathy in pregnancy and caesarean section: Four case reports. International Journal of Anesthesia 16:68–73

Rahimy M C, Gangbo A, Adjou R et al 2000 Effect of active prenatal management on pregnancy outcome in sickle cell disease in an African setting. Blood 96(5):1685–1689

Raja S G, Basu D 2005 Pulmonary hypertension in congenital heart disease. Nursing Standard 19(50):41–49

Ramsay M 2006 Management of the puerperium in women with heart disease. In: Steer P J, Gatzoulis M A, Baker P (eds) Heart disease in pregnancy. RCOG Press, London

Ramsay M M (ed.) 2000 Normal values in pregnancy, 2nd edn. Saunders, London

Rashid M, Rashid M H 2007 Obstetric management of thyroid disease. Obstetrical and Gynecological Survey 62(10):680–688

Rasmussen K N 2001 Is there a causal relationship between iron deficiency or iron-deficiency anaemia and weight at birth, length of gestation and perinatal mortality? Journal of Nutrition 131(25–22):590S–603S

Ray P, Murphy G J, Shutt L E 2004 Recognition and management of maternal cardiac disease in pregnancy. British Journal of Anaesthesia 93(3):428–439

Rees J 2005 ABC of asthma – Prevalence. British Medical Journal 331:443–445

Reddy D S 2007 Perimenstrual catamenial epilepsy. Women's Health 3(2):195–206

Rowe S M, Miller S, Sorscher E J 2005 Mechanisms of disease – cystic fibrosis. New England Journal of Medicine 352 (19):1992–2001

Royal College of Physicians/The National Collaborating Centre for Chronic Conditions 2006 Tuberculosis. Clinical diagnosis and management of tuberculosis, and measures for its prevention and control. RCP, London

Ruiz-Irastorza G, Khamashta M A, Castellino G et al 2001 Systemic lupus erythematosus. Lancet 357:1027–1032

Sergeant G R, Look Loy L, Crowther M et al 2004 Outcome of pregnancy in homozygous sickle cell disease. American College of Obstetricians and Gynecologists 103(6):1278–1285

Schatz M, Dombrowski M P, Wise R et al 2006 Spirometry is related to perinatal outcomes in pregnant women with asthma. American Journal of Obstetrics and Gynecology 194:120–126

Scholl T, Reilly T 2000 Anaemia, iron and pregnancy outcome. Journal of Nutrition 130:443S–447S

SIGN (Scottish Intercollegiate Guidelines Network) 2001 Management of diabetes in pregnancy. SIGN, Edinburgh

SIGN (Scottish Intercollegiate Guidelines Network) 2003 Diagnosis and management of epilepsy in adults. SIGN, Edinburgh

Sharma P, Thapa L 2007 Acute pyelonephritis in pregnancy: a retrospective study. Australian and New Zealand Journal of Obstetrics and Gynaecology 47:313–315

Sheffield J S, Cunningham F G 2004 Thyrotoxicosis and heart failure that complicates pregnancy. American Journal of Obstetrics and Gynecology 190:211–217

Siu S C, Colman J M 2001 Heart disease and pregnancy. Heart 85:710–715

Smaill F, Vazquez J C 2007 Antibiotics for asymptomatic bacteriuria in pregnancy. Cochrane Database of Systematic Reviews, Issue 2:CD000490. Online. Available: www. cochranedatabase.co.uk

Stoneman A 2005 Mother in mind. Epilepsy Action, Leeds. Online. Available:www.epilepsy.org.uk

Strong J 2006 Anaemia and white blood cell disorders. In: James D K, Steer P J, Weiner C P et al (eds) High risk pregnancy management options, 3rd edn. W B Saunders, Philadelphia

Stuart G 2006 Maternal endocarditis. In: Steer P J, Gatzoulis M A, Baker P, Heart disease and pregnancy. RCOG Press, London

Sun P M, Wilburn W, Raynor B D et al 2001 Sickle cell disease in pregnancy: Twenty years of experience at Grady Memorial Hospital, Atlanta, Georgia. American Journal of Obstetrics and Gynecology 184(6):1127–1130

SVD (Saint Vincent declaration) Working Party 1990 Diabetes care and research in Europe: the St Vincent declaration. Diabetic Medicine 7:360

Tan J 1999 Diagnosis of unsuspected heart disease in pregnancy. Contemporary Reviews in Obstetrics and Gynaecology 10(2):85–91

Taylor M 2000 Managing epilepsy: a clinical handbook. Blackwell Science, Oxford

Temple R 2007 Hypoglycaemia during pregnancy. Diabetes update. Diabetes UK Autumn:38–42

Thomas V J, Taylor L M 2002 The psychosocial experience of people with sickle cell disease and its impact on the quality of life: qualitative findings from focus groups. British Journal of Psychology 7(3):345–363

Thorne S, MacGregor A, Nelson-Piercy C 2006 Risks of contraception and pregnancy in heart disease. Heart 92:1520–1525

Tincani A, Bompane D, Danieli E et al 2006 Pregnancy, lupus and antiphospholipid syndrome (Hughes Syndrome). Lupus 15:156–160

Tomson T, Hiilesmaa V 2007 Epilepsy in pregnancy. British Medical Journal 335:769–773

UKNSPC (UK Newborn Screening Programme Centre) 2005 Health professional handbook for newborn blood spot screening in the UK. UKNSPC, London. Online. Available: www.newbornscreening-bloodspot.org.uk

Vazquez J C, Villar J 2003 Treatments for symptomatic urinary tract infections during pregnancy. Cochrane Database of Systematic Reviews, Issue 4:CD002256. Online. Available: www.cochranedatabase.co.uk

Virjee S, Robinson S, Johnston D G 2001 Screening for diabetes in pregnancy. Journal of the Royal Society of Medicine 94:502–509

WHO (World Health Organization) 1999 Definition, diagnosis and classification of diabetes mellitus and its complications. Report of a WHO consultation. Part 1: diagnosis and classification of diabetes mellitus. WHO, Geneva

WHO (World Health Organization) 2001 Iron deficiency anaemia: assessment, prevention and control. A guide for programme managers. WHO, Geneva

Witcher P M, Harvey C J 2006 Modifying labor routines for the woman with cardiac disease. Journal of Perinatal & Neonatal Nursing 20(4):303–310

Yasmeen S, Wilkins E E, Field N T et al 2001 Pregnancy outcomes in women with systemic lupus erythematosus. Journal of Maternal Fetal Medicine 10(2):91–96

Yip R 1996 Iron supplementation in pregnancy: is it effective? American Journal of Clinical Nutrition 63:853–855

Zack-Williams D 2007 Sickle cell anaemia in pregnancy and the neonates: ethical issues. British Journal of Midwifery 14(4):205–209

FURTHER READING

Blackburn S T, Loper D L 2007 Maternal, fetal and neonatal physiology: a clinical perspective, 3rd edn. W B Saunders, Philadelphia

Greer I A, Nelson Piercy C, Walters B (eds) 2007 Maternal medicine: medical problems in pregnancy. Churchill Livingstone, London

de Swiet M (ed.) 2002 Medical disorders in pregnancy, 4th edn. Blackwell, London

Nelson Piercy C 2006 Handbook of obstetric medicine, 3rd edn. Taylor Francis, London

Robson S E, Waugh J N S (eds) 2008 Medical disorders in pregnancy: a manual for midwives. Blackwell, Oxford

22 Hypertensive disorders of pregnancy

Carmel Lloyd

CHAPTER CONTENTS

The hypertensive disorders of pregnancy represent the most significant complication of pregnancy affecting approximately 5% of all pregnancies and 11% of all first pregnancies (Villar et al 2003). They continue to be a major cause of maternal, fetal and neonatal morbidity and mortality. Between 40000–70000 maternal deaths annually worldwide are due to severe pre-eclampsia and eclampsia (Chhabra & Kakani 2007, Villar et al 2004). The majority of these deaths occur in the developing world due to lack of technological and therapeutic interventions. In the last triennial report of maternal deaths in the UK, pre-eclampsia and eclampsia caused 18 deaths and remains the second most common cause of direct maternal death. The majority of women died from intracranial haemorrhage, and inadequate antihypertensive therapy was the most common source of sub-standard care (Lewis 2007). The risk to the fetus includes growth restriction secondary to placental insufficiency and prematurity, accounting for approximately 25% of all infants with very low birth weight (<1500g). Despite continued investigation throughout the world there is still limited understanding of the cause, pathophysiology and thus prevention of the hypertensive disorders which include a variety of vascular disturbances, such as gestational hypertension, pre-eclampsia, HELLP syndrome, eclampsia and chronic hypertension.

The chapter aims to:

- list the classifications for hypertensive disorders in pregnancy including the main differentiating characteristics
- outline the aetiology and pathophysiology as currently understood

- describe the signs, symptoms and potential sequelae of the hypertensive disorders
- provide an overview of the medical and therapeutic regimens that may be utilized in the treatment of hypertensive disorders
- identify the midwifery care and support required by a woman with a hypertensive disorder.

Definition and classification

The definition and classification of the hypertensive disorders are complex as the pathophysiology remains poorly understood and there is considerable clinical variation in their presentation. It is important to recognize the distinction between a woman whose hypertension antedates pregnancy (pre-existing hypertension) and one who develops increased blood pressure during pregnancy (new hypertension). Work undertaken by the National High Blood Pressure Education Programme (NHBPEP), Working Group on High Blood Pressure in Pregnancy (2000) and the Pre-eclampsia Community Guideline Development Group (PRE-COG 2004) describe the following main categories of hypertension during pregnancy:

1. *Pre-existing or chronic hypertension* This is known as hypertension before pregnancy or a diastolic blood pressure of 90 mmHg pre-pregnancy or before 20 weeks' gestation. The diagnosis is confirmed if pre-eclampsia has not developed and the blood pressure has not returned to normal by 12 weeks postpartum.

2. *New, gestational or pregnancy-induced hypertension* This is the development of hypertension at or after 20 weeks' gestation when the woman's diastolic blood pressure was <90 mmHg before 20 weeks. There are no other signs of pre-eclampsia. It is diagnosed when, after resting, the woman's blood pressure rises above 140/90 mmHg, on at least two occasions, no more than 1 week apart after the 20th week of pregnancy in a woman known to be normotensive. The blood pressure usually returns to normal by 6 weeks postpartum.

3. *New proteinuria* This is the presence of proteinuria defined as 1+ (300 mg/L or more) on dipstick testing, a protein:creatinine ratio of ≥30 mg/mmol on a random sample, or a urine protein excretion of ≥300 mg/24 hrs. Significant proteinuria is defined as urine protein excretion ≥300 mg/24 hrs.

4. *Pre-eclampsia* This is diagnosed on the basis of new hypertension with significant proteinuria at or after 20 weeks' gestation. Pre-eclampsia is a multisystem disorder, which can affect the placenta, kidney, liver, brain and other organs. In the absence of proteinuria, pre-eclampsia is suspected when hypertension is accompanied by symptoms including headache, blurred vision, upper abdominal pain, or altered biochemistry; specifically, raised urates, low platelet counts and abnormal liver enzyme levels (i.e. alanine aminotransferase (ALT), aspartate aminotransferase (AST) and γ-glutamyl transpeptidase (GGT)). These signs and symptoms, together with blood pressure >160 mmHg systolic or >110 mmHg diastolic and proteinuria of 2+ or 3+ on a dipstick, demonstrate the more severe form of the disorder.

5. *Eclampsia* This is defined as the new onset of seizures during pregnancy or postpartum, unrelated to other cerebral pathological conditions, in a woman with pre-eclampsia.

6. *Superimposed pre-eclampsia* The development of pre-eclampsia in women with pre-existing hypertension and or pre-existing proteinuria.

An incremental rise in blood pressure is not included in this classification system. However, the working group considered that women who have a rise of 30 mmHg systolic or 15 mmHg diastolic blood pressure require close observation especially if proteinuria and hyperuricaemia (raised uric acid level) are also present.

Aetiology

The development of pre-eclampsia is generally considered to occur in two stages. The placenta is thought to be the primary cause of the hypertensive disorders of pregnancy as following birth of the baby the disease regresses. Early studies by Roberts & Redman (1993) indicated that abnormal placentation may be one of the initial events in the disease process. In normal pregnancy placentation involves invasion of the decidua by the syncytiotrophoblast. During early pregnancy, the muscular walls and endothelium of the spiral arteries are eroded and replaced by trophoblast to ensure an optimum environment for the developing blastocyst. A second phase of this invasive process occurs between 16 and 20 weeks' gestation when the trophoblast erodes the myometrium of the spiral arteries. The loss of this musculoelastic tissue results in dilated vessels that are incapable of vasoconstriction; hence a system of low pressure and high blood flow into the placenta is produced with maximal placental perfusion (Sheppard & Bonnar 1989). In pre-eclampsia, trophoblastic invasion of the spiral arteries is thought to be inhibited resulting in decreased placental perfusion, which may ultimately lead to early placental hypoxia and oxidative stress (Borzychowski et al 2006). This first stage of the disease process occurs early in pregnancy and is difficult to detect clinically.

Stage two follows when the oxidatively stressed placenta triggers the release of one or more factors that damage the endothelial cells in the maternal circulation. Endothelial cells form the endothelium, which lines the cardiovascular system and serous cavities of the body. The subsequent maternal systemic inflammatory response and endothelial cell dysfunction results in the clinical signs of pre-eclampsia seen after 20 weeks' gestation (Redman & Sargent 2003). Endothelial cells play an important role in regulating capillary transport, controlling plasma lipid contact and modulating vascular smooth muscle reactivity in response to various stimuli. They also synthesize several substances, two of which – prostacyclin and nitric oxide – are mediators in vasodilation and inhibit platelet aggregation, thus preventing blood clot formation. Damage to the endothelial cells with widespread inflammation will:

- reduce the production of prostacyclin and nitric oxide
- increase the production of thromboxane (Tx), a potent vasoconstrictor
- increase vascular sensitivity to angiotensin II (a substance that controls blood pressure and the excretion of salt and water from the body)
- activate the coagulation cascade and trigger abnormal intravascular coagulation

- increase the production of lipid peroxides and decrease antioxidant production, known as 'oxidative stress' (Noris et al 2005, Redman & Sargent 2003).

Several epidemiological studies suggest that the abnormal placentation is caused by a genetically pre-determined maternal immune response to fetal antigens, derived from the father, and expressed in normal placental tissue (Redman et al 1999, Robillard 2002). Additional evidence for the immune response theory includes the high incidence of hypertensive disease in primigravidae, increased inflammatory substances in the maternal circulation (Redman & Sargent 2003) and partner specificity (Li & Wi 2000).

Some women are thought to be more sensitive to endothelial cell dysfunction or have pre-existing endothelial cell dysfunction seen in conditions with associated microvascular disease such as diabetes, hypertension or thrombophilia. In addition it is more likely to occur where there is a large placental mass such as in multiple pregnancy or gestational trophoblastic disease (hydatidiform mole). Women with these conditions are at an increased risk of developing pre-eclampsia (Roberts & Redman 1993).

The combined effect of these events will cause:

- vasospasm and increased blood pressure
- abnormal coagulation and thrombosis
- increased permeability of the endothelium leading to oedema, proteinuria and hypovolaemia.

These are the characteristic features of pre-eclampsia, which become manifest throughout the body resulting in pathological changes consistent with a multisystem disorder (Dekker & Sibai 2001).

Pathological changes

Cardiovascular system

Hypertension together with endothelial cell damage affects capillary permeability. Plasma proteins leak from the damaged blood vessels causing a decrease in the plasma colloid pressure and an increase in oedema within the extracellular space. The reduced intravascular plasma volume causes hypovolaemia and haemoconcentration, which is reflected in an elevated haematocrit. In severe cases the lungs become congested with fluid and pulmonary oedema develops, oxygenation is impaired and cyanosis occurs. With vasoconstriction and disruption of the vascular endothelium the coagulation cascade is activated.

Coagulation system

Activation of the coagulation cascade results in formation of fibrin clots which trap platelets. This consumption of platelets produces thrombocytopenia. This process of disseminated intravascular coagulation (DIC) is characterized by low platelets, prolonged prothrombin time and low fibrinogen levels. As the process progresses fibrin and platelets are deposited, which will occlude blood flow to many organs, particularly the kidneys, liver, brain and placenta.

Kidneys

In the kidney, hypertension leads to vasospasm of the afferent arterioles resulting in a decreased renal blood flow, which produces hypoxia and oedema of the endothelial cells of the glomerular capillaries. Glomeruloendotheliosis (glomerular endothelial damage) allows plasma proteins, mainly in the form of albumin, to filter into the urine, producing proteinuria. Renal damage is reflected by reduced creatinine clearance and increased serum creatinine and uric acid levels. Oliguria develops as the condition worsens, signifying severe renal vasoconstriction.

Liver

Vasoconstriction of the hepatic vascular bed will result in hypoxia and oedema of the liver cells. In severe cases, oedematous swelling of the liver causes upper abdominal pain and can lead to intracapsular haemorrhages and, in very rare cases, rupture of the liver. Altered liver function is reflected by falling albumin and a rise in liver enzyme levels.

Brain

Hypertension, combined with cerebrovascular endothelial dysfunction, increases the permeability of the blood–brain barrier resulting in cerebral oedema and microhaemorrhaging. Clinically, this is characterized by the onset of headaches, visual disturbances and convulsions. Where the mean arterial pressure

(MAP, i.e. the systolic blood pressure plus twice the diastolic pressure divided by 3) exceeds 125 mmHg, the autoregulation of cerebral flow is disrupted resulting in cerebral vasospasm, cerebral oedema and blood clot formation. This is known as *hypertensive encephalopathy*, which if left untreated can progress to cerebral haemorrhage and death (Vaughan & Delanty 2000).

Fetoplacental unit

In the uterus, vasoconstriction caused by hypertension reduces the uterine blood flow which can result in placental abruption and placental scarring. Reduction in blood flow to the choriodecidual spaces diminishes the amount of oxygen that diffuses through the cells of the syncytiotrophoblast and cytotrophoblast into the fetal circulation within the placenta. The result is that the placental tissue becomes ischaemic, the capillaries in the chorionic villi thrombose and infarctions occur, leading to fetal growth restriction (Odegard et al 2000). Hormonal output is also impaired with reduced placental function and this has serious implications for the survival of the fetus. This combination of factors often results in preterm labour and birth.

The midwife's role in assessment and diagnosis

As the hypertensive disorders are unlikely to be prevented, early detection and referral by the midwife is crucial so that monitoring and treatment can be implemented to minimize the severity of the condition (PRECOG 2004, Sallah 2004). All women, particularly those from disadvantaged and vulnerable groups, must receive appropriate antenatal care (NICE 2008); women who do not receive antenatal care are more likely to die from complications related to the hypertensive disorders of pregnancy (Lewis 2007, Lewis & Drife 2001). The midwife is in a unique position to identify those women who are more likely to develop pre-eclampsia; a comprehensive history taking at their first meeting will identify the following risk factors (Duckitt & Harrington 2005):

- nulliparity
- previous history of pre-eclampsia

- raised blood pressure at booking (diastolic ≥80mmHg, systolic ≥130mmHg)
- raised body mass index (BMI ≥35kg/m^2) before pregnancy or booking
- maternal age ≥40 years
- an interval of >10 years since a previous pregnancy
- the presence of underlying medical disorders for example: pre-existing hypertension, renal disease, diabetes, antiphospholipid syndrome and auto-immune disease such as lupus.

On subsequent visits the midwife must take note of any further pregnancy-associated risk factors such as multiple pregnancy. The two essential features of pre-eclampsia, hypertension and proteinuria, are assessed for at regular intervals throughout pregnancy and diagnosis is usually based on the rise in blood pressure and the presence of proteinuria after 20 weeks' gestation.

Blood pressure measurement

In order to detect increases in blood pressure, the midwife should take the woman's blood pressure early in pregnancy and compare this with all subsequent recordings, taking into account the normal pattern in pregnancy (see Ch. 14). It is important to consider several factors in assessing blood pressure.

Blood pressure machines should be calibrated for use in pregnancy and regularly maintained. Mercury sphygmomanometry is still considered the gold standard for blood pressure measurement although the use of mercury for clinical purposes has been phased out in the UK. This raises problems with regard to the accurate assessment of blood pressure in pregnancy. If automated and ambulatory blood pressure monitoring devices are used they should be validated for use in pregnancy. In addition, automated blood pressure measuring devices such as the Dinamap need to be calibrated and checked regularly as they can systematically underestimate blood pressure by at least 10mmHg in pre-eclampsia (Lewis & Drife 2004, Pomini et al 2001).

Blood pressure should not be taken immediately after a woman has experienced anxiety, pain, a period of exercise or has smoked. A 10min rest period is recommended before measuring the blood pressure

in these circumstances. The position of the person in whom the blood pressure is measured is important in pregnancy. The supine and right lateral positions are not recommended in view of the effect of the gravid uterus on venous return resulting in postural hypotension. Women should be seated or lying in the left lateral position at an angle of 45°, with the sphygmomanometer cuff approximately level with the heart (Duley et al 2006). Blood pressure can be overestimated as a result of using a sphygmomanometer cuff of inadequate size relative to the arm circumference. The length of the bladder should be at least 80% of the arm circumference. Appropriately sized cuffs should be available with inflation bladders of 35cm (standard size), 41cm (large size) and >42cm (thigh size) (PRECOG 2004).

The rounding off of the blood pressure measurements should be avoided and an attempt made to record the blood pressure as accurately as possible to the nearest 2mmHg. The use of Korotkoff V (disappearance of heart sounds) as a measure of the diastolic blood pressure has been found to be easier to obtain, more reproducible and closer to the intra-arterial pressure in pregnancy. This reading should be used unless the sound is near zero, in which case Korotkoff IV (muffling sound) should also be recorded (PRECOG 2004).

Urinalysis

Proteinuria in the absence of urinary tract infection is indicative of glomerular endotheliosis. The amount of protein in the urine is frequently taken as an index of the severity of pre-eclampsia. A significant increase in proteinuria coupled with diminished urinary output indicates renal impairment. Interobserver variation in the assessment of proteinuria and a high proportion of false positive and false negative results by dipstick analyses have been well documented (Gangaram et al 2005). It is important therefore to follow the instructions provided with the dipsticks in order to reduce the likelihood of error. Studies show that in routine clinical practice 'nil' or 'trace' proteinuria will miss significant proteinuria in one out of eight hypertensive women. Accuracy can be improved by using an automated device for dipstick analysis (Waugh et al 2005). Vaginal discharge, blood, amniotic fluid and bacteria can contaminate the specimen and give a false positive reading.

A 24 hrs urine collection for total protein measurement will be required to be certain about the presence or absence of proteinuria and to provide an accurate quantitative assessment of protein loss (PRECOG 2004) . A finding of >300 mg/24 hrs is considered to be indicative of mild-moderate pre-eclampsia, and >3 g/24 hrs is considered to be severe.

Oedema and excessive weight gain

These used to be included in the diagnostic criteria for pre-eclampsia but both are variable findings and nowadays, are usually considered only when a diagnosis of pre-eclampsia has been made based on other criteria. Clinical oedema may be mild or severe in nature and the severity is related to the worsening of the pre-eclampsia. Oedema of the ankles in late pregnancy is a common occurrence. It is of a dependent nature, usually disappears overnight and is not significant in the absence of raised blood pressure and proteinuria. However, the sudden severe widespread appearance of oedema is suggestive of pre-eclampsia or some other underlying pathology and further investigations are necessary. This oedema pits on pressure and may be found in non-dependent anatomical areas such as the face, hands, lower abdomen, vulval and sacral areas.

Laboratory tests

These now make a significant contribution to the assessment and diagnosis of pre-eclampsia, particularly when the presentation is atypical and hypertension or proteinuria, or both, are absent. The expected normal blood values in pregnancy are outlined in Table 22.1. It is important to state that the data are limited and therefore the quoted normal range may vary (Nelson-Piercy 2006, Ramsay et al 2000). The following alterations in the haematological and biochemical parameters are suggestive of the onset of pre-eclampsia:

- increased haemoglobin and haematocrit levels
- thrombocytopenia (platelet count $<150 \times 10^9$/L)
- prolonged clotting times
- raised serum creatinine (>90 mmol/L) and urea levels

Table 22.1   Normal blood values in pregnancy

Full blood count[a]	
Haemoglobin	11.1–12 g/dL
Haematocrit	33–39%
Platelets	150–400 × 10^9/L
Fibrinogen	3.63–4.23 g/L
Renal function[b]	
Creatinine	44–73 μmol/L
Urate	2.4–4.2 mmol/L
Uric acid	0.14–0.38 mmol/L
Liver function[c]	
ALT	10–30 IU/L
AST	6–32 IU/L
GGT	5–43 IU/L
Albumin	28–35 g/L
Total protein	48–65 g/L

[a]Ramsay et al 2000;
[b]Nelson-Piercy 2006;
[c]Girling et al 1997, Ramsay et al 2000.

- raised serum uric acid level (> mean for gestational age + 2 SD)
- abnormal liver function tests, particularly raised aspartate transaminase (AST) and alanine aminotransferase (ALT) (>50 U/L).

Symptoms may contribute to the diagnosis as described earlier, but these are rarely experienced by the woman until the disease has progressed to an advanced stage.

Care and management

The aim of care is to monitor the condition of the woman and her fetus and if possible to prevent the hypertensive disorder worsening by using appropriate interventions and treatment. The ultimate aim is to prolong the pregnancy until the fetus is sufficiently mature to survive, while safeguarding the mother's life. The maternal and fetal condition, together with the plan of care, need to be discussed with the woman and her partner and family. Helping the woman and her partner to interpret the situation, in particular the prognosis for the pregnancy and the potential for perinatal loss, is an important consideration (Kidner & Flanders-Stephans 2004).

The midwife should be sensitive to the needs of the family if the woman requires admission to hospital, particularly if she is feeling well enough to be at home. She is likely to be anxious about the well-being of her children and visiting should be encouraged to allay her fears. The woman and her partner will be concerned for the current pregnancy; sensitive support and encouragement will be required of the midwife. The midwife has a key role in providing psychosocial support for these women (Hodnett 2000). Good communication with the multidisciplinary team involved in the care of the woman and her baby is essential (Mander 2001).

Antenatal care

If the midwife diagnoses hypertension or pre-eclampsia during pregnancy, the woman should be referred to a doctor or directly to a maternity unit for assessment. Gestational hypertension will require close monitoring and if pre-eclampsia develops, then admission to hospital and more therapeutic interventions will be required. Care and management will vary depending on the degree of pre-eclampsia. Guidelines for the management of severe pre-eclampsia have been outlined by Lewis & Drife (2001) and Tufnell et al (2006) and these have been incorporated below.

Rest

Women are advised to rest as much as possible, but rest does not prevent the development of pre-eclampsia. Admitting women to hospital to facilitate this has not been found to be cost-effective, can be disruptive to family life and Meher et al (2005) found that in-patient care does not improve outcomes, nor prevent the development of proteinuria. It is recommended that women attend a day assessment unit as a means of reducing the need for antenatal admissions and the number of medical interventions. It is preferable for the woman to rest at home and to have regular visits by the midwife or GP and in some instances, this can be highly effective where there is the availability of distance monitoring. When proteinuria develops in addition to hypertension the risks to the mother and fetus are considerably increased. Admission to hospital is required to monitor and evaluate the maternal and fetal condition.

Diet

There is little evidence to support dietary intervention for preventing or restricting the advance of pre-eclampsia. As for any pregnant woman, a diet rich in protein, fibre and vitamins may be recommended. There is some evidence to suggest that prophylactic fish oil in pregnancy may act as an anti-platelet agent, thereby preventing hypertension and proteinuric pre-eclampsia (Roberts & Redman 1993). Calcium supplementation has also been investigated and appears to be beneficial for women at high risk of developing hypertension in pregnancy and in communities with low dietary calcium intake (Hofmeyr et al 2007). Studies have been undertaken to find out whether the use of antioxidant Vitamin C and E supplements could reduce the incidence of pre-eclampsia. However the Vitamins in Pre-eclampsia (VIP) Trial Consortium found that supplementation with vitamins C (1000 mg) and E (400 IU) does not prevent pre-eclampsia in women at risk, but does increase the rate of babies born with low birth weight. Therefore, these high dose antioxidants should not be given in pregnancy (Poston et al 2006).

Weight gain

The value of routine weighing during antenatal visits has been questioned and in many areas has now been abandoned as a form of antenatal screening for pre-eclampsia. However, weight gain may be useful for monitoring the progression of pre-eclampsia in conjunction with other parameters. The initial BMI (see Ch. 13) is considered a more useful predictor of hypertension in pregnancy, since this is higher in women who subsequently develop pre-eclampsia (Duckitt & Harrington 2005).

Blood pressure and urinalysis

If hypertension is detected during pregnancy, the blood pressure is monitored daily at home or every 4 hrs when in hospital. Urine should be tested for protein daily. If the woman or midwife identifies protein in a midstream specimen of urine, a 24 hrs urine collection is required in order to determine the amount of proteinuria. The level of protein indicates the degree of vascular damage. Reduced kidney perfusion is indicated by proteinuria, reduced creatinine clearance and increased serum creatinine and uric acid.

Abdominal examination

Abdominal examination is carried out daily. Any discomfort or tenderness should be recorded and reported immediately to a doctor, as this may be a sign of placental abruption. Upper abdominal pain is highly significant and indicative of HELLP syndrome associated with fulminating (rapid onset) pre-eclampsia.

Doppler assessment of uterine arteries

Doppler assessment of uterine arteries can demonstrate increased placental vascular resistance as a result of failure of the trophoblastic invasion of the spiral arteries early in pregnancy (<20 weeks).

Fetal assessment

Biophysical profile assessment is recommended in order to determine fetal health and well-being. This can be done by the use of the following: fetal movement charts, CTG monitoring, serial ultrasound scans to check for fetal growth, assessment of liquor volume and fetal breathing movements and umbilical artery Doppler blood flow (see Ch. 18).

Laboratory studies

These are often referred to as 'PET' bloods and include full blood count (haemoglobin, haematocrit and platelet count), urea and electrolytes, serum creatinine level, serum uric acid level, liver function tests including albumin levels, clotting studies if platelet count $<100 \times 10^9$/L. In severe pre-eclampsia, there should be blood studies undertaken every 12–24 hrs (Lewis & Drife 2001).

Antihypertensive therapy

The use of antihypertensive therapy as prophylaxis is controversial, as this shows no benefit in significantly prolonging pregnancy or improving maternal or fetal outcome in women with mild to moderate hypertension (Abalos et al 2007). Its use is, however, advocated as short-term therapy in order to prevent an increase in blood pressure and the development of severe hypertension (diastolic of 110 mmHg and systolic of 170 mmHg), thereby reducing the risk to the mother of cerebral haemorrhage (Duley et al 2007). The aim of treatment is to gradually reduce the blood pressure to a level that is safe for both

mother and fetus and to maintain the systolic blood pressure between 140–155 mmHg and the diastolic 90–100 mmHg. A review undertaken by Duley et al (2006) concludes that there is no one antihypertensive which is preferable to others and clinicians should use the one/s with which they are familiar.

Methyldopa is the most widely used drug in women with mild to moderate gestational hypertension. Drowsiness is a common side effect and it can cause depression, however it is considered to be safe and effective for both mother and fetus. An α- and β-blocker such as labetalol is an alternative and is considered safe in pregnancy except for women with asthma or congestive heart failure. Atenolol used over the long term is not recommended as this is linked with fetal growth restriction and the use of angiotensin-converting enzyme (ACE) inhibitors are contraindicated in pregnancy. Calcium channel blockers such as nifedipine, are increasingly used to treat severe hypertension in pregnancy (Duley et al 2006). These act on arteriolar smooth muscle to induce vasodilation by blocking calcium entry into cells thus decreasing cerebral vasospasm and increasing urinary output and uteroplacental blood flow. Maternal side-effects include tachycardia, palpitations and headache (Frishman et al 2005).

Antithrombotic agents

Early activation of the clotting system may contribute to the later pathology of pre-eclampsia and as a result the use of anticoagulants or antiplatelet agents has been considered for the prevention of pre-eclampsia and fetal growth restriction. Aspirin is thought to inhibit the production of the platelet-aggregating agent thromboxane A_2. The PARIS (Perinatal Antiplatelet Review of International Studies) Collaboration systematic review and meta-analysis found that women receiving antiplatelet agents had a 10% reduced risk of: developing pre-eclampsia, pre-term birth before 34 weeks' gestation and having a pregnancy with serious adverse outcome (Askie et al 2007).

Intrapartum care

Timing and mode of delivery is dependent on the maternal and fetal condition as well as the gestation of the pregnancy. Where possible, spontaneous onset of labour and vaginal birth is preferable (NHBPEP Working Group 2000). The midwife should remain with the woman throughout the course of labour as pre-eclampsia can suddenly worsen at any time. It is essential to monitor the maternal and fetal condition carefully. Marked deviations should be noted and medical assistance sought. The woman with gestational or mild pre-eclampsia will require less intensive care than a woman with severe pre-eclampsia or eclampsia.

Vital signs

Blood pressure is measured half-hourly, 15–20 min in severe pre-eclampsia. Because of the potentially rapid haemodynamic changes in pre-eclampsia, a number of authors recommend the measurement of the MAP. As mentioned earlier this can be calculated manually or by the use of an automated blood pressure recorder such as the Dinamap. MAP reflects the systemic perfusion pressure, and therefore the degree of hypovolaemia, whereas manual measurement of diastolic pressure alone is a better indicator of the degree of hypertension (Churchill & Beevers 1999). Observation of the respiratory rate (>14/min) will be complemented with pulse oximetry in severe pre-eclampsia; this is a non-invasive measure of the saturation of haemoglobin with oxygen and gives an indication of the degree of maternal hypoxia. Temperature should be recorded as necessary. In severe pre-eclampsia, examination of the optic fundi can give an indication of optic vasospasm and papill-oedema. Cerebral irritability can be assessed by the degree of hyper-reflexia or the presence of clonus (significant if more than three beats).

Fluid balance

The reduced intravascular compartment in pre-eclampsia together with poorly controlled fluid balance can result in circulatory overload, pulmonary oedema, adult respiratory distress syndrome and ultimately death (Lewis & Drife 2001). In severe pre-eclampsia, a central venous pressure (CVP) line may be considered in order to monitor the fluid status more effectively (see Ch. 33). If the value is >10 mmHg, then 20 mg furosemide (frusemide), a diuretic drug, should be considered. Intravenous fluids are administered using infusion pumps and the total recommended fluid intake in severe pre-eclampsia is 85 mL/hr. Oxytocin should be administered with caution as it has an antidiuretic effect. Urinary output should be monitored closely and urinalysis undertaken every 4 hrs to detect the presence of protein, ketones and glucose. In severe pre-eclampsia a urinary catheter should be *in situ* and urine output is measured hourly; a level >30 mL/hr reflects adequate renal function.

Plasma volume

Although women with pre-eclampsia have oedema, they are hypovolaemic. The blood volume is low, as shown by a high haemoglobin concentration and a high haematocrit level. This results in movement of fluid into the extravascular compartment causing oedema. The oedema initially occurs in dependent tissues, but as the disease progresses oedema occurs in the liver and brain giving rise to the symptoms described previously. Nevertheless, this cannot be corrected simply by plasma volume expansion. Treatment is controversial as colloids can seep into the tissues and 'hold' fluid there and they can thus cause even worse pulmonary oedema than crystalloids. Any fluids are therefore given with caution.

Pain relief

Epidural analgesia may procure the best pain relief, reduce the blood pressure and facilitate rapid caesarean section should the need arise. It is important to ensure a normal clotting screen and a platelet count $>100 \times 10^9$/L prior to insertion of the epidural.

Fetal condition

The fetal heart rate should be monitored closely and deviations from the normal reported and acted upon.

Birth plan

When the second stage commences, the obstetrician and paediatrician should be notified. The midwife will continue her care of the woman and will usually assist the woman during the birth. A short second stage may be preferred depending on the maternal and fetal conditions; in this instance a ventouse extraction or forceps delivery will be performed by the obstetrician. If the maternal or fetal condition shows significant deterioration during the first stage of labour, a caesarean section will be undertaken. Oxytocin is recommended for the management of the third stage of labour. Ergometrine and Syntometrine will cause peripheral vasoconstriction and increase hypertension and therefore should not normally be used in the presence of any degree of pre-eclampsia unless there is severe haemorrhage.

Postpartum care

The maternal condition should continue to be monitored at least every 4 hrs for at least the next 24 hrs following childbirth, as there is still the potential danger of the mother developing worsening pre-eclampsia or eclampsia. The blood pressure may initially rise after delivery but should gradually return to normal by the end of the first postnatal week. Persistent hypertension will need to be treated. Methyldopa should be avoided postpartum because of the risk of postpartum depression; the drug of choice is atenolol and/or nifedipine. Most antihypertensive drugs are compatible with breastfeeding (James & Nelson-Piercy 2004).

Signs of impending eclampsia

The signs and symptoms described in Box 22.1 will signal the onset of eclampsia. The midwife should be alert to any of these signs and summon medical assistance immediately. The aim of care at this time

> **Box 22.1** Signs of impending eclampsia
>
> - A sharp rise in blood pressure
> - Headache, which is usually severe, persistent and frontal in location (cerebral vasospasm)
> - Drowsiness or confusion (cerebral vasospasm)
> - Visual disturbances, such as blurring of vision or blindness (cerebral vasospasm)
> - Diminished urinary output ± increase in proteinuria (renal failure)
> - Upper abdominal pain (liver oedema) ± nausea and vomiting.

is to preclude death of the mother and fetus by controlling hypertension, inhibiting seizures and preventing coma.

HELLP syndrome

The syndrome of haemolysis (H), elevated liver enzymes (EL) and low platelet count (LP) was first described by Weinstein in 1982 and is generally thought to represent a variant of the pre-eclampsia/eclampsia syndrome but can occur on its own or in association with pre-eclampsia. The incidence of the disease is reported as being 0.17–0.85% of all livebirths (Rath et al 2000).

Clinical presentation

HELLP syndrome typically manifests itself between 32 and 34 weeks' gestation and 30% of cases will occur postpartum. With postpartum presentation, the onset is typically within the first 48 hrs following birth. Women with HELLP syndrome often complain of malaise, nausea and vomiting, upper abdominal pain with tenderness; some will have non-specific viral-syndrome-like symptoms. Hypertension and proteinuria may be minimal or absent (Rath et al 2000) (see Sharon's story, Box 22.2).

Diagnosis

Early diagnosis of HELLP syndrome is critical; any woman presenting with the above symptoms should have a full blood count, platelet count and liver function tests, irrespective of maternal blood pressure. Haemolysis with elevated lactate dehydrogenase (LDH) and raised bilirubin levels, low ($<100 \times 10^9$/L) or falling platelets and elevated liver transaminases (AST, ALT and GGT) assist in confirming the diagnosis of HELLP syndrome (Knappen et al 1999). A positive D-dimer test (indicator of coagulopathy) in conjunction with pre-eclampsia has also been found to be predictive of women who will develop HELLP syndrome (Padden 1999).

HELLP syndrome may be classified as partial (one or two features of the syndrome) or full (all three features). It may also be classified on the basis of the platelet count: Class I $<50 \times 10^9$/L, Class II $50–100 \times 10^9$/L,

Box 22.2 Sharon's story

At 31 weeks pregnant, I felt really good. Ten days later I was attending an aquanatal class in which I really struggled to bend my ankles to swim. The following day I saw my midwife who after taking my blood pressure phoned the hospital as my readings were of concern and I had protein in my urine.

I was admitted to the maternity ward, my blood pressure was taken regularly and I was told to rest. I found this quite difficult, as I felt a fraud being on the ward as I felt well. How naive was I.

Late one evening the midwife took my blood pressure and was alarmed by the reading, 'I can't fit it on the chart', she said, so after a few minutes she re-took it with a manual pump. The second readings were the same, so at around midnight I was wheeled down to the labour ward. Still at this stage I didn't realize how serious this was. I was monitored all night and my baby was monitored as well. The doctors wanted to take blood but my hands and forearms had now swollen up, so trying to extract blood from me was very difficult, so the decision was taken that I should have a central venous pressure line with three parts. This was quite uncomfortable in my neck, and heavy with all the parts coming out to the machines.

The doctors wanted to induce me, so they broke my waters. Some hours passed and I was only 3 cm, I had an epidural but nothing seemed to ease the blood pressure. Then my baby's heart rate dropped, so I was taken for an emergency caesarean section.

In the early hours of the following morning and 6 weeks premature, I had a baby boy weighing 3 lb 5 oz. I saw him briefly but he was rushed into the neonatal intensive care unit. I was then taken back to high dependency, where I had further complications. My blood was taken every 6 hrs to monitor the platelets in my red blood cells, as they were getting very low, down to 30 at it lowest stage. Platelets had been ordered in preparation for a transfusion, but luckily after 2 days they started to increase. After 7 days, I was transferred to the postnatal ward where I stayed for a further 5 days.

The hardest thing of all was that it was 36 hrs after birth before I got to see my son and this was only for 1 hr. The following 4 weeks were also very difficult, as my husband was at home and work, I was in the postnatal ward and our son was on the neonatal unit. We both felt as if we were renting our own son from the hospital and the house felt so empty when we got home.

Now that we are both well, I can reflect on what happened. I didn't realize how serious pre-eclampsia and HELLP syndrome were or what the implications could have been for me and my baby.

Class III 100–150 × 10^9/L. Women with Class I HELLP syndrome are at increased risk for maternal and perinatal morbidity and mortality (Padden 1999).

Complications

Serious maternal complications include abruptio placentae, disseminated intravascular coagulation (DIC), eclampsia, acute renal failure and subcapsular haematoma of the liver (Deruelle et al 2006, Haddad et al 2000, Vigil-De 2001). Rupture of the liver is a very rare but potentially fatal complication of the HELLP syndrome and usually presents with severe upper abdominal, neck and shoulder pain, which may persist for several hours. Radiographic imaging of the liver is required to assess the extent of the damage; surgical intervention and/or liver transplantation, may be required to prevent haemorrhagic shock and liver failure (Reck et al 2001). Infants whose mothers have HELLP syndrome are often small for gestational age and are at risk of perinatal asphyxia (Rath et al 2000).

Treatment

Prompt recognition of HELLP syndrome and initiation of therapeutic interventions are essential to ensure the best outcome for mother and fetus. Women with the HELLP syndrome should be admitted to a consultant unit with intensive or high dependency care facilities available. Treatment and interventions are based on the gestational age and the health of the mother and fetus. Corticosteroids may stabilize some of the abnormal biochemical and clinical parameters, as well as aid fetal lung maturity (Clenney & Viera 2004). However, further research is required to determine if maternal and perinatal morbidity and mortality is significantly reduced (Matchaba & Moodley 2004). In term pregnancies, or where there is a deteriorating maternal or fetal condition, immediate delivery is recommended (Curtain & Weinstein 1999). A significant number of women with HELLP syndrome also require blood product transfusions to correct the coagulation abnormalities (Deruelle et 2006, Haddad et al 2000, Padden 1999).

Eclampsia

Eclampsia is rarely seen in developed countries today, especially if there are good facilities for antenatal care. Leith et al (1997) demonstrated that over a 60-year period, the incidence of eclampsia had fallen from 74 to 7.4 per 10000 deliveries. More recently, the reported rate of eclampsia in Europe and other developed countries is 1 in 2000–3000 deliveries (Mattar & Sibai 2000). In the UK, there was an incidence of 4.8/10000 maternities (Lewis & Drife 2004) but a more recent UKOSS (UK Obstetric Surveillance System) study found an incidence of 2.1/10000 births (UKOSS 2006). Usually pre-eclampsia is diagnosed and treatment instituted to prevent eclampsia but occasionally pre-eclampsia is so rapid in onset and progress that eclampsia ensues before any action can be taken. In this situation, pre-eclampsia is termed 'fulminating' (Katz et al 2000).

Eclampsia is associated with increased risks of maternal and perinatal morbidity and mortality. Significant maternal life-threatening complications as a result of eclampsia include placental abruption and haemorrhage, DIC, pulmonary oedema, multi-organ failure including cardiac, renal and liver, HELLP syndrome and brain haemorrhage (Lewis & Drife 2001, 2004).

There is a proposed link between the hypertension in eclampsia, which may not be extreme, and cerebral disease; Vaughan & Delanty (2000) identify the clinical similarities between eclampsia and hypertensive encephalopathy. A significant finding, however, is that hypertension is not necessarily a precursor to the onset of eclampsia but will almost always be evident following a seizure (Sibai 2005). MRI studies suggest that there is cerebral vasospasm causing ischaemia and cellular oedema, especially in the territory of the posterior cerebral arteries.

Detecting and managing imminent eclampsia is also made more difficult in that, unlike other types of seizure, warning symptoms are not always present before onset of the convulsion. Variations also exist according to the gestational period with 38–53% occurring antenatally, 18% intrapartum and 28–44% postpartum (Douglas & Redman 1994, Mattar & Sibai 2000). Late postpartum eclampsia has also been described, where eclampsia can occur between 48hrs and 4 weeks after birth (Chames et al 2002, Munjuiuri et al 2005).

In fulminating pre-eclampsia or eclampsia, delivery of the mother should take place as soon as possible once the condition has been stabilized by the following measures.

Care of a woman with eclampsia

The aims of immediate care are to:

- summon medical aid
- clear and maintain the mother's airway – this may be achieved by placing the mother in a semiprone position in order to facilitate the drainage of saliva/vomit
- ensure maternal oxygenation – during the convulsive episode, hypoventilation and respiratory acidosis may occur therefore oxygen should be administered via a face mask at 8–10L/min and oxygen saturation monitoring commenced
- prevent maternal injury
- determine the fetal heart rate – fetal compromise secondary to maternal hypoxaemia or placental abruption will indicate the need for an emergency caesarean section under general anaesthesia once the maternal condition has been stabilized (Levy 2003, Sibai 2005).

The midwife must remain with the mother constantly and provide assistance with medical treatment. In the first instance, all effort is devoted to the preservation of the mother's life and the well-being of the baby is secondary. This may seem arbitrary, but if the mother dies then fetal death is inevitable. The woman will require intensive/high dependency care as she may remain comatose for a time following the seizure or may be sleepy. Clinical observations should be measured and recorded. The midwife must observe for periodic restlessness associated with uterine contraction, which indicates that labour has commenced. The woman's partner should be kept informed and the midwife will need to give emotional support through this unexpected and anxious time. It is usual to deliver the baby as soon as possible when eclampsia occurs, initial seizures are usually of short duration but may become prolonged while the woman remains pregnant; in this instance caesarean section is the usual mode of delivery. The following therapeutic interventions are essential (Tufnell et al 2006).

Anticonvulsant therapy

Magnesium sulphate ($MgSO_4$) is now the recommended drug of choice to treat and prevent eclampsia rather than diazepam or phenytoin. It is thought to aid vasodilation thereby reducing cerebral oedema and preventing seizures. There is a reduction in the incidence of pneumonia, artificial ventilation and admission to intensive care in women treated with $MgSO_4$ compared with those treated with diazepam (ETCG 1995, Lewis & Drife 2001, 2004, Magpie Trial Collaborative Group 2002). Diazepam is used to control other types of seizures and has a sedative effect and should only be used in the treatment of pre-eclampsia if $MgSO_4$ is not available.

$MgSO_4$ is administered intravenously according to a protocol. The Confidential Enquiries into Maternal Deaths (Lewis & Drife 2001) recommend that a loading dose of 4g is given over 5–10min i.v. followed by a maintenance dose of 5g/500 mL normal saline given as an i.v. infusion at a rate of 1–2g/hr until 24 hrs following delivery or the last seizure. Recurrent seizures should be treated with a further bolus of 2g. Continuous infusion of $MgSO_4$ can be toxic particularly in women with renal insufficiency. Early signs and symptoms of toxicity include nausea, weakness, slurred speech, double vision and loss of patellar reflexes. In more severe cases muscular paralysis, respiratory arrest and cardiac arrest ensue. The respiratory rate (>14/min) and oxygen saturation levels (>95%) and deep tendon reflexes should be monitored hourly.

In women with oliguria, serum magnesium levels should be monitored and maintained within the therapeutic range (2–3mmol/L). In the event of toxicity, the $MgSO_4$ infusion should be stopped and ventilatory and circulatory support given as required. Calcium gluconate (10–20mL of 10% solution) is the antidote for magnesium toxicity and should be readily available.

Treatment of hypertension

Severe hypertension is defined as >160/110mmHg or a mean arterial pressure >125mmHg. The aim of treating severe hypertension is to avoid the loss of cerebral autoregulation and prevent cerebral haemorrhage without significantly reducing cerebral perfusion or uteroplacental blood flow. Intravenous hydralazine is the most useful agent to gain control of the blood pressure quickly; 5–10mg should be administered slowly intravenously and the blood pressure measured at 5min intervals until the diastolic pressure reaches 90–100mmHg. The diastolic blood pressure may be maintained at this level by titrating the infusion of hydralazine against the blood pressure. Labetalol may be used in preference to hydralazine, in which case 20 mg is given i.v. followed at 10-min intervals by 40mg, 80mg and 80mg up to a cumulative dose of 300mg (Lewis & Drife 2001, p 92). Care should be taken when using nifedipine in conjunction with $MgSO_4$ as this may result in excessive calcium channel blockade and potentiate hypotension.

Fluid balance

Care must be taken not to overload the maternal system with intravenous fluids as discussed in the management of pre-eclampsia. Frequent assessment of the fluid intake (intravenous, oral and blood products) and urine output, as well as monitoring by pulmonary function (pulse oximetry and respirations) is essential (Lewis 2007, Lewis & Drife 2001, 2004).

Anaesthesia

Use of anaesthesia in eclampsia is difficult, as the condition of women with eclampsia varies considerably. Both general and regional (epidural/spinal) anaesthesia carry a degree of risk (Levy 2003); epidural is preferred in eclamptic women who are conscious, haemodynamically stable and cooperative (Moodley et al 2001).

Postnatal care

As soon as the baby is born, the woman's partner should be encouraged to hold him and accompany him to the neonatal intensive care unit if that is where he will be cared for. It is important that the partner has early interaction with the baby so that an account can be given of the baby's progress from the time of birth. Likewise, the midwife should liaise with the neonatal unit staff and explain the treatment given to the baby and the likely prognosis. A photograph should be taken of the baby so that the mother can see him as soon as she recovers. Postpartum care should be given, as recommended by NICE (2006) and as soon as the mother's condition permits, she should be taken in her bed or a chair to see her baby. Alternatively, if the baby's condition is good, he may be returned to his mother.

As almost half of eclamptic seizures occur following childbirth, intensive surveillance of the woman is required in a high dependency or intensive care unit. Parameters to monitor are: a return to normal blood pressure, an increase in urine output, reduction in proteinuria, a reduction in oedema and a return to normal laboratory indices. Antithrombotic agents and the use of thromboelastic stockings will prevent deep vein thrombosis. Antihypertensive therapy should be maintained and gradually reduced as the blood pressure returns to normal; this may take up to 12 weeks. Most antihypertensive drugs are compatible with breastfeeding.

Future care and management following hypertensive disease

There is no indication that the hypertensive disorders of pregnancy cause later hypertensive disease but it can bring to the fore an inherent disposition towards hypertension. Women with a history of severe pre-eclampsia before 32 weeks' gestation have a 5% risk of recurrence by this gestational age and a 15% risk of recurrence overall (Mattar & Sibai 2000). Recent studies have also identified that women who have a history of pre-eclampsia are more likely to develop cardiovascular disease in later life (Manton et al 2007, Wilson et al 2003).

Usually the blood pressure returns to normal within several weeks but the proteinuria may persist for a longer period. Six weeks after the birth of her baby, the mother is examined by the obstetrician and if all is well, she will be discharged and advised to seek advice as soon as a subsequent pregnancy occurs. Referral to voluntary organizations, such as Action on Pre-eclampsia (www.apec.org.uk) may provide additional information, advice and support following a pregnancy complicated by hypertensive disorders.

The mother may have very little recollection of the birth and the events surrounding it if she was unconscious or heavily sedated at the time. It is essential that the midwife enquire further if a mother gives no clear history of a previous birth or if she says that she was ill. It is advisable to obtain the previous case notes where possible. In this way good care can be provided and prophylactic management established where indicated.

Pre-existing (chronic) hypertension

Pre-existing (chronic) hypertension has the following possible causes:

1. It may be a long-term problem, present before the beginning of the pregnancy and accounts for 5% of the cases of hypertension in pregnancy.
2. It may be secondary to existing medical problems, such as:
   - renal disease
   - SLE
   - coarctation of the aorta
   - Cushing's syndrome
   - phaeochromocytoma, which is a rare but dangerous tumour of the adrenal medulla.

Diagnosis

Consistent blood pressure recordings of $\geq 140/90$ mmHg, on two occasions more than 24 hrs apart during the first 20 weeks of pregnancy, suggest that the hypertension is pre-existing and unrelated to the pregnancy. The diagnosis may be difficult to make because of the changes seen with blood pressure in pregnancy. This is a particular problem in women who present late in their pregnancy with no baseline blood pressure measurement. These women may appear normotensive in early pregnancy and hypertension identified later in pregnancy is considered gestational. The diagnosis may only be made when the blood pressure remains elevated at 12 weeks postpartum.

Investigation

When taking a history, the midwife may identify potential or existing medical problems. Women with pre-existing (chronic) hypertension tend to be older, parous and have a family history of hypertension.

Accurate measurement of blood pressure is important and the midwife needs to consider the guidelines mentioned earlier. Serial blood pressure recordings should be made in order to determine the true pattern as even normotensive women show occasional peaks.

The doctor's physical examination of the woman may reveal the long term effects of hypertension such as retinopathy, ischaemic heart disease and renal damage. Renal function tests may be performed although alterations in the physiological norms may affect clinical interpretation in pregnancy. Elevated serum uric acid levels may assist in identifying women with chronic hypertension. Admission to a hospital or day assessment unit for initial assessment may be necessary.

Complications

The perinatal outcome in mild pre-existing (chronic) hypertension is good. However, the perinatal morbidity and mortality are increased in those women who develop severe chronic hypertension or superimposed pre-eclampsia. Other complications are independent of pregnancy and include renal failure and cerebral haemorrhage. In 1–2% of cases, hypertensive encephalopathy may develop if the blood pressure suddenly rises above 240/140mmHg; this is a hypertensive emergency requiring admission to an intensive care unit (Vidaeff et al 2005). Maternal mortality is high if phaeochromocytoma is not diagnosed and left untreated.

Management

Mild pre-existing (chronic) hypertension

This is defined as a systolic blood pressure of <160 mmHg and a diastolic blood pressure of <110mmHg. All women with pre-existing (chronic) hypertension should be referred to a specialist either preconception or early in pregnancy in order to arrange shared care, review the diagnosis and review their medication. Women who are already taking antihypertensive therapy will need to discontinue those drugs which may be harmful to the fetus, e.g. ACE inhibitors and atenolol and replace them with medications considered to be safe in pregnancy. Most of these women are at low risk of pregnancy complications and are unlikely to need antenatal admission to hospital. The woman's condition should be carefully monitored in the community by the midwife and GP in order to identify if superimposed pre-eclampsia develops.

Severe pre-existing (chronic) hypertension

The systolic blood pressure is >160mmHg and the diastolic blood pressure is >110mmHg. The woman should be cared for by the obstetric team in conjunction with a physician. Frequent antenatal visits are recommended in order to monitor the maternal condition. This includes blood pressure monitoring, urinalysis to detect proteinuria and blood tests to measure the haematocrit and renal function. Antihypertensive therapy is used in order to prevent maternal complications but has no proven benefit for the fetus and does not stop the development of pre-eclampsia. The midwife may do much to settle anxiety by the use of counselling skills and by mobilizing resources to meet social needs if required. In the rare event of a phaeochromocytoma being present, the blood pressure will be treated with appropriate antihypertensive drugs during the pregnancy and the tumour resected postnatally.

Monitoring of fetal well-being and of placental function should be carried as there is an increased risk of placental abruption and growth restriction (see Ch. 18). If the maternal or fetal condition causes concern, the woman will be admitted to hospital.

The timing and mode of the birth is planned according to the needs of mother and fetus, if early delivery is required, induction of labour is preferred to caesarean section. Postnatally, the woman should be seen by a physician to review the management and treatment of persistent hypertension and renal function should also be reassessed. The midwife who is advising the woman on family planning should be aware of the hypertensive effect of the combined oral contraceptive pill.

REFERENCES

Abalos E, Duley L, Steyn D W et al 2007 Antihypertensive drug therapy for mild to moderate hypertension in pregnancy (review). Cochrane Database of Systematic Reviews, Issue 1: CD002252. Online. Available: www.cochrane.org

Askie L M, Duley L, Henderson-Smart D J et al 2007 Antiplatelet agents for prevention of pre-eclampsia: a meta-analysis of individual patient data. Lancet 369:1791–1798

Borzychowski A M, Sargent I L, Redman C W G 2006 Inflammation and pre-eclampsia. Seminars in Fetal and Neonatal Medicine 11:309–316

Chames M C, Livingston J C, Investor T S et al 2002 Late postpartum eclampsia: a preventable disease? American Journal of Obstetrics and Gynecology 186:1174–1177

Chhabra S, Kakani A 2007 Maternal mortality due to eclamptic and non-eclamptic hypertensive disorders: a challenge. Journal of Obstetrics and Gynaecology 27(1):25–29

Churchill D, Beevers D G 1999 Hypertension in pregnancy. BMJ Books, London.

Clenney T L, Viera A J 2004 Corticosteroids for HELLP (haemolysis, elevated liver enzymes, low platelets) syndrome. British Medical Journal 329:270–272

Curtain W M, Weinstein L 1999 A review of HELLP syndrome. Journal of Perinatology 19(2):138–143

Dekker G, Sibai B 2001 Primary, secondary and tertiary prevention of pre-eclampsia. Lancet 357:209–215

Deruelle P, Coudoux E, Ego A et al 2006 Risk factors for post-partum complications occurring after pre-eclampsia and HELLP syndrome. A study of 453 consecutive pregnancies. European Journal of Obstetrics and Gynaecology and Reproductive Biology 125:59–65

Douglas K A, Redman C W 1994 Eclampsia in the United Kingdom. British Medical Journal 309:1395–1400

Duckitt K, Harrington D 2005 Risk factors for pre-eclampsia at antenatal booking: a systematic review of controlled studies. British Medical Journal 330:565–573

Duley L, Meher S, Abalos E 2006 Management of pre-eclampsia. British Medical Journal 332(7539):463–468

Duley L, Henderson-Smart D J, Meher S 2007 Drugs for treatment of very high blood pressure during pregnancy (review). Cochrane Database of Systematic Reviews, Issue 3: CD001449. Online. Available: www.cochrane.org

ETCG (Eclampsia Trial Collaborative Group) 1995 Which anticonvulsant for women with eclampsia? Evidence from the Collaborative Eclampsia Trial. Lancet 345:1455–1463

Frishman W H, Schlocker M D, Awad K et al 2005 Pathophysiology and medical management of systemic hypertension in pregnancy. Cardiology in Review 13(6): 275–284

Gangaram R, Ojwang P J, Moodley J et al 2005 The accuracy of dipsticks as a screening test for proteinuria in hypertensive disorders of pregnancy. Hypertension in Pregnancy 24(2):117–123

Girling J C, Dow E, Smith J H 1997 Liver function tests in pre-eclampsia: importance of comparison with a reference range derived for normal pregnancy. British Journal of Obstetrics and Gynaecology 104:246–250

Haddad B, Barton J R, Livingston J C et al 2000 Risk factors for adverse maternal outcomes among women with HELLP (haemolysis, elevated liver enzymes and low platelet count) syndrome. American Journal of Obstetrics and Gynecology 183(2):444–448

Hodnett 2000 Support during pregnancy for women at increased risk. Cochrane Database of Systematic Reviews, Issue 1. Online. Available: www.cochrane.org

Hofmeyr G J, Duley L, Atallah A 2007 Dietary calcium supplementation for prevention of pre-eclampsia and related problems: a systematic review and commentary. British Journal of Obstetrics and Gynaecology 114:933–943

James P R, Nelson-Piercy C 2004 Management of hypertension before, during and after pregnancy. Heart 90:1499–1504

Katz V L, Farmer R, Kuller J A 2000 Preeclampsia into eclampsia: toward a new paradigm. American Journal of Obstetrics and Gynecology 182(6):1389–1396

Kidner M C, Flanders-Stephans M B 2004 A model for the HELLP syndrome: the maternal experience. Journal of Obstetric, Gynaecological & Neonatal Nursing 33(1):44–53

Knappen M F C M, Peters W H M, Steegers E A P 1999 Liver function tests in pregnancies complicated by hypertensive disorders of pregnancy or the HELLP syndrome. Contemporary Reviews in Obstetrics and Gynaecology 10(2):105–112

Leith C R, Cameron A D, Walker J J 1997 The changing pattern of eclampsia over a 60-year period. British Journal of Obstetrics and Gynaecology 104:917–922

Levy D M 2003 Hypertensive disorders of pregnancy. World Anaesthesia 17(8):1–10

Lewis, G (ed.) (2007) The Confidential Enquiry into Maternal and Child Health (CEMACH). Saving mothers' lives: reviewing maternal deaths to make motherhood safer 2003–2005. The seventh report on Confidential Enquiries into Maternal Deaths in the United Kingdom. London: CEMACH

Lewis G, Drife J 2001 The 5th Report of the Confidential Enquiries into Maternal Deaths in the United Kingdom. RCOG Press, London

Lewis G, Drife J (eds) 2004 Why mothers die 2000–2002. The Sixth Report of the Confidential Enquiries into Maternal Deaths in the United Kingdom. RCOG Press, London

Li D K, Wi S 2000 Changing paternity and the risk of pre-eclampsia/eclampsia in the subsequent pregnancy. American Journal of Epidemiology 151:57–62

Mander R 2001 Supportive Care and Midwifery. Blackwell Science, Oxford

Magpie Trial Collaborative Group 2002 Do women with pre-eclampsia, and their babies, benefit from magnesium sulphate? The Magpie Trial: a randomised placebo-controlled trial. Lancet 359:1877–1890

Manton G T R, Sikkena M J, Voorbij H A M et al 2007 Risk factors for cardiovascular disease in women with a history of pregnancy complicated by pre-eclampsia or intrauterine growth restriction. Hypertension in Pregnancy 26(1):39–50

Matchaba P, Moodley J 2004 Corticosteroids for HELLP syndrome in pregnancy. Cochrane Database of Systematic Reviews, Issue 1. Online. Available: www.cochrane.org

Mattar F, Sibai B M 2000 Eclampsia VIII. Risk factors for maternal morbidity. American Journal of Obstetrics and Gynecology 182(2):307–312

Meher S, Abalos E, Carroli G 2005 Bed rest with or without hospitalization for hypertension during pregnancy (review). Cochrane Database of Systematic Reviews, Issue 4. Online. Available: www.cochrane.org

Moodley J, Jjuuko G, Rout C 2001 Epidural compared with general anaesthesia for caesarean delivery in conscious women with eclampsia. British Journal of Obstetrics and Gynaecology 108(4):378–382

Munjuiuri N, Lipman M, Valentine A et al 2005 Postpartum eclampsia of late onset. British Medical Journal 331:1070–1071

Nelson-Piercy C 2006 Handbook of obstetric medicine, 3rd edn. Taylor & Francis, London

NHBPEP (National High Blood Pressure Education Program) Working Group on High Blood Pressure in Pregnancy 2000 Report of the working group on high blood pressure in pregnancy. American Journal of Obstetrics and Gynecology 183:S1–S22

NICE (National Institute for Health and Clinical Excellence) 2008 Antenatal care: routine care for healthy pregnant women. NICE, London. Online. Available: www.nice.org.uk

NICE (National Institute for Health and Clinical Excellence) 2006 Postnatal care: routine postnatal care of women and their babies. NICE, London. Online. Available: www.nice.org.uk

Noris M, Perico N, Remuzzi G 2005 Mechanisms of disease: Pre-eclampsia. Nature Clinical Practice. Nephrology 1(2): 98–114

Odegard R A, Vatten L J, Nilsen S T 2000 Risk factors and clinical manifestations of pre-eclampsia. British Journal of Obstetrics and Gynaecology 107(11):1410–1416

Padden M 1999 HELLP Syndrome: Recognition and perinatal management. American Family Physician 60:829–836, 839

Pomini F, Scavo M, Ferrazzani S et al 2001 There is poor agreement between manual auscultatory and automated oscillometric methods for the measurement of blood pressure in normotensive women. Journal of Maternal Fetal Medicine 10(6):398–403

Poston L, Briley A L, Seed P T et al 2006 Vitamin C and Vitamin E in pregnant women at risk for pre-eclampsia (VIP trial): randomized placebo-controlled trial. Lancet 357 (9517):1145–1154

PRECOG Development Group 2004 Pre-eclampsia Community Guideline (PRECOG). Action on Pre-eclampsia (APEC). Online. Available: www.apec.org.uk

Ramsay M M, James D K, Steer P J, et al (eds) 2000 Normal values in pregnancy. W B Saunders, London

Rath W, Faridi A, Dudenhausen J W 2000 HELLP syndrome. Journal of Perinatal Medicine 28(4):249 260

Reck T, Bussenius-Kammerer M, Ott R et al 2001 Surgical treatment of HELLP syndrome associated liver rupture – an update. European Journal of Obstetric Gynaecological Reproductive Biology 99(1):57–65

Redman C W G, Sacks G P, Sargent I L 1999 Pre-eclampsia: an excessive maternal inflammatory response to pregnancy. American Journal of Obstetrics and Gynecology 180(2):499–506

Redman C W G, Sargent I L 2003 Pre-eclampsia, the placenta and the maternal systemic inflammatory response – a review. Placenta 24:S21–S27

Roberts J M, Redman C W G 1993 Pre-eclampsia: more than pregnancy-induced hypertension. Lancet 341:1447–1451

Robillard P Y 2002 Interest in preeclampsia for researchers in reproduction. Journal of Reproductive Immunology 53(1):279–287

Sallah K 2004 Issues for Midwives. In: Lewis G, C (ed) Why mothers die 2000–2002. The Sixth Report of the Confidential Enquiries into Maternal Deaths in the United Kingdom. CEMACH, London

Sheppard B L, Bonnar J 1989 The maternal blood supply to the placenta. In: Studd J (ed.) Progress in Obstetrics and Gynaecology, Vol. 7. Churchill Livingstone, Edinburgh

Sibai B M 2005 Diagnosis, prevention and management of eclampsia. American Journal of Obstetrics and Gynecology 105(2):402–410

Tufnell D J, Shennan A H, Waugh J J S et al 2006 The management of severe pre-eclampsia/eclampsia. RCOG Green-top Guideline No. 10(A). Online. Available: www. rcog.org

UKOSS 2006 Abstract. Online. Available: www.npeu.ox.ac.uk? UKOSS/index.php?content=completed_surveillance.inc

Vaughan C J, Delanty N 2000 Hypertensive emergencies. Lancet 356:411–417

Vidaeff A C, Carroll M A, Ramin S M 2005 Acute hypertensive emergencies in pregnancy. Critical Care Medicine 33(10): S307–S312

Vigil-De G P 2001 Pregnancy complicated by pre-eclampsia-eclampsia with HELLP syndrome. International Journal of Obstetrics and Gynaecology 72(1):17–23

Villar J, Say L, Gulmezoglu M et al 2003 Eclampsia and pre-eclampsia: a worldwide health problem since 2000 years. In: Critchley H O D, Poston L, Walker J J (eds) Pre-eclampsia. RCOG Press, London

Villar J, Say L, Shennan A et al 2004 Methodological and technical issues related to the diagnosis, screening, prevention and treatment of pre-eclampsia and eclampsia. International Journal of Gynaecology and Obstetrics 85: S28–S41

Waugh J J, Bell S C, Kilby M D et al 2005 Optimal bedside urinalysis for the detection of proteinuria in hypertensive pregnancy: a study of diagnostic accuracy. British Journal of Obstetrics and Gynaecology 112(4):412–417

Weinstein L 1982 Syndrome of haemolysis, elevated liver enzymes and low platelet count: a severe consequence of hypertension in pregnancy. American Journal of Obstetrics and Gynecology 142:159–167

Wilson B J, Watson M S, Prescott G L et al 2003 Hypertensive disease of pregnancy and risk of hypertension and stroke in later life: results from a cohort study. British Medical Journal 326:845–885

23 Sexually transmissible and reproductive tract infections in pregnancy

Susan Dapaah   Victor E. Dapaah

This chapter presents an overview of issues relating to sexual health. The clinical features, diagnosis and management of the common types of sexually transmissible and reproductive tract infections and their relevance in pregnancy are described. Specialist detail on these infections can be obtained from other sources such as Holmes et al (1999). Treatment regimens are stated but drug dosages have intentionally been omitted as these should be obtained from regularly updated pharmaceutical publications.

The chapter aims to:

- consider the challenges facing health professionals with the rising trends of HIV and sexually transmissible infections (STIs)
- discuss the significance and management of STIs in pregnancy
- discuss the role of the midwife in caring for women with STIs during pregnancy

Genitourinary medicine (GUM) clinics specialize in the holistic management of individuals with HIV and STIs. Midwives should be aware of sexual health services so that pregnant women are appropriately referred for management and treatment.

Introduction

HIV and STIs are associated with considerable levels of morbidity and mortality. They are thus a major public health concern in the UK and present a serious

415

challenge to health professionals and healthcare provision. High priority has been given to the improvement of sexual health services. In 2001, the National Strategy for Sexual Health and HIV was launched in England (DH 2001). Similar strategies have been produced in the rest of the UK. The strategy has been augmented by an action plan (DH 2002) and more recently by the White Paper 'Making Healthier Choices Easier' (DH 2004a).

The successful control of STIs requires a range of activities that includes screening programmes, effective treatment regimens, partner notification and referral, health education, and counselling and voluntary testing for HIV. Health professionals have a role in promoting public health and may contribute to the sexual health strategy by raising awareness and helping people to access services and information.

The diagnosis, treatment and care of women with STIs during pregnancy requires health professionals to work collaboratively to meet individual needs and improve pregnancy outcomes and lower maternal and neonatal morbidity and mortality. Joint management between an obstetrician and a GUM physician is essential for women with STIs during pregnancy and a paediatrician is required to care and manage the neonate infected through vertical transmission. The midwife plays a vital role in caring for the mother and her family in the provision of individualized care during childbirth. This is particularly important for women diagnosed with an STI during pregnancy who have the extra burden of worrying about the well-being of their babies.

Epidemiological trends

There have been significant changes in the epidemiology of HIV and other STIs over the last 25 years, in particular during the decade 1996–2005.

The prevalence of HIV continues to increase. At the end of 2005 it was estimated that 63 500 adults in the UK aged between 15 and 59 were suffering from HIV infection, 32% of whom were unaware of their HIV status (Health Protection Agency (HPA) 2006). This contrasts with an estimated 30 000 cases in 2000. The annual number of new diagnoses of HIV rose by 175% from 2707 in 1996 to 7450 in 2005. However,

the high number in 2005 is comparable to the numbers diagnosed in 2003 and 2004 suggesting that the incidence may be stabilizing.

The number of new diagnoses of other STIs in UK GUM clinics rose by 60% during the same period. Chlamydia and gonorrhoea, two of the most common STIs showed considerable increases. The number of uncomplicated genital chlamydial infections trebled, rising by 207% from 35 840 cases to 109 958. Gonorrhoea increased by 54% from 12 579 cases to 19 392. The incidence peaked in 2002 at 25 599 cases, but a gradual decline has since been observed. However, the level of antibiotic resistance to gonorrhoea has increased throughout the UK (HPA 2006).

There has been a dramatic rise of 1954% in the incidence of infectious syphilis. Cases increased from 290 in 1996 to 3712 in 2005 with a reported six-fold increase in the diagnosis of early latent syphilis (HPA 2006).

The incidence of viral STIs also increased. The number of first attack genital warts rose by 26% from 64 178 cases in 1996 to 81 137 in 2005. During the same period the number of first attack herpes increased by 18% from 16 811 to 19 837 cases.

The burden of HIV and STIs falls disproportionately on marginalized groups. The highest infection rates are found in women, gay men, teenagers, young adults and black and minority ethnic groups (House of Commons Health Committee 2003). Additionally, direct links between sexual ill-health and poverty, poor housing, unemployment and other forms of social exclusion have been recognized (DH 2003). Statistics show that females account for most cases of uncomplicated chlamydia and first attack herpes, and males account for most cases of primary/secondary syphilis and uncomplicated gonorrhoea. The number of cases of first attack genital warts is higher in males than females (HPA 2006). The highest rates of gonorrhoea, genital warts and chlamydial infections are found in the 16–19 year age group in women, and the 20–24 year age group in women and men.

A number of factors are thought to contribute to the increase in the incidence of HIV and STIs. The rise in the number of diagnoses may be due to the increased availability and sensitivity of tests and greater public awareness of the services available. In addition, there is evidence of changes in attitudes and patterns of sexual behaviour. The second 'National Survey of Sexual Attitudes and Lifestyles' also known as NATSAL 2000 (Johnson et al 2001) reported a wide range of behaviours associated with increased risk of HIV and STI transmission. The mean number of sexual partners in a lifetime and the proportion of people having concurrent sexual relationships have increased. The average age at first intercourse has fallen from 17 to 16 years. Although the use of condoms has increased, a greater proportion of people with two or more partners reported inconsistent use.

Risky sexual behaviours are probably influenced by several factors including low self esteem, lack of skills and confidence to negotiate safer sex and a lack of knowledge about the risks of different sexual behaviours. Peer pressure, the attitudes and prejudices of society and the availability of sexual health services are also contributory factors (Ellis et al 2003).

GUM clinics provide important surveillance data for STIs and sexual health in the UK. However, family planning, gynaecology and antenatal clinics, general practice, prison health services and schools also contribute to sexual health. In addition, many infections are often asymptomatic and are consequently not diagnosed. The total number of STI diagnoses is therefore likely to be underestimated (PHLS 2000).

Psychosocial aspects of STIs

Health professionals need to be aware of the broad range of psychological and social responses to STIs. Two general themes appear in the literature. The first is the range of psychological responses often manifest by individuals on initial diagnosis. These include shock, embarrassment, disbelief, distress, anxiety, feeling dirty/contaminated and worry about future health. The second relates to specific areas of concern. These include stigma, guilt/blame for the infection, concerns about transmitting the infection to others and anxiety and fear about disclosure to sexual partners, family and friends (Maissi et al 2004, McCaffery et al 2006). Stigma, shame and ostracism have historically been associated with STIs and are still thought to be important barriers that prevent individuals from seeking diagnosis and treatment (Cunningham et al 2002, Scoular et al 2001). Prejudice

and discrimination pose real threats to individuals suffering from STIs, in particular, those with HIV (Terence Higgins Trust 2001).

Good communication skills are essential as individuals who have or are at risk of an STI need to be approached in a sensitive, tactful and non-judgemental manner (Peate 2005). A full sexual history is vital for accurate diagnosis, treatment and risk-assessment, but many patients find discussing sexually related matters difficult and embarrassing. Health professionals therefore must establish trust and rapport with patients and provide a comfortable, friendly and relaxed environment in which to discuss these issues (French 2004). The assurance of confidentiality is a vital component in the promotion of mutual trust, respect and effective partnerships. Healthcare professionals have a professional and a legal duty to ensure the confidentiality and security of all information gained in the course of professional practice (Dimond 2002). In relation to individuals with STIs, particularly HIV, the maintenance of confidentiality is a common source of worry. Midwives should therefore assure their clients that sensitive information will not be disclosed to others without their consent or other lawful exception.

Psychosocial responses to STIs may vary according to the type of infection, the circumstances in which it was acquired, associated sequelae and the likely effect on future lives. Whereas many STIs are curable, some such as HIV and genital herpes cannot be eradicated and require long term management. There have been marked improvements in the treatment of HIV and AIDS but they still carry significant morbidity and mortality. Genital herpes is a lifelong chronic infection with the possibility of recurrences. Women with chlamydial infection are fearful of the possible adverse effects on their reproductive capacity. Victims of sexual abuse and/or assault can experience a wide range of psychological and emotional disorders. It is therefore imperative that these groups of patients receive appropriate specialist management. Some patients are likely to suffer psychological maladjustment and will require psychological/psychiatric assessment and treatment. Psychological support and correct information can help people to come to terms with their conditions (Chippindale & French 2001).

Types of genital infections

Trichomoniasis

Trichomoniasis is one of the most common sexually transmitted infections. It is caused by *Trichomonas vaginalis*, a round/oval flagellated protozoal parasite. The World Health Organization (WHO) estimates that about 170 million new cases occur annually (Mabey et al 2006). Although 10–50% of women are asymptomatic, common symptoms include vaginal and urethral discharge, vulval pruritus and inflammation. Vaginal discharge is present in up to 70% of cases and can range from thin and scanty to profuse and thick and may be malodorous. A classic frothy yellow-green discharge occurs in 10–30% of women. Dyspareunia, mild dysuria and lower abdominal pain may also be experienced (Sherrard 2007).

Trichomoniasis in pregnancy

Trichomoniasis has been linked with a small risk of pre-term delivery and low birth weight, and an increase in the risk of HIV via sexual intercourse. Trichomoniasis may be acquired perinatally and occurs in about 5% of babies born to infected mothers (Sherrard 2007).

Diagnosis and treatment

In women, 95% of cases can be diagnosed by cultures and 40–80% by microscopy of a high vaginal swab. Other diagnostic tests include a latex agglutination test and polymerase chain reaction (PCR). UK guidelines state that metronidazole and related drugs achieve a 95% cure rate (Sherrard 2007). The recommended treatment is metronidazole daily for 5–7 days or in a single dose. Although contraindicated in pregnancy, meta-analyses have concluded that there is no evidence of teratogenicity from its use during the first trimester. However, it is not known whether this treatment will have any effect on pregnancy outcomes (Gülmezoglu 2002). Clotrimazole pessaries daily for 7 days can be used in early pregnancy. High single dose regimens should be avoided during pregnancy and breastfeeding. It is usual to treat the partner(s) and advise against sexual intercourse until the treatment is completed. In addition, patients should be advised not to consume alcohol during the treatment and for at least 48 hrs afterwards as this may cause nausea and vomiting.

Vulvovaginal candidiasis (thrush)

Candidiasis is a common cause of vaginal discharge, vulvitis and vaginitis and it is responsible for 20–30% of all vaginal infections. The main causative organism is *Candida albicans*, a fungal parasite, but other candidal species for example *Candida glabrata*, account for 10% of genital yeast infections (Schwebke & Hillier 2005). *Candida albicans* is often found as a commensal in the flora of the mouth, gastrointestinal tract and probably the vagina (Hay 2005). It is not thought to be sexually transmitted. During the reproductive years women are prone to develop vulvovaginal candidiasis because oestrogens encourage *Candida albicans* to flourish. Most women will probably develop candidiasis at some point during their adult life and <5% will experience recurrent vulvovaginal candidiasis defined as four or more episodes a year. Some 10–20% of women harbour *Candida* species but remain asymptomatic and do not require treatment (Daniels & Forster 2002).

Several factors are thought to predispose to *Candida albicans* infections. These include:

- changes to the vaginal flora (e.g. antibiotics, spermicides)
- immunosuppressant disease or treatment (e.g. AIDS, chemotherapy)
- poor diabetic control
- pregnancy.

The signs and symptoms of candidiasis include intense vulval itching and soreness and usually a non-offensive, thick, white curdy discharge. On examination the vulva, vagina and cervix may be erythematous and oedematous, and white plaques are noted. Superficial dyspareunia and external dysuria may also be experienced.

Diagnosis and treatment

Microscopy and culture of a high vaginal swab are the most sensitive methods currently available for detecting candida cells. However, diagnosis is often based on clinical signs and symptoms. Candidiasis may be treated with topical preparations such as clotrimazole pessaries or nystatin gel, or oral preparations such as fluconazole. All therapies effect high cure rates (Daniels & Forster 2002). Fluconazole

(Diflucan) is available over the counter but has not been tested in pregnancy and therefore cannot be assumed to be safe. It should also be used with caution whilst breastfeeding owing to toxic effects in high doses.

A Cochrane systematic review of topical treatments for vaginal candidiasis in pregnancy concluded that topical imidazole drugs are more effective than nystatin; that single dose treatments are less effective than 3–4 day treatments; and that treatment lasting for 4 days is less effective than treatment for 7 days (Young & Jewell 2001).

Treatment failure can occur in up to 20% of women. It may be helpful to advise on general and genital hygiene such as the avoidance of local irritants e.g. perfumed products, the wearing of tight-fitting synthetic clothing and washing and wiping the genitals from front to back. It is not necessary to treat asymptomatic partners (Daniels & Forster 2002).

Bacterial infections

Bacterial vaginosis

Bacterial vaginosis (BV) is the most common cause of vaginal discharge in women of childbearing age. It does not appear to be sexually transmitted but may be associated with sexual activity and often co-exists with other sexually transmitted infections such as gonorrhoea and chlamydia. It can arise and remit spontaneously. It is more common in black than white women, those with an intrauterine contraceptive device and those who smoke (Hay 2006). The incidence of BV is high in women with pelvic inflammatory disease (PID) and some populations of women undergoing elective termination of pregnancy (TOP). It is also associated with post-TOP endometritis.

The aetiology is unknown but BV is associated with a change in vaginal ecology. The normal lactobacilli-predominant vaginal flora is replaced with an overgrowth of predominantly anaerobic bacteria including *Gardnerella vaginalis*, *Prevotella* species, *Mobiluncus* species and *Mycoplasma hominis*. The vaginal epithelium is not inflamed, hence the term 'vaginosis' rather than 'vaginitis'. The main symptom is a malodorous and greyish watery vaginal discharge, although approximately 50% of women are asymptomatic. The odour is usually more pronounced following sexual intercourse owing to the release of amines by the alkaline semen.

Bacterial vaginosis in pregnancy

BV is present in up to 20% of women during pregnancy, the majority of whom will be asymptomatic (McDonald et al 2007). Flynn et al (1999) found in a review of case-control and cohort studies that women with BV infections were 1.85 times more likely to deliver pre-term than women without BV. Other adverse outcomes of pregnancy include late miscarriage, pre-term premature rupture of membranes and postpartum endometritis (Hay 2006).

Diagnosis and treatment

The two most common approaches used to diagnose BV are the use of Amsel's criteria or evaluation of a Gram-stained vaginal smear. A diagnosis of BV is confirmed by fulfilling three out of four criteria (Amsel et al 1983):

- a thin, white to grey, homogenous discharge
- 'clue cells' on microscopy
- a vaginal pH of >4.5
- the release of a fishy odour when adding potassium hydroxide to a sample of the discharge.

An alternative test is the evaluation of a Gram-stained vaginal smear using the Ison-Hay scoring system (Ison & Hay 2002). This method grades the vaginal flora and correlates well with Amsel's criteria, and has been endorsed by the Bacterial Special Interest Group of the British Association for Sexual Health and HIV (BASHH).

A Cochrane systematic review assessing the effects of antibiotic therapy on BV in pregnancy concluded that although it was effective at eradicating infection, it did not reduce the number of pre-term births (McDonald et al 2007). The treatment regimen is the same as for trichomoniasis. Alternative treatments include oral clindamycin or tinidazole or intravaginal clindamycin cream or metronidazole gel. All these treatments have been shown in controlled trials to achieve cure rates of 70–80% after 4 weeks, but recurrences of infection are common. Women should be advised to avoid vaginal douching, use of shower gel and antiseptic agents in the bath (Hay 2006). There is insufficient evidence to recommend the routine screening of pregnant women and the treatment of asymptomatic BV (National Institute for Health and Clinical Excellence (NICE) 2003).

Chlamydia

Chlamydia trachomatis is an intracellular bacterium. It is one of the most prevalent STIs worldwide and the most common cause of sexually transmitted bacterial infection in the UK (Fletcher & Ball 2006). Serotypes D to K are sexually transmitted and are important causes of morbidity in both sexes. Serotypes A, B and C cause trachoma and blindness, and serotypes L1 to L3 cause the genital disease lymphogranuloma venereum.

Genital chlamydial infection is asymptomatic in at least 70% of women and 50% of men (HPA 2006). The clinical signs and symptoms include post-coital or intermenstrual bleeding, a purulent vaginal discharge, mucopurulent cervicitis and/or contact bleeding, dyspareunia and lower abdominal pain. Dysuria, bartholinitis and Fitz–Hugh–Curtis syndrome (perihepatitis) may also be experienced (Fletcher & Ball 2006, Horner & Boag 2006).

Chlamydial infection of the cervix is found in 15–30% of women attending GUM clinics, and concurrently in 35–40% of women with gonorrhoea (Schachter et al 1998). Significant factors associated with infection include those aged less than 25 years, a new sexual partner or more than one sexual partner in the past year, lack of consistent use of condoms and those attending GUM clinics (Adams et al 2004, Horner & Boag 2006). In untreated cases the complications among women may include PID and its associated sequelae.

Chlamydia in pregnancy

Infection rates in pregnancy range from approximately 2–13% (Adams et al 2004, Shankar et al 2006). *C. trachomatis* is associated with pre-term delivery, pre-labour rupture of membranes, chorioamnionitis and postpartum endometritis.

Fetal and neonatal infections

The major risk to the infant is from passing through an infected cervix during birth although intrauterine infection may occur. This can lead to neonatal conjunctivitis (ophthalmia neonatorum, a notifiable condition in the UK) and a characteristic pneumonia. Chlamydial ophthalmia neonatorum is more common than that of gonococcal aetiology. In practice, the conditions are indistinguishable and may occur together. The incubation period of chlamydial ophthalmia is 6–21 days, compared with 48 hrs for gonococcal ophthalmia. Chlamydial pneumonia usually occurs between the 4th and 12th week of life. It affects about half the babies who develop conjunctivitis but is not always preceded by it. It is thought that children affected by chlamydial pneumonia are more likely to develop obstructive lung disease and asthma than those who have had pneumonia from other causes. The pharynx, middle ear, rectum and vagina are also targets for infection, with a delay of up to 7 months before cultures become positive.

The routine screening of pregnant women for asymptomatic chlamydia is not currently recommended in the UK (NICE 2003). However, there is growing evidence that the substantial morbidity associated with chlamydial infections can be reduced through the targeted screening of at-risk populations. In 2002 a National Chlamydia Screening Programme was launched in the UK.

Diagnosis and treatment

Nucleic acid amplification tests (NAATs) are recommended as the most reliable means to diagnose chlamydia (Horner & Boag 2006). Three commercial tests are now available:

- Polymerase chain reaction (PCR)
- Strand displacement amplification (SDA)
- Transcription mediated amplification (TMA).

These tests have high rates of sensitivity and specificity. Less sensitive methods of diagnosis include tissue culture, enzyme immunoassays (EIAs) and direct fluorescent antibody (DFA).

Genital chlamydial infections are sensitive to three classes of antibiotics. These are the tetracyclines, the macrolides (e.g. erythromycin) and the fluoroquinolones, especially ofloxacin. The tetracyclines and the fluoroquinolones are contraindicated in pregnancy. Despite the side-effects of nausea and vomiting, erythromycin is considered to be the first line treatment in pregnancy. Erythromycin is also used for chlamydial infections in infants, young children and lactating women. Although available data indicate the safety of azithromycin in pregnancy and lactation (Brocklehurst & Rooney 2000), UK guidelines recommend its use only if no alternative exists (Horner & Boag 2006). Women and partners should be advised to abstain from sexual intercourse until treatment is complete. A test of cure is not routinely recommended but should be performed in pregnancy to identify treatment failure or re-infection.

Gonorrhoea

Gonorrhoea is caused by infection with *Neisseria gonorrhoeae*, a Gram-negative, intracellular diplococcus. The mode of transmission is almost exclusively by sexual contact. This organism adheres primarily to the mucous membranes of the urethra, endocervix, rectum, pharynx and conjunctiva. Gonorrhoea may co-exist with other genital mucosal pathogens, notably *C. trachomatis*, *T. vaginalis* and *C. albicans*. Up to 80% of initial cases of PID are caused by *N. gonorrhoeae* or *C. trachomatis*, or both. Although uncommon, gonorrhoea may also cause disseminated systemic disease and arthritis.

The most common symptom is an increased or altered vaginal discharge although up to 50% of women are asymptomatic. Lower abdominal pain, dysuria, intermenstrual bleeding and menorrhagia may also be experienced, ranging in intensity from minimal to severe (Bignell 2005).

Gonorrhoea in pregnancy

Infection with *N. gonorrhoeae* has been associated with adverse pregnancy outcomes. These include low birthweight, pre-term rupture of membranes, pre-term birth, chorioamnionitis and postpartum endometritis and salpingitis. Other possible complications are spontaneous miscarriage and secondary infertility (Herbert & Impey 2005, Mitchell 2004).

Neonatal infection

N. gonorrhoeae is usually transmitted from the mother's genital tract to the baby at the time of birth although occasionally it may occur in utero when there is prolonged rupture of the membranes. The risk of transmission from an untreated mother is about 30–50% (Mitchell 2004). Infection usually manifests as ophthalmia neonatorum (see Plate 23) with a purulent discharge usually evident within 2–5 days of birth. It can be diagnosed by microscopy and culture of an eye swab. The eyes may be cleaned with saline but systemic antibiotics are required. If left untreated the condition can lead to corneal ulceration and perforation with permanent loss of vision. Occasionally the neonate may develop gonococcal arthritis and/or disseminated infection.

Diagnosis and treatment

The methods used to diagnose gonorrhoea consist of:

- microscopy of a suitably stained specimen
- culture for *N. gonorrhoeae* on a medium with antimicrobial agents
- nucleic acid hybridization or amplification tests.

In women, microscopic examination of Gram-stained endocervical smears is the first-line in diagnosis. Specificity is high (>99%) when screened by trained personnel. Microscopy is unsuitable for pharyngeal and rectal specimens because of the presence of other Gram-negative cocci (Bignell et al 2006).

Culture for *N. gonorrhoeae* can be undertaken with specimens from all sites. This method provides a viable organism for antibiotic sensitivity testing. Culture has been reported to have a sensitivity of 85–95% for urethral and endocervical infection (Bignell et al 2006). Nucleic acid hybridization or amplification tests are not currently recommended for use in GUM clinics because of the inability to assess antibiotic sensitivity.

Penicillin has been used as a first-line therapy for gonorrhoea for many years. However, surveillance data in the UK show that *N. gonorrhoeae* is becoming resistant to penicillin, tetracyclines and ciprofloxacin (a quinolone) (Gonococcal Resistance to Antimicrobials Surveillance Programme (GRASP) 2004). Nevertheless, local patterns of antimicrobial sensitivity should be taken into account when prescribing treatment. If antimicrobial sensitivity to the above antibiotics is known then ciprofloxacin, ofloxacin and ampicillin plus probenecid may be prescribed in oral, single doses. Otherwise, third-generation cephalosporins such as ceftriaxone or cefixime should be prescribed orally or intramuscularly in single doses.

Spectinomycin may also be given in a single oral dose. Pregnant women should not be treated with quinolone or tetracycline (Bignell 2005).

Group B streptococcus

Group B streptococcus (GBS) (*Streptococcus agalactiae*) is a Gram-positive bacterium that naturally colonizes the body. It is harboured in the genital and gastrointestinal tracts and carried asymptomatically in up to 40% of adults. GBS is not considered to be sexually transmitted but infection increases with sexual activity and rates are highest in women attending genitourinary clinics. Approximately 12–26% of pregnant women are colonized with the organism (Herbert & Impey 2005).

Group B streptococcus in pregnancy

In pregnant women colonized with GBS, high risk factors associated with vertical transmission include: preterm delivery, prolonged rupture of membranes, maternal pyrexia during labour, GBS cultured in a urine sample, known carriage of GBS or a history of a GBS infection in a previous pregnancy (Feldman 2001, Smaill 2001). GBS is able to infiltrate the amniotic cavity, whether or not the membranes are intact, and infect the fetus through the lung epithelium. Postpartum endometritis and post-caesarean wound infection may also occur in the mother.

Fetal and neonatal infections

GBS is the leading cause of serious neonatal infection in the UK (NICE 2003). The prevalence of early onset GBS disease in the UK is estimated to range from 0.5/1000 to 1.15/1000 live births (Oddie & Embleton 2002). Early onset is when symptoms develop within the first 5 days of life (average 20 hrs) suggesting that the infection started in utero. Late onset usually presents between 7 days and 3 months of age in previously healthy babies.

Diagnosis and treatment

The identification of women colonized with GBS can reliably be undertaken with vaginal and rectal swabs. In the USA, pregnant women are screened in the third trimester for GBS and are treated prophylactically with intrapartum penicillin if identified as high risk

of transmitting the infection. However, pregnant women in the UK are not routinely screened because evidence of clinical and cost-effectiveness remain uncertain (NICE 2003, Woodgate et al 2004).

Syphilis

Syphilis is an acute and chronic sexually transmitted infection caused by the bacterium *Treponema pallidum*, a spirochaete. It can also be transmitted transplacentally to the fetus from the 9th week of gestation onwards (Genç & Ledger 2000). It is a common infection worldwide with an estimated 12 million diagnosed new cases each year (Adler & French 2004). Syphilis is a complex systemic disease that can involve virtually any organ in the body. Acquired syphilis is classified into the following stages (Winter 2006):

Early (infectious) syphilis:

- *Primary:* 9–90 days after exposure (mean 21 days)
- *Secondary:* 6 weeks-6 months after exposure (4–8 weeks after primary lesion)
- *Latent (early):* <2 years after exposure.

Late (non-infectious) syphilis:

- *Latent (late):* > 2 years after exposure with no symptoms or signs
- *Tertiary, gummatous, cardiovascular, neurosyphilis:* 3–20 years after exposure.

Syphilis in pregnancy

WHO figures estimate that maternal syphilis adversely affects 1 million pregnancies each year, with 460000 resulting in abortion or perinatal death, 270000 babies being born with congenital syphilis and 270000 being born premature or with low birthweight (Walker & Walker 2002). In the UK, antenatal screening for syphilis is routine and the incidence of infectious syphilis is low although there is no systematic national surveillance for the number of cases diagnosed during pregnancy (NICE 2003, Simms & Ward 2006). Herbert and Impey (2005) report an incidence of 0.2% in London and 0.02% in the rest of the UK. The prevalence in Northern Europe is between 0.02% and 4.5% (Genç & Ledger 2000).

Vertical transmission may occur at any time during pregnancy in untreated early syphilis but the risk of transmission diminishes as maternal syphilis advances. The rate of vertical transmission in untreated women is 70–100% for primary syphilis, 40% for early latent syphilis and an estimated 10% for mothers with late latent syphilis (Doroshenko et al 2006).

Congenital syphilis

The prevalence of congenital syphilis in the UK is estimated as very low. It is classified into early or late congenital syphilis depending on whether it presents before or after 2 years of age. It is associated with serious neurological, developmental and musculoskeletal sequelae and the prognosis is considered poor if symptoms present in the first few weeks of life (French 2007, Saloojee et al 2004). Diagnosis may be complicated because more than half of all infants are asymptomatic at birth, and signs in symptomatic infants may be subtle and non-specific. Characteristically, prematurity, low birthweight, hepatomegaly with or without splenomegaly and failure to thrive are some of the findings of early syphilis, although these signs are also seen in other congenital infections (Saloojee et al 2004). Serological tests should be performed on the baby's blood not cord blood. A positive antitreponemal EIA IgM is consistent with a diagnosis of congenital infection although positive tests should be repeated to confirm this. A negative IgM test should be repeated at 4, 8 and 12 weeks as the IgM response could be delayed or suppressed (Goh 2002).

Babies born to mothers treated antenatally for syphilis should be managed jointly with paediatricians and followed up at 3 months, 6 months and 1 year. UK guidelines suggest that older siblings should also be screened for congenital syphilis (Goh 2002). Treatment is usually with penicillin.

Diagnosis and treatment

Women in the UK are screened for syphilis at antenatal booking and treated if needed in the same way as non-pregnant women. However, this does not detect those who acquire the infection during pregnancy, or are incubating syphilis at the time of serological testing. There are two main classifications of serological tests for syphilis (French 2007):

Non-treponemal tests which detect non-specific treponemal antibodies:

- Venereal Diseases Research Laboratory (VDRL)
- Rapid plasma reagin (RPR) tests.

Treponemal tests which detect specific treponemal antibodies:

- Enzyme immunoassays (EIAs)
- *T pallidum* haemagglutination assay (TPHA)
- *T pallidum* particle agglutination assay (TPPA)
- Fluorescent treponemal antibody-absorbed test (FTA-abs).

If syphilis is suspected on the basis of clinical findings, dark-field microscopic examination or fluorescent antibody staining of a specimen taken from a lesion should be undertaken (see Plate 4) (Goh 2002). A Cochrane systematic review of antibiotics for syphilis diagnosed during pregnancy concluded that penicillin is effective in the treatment of syphilis and the prevention of congenital syphilis but more research is needed on the best dosage and duration of treatment (Walker 2001). The management of pregnant women with syphilis should be undertaken jointly between a GUM physician and obstetricians and midwives. In the case of penicillin allergy, tetracycline is the second-line treatment but this is contraindicated in pregnancy. Erythromycin or azithromycin are alternatives but these may be ineffective in treating pregnant women (NICE 2003). Desensitization to penicillin should therefore be considered as an option. Breastfeeding is safe unless an infectious lesion is present on the breast (Genç & Ledger 2000).

Patients should be warned of possible reactions to treatment with penicillin. The Jarisch–Herxheimer reaction is an acute febrile illness characterized by fever, chills, myalgia, headache, hypotension and tachycardia that occurs in up to 45% of pregnant women after treatment for early syphilis. The release of pro-inflammatory cytokines in response to dying organisms is thought to induce this reaction. Symptoms may occur within several hours of treatment but resolve within 24–36 hrs. In pregnant women, it can cause uterine contractions, fetal distress and precipitate pre-term labour. For this reason some recommend that the mother is admitted to hospital for the first 24 hrs of treatment (Genç & Ledger 2000).

Women who are known to have been treated for syphilis in the past do not require treatment in subsequent pregnancies if there is no clinical or serological evidence of infection but the baby should be tested to exclude congenital syphilis (Goh 2002).

Viral infections

Genital warts

Genital warts (condyloma acuminatum) are caused by the human papillomavirus (HPV). Although there are over 100 subtypes of HPV, several of which can cause genital warts, they are most commonly caused by types 6 and 11. Transmission is primarily by sexual contact but infants and young children may develop laryngeal papillomas after being infected from maternal genital warts at delivery (Adler 2004). The rate of first attack genital warts has been rising since 1996 with the highest rates seen in women in the 16–19 and 20–24 year age-groups. Most genital warts are asymptomatic and painless and many resolve spontaneously in healthy women. They may occasionally cause irritation and soreness, but essentially they are more of a cosmetic problem often causing psychological and psychosexual distress (Maw 2006). In pregnancy they tend to multiply and grow faster as a result of changes in local cellular immunity and may appear like cauliflower-like masses (see Plate 3) (Mitchell 2004).

Viral eradication is not possible; therefore treatment is aimed at removing the warts (Peate 2006). Treatment can be difficult and time consuming and often depends on patient compliance and skilled health professionals. Warts are usually treated with locally applied caustic agents such as podophyllum. However, this is contraindicated in pregnancy because of possible teratogenicity. Treatment is not recommended during pregnancy, but in exceptional circumstances trichloroacetic acid, cryotherapy, diathermy, laser therapy or surgery may be appropriate (Adler 2004; Peate 2006). Women presenting with genital warts should be fully investigated to exclude other sexually transmitted infections. In addition, colposcopy should be performed to exclude flat warts on the cervix. Most genital warts are benign, but cervical intraepithelial neoplasia is strongly associated with HPV

types 16, 18, 31, 33 and 35, therefore an annual cervical smear is recommended (Adler 2004).

Prophylactic vaccines to prevent primary infection with HPV and reduce the incidence of related conditions such as cervical cancer and genital warts are being developed. Trial data point towards the potential for protecting young uninfected girls from cervical cancer (Cadman 2006; HPA 2006).

Hepatitis B virus

Hepatitis B virus (HBV) is an hepadnavirus belonging to a family of DNA viruses that cause acute infection of the liver. HBV can be transmitted sexually, parenterally or vertically from mother to fetus (Gilson & Brook 2006). Body fluids such as saliva, menstrual and vaginal fluid, serous exudates, seminal fluid and breastmilk have been implicated in the spread of infection, but infectivity is largely related to blood and body fluids contaminated with blood. Transmission occurs in injecting drug-users sharing needles and syringes, tattooing or acupuncture, or as a consequence of needle-stick injury in healthcare workers (Brook 2005).

Acute infection with HBV is asymptomatic in 10–50% of adults and virtually all infants and children. In typical cases there are two phases of symptoms:

- the prodromal phase (3–10 days) characterized by flu-like symptoms of malaise, myalgia and fatigue, often accompanied by pain in the right hypochondrium
- the icteric phase (7–21 days) characterized by jaundice, anorexia, nausea and fatigue. In a small number of cases, symptoms can persist for 12 or more weeks (cholestatic symptoms of itching and deep jaundice).

The diagnosis of HBV relies on serological tests. Acute HBV is diagnosed by the presence of IgM antibodies to the HBV core (anti-HBc IgM). Hepatitis B surface antigen (HBsAg) is detectable during the acute phase. Patients who remain HBsAg positive after six months are classified as persistent virus carriers. Another serological marker is the hepatitis Be antigen (HBeAg) which can be detected during the acute phase but disappears quickly unless the individual becomes a carrier. The appearance of anti-HBs in the serum indicates immunity.

Chronic infection occurs in 5–10% of symptomatic cases but higher rates are seen in immuno-compromised patients with HIV infection, chronic renal failure and those receiving immunosuppressive therapy (Brook 2005). In the UK about 1 in 1000 of the population carries the hepatitis B virus. HBeAg positive carriers are much more likely to transmit the infection during sexual contact or from mother to baby at birth (Gilson 2004). More than 90% of infants born to HBeAg positive mothers will also become chronic carriers unless immunized.

The prevalence of infection (HBsAg) among pregnant women ranges from 0.5% to 1%. All pregnant women should be offered antenatal screening for HBV and babies born to infected mothers should be vaccinated at birth (NICE 2003). In addition, the babies of mothers who have become infected with HBV during pregnancy and those who do not have anti-HBe antibodies should also receive hepatitis B specific immunoglobulin (HBIg) (Lee et al 2006). This confers immediate immunity and reduces vertical transmission by 90%. Infected mothers should continue to breastfeed as there is no additional risk of transmission (Brook 2005).

Hepatitis C virus

Hepatitis C virus (HCV) infection is a global health problem with a worldwide prevalence of between 0.5% and 15% (Fischler 2007). In the UK it ranges from 0.06% in blood donors to over 60% in intravenous drug users (Brook 2005). Acute HCV infection is usually asymptomatic. Approximately 50–85% of infected individuals will develop a chronic infection leading to severe liver damage, liver cirrhosis, and hepatocellular carcinoma (Thomas 2005). The principal route of transmission is by percutaneous inoculation of blood and/or blood products, intravenous drug use, tattooing, body piercing and mother-to-child transmission (NICE 2003). Vertical transmission rates are low, occurring at <5%, but co-infection with HIV has consistently been associated with a greater likelihood of transmitting HCV to the fetus. Breastfeeding does not pose an important risk of transmission if the nipples are not traumatized and maternal HCV infection is quiescent (Roberts & Yeung 2002). Sexual transmission rates are very low but these are increased in high risk groups such as female sex workers and those with multiple sexual partners (Brook 2005). At present, there is a lack of effective intervention strategies to prevent vertical transmission and the routine screening of pregnant women for HCV is not recommended (Fischler 2007; NICE 2003).

Herpes simplex virus

There are two herpes simplex virus (HSV) subtypes. Type 1 (HSV-1) causes the majority of orolabial infections, and is often acquired during childhood through direct physical contact with oral secretions. Type 2 (HSV-2) is almost entirely associated with genital disease and is acquired through contaminated secretions during sexual contact. Genital HPV-1 can be acquired through orogenital contact and the incidence of genital HSV-1 infection is increasing, especially in young women (Vyse et al 2000). Genital herpes is a lifelong infection. Once acquired, the virus becomes latent in sensory nerve ganglia and reactivates periodically. Infected people shed the virus regardless of whether or not lesions are present. Infections may be primary, when an HSV seronegative person acquires HSV-1 or HSV-2, or initial non-primary when a person with antibody against one virus type acquires the opposite type (Geretti 2006). Previous oral infection with HSV-1 provides a high level of protection against genital HSV-1 infection but not against genital HSV-2 infection. Nevertheless, it usually prevents the severe symptoms associated with primary HSV-2 infections (Vyse et al 2000).

In adults, primary genital HSV infection may be asymptomatic, but painful, vesicular or ulcerative lesions on the vulva, perineum, vagina and cervix frequently occur. Dysuria and vaginal or urethral discharge may also occur (Barton et al 2001). There may be systemic symptoms of fever, headache and myalgia. Symptoms tend to be more severe in women than in men (Sissons 2005).

HSV in pregnancy

Neonatal herpes is a severe systemic viral infection with a high morbidity and mortality (RCOG 2002). The incidence in the UK is about 1.65 in 100 000 births and can be caused by either HSV-1 or HSV-2 (Khare 2005). Women who have had herpes prior to pregnancy will have developed antibodies to the virus.

The fetus will also develop these antibodies and consequently at birth will have passive immunity. The greatest risk to the fetus is therefore if the mother acquires a primary infection during late pregnancy and the baby is born before the development of maternal antibodies (RCOG 2002). Primary infection in early pregnancy can lead to congenital HSV infection which although rare can cause severe congenital abnormalities. About 70% of cases of neonatal HSV infection are caused by HSV-2 and result from contact with maternal genital secretions during delivery. Neonatal herpes may be acquired from an ascending infection following rupture of the membranes. The risk of neonatal infection is about 50% with symptomatic primary infection and 20% from a woman with clinically evident recurrent HSV-2 infection (Sissons 2005).

Diagnosis

HSV infections are usually diagnosed clinically. HSV DNA detection by PCR is the preferred diagnostic method for genital herpes. Viral cultures from open lesions are used routinely in the UK. Other methods of diagnosis include direct immunofluorescence assay (IFA) or enzyme immunoassay (EIA). Serological tests for HSV specific antibody can be used to diagnose HSV infection in asymptomatic individuals. The presence of HSV-2 antibodies is indicative of genital herpes but HSV-1 antibodies do not provide any distinction between genital and oropharyngeal infection (Geretti 2006).

Management of HSV infection in pregnancy

A referral to a genitourinary physician should be made for any pregnant woman in whom a first-episode herpes infection is suspected. Primary infection acquired during the first or second trimester should be treated with acyclovir. Acyclovir reduces viral shedding, reduces pain and promotes the healing of lesions. Evidence from the Acyclovir Pregnancy Registry has shown there is no clinical or laboratory evidence of maternal or fetal toxicity (RCOG 2002). Caesarean section is recommended for all women presenting with first-episode genital herpes lesions at the time of delivery as the risk of viral shedding and vertical transmission is high. It should also be considered for women with first-episode genital herpes lesions within 6 weeks of the expected date of delivery or onset of pre-term labour (RCOG 2002). For women with recurrent genital herpes lesions at the time of delivery the risks to the baby of neonatal herpes are small therefore they should be weighed against the risks to the mother of caesarean section. Continuous acyclovir in the last 4 weeks of pregnancy may reduce the risk of clinical recurrence at term but there is insufficient evidence to recommend this practice routinely. It has been proposed that specific antibody testing be undertaken in the latter half of pregnancy in order to identify babies at risk of infection. However, it has been concluded that the low incidence of neonatal herpes in the UK would not make this a cost-effective measure.

Human cytomegalovirus

Human cytomegalovirus (HCMV) is a member of the herpes virus family and humans are the only reservoir. It is found universally throughout all geographic locations and in all socioeconomic groups (Ornoy & Diav-Citrin 2006). About 75% of pregnant women in developed countries are immune and about 1–4% of women acquire a primary infection in pregnancy (Herbert & Impey 2005). Most HCMV infections are asymptomatic. Primary infection may cause generally mild mononucleosis-type symptoms such as myalgia and fever in immunocompetent adults, whereas it is particularly pathogenic among immunosuppressed and immunodeficient individuals. Following primary infection HCMV persists for life as a latent infection with periodic viral shedding in saliva, breastmilk, urine, semen and cervical secretions (Sissons 2005). The source of maternal HCMV infection is therefore likely to be close contact with an asymptomatic child or sexual partner (Pass et al 2006).

HCMV infection in pregnancy

The most severe congenital infections are associated with a primary maternal infection during pregnancy. If contracted in early gestation, approximately 50% of fetuses will become infected, half of whom will have symptoms at birth. Babies born to mothers who are immune before pregnancy are rarely symptomatic or severely affected. If affected it is likely that a latent infection has been reactivated but it is also possible that the mother has been re-infected with a new virus strain. The congenital infection rate of babies to mothers with prior immunity is between 0.2 and 2% (Adler et al 2007).

The modes of transmission are incompletely understood but it is assumed that the fetus can be infected with HCMV transplacentally or during birth via cervical secretions or blood, and the neonate can be infected postnatally from breastmilk. Between 5% and 20% of babies with congenital HCMV are symptomatic at birth. The higher rates are associated with primary infection, particularly in the first trimester. The prognosis is poor with 80% likely to suffer serious neurological sequelae and psychomotor retardation. The majority of congenital infections are asymptomatic and only 5–15% subsequently develop sequelae on long term follow-up of which the commonest is sensorineural hearing impairment (Sissons 2005).

Diagnosis and treatment

HCMV infections can be diagnosed by a variety of methods. Maternal seroconversion of HCMV-IgG and IgM antibodies is highly accurate in the diagnosis of immunocompetent individuals in pregnancy. Fetal infection can be diagnosed by viral cultures or DNA analysis of amniotic fluid by PCR, or HCMV-IgM antibody activity in cord blood. Congenital infection can be diagnosed through isolation of the virus from urine, DNA analysis by PCR of urine, blood, saliva and CSF. The demonstration of IgM antibodies in the neonate is indicative of congenital infection (Malm & Engman 2007).

There are currently no vaccines available or prophylactic therapies to prevent the transmission of HCMV other than simple hygiene measures such as handwashing. Antenatal screening is thought to be inappropriate. In addition, there is no evidence to recommend the administration of antiviral treatments to neonates with congenital HCMV infection (Malm & Engman 2007, NICE 2003).

Human immunodeficiency virus

There are two types of human immunodeficiency virus (HIV) which belong to the lentivirus subfamily of retroviruses that cause AIDS (acquired immunodeficiency syndrome). HIV-1 is the cause of the world pandemic of AIDS, whereas HIV-2 is largely confined to West Africa. HIV is transmitted sexually, in blood, blood products and perinatally.

Two to six weeks after exposure to HIV, 50–70% of those infected develop a transient non-specific illness (primary infection or seroconversion illness) with fever, myalgia, malaise, lymphadenopathy, pharyngitis and a rash. This coincides with the development of serum antibodies to the core and surface proteins of the virus. The illness begins abruptly and usually lasts for 1–2 weeks but can be more protracted. Without antiretroviral therapy, seroconversion is followed by a clinically latent phase of about 10 years. During this period there is intense viral and lymphocyte turnover with worsening immunodeficiency. Approximately one-third of patients will experience persistent generalized lymphadenopathy. The average time for progression from HIV to AIDS is between 5 and 20 years (Luzzi et al 2005).

Diagnosis

Over 90% of seroconversions occur within 3 months of infection. In a minority of cases seroconversion may be delayed to more than 6 months. Therefore negative diagnostic tests need to be repeated 3 months after possible exposure and at 6–9 months where there has been a high risk of transmission. Following seroconversion, antibody persists indefinitely in the serum and forms a highly specific test for HIV infection (Luzzi et al 2005).

In the UK, several HIV antibody tests with high sensitivities and specificities are available. These include enzyme immunoassays (EIA) for screening, and PCR which can detect the viral RNA/DNA before antibodies become detectable (Smit 2006). Positive screening tests should be repeated before referral to a specialist laboratory for confirmation of the diagnosis.

Routine antenatal testing for HIV was introduced in the UK in 2000. Antenatal HIV antibody testing should be voluntary and subject to explicit informed consent. Evidence suggests that most women are now offered and accept the test (RCPCH 2006).

HIV in pregnancy

As the incidence of HIV infection in women increases so does the problem of vertical transmission. Worldwide, millions of children are infected primarily through mother-to-child transmission during pregnancy or breastfeeding (Volmink et al 2007). By the end of 2005, 1765 children aged <16 years when diagnosed with HIV had been reported in the UK, of which 82% were infected from their mother (HPA 2006). In 2004 the prevalence of HIV infection among pregnant women was greatest in London at 0.45% and 0.11% elsewhere in the UK. The rate reported for women born in sub-Saharan Africa was 2.2% compared with 0.07% for women born in the UK (RCPCH 2006).

HIV infection during pregnancy is associated with an increase in the risk of stillbirth, pre-term delivery and intrauterine growth restriction (Brocklehurst & French 1998). A systematic review of the literature suggested that pregnancy might have a small but detrimental effect on the progression of HIV infection (Brocklehurst & French 1998). The immunosuppressant effect of pregnancy may predispose the woman to opportunistic infections and confuse the clinical picture (Herbert & Impey 2005). Non-specific symptoms relatively common in pregnancy such as breathlessness, tiredness and nausea may lead to a delay in the detection and treatment of a serious problem, thus highlighting the importance of knowledge of HIV status in pregnancy.

Management and treatment of HIV in pregnancy

The incidence of vertical transmission can be significantly reduced if the mother is diagnosed antenatally. A systematic review of antiretroviral therapies for reducing the risk of vertical transmission of HIV confirmed that short treatment regimens are effective and that they are not associated with any safety concerns in the short term. Antiviral drugs include zidovudine, lamivudine and nevirapine. Regimens involve different combinations over different periods of time. They may be given to women antepartum, intrapartum and postpartum and prophylactically to babies. Highly active antiretroviral therapy (HAART) has reduced vertical transmission rates to around 1–2% in affluent countries but is not widely available in poorer ones (Volmink et al 2007).

HIV-positive women should be offered an elective caesarean section because it is an effective way of reducing vertical transmission among infected women not taking antiretrovirals or only taking zidovudine (NICE 2004; Read & Newell 2005). In the event of labour and vaginal birth the following high risk activities known to predispose to vertical transmission of HIV should be avoided: CTG monitoring through scalp clips, fetal blood sampling, prolonged membrane-rupture-delivery interval, episiotomy and instrumental delivery. Amniotomy is contraindicated (de Ruiter & Brocklehurst 1998).

In relation to the risk of vertical transmission in a mother with a low viral load, it is unclear whether a caesarean section is more or less effective than a vaginal birth (Read & Newell 2005).

Breastfeeding contributes significantly to vertical transmission of HIV. It is therefore recommended that breastfeeding be avoided if safe and affordable alternatives are available. The midwife has an important duty to provide women with information about the risks of breastfeeding and help them to choose what is appropriate for them (DH 2004b). It is possible that in many developing countries the high expense and rates of infant morbidity and mortality associated with alternative feeding methods outweigh the benefits of reduced vertical transmission. Babies born to infected mothers are likely to have maternal HIV antibody. A specific test such as PCR can confirm HIV infection in 95% of infected infants by 1 month of age (Luzzi et al 2005).

HIV testing and counselling in pregnancy

The provision of pre- and post-test information, counselling and support for pregnant women is vitally important and should be undertaken by specialist counsellors or midwives who have received appropriate training (RCM 1998). Issues for discussion include the client's risk of HIV infection, the likelihood and meaning of positive, negative and indeterminate results, confidentiality and the difference between HIV (the virus) and AIDS (the clinical condition). The impact that the diagnosis of HIV may have on a pregnant woman must be appreciated. It is important that adequate time is allowed to handle emotional distress and provide an opportunity for questions. Issues for discussion include the natural history of the infection, treatment options and safe sex to avoid transmission to an HIV negative partner(s) and acquisition of other STIs.

A pregnant woman who is diagnosed with HIV infection should be managed and treated by the appropriate specialist teams. It is recommended that every maternity unit should have an appropriately trained multidisciplinary team to manage HIV in pregnancy (RCPCH 2006). Women should be encouraged to allow disclosure of their diagnosis to the primary care team in order to avoid conflicting advice and to ensure they receive appropriate information.

Conclusion

The health, social and economic consequences associated with HIV and other STIs are considerable. They constitute a major worldwide public health problem and their control represents a serious challenge for health professionals. The midwife has a particular role to play in the sexual health of pregnant women and the effect on their babies. Health education about the transmission of STIs, sexual behaviour and attitudes, and safe sexual practice is a primary prevention strategy. Screening programmes leading to early diagnosis and treatment of infections, together with the tracing and treatment of sexual contacts, form important aspects of secondary prevention.

REFERENCES

Adams E J, Charlett A, Edmunds W J et al G 2004 Chlamydia trachomatis in the United Kingdom: a systematic review and analysis of prevalence studies. Sexually Transmitted Infections 80:354–362

Adler M 2004 Genital growths. In: Adler M W, Cowen F, French P et al 2004 ABC of sexually transmitted infections, 5th edn. BMJ Books, London, p 56–59

Adler M, French P 2004 Syphilis-clinical features, diagnosis and management. In: Adler M W, Cowen F, French P et al 2004 ABC of sexually transmitted infections, 5th edn. BMJ Books, London, p 49–55

Adler S P, Nigro G, Pereira L 2007 Recent advances in the prevention and treatment of congenital cytomegalovirus infections. Seminars in Perinatology d.o.i.:10.1053/j. semperi.2007.01.002

Amsel R, Totten P A, Spiegel C A et al 1983 Diagnostic criteria and microbial and epidemiologic associations. American Journal of Medicine 74(1):14–22

Barton S, Brown D, Cowan F M et al 2001 National guideline for the management of genital herpes. Clinical Effectiveness Group, British Association for Sexual Health and HIV Online. Available: http://www.bashh.org

Bignell C 2005 National guideline on the diagnosis and treatment of gonorrhoea in adults. Clinical Effectiveness Group, British Association for Sexual Health and HIV. Online. Available: http://www.bashh.org

Bignell C, Ison C A, Jungmann E 2006 Gonorrhoea. Sexually Transmitted Infections 82(Suppl IV):iv6–iv9.doi:10.1136/ sti.2006.023036

Brocklehurst P, French R 1998 The association between maternal HIV infection and perinatal outcome: a systematic review of the literature and meta-analysis. British Journal of Obstetrics and Gynaecology 105:836–848

Brocklehurst P, Rooney G 2000 Interventions for treating genital chlamydia trachomatis infection in pregnancy. Cochrane Database of Systematic Reviews 2000(2): CD000054

Brook G 2005 United Kingdom National guideline on the management of the viral hepatitides A, B & C. Clinical Effectiveness Group, British Association for Sexual Health and HIV Online. Available: http://www.bashh.org

Cadman L 2006 Human papillomavirus. Practice Nursing 17 (2):393–395

Chippindale S, French L 2001 HIV counselling and the psychosocial management of patients with HIV or AIDS. British Medical Journal 322:1533–1535

Cunningham S D, Tschann J, Gurvey J E et al 2002 Attitudes about sexual disclosure and perceptions of stigma and shame. Sexually Transmitted Infections 78:334–338

Daniels D, Forster G 2002 National Guideline on the management of vulvovaginal candidiasis. Clinical Effectiveness Group, British Association for Sexual Health and HIV. Online. Available: http://www.bashh.org

de Ruiter A, Brocklehurst P 1998 HIV infection and pregnancy. International Journal of STD & AIDS 9:647–655

Department of Health 2001 The national strategy for sexual health and HIV. HMSO, London

Department of Health 2002 The national strategy for sexual health and HIV: Implementation Action Plan. DH, London

Department of Health 2003 Effective sexual health: a toolkit for primary care trusts and others working in the field of providing good sexual health and HIV prevention. HMSO, London

Department of Health 2004a Choosing health: making healthier choices easier. HMSO, London

Department of Health 2004b HIV and infant feeding: Guidance from the UK Chief Medical Officers' Expert Advisory Group on AIDS. HMSO, London

Dimond B 2002 Legal aspects of midwifery, 2nd edn. Books for Midwives, Edinburgh, p 139–161

Doroshenko A, Sherrard J, Pollard A J 2006 Syphilis in pregnancy and the neonatal period. International Journal of STD & AIDS 17(4):221–226

Ellis S, Barnett-Page E, Morgan A et al (2003) HIV prevention: a review of reviews assessing the effectiveness of interventions to reduce the risk of sexual transmission. Health Development Agency, London

Feldman R G 2001 Group B streptococcus prevention of infection in the newborn. Practising Midwife 4:16–18

Fischler B 2007 Hepatitis C virus infection. Seminars in Fetal and Neonatal Medicine doi:10.1016/j.siny.2007.01.008

Fletcher J, Ball G 2006 Chlamydia screening in pregnancy: A missed opportunity? British Journal of Midwifery 14 (7):390–392

Flynn C A, Helwig A L, Meurer L N 1999 Bacterial vaginosis in pregnancy and the risk of prematurity: a meta-analysis. Journal of Family Practice 48:885–892

French P 2004 The clinical process. In: Adler M W, Cowen F, French P et al 2004 ABC of sexually transmitted infections, 5th edn. BMJ Books, London, p 11–14

French P 2007 Syphilis. British Medical Journal 334:143–147

Genç M, Ledger W J 2000 Syphilis in pregnancy. Sexually Transmitted Infections 76:70–73

Geretti A M 2006 Genital herpes. Sexually Transmitted Infections 82(Suppl IV):iv31–iv34.doi:10.1136/sti.2006.023200

Gilson R 2004 Viral hepatitis. In: Adler M W, Cowen F, French P et al 2004 ABC of sexually transmitted infections, 5th edn. BMJ Books, London, p 62–67

Gilson R, Brook M G 2006 Hepatitis A, B, and C. Sexually Transmitted Infections 82(Suppl IV):iv35–iv39.d.o.i.:10.1136/sti.2006.023218

Goh B 2002 UK National guidelines on the management of early syphilis. Online. Clinical Effectiveness Group, British Association for Sexual Health and HIV. Online. Available: http://www.bashh.org

GRASP The Gonococcal Resistance to Antimicrobials Surveillance Programme – Annual Report 2004. Health Protection Agency, London. Online. Available: http://hpa.org.uk

Gülmezoglu A M (2002) Interventions for trichomoniasis in pregnancy. Cochrane Database of Systematic Reviews 2002, issue 3. Art. No: CD000220.d.o.i.:10.1002/14651858. Cd000220

Hay P 2006 National guideline for the management of bacterial vaginosis. Clinical Effectiveness Group, British Association for Sexual Health and HIV Online. Available: http://www.bashh.org

Hay R J 2005 Fungal infections. In: Warrell D, Cox T M, Firth J D (eds) 2005 Oxford textbook of medicine, 4th edn. Oxford University Press, Oxford, Vol. 1, p 689–703

Health Protection Agency 2006 A complex picture: HIV and other sexually transmitted infections in the United Kingdom. Health Protection Agency, Centre for Infections, London

Herbert M, Impey L (2005) Infections in pregnancy. In: Warrell D, Cox T M, Firth J D (eds) 2005 Oxford Textbook of Medicine, 4th edn. Oxford University Press, Oxford, Vol. 2, p 449–455

Holmes K K, Sparling P F, Mårdh P A et al 1999 Sexually transmitted diseases, 3rd edn. McGraw-Hill, New York

Horner P J, Boag F 2006 UK National guideline for the management of genital tract infection with chlamydia trachomatis. Clinical Effectiveness Group, British Association for Sexual Health and HIV. Online. Available: http://www.bashh.org

House of Commons Health Committee 2003 Sexual health. Third Report of Session 2002–3, Vol. 1. HMSO, London

Ison C A, Hay P E 2002 Validation of a simplified grading of Gram-stained vaginal smears for use in genitourinary medicine clinics. Sexually Transmitted Infections 78 (6):413–415

Johnson A M, Mercer D C, Erens B et al (2001) Sexual behaviour in Britain: partnerships, practices, and HIV risk behaviours. Lancet 358(9296):1835–1842

Khare M M 2005 Infectious disease in pregnancy. Current Obstetrics and Gynaecology 15:149–56

Lee C, Gong Y, Brok J et al 2006 Hepatitis B immunization for newborn infants of hepatitis B surface antigen-positive mothers. Cochrane Database of Systematic Reviews 2006, issue 2, Art. No: CD004790.d.o.i.10.1002/14651858. CD004790.pub2

Luzzi G A, Teto T E A, Weiss R et al 2005 HIV and AIDS. In: D, Cox T M, Firth J D (eds) 2005 Oxford Textbook of Medicine, 4th edn. Oxford University Press, Oxford, 1: p 423–442

Mabey D, Ackers J, Adu-Sarkodie Y (2006) Trichomonas vaginalis infection. Sexually Transmitted Infections 82(Suppl IV): iv26–iv27

Maissi E, Marteau T M, Hankins M et al 2004 Psychological impact of human papillomavirus testing in women with borderline or mildly dyskaryotic cervical smear test results: cross sectional questionnaire study. British Medical Journal 328:1293

Malm G, Engman M L 2007 Congenital cytomegalovirus infections. Seminars in Fetal & Neonatal Medicine doi:10.1016/j.siny.2007.01.012

Maw R 2006 Anogenital warts. Sexually Transmitted Infections 82(Suppl IV):iv40–iv41.d.o.i. 10.1136/sti.2006.023226

McCaffery K, Waller J, Nazroo J et al 2006 Social and psychological impact of HPV testing in cervical screening: a qualitative study. Sexually Transmitted Infections 82:169–174

McDonald H M, Brocklehurst P, Gordon A 2007 Antibiotics for treating bacterial vaginosis in pregnancy. Cochrane Database of Systematic Reviews 2007, Issue 1. Art. No. CD000262d.o.i.10.1002/14651858.CD000262.pub3

Mitchell H 2004 Sexually transmitted infections in pregnancy. In: Adler M W, Cowen F, French P et al 2004 ABC of sexually transmitted infections, 5th edn. BMJ Books, London, p 34–38

National Institute for Health and Clinical Excellence 2003 Antenatal care: Routine care for the healthy pregnant woman. Clinical Guideline 6, NICE, London

National Institute for Health and Clinical Excellence 2004 Caesarean section, clinical guideline. RCOG Press, London

Oddie S, Embleton N D 2002 Risk factors for early onset neonatal group B streptococcal sepsis: case-control study. British Medical Journal 325:308–312

Ornoy A, Diav-Citrin O 2006 Fetal effects of primary and secondary cytomegalovirus infection in pregnancy. Reproductive Toxicology 21:399–409. Online. Available: http://www.sciencedirect.com

Pass R F, Fowler K B, Boppana S et al 2006 Congenital cytomegalovirus infection following first trimester maternal infection: Symptoms at birth and outcome. Journal of Clinical Virology 35:216–220

Peate I 2006 Nursing care and treatment of the patient with human papillomavirus. British Journal of Nursing 15 (19):1063–1069

Peate I 2005 Manual of sexually transmitted diseases. Whurr Publishers, London.

PHLS (Public Health Laboratory Service), DHSS&PS and the Scottish ISD(D)5 Collaborative Group 2000 Trends in sexually transmitted infections in the United Kingdom 1990–1999. PHLS, London

Read J S, Newell M L 2005 Efficacy and safety of caesarean delivery for prevention of mother-to-child transmission of HIV-1. Cochrane Database of Systematic Reviews 2005, (issue 4). Art. No. CD005479.d.o.i.10.10002/14651858.CD005479

Roberts E A, Yeung L 2002 Maternal-infant transmission of hepatitis C virus infection. Hepatology 36(5):107–113

Royal College of Midwives 1998 HIV & AIDS. Position paper 16a. RCM, London

Royal College of Obstetricians and Gynaecologists 2002 Management of genital herpes in pregnancy. Clinical guideline No. 30. RCOG, London

Royal College of Paediatrics and Child Health (RCPCH) 2006 Reducing mother to child transmission of HIV infection in the United Kingdom: Update Report of an Intercollegiate Working Party. RCPHC, London

Saloojee H, Velaphi S, Goga Y et al 2004 The prevention and management of congenital syphilis: an overview and recommendations. Bulletin of the World Health Organization 82 (6):424–432

Schachter J, Ridgeway G L, Collier L 1998 Chlamydia diseases. In: Hausler W J, Sussman M (eds) Topley and Wilson's microbiology and microbial infections. Arnold, London, Vol. 3, p 977–994

Schwebke J, Hillier S L 2005 Vaginal discharge. In: Warrell D, Cox T M, Firth J D (eds) 2005 Oxford Textbook of Medicine, 4th edn. Oxford University Press, Oxford, Vol. 3, p 486–488

Scoular A, Duncan B, Hart G 2001 'That sort of place...where filthy men go...' a qualitative study of women's perceptions of genitourinary medicine services. Sexually Transmitted Infections 77:340–343

Shankar M, Dutta R, Gkaras A et al 2006 Prevalence of *Chlamydia trachomatis* and bacterial vaginosis in women presenting to the early pregnancy unit. Journal of Obstetrics and Gynaecology 26(1):15–19

Sherrard J 2007 UK National Guideline on the Management of Trichomonas vaginalis, Clinical Effectiveness Group, British Association for Sexual Health and HIV. Online. Available: http://www.bashh.org

Simms I, Ward H 2006 Congenital syphilis in the United Kingdom. Sexually Transmitted Infections 82:1

Sissons J G P 2005 Herpes viruses. In: Warrell D, Cox T M, Firth J D (eds) 2005 Oxford Textbook of Medicine, 4th edn. Oxford University Press, Oxford, Vol. 1, p 327–341

Smaill F 2001 Intrapartum antibiotics for Group B streptococcal colonization. Cochrane Database of Systematic Reviews, issue 1. Art. No. CD000115.d.o.i.:10.1002/14651858.CD000115

Smit E J 2006 HIV. Sexually Transmitted Infections 82(Suppl IV):iv42–iv45.doi:10.1136/sti.2006.023234

Terence Higgins Trust 2001 Prejudice, Discrimination and HIV: A Report. Terence Higgins Trust

Thomas D L 2005 Hepatitis C virus. In: Warrell D, Cox T M, Firth J D (eds) 2005 Oxford Textbook of Medicine, 4th edn. Oxford University Press, Oxford, Vol. 1, p 419–423

Volmink J, Siegfried S, van der Merwe L et al 2007 Antiretrovirals for reducing the risk of mother-to-child transmission of HIV infection. Cochrane Database of Systematic Reviews 2007, issue 1. Art. No: CD003510.d.o.i.:10.102/14651858.CD003510.pub2

Vyse A J, Gay N J, Slomka M J et al 2000 The burden of infection with HSV-1 and HSV-2 in England and Wales: implications for the changing epidemiology of genital herpes. Sexually Transmitted Infections 76:183–187

Walker G J A 2001 Antibiotics for syphilis diagnosed during pregnancy Cochrane Database of Systematic Reviews, issue 3. Art. No: CD001143.d.o.i.:10.1002/14651853. CD001143

Walker D G, Walker G J A 2002 Forgotten but not gone: the continuing scourge of congenital syphilis. The Lancet Infectious Diseases 2:432–436

Winter G 2006 Syphilis: 'Cupid's disease' makes a comeback. Practice Nursing 17(12):611–614

Woodgate P, Flenady V, Steer P 2004 Intramuscular penicillin for the prevention of early onset group B streptococcal infection in newborn infants. Cochrane Database of Systematic Reviews 2004, issue 2. Art. No: DC003667.d.o.i.:10.1002/14651858.DC003667.pub2

Young G L, Jewell D 2001 Topical treatment for vaginal candidiasis in pregnancy (Cochrane review). In: The Cochrane Library, issue 3. Update Software, Oxford

FURTHER READING

This chapter has concentrated on sexually transmissible infections in pregnancy. The reader is directed to the following texts for more general detail about the presentation, diagnosis, treatment and management of these infections:

Adler M W, Cowen F, French P, Mitchell H, Richens J 2004 ABC of sexually transmitted infections, 5th edn. BMJ Books, London

Holmes K K, Sparling P F, Mårdh P A et al 1999 Sexually transmitted diseases, 3rd edn. McGraw-Hill, New York

24 Multiple pregnancy

Margie Davies

The term 'multiple pregnancy' is used to describe the development of more than one fetus *in utero* at the same time. Families expecting a multiple birth have different health needs, requiring extra practical support and understanding throughout pregnancy, the postnatal period and the early years. Information and support from well-informed health care professionals from the time the multiple pregnancy is diagnosed will help to prepare the parents and avoid potential problems.

The chapter aims to:

- describe how types of multiple pregnancy may be distinguished
- consider the diagnosis and management of twin pregnancy, the labour and the care of the mother and babies after birth
- give an overview of the problems particularly associated with twins and higher order births and the fetal anomalies unique to the twinning process
- explain the special needs of the parents and identify the sources of help available.

Incidence

The incidence of multiple births in the UK continues to rise; in 2006 there were 11,165 sets of twins born, that is 15.06/1000 (Table 24.1) or 1 in 66. In the 1940s and 1950s, the incidence was 1 in 80 but then fell to 1 in 104 in 1979 (Fig. 24.1). The full explanation for the fall is unknown. The current rise is probably due to the increased use of various kinds of treatments for infertility.

The number of triplets born more than trebled in the 15 years up to 2001 (Botting et al 1990). The highest number in any 1 year was 323 in 1998; this was due

Table 24.1 Multiple birth rates/1000 maternities 1995–2006

	1995	1996	1997	1998	1999	2000	2001	2002	2003	2004	2005	2006
England and Wales	14.10	13.80	14.50	14.40	14.46	14.68	14.77	15.00	14.82	15.02	14.91	15.29
Northern Ireland	14.1	13.3	13.7	13.3	14.95	14.98	15.65	15.43	14.41	15.25	13.56	13.71
Scotland	14.2	14.1	13.8	14.6	13.72	14.39	15.22	15.02	15.76	14.29	15.81	15.75
Whole of UK	14.10	13.80	14.40	14.40	14.42	14.67	14.83	15.02	14.88	14.97	14.94	15.28

Sources: Office of National Statistics London, General Register Office Northern Ireland, General Register Office Scotland.
Note: Figures include live and stillbirths.

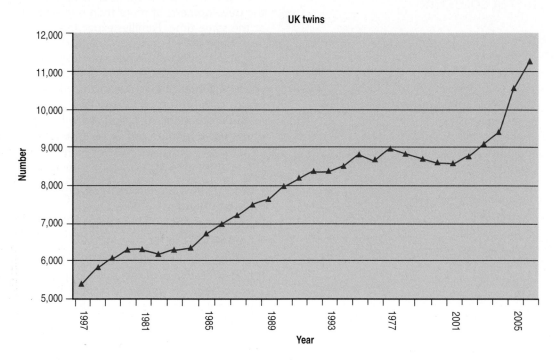

Figure 24.1   UK Twinning rates 1977–2006. (Data from Office of National Statistics.)

to the rise in treatments for infertility such as IVF and ovulation-stimulating drugs, like clomifene citrate and gonadotrophins. In 2006 there were 149 sets of triplets and seven sets of quadruplets born in the UK. The decrease in numbers is due to the code of practice now being to replace a maximum of two embryos in women under 40. The birth of triplets or more puts a considerable burden on the families, the health services and society (Mugford & Henderson 1995).

In other parts of the world the incidences are different: in West Africa, they are much higher and in Japan, much lower. Triplets in the UK occur in about 1 in 4500 pregnancies and quadruplets 1 in 700000.

Naturally occurring quadruplets and more are rare, but when IVF treatments were first introduced, with no limit to the number of embryos that could be replaced, the incidence of quintuplets, sextuplets and septuplets increased. Survival rates in such pregnancies, however, were poor.

The Human Fertilization & Embryo Authority (HFEA) Act 1990 requires all centres providing IVF, using donated gametes (egg and sperm) in treatment, storing gametes and using human embryos in research to be licensed by the HFEA. In 2004, 1854 sets of twin births and 23 triplets resulted from IVF and ICSI (HFEA 2006), giving a live multiple birth rate of 22.7. The HFEA code of practice states that in normal circumstances only two embryos should be replaced, but there is now discussion on whether this number should be further reduced to one (http://www.HFEA.gov.uk).

Twin pregnancy

Types of twin pregnancy

Twins will be either *monozygotic* (MZ) or *dizygotic* (DZ). Monozygotic or uniovular twins are also referred to as 'identical twins'. They develop from the fusion of one oocyte and one spermatozoon, which after fertilization splits into two. These twins will be of the same sex and have the same genes, blood groups and physical features, such as eye and hair colour, ear shapes and palm creases. However, they may be of different sizes and often have very different personalities and characters.

Dizygotic or binovular twins develop from two separate oocytes that are fertilized by two different spermatozoa, and are often referred to as 'non-identical twins'. They are no more alike than any brother or sister and can be of the same or different sex. Because in any pregnancy there is a 50:50 chance of a girl or boy, half of dizygotic twins will be boy-girl pairs. A quarter of dizygotic twins will be both boys and a quarter both girls. Of all twins born in the UK, two-thirds will be dizygotic and one-third monozygotic. Therefore, approximately one-third of twins are girls, one-third boys and one-third girl-boy pairs.

Superfecundation is the term used when twins are conceived from sperm from different men if a woman has had more than one partner during a menstrual cycle. It is not known how often this happens, but if suspected, then paternity can be checked by DNA testing (Terasaki et al 1978).

Superfetation is the term used for twins conceived as the result of two coital acts in different menstrual cycles. This is thought to be very rare (Rhine & Nance 1976).

Determination of zygosity and chorionicity

Midwives must understand the differences between the two terms (Table 24.2) and why it is important.

Table 24.2 Relationship between zygosity and chorionicity

Dichorionic	Monochorionic
Two placentae (may be fused)	One placenta
Two chorions	One chorion
Two amnions	Two amnions (one amnion in monoamniotic twins is very rare)
These twins can be either dizygotic or monozygotic	These twins can only be monozygotic

Determination of zygosity means determining whether or not the twins are monozygotic (identical) or dizygotic (non-identical). In about one-third of all twins born, it will be obvious as the children will be of a different sex. Of the remaining same-sex twins, zygosity will usually be apparent from physical features by the time the children are 2 years old, although parents are not usually prepared to wait this long. By the age of two, parents will know their children so well and see the differences in character and personalities that they find it difficult to believe they can be identical. At birth, monochorionic twins tend to have a greater weight variation than dichorionic ones. In approximately two-thirds of monozygotic twins, a monochorionic diamniotic placenta (MCDA) will confirm monozygosity. If the babies have a single outer membrane, the chorion, they must be monochorionic and so monozygotic (Fig. 24.2). In one-third of monozygotic twins, the placenta will have two chorions and two amnions (DCDA), and either fused placentae (Fig. 24.2C) or two separate placentae (dichorionic) (Fig. 24.2A), which is indistinguishable from the situation in dizygotic twins.

With monozygotic twins the type of placenta produced is determined by the time at which the fertilized oocyte splits:

- 0–4 days: dichorionic diamniotic placenta DCDA (approx. 33% – 1/3 cases) (Fig. 24.2A,C)
- 4–8 days: monochorionic diamniotic placenta MCDA (approx. 66% – 2/3 cases) (Fig. 24.2B)
- 8–12 days: monochorionic monoamniotic placenta MCMA (approx. 1% of cases) (Fig. 24.2D)

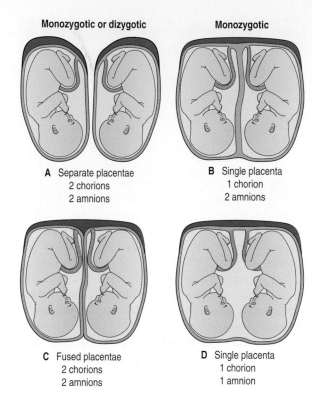

Monozygotic or dizygotic

A Separate placentae
2 chorions
2 amnions

C Fused placentae
2 chorions
2 amnions

Monozygotic

B Single placenta
1 chorion
2 amnions

D Single placenta
1 chorion
1 amnion

Figure 24.2 Placentation of twins. (After Bryan 1984, with permission of Edward Arnold.)

- 12–13 days: (very rare indeed) conjoined twins can develop when the division is incomplete (Bomsel-Helmreich & Mufti 2005).

Despite the well-established facts about placentation and zygosity, there is still misinformation given to parents who are told that if same-sex twins are dichorionic they must be non-identical, which of course is incorrect.

Chorionicity: why is it important to know?

This knowledge is important clinically because monochorionic twin pregnancies have a 3–5 times higher risk of perinatal mortality and morbidity than dichorionic twin pregnancies (Pasquini et al 2004).

Prenatally the chorionicity is determined by ultrasound examination. Preferably this should be performed during the first trimester, as the differences between the two types of placentation are more pronounced. The chorions forming the septum between the amniotic sacs can be seen more clearly in the first trimester of pregnancy. If the septum has a mean thickness of 2.4 mm or more, then it is usually a dichorionic twin pregnancy; if it is a thin septum with a mean thickness of 1.4 mm, then it is more likely to be a monochorionic pregnancy (Winn et al 1989).

Another method of determining chorionicity is by studying the septum at its base, adjacent to the placenta. A tongue of placental tissue is seen ultrasonically between the two chorions and this is termed the 'twin peak' (Finberg 1992) or 'lambda sign' (Kurtz et al 1992).

Zygosity determination after birth

The most accurate method of determining zygosity is to compare DNA. The DNA can be extracted from cells taken from a cheek swab from inside the mouth. Specific genetic markers extracted from different chromosomes are compared and the results are up to 99.99% accurate.

Zygosity determination should be routinely offered to all same-sex twins for the following reasons:

- Most parents will want to know whether or not their twins are identical, so they can answer the most commonly asked question: 'Are they identical?'; also as the twins get older they usually want to know.

- If parents are considering further pregnancies, they will want to know the risk of having twins again. DZ twins tend to run in families and the increased likelihood is approximately five-fold, usually on the female side though not in all cases. MZ twins do not run in families and the likelihood does not change (except in rare families who carry a dominant gene for monozygotic twinning). The chance of any fertile woman having MZ twins is approximately 1 in 350–400.

- It will help the twins in establishing their sense of identity; it will influence their life and family relationships.

- The information is important for genetic reasons, not just with monogenic disorders but with any serious illness later in life.

- Twins are frequently asked to be involved in research where knowledge of zygosity is essential.

Diagnosis of twin pregnancy

This is usually through ultrasound examination. Diagnosis can be made as early as 6 weeks into the pregnancy or later, and at the routine detailed structural scan between the 20th and 22nd weeks. When booking a woman in the antenatal clinic a family history of twins should alert the midwife to the possibility of a multiple pregnancy. If the pregnancy is diagnosed at 6 weeks, the woman should be told about 'vanishing twin syndrome' (Landy & Nies 1995). Occasionally one fetus may die in the second trimester and become a fetus papyraceous (Fig. 24.3), which then becomes embedded in the placenta and expelled with the placenta at delivery. This is very rare and probably occurs in 1 in 12 000 live births.

The news that a woman is expecting a multiple birth should be broken to the parents in a sensitive manner (Spillman 1985). As soon as a multiple pregnancy has been diagnosed, the mother must be given relevant information about the pregnancy, including telephone numbers of local and national support organizations (see Useful addresses, below). Many parents can spend weeks of unnecessary anxiety through ignorance of the help available (Spillman 1987).

Since the advent of routine ultrasound scanning, it is very rare for a woman to get to term with undiagnosed twins, but this will not apply in areas where this technology is unavailable, or where the mother declines.

Abdominal examination

Inspection

On inspection, the size of the uterus may be larger than expected for the period of gestation, particularly after the 20th week. The uterus may look broad or round and fetal movements may be seen over a wide area, although the findings are not diagnostic of twins. Fresh striae gravidarum may be apparent. Up to twice the amount of amniotic fluid is normal in a twin pregnancy but polyhydramnios is not an uncommon complication of a twin pregnancy, particularly with monochorionic twins.

Palpation

On palpation, the fundal height may be greater than expected for the period of gestation. The presence of two fetal poles (head or breech) in the fundus of the uterus may be revealed on palpation and multiple fetal limbs may also be palpable. The head may be small in relation to the size of the uterus and may suggest that the fetus is also small and that there may therefore be more than one present. Lateral palpation may reveal two fetal backs or limbs on both sides. Pelvic palpation may give findings similar to those on fundal palpation, although one fetus may lie behind the other and make detection difficult. Location of three poles in total is diagnostic of at least two fetuses.

Auscultation

Hearing two fetal hearts is not diagnostic as one can often be heard over a wide area in a singleton pregnancy. If simultaneous comparison of the heart rates reveals a difference of at least 10 b.p.m., it may be assumed that two hearts are being heard.

The pregnancy

A multiple pregnancy tends to be shorter than a single pregnancy. The average gestation for twins is 37 weeks, for triplets 34 weeks and for quadruplets, 33 weeks.

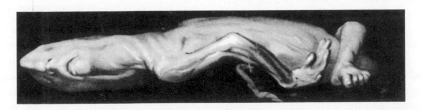

Figure 24.3   Fetus papyraceous.

Effects of pregnancy

Exacerbation of common disorders

The presence of more than one fetus *in utero* and the higher levels of circulating hormones often exacerbate the common disorders of pregnancy. Sickness, nausea and heartburn may be more persistent and more troublesome than in a singleton pregnancy.

Anaemia

Iron deficiency and folic acid deficiency anaemias are common in twin pregnancies. Early growth and development of the uterus and its contents make greater demands on the maternal iron stores; in later pregnancy (after the 28th week), fetal demands may lead to anaemia. Routine oral iron supplementation remains a controversial issue, research suggesting that iron and folic acid supplements prescribed routinely are not necessary; only mothers with evidence of significant anaemia should be treated (Mahomed 2000).

Polyhydramnios

This is also common and is particularly associated with monochorionic twins and with fetal abnormalities. Polyhydramnios will add to any discomfort that the woman is already experiencing. If acute polyhydramnios occurs, it can lead to miscarriage or premature labour.

Pressure symptoms

The increased weight and size of the uterus and its contents may be troublesome. Impaired venous return from the lower limbs increases the tendency to varicose veins and oedema of the legs. Backache is common and the increased uterine size may also lead to marked dyspnoea and indigestion.

Other

There can be an increase in complications of pregnancy (see Chs 20 and 22).

Antenatal screening

- The recommended method of screening is by measurement of the nuchal translucency, preferably in combination with biochemistry (UK National Screening Committee 2007).

- Nuchal translucency for Down syndrome is accurate only if performed between 11 and 13 weeks and 6 days.
- Chorionic villus sampling (CVS) is not usually recommended in multiple pregnancy as loss rates are high.
- Amniocentesis can be performed in twin pregnancies, usually between 15 and 20 weeks. It should be performed in a specialist fetal medicine unit. Most obstetricians prefer to do a dual needle insertion so there is no chance of contamination between the two sacs.
- Chorionicity should be determined in the first trimester.
- All monozygotic twins should have echocardiography performed at approximately 24 weeks' gestation, as there is a much higher risk of cardiac anomalies in these babies. In the UK at present the incidence is 32/1000.

Ultrasound examination

- Monochorionic twin pregnancies should be scanned every 2 weeks from diagnosis to check for discordant fetal growth and signs of twin-to-twin transfusion syndrome (TTTS). A cardiac anomaly scan should be performed at 24 weeks.
- Dichorionic twin pregnancies should be scanned at 20 weeks for anomalies, as with a singleton, and then usually every 4 weeks.

Antenatal preparation

Early diagnosis of a twin pregnancy and of chorionicity is extremely important in order to prepare the parents by giving them the specialist support and advice they will need.

Parent education

When a multiple pregnancy is diagnosed, written information on multiple pregnancy should be given to the mother. This should include contact phone numbers of any local support organizations, local twins club, the national twin organizations (see Useful addresses, below), and details of special parent education classes that may be available. The news they are expecting twins or more can come as a considerable shock and the midwife should give them the opportunity to discuss any worries or problems they may have, as two babies will add a considerable financial burden to any family's income (Leonard & Denton 2006).

Routine parent education classes should start earlier for twin mothers than for singleton mothers, ideally at 24–26 weeks' gestation or even earlier if a mother's work commitments allow. A specialist class for couples expecting a multiple birth should be offered at 28–30 weeks; usually one session is enough. In most Trusts these classes are held monthly, but a course of two or three held every 2 or 3 months may be preferred (Davies 1995). When planning these classes, contact with a local twins club can provide a valuable source of practical information. Mothers from twins clubs are usually delighted to participate in the classes and talk on the more practical issues such as coping with two or more babies, equipment and breastfeeding (Denton & Bryan 1995). Suggestions for class topics are listed in Box 24.1.

Preparation for breastfeeding

Mothers will inevitably give a lot of thought to how they are going to feed their babies, not only from the nutritional but also from the practical point of view,

---

Box 24.1 Topics for parent education classes

- Facts and figures on twins and twinning
- Diet and exercise
- Parental anxieties about obstetric complications
- Labour, pain relief and the birth
- Possibilities of premature labour and birth and the outcome
- Visit to the neonatal unit
- Breastfeeding and bottle-feeding
- Zygosity
- Equipment (prams and buggies, car seats, layette, etc.)
- Coping with newborn twins or more
- Development of twins including individuality and identity
- Sources of help.

Box 24.2 Support needed by the breastfeeding mother of twins or more

- Consistent professional advice
- Reassurance of her ability to produce enough milk to satisfy her babies
- Encouragement from professionals and family in her ability to cope with feeding two or more
- Support from her partner
- Help at home with household chores
- Help with older siblings
- A high calorie and high protein diet.

---

as feeding will take up a large amount of their time during the first 6 months. Mothers should be encouraged right from the beginning that it is not only possible to breastfeed two, and in some cases three babies, but it is the best way for her to feed her babies nutritionally and it can be a very rewarding experience for her as well (see Plates 24.1 and 24.2, p. 452, 453). Many sets of twins have been entirely breastfed, some beyond their first birthdays. Very few sets of triplets are totally breastfed (Fiducia 1995) but many manage to combine breast- and bottle-feeding very successfully.

Early in the antenatal period the mother should be given as much information and advice as possible about both breast- and bottle-feeding, so she can make an informed choice on how to feed her babies. Both parents should have the opportunity to ask questions and be encouraged to meet another mother who is successfully breastfeeding her babies (Box 24.2). Introductions can usually be made through a local twins group.

Labour and the birth

Onset

The more fetuses the mother is carrying, the earlier labour is likely to start. Term for twins is usually considered to be 37 weeks rather than 40, and approximately 50% of twins are born pre-term, that is before 37 weeks' gestation. In addition to being pre-term, the babies may be small for gestational age and therefore prone to the associated complications of both conditions. If spontaneous labour begins very early, the chances of survival outside the uterus are small and the mother will usually be given drugs to inhibit uterine activity. Intravenous salbutamol and sulindac tablets are the drugs most commonly used. Known causes of pre-term labour must, if at all possible, be diagnosed and treated quickly, for example urinary tract infection should be treated with antibiotics.

It is very unusual for a twin pregnancy to last more than 40 weeks; many obstetricians advise induction of labour at 38 weeks. If the first twin is in a cephalic presentation, labour is usually allowed to continue normally to a vaginal birth, but if the first twin is presenting in any other way (Fig. 24.4), an elective caesarean section is usually recommended. The

incidence of caesarean sections is approximately 60% with a twin pregnancy (RCOG 2001). More monochorionic twin pregnancies are now being delivered by elective caesarean section due to the risks of TTTS and premature separation of placenta before the birth of the second twin.

Management of labour

During the antenatal classes the mother must be warned that a multiple birth is less common and, for educational purposes, a number of people may ask to observe the birth. If the mother has any objection to this, her wishes must be respected and a record made in her notes that she wants only those concerned with her care to be present.

Induction of labour usually occurs around 38 weeks' gestation for DCDA twins (Box 24.3) and

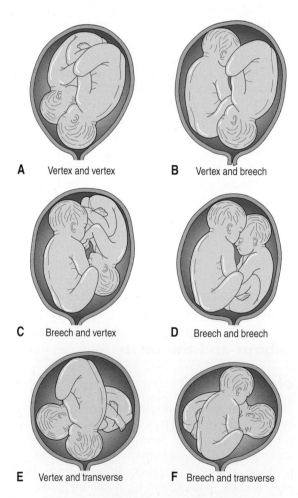

A Vertex and vertex   **B** Vertex and breech

C Breech and vertex   **D** Breech and breech

E Vertex and transverse   **F** Breech and transverse

Figure 24.4 Presentation of twins before birth. (After Bryan 1984, with permission of Edward Arnold.)

> **Box 24.3** Case history 1
>
> A 34-year-old para 1 was diagnosed with DCDA twins, no family history, so it was a complete shock. At the ultrasound department, a leaflet with local twin organizations and contacts was given to the mother. Through the hospital specialist, multiple birth midwife and twins club, the mother started to come to terms with the prospect of twins. She knew she was expecting two boys and began to wonder if they were identical or not, but would have to wait until they were born and have DNA tests if they looked alike. She had a straightforward birth with her first child, so she was keen to have a vaginal birth again, but felt there was pressure on her to have an elective caesarean section. The pregnancy progressed normally and with support from the specialist midwife, she wrote her birth plan. The presenting baby was cephalic, and at 38 weeks labour was induced. The woman had an epidural and progressed to birth both babies vaginally after a short labour. Both babies were put to her breast in the labour suite; twin one sucked well but twin two was not interested. As establishing feeding was more problematic than she expected and she felt she needed a lot of help from the midwives, she stayed in hospital until day 5. Both babies were sucking well on return home, although twin two did occasionally need a 'top up' from the bottle.

36–37 weeks for MCDA twins (RCOG 2006). The presence of complications such as pregnancy-induced hypertension, intrauterine growth restriction or twin-to-twin transfusion syndrome may be reasons for earlier induction.

The majority of women expecting twins will go into labour spontaneously. Theoretically the duration of the first stage of labour should be no different from that of a single pregnancy. However, there is an increased incidence of dysfunctional labour in twin pregnancies, possibly because of over-distension of the uterus.

Labour in the mother of twins must be recognized as high risk and continuous fetal heart monitoring of both fetuses is advocated. This can be achieved either with two external transducers or, once the membranes are ruptured, a scalp electrode on the presenting twin and an external transducer on the second. If a 'twin monitor' is available, both heartbeats can be monitored simultaneously to give a more reliable reading. Uterine activity will also need to be monitored.

If cardiotocography is not available, use of the Doptone or Sonicaid may give more accurate recordings of the fetal heart rates than a fetal stethoscope. If the latter has to be used, two people must auscultate simultaneously, so that fetal heart rates are counted over the same minute.

While in labour, the mother should be encouraged to adopt whichever position she finds most comfortable. A foam rubber wedge under the side of the mattress will help to prevent supine hypotensive syndrome by giving a lateral tilt. It may be preferable for her to adopt a semiprone position, well supported by pillows or a beanbag. A birthing chair or a reclining chair, if available, may be more comfortable than a conventional labour ward bed.

Regional epidural block provides excellent analgesia and, if necessary, allows easier instrumental deliveries and also manipulation of the second twin. The use of Entonox analgesia may be helpful, either before the epidural is *in situ* or during the second stage, if the effect of the epidural is wearing off.

The mother should be encouraged to use whatever form of relaxation she finds helpful. If she chooses to use drugs only after other methods have failed, her wishes should be respected. The midwife should explain that, if complications arise, intervention and the use of drugs may be necessary. This should be discussed long before the onset of labour.

If fetal compromise occurs during labour, the birth will need to be expedited, usually by caesarean section. Action may also need to be taken if the mother's condition gives cause for concern.

If uterine activity is poor, the use of intravenous oxytocin may be required once the membranes have been ruptured. Artificial rupture of the membranes may be sufficient to stimulate good uterine activity but may need to be used in conjunction with intravenous oxytocin. The cardiotocograph will give a good indication of the pattern of uterine activity, whether the labour is induced or spontaneous. The response of the fetal hearts to uterine contractions can be observed on the graph paper.

If the babies are expected to be premature, and of low birth weight, or known to have any other problems, the neonatal unit must be informed that the woman is in labour so they can make the necessary preparations to receive the babies. When the delivery is imminent, the paediatric team should be summoned.

Throughout labour, the emotional and general physical condition of the mother must be considered. She requires support from her midwife and may be apprehensive about the delivery. The presence of her partner or companion will be helpful and the midwife should encourage her to ask questions and express her feelings.

Management of the birth

The onset of the second stage of labour should be confirmed by a vaginal examination. The obstetrician, paediatric team and anaesthetist should be present for the birth as there is a risk of complications.

If epidural analgesia has been used it may be 'topped up' prior to the birth. The possibility of emergency caesarean section is ever present and the operating theatre should be ready to receive the mother at short notice. Monitoring of both fetal hearts should continue until birth. Provided that the first twin is presenting by the vertex, the birth can be expected to proceed normally, as with a singleton pregnancy. When the first twin is born, the time of birth and the sex are noted. This baby and cord must be labelled as 'twin one' immediately. The identity bracelets should be checked with the mother or father before they are applied to the infant's wrist and ankle. The baby may be put to the breast as sucking stimulates uterine contractions.

After the birth of the first twin, abdominal palpation is made to ascertain the lie, presentation and position of the second twin and to auscultate the fetal heart. If the lie is not longitudinal, an attempt may be made to correct it by external cephalic version (see Ch. 31). If it is longitudinal, a vaginal examination is made to confirm the presentation. If the presenting part is not engaged it should be pushed into the pelvis by fundal pressure before the second sac of membranes is ruptured. The fetal heart must be auscultated again and a scalp electrode applied once the membranes are ruptured. If uterine activity does not recommence, intravenous oxytocin may be used to stimulate it.

When the presenting part becomes visible, the mother should be encouraged to push with contractions to birth the second twin. The midwife should be aware that, owing to the reduced size of the placental site following the birth of the first twin, the second fetus may be deprived of oxygen. The birth will proceed as normal if the presentation is vertex, but if the fetus presents by the breech and the midwife is not experienced in breech births she may need a doctor's assistance.

The birth of the second twin should ideally be completed within 45 min of the first twin but, as long as there are no signs of fetal distress in the second twin, it may be allowed to continue longer; if there are, the delivery must be expedited and the second twin may need to be born by caesarean section. A uterotonic drug (usually Syntocinon or Syntometrine) is usually given intramuscularly or intravenously, depending on local policy, after the birth of the anterior shoulder as with a singleton pregnancy. This baby and cord are labelled as 'twin two'. The time of birth and sex of child must be noted. The risk of asphyxia is greater for the second twin and the paediatric team may need to actively resuscitate this infant. If so, he may need to be transferred to the neonatal unit for observation, in which case his mother should have a chance to see him first and, if at all possible be allowed a cuddle with him.

Once the uterotonic drug has taken effect, controlled cord traction is applied to both cords simultaneously and the placentae delivered without delay. Emptying the uterus enables bleeding to be controlled and postpartum haemorrhage prevented.

The placenta(e) should be examined and the number of amniotic sacs, chorions and placentae noted (Fig. 24.2). If the babies are of different sexes, they are dizygotic. If the placenta is monochorionic (MCDA), they must be monozygotic. If they are of the same sex and the placenta is dichorionic (DCDA), then further tests will be needed (see above).

The umbilical cords should also be examined and the number of cord vessels and the presence of any abnormalities noted.

Complications associated with multiple pregnancy

The higher perinatal mortality associated with twinning is largely due to complications of pregnancy, such as the premature onset of labour, intrauterine growth restriction and complications at birth. The management of multiple pregnancy is concerned with the prevention, early detection and treatment of these complications.

Polyhydramnios

Acute polyhydramnios may occur as early as 16 weeks. It may be associated with fetal abnormality but is more likely to be due to TTTS, which can also be known as fetofetal transfusion syndrome (FFTS).

Twin-to-twin transfusion syndrome

Twin-to-twin transfusion syndrome (TTTS) can be acute or chronic. The acute form usually occurs during labour and is the result of blood transfusing from one fetus (donor) to the other (recipient) through vascular anastomosis in a monochorionic placenta. Both fetuses may die of cardiac failure if not treated urgently.

Chronic TTTS occurs in about 15% of monochorionic twin pregnancies (Dennes et al 2006) and accounts for 15% of perinatal mortality in twins (Yamamoto & Ville 2006). The placenta in TTTS transfuses blood from one twin fetus to the other. These cases are characterized by one or more deep unidirectional arteriovenous anastomoses. This results in anaemia and growth restriction in the donor twin (the term 'stuck twin' may be used) and polycythaemia with circulatory overload in the recipient twin (hydrops). The fetal and neonatal mortality is high but infants may be saved by early diagnosis and prenatal treatment with either amnioreduction, which may have to be repeated regularly as fluid can reaccumulate rapidly (Box 24.4), or laser ablation therapy of communicating placental vessels, or septostomy (MBF Monochorionic Pregnancy booklet 2008).

The midwife should always be alerted to the mother who complains of a rapid increase in her abdominal girth in the second trimester, as well as a uterus that feels hard and uncomfortable continuously. This may be due to polyhydramnios and if not treated urgently can cause premature labour. This usually occurs in women who have a monochorionic pregnancy.

Fetal abnormality

This is particularly associated with monochorionic twins.

Conjoined twins

This extremely rare malformation of monozygotic twinning results from the incomplete division of the fertilized oocyte; it occurs once in 50 000 births and over half the cases are stillborn. Delivery has to be by caesarean section. Separation of the babies is sometimes possible and will depend on how they are joined and which internal organs are involved. The site and extent of fusion of the fetuses are infinitely variable. Thoracopagus is the commonest form of fusion (over 70% of cases). The feasibility of separating conjoined twins depends on the site and extent of fusion and the degree to which organs are shared (Creinin 1995). Many conjoined twins can now be successfully separated. Others pose major ethical dilemmas – particularly if one can be saved at the expense of the other (Mifflin 2001).

Twin reversed arterial perfusion

Twin reversed arterial perfusion (TRAP) occurs in about 1 in 30000 births. In TRAP, one twin presents without a well-defined cardiac structure and is kept alive through placental anastomoses to the circulatory system of the viable fetus (Sebire & Sepulveda 2006).

Fetus-in-fetu

In fetus-in-fetu (endoparasite), parts of a fetus may be lodged within another fetus; this can happen only in MZ twins (Eng et al 1989).

Malpresentations

Although the uterus is large and distended, the fetuses are less mobile than may be supposed. They can restrict each other's movements, which may result in malpresentations, particularly of the second twin. After the birth of the first twin, the presentation of the second twin may change.

Box 24.4 Case history 2

A 26-year-old primigravida's early scan showed MCDA twins. The mother read on the Internet that problems can be associated with MCDA pregnancy and was very worried about TTTS.

From 16 weeks, she had 2-weekly scans for signs of TTTS and growth discordancy. At 22 weeks, she noticed a rapid increase in abdominal size and her tummy was hard and uncomfortable. Her local hospital referred her to the Centre for Fetal Care (CFC) at a tertiary level hospital, where type 2 TTTS was diagnosed. Immediate treatment was amnioreduction of over 2L and care transferred to CFC for weekly scans. Here she saw mainly doctors and felt she missed out on midwife contact. Regular amnioreductions were needed. At 32 weeks TTTS was diagnosed as type 3, with very abnormal Dopplers in the donor twin. Steroid injections were given and an emergency caesarean section was performed at 33 weeks. Both babies were born in a fair condition and were admitted to the NNU. The mother was encouraged to hand express her milk as soon as she felt well enough, to continue 2–3-hourly during the day and on 6th day she started expressing using an electric pump. The twins were able to go to the breast after 2 weeks and started sucking for very short periods. Progress continued and both babies were discharged home at 5 weeks of age, fully breastfeeding.

Premature rupture of the membranes

Malpresentations due to polyhydramnios may predispose to pre-term rupture of the membranes.

Prolapse of the cord

This, too, is associated with malpresentations and polyhydramnios and is more likely if there is a poorly fitting presenting part. The second twin is particularly at risk of cord prolapse.

Prolonged labour

Malpresentations are a poor stimulus to good uterine action and a distended uterus is likely to lead to poor uterine activity and consequently prolonged labour.

Monoamniotic twins

Approximately 1% of twins share the same sac. Monoamniotic (MCMA) twins risk cord entanglement with occlusion of the blood supply through the umbilical cords to one or both fetuses. These can be treated with sulindac taken by the mother to reduce amniotic fluid levels and are usually delivered at around 32–34 weeks and by elective caesarean section.

Locked twins

This is a very rare but serious complication of twin pregnancy. There are two types. One occurs when the first twin presents by the breech and the second by the vertex; the other when both are vertex presentations (Fig. 24.5). In both instances, the head of the second twin prevents the continued descent of the first. Primigravidae are more at risk than multiparous women.

Delay in the birth of the second twin

After the birth of the first twin, uterine activity should recommence within 5min. Ideally the birth of the second twin should be completed within 45min of the first twin being born but with close monitoring can be extended if there are no signs of fetal compromise. Poor uterine action as a result of malpresentation may be the cause of delay. The risks of such delay are intrauterine hypoxia, birth asphyxia following premature separation of the placenta and sepsis as a result of ascending infection from the first umbilical cord, which lies outside the vulva. After the birth of the first twin the lower uterine segment begins to reform and the cervical canal may have to dilate fully again.

The midwife may need to 'rub up' a contraction and put the first twin to the breast to stimulate uterine activity. If there appears to be an obstruction, medical aid is summoned and a caesarean section may be necessary. If there is no obstruction, oxytocin infusion may be commenced or forceps delivery considered.

Premature expulsion of the placenta

The placenta may be expelled before the birth of the second twin. In dichorionic twins with separate placentae, one placenta may be delivered separately; in monochorionic twins the shared placenta may be expelled. The risks of severe asphyxia and death of

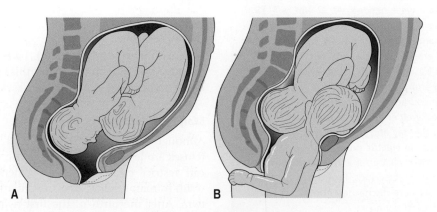

Figure 24.5 Locked twins.

the second twin are very high. Haemorrhage is also likely if one twin is retained *in utero* as this prevents adequate retraction of the placental site.

Postpartum haemorrhage

Poor uterine tone as a result of overdistension or hypotonic activity is likely to lead to postpartum haemorrhage. There is also a much larger placental site to contract down.

Undiagnosed twins

The possibility of an unexpected, undiagnosed second baby (though this is unlikely with ultrasound scanning) should be considered if the uterus appears larger than expected after the birth of the first baby or if the baby is surprisingly smaller than expected. If an uterotonic drug has been given after the birth of the anterior shoulder of the first baby, the second baby is in great danger of birth asphyxia and his birth should be expedited. The midwife must break the news of undiagnosed twins gently to the parents. These parents will require special support and guidance during the postnatal period.

Delayed interval delivery of the second twin

There have been several reported cases where the first twin has been born, often very prematurely, and there has been a long gap before labour recommences; it can be days or even weeks before the second twin is born (Zhang et al 2004). This opportunity can be used to give betamethasone to the mother to help mature the lungs of the second twin. Careful observations of the mother's condition must be made during this time for signs of infection and fetal compromise. The mother will need additional support from the midwives to cope with her anxieties for her premature baby on the NNU, which may not survive, or time to grieve if the baby has died, as well as still being pregnant and her concerns for the outcome of her pregnancy.

Postnatal period

Care of the babies

Immediate care after the birth is the same as for a single baby. Maintenance of body temperature is vital, particularly if the babies are small; use of overhead heaters will help to prevent heat loss. Identification of the babies should be clear and the parents given the opportunity to check the identity bracelets and cuddle them. The babies may need to be admitted directly to the neonatal unit (NNU) from the labour suite, in which case the father should accompany them; otherwise they will be transferred to the postnatal ward with their mother.

Temperature control

Maintenance of a thermoneutral environment is essential, particularly for babies in the neonatal unit. American studies have shown that a sick baby can benefit from sharing the incubator with his twin (Hedberg Nyquist & Lutes 1998). Clothing should be light but warm and allow air to circulate.

Nutrition

The mother may choose to feed her babies by breast or with formula milk but whatever her choice, the midwife must support her in her decision. With breastfeeding both babies may be breastfed separately or simultaneously. In the immediate postnatal days, it is recommended the mother breastfeeds her twins separately, as this gives her time to get to know each baby and to feel confident in her ability to cope. If the babies are small for gestational age or pre-term, the paediatricians may recommend that the babies be 'topped up' after a breastfeed. Expressed breastmilk is best for these babies. If the babies are not able to suck adequately at the breast the mother should be encouraged to express her milk regularly. If she does not have sufficient milk for them, milk from a human milk bank can be used; this is preferable for pre-term babies, (Lucas & Cole 1990) and reduces the risk of necrotizing enterocolitis (NEC) (Beeby & Jeffrey 1992). As twin babies are more likely to be pre-term or small for gestational age, their ability to coordinate the sucking and swallowing reflexes may be poor. If so, they may need to be fed intravenously or by nasogastric tube, or cup-fed (Lang 1995), depending on their size and general condition. The mother should be encouraged to participate in whatever method is used. Careful monitoring of weight gain is required. Hypoglycaemia may occur and regular capillary blood glucose estimations may be needed.

In the early postnatal days, mothers may worry that their milk supply is inadequate for two babies, the midwife should reassure her that lactation responds to the demands made by the babies sucking at the breast. The more stimulation the breasts are given, the more plentiful is the milk supply. At feeding times, the midwife must be with the mother to offer support and advice on positioning and fixing the babies (Fig. 24.6), as well as encouraging her in her ability to breastfeed two babies.

Breastfeeding

The advantages of breastfeeding are the same as for single babies, but as twins have a higher tendency to be born prematurely and small for gestational age, it is even more important that they should be

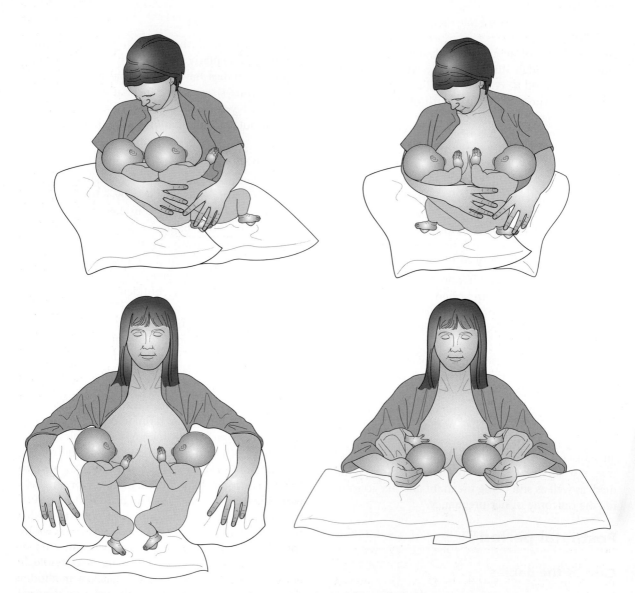

Figure 24.6 Breastfeeding positions for twins.

breastfed. As well as the medical and nutritional advantages, there are practical reasons too:

- It is cheaper, and breastmilk is available 24 hrs a day at the correct temperature.
- There are no bottles to wash, no sterilizing to organize or feeds to make up, all of which take time. Time is limited for a mother of twins in the early days.
- Twins can be breastfed together or separately. If the babies are to be fed together, then the feeds will take only a little longer than with a single baby.

The mother must be encouraged to be organized before she starts feeding. The ideal place to sit is either in bed or on a sofa, so there is room to put the babies down while getting ready. In the early days a mother will need help to position the babies. If she wants to feed them both together, it is advisable to try this before being transferred home from hospital, so that the midwife can stay with her throughout the entire feed, providing advice, support and another pair of hands.

Using pillows to support the babies, the mother is able to get herself into a comfortable sitting position (Fig. 24.6). She will need to have plenty of pillows to take the weight of the babies, so not putting stain on her arms or back causing her pain.

Mothers of twins always complain that there is never enough time for cuddling; breastfeeding together is the only way for her to hold and feed both babies together at the same time.

The main advantage of bottle-feeding is that someone else can always help, although this can be done with expressed breastmilk.

Routine is the key to coping with two or more babies. It may take 4–6 weeks for a feeding routine to get established (MBF Feeding booklet 2006).

Mother–baby relationships

Mothers who have a multiple birth often find it more difficult to bond with both babies equally. This is quite common and reassurance that their feelings are not unusual should be given. Very quickly this changes as they get to know their babies. If, for example, they are of markedly different sizes, a mother may favour one over the other, or if one baby is in the neonatal unit while the other is on the postnatal ward with her, she may find she bonds with the one on the ward much more quickly. In such cases the mother should be encouraged to spend as much time as possible with the baby on the NNU and to visit as soon after the birth as she feels able. If she has had an operative birth, she may find it difficult to care for two babies and extreme tiredness or anaemia will exacerbate the situation. She may have feelings of guilt if the birth and immediate postnatal period have not gone as she had planned. The midwife should be alert for such circumstances and help the mother to divide her attention between both babies and to give plenty of reassurance that she is not the first mother to feel the same way.

Mother–partner relationships

A mother who has had twins or more will inevitably turn to her partner for help with the care of the babies, and many families work well together in the care and upbringing of their children, despite the added strains and stresses a multiple birth puts on a family. In some cases her partner may feel that she is devoting too much time to the babies and not enough to him, thus making him feel excluded, especially if when he comes home from work she is too exhausted to take any interest in him. The strain on any relationship when a new baby is born can be quite difficult for the couple to adjust to, but with a multiple birth it is even worse. The midwife should always encourage the father to be involved in the daily care of the babies, either in hospital or at home.

Care of the mother

Involution of the uterus will be slower because of its increased bulk. 'After pains' may be troublesome and analgesia should be offered. A good diet is essential and if the mother is breastfeeding she requires a high protein, high calorie diet. It is quite common for breastfeeding mothers to feel hungry between meals and they should be encouraged to keep sensible snacks to hand for such times. A dietician may be able to offer help. The physiotherapist or midwife should instruct the mother in her postnatal exercises (see Ch. 16).

The midwife must give the mother of twins extra support. Teaching her simple parenting skills and encouraging her to carry them out with increasing assurance will build up her confidence.

The mother may feel 'in the way' if the babies are in the neonatal unit and require a lot of intensive care from the medical and nursing staff. She may also have feelings of guilt because of their prematurity and feel it was something she did or did not do that they were born early. In this situation she will need time to talk her feelings through. While on the neonatal unit she should always be kept up-to-date with the care and condition of her infants. Most units now have a named nurse caring for each baby so parents know who to talk to. If one infant is very ill or dies, the mother will experience additional psychological problems.

It is very unusual for the babies to be discharged home from the NNU at different times but there are occasions when this happens. When it does, greater demands are placed on the mother, as she has to care for one baby at home and still visit the sick baby in hospital. Most units have a rooming-in policy so mothers can stay in the hospital with their babies for two or three nights before they are transferred home, to give them a chance to take over their total care and prepare them for coping at home. It is advisable for a new mother of twins or more to organize help at home for the first 2–3 weeks after discharge. Initially, this may be in the form of her partner taking time off work. If relations or friends have offered to help, the mother should be sure to let them know what kind of help she is expecting from them before it is needed. If the parents are fortunate enough to be able to afford paid help, then they can say exactly what it is they expect to be done. There is no statutory help available for twins or triplets in England and Wales. One excellent source of free help are nursery nurse students, who in their final year need practical placements in families. Local colleges of further education will be able to put midwives or mothers in contact with these courses.

The community midwife will contact the mother after discharge from hospital to arrange home visits. The health visitor will also arrange to see the mother and her babies after the community midwife has discharged them.

Once the mother is at home, she must be encouraged to rest and catch up on her sleep during the day as much as possible, and eat a well-balanced diet in order to recover her strength and ability to cope with her family. A good routine is the only way of coping with new babies and all mothers should be encouraged to establish one as soon as possible.

It may be wise to discourage visitors in the first week at home while the mother adjusts to the new circumstances. The father should be encouraged to help as much as possible.

Isolation can be a real problem for new mothers. The thought of getting two babies ready to go out can be quite fearful. Studies have shown the incidence of postnatal depression to be significantly higher in mothers of twins (Thorpe et al 1991). Stress, isolation and exhaustion are all significant precipitants of depression; mothers of twins are therefore more vulnerable.

Development of twins

Twins in most respects will do as well as a single baby, but the one area in which they can fall behind is language. With twins, the mother tends to talk to both of them together, so there is less one-to-one communication. Inevitably, she will be much busier and the temptation to leave the twins to amuse themselves is much greater. Talking to each other, the twins act as each other's role model for language (unlike the singleton baby, who has his mother). If one child speaks a word incorrectly the twin will copy it, reinforcing the mistake. This is how the so-called 'secret language' of twins develops, otherwise known as 'cryptophasia' or 'idioglossia'. It is essential that each twin is spoken to individually as much as possible. Eye contact is vital in any relationship. If one twin is more responsive and makes eye contact more easily than the other, the mother may respond much more readily to this twin without realizing it.

Identity and individuality

Parents of twins should be encouraged to think of their children as individuals. Often parents feel a special pride in having twins and buy the same style of clothes, but in different colours. The distinction between twins can start in the postnatal ward with differently coloured blankets, or different small soft toys. As they grow up, giving them different hair-styles can make children individual. People should be encouraged to refer to the children by name, or 'the girls' or 'boys' and not 'the twins'. At birthdays or Christmas, separate cards and different presents help to retain individuality. The twins should also be given the opportunity to spend time apart.

Siblings of multiples

An elder brother or sister of twins may find their arrival very difficult, especially if they have had a number of years of undivided parental attention. Parents must be alert to the feelings of their other children and include them as much as possible in all activities with the twins. A single older sibling may see the parents as a pair, the twins as a pair, while he or she is on her own. It can be very helpful to find a 'special friend' for the older child, for instance a godparent, or teenage friend. It can be helpful if the parents arrange for the twins to have a present for the older child and also for the child to have a present to give to each of the twins. Two different small cuddly toys as the first presents the twins receive can become very special gifts.

Triplets and higher order births

The increasing number of surviving triplets and higher order births (Fig. 24.7) will produce many more families needing special advice and support from healthcare workers. The UK Triplet Study by Botting et al (1990) revealed that the problems these families face are even greater than were previously realized.

A woman expecting three or more babies is at risk of all the same complications as one expecting twins, but more so. She is more likely to have a period in hospital resting before the babies are born and they will almost certainly be born prematurely. Perinatal mortality rates are higher for triplets than twins and the incidence of cerebral palsy is also increased (Patterson et al 1990).

Triplets or more are almost always delivered by caesarean section. The midwives must be prepared to receive several small babies within a very short time span. It is essential the paediatric team be present as specialist care may be required. The dangers associated with these births are asphyxia, intracranial injury and perinatal death.

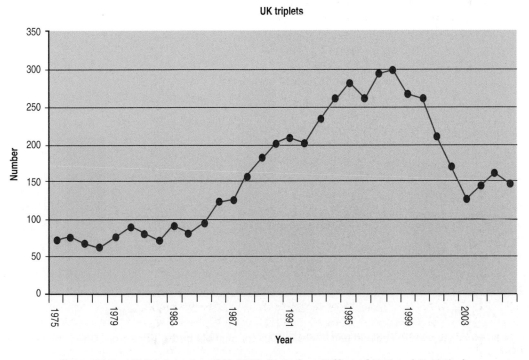

Figure 24.7 UK Triplet rates 1975–2006. (Data from Office of National Statistics.)

The main difficulties these families experience are insufficient practical and financial help and the lack of awareness of their problems by professionals. All mothers of triplets or more should arrange for extra help at home before the babies are born. The emotional stress and anxiety of the birth, having babies in the NNU and the worries of coping with the babies when they go home will seem overwhelming if no arrangements for extra help have been made beforehand. A mother should never be expected to manage by herself. A study by the Australian Multiple Births Association (AMBA 1984) showed that it took 197.5 hrs/week to care adequately for 6-month-old triplets and do the basic household tasks. Unfortunately, there are only 168 hrs in a week, taking no account of the mother's need to sleep!

Taking triplets out for a walk or any expedition can need major organization, even without the parents having to cope with uninvited comments from passers-by. Some of these can be insensitive and hurtful, making inferences about fertility and the parents bringing extra work on themselves.

The midwife must ensure that the mother's health visitor and, if necessary, a social worker are involved in her care. If the family needs extra outside help, this must be organized before the babies are born.

Applications to the council for rehousing may also be needed.

Disability and bereavement

Perinatal mortality and long-term morbidity are both more common among multiple births than singletons. The perinatal mortality rate for twins is about four times that of singletons, and triplets, 12 times (Fig. 24.8).

The grief of parents following the death of one of a multiple set is often underestimated. The specific problems they face are ill understood and their needs poorly met. It often feels 'easier' to concentrate on the survivor(s), thus denying the parents essential time and space to grieve. All too often people say that they are lucky because they still have one healthy child (or more). No-one ever says that to parents who lose one of their two or three singleton children (Bryan 1986). The conflicting emotions the parents will feel and the need to grieve for the child who has died, while wanting to rejoice at the birth of the healthy twin, can be confusing. Birthdays and anniversaries and the constant presence of the survivor(s) are all reminders of the dead child. The

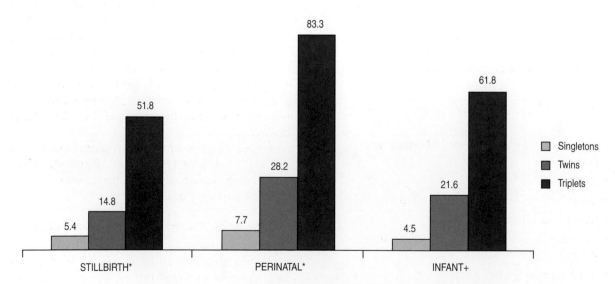

Figure 24.8 Mortality rates in England and Wales in 2004 for multiple births. (Data from Office for National Statistics.)

parents may need help in relating to the survivor(s). Addresses of organizations that offer such support should be made available to the parents. Where one or more of a multiple set has a disability it is often the healthy child who needs special attention. He may feel guilt that it was something he did that caused the twin's disability and may be resentful of the attention that the other one needs, or of the loss of twinship. Any of these may lead to emotional and behavioral problems if not addressed early on.

Multifetal pregnancy reduction (MFPR)

This is the reduction of an apparently healthy higher order multiple pregnancy down to two or even one embryo so the chances of survival are much higher. It may be offered to parents who have conceived triplets or more, whether spontaneously or as a result of assisted reproduction (see Ch. 13).

The procedure is usually carried out between the 10th and 12th week of the pregnancy. Various techniques may be used, either inserting a needle under ultrasound guidance via the vagina or, more commonly, through the abdominal wall into the fetal thorax. Potassium chloride is usually used, although some doctors prefer saline. Whichever technique is used, all embryos remain in the uterus until delivery. Usually the pregnancy is reduced to two embryos, but in some cases to three or even one (Wimalasundera 2006). Any parents who have been offered this treatment must be given counselling, which should include:

- the advantages and disadvantages of reducing the pregnancy
- the risks of continuing with a higher multiple pregnancy
- the risks of MFPR
- the effects on the surviving children
- how the parents may feel afterwards
- help for the parents to reach the right decision for them
- organizations who can help them
- the offer of long-term support if and when required.

Selective feticide

This may be offered to parents with a multiple pregnancy, where one of the babies has a serious abnormality. The affected fetus is injected as described in MFPR, but this is not usually performed until much later in the pregnancy so allowing the healthy fetus time to grow and develop normally. Counselling must again be offered to the parents. The full impact of either of these procedures and their bereavement will often not be felt until the birth of all their babies (including the dead baby) often many weeks later. Moreover, unlike the termination of a single pregnancy, the parents will be more aware of what could have been as they watch the survivor(s) grow up. When it comes to the labour, midwives must be ready to offer the appropriate care and understanding of the parents' bereavement. The bereavement should be clearly indicated in the notes so it is not forgotten when the mother comes back for her postnatal check and for future pregnancies.

Sources of help

In the UK, there is at present no statutory obligation to provide any extra help for families with twins, triplets or more. The support provided by social services varies greatly so it is always advisable for families with triplets to apply. Healthcare workers should be prepared to write letters supporting any applications these families have made. In the UK, a child allowance is paid to all children born. The firstborn child receives a higher allowance than subsequent children. In multiple pregnancies, it is only the firstborn child that receives the higher allowance.

Parents should be advised to contact organizations such as Home Start (see Useful addresses), or the local colleges with nursery training courses, both of which may be able to offer assistance.

TAMBA (Twins and Multiple Births Association)

This is the umbrella organization for the 150+ local twins clubs throughout the country. The clubs are run by parents of twins and are the best source of practical advice and support for parents expecting twins or more.

TAMBA also run the following specialist groups: Supertwins (triplets or more); Single parent group; Bereavement group; Special needs group; Health and education group; Infertility group; Adoptive parents group; and TAMBA Twinline, which is a national, confidential listening and information telephone service for all parents of twins, triplets and more (see Useful addresses).

The Multiple Births Foundation (MBF)

The MBF offers advice and support to families as soon as their multiple pregnancy is diagnosed, as well as to couples considering treatment for infertility. It offers information through its antenatal meetings for couples and professionals. The MBF also provides information and support to professionals through its education programme – study days, courses, lectures and the following publications:

Guidelines for professionals

Multiple births and their impact on families is a series of publications for professionals. It comprises a set of five books, which can be bought together or individually:

- *Facts about multiple births*
- *Multiple pregnancy*
- *Bereavement*
- *Special needs in twins*
- *Twins and triplets: the first five years and beyond.*

Other booklets

These include:

- *Multiple pregnancy and multiple birth – information for couples considering treatment for infertility*
- *Are they identical? – zygosity determination for twins, triplets and more*
- *Monochorionic twins – when twins share a placenta*
- *Preparing for twins and triplets*
- *Higher multiple pregnancies – fetal reduction*
- *Multiple pregnancy – selective feticide*
- *Feeding twins or more*
- *When a twin or triplet dies*
- *How to get twins (or more) to sleep.*
  (see Useful addresses)

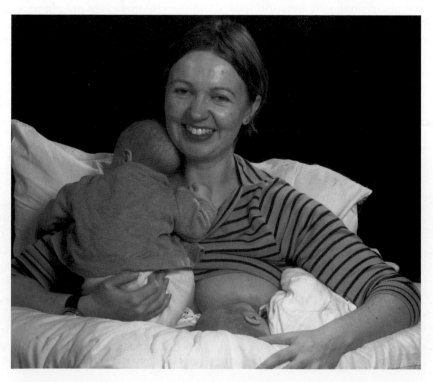

Plate 24.1

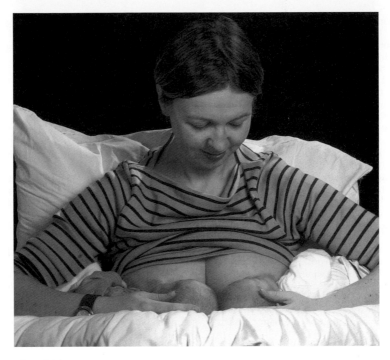

Plate 24.2

REFERENCES

AMBA (Australian Multiple Births Association) 1984 Proposal submitted to the Federal Government concerning 'act of grace' payments for triplets and quad families. Coogee, Australia

Beeby P J, Jeffrey H 1992 Risk factors for necrotizing enterocolitis: the influence of gestational age. Archives of Disease in Childhood 67:432–435

Bomsel-Helmreich O, Al Mufti W 2005 Multiple pregnancy: epidemiology, gestation and perinatal outcome. Informa Healthcare, New York, p 94–100

Botting B, Macfarlane A J, Price F V 1990 Three four and more: a study of triplets and higher order births. HMSO, London

Bryan E M 1984 Twins in the family (a parents guide). Constable, London

Bryan E M 1986 The death of a newborn twin. How can support for parents be improved? Acta Geneticae Medicae et Gemellologiae 5:166–170

Creinin M 1995 Conjoined twins. In: Keith L G, Papiernik E, Keith D (eds) Multiple pregnancy, epidemiology, gestation and perinatal outcome. Parthenon, New York, 93–112

Davies M E 1995 Managing multiple births, supporting parents. Modern Midwife 5(11):10–14

Dennes W J B, Sullivan M F H, Fisk N M, 2006 Scientific basis of twin-to twin transfusion syndrome In: Kilby M, Baker P, Critchley H et al (eds) Multiple pregnancy. RCOG Press, London, p. 167–181

Denton J, Bryan E M 1995 Prenatal preparation for parenting twins, triplets or more: the social aspect. In: Whittle M, Ward R H (eds) Multiple pregnancy. RCOG Press, London, p. 119

Eng H L, Chuang J H, Lee T Y 1989 Fetus-in-fetu, a case report and review of the literature. Journal of Pediatric Surgery 24:296–299

Fiducia A 1995 Breast-feeding three babies at once. Twins, Triplets and More Magazine 6(3):10–11

Finberg H J 1992 The 'twin peak' sign: reliable evidence of dichorionic twinning. Journal of Ultrasound in Medicine 11:571–577

Hedberg Nyquist K, Lutes L M 1998 Co-bedding twins: A developmentally supportive care strategy. Journal of Obstetrics, Gynecology and Neonatal Nursing 27(4):450–456

HFEA (Human Fertilisation and Embryology Authority) 2006 A long-term analysis of the HFEA register data 1991–2006. HFEA, London

HFEA (Human Fertilisation and Embryology Authority) Act 1990. HMSO, London

Kurtz A B, Wapne R J, Mata J et al 1992 Twin pregnancies: accuracy of first trimester abdominal ultrasound in predicting chorionicity and amnionicity. Radiology 185:759–762

Landy H J, Nies B M 1995 The vanishing twin. In: Keith L, Papiernik E, Keith D et al (eds) Multiple pregnancy, epidemiology, gestation and perinatal outcome. Parthenon, New York, p 59

Lang S 1995 Cup feeding alternate method. Midwives Chronicle 107:171–176

Leonard L G, Denton J 2006 Preparation for parenting multiple birth children. Early Human Development 82:371–378

Lucas A, Cole T J 1990 breastmilk and neonatal necrotising enterocolitis. Lancet 336:1519–1523

Mahomed K. 2000 Iron and folate supplementation in pregnancy. Cochrane Database System Review, Issue 2:CD001135

MBF (Multiple Births Foundation) 2006 Feeding Twins Triplets & More. MBF, London

MBF (Multiple Births Foundation) 2008 Monochorionic Pregnancy booklet, MBF, London

Mifflin P C 2001 Jodie and Mary, ethical and legal implications of separating conjoined twins. Practising Midwife 4(7):48–49

Mugford M, Henderson J 1995 Resource implications of multiple births. In: Humphrey Ward R, Whittle M (eds) Multiple pregnancy. RCOG Press, London, p 334–345

Pasquini L, Wimalasundera R C, Fisk N M 2004. Management of other complications specific to monochorionic twin pregnancies. Clinical Obstetrics and Gynaecology 5:576–599

Patterson B, Stanley F, Henderson D 1990 Cerebral palsy in multiple births in Western Australia. American Journal of Medical Genetics 37:346–351

RCOG (Royal College of Obstetricians and Gynaecologists) 2006 Multiple pregnancy. Consensus views arising from the 50th Study Group. RCOG, London, p 283–286

RCOG (Royal College of Obstetricians and Gynaecologists) 2001 Clinical Effectiveness Support Unit. The National Sentinel Caesarian Section Audit Report. RCOG, London

Rhine S A, Nance W E 1976 Familial twinning: case of superfetation in man. Acta Geneticae Medicae et Gemellologiae 25:66–69

Spillman J R 1985 'You have a little bonus my dear'. The effect on mothers of the diagnosis of multiple pregnancy. British Medical Ultrasound Society Bulletin 39:6–9

Spillman J R 1987 The emotional impact of multiple pregnancy: the midwives' role in supporting the family. Midwives Chronicle 100:58–62

Sebire N J, Sepulveda W, 2006 Management of twin reversed arterial perfusion TRAP) sequence. In: Kilby M, Baker P, Critchley H et al (eds) Multiple pregnancy. RCOG Press, London, p 199–222

Terasaki P I, Gjertson D, Bernoco D et al 1978 Twins with two different fathers identified by HLN. New England Journal of Medicine 299:590–592

Thorpe K, Golding J, MacGillivray I et al 1991 Comparisons of prevalence of depression in mothers of twins and mothers of singletons. British Medical Journal 302:875–878

UK National Screening Committee 2007. Screening for Down's syndrome in multiple pregnancy. UK National Screening Committee, London

Wimalasundera R, 2006 Selective reduction and termination of multiple pregnancies. In: Kilby M, Baker P, Critchley H et al (eds) Multiple pregnancy. RCOG press, London, p 95–108

Winn H N, Gabrielli S, Reece E A et al 1989 Ultrasonographic criteria for the prenatal diagnosis of placental chorionicity in twin gestations. American Journal of Obstetrics and Gynecology 161:1540–1542

Yamamoto M, Ville Y. 2006 Twin-to-twin transfusion syndrome. In: Kilby M, Baker P, Critchley H et al (eds) Multiple pregnancy. RCOG press, London, p 183–197

Zhang J, Hamilton B, Martin J et al 2004 Delayed interval delivery and infant survival: a population – based study. American Journal of Obstetrics and Gynecology 191(2):470–476

FURTHER READING

Cooper C 2004 Twins and multiple births. Vermilion, London

A GP and mother of twins gives practical advice on coping with twins and more. Suitable for parents and professionals alike.

Lyons S 2001 Finding our way – life with triplets, quadruplets and quintuplets. A collection of experiences. Triplets, Quadruplets and Quintuplets Association, Mississanga, Ontario, Canada

Written by a group of Canadian parents who have had triplets and more giving a fantastic insight into life with higher order multiples, with comments and advice by medical professionals.

Multiple Pregnancy 2006 RCOG Press, London

Written by specialists in multiple pregnancy and includes all the latest guidelines.

USEFUL ADDRESSES

Homestart UK
2 Salisbury Rd, Leicester LE1 7QR
Tel: 01162 339955

Multiple Births Foundation (MBF)
4th floor, Hammersmith House,
Queen Charlottes and Chelsea Hospital,
Du Cane Rd, London W12 0HS
Tel: 020 8383 3519
Fax: 020 8383 3041

e-mail: mbf@imperial.nhs.uk
www.multiplebirths.org.uk

TAMBA (Twins and Multiple Births Association)
2 The Willows, Gardner Road,
Guildford GU1 4PG
Tel: 01483 304 442
Tamba Twinline:
Tel: 0800 138 0509

4

Section 4
Labour

SECTION CONTENTS

25

The first stage of labour: physiology and early care

Carol McCormick

The transition from pregnancy to labour is a sequence of events that often begins gradually. The first stage of labour, although difficult to diagnose, is usually recognized by the onset of regular uterine contractions and finally culminates in complete effacement and dilatation of the cervix.

The chapter aims to:

- encourage midwives to consider the onset and diagnosis of labour, and how it can be recognized by both the woman and the midwife
- describe some of the physical changes taking place as labour progresses
- reflect on interventions and timing of care in order to optimize the well-being of the woman and her fetus during the course of labour.

Changes during the last few weeks of pregnancy

The physiological transition from being a pregnant woman to becoming a mother means an enormous change for each woman, both physically and psychologically. Every system in the body is affected and the experience, although unfortunately not joyous for all, represents a major transition in a woman's life.

During the last few weeks of pregnancy, a number of physical and psychological changes may occur:

- Mood swings are common and a surge of energy may be experienced.
- 2–3 weeks before the onset of labour the lower uterine segment expands and allows the fetal head

to sink lower and it may engage in the pelvis, particularly in first-time mothers. When this happens, the fundus of the uterus descends and there is more room for the lungs, breathing is easier, and the heart and stomach can function more easily. The woman may experience relief, which is historically known as *lightening*. Under hormonal influence, the symphysis pubis widens and the pelvic floor becomes more relaxed and softened, allowing the uterus to descend further into the pelvis. There is engagement of the fetal head (Fig. 25.1).

- Walking may become more difficult for some women at the end of pregnancy because the symphysis pubis is more mobile and relaxation of the sacroiliac joints may give rise to backache. Conditions such as pelvic girdle pain are increasingly being recognized and treated.

- Relief of pressure at the fundus results in an increase in pressure within the pelvis, which may be accounted for by the presence of the fetal head causing venous congestion of the whole pelvis. Vaginal secretions may also increase at this time. The presence of the fetal head in the pelvis can, in some women, also give rise to frequency of micturition, urgency and some degree of stress incontinence.

In a healthy pregnancy, the placenta nourishes and protects the growing fetus; the body of the uterus remains relaxed and the cervix closed. As birth approaches, the non-progressive Braxton Hicks contractions experienced during pregnancy alter and intensify to become the progressive form of labour. The cervix, which has remained firm and closed, becomes soft and able to dilate. Accompanying the physical changes the woman may have feelings of great intensity varying from excited anticipation to fearful expectancy. The midwife and other supporters must exercise great sensitivity at this time in order to meet the specific needs and hopes of the woman.

Labour, purely in the physical sense, may be described as the process by which the fetus, placenta and membranes are expelled through the birth canal – but of course, labour is much more than a purely physical event. What happens during labour can affect the relationship between mother and baby and can influence the likelihood of future pregnancies.

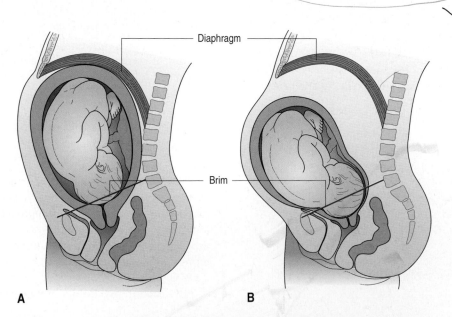

A   **B**

Figure 25.1 (A) *Prior to lightening*. The fundus crowds the diaphragm. The lower uterine segment has not stretched to accommodate the fetal head, which therefore remains high. The lower segment is 'V' shaped. (B) *After lightening*. The fundus sinks below the diaphragm and breathing is easier. The lower segment is 'U' shaped; it has softened and dilated so that the head sinks down into it and may partly enter the pelvic brim.

Traditionally, a human pregnancy is considered to last approximately 40 weeks (see Ch. 17). Normal labour occurs between 37 and 42 weeks' gestation.

The World Health Organization (WHO 1997) defines normal labour as: low risk throughout, spontaneous in onset with the fetus presenting by the vertex, culminating in the mother and infant in good condition following birth. All definitions of labour appear to be purely physiological and do not encompass the psychological well-being of the parents.

Once physiological labour commences, its progress is measured by descent of the head and dilatation of the cervix. The expected rate of cervical dilatation in labour was based on work by Friedman during the 1950s, but more recent research demonstrates that the process of labour in terms of cervical dilatation should not be strictly timed and may last longer than some clinicians expect. The criteria for distinguishing normal labour from abnormal labour based on time limits needs revision (Albers 1999, Lavender et al 2006).

Traditionally, three stages of labour are described: the first, second and third stage. But this is a rather pedantic view, as labour is obviously a continuous process. There is increasing acknowledgement that there are not just three clear phases of normal labour. Sherblom Matteson (2001) gives a full description of this view of more than three stages to labour, along with not only the physical changes but the emotional effects observed in women at this time.

First stage

- The latent phase is prior to active first stage of labour and may last 6–8hrs in first time mothers when the cervix dilates from 0 cm to 3–4 cm dilated (Stables 1999) and the cervical canal shortens from 3cm long to <0.5cm long (Arulkumaran 1996).
- The active first stage is the time when the cervix undergoes more rapid dilatation. This begins when the cervix is 3–4 cm dilated and, in the presence of rhythmic contractions, is complete when the cervix is fully dilated (10 cm).
- The transitional phase is the stage of labour when the cervix is from around 8cm dilated until it is fully dilated (or until the expulsive contractions during second stage are felt by the woman). There

is often a brief lull in the intensity of uterine activity at this time (Sherblom Matteson 2001, Woods 2006).

Second stage

- The second stage is that of expulsion of the fetus. It begins when the cervix is fully dilated; in physiological labour the woman usually feels the urge to expel the fetus. It is complete when the baby is born.

Third stage

- The third stage is that of separation and expulsion of placenta and membranes; it also involves the control of bleeding. It lasts from the birth of the baby until the placenta and membranes have been expelled.

The onset of spontaneous physiological labour

Women should have adequate information prior to labour to ensure comprehension of the changes labour will bring. This information is also needed to allow women to make their own choices based on good unbiased evidence. The complex physical, psychological and emotional experience of labour affects every woman differently and midwives must have sound knowledge as well as a range of different experiences to ensure the woman has some control over the birth of her baby. Women in labour should be encouraged to trust their own instincts, listen to their own body and verbalize feelings in order to get the help and support they need. Anxiety can increase the production of adrenaline (epinephrine), which inhibits uterine activity and may in turn prolong labour (Niven 1992, Seitchik 1987, Wuitchik et al 1989). The attitude of the midwife and the advice and guidance she gives during pregnancy influence the progress of labour and the attitudes of both the partners to each other and to their baby after it is born (Fisher et al 2006, Halldorsdottir & Karlsdottir 1996, Nolan 1995).

Recognition of the onset of normal spontaneous labour is not always easy. A woman may construe herself to be labouring, whereas sound midwifery judgement and understanding of the physiology of the first stage of labour may lead the midwife to the diagnosis of the latent phase of labour. Both the woman and midwife being aware of the latent phase of labour and allowing this time to pass with no intervention may prevent the medical diagnosis of 'poor progress' or 'failure to progress' later in labour. In a hospital setting, it is good practice not to commence the partogram until active labour has commenced.

Spurious labour

Many women experience contractions before the onset of labour; these may be painful and may even be regular for a time, causing a woman to think that labour has started. The two features of true labour that are absent in spurious labour are effacement and dilatation of the cervix (see below). It is important to note that the discomfort or even pain that the woman is conscious of is not false; the contractions she is experiencing are real but have not yet settled into the rhythmic pattern of 'true' labour and are not having an effect on the cervix. Reassurance should be given; discussion of this potential situation earlier in the pregnancy will have allowed the woman and her partner to prepare for such a scenario.

Cervical effacement (taking up of the cervix)

Here the cervix is drawn up and gradually merges into the lower uterine segment (Fig. 25.2). In the primiparous woman, this may result in complete effacement of the internal and external cervical os. But in the multiparous woman a perceptible canal may remain.

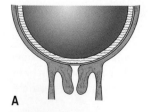 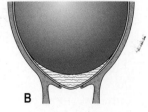

A   **B**

Figure 25.2 (A) The cervix before effacement. (B) The cervix after effacement. The cervical canal is now part of the lower uterine segment.

The onset of labour is determined by a complex interaction of maternal and fetal hormones and is not fully understood. It would appear to be multifactorial in origin, being a combination of hormonal and mechanical factors. Levels of maternal oestrogen rise sharply during the last weeks of pregnancy, resulting in changes that overcome the inhibiting effects of progesterone. High levels of oestrogens cause uterine muscle fibres to display oxytocic receptors and form gap junctions with each other. Oestrogen also stimulates the placenta to release prostaglandins that induce a production of enzymes that will digest collagen in the cervix, helping it to soften (Tortora & Grabowski 2000). The process is unclear but it is thought that both fetal and placental factors are involved. There is no clear evidence that concentrations of oestrogens and progesterone alter at the onset of labour, but the balance between them does facilitate myometrial activity.

Uterine activity may also result from mechanical stimulation of the uterus and cervix. This may be brought about by overstretching, as in the case of a multiple pregnancy, or pressure from a presenting part that is well applied to the cervix (Allman et al 1996, Beazley 1995).

The onset of labour is a process, not an event; therefore it is very difficult to pinpoint exactly when the painless (sometimes painful) contractions of pre-labour develop into the progressive rhythmic contractions of established labour.

Diagnosing the onset of labour is extremely important, since it is on the basis of this finding that decisions are made that will affect the management of labour (Gee & Olah 1993, Gharoro & Enabudoso 2006, O'Driscoll & Meagher 1993).

It is part of the remit of the midwife to ensure that women have sufficient information to assist them to recognize the onset of true labour. Contact with the midwife should be made when regular, rhythmic, uterine contractions are experienced, and these are perceived by the woman as uncomfortable or painful.

When in labour, contractions will often be accompanied or preceded by a bloodstained mucoid 'show'. Occasionally, the membranes will rupture; a midwife may want to be assured that there are no changes in the fetal heart rate due to the rare complication of cord prolapse and that meconium is not present in the liquor.

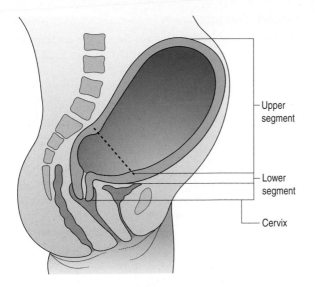

Figure 25.5 Birth canal before labour begins.

A Bandl's ring may be associated with fetal compromise. (Lauria et al 2007).

The physiological ring gradually rises as the upper uterine segment contracts and retracts and the lower uterine segment thins out to accommodate the descending fetus. Once the cervix is fully dilated and the fetus can leave the uterus, the retraction ring rises no further.

Cervical effacement

'Effacement' refers to the inclusion of the cervical canal into the lower uterine segment. According to conventional obstetric belief this process takes place from above downward; that is, the muscle fibres surrounding the internal os are drawn upwards by the retracted upper segment and the cervix merges into the lower uterine segment. The cervical canal widens at the level of the internal os, whereas the condition of the external os remains unchanged (Cunningham et al 1989, O'Driscoll & Meagher 1993) (Fig. 25.2).

However, an alternative mechanism of cervical effacement has been suggested, in which the tissues in the region of the external os are taken up first. By an outward unrolling movement, the cervix thins from the external os upwards, leaving the internal os to be affected last (Beazley 1995, Olah et al 1993).

Effacement may occur late in pregnancy, or it may not take place until labour begins. In the nulliparous woman the cervix will not usually dilate until effacement is complete, whereas in the parous woman effacement and dilatation may occur simultaneously and a small canal may be felt in early labour. This is often referred to by midwives as a 'multips os'.

Cervical dilatation

Dilatation of the cervix is the process of enlargement of the os uteri from a tightly closed aperture to an

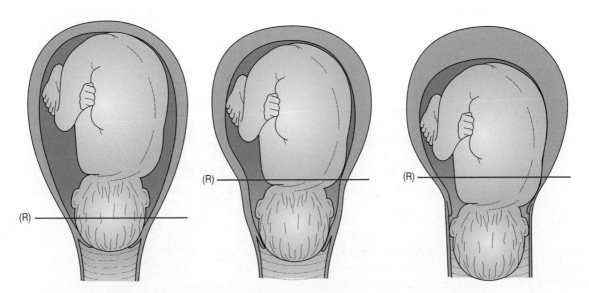

Figure 25.6 Diagram showing the retraction ring between the upper and lower uterine segments.

opening large enough to permit passage of the fetal head. Dilatation is measured in centimetres and full dilatation at term equates to about 10cm.

Dilatation occurs as a result of uterine action and the counterpressure applied by either the intact bag of membranes or the presenting part, or both. A well-flexed fetal head closely applied to the cervix favours efficient dilatation. Pressure applied evenly to the cervix causes the uterine fundus to respond by contraction and retraction (Beazley & Lobb 1983, Ferguson 1941).

Show

As a result of the dilatation of the cervix, the operculum, which formed the cervical plug during pregnancy, is lost. The woman may see a bloodstained mucoid discharge a few hours before, or within a few hours after, labour starts. The blood comes from ruptured capillaries in the parietal decidua where the chorion has become detached from the dilating cervix. There should never be more than bloodstaining; frank fresh bleeding is not normal at this stage – though, as the first stage ends, during the transitional period there is often a small loss of bright red blood that heralds the second stage. Both are referred to as a 'show'.

Mechanical factors

Formation of the forewaters

As the lower uterine segment forms and stretches, the chorion becomes detached from it and the increased intrauterine pressure causes this loosened part of the sac of fluid to bulge downwards into the internal os, to the depth of 6–12 mm. The well-flexed head fits snugly into the cervix and cuts off the fluid in front of the head from that which surrounds the body. The former is known as the 'forewaters' and the latter the 'hindwaters'. In early labour, it is often possible to feel intact forewaters bulging even when the hindwaters have ruptured, making ruptured membranes a difficult diagnosis at times.

The effect of separation of the forewaters prevents the pressure that is applied to the hindwaters during uterine contractions from being applied to the forewaters. This may help keep the membranes intact during the first stage of labour and be a natural defence against ascending infection.

General fluid pressure

While the membranes remain intact, the pressure of the uterine contractions is exerted on the fluid and, as fluid is not compressible, the pressure is equalized throughout the uterus and over the fetal body; it is known as 'general fluid pressure' (Fig. 25.7). When the membranes rupture and a quantity of fluid emerges, the fetal head, and the placenta and umbilical cord are compressed between the uterine wall and the fetus during contractions and the oxygen supply to the fetus is diminished. Preserving the integrity of the membranes, therefore, optimizes the oxygen supply to the fetus and also helps to prevent intrauterine and fetal infection, especially in longer labours.

Rupture of the membranes

The optimum physiological time for the membranes to rupture spontaneously is at the end of the first stage of labour after the cervix becomes fully dilated and no longer supports the bag of forewaters. The uterine contractions are also applying increasing expulsive force at this time.

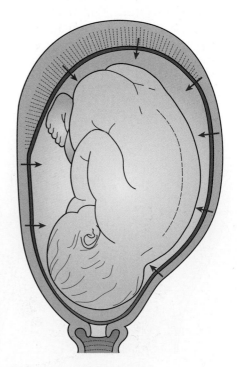

Figure 25.7 General fluid pressure.

The membranes may sometimes rupture days before labour begins or during the first stage. If for any reason there is a badly fitting presenting part and the forewaters are not cut off effectively then the membranes may rupture early. But in most cases there is no apparent reason for early spontaneous membrane rupture. Occasionally the membranes do not rupture even in the second stage and appear at the vulva as a bulging sac covering the fetal head as it is born; this is known as the 'caul'.

Early rupture of membranes may lead to an increased incidence of variable decelerations on cardiotocograph (CTG), which may lead to an increase in caesarean section rate if fetal blood sampling is not available (Goffinet et al 1997). A large meta-analysis (Brissen-Carroll et al 1997) suggests that routine artificial rupture of membranes (ARM) may decrease the overall length of labour by 60–120min. ARM does not reduce the overall caesarean section rate. It was concluded in this study that routine ARM should be reserved for women who are progressing slowly in labour or have abnormalities in the CTG.

All women need to give consent for this intervention and the practitioner should have a positive indication for performing ARM, which should be recorded in the notes.

Fetal axis pressure

During each contraction, the uterus rises forward and the force of the fundal contraction is transmitted to the upper pole of the fetus, down the long axis of the fetus and applied by the presenting part to the cervix. This is known as 'fetal axis pressure' (Fig. 25.8) and becomes much more significant after rupture of the membranes and during the second stage of labour.

Recognition of the first stage of labour

Ideally, the woman should know her own midwife and be able to contact her when labour starts. Where this is not possible, it is crucial that the first meeting between the midwife, the labouring woman and her partner establishes a rapport, which sets the scene for the remainder of labour. If the woman is planning to birth in hospital, she may worry about the reception she and her companion will receive and the attitude of the people attending her. In addition, an unfamiliar environment may provoke feelings of vulnerability and undermine her confidence. Comfortable surroundings, a welcoming manner and a midwife who greets the woman as an equal in a partnership will engender feelings of mutual respect, thus enabling the woman to relax and respond positively to the amazing forces of labour (Berry 2006, Raphael-Leff 1993).

Recognition of labour by the woman

It is the woman herself who usually diagnoses the onset of normal labour and many women and their partners are apprehensive in case the labour is very quick, resulting in an unattended birth. Education during the prenatal period is important to enable the woman to recognize the beginning of labour and understand the latent phase.

Women should be aware of what a 'show' is like, and know that in late pregnancy vaginal secretions

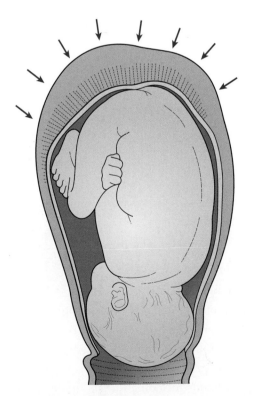

Figure 25.8 Fetal axis pressure.

are increased but should not be bloodstained. A 'show' in early labour or prior to the onset of labour is quite common. It is usually a pink or bloodstained jelly-like loss; labour may be imminent or under way. Women who are examined vaginally in late pregnancy should be made aware that there may be some slight blood loss after this procedure.

Braxton Hicks contractions are more noticeable in late pregnancy and some women experience them as painful. They are usually irregular or their regularity is not maintained for long spells of time. They seldom last more than 1 min. In true labour, contractions exhibit a pattern of rhythm and regularity, usually increasing in length, strength and frequency as time goes on. When the woman first feels contractions she may be aware only of backache but if she places a hand on her abdomen she may perceive simultaneous hardening of the uterus. Contractions will often be short initially, lasting 30–40 secs, and may be as much as 30 min apart. If the pregnancy is problem free, with a normal birth anticipated, the midwife should advise the woman to stay in her own surroundings, continue with her normal activities, to eat, be active and upright.

It is often difficult to be sure whether or not the membranes have ruptured spontaneously prior to labour or in early labour. The woman may be experiencing some degree of stress incontinence, so she may be unsure if it is liquor or urine that she is passing. If there is any doubt, the woman should contact her midwife. The midwife may decide to pass a speculum and look for amniotic fluid in the vagina. Digital examination should be avoided if the woman is not in labour as it will increase the risk of ascending infection and chorioamnionitis.

Initial meeting with the midwife and care in labour

Communication

When a woman begins to labour, she may have a mixture of emotions. Most women anticipate labour with a degree of excitement, anxiety, fear and hope. Many other emotions are influenced by cultural expectations and previous life experiences. The state of the woman's knowledge, her fears and expectations are also influenced by her companions during labour. By the time labour starts, a decision will have been reached about where the woman plans to give birth. Some women may choose to give birth at home, some in hospital and some may wish to labour as long as possible at home but give birth in hospital. Whatever choice the woman makes, she must be the focus of the care, should be able to feel she is in control of what is happening to her and be able to make decisions about her care (DH 2007, Sinivaara et al 2004).

Providing that there are no complications and labour is not well advanced, the woman may remain at home as long as she feels comfortable and confident. If labour is pre-term, however, admission to hospital is always advised (see Ch. 26).

The initial examination will include details of when labour started, whether the membranes have ruptured and the frequency and strength of the contractions. The midwife should remember that the woman will be very conscious of her body and may therefore be unable to pay attention or respond while experiencing a contraction. Since the woman has embarked on an intensely energy-demanding process, inquiry should be made as to whether she has been deprived of sleep and also what food she has recently eaten. If still in early labour with a problem-free pregnancy, she should be advised to eat or drink if she wishes and remain mobile, maybe to bathe if she would find this relaxing (Champion & McCormick 2002).

Thought should be given to the social circumstances, particularly the care of other children and whether a birthing partner is available and has been contacted.

Past history

Of particular relevance at the onset of labour are:

- the birth plan
- parity and age
- gestational age and outcomes of previous labours
- weights and condition of previous babies
- if she has attended any specialist clinics
- any known problems – social or physical
- blood results including Rhesus isoimmunization and haemoglobin.

Birth plan

Most women currently give birth in hospital. Admission to hospital of a woman in labour provides the opportunity for the midwife to discuss with each woman and her partner any plans that may have already been prepared by them. An outline may be present in the case notes, or the couple may bring a birth plan with them. Some women will not have prepared a birth plan and, if this is the case, the midwife can encourage the couple to consider any preferences that they may have. A birth plan simply means that a pregnant woman has (usually) written down, and may have discussed with her midwife, the kind of birth she would like. Frequently, the partner is involved in this forward planning, which should be a flexible proposal that can be reviewed and revised during labour (DH 2007). To welcome the woman who is being admitted in labour, to introduce oneself and to ascertain how she would like to be addressed should help the midwife establish a trusting relationship. Whether or not they are already identified in a birth plan, she should explore the following issues:

- the woman's chosen birth companion(s)
- her choice of clothes for labour
- ambulation and fetal monitoring (intermittent, electronic or a mixture)
- pain relief
- position for labour and birth
- natural or managed third stage
- cutting the umbilical cord
- skin to skin contact and feeding the baby after birth.

The midwife should also offer to explain anything the woman or her partner wishes to know, and document all requests.

Midwife's initial physical examination of the mother

Prior to touching the woman, a sound explanation of the proposed examination and their significance should be given. Verbal consent should be obtained and recorded in the notes. The midwife must be aware that a competent woman, with a capacity to make decisions, is within her rights to refuse any treatment regardless of the consequences to her and her unborn baby. She does *not* have to give a reason.

Basic observations including pulse rate, temperature and blood pressure are taken and recorded. The woman's hands and feet are usually examined for signs of oedema. Slight swelling of the feet and ankles is normal, but pretibial oedema or puffiness of the fingers or face is not.

A detailed abdominal examination including symphysis fundal height as described in Ch. 17 should be carried out and recorded. Initial observations form a baseline for further examinations carried out throughout labour. The abdominal examination may be repeated at intervals in order to assess descent of the head. This is measured by the number of fifths palpable above the pelvic brim and should be recorded on the partogram.

Vaginal examination

Physical examination of the cervix is not the only way to assess labour; skills of listening watching and communicating with the woman should be used in conjunction with vaginal examination. Generally, the trend is away from routine four-hourly vaginal examinations and justification for a vaginal examination should always be recorded, a vaginal examination should be preceded by an abdominal examination, an explanation and the obtaining of verbal consent from the woman. The woman's bladder should be empty as the head may be displaced by a full bladder as well as being very uncomfortable for the woman. With the combination of external and internal findings, the skilled midwife will have a very detailed picture of the labour and subsequent progress of labour.

Indications for vaginal examination

These are to:

- make a positive identification of presentation
- determine whether the head is engaged in case of doubt
- ascertain whether the forewaters have ruptured, or to rupture them artificially
- exclude cord prolapse after rupture of the forewaters, especially if there is an ill-fitting presenting part or the fetal heart rate changes

- assess progress or delay in labour
- confirm full dilatation of the cervix
- confirm the axis of the fetus and presentation of the second twin in multiple pregnancy, and if necessary in order to rupture the second amniotic sac.

The midwife should realize that a vaginal examination is not always the only way of obtaining this information and that careful, continuous observation of the labouring mother will enable her to avoid making unnecessary vaginal examinations, which should be kept to a minimum. Under no circumstances should a midwife make a vaginal examination if there is any frank bleeding unless the placenta is positively known to be in the upper uterine segment.

Method

A vaginal examination during labour is an aseptic procedure. The midwife should first explain the procedure carefully to the woman and give her an opportunity to ask questions. In order to obtain the most information, the woman is usually asked to lie on her back but the technique can be easily adapted to accommodate other positions that suit the woman better. During the examination the woman's dignity and privacy need to be considered; to avoid unnecessary exposure, the woman can be asked to move and uncover herself when the midwife is ready to begin. It appears that there is no increased risk of infection to mothers and babies if the midwife does not swab the vulva with antiseptic solution or use sterile vaginal packs (McCormick 2001); what is important is using a good hand-washing technique and wearing sterile gloves.

Findings

The midwife should observe the labia for any sign of varicosities, oedema or vulval warts or sores (see Ch. 23). She notes whether the perineum is scarred from a previous tear or episiotomy. Some cultures practise female genital mutilation (excision of the clitoris and the labia minora); scarring from this operation would be evident. The midwife should also note any discharge or bleeding from the vaginal orifice. If the membranes have ruptured the colour and odour of any amniotic fluid or discharge are noted. Offensive liquor suggests infection and green fluid indicates the presence of meconium, which may be a sign of fetal compromise or postmaturity.

Particularly in a multiparous woman, a cystocele may be found. A loaded rectum may also be felt through the posterior vaginal wall. If time allows, a suppository or microenema may be offered. Many women have some degree of loose bowels in early labour though, which reduces the need for enema or suppositories in most spontaneous labours.

As the examining fingers reach the end of the vagina they are turned so that their sensitive pads face upwards and come into contact with the cervix. Palpate around the fornices and sense the proximity of the presenting part of the fetus to the examining finger. The os uteri is located by gently sweeping the fingers from side to side. It will normally be situated centrally, but sometimes in early labour, it will be very posterior. In the rare event of a sacculated retroverted gravid uterus the cervix may be located in an extreme anterior position.

The midwife must assess the length of the cervical canal. A long, tightly closed cervix indicates that labour has not yet started. The cervical canal may be partially or completely obliterated depending on the degree of effacement (see above). In a primigravida, the cervix may be completely effaced but still closed; in this case, it will be closely applied to the presenting part and can easily be confused with a completely dilated cervix until the small tell-tale depression in the centre is found.

The consistency of the cervix is noted. It should be soft, elastic and applied closely to the presenting part.

Dilatation of the cervix, that is the distance across the opening, is estimated in centimetres (Fig. 25.9); 10 cm dilatation equates to full dilatation (Fig. 25.10). In preterm labours the smaller fetal head will pass through the os at a smaller diameter. At the point where the maximum diameters of the fetal head have passed through the os, the cervix can no longer be felt.

The midwife should always take care to feel for the cervix in every direction as a lip of cervix frequently remains in one quarter only, usually anteriorly (see also Bishop's score, Ch. 30).

Intact membranes can be felt through the dilating os. When felt between contractions they are slack but will become tense when the uterus contracts

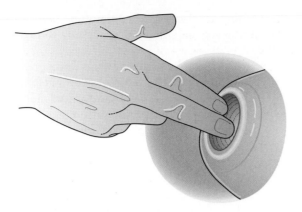

Figure 25.9 Cervix 4 cm dilated.

and the fluid behind them is then more readily appreciated. The consistency of the membranes can be likened to 'Cling film'. When the forewaters are very shallow it may be difficult to feel the membranes.

If the presenting part does not fit well, some of the fluid from the hindwaters escapes into the forewaters, causing the membranes to protrude through the cervix. This will be more exaggerated in obstructed labour. Bulging membranes are more

likely to rupture early and in this case they will not be felt at all. Following rupture of the membranes the midwife needs to satisfy herself that the cord has not prolapsed by listening to the fetal heart through a contraction.

If the forewaters are felt following a leakage of amniotic fluid it may be supposed that the hindwaters have ruptured.

The presenting part is defined as the part of the fetus lying over the uterine os during labour. In order to assess the descent of the fetus in labour, the level of the presenting part is estimated in relation to the maternal ischial spines. The distance of the presenting part above or below the ischial spines is expressed in centimetres (Fig. 25.11). As a caput succedaneum (see Ch. 45) may form over the presenting part, care must be taken to relate the bony part of the fetus to the ischial spines and not to the oedematous swelling. Moulding of the fetal skull can also result in the presenting part becoming lower without any appreciable advance of the head as a whole. The midwife must bear in mind that the fetus follows the curve of Carus (see Ch. 8) and it is impossible to judge the station precisely. The purpose of making this estimate is to assess progress

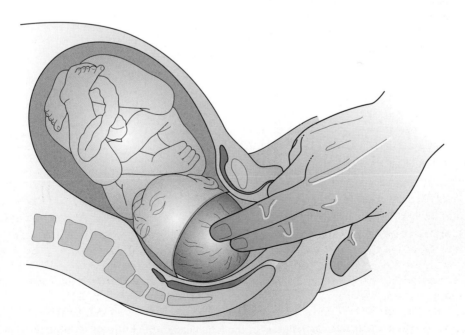

Figure 25.10 Cervix fully dilated.

and it is therefore valuable for the same person to make all the vaginal examinations on any particular mother.

In 96% of cases, the vertex presents and is recognized by feeling the hard bones of the vault of the skull and the fontanelles and sutures in relation to the maternal pelvis. For details of the findings in face, brow, breech and shoulder presentations see Ch. 31.

By feeling the features of the presenting part, the midwife can deduce the position of the presentation. The vertex has the fewest diagnostic features but, being the most common presentation, is the one with which she must become most familiar.

Commonly, the first feature to be felt, even in early labour, is the sagittal suture. Its slope should be noted; most frequently it will be in the right or left oblique diameter of the maternal pelvis, or it may be transverse. Later it rotates into the anteroposterior diameter of the maternal pelvis (Fig. 25.12).

The sagittal suture should be followed with the finger until a fontanelle is reached. If the head is well

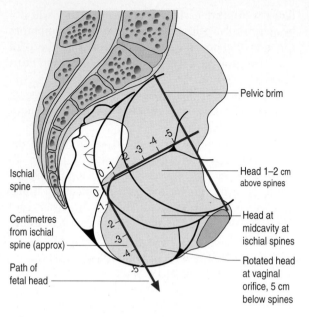

Figure 25.11 Diagram to show stations of the fetal head in relation to the pelvic canal.

Labels in figure: Pelvic brim; Head 1–2 cm above spines; Head at midcavity at ischial spines; Rotated head at vaginal orifice, 5 cm below spines; Ischial spine; Centimetres from ischial spine (approx); Path of fetal head

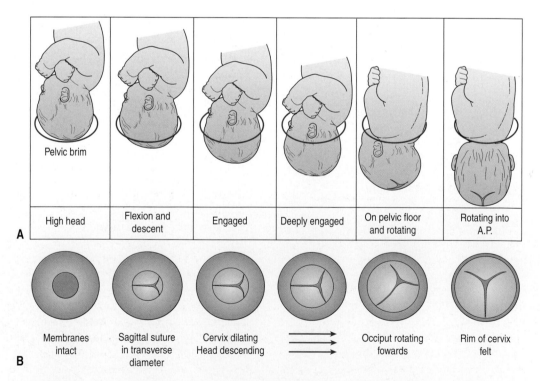

A: High head | Flexion and descent | Engaged | Deeply engaged | On pelvic floor and rotating | Rotating into A.P.

Pelvic brim

B: Membranes intact | Sagittal suture in transverse diameter | Cervix dilating Head descending | | Occiput rotating fowards | Rim of cervix felt

Figure 25.12 (A) Diagrams showing descent of the fetal head through the pelvic brim. (B) Diagrams showing dilatation of the cervix and rotation of the fetal head as felt on vaginal examination.

flexed, this will be the posterior fontanelle, which is recognized because it is small and triangular with three sutures leaving it. The anterior fontanelle is diamond shaped, covered with membrane and with four sutures leaving it. The location of the fontanelle in relation to the maternal pelvis will give information about the whereabouts of the fetal occiput.

Moulding (see Ch. 12)

This can be judged by feeling the amount of overlapping of the skull bones; it can also give additional information as to position. The parietal bones override the occipital bone and the anterior parietal bone overrides the posterior.

An understanding of the mechanism of labour (see Ch. 28) will help the midwife to appreciate the significance of flexion, rotation and descent as determinants of progress in labour.

Although the capacity of the pelvis may have been assessed antenatally, the midwife should take the opportunity to assure herself of its adequacy as she completes her vaginal examination. She may be able to feel the ischial spines, which should be blunt, and note the size of the subpubic angle, which should be about 90° and accommodate the two examining fingers. Prominent ischial spines and a reduced subpubic angle are unfavourable features associated with the android pelvis.

Keeping the woman fully informed in labour shows sensitivity to her needs and is an essential, integral component of the support provided by the midwife.

Cleanliness and comfort

Bowel preparation

If there has been no recent bowel action (depending on the woman's normal bowel habits) or the rectum feels loaded on vaginal examination, the woman should be consulted and asked if she would like an enema or suppositories. This is never done as a routine procedure. A small, low volume disposable enema may be administered, or two glycerine suppositories. There is no evidence to suggest a full rectum causes delay in the progress of labour (Drayton 1990), but the woman may be embarrassed if she feels she is likely to pass faeces during labour.

Perineal shave

Routine perineal shaving has not been carried out in the UK for some years. Research has shown that perineal shaving is unnecessary and does not improve infection rates. Dislike of the procedure and abrasions sustained cause discomfort for many women and detract from the positive experience of labour (Drayton 1990).

Bath or shower

If a woman has had no access to a bath or shower at home, she may wish to use these facilities on admission to the hospital. For women in normal labour, a warm bath (or birthing pool) can be an effective form of pain relief that allows increased mobility with no increased incidence of adverse outcome for mother or baby (Alderdice et al 1995, Gilbert & Tookey 1999). The woman may choose to rest in the bath for a long time. The midwife should invite the mother who is mobile to have a bath or shower whenever she wishes during normal labour.

Clothing

It is entirely up to the individual woman what she wears in labour. If in hospital she may prefer to wear the loose gown offered or she may feel more comfortable wearing her own choice of clothing. As long as she is aware that the garment may become wet and bloodstained and that she may require more than one, there is no reason to restrict her choice.

Records

Midwifery is becoming increasingly litigious. The midwife's record of labour is a legal document and must be kept meticulously. The records may be examined by any court for up to 25 years, they may go before the Nursing and Midwifery Council professional conduct or health committee, and will usually be examined in the audit process of statutory supervision or on behalf of the Clinical Negligence Scheme for Trusts. The midwives rules and standards (NMC 2004) and guidelines for records and record keeping (NMC 2005) both reiterate that records should be as contemporaneous as is reasonable, and must be authenticated with the midwife's full signature; it is good practice to print the author's name under the signature. A midwife must not destroy or arrange for destruction of these records and must be satisfied they are stored securely.

The records are created to give comprehensive and concise information regarding the woman's observations, her physical, psychological and sociological state, and any problem that arises as well as the midwife's response to that problem, including any interventions. They are there to serve the interest of the woman and to demonstrate that the midwife has understood and carried out her duty of care as a reasonable midwife should.

An accurate record during labour provides the basis from which clinical improvements, progress or deterioration of the mother or fetus can be judged. For this reason, the notes should be kept in chronological order.

The maternity record is shared between the midwife and the obstetrician. The obstetrician makes notes of his or her findings, timing of visits and any prescriptions made. The same standards apply to all practitioners. The midwife usually enters the summary of labour and initial details about the baby.

In recent years, the partogram or partograph has been widely accepted as an effective means of recording the progress of labour. It is a chart on which the salient features of labour are entered in a graphic form and therefore provides the opportunity for early identification of deviations from normal. Figure 25.13 shows one example of a partogram, which is a visual means of recording all observations and includes a pictorial record of the rate of cervical dilatation. The charts are usually designed to allow for recordings at 15 min intervals and include:

- fetal heart rate
- maternal temperature
- pulse
- blood pressure
- details of vaginal examinations
- strength of contractions
- frequency of contractions in terms of the number in 10 min
- fluid balance

- urine analysis
- drugs administered.

The cervicograph is the diagrammatic representation of the dilatation of the cervix charted against the hours in labour. Some studies (Friedman & Sachtleben 1965, Pearson 1981) have shown that the cervical dilatation time of normal labour has a characteristic sigmoid curve. This curve can be divided into two distinct parts – the latent phase and the active phase. The active phase has been said to proceed at a rate 0.5–1 cm/hr, but more recent work has challenged this rigid view (Albers 1999, Lavender et al 2006). The disadvantage of using such prescribed parameters of normal is the temptation to make all women fit predetermined criteria for normality. The rate of progress in labour must be considered in the context of the woman's total well-being and choice.

If it becomes necessary to confer with an obstetrician, paediatrician or other practitioner, the midwife records the times and the nature of the consultation, including whether the practitioner was informed, consulted or asked to be present.

Medicine records

Midwives have an exemption from needing a prescription for specific medicines used for the care of women in normal labour (see Ch. 49). Even so, most NHS Trusts also have locally agreed patient group directions to which the midwife should adhere; these usually guide the midwife as to which medicines are preferred and what doses and frequency are to be used within that Trust. If the midwife is practising outside the area in which she has notified her intention to practise, she should consult the supervisor of midwives regarding any matters relating to the supply, administration, storage or surrender of controlled drugs or medicines (NMC 2004).

As well as being entered on the partogram, doses of drugs are recorded on the prescription sheet, in the summary of labour and, in the case of controlled drugs, in the Controlled Drug Register.

Box 25.1 lists key points for care in the first stage of labour.

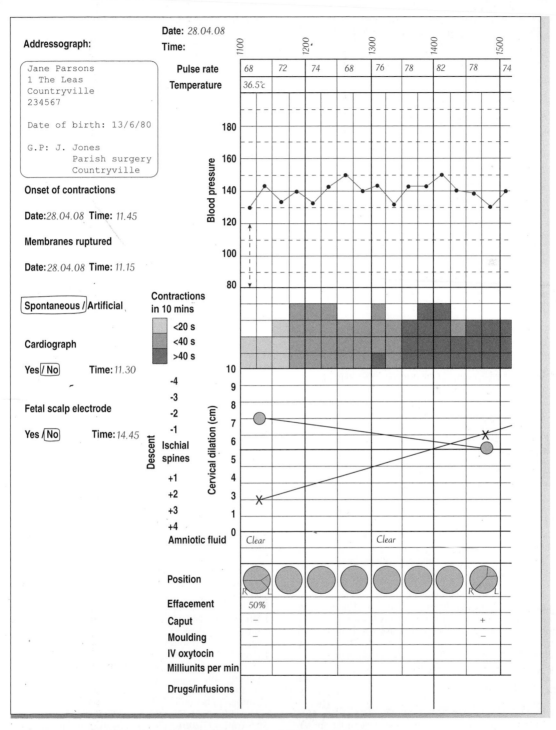

Figure 25.13   Example of a partogram.

Box 25.1 Key points for the first stage of labour

- Women should have adequate and unbiased information to make choices for their labour and birth including place of birth
- Good communication and constant individualized care will improve outcomes of women and their babies
- The midwife should assess the woman with a problem-free pregnancy at home to diagnose labour regardless of planned place of birth
- Midwives should ensure women are aware of the latent phase of labour
- Women in normal labour should remain mobile and in their own surroundings as long as possible when booked for hospital birth
- Labour is a continuous process that may not always progress as obstetric curves currently suggest
- It is the responsibility of the midwife to ensure all maternity records that she completes meet legal and professional standards.

REFERENCES

Albers L L 1999 The duration of labor in healthy women. Journal of Perinatology 19(2):114–119

Alderdice F, Renfrew M, Marchant S et al 1995 Labour and birth in water in England and Wales. Report of a survey funded by the Department of Health into the safety of water birth. British Medical Journal 310(6983):837

Allman A C J, Genevier E S, Johnson M R et al 1996 Head to cervix force: an important physiological variable in labour. 1. The temporal relation between head to cervix force and intrauterine pressure during labour. British Journal of Obstetrics and Gynaecology 103:763–768

Arulkumaran S 1996 Poor progress in labour including augmentation, malpositions and malpresentations. In: James D, Steer P, Gonik B (eds.) High risk pregnancy. W B Saunders, London, p 1063

Beazley J M 1995 Natural labour and its active management. In: Whitfield C (ed.) Dewhurst's textbook of obstetrics and gynaecology for postgraduates, 5th edn. Blackwell Science, Oxford, Ch. 21

Beazley J M, Lobb M O 1983 Aspects of care in labour. Churchill Livingstone, New York

Berry D 2006 Health communication: theory and practice. Open University Press, Maidenhead, p 151

Brissen-Carroll G, Fraser W, Breart G et al 1997 The effect of routine early amniotomy on spontaneous labour: a meta analysis. The Cochrane Collaboration, Issue 4. Update Software, Oxford

Champion P, McCormick C 2002 Eating and drinking in labour. Books for Midwives, Oxford

Cunningham F G, MacDonald P C, Grant N F 1989 Williams obstetrics, 18th edn. Prentice-Hall, London

DH (Department of Health) 2007 Maternity matters: Choice, access and continuity of care in a safe service. DH, London

Drayton S 1990 Midwifery care in the first stage of labour. In: Alexander J, Levy V, Roch S (eds) Intrapartum care: a research based approach. Macmillan, Basingstoke

Ferguson J K 1941 A study of the motility of the intact uterus at term. Surgery, Gynecology and Obstetrics 73:359–366

Fisher C, Hauck Y, Fenwick J 2006 How social context impacts on women's fears of childbirth: a Western Australian example. Social Science and Medicine 63(1):64–75

Friedman E A, Sachtleben M R 1965 Station of the fetal presenting part. American Journal of Obstetrics and Gynecology 93(4):522–529

Gee H, Olah K S 1993 Failure to progress in labour. In: Studd J (ed.) Progress in obstetrics and gynaecology. Churchill Livingstone, New York, Ch. 10

Gharoro E P, Enabudoso E J 2006 Labour management: an appraisal of the role of false labour and latent phase on the delivery mode. Journal of Obstetrics and Gynaecology 26(6):534–537

Gilbert R E, Tookey P A 1999 Perinatal mortality and morbidity among babies delivered in water: surveillance study and postal survey. British Medical Journal 319(7208):483–487

Goffinet F, Fraser W, Marcoux S et al 1997 Early amniotomy increases the frequency of fetal heart rate abnormalities. British Journal of Obstetrics and Gynaecology 104:548–553

Gross M M, Hecker H, Matterne A et al 2006 Does the way that women experience the onset of labour influence the duration of labour?. British Journal of Obstetrics and Gynaecology 113(3):289–294

Halldorsdottir S, Karlsdottir S I 1996 Journeying through labour and delivery: perceptions of women who have given birth. Midwifery 12:48–61

Lauria M R, Barthold J C, Zimmerman R A et al 2007 Pathologic uterine ring associated with fetal head trauma and subsequent cerebral palsy. Obstetrics and Gynecology 109(2):495–497

Lavender T, Alfirevic Z, Walkinshaw S 2006 Effect of different partogram action lines on birth outcomes: a randomized controlled trial. Obstetrics and Gynecology 108(2):295–302

McCormick C 2001 Vulval preparation in labour: use of lotions or tap water. British Journal of Midwifery 9(7):453–455

Niven C 1992 Psychological care for families: before, during and after birth. Butterworth Heinemann, Oxford

NMC (Nursing and Midwifery Council) 2004 Midwives rules and standards. NMC, London

NMC (Nursing and Midwifery Council) 2005 Guidelines for records and record keeping. NMC, London

Nolan M 1995 Supporting women in labour: the doula's role. Modern Midwife 5(3):12–15

O'Driscoll K, Meagher D 1993 Active management of labour, 3rd edn. Mosby, London

Olah K S, Brown J S, Gee H 1993 Cervical contractions: the response of the cervix to oxytocic stimulation in the latent phase of labour. British Journal of Obstetrics and Gynaecology 100:635–640

Pearson J 1981 Partography. Nursing Mirror 153(2):xxv–xxix

Raphael-Leff J 1993 Pregnancy: the inside story. Sheldon, London

Seitchik J 1987 The management of functional dystocia in the first stage of labour. Clinical Obstetrics and Gynecology 30 (1):42–49

Sherblom Matteson P 2001 Women's health during the childbearing years: A community based approach. Mosby, New York, p 358–359

Sinivaara M, Suominen T, Routasolo P et al 2004 How delivery ward staff exercise power over women in communication. Journal of Advanced Nursing 46(1):33–41

Stables D 1999 Physiology in childbearing. Baillière Tindall, London, p 450

Tortora G, Grabowski S 2000 Principles of anatomy and physiology, 9th edn. John Wiley, New York, p 1039–1040

WHO (World Health Organization) Department of Reproductive Health and Research 1997 Care in normal labour. A practical guide. WHO, Geneva

Woods T 2006 The transitional stage of labour. MIDIRS Midwifery Digest 16(2):225–228

Wuitchik M, Bakal D, Lipshitz J 1989 The clinical significance of pain and cognitive activity in latent labour. Obstetrics and Gynecology 73(1):25–41

FURTHER READING

National Institute for Health and Clinical Excellence: Intrapartum guidelines. Online. Available: www. nice.org.uk

26 Active first stage of labour

Carol McCormick

Labour, the culmination of pregnancy, is an event with great psychological, social and emotional meaning for the mother and her family. In addition, many women experience stress and physical pain. The midwife and all other supporters should display tact and sensitivity, respect the needs and choices of the individual woman and provide an environment which enables her to labour and give birth with dignity.

The chapter aims to:

- stress the importance of women's environment in relation to choice, control, comfort, companionship and communication during labour
- describe the principles of consent and record keeping
- describe the process of monitoring, both the progress of labour and the condition of the mother and fetus
- briefly describe the current principles used in the management of pre-term labour.

Communication and environment

In Europe, the vast majority of women opt to give birth in hospital or a birth centre. However, some may choose to give birth in their own home where they may feel they have more control over the environment so reducing fear.

The woman should decide where to give birth only after full and unbiased discussion of her options and the associated benefits and potential risks in terms of outcomes. There are times, when the midwife should advise the woman in individual circumstances (Sinivaara et al 2004). Once a decision has been made, her choice should be supported.

Currently in the UK most births occur in hospital, therefore the atmosphere and environment of hospital birthing rooms are important (Sullivan & McCormick 2007). Soft furnishings, the use of colour and the arrangement of appropriate furniture can help to soften a hospital atmosphere with its implications of sickness and institutional rules. The attitude of the staff, however, is much more important than physical surroundings. The Royal College of Obstetricians and Gynaecologists and the Royal College of Midwives in their joint report 'Towards safer childbirth' (RCOG/RCM 1999) make specific recommendations regarding making 'delivery' rooms more homely. This includes furnishings that allow women to adopt a variety of positions in labour, as well as the provision of dedicated bereavement rooms.

Good communication on labour wards between women and midwives, midwives and doctors, and doctors and women can have enormous impact (Crofts et al 2006, Hunter 2006, Lewis 2007). Labour ward staff having a shared philosophy and communicating well in multidisciplinary forums are helpful in improving the culture of busy labour wards. Improvement of multidisciplinary communication should be actively sought. Risk management issues and statutory supervision must be dealt with in a way that positively develops and supports staff. Communication is not only the content of what is said but includes non-verbal communication, written birth plans and involvement of the whole team in decision making. The 8th annual report from the Confidential Enquiry into Stillbirths and Deaths in Infancy (CESDI 2001) reiterated that all healthcare professionals involved in maternity care should be vigilant in identifying and communicating risk factors to specialist services, and that plans for both antenatal and intrapartum care should be made. Lewis (2007) also cites lack of communication, teamwork and cross-agency working as contributory factors in maternal death.

Prior to admission to a hospital, the woman should have been given good information about the physical process of labour and should have considered what strategies she may use to cope during the birth. It is essential that the labouring woman is welcomed and encouraged to feel at ease, and most of all that the midwife spends time actively listening as the woman recounts the details of the onset of labour.

Emotional support

The midwife has a defined role to fulfil which includes both physical and emotional assessment. Emotional support is provided by exercising skill in imparting confidence, expressing caring and dependability as well as being an advocate for her if needed. Clinical assessment includes the progress of labour and the physical status of mother and fetus. The midwife should display a tolerant non-judgemental attitude, ensuring that the woman is accepted whatever her reactions to labour may be.

Companion in labour

For more than 20 years, research has consistently shown that continuous one-to-one support of a woman during labour creates a strong feeling of security and satisfaction as well as having a positive effect on outcomes (Ball 1994, Hodnett & Osborn 1989a,b, Langer et al 1998, Madi et al 1999). A meta-analysis by Hodnett (2001) demonstrates a number of benefits of one-to-one care for mothers and babies. These include reduction in pain relief, in operative vaginal delivery and caesarean section as well as in length of labour; there were no harmful effects demonstrated. Women greatly value companionship and social support in labour (Price et al 2007).

The woman herself is central to all the decisions made about care during labour. Her chosen companion, whether sexual partner, friend or family member, should understand this. Ideally the companion should be involved in pre-labour preparation and decision-making. The companion should have participated in compiling a birth plan and any contingency plans drawn up in the event of change.

Admission to hospital labour wards is often an unknown entity and the company of a supportive companion can help reduce anxiety. During labour, the companion can keep the woman company, walk with her if she is ambulant, support her decisions about pain relief and encourage her with whatever she has chosen as her coping mechanism. Providing encouragement and reassurance that labour is progressing is also important, as is helping with physical comfort. In some areas a midwife will be able to remain with one woman through her entire labour but due to the unpredictable workloads on busy labour wards this is not always possible. Students can play an invaluable role in providing support.

The midwife should appreciate that the companion may also need direct support at times. This is particularly evident when a sudden emergency develops. If, for instance, a caesarean section becomes necessary, the midwife should delegate someone to keep the companion as informed as the woman wishes and ensure that he or she is not left feeling abandoned or uncared for.

Consent and information giving

Consent

Common law in the UK has developed rules that require patients to agree in meaningful terms to any recommended treatment. As Lord Donaldson has said (Re F 1990) 'The ability of the ordinary adult to exercise free choice in deciding whether to accept or refuse medical treatment... is a crucial factor in relation to all medical treatment'. It can therefore be concluded that patient autonomy is protected only when there is a meaningful choice made by the patient on the basis of adequate information and comprehension of that information.

Women need sufficient information before they can decide whether to give their consent, for example information about the benefits and risks of the proposed treatment, and alternative treatments. If she is not offered as much information as she reasonably needs to make her decision, and in a way she can understand, then consent may not be valid.

Consent must be given voluntarily, not under any form of duress or undue influence from health professionals, family or friends. It can be written or verbal. It is a common misunderstanding that a patient's signature on a consent form proves the consent is valid. This is not always the case. In an absolute emergency, it may be more appropriate to take witnessed verbal consent as more time can be spent on discussion and explanation and less on paperwork. In this scenario, it must be carefully documented in the case notes.

Under common law, a competent adult, including a competent pregnant woman, has the right to refuse medical treatment, however unreasonable this is deemed to be, even when the life of herself or her fetus is at risk. This is true whether the reason is rational or irrational, or even when there is no reason at all. The courts have no jurisdiction to declare non-consensual treatment of competent women (women that have capacity) to be lawful. Only when a baby has been born does it acquire rights.

There are exceptions to this rule, e.g. where the treatment is for a mental disorder and the patient is detained under the Mental Health Act of 1983.

A person lacks capacity if some impairment or disturbance of mental functioning renders that person unable to make a decision about treatment. This will occur when the person is unable to comprehend and retain the information material to the decision, or when the person is unable to retain information and weigh it in the balance as part of the process of arriving at a decision. Incapacity may be temporary, for instance if caused by shock, pain, fatigue, confusion, or panic induced by fear. If a healthcare professional fears a patient's decision-making (capacity) is impaired they should ask for help is assessing capacity. The Law Commission is keen to ensure that any decisions taken do not violate the European Convention on Human Rights. It is envisaged that, in the future, statutory protection will be given to the informal way decisions are currently made on behalf of incapacitated adults.

Midwives must provide support by giving information that ensures the woman understands events, feels free to ask questions and is aware of how labour is progressing. Before performing any examination, verbal permission should be sought, and explanations should be given of what is about to be done and why. Following any procedures, the midwife should provide feedback and verbal reinforcement; she can only then involve the woman in making further decisions about care. Relatives cannot give consent on behalf of a competent woman; it is only the woman herself who can give consent. It is an important principle that a midwife remembers no one else can consent on behalf of a competent adult.

Prevention of infection

Hospitals are notorious sources of infection, which can be resistant to antibiotic treatment. Effective cleaning will reduce the transfer of airborne organisms.

A balance between encouraging visitors and accommodating lots of unnecessary people in a birthing environment should be considered. Where the birth is not occurring at home, baths, sinks and toilets should be scrupulously cleaned and disinfected between users as necessary. Beds and rooms must also be cleaned thoroughly after use. It is part of ensuring a safe environment for the midwife to ensure that high standards of cleanliness are maintained even if she does not have managerial control over domestic services.

Personal hygiene is important for both mothers and their attendants. The woman should be encouraged to bathe and wash as she wishes to maintain personal freshness and the midwife must wash her hands before and after examining the mother and wear gloves when handling used sanitary pads, bloodstained linen or body fluids.

In the healthy woman, the immune system is the body's defence against not only bacteria and viruses but also other foreign organisms or harmful chemicals. It is very complex and it has to work properly to protect us from harmful bacteria and other organisms. Women with problems during pregnancy may have less resistance to combat infection. Some women will need very specialized care, especially women with any transmissible infection such as gastroenteritis, hepatitis or HIV infection.

Women with problem-free pregnancies and labours should be encouraged to stay in their own environment as long as possible, thus reducing the time spent in hospital. If a woman in normal labour is able to stay at home during the latent phase of labour this may also reduce the diagnosis of prolonged labour.

True prolonged labour increases the risk of infection and haemorrhage. Once the woman is admitted to hospital, invasive procedures should be kept to a minimum as an intact skin provides an excellent barrier to organisms.

The fetal membranes should also be preserved intact unless there is a positive indication for their rupture that would outweigh the advantage of their protective functions (Clements 2001). Certain invasive techniques, such as the performance of vaginal examinations, may be deemed necessary during labour. However, the midwife should ensure that she has a sound reason before embarking on any procedure. Women whose labours are prolonged are at particular risk of infection and are often subjected to a number of invasive procedures including the administration of intravenous fluids, repeated vaginal examinations, epidural analgesia and fetal blood sampling.

Pre-labour rupture of fetal membranes at term

The incidence of pre-labour rupture of membranes (PROM) at term (>37 weeks) is between 8–10% of all pregnancies (NICE 2008), and most women with PROM will labour spontaneously within 24 hrs. Following PROM with no signs of labour and no obvious liquor draining, digital examination should be avoided owing to an increased risk of ascending infection. If there is any uncertainty regarding the status of the membranes and in the absence of any pathology (including meconium staining), a woman may wear a pad for an hour or two then, with the midwife, reassess the clinical findings. Where there are facilities and the diagnosis of ROM is ambiguous, one sterile speculum examination should be performed to try and visualize pooling of liquor in the posterior fornix. Endocervical swabs may also be taken at this time.

Management of rupture of membranes

Active management has been shown to slightly reduce maternal infectious morbidity and admissions of babies to neonatal intensive care though neonatal infection rates were not increased (Dare 2006). Active management should most commonly be with the use of vaginal prostaglandins but may alternatively be via intravenous oxytocin depending on individualized care. Women with pre-labour ruptured membranes who opt for expectant management should have their temperature monitored and auscultation of the fetal heart to exclude a fetal tachycardia or other signs of fetal compromise associated with infection. This observation does not necessitate hospital admission in an otherwise uncomplicated pregnancy. Women should be given adequate information to decide between expectant management or active management of labour following pre-labour rupture of membranes.

Pre-term pre-labour rupture of membranes

In pre-term pregnancies, complicated by pre-labour rupture of membranes the presentation is often not cephalic. Transfer to a hospital with appropriate neonatal facilities is required. Corticosteroids reduce the incidence of respiratory distress syndrome and neonatal death. The use of antibiotics (specifically erythromycin) reduces neonatal treatment and is associated with prolongation of pregnancy (Kenyon et al 2001). Expectant management is usually considered until 34 weeks when individualized decisions would be made (RCOG 2006).

Position and mobility

A prospective RCT (de Jong et al 1997) demonstrated that women who adopt an upright position during labour experience significantly less pain and suffer less perineal trauma. Lateral and posterior position of the fetal presenting parts may be associated with more painful, prolonged or obstructed labour and difficult birth. It is possible that maternal posture may influence fetal position (Hofmeyr & Kulier 2001).

Women should be encouraged to give birth in the position they find most comfortable. Sutton & Scott (1995) have written and taught much on optimal fetal positioning. The benefits and risks of various labour and birthing positions need to be examined to ensure greater certainty. When methodologically stringent trials data are available, then women should be encouraged to use this information to make informed choices about the birth positions they might wish to assume. Midwives must be flexible in their approach to positions that women adopt as well as considering their own health, for example when assuming positions such as leaning to one side for sustained periods to assist women giving birth in a semi-sitting position on a labour ward bed.

Analgesia

Women should be aware of the advantages and disadvantages of all methods of analgesia available to them in their chosen birth environment. This is an essential part of antenatal education and the chosen method of analgesia may affect outcomes (see Ch. 27). Epidural analgesia gives the most effective pain relief in labour but is associated with increased rates of instrumental birth. The Comparative Obstetric Mobile Epidural Trial (COMET) study group (2001) reported a normal delivery rate of 35.1% with 'traditional epidural' and 42.7% with low dose (mobile) epidural.

Monitoring the fetus

The National Institute for Health and Clinical Excellence (NICE 2001b) has recommended that women with an uncomplicated pregnancy should not have electronic fetal monitoring (EFM) as a routine, but that intermittent auscultation with a Pinard stethoscope or handheld Doppler device should be the monitoring of choice. In this group of women there is no evidence to support an admission cardiotocograph (CTG); it should therefore not be done as routine.

The term 'intermittent auscultation' is used when the fetal heart is auscultated at intervals using a monaural fetal stethoscope (Pinard's) or a handheld Doppler device. Doppler apparatus can be used throughout a contraction, but listening during a contraction with a monaural stethoscope (Pinard) is uncomfortable for the woman and the fetal heart sounds may be inaudible. Using a Pinard the midwife can listen in to the fetal heart rate as the contraction is finishing to detect any slow recovery of the fetal heart rate back to the baseline.

The baseline rate should be between 110 and 160 b.p.m.

Normally the baseline rate is maintained during a contraction and immediately after it. However, in late labour some decelerations with contractions that recover quickly may be due to cord compression or compression of the fetal head and are normal.

Variability of >5 b.p.m. should be maintained throughout labour. The rate of the fetal heart should be counted over 1 complete minute in order to listen for the beat-to-beat variation. Variability can be confirmed by counting the number of fetal heartbeats heard in a 5s interval repeating this exercise for one minute. The fetal heart should be auscultated every 15 min when the woman is in established labour. If decelerations are heard in the first stage of labour with a Pinard or Doppler instrument, then electronic monitoring may be indicated to assess the extent of decelerations.

Electronic fetal monitoring

Electronic fetal monitoring (EFM) was introduced in the 1970s with the aim of reducing cerebral palsy. However, a reduction has not been demonstrated and the rate of cerebral palsy remains 2–3/10 000 live births (Parkes et al 2001). What has been demonstrated by the use of continuous EFM is an increase in obstetric intervention.

For women with problems in their pregnancy or other risk factors including the use of oxytocin, or epidural analgesia, EFM is appropriate.

The use of a CTG may appear to limit the choice of position, but telemetric apparatus allows the woman to walk around freely, provided that she remains within a given range. A conventional CTG (Fig. 26.1) does not necessarily confine the woman to bed but accurate external monitoring of uterine contractions may be difficult if she is very mobile.

Interpretation of CTG

Hospitals should ensure that staff who are performing and interpreting CTG traces have received training and assessment of their skills to ensure these are up-to-date (NICE 2001). The Clinical Negligence Scheme for Trusts has also set a standard for 6-monthly updating.

Only four variables are considered when interpreting a CTG. The CTG provides information on:

- baseline fetal heart rate
- baseline variability
- accelerations from the baseline rate
- decelerations from the baseline rate.

Baseline fetal heart rate

This is the fetal heart rate between uterine contractions. A rate more rapid than 160 b.p.m. is termed baseline tachycardia; a rate slower than 110 b.p.m. is baseline bradycardia. Either may be indicative of fetal compromise due to a number of causes. If the baseline is outside the stated normal range then referral to an obstetrician is appropriate.

Baseline variability

Electrical activity in the fetal heart results in minute variations in the length of each beat. This causes the tracing to appear as a jagged rather than a smooth line (Fig. 26.2). The baseline rate should vary by at least 5 beats over a period of 1 min. Loss of this variability (Fig. 26.3) may indicate fetal compromise. Reduced variability may be noted for a short period after the administration of maternal diamorphine/pethidine, which depress the fetal brain. Periods of 'fetal sleep' also cause a reduction in variability and commonly last for 20–30 min even in advanced labour (Gibb 1988, Lowe & Reiss 1996).

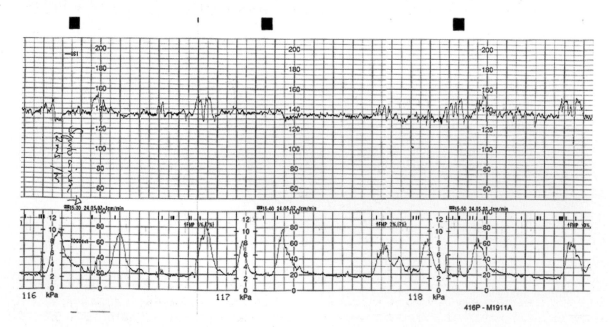

Figure 26.1 Normal CTG showing baseline variability.

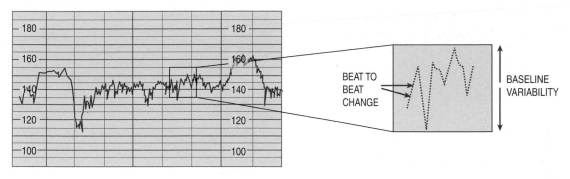

Figure 26.2 Baseline variability.

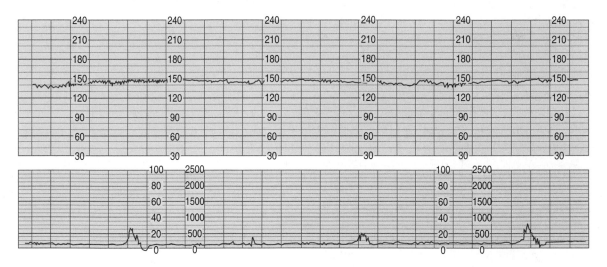

Figure 26.3 Uncomplicated loss of baseline variability: normal rate, no decelerations.

An acceleration is a brief rise in the fetal heart rate of at least 15 beats, for at least 15 s.

A deceleration is a drop from the baseline of 15 beats for >15 s but <3 min.

A deceleration of the fetal heart rate lasting longer than 3 min is referred to as a bradycardia.

Response of the fetal heart to uterine contractions

The fetal heart rate will normally remain steady or accelerate during uterine contractions during the first stage of labour. In order to assess the significance of fetal heart rate decelerations accurately, their exact relationship to uterine contractions, size, shape and uniformity must be noted. Compression of the umbilical cord, or fetal head, will result in some decelerations, particularly if the membranes are not intact. These would be early or variable decelerations lasting <3 min with good recovery to pre-deceleration rate.

This analysis of the fetal heart rate makes a CTG interpretable into the three categories recommended by NICE (2001) (Fig. 26.4):

- normal
- suspicious (non-reassuring)
- pathological (abnormal).

This is of course a rather simplistic view, as the whole picture of labour must be taken into account, including the gestation, any complications, particularly if the baby is not well grown and is presumed to have less reserves, as well as the stage and length

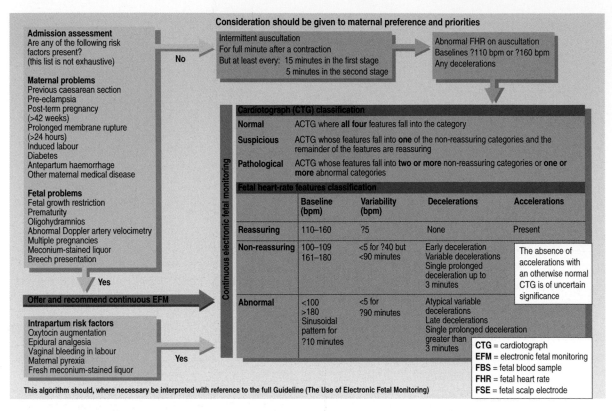

Figure 26.4 Guidelines for fetal monitoring in labour. (From NICE 2001, with permission.)

of that specific labour. These guidelines are an aid to clinical judgement with the exception of clearly pathological traces.

All CTG traces should be secured in the notes and kept for a minimum of 25 years, along with all other maternity records.

Fetal blood sampling

Units that use electronic fetal monitoring should have 24 hrs access to fetal blood sampling (FBS) facilities. When the fetal heart rate pattern is suspicious or pathological and fetal acidosis is suspected, then FBS should always be carried out NICE (2001). The procedure should be carried out with the woman in the left lateral position as a lithotomy position is more distressing for both mother and fetus (Fig. 26.5). If imminent delivery is clearly indicated by a severely pathological CTG, then no time should be wasted performing an FBS. This would be the clinical decision of a senior obstetrician. A fetal

blood sample result of ≤7.25 should be repeated usually within 30 min to 1 hr. An FBS <7.20 indicates that the baby should be delivered.

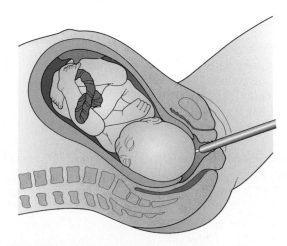

Figure 26.5 Fetal blood sampling. Access to fetal scalp via amnioscope passed through the cervix.

Nutrition

Despite food and drink nowadays being more freely available to most women in labour, once in established labour, most women have no desire to eat, though some fluids should be encouraged. A large amount of women feel nauseated or too distracted to eat. But for those who do not, particularly in the latent phase, women may have a desire for energy rich foods and carbohydrate. Low fat foods, such as toast, breakfast cereal, yoghurt, fruit juice, tea, plain biscuits and clear broth are easily digested. Ice cream and jelly may also be refreshing. Fluids may be taken freely, although women tend to reduce their drinking as labour progresses (Roberts & Ludka 1994).

Intake in normal labour

Opinions are divided and policies vary between hospitals. Most low risk women in spontaneous labour have little risk of requiring an emergency general anaesthetic. Therefore most hospitals will allow such women to take a low fat, low residue diet according to appetite, in order to give her energy and ensure that she is not hungry. However, in some centres, women receive nothing to eat after labour is established and are allowed only ice chips to suck. The latter policy stems from 'the widespread concern that eating and drinking during labour will put women at an increased and unacceptable risk of regurgitation and aspiration of gastric contents' (Johnson et al 1989, p 827). Aspirated contents from the stomach may contain undigested food and predispose to airway obstruction. But if the woman has been fasting, the strongly acidic gastric juice can cause a chemical pneumonitis if inhaled (Mendelson's syndrome). The cardiac sphincter, rendered less efficient by the effects of progesterone, allows a passive leak of stomach contents into the pharynx when loss of consciousness is induced with general anaesthesia. This, combined with the oedema of the pharynx so often present in pregnancy, makes intubation by the anaesthetist a difficult procedure. The answer clearly is to reduce the risk of general anaesthetic and use cricoid pressure during induction of such emergency anaesthetics (see Ch. 32).

Different foods and fluids empty from the stomach at different rates and gastric emptying is prolonged following the administration of narcotic analgesia. Johnson and colleagues point out that there is, however, 'no guarantee that withholding food and drink during labour will ensure that the stomach will be empty in the event that general anaesthesia should become necessary' (Johnson et al 1989, p 829). In an effort to reduce gastric volume and decrease the gastric acidity of the labouring woman, prophylactic antacids may be administered (see Ch. 32).

Glycogenic and fluid requirements

The vigorous muscle contractions of the uterus during labour demand a continuous supply of glucose. If this is not obtained from the diet, the body will start to metabolize protein and fat stores in an effort to provide glucose (gluconeogenesis) without which uterine muscle inertia will occur. This relatively inefficient method of producing glucose results in the occurrence of ketoacidosis. High concentrations of intravenous glucose may artificially increase fetal blood glucose levels, thereby causing fetal hyperinsulinism and resulting in hypoglycaemia of the neonate (Lowe & Reiss 1996, Steele 1995).

For women at increased risk of a general anaesthetic, giving small volumes of water or a weak fruit cordial may be acceptable. If the woman is permitted to follow her inclinations about drinking she is unlikely to become dehydrated. Simple measures such as brushing her teeth or using a mouthwash can help relieve the discomfort of a dry and uncomfortable mouth.

Bladder care

The woman should be encouraged to empty her bladder every 1–2 hrs during labour. The midwife should not rely on the mother to request to use the toilet as the sensation of needing to micturate may be reduced, particularly if there is an effective epidural block in progress. If the woman is mobile she may visit the toilet. In women who suffer pregnancy complications and have fluids restricted or an intravenous infusion the quantity of urine passed should be measured and a specimen obtained for testing. As urine in the bladder is a non-compressible mass, it may interfere with descent of the presenting part or reduce the capacity of the uterus to contract, increasing the risk of postpartum haemorrhage.

A full bladder may initially prevent the fetal head from entering the pelvic brim. In all cases of delay in labour, the midwife should ascertain whether the bladder is full and encourage the woman to void regularly. If it is not possible for the woman to use the toilet, the midwife should provide privacy and ensure maximum comfort by placing the bedpan on a stool or chair or encouraging the woman to adopt a squatting position on the bed. The sound or feel of water can also help to trigger the micturition reflex. If the bladder is incompletely emptied or the woman is unable to void for some hours, it may become necessary to pass a catheter.

Observations

The mother

Reaction to labour

As with other major life events, women vary in their reactions to labour. Some may view the contractions experienced as a positive, motivating, life-giving force. Others may feel them as pain and resist them. One woman may welcome the event with excitement because soon she will see her baby; another may be glad the pregnancy is over and with it the cumbersome ungainliness she experienced. However she views labour, the preparatory phase of pregnancy is at an end and within a relatively short period, a baby will be born. There may be feelings of apprehension, fear and worry in case she does not conform to the social expectations of her culture. She may experience anxiety in case childbirth is painful and have concerns about her ability to control pain (Niven 1992). As labour progresses she may feel less confident in her ability to cope with the relentless nature of the contractions that control her body. The midwife, with her skillful observations, advice and assistance, can do much to help her. She can encourage and help the woman and when possible give her one-to-one care. Accurate and easy-to-understand information given to the woman about the progress of labour will provide encouragement. Consultation about methods of pain relief will increase feelings of being in control (Ball 1994, Lovell 1996). The management of pain is discussed in Ch. 27.

Pulse rate

If the rate increases to >100 b.p.m. it may be indicative of anxiety, pain, infection, ketosis or haemorrhage. It is usual to record the pulse rate every 1–2 hrs during early labour and every 30 min when labour is more advanced.

Respiratory rate

Respiratory rate is a good indicator of the general physical condition of the woman. It should be recorded at least every 4 hrs. The rate may be over 20 respirations/min in severe anxiety or other pathologies. Some breathing techniques used in labour by women may make it difficult to monitor. In late labour and second stage, respiratory rates will vary because of the physical effort and strategies for second stage.

Temperature

This should remain within the normal range. Pyrexia is indicative of infection or ketosis, or may be associated with epidural analgesia. In normal labour, the maternal temperature should be recorded at least every 4 hrs and additionally when there is a clinical indication.

Blood pressure

Blood pressure is measured every 2–4 hrs unless it is abnormal, in which case, more frequent recordings will be necessary depending on the individual situation. The blood pressure must also be monitored very closely following epidural or spinal anaesthetic (see Ch. 27). Hypotension may be caused by the supine position, shock or as a result of epidural anaesthesia.

In a woman who has had pre-eclampsia or essential hypertension during pregnancy, labour may further elevate a raised blood pressure.

Urinalysis

Urine passed during labour should be tested for glucose, ketones and protein. Ketones may occur as a result of starvation or maternal distress when all available energy has been utilized. A low level of ketones is very common during labour and thought not to be significant. Unless the non-diabetic mother has recently eaten a large quantity of carbohydrate or sugar, glucose is found in the urine only following intravenous administration of glucose.

A trace of protein may be a contaminant following rupture of the membranes or a sign of a urinary infection, but more significant proteinuria may indicate pre-eclampsia.

Fluid balance

A record should be kept of all urine passed to ensure that the bladder is being emptied. If an intravenous infusion is in progress, the fluids administered must be recorded accurately. It is particularly important to note how much fluid remains if a bag is changed when only partially used.

Abdominal examination

An initial abdominal examination is carried out when the midwife first examines the mother. This should be repeated at intervals throughout labour in order to assess the length, strength and frequency of contractions and the descent of the presenting part. The method is described in Ch. 17.

Contractions

The frequency, length and strength of the contractions should be noted. When a uterine contraction begins, it is painless for a number of seconds and painless again at the end. The midwife, when feeling for contractions, is aware of the beginning of the contraction before the woman feels it. This knowledge can be utilized when giving inhalational analgesia or using other coping mechanisms (see Ch. 27). The uterus should always feel softer between contractions. Contractions, which are unduly long or very strong and in quick succession give cause for concern as fetal hypoxia may develop. Hyperstimulation should be considered if oxytocin is being infused. It should be stopped if fetal compromise or hyperstimulation is apparent.

Descent of the presenting part

During the first stage of labour, descent can be followed almost entirely by abdominal palpation. It is usual to describe the level in terms of the fifths of the head, which can still be palpated above the pelvic brim (see Ch. 17 and Ch. 25).

In the primiparous woman, the fetal head is usually engaged before labour begins. If this is not the case, the level of the head must be estimated frequently by abdominal palpation in order to observe whether the head will pass through the brim with the aid of good contractions.

When the head is engaged, the occipital protuberance can be felt only with difficulty from above but the sinciput may still be palpable, owing to increased flexion of the head, until the occiput reaches the pelvic floor and rotates forwards.

Vaginal examination and progress in labour

Although it is not essential to examine the woman vaginally at frequent intervals, it may be useful to do so when progress is in doubt or another indication arises (see Ch. 25). The features that are indicative of progress are effacement and dilatation of the cervix, and descent, flexion and rotation of the fetal head. There do not appear to be many research-based recommendations on the timing and frequency of carrying out a vaginal examination in labour. As this intervention can be extremely distressing to some women, alternative methods of assessment should be considered (Nolan 2001); routine examinations in normal labour should be abandoned and an individualized approach taken. All examinations should be recorded on the labour record.

The minimal standard of recording should include:

- effacement and dilatation of the cervix
- whether the membranes are present or absent (if absent the colour of liquor draining)
- the presenting part and its position in relation to the ischial spines
- the position of the fetal head as defined by the occiput including flexion.

Effacement and dilatation of the cervix. In normal labour, the primiparous cervix effaces before dilating, whereas in the parous woman, these two events often occur simultaneously. The latent phase of labour is usually defined as up to 3–4 cm dilated (see Ch. 25). There is no agreed 'starting point' for the onset of labour. However, acknowledging the latent phase and not commencing a partogram too early will reduce the overdiagnosis of 'failure to progress' later in labour.

Progressive dilatation is monitored as labour continues and charted on either the partograph or the cervicograph. This will allow for early detection of abnormal progress and indicate when intervention is likely. The use of cervograms to monitor labour has limitations and must be understood and applied appropriately (Gee 2000) (see also Ch. 25).

Descent

When assessed vaginally, the level or station of the presenting part is estimated in relation to the ischial spines, which are fixed points at the outlet of the bony pelvis. During normal labour the head descends progressively. The midwife must be aware, while estimating whether the head is lower than previously, that marked moulding or a large caput succedaneum will give a false impression of the level of the fetal head.

Flexion

In vertex presentations, progress depends partly on increased flexion. When the head is driven down on to the pelvic floor it encounters resistance: the lever principle causes the anterior part of the head to flex because there is less counterpressure. The midwife assesses flexion by the position of the sutures and fontanelles. If the head is fully flexed, the posterior fontanelle becomes almost central; if the head is deflexed, both anterior and posterior fontanelles may be palpable.

Rotation

Rotation is assessed by noting changes in the position of the fetus between one examination and the next. The sutures and fontanelles are palpated in order to determine position. Even if insufficient information is gained to make a definitive diagnosis, a record is made of what is felt and the findings will be evaluated with the abdominal findings at the time and compared with the findings of earlier or later vaginal examinations.

The fetus

Fetal condition during labour can be assessed by obtaining information about the fetal movements, heart rate patterns, the pH of the fetal blood and the colour and amount of amniotic fluid.

The fetal heart

The fetal heart rate may be assessed intermittently by a Pinard stethoscope or handheld Doppler device or continuously using EFM as appropriate.

Amniotic fluid

Amniotic fluid escapes from the uterus continuously following rupture of the membranes. This fluid should normally remain clear. If the fetus becomes hypoxic, meconium may be passed as hypoxia causes relaxation of the anal sphincter. The amniotic fluid becomes green as a result of meconium staining. Amniotic fluid that is a muddy yellow colour or is only slightly green may signify a previous event from which the fetus has recovered, but is common and may be of no significance in post-dates babies.

If the breech is presenting and is compacted in the pelvis, the fetus may pass frank thick meconium because of the compression of the abdomen; a fetus presenting by the breech is also prone to fetal compromise and may pass meconium as a result of hypoxia.

In the rare case of a fetus that is severely affected by Rhesus isoimmunization, the amniotic fluid may be golden-yellow owing to an excess of bilirubin.

Bleeding of sudden onset at the time of rupture of the membranes may be the result of ruptured vasa praevia and is an acute emergency (see Ch. 33).

Fetal compromise

'Fetal distress' is a term that should no longer be used; suspected fetal compromise should be favoured. If the fetus suffers as a result of an intrapartum event resulting in oxygen deprivation then the following signs may be present:

- fetal tachycardia
- a pathological CTG and corresponding poor FBS result
- fetal bradycardia or a severe change in fetal heart rate or decelerations related to uterine contractions, or both
- passage of meconium-stained amniotic fluid.

Midwife's management of fetal compromise. If signs of suspected fetal compromise are apparent, a midwife must call an appropriately trained obstetrician. If oxytocin is being administered, it should be stopped and the woman placed in a favourable position, usually on her left side. In cases of maternal oxygen lack, such as eclampsia or shock due to antepartum haemorrhage, oxygen may be given via a face mask. Prolonged oxygen administration will not benefit the fetus. The doctor may wish to take a sample of fetal blood for testing and arrangements should be made for this or delivery will be expedited depending on the clinical situation. In the first stage of labour this will necessitate caesarean section. In the second stage of labour a forceps delivery or ventouse extraction may be performed. When it is necessary to expedite delivery, the presence of a neonatologist or appropriately qualified health professional is desirable (NMC 2004).

Pre-term labour

Pre-term labour (for causes of this, see Ch. 42) is defined as labour occurring before the 37th completed week of pregnancy, regardless of birth weight (WHO 1969). A fetus is legally viable from 24 weeks' gestation. If a fetus is expelled from the uterus prior to 24 weeks and shows no sign of life, it is classified in the UK as a miscarriage (abortion). The World Health Organization recommends recording all deliveries of >500g birth weight.

Pre-term labour is associated with significant long-term disability and morbidity. After 29–30 weeks' gestation, the birth weight is a good predictor of survival. Prior to 29 weeks' gestation, the birth weight, gender, multiple pregnancy and gestation are all considered in the equation of risks of morbidity and mortality. The incidence of pre-term birth is increasing, but currently stands at around 8%, although with wide racial differences (Atalla et al 2000, p 113).

Increased perinatal survival, which is attributed to increased neonatal intensive care facilities and appropriately trained personnel, has altered policies towards management of the woman in pre-term labour. A woman who is at risk of delivering prematurely should be transferred to a maternity unit with intensive neonatal facilities, preferably with the fetus in utero. Tocolytic drugs may be used in very early labour to delay delivery until transfer to such a unit. Antenatal administration of corticosteroids has been shown to reduce the incidence of hyaline membrane disease, intraventricular haemorrhage and necrotizing enterocolitis in fetuses of 26–34 weeks' gestation. Two doses given over 24hrs last for at least 7 days.

The 8th Annual CESDI (2001) report on the project of 27/28 week-gestation babies states that 88% of these survive – almost double that of 15 years previously.

Management of pre-term labour

The gestation of the pregnancy in pre-term labour influences the management. Generally, the earlier the gestational age the higher is the possibility of an infective cause, which is often followed by rapid labour and delivery. Caesarean section of cephalic pre-term infants offers no reduction in fetal morbidity or trauma and is associated with its own morbidity. It is generally accepted that the mode of delivery of gestations <26 weeks does not alter the outcome. Prolonging pregnancies beyond 34 weeks does not improve neonatal outcomes, therefore in practice no attempt is usually made to arrest labour if pregnancy has advanced to 34 weeks' gestation.

Skilled care is required for the woman and the fetus during labour. The mother is faced with an unexpected emotional crisis because of the interruption of the normal progress of pregnancy. In extreme prematurity (22–25 weeks), a high perinatal mortality rate means the woman and her partner have to face the possibility of the death or disability of their baby. Full discussion regarding possible outcomes and whether or not to attempt resuscitation should be carried out with the senior clinicians involved in the care, and of course the parents. Continuous electronic heart rate monitoring is difficult to interpret at <30 weeks' gestation and should therefore be used and interpreted with caution. Baseline variability may be reduced on the CTG.

Records

Midwives are subject to statutory supervision and the Midwives Rules. The Nursing and Midwifery Council has set out how midwives' records should be kept, stored, handled and supervised. Rule 9 of the Midwives Rules and Standards (NMC 2004) sets out stipulations in relation to the keeping of midwifery records. Rule 10 requires midwives to permit the inspection of their records by the supervisor, the local supervising authority and the NMC (Dimond 2005). The content of these records should pertain to both the woman's physical and psychological condition and the condition of her fetus (see Ch. 25). Records must be legible in ink that can be reliably photocopied; they must also be dated and signed. The purpose of records is to serve the interest of the woman, to demonstrate the chronology of events as well as all significant consultations, assessments, observations, decisions, interventions and outcomes.

A written individualized care plan should be recorded in labour following examination and consultation with the woman. This should attempt to fit nicely with the birth plan that was devised in pregnancy and address anything that has changed. If the woman changes her mind as her labour progresses, or the situation changes, adjustments can and sometimes must be made. Whether or not a formal birth plan has been prepared, the midwife who is with the woman should communicate effectively with her, evaluate whether the labour is proceeding as expected and listen to her requests. A comprehensive record of the discussions that take place about changes in the plan or about proposed measures will ensure that the closest possible attention is paid to achieving the outcome that the parents are hoping for and will also provide an excellent documented history of the labour and improve communication. The midwife must

> **Box 26.1** Best practice points
>
> - Women should be well informed and choice offered on evidence-based information where possible
> - A competent woman can give or withhold consent for any procedure
> - Another adult cannot consent or withhold consent on behalf of a competent woman
> - Good communication between women, midwives and between professionals is a fundamental component of maternity services
> - The latent phase of labour should be more widely acknowledged in hospital settings
> - The use of strict time limits for first and second stage of labour should be reviewed in problem-free pregnancies
> - Good record-keeping and care plans are an essential aspect of care.

also record reasonable observations and examinations as contemporaneously as possible.

Box 26.1 lists best practice points for this stage of labour.

REFERENCES

Atalla R, Kean L, McParland P 2000 Preterm labour and prelabour rupture of fetal membranes. In: Kean L, Baker P, Edlestone D (eds) Best practice in labour ward management. W B Saunders, London, p 113, 129

Ball J A 1994 Reactions to motherhood, 2nd edn. Books for Midwives Press, Hale

Clements C 2001 Amniotomy in spontaneous, uncomplicated labour at term. British Journal of Midwifery 9(10):629–634

CESDI (Confidential Enquiry into Stillbirths and Deaths in Infancy) 2001 8th annual report. Maternal and Child Health Research Consortium, London

COMET (Comparative Obstetric Mobile Epidural Trial) Study Group UK 2001 Effect of low dose mobile versus traditional epidural techniques on mode of delivery: a randomized controlled trial. Lancet 358(9275):19–23

Crofts J F, Bartlett C, Ellis D et al 2006 Training for shoulder dystocia: a trial of simulation using low-fidelity and high-fidelity mannequins. Obstetrics and Gynecology 108(6):1477–1485

Dare M R, Middleton P, Crowther C A et al 2006 Planned early birth versus expectant management (waiting) for prelabour rupture of membranes at term (37 weeks or more). Cochrane Database of Systematic Reviews, Issue 1

de Jong P R, Johanson R B, Baxen P et al 1997 Randomised controlled trial comparing the upright and supine positions for second stage of labour. British Journal of Obstetrics and Gynaecology 104:567–571

Dimond B 2005 Midwifery records and legal issues surrounding them. British Journal of Nursing 14(20):1076–1078

Gee H 2000 Abnormal patterns of labour and prolonged labour. In: Kean L H, Baker P, Edleston D I (eds) Best practice in labour ward management. W B Saunders, London

Gibb D 1988 A practical guide to labour management. Blackwell Scientific, Oxford

Hodnett E D 2001 Caregiver support for women during childbirth. In: The Cochrane Library, Issue 3. Update Software, Oxford

Hodnett E D, Osborn R W 1989a Effects of continuous intrapartum professional support on childbirth outcomes. Research in Nursing and Health 12:289–297

Hodnett E D, Osborn R W 1989b A randomized trial of the effects of support during labour: mothers' views two to four weeks postpartum. Birth 16(4):177–183

Hofmeyr G, Kulier R 2001 Hands/knees posture in late pregnancy or labour for fetal malposition (lateral or posterior). In: The Cochrane Library, Issue 3. Update Software, Oxford

Hunter L P 2006 Women give birth and pizzas are delivered: language and Western childbirth paradigms. Journal of Midwifery and Women's Health 51(2):119–124

Johnson C, Keirse M J N C, Enkin M et al 1989 Nutrition and hydration in labour. In: Chalmers I, Enkin M, Keirse M J N C (eds) Effective care in pregnancy and childbirth. Oxford University Press, Oxford, p 827–832

Kenyon S L, Taylor D J, Tarnow-Mordi W et al 2001 Broad-spectrum antibiotics for preterm, prelabour rupture of fetal membranes: the ORACLE I randomised trial. Lancet 357 (9261):979–988

Langer A, Campero L, Garcia C et al 1998 Effects of psychosocial support during labour and childbirth on breastfeeding, medical interventions, and mothers' wellbeing in a Mexican public hospital: a randomised clinical trial. British Journal of Obstetrics and Gynaecology 105(10):1056–1063

Lewis G (ed.) (2007) The Confidential Enquiry into Maternal and Child Health (CEMACH). Saving mothers' lives: reviewing maternal deaths to make motherhood safer 2003–2005. The 7th report on Confidential Enquiries into Maternal Deaths in the United Kingdom. CEMACH, London

Lovell A 1996 Power and choice in birthgiving: some thoughts. British Journal of Midwifery 4(5):268–272

Lowe N K, Reiss R 1996 Parturition and fetal adaptation. Journal of Obstetric, Gynecological and Neonatal Nursing 25 (4):339–349

Madi B C, Sandall J, Bennett R et al 1999 Effects of female relative support in labour: a randomized controlled trial. Birth 26(1):4–8

NICE (National Institute for Clinical Excellence) 2008 Clinical guideline No. 70: Induction of labour. RCOG Press, London

NICE (National Institute for Clinical Excellence) 2001 The use of electronic fetal monitoring: the use and interpretation of cardiotocography in intrapartum fetal surveillance. NICE, London

Niven C 1992 Psychological care for families: before, during and after birth. Butterworth-Heinemann, Oxford

NMC (Nursing and Midwifery Council) 2004 Midwives rules and standards. NMC, London

Nolan M 2001 Vaginal examinations in labour: expert view. Practising Midwife 4(6):22

Parkes J, Dolk H, Hill N et al 2001 Cerebral palsy in Northern Ireland: 1981–1993. Paediatric and Perinatal Epidemiology 15(3):278–286

Price S, Noseworthy J, Thornton J 2007 Women's experience with social presence during childbirth. American Journal of Maternal Child Nursing 32(3):184–191

RCOG/RCM (Royal College of Obstetricians and Gynaecologists/ Royal Colleges of Midwives) 1999 Towards safer childbirth. RCOG/RCM, London

RCOG 2006 Guideline No. 44 Preterm prelabour rupture of membranes. RCOG, London

Re F (Mental Patient:Sterilisation) [1990] 2 AC 1.

Roberts C C, Ludka L M 1994 Food for thought. Childbirth Instructor Magazine Spring:25–29

Sinivaara M, Suominen T, Routasolo P et al 2004 How delivery ward staff exercise power over women in communication. Journal of Advanced Nursing 46(1):33–41

Steele R 1995 Midwifery care during the first stage of labour. In: Alexander J, Levy V, Roch S (eds) Aspects of midwifery practice: a research-based approach. Macmillan, Hampshire, Ch. 2

Sullivan A, McCormick C 2007 In: Liu D (ed.) Labour ward manual. Churchill Livingstone, Edinburgh, p 19–22

Sutton J, Scott P 1995 Understanding and teaching optimal foetal positioning. Birth concepts, New Zealand, p 11

WHO (World Health Organization) 1969 Prevention of perinatal morbidity and mortality. Public Health Papers No. 42. WHO, Geneva

27

Comfort and support in labour

Adela Hamilton

This chapter will explore the variety of means used
by the midwife to achieve, for each woman and her
partner, a birth experience that they can regard as
positive.

The chapter aims to:

- present an overview of factors affecting women's
  perceptions of labour (language, environment)
- discuss how methods such as support and reassurance, encouragement, information giving and
  the provision of a relaxing environment can
  impact positively on the birth experience of
  women
- describe how strategies that use the body's own
  mechanisms to facilitate the progress and process
  of labour work
- consider the pharmacological methods of relieving pain in labour.

A variety of factors affect the woman's experience
of labour and the progress made. These include:

- her coping mechanisms
- her own individual meaning of discomfort or
  pain of labour
- the cultural characteristics of the woman
- the labouring environment – whether at hospital
  or at home, etc.

Factors influencing women's perceptions and experience of labour

The biological, psychological, social, spiritual, cultural and educational dimensions of each woman
have an impact on how they express themselves

and, indeed, how they experience labour. The challenge for midwifery is to provide adequate and adapted care for each childbearing woman. The essence of midwifery is to be 'with woman', providing comfort and support to women in labour. Historically, the provision of care has been the role of women (Kitzinger 2000). Women have, throughout the ages, supported and helped each other during the process of birth. There is much literature to venerate the presence of the doula, midwife or friend of the birthing woman and the positive effect of the presence of this person on the outcome of labour.

One-to-one support in labour

Much midwifery and medical research has indicated that the one-to-one support by a midwife in labour reduces the need for analgesia and improves the birth experience of the mother. It also shortens the length of the labour (Haines & Kimber 2005, RCM 2006). This is reaffirmed in the *Modernizing Maternity Care* document (MCWP 2006), which concludes that maternity services should develop the capacity for every woman to have a designated midwife to provide care in established labour for 100% of the time. Continuous one-to-one support during labour can both reduce intervention rates and improve maternal and neonatal outcomes. The relationship between the woman and the midwife is important and can also impact on how the woman perceives the pain of labour (Lundgren & Dahlberg 2005).

The language of childbirth

The terms 'pain' and 'labour' are suggestive of difficulty and trouble. 'The skill of *watching what you are saying* is essential' (Robertson 2003, p 63), when dealing with women during childbirth. A huge difference is made if sensitivity is used when explanations are provided or when information is given, to women. A lot of the terminology is medical, masculine and negative (Robertson 2003). The midwife is now able to rely on research, evidence and her/his decision-making skills to provide care. The word 'delivery' today is replaced by the term birthing or birth and this is more suitable when talking about the concept and practice of normality within midwifery. Care must be taken to use appropriate and adapted language which is woman-friendly.

Understanding childbirth processes

As pain is caused by an ailment such as a burn, fracture or cut and not caused by a physiological process, these pathological notions cannot be readily employed or drawn upon, for midwifery purposes, or to explain what occurs during labour. The discomfort of labour is caused by the descent of the fetal head further into the pelvis. It is also caused by pressure on the cervix and the stretching of the vaginal walls and pelvic floor muscles, as descent of the presenting part occurs. The large uterine muscle is contracting more strongly, more frequently and for a longer duration, as labour progresses. This also increases the discomfort felt by the woman. It is therefore not suitable to use pain-relieving measures used in other medical circumstances, as the purpose is not to stop or impair the birth process (or contractions), but to let the labour progress normally, with the descent of the presenting part and with the rotation of this.

The object behind providing relief for the childbearing woman is to work with the contractions and the discomfort caused by these and the descending presenting part. The reactions of the woman to labour and to the discomfort of this varies greatly. So then must the response of the midwife. Answers and solutions are needed to support and enable the woman to cope with the birthing process.

Normal birth is a physiological process characterized by non-intervention, a supportive environment and empowerment of the woman (Anderson 2003). The midwife is a key figure in this process, supporting and assisting women through childbirth. Women state that they need someone who cares about them, rather than the use of supportive technology, to help them during childbirth (Walsh et al 2004). The needs of women must be addressed rather than prioritizing the needs of the service (Deery & Kirkham 2006). One study describes the midwife as 'anchored companion' (Lundgren & Dahlberg 2005). Midwives stated that listening to the woman, giving the woman the opportunity to participate and take responsibility, developing a trusting relationship, reading the bodily expressions and following the woman through childbirth, were all very important aspects to ensure an optimal birth experience. Time, waiting and following the woman are important elements of care. The idea of patience and supporting the woman on her journey, giving meaning and sense to the pain of labour is paramount.

It is more convenient to think in terms of facilitating the birthing process. The campaign for normal birth launched by the Royal College of Midwives (RCM) (Day-Stirk 2005) has the following intended outcomes:

- midwives to be energized and confident in practices that facilitate normal birth
- birth experiences for women and job satisfaction for midwives to be improved
- greater rates of normal birth and decrease in unnecessary intervention rates to be achieved.

From this it is clear that the needs of the women who are giving birth are at the centre and the focus of the midwife's attention. Not only will this ensure that care is optimal, but the midwife will enjoy providing care for women.

The MCWP (2006, p 10) reiterates this sentiment proposing a course of action that all '... Maternity services develop the capacity for every woman to have a designated midwife to provide care for them when in established labour for 100% of the time'.

Mobility and positioning in labour

Studies carried out on ambulation, mobility and positioning during labour confirm that mobility during labour improves both the woman's experience and the outcome of labour (Deakin 2001, Downe et al 2001, Haines & Kimber 2005). The uterine action is more effective, labour is shortened, there is a reduced need for pharmacological analgesia and oxytocin augmentation. The risk of fetal compromise is lowered.

It is documented that recumbent positions result in supine hypotension, diminished uterine activity and a reduction in the dimensions of the pelvic outlet (Walsh 2000). Women who take up an erect position during labour experience less pain, have significantly less perineal trauma and have fewer episiotomies. Restriction of movement can actually compromise labour (Gould 2000).

Culture, movement and positioning

Kitzinger (2000, p 749) would go as far as pronouncing that 'birth is movement'. Gould (2000) would agree, saying that movement is a significant characteristic of normal labour. Cultures where women are constrained and limited in their posture and positioning during labour, are in fact the exception, rather than the rule. Many cultures use movement, dance, physical contact and massage to encourage and sustain the process of labour. Writers now provide valuable reports and evidence of the engineering and movements made by some mothers in Africa, Japan and Fiji, which actually employ physiological responses of the woman, including turning, moving and dancing. These enhance the experience and facilitate the process of labour. There is much to be said for such an approach where the woman dictates the course of events and adapts to the activity of the uterus. One author also remarks how women move and swing their pelvis, thereby accommodating the passage of the fetal head through it (Kitzinger 2000). Walsh (2000) mentions that the compelling logic of gravity, meaning birthing in an upright position, should make us wonder how it has become routine practice to birth in a semi-recumbent position.

Henley-Einion (2007) discusses the value of the Five Rhythms method. Movements described as flowing, staccato, chaos, lyrical and stillness, which are a combination of expressive movements, rather than a set of routine exercises, are employed to provide dance and the music defines, guides, inspires and prompts the body. This is explained by Henley-Einion (2007, p 20) as the dance, beginning '... with the head and then move the shoulders, elbows, hands, spine, hips, knees and feet. These body parts are used to "lead" the dance and to understand the connections between the body's elements and how they blend together'. Such a strategy would be a fitting one to use during the birthing process.

The birth plan

The birth plan is a document that describes the woman's requests in relation to her antenatal, intrapartum and postnatal care. This may be adjusted and changed as necessary to meet the needs of the woman during the pregnancy, labour, birth and postpartum period. It is a valuable tool for midwives and facilitates the provision of holistic, individualized care. Requests are written down and are kept in the handheld notes of the woman. It may also be useful to confirm the contents of the plan with her as labour commences. It must also be made clear that these are the personal choices of the woman in labour, and may well change as labour progresses, the unpredictable nature of labour being as it is. It may be useful for providing an insight into how the woman has viewed her pain relief at the beginning of pregnancy, and on commencing labour. The midwife may use this information to tailor and plan suitable care for the woman.

Nolan (2005) warns of the harm, which can be caused by the birth plan. In one study (Jones et al 1998), findings revealed that far from improving relationships between mothers and obstetric and midwifery staff, birth plans caused annoyance and actually affected the outcome of these labours negatively, with high intervention rates.

Women's control of pain during labour

Pain control during labour should be a woman-centred strategem and not a medically oriented one. There is much evidence to suggest that women are not always more satisfied by a birth experience that is pain free (Fairlie et al 1999). Midwives are therefore required to give control of the pain to women rather than eradicating it. A clear differentiation must be made between the traditional goal of pain relief and the control of pain in labour.

The role of pain in labour is an important one and an empowering process, whereby the woman triumphs, by giving birth. The midwife must realize the importance of her own attitude to 'pain relief' in labour, as this is frequently informed by the medical model.

The role of the midwife is to encourage and assist women to 'anticipate positively' the birth of their baby. Two researchers in Japan revealed in their study on the intensity of memorized labour pain (Kabeyama & Miyoshi 2001, p 51) that 'Self-control is the most important predictor of satisfactory childbirth experience for mothers'. They state that women who viewed labour as a challenge, in their attempt to control their breathing and relaxation, had much better outcomes. These active attitudes are supposed to reflect the positive attitudes to everything in daily life by the individual. The study goes on to say that not only does the removal of excessive fear and anxiety make a birth experience more satisfactory but that it also increases the mother's pride and self-confidence. A greater motivation for constructing good mother–baby relationships also comes about.

Pain perception and somatosensory sensation

Many writers and researchers now agree that emotions such as fear, confidence, and also cognition, affect the person's perception of pain (Leap & Anderson 2004, Mander 1998). More than any other type of sensation, pain can be modified by past experience, anxiety, emotion and suggestion. Lack of food, rest and sleep also impact on the woman's perception of pain. The midwife must take into account not only the level or extent of the pain, but also all other subjective or illusory aspects of this.

The physiology of pain

Pain stimulus and pain sensation

Pain is caused by a stimulus; this stimulus may cause, or be on the verge of causing, tissue damage. Pain sensation may therefore be distinguished from other sensations, although emotions such as fear and anxiety are also experienced at the same time, thereby affecting the person's perception of pain. It must also be remembered that a painful stimulus may also induce such changes by the sympathetic nervous system as increased heart rate, a rise in blood pressure, release of adrenaline (epinephrine) into the bloodstream and an increase in blood glucose levels. There is also a decrease in gastric motility and a reduction in the blood supply to the skin, causing sweating. Thus, stimuli that cause pain result in a *sensory* incident or occurrence.

Pain transmission

The pain pathway or ascending sensory tract originates in the sensory nerve endings at the site of trauma. The impulse travels along the sensory nerves to the dorsal root ganglion of the relevant spinal nerve and into the posterior horn of the spinal cord. This is known as the *first neuron*. The *second neuron* arises in the posterior horn, crosses over within the spinal cord (the sensory decussation) and transmits the impulse via the medulla oblongata, pons varolii and the mid-brain to the thalamus. From here, it travels along the *third neuron* to the sensory cortex (Fig. 27.1).

In cases of *acute pain*, sensations are transmitted along *Aδ fibres*, which are large diameter nerve fibres. This type of pain is perceived as being a pricking pain that is readily localized by the sufferer. The pathway for *chronic pain* is slightly different, the nerve fibres involved are of smaller diameter and are called *C fibres*. Chronic pain is often described as a burning pain that is difficult to localize.

Somatosensory function

'Somatic sensation' refers to the sensory function of the skin and body walls. This is moderated by a variety of somatic receptors. There are particular receptors for each sensation, such as heat, cold, touch, pressure, etc. On entering the central nervous system, the afferent nerve fibres from somatic receptors form synapses with interneurons that comprise the specific ascending pathways going to the somatosensory cortex via the brain stem and the thalamus.

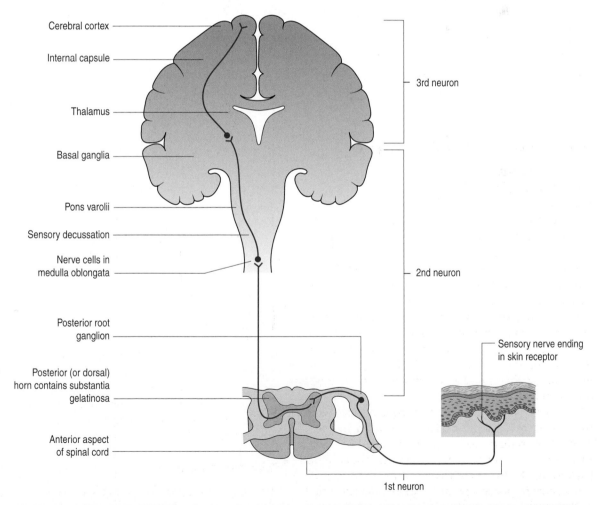

Figure 27.1 The sensory pathway showing the structures involved in the appreciation of pain. (From Bevis 1984 with permission from Baillière Tindall.)

An *afferent neuron*, with its receptor, makes up a sensory unit. Usually the peripheral end of an afferent neuron branches into many receptors. The receptors whose stimulation gives rise to pain are situated in the peripheries of small unmyelinated or slightly myelinated afferent neurons. These receptors are known as *nociceptors* because they detect injury (*Noci*, from the Latin: harm, injury). The primary afferents coming from nociceptors form synapses with interneurons after entering the central nervous system. Substance P is a *neurotransmitter* that is liberated at some of these synapses when there is a pain impulse; it facilitates information about pain, which is transmitted to the higher centres.

The stretching of the muscles and ligaments of the pelvic cavity and the pressure of the descending fetus during the birthing process causes, to varying degrees, pain in labour (Fig. 27.2). This sensation is transmitted by afferent or visceral sensory neurons, visceral pain being caused by the stretching or irritation of the viscera. Afferent neurons convey both autonomic sympathetic and parasympathetic fibres. Pain fibres from the skin and the viscera run adjacent to each other in the spinothalamic tract. Therefore pain from an internal organ, such as the uterus, may be perceived or felt as if it was coming from a skin area supplied by the same section or part of the spinal cord. Pain from the uterus may be perceived or felt in the back or the labia. When this sort of pain occurs or is experienced, it is commonly called *referred pain*.

One physiological explanation for the differing views, attitudes and perceptions of pain is that

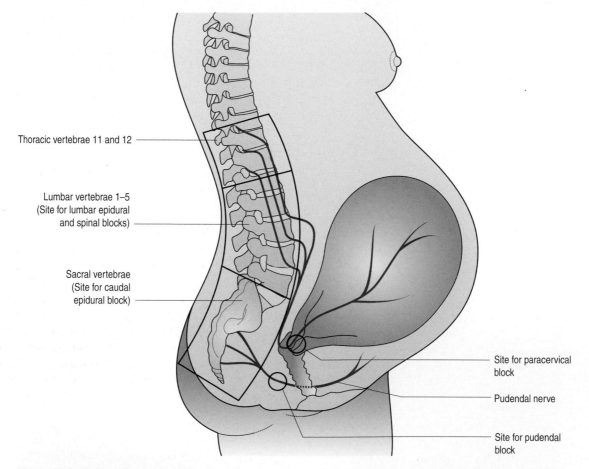

Figure 27.2   Pain pathways in labour showing the sites at which pain may be intercepted by local anaesthetic techniques. (From Bevis 1984 with permission of Baillière Tindall.)

offered by Martini (2001, p 93) who states that: 'Due to the facilitation that results from glutamate and substance P release, the level of pain experienced can be out of proportion to the amount of painful stimuli. This effect can be one reason why people differ so widely in their perception of pain associated with childbirth'.

Endorphins and enkephalins

Endorphins are described as being opiate-like peptides, or *neuropeptides*, which are produced naturally by the body at neural synapses at various points in the central nervous system pathways. They modulate the transmission of pain perception in these areas. Endorphins are found in the limbic system, hypothalamus and reticular formation (Martini 2001). They bind to the presynaptic membrane, inhibiting the release of substance P. Therefore they inhibit the transmission of pain. *Enkephalins* are also neuropeptides; they have the ability to inhibit neurotransmitters along the pathway of pain transmission, thereby reducing it. These act like a natural pain relieving substance.

Theories of pain

Many theories of pain have been presented in the literature. These are not always applicable in the situation mentioned here (i.e. pain and labour). These theories include specificity, pattern, affect and psychological/behavioural theory (Mander 1998). The most widely used and accepted theory is that of Melzack & Wall (1965). These researchers have established that gentle stimulation actually inhibits the sensation of pain (Mander 1998). Their *gate-control theory* declares that a neural or spinal gating mechanism occurs in the substantia gelatinosa of the dorsal horns of the spinal cord. The nerve impulses received by nociceptors, the receptors for pain in the skin and tissue of the body, are affected by the gating mechanism. It is the position of the gate that determines whether or not the nerve impulses travel freely to the medulla and the thalamus, thereby transmitting the sensory impulse or message, to the sensory cortex. If the gate is closed, there is little or no conduction. If the gate is open, the impulses and messages pass and are transmitted freely (Fig. 27.2). Therefore, when the gate is open, pain and sensation are experienced.

Physiological responses to pain in labour

Several of the body's systems are affected by labour. Pain of labour is associated with an *increased respiratory rate*. This may cause a decrease in the $PaCO_2$ level, with a corresponding increase in the pH. The fetus is then affected and a subsequent drop in the fetal $PaCO_2$ ensues. This may be suspected by the presence of late decelerations on the cardiotocograph. The acid–base equilibrium of the system may be altered by hyperventilation and breathing exercises. Alkalosis may then affect the diffusion of oxygen across the placenta, leading to a degree of fetal hypoxia.

Cardiac output increases during the first and second stages of labour. This can be by up to 20% and 50%, respectively. The augmentation is caused by the return of uterine blood to the maternal circulation, about 250–300 ml with each contraction. Pain, apprehension and fear may cause a sympathetic response, thereby producing a greater cardiac output.

Both the above systems are affected by catecholamine release. Adrenaline (epinephrine), which comprises about 80% of this, has the effect of reducing the uterine blood flow. This may in turn lead to a reduction of uterine activity.

Non-pharmacological methods of pain control

Homeopathy (see Ch. 50)

The aim of homeopathy is to reinforce the body's physiological response. It attempts to 'cure like with like' (Alexander et al 1990). Homeopathic remedies are prepared from plant extracts and from minerals. Professional advice is recommended during pregnancy as the holistic approach of this method entails a consideration of all the facets and the requirements of the individual. Castro (1992) recommends such solutions as Aconitum to relieve anxiety and Kali Carbonicum to alleviate back pain during labour.

Hydrotherapy

Immersion in water during labour as a means of analgesia has been used for years (Forde et al 1999). Garland & Jones (1994) state that the effectiveness of hydrotherapy is due to two factors. Heat relieves muscle spasm, and therefore pain, and 'hydrokinesis' does away with the effects of gravity and also the discomfort and strain on the pelvis. Mander (1998) suggests that there is relatively little reliable and valid evidence to prove that bathing during labour increases maternal or neonatal infection. Other writers agree with this (Forde et al 1999). Advantages such as less augmentation by oxytocics and a reduction of analgesia used, were reported (Forde et al 1999, Mander 1998). Forde et al (1999) maintain that hydrotherapy has other benefits such as a reduction in the length of labour and a lower incidence of genital tract trauma. It is difficult to establish the evidence for hydrotherapy, because of the increase in pool births. However, these two –hydrotherapy used as analgesia, and, birthing in the pool, when the birth is carried out in water – are different.

Hydrotherapy during childbirth has the following outcomes:

- mothers require less augmentation of labour
- the mother's experience was positively affected by hydrotherapy
- the use of analgesia was consistently lower in this group
- the need for pethidine and Entonox was significantly reduced.

There is however some contention regarding the use of water during labour and birth. A study by Burns (2001) shows that water immersion has been highly rated by both women and midwives and was valued by both multiparous and first time mothers (Box 27.1, Aly's story). Benjoya Miller (2006, p 484) agrees that 'the calming atmosphere of a pool room benefits everyone involved'. The woman is less anxious and therefore feels less pain. Most women (95%) who used the pool had a normal vaginal birth (Baxter 2006).

One randomized controlled trial showed that pain increased less markedly in women who used hydrotherapy (Cammu et al 1994). One Swiss hospital (Geissbuhler & Eberhard 2000) is able to offer hydrotherapy to all birthing women and this without harmful consequences.

Music therapy

Many birthing rooms are equipped with radio or CD apparatus and this is often a useful strategem to help

---

Box 27.1 Aly's story of Reuben's birth

My waters broke at home at 2.45 a.m. (in two bursts) and my contractions started with gentle flutterings. The advice from our antenatal class was to stay at home as long as possible, ideally until the contractions were 2 every 10 min.

By 8.15 a.m., this was the case, and we were driving through rush hour traffic with me on all fours in the back of the car!

At the hospital, we were shown to the birthing pool room and I was examined at 9.00 a.m. to find I was 3 cm. The contractions continued to come stronger and closer together. I managed the pain with a TENS machine and some well taught yoga breathing, while sitting on an exercise ball!

At the point of needing something stronger, it was suggested I got into the pool; wow, it felt great, my whole body instantly felt calmer and with the aid of gas and air, I was ready to push. An hour later at 1.14 p.m. out came a beautiful, sleeping little boy.

We were so lucky with our birth, the support from the midwives was invaluable as even with a straightforward labour they are still an essential ingredient. Together with the imagery a pool birth creates, the day will always be a positive memory for us.

---

women relax, be entertained and find some distraction while birthing. This is especially useful during the early stages of labour. Many types of music are available for relaxation, some are provided specifically for the birthing woman. Henley-Einion (2007) recounts that music has a positive effect on the body, mind and spirit of the woman. It provides empowerment and an enabling effect.

TENS

Transcutaneous electrical nerve stimulation (TENS) is a widely used, well-appreciated and effective method of pain relief. This effectiveness is related to the action of TENS, which stimulates the production of natural endorphins and enkephalins and also its ability to impede incoming pain stimuli. One of its distinct advantages is that it includes the partner in the events surrounding the birth. Much documentary evidence suggests that when using TENS many husbands and birth partners feel able to assist and support their partner in labour and childbirth to a much greater degree. Partners feel a purposeful role and are able to help in managing the device. A reduction in the demand for pethidine and other pain relief was also found when TENS was employed (Poole 2007).

Technique

TENS is a small device which distributes low intensity electrical charges across the skin (de Ferrer 2006). These signals are said to prevent pain signals from the uterus, vagina and cervix arriving at the brain. The body's own pain relief, the endorphins, are then released. TENS works by stimulating low threshold afferent fibres from, for example, the fibres of touch receptors. This then leads to inhibition of neurons in the pain pathways. As pathways activated by the touch receptors add a synaptic input into the pain pathways, people may rub or massage a painful area to relieve the pain; TENS functions in the same way.

The apparatus consists of four electrodes and four flexes that connect these to the TENS unit, which has controls to alter the frequency and the intensity of the impulse. The electrodes are positioned at the level of T10 and L1 on the mother's back. These have been found to be effective for the control of pain during the first stage of labour. The other two electrodes are situated between S2 and S4 and provide control of pain during the second stage of labour. A boost control button conveys high intensity and high frequency patterns of stimulation of the dermatomes, thereby controlling pain during the uterine contraction and providing relief.

There are few contraindications to the utilization of TENS in labour (Walsh 1999). There is a slight risk of interference with the fetal monitor. Skin allergies may be caused by the electrodes or by the tape used. Finally, clients who have pacemakers may not employ this mode of pain control.

TENS is often more effective when started in early labour, and this fact is upheld by the literature (Johnson 1997, Walsh 1999). An important factor regarding TENS is that it is preferred by women. This is probably due to the fact that TENS enhances their control over the birth process.

The research on TENS reveals the paucity of scientific evidence to substantiate the fact that women in labour do find the application of this method effective (Juman Blincoe 2007). The reality is that it is used in conjunction with other methods of pain relief, and this makes the method very difficult for researchers to verify the evidence. There is, however, evidence of the usefulness of TENS as a pain relieving strategy in labour. In one study by Johnson (1997), 71% of the respondents out of a population of 10 077 stated having had either good or excellent pain relief from the TENS. Although Johnson (1997) cautions against an over simplistic interpretation of these results, as many of the participants used other methods of pain relief in conjunction with TENS, it can still be observed that many women find TENS suitable, effective and beneficial.

Pharmacological methods of pain control

Opiate drugs

The pain of labour is only partially amenable to opiates. Because of the episodic nature of labour pain, the mother tends to receive little benefit during contractions but may become over-sedated at other times.

(Collis 2000, p 365)

Opiate drugs are frequently used during childbirth because of their powerful analgesic properties. The action of these drugs lies in their ability to bind with receptor sites in the central nervous system. The receptor sites are mainly found in the substantia gelatinosa of the dorsal horn of the spinal cord. Others are located in the midbrain, thalamus and hypothalamus.

Three systemic opioids are commonly used for pain relief in labour. Pethidine (meperidine in the USA) is the most popular but some units prefer diamorphine or meptazinol (Meptid). All have similar pain-relieving properties but they also have side-effects. These include nausea, vomiting and drowsiness in the mother and depression of the baby's respiratory centre at birth. An antiemetic agent is sometimes given at the same time to reduce the nausea effect. Opioids given to the mother in labour can make breastfeeding more difficult to establish as the baby tends to be sleepy (Ransjo-Arvidson et al 2001). The side-effects are, however, variable and are influenced by maternal metabolism of drugs, the degree and speed of transfer of drugs and metabolites from maternal to fetal circulation and the ability of the fetus to process and excrete both. It is therefore important to ensure that the mother is fully informed antenatally so that she can make informed decisions about pain relief. A systematic review by Elbourne & Wiseman (2000) to compare different types of opioids concluded that no strong preference could be recommended.

Pethidine

Pethidine is the most frequently used systemic narcotic analgesic in England. This is possibly because it is of low cost and midwives have been administering pethidine for many years. It is a synthetic compound and acts on the receptors in the body. It is usually administered intramuscularly in doses of 50–150 mg (taking the size of the woman into account) and takes about 20 min to have an effect. Pethidine can be administered intravenously for a faster effect and some units use a machine to allow patient-controlled analgesia (PCA), but this is less common.

Pethidine delays stomach emptying and women may not use the birthing pool if they have been given an opiate drug. Some reports show that pethidine slows down the process of labour. Carson (1996) states that this may be due to the effect of opioids on the myometrium, relaxing it by their action on calcium ions, and also the effect of opioids on the hypothalamus, inhibiting the release of oxytocin from the posterior pituitary gland.

There is evidence to show that pethidine is reported as being less effective, or even not effective at all (Ranta et al 1994), when compared to nitrous oxide and oxygen (Entonox) and that sedation was wrongly assumed to be analgesia.

Diamorphine

Diamorphine has been found to provide effective analgesia for up to 4 hrs in labour. It is also said to be more rapidly eliminated from maternal and neonatal plasma (Freeman et al 1982). Diamorphine is used far less commonly than other opiates in labour, even though some claim it gives better pain relief and hence more comparative studies are needed (Fairlie et al 1999). It is possible that its lack of use

in normal labour might be due to fears of the potentially addictive nature of diamorphine.

Meptazinol

Meptazinol is usually given in doses of 100–150 mg intramuscularly. It is fast acting and is effective for about 4 hrs. Meptazinol may be associated with an increased incidence of nausea and vomiting (Carson 1996). It has failed to replace pethidine in most maternity units in England.

Inhalation analgesia

A premixed gas made up of 50% nitrous oxide (N_2O) and 50% oxygen administered via the Entonox apparatus is the most commonly used inhalation analgesia in labour. Nitrous oxide, like many other forms of analgesia, acts by limiting the neuronal and synaptic transmission within the central nervous system. Evidence shows that N_2O induces opioid peptide release in the periaqueductal grey area of the mid-brain leading to the activation of the descending inhibitory pathways, which results in modulation of the pain/nociceptive processing in the spinal cord (Fujinaga & Maze 2002). The mixture (of gases) is stable at normal temperature, but separates under the temperature of $-7°C$. In many large obstetric units the gas is piped, (this is stored in a bank) or alternatively is available in cylinders. Hospitals take responsibility for the safe storage of cylinders but in community practice midwives should store cylinders on their side, rather than upright. This is because nitrous oxide is heavier than oxygen and the horizontal position reduces the risk of delivering a severely hypoxic mixture. The cylinders must be brought into a warm room if they have been exposed to cold temperatures, and the gases remixed by inverting the cylinder at least three times before use.

Entonox apparatus is usually manufactured by the British Oxygen Company (BOC). Both the apparatus and the cylinder are made so that they do not fit on to other equipment. These fit together by a pin index system. The cylinder is blue with a blue and white shoulder. The one-way valve opens on inspiration and the mother needs to be adequately informed of the functioning of the apparatus, being advised that optimal analgesia is obtained by closely applying the lips around the mouthpiece (Fig. 27.3) or, in some cases, firmly applying the mask to the face.

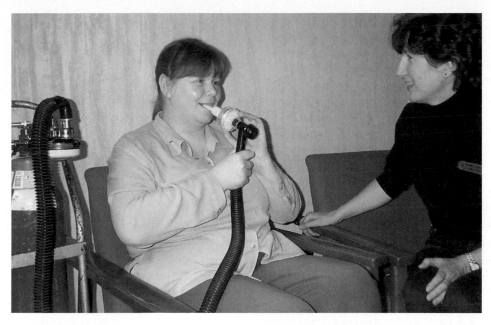

Figure 27.3 Midwife explaining the use of Entonox apparatus. Note the mouth piece and filter.

The gases take effect within 20s; it is therefore important that the woman uses it before a contraction. The maximum efficacy of the gases occurs after about 45–50s and, if the timing is right, this should happen with the height of the contraction, providing maximum relief for the woman. This method of pain control is useful in that the woman is able to administer it herself. The effectiveness of it relies on the woman's prior instruction and ability to follow this.

Some reports state that teratogenic and other side-effects exist among staff who are exposed to high levels of nitrous oxide (Ahlborg et al 1996). The main one of these is that of sub-fertility. Scavenging equipment, to extract expired gases, is recommended for all birthing rooms.

Regional (epidural) analgesia

More women are now requesting a pain-free labour and ask for epidural analgesia as soon as labour is established. Women who find alternative methods of pain relief inadequate once experiencing strong contractions might decide to request an epidural when labour is well advanced. This makes explanation of epidural analgesia antenatally even more important. The pain relief from an epidural is obtained by blocking the conduction of impulses along sensory nerves as they enter the spinal cord. When epidural block in labour was first introduced in the 1970s most attention was focused on the technique and less on the problems it caused in relation to normal birth. In those early years, as well as providing the required sensory block, the blockade of motor and sympathetic nerves caused loss of bladder sensation and function, complete numbness of the legs, significant hypotension, relaxation of pelvic floor muscles and impairment of expulsive efforts in the second stage of labour.

Preparation of the woman

The woman and her partner must receive clear explanations of the procedure and the woman's consent must be obtained. An intravenous infusion of crystalloid fluids is commenced prior to siting the epidural. The need for 'preloading' has reduced now that low dose epidural blockades are used, reducing the risk of hypotension. Frequently the mother is positioned in the left lateral position for the procedure. This is partly because of the risk of supine hypotension and also because the mother may well be more comfortable in this position when in labour. Some may prefer to ask the mother to sit up and flex the spine, in an effort to separate the vertebrae, thus facilitating the management of the procedure. The position of the mother is very important, and this should be discussed and negotiated with her. The fetal heart rate and the woman's blood pressure must be recorded throughout, especially in the case of pregnancy-induced hypertension, or in any case of suspicion of fetal compromise.

Epidural technique

A local anaesthetic is injected into the epidural space of the lumbar region, usually between vertebrae L1 and L2, or between L2 and L3, or between L3 and L4. The procedure is usually carried out by an experienced (obstetric) anaesthetist, under strict aseptic conditions. A small amount of local anaesthetic is used before inserting a Tuohy needle into the epidural space (Fig. 27.4). To locate the epidural space the anaesthetist advances the needle cautiously. The Tuohy needle, usually 16g, is introduced little by little until the resistance of the ligamentum flavum is encountered. At this point a syringe is attached to the Tuohy needle, after removal of the stilette. The needle is then inserted further, cautiously, until it enters the epidural space. This is recognized by the loss of resistance when pressure is applied to the

plunger of the syringe (loss of resistance to saline is sometimes a preferred technique). It is particularly important that the woman keeps very still at this stage as the subarachnoid space is a few millimetres deeper. A slight movement by the woman could result in the Tuohy needle inadvertently puncturing the meninges and causing a 'dural tap'.

Once confident that the Tuohy needle is in the epidural space and there has been no leakage of blood or CSF, a catheter is threaded through the needle to facilitate bolus top-ups or a continuous infusion. A test dose of the local anaesthetic lidocaine (lignocaine), of about 4 ml, may then be given – although some anaesthetists prefer to inject the first dose of bupivacaine (Marcain) very slowly whilst observing for any adverse reactions. Continuous infusion of dilute bupivacaine and opioids (usually fentanyl) has permitted significant reductions in the amount of local anaesthetic used whilst ensuring rapid analgesia. A further advantage of this regimen lies in the mother's ability to move about and bear down in the second stage of labour because of the minimal motor block effect. The Comparative Obstetric Mobile Epidural Trial (COMET Study Group UK 2001) found that low dose infusion epidurals resulted in a lower incidence of instrumental vaginal deliveries compared with traditional bolus epidurals.

An antibacterial filter is attached to the end of the catheter. The catheter is then secured to the mother's

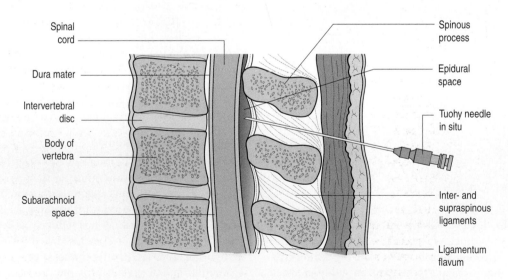

Figure 27.4 Sagittal section of the lumbar spine with Tuohy needle in position.

back with strapping and a syringe pump set up by the anaesthetist if there is to be a continuous infusion.

Observations and care by the midwife

After the administration of the first dose of bupivacaine and any subsequent top-up doses of local anaesthetic, the blood pressure and pulse should be measured and recorded every 5 min for 20–30 min and then every 30 min. The mother may sit up in bed once it has become established that her blood pressure is stable, but should be tilted to one side to prevent aortocaval compression.

Throughout labour the mother should be assisted to change her position regularly to avoid soft tissue damage. The fetal heart is usually monitored electronically. The mother may be unaware of a full bladder, so the midwife must ensure that the woman is encouraged to empty her bladder regularly. Similarly she will not feel uterine contractions, or a desire to bear down in the second stage of labour, so close observation is necessary. Uterine activity may be electronically monitored.

The spread of the block is checked regularly by the midwife. Units vary in whether they use a cold object or ethyl chloride spray to test the extent to which the mother has lost sensation.

The epidural top-up

Midwives top-up the epidural block by giving a further dose as prescribed by the anaesthetist. The prescription should indicate clearly the dosage and frequency of the drugs to be given, and the positioning of the woman. The midwife is personally responsible for ensuring that she is competent to carry out the procedure. The same observations are made as with the initial dose. The midwife should be aware of the possible complications and their immediate treatment. It is important to prevent aortocaval occlusion since this would compound the effects of any hypotension occurring as a result of the epidural block.

Complications of epidural analgesia

The use of low dose bupivacaine solutions for analgesia in labour has limited the risks of hypotension and local anaesthetic toxicity. The complications of epidurals may include:

- dural puncture and consequent headache
- total spinal leading to respiratory arrest
- local anaesthetic toxicity leading to cardiac arrest
- fetal compromise (resulting from hypotension or local analgesic toxicity)
- loss of bladder sensation (need for catheterization)
- increased need for assisted vaginal birth
- neurological sequelae (serious damage extremely rare; weakness/sensory loss is uncommon but soon resolves).

For most women, the side-effects following epidural are minimal and backache is more likely to be due to localized bruising and immobility than epidural analgesia. The increased use of epidural analgesia has in particular resulted in an increase in assisted vaginal birth. According to Thorp et al (1993), intervention is much less likely to occur if the epidural has been sited after 5 cm of dilatation of the cervical os, but this view remains contentious. Thorp's study is in keeping with the view of Sutton (2000), who puts forward the notion that the birth process necessitates the 'opening of the mother's back'. This means the lifting up of the lower lumbar vertebrae and the sacrum to facilitate the passage and birth of the baby. It is argued that today's lifestyle, e.g. the way women sit with their legs crossed or in a car seat position, with their knees higher than the pelvis, does not increase the available space for the fetus to descend, therefore making it difficult for the head to enter the pelvis.

The fact that more forceps births are carried out if the cervical dilatation is <5 cm when the epidural is sited also supports the above view. If the head is engaged and below the ischial spines, the head is likely to be well flexed and satisfactory progress will be made. The effect of the local anaesthetic reduces the muscle tone of the pelvic floor, which needs to remain firm, to aid flexion and rotation of the fetal head, before allowing the fetal head to advance. The fetal head then, in the case of an epidural, may not fully flex and progression may be arrested. Intervention then follows.

Post-dural puncture headaches and dural tap

If there has been a 'dural tap' during the procedure, women are likely to develop a severe postural headache caused by leakage of CSF. Headaches from a dural tap can also follow spinal anaesthesia for operative deliveries. However, needles used for deliberate spinal injection are much finer than Tuohy needles and the use of smaller gauge 'pencil point' needles has greatly reduced the leakage of CSF. Severe headache following a 'dural tap' is treated by epidural injection of 10–20 ml of maternal blood (a 'blood patch'), to seal the puncture and relieve the headache.

Hypotensive incident

Local analgesia affects the sympathetic nervous system by causing vasodilatation and a fall in blood pressure. For most women the fall is minimal. However, if the mother's systolic blood pressure falls below 75% of baseline (e.g. from 120 to 90 mmHg) she should be given oxygen and turned on her side while waiting for the anaesthetist. Hartmann's solution is normally infused rapidly if the blood pressure remains low. The lateral position should be assumed to prevent this happening. Adrenaline (epinephrine), a vasopressor, may be used if required to raise maternal blood pressure, increase cardiac output and the heart rate.

Patchy blocks

The epidural may be more effective on one side or in certain areas of the woman's body. It may be extremely difficult for the anaesthetist to produce an even, effective block. The anaesthetist must be kept informed and will attempt to render the block more efficient, by re-siting it, changing the position of the woman or injecting more local anaesthetic.

The responsibilities of the midwife

The midwife has an important enabling and facilitating role to help the woman during childbirth. Careful administration of drugs and monitoring the effects of these is essential to the provision of quality care. Accurate and detailed records of all care given will provide a good basis from which proper decisions may be made concerning the progress and the needs of the woman.

REFERENCES

Ahlborg G, Axelsson J, Bodin L 1996 Shift work nitrous oxide exposure and subfertility among Swedish midwives. International Journal of Epidemiology 25(4):783–790

Alexander J, Levy V, Roch S 1990 Intrapartum care: a research-based approach. MacMillan, London

Anderson G 2003 A concept analysis of normal birth. Evidence-based Midwifery 1(2):48–54

Baxter L 2006 What a difference a pool makes: Making choice a reality. British Journal of Midwifery 16(6):368–372

Benjoya Miller J 2006 All women should have the choice of waterbirth. British Journal of Midwifery 14(8):484

Bevis R 1984 Anaesthesia in midwifery. Baillière Tindall, London

Burns E 2001 Waterbirth. MIDIRS Midwifery Digest 11:S10–S13

Cammu H, van Classen K, Wettere L et al 1994 'To bathe or not to bathe' during the first stage. Acta Obstetricia et Gynecologica Scandinavica 73(6):468

Carson R 1996 The administration of analgesics. Modern Midwife 6:12–16

Castro M 1992 Homeopathy for mother and baby. MacMillan, London

Collis R 2000 Pain relief and anesthesia. In: Kean L, Baker P, Edelstone D (eds) 2000 Best practice in labor ward management. W B Saunders, London

COMET (Comparative Obstetric Mobile Epidural Trial) Study Group UK 2001 Effect of low-dose mobile versus traditional epidural techniques on mode of delivery: a randomised controlled trial. Lancet 358:19–23

Day-Stirk F 2005 The big push for normal birth. Midwives 8:18–20

Deakin B-A 2001 Alternative positions in labour and childbirth. British Journal of Midwifery 9(10):620–625

Deery R, Kirkham M 2006 Supporting midwives to support women. In: Page L, McCandlish (eds) The new midwifery, 2nd edn. Churchill Livingstone, London, Ch. 6

de Ferrer G 2006 TENS: Non-invasive pain relief for the early stages of labour. British Journal of Midwifery 14(8):480–482

Downe S, McCormick C, Beech B L et al 2001 Labour interventions associated with normal birth. British Journal of Midwifery 9(10):602–606

Elbourne D, Wiseman R A 2000 Types of intra-muscular opioids for maternal pain relief in labour. Cochrane Database System Reviews, Issue 2:CD001237

Fairlie F M, Marshall L, Walker J J et al 1999 Intramuscular opioids for maternal pain relief in labour: a randomised controlled trial comparing pethidine with diamorphine. British Journal of Obstetrics and Gynaecology 106:1181–1187

Forde C, Creighton S, Batty A et al 1999 Labour and delivery in the birthing pool. British Journal of Midwifery 7(3):165–171

Freeman R M, Moreland T A, Blair A W 1982 Diamorphine, the obstetric analgesia: a neurobehavioural and pharmacokinetic study in the neonate. Journal of Obstetrics and Gynaecology 3:102–106

Fujinaga M, Maze M 2002 Neurobiology of nitrous oxide-induced antinociceptive effects. Molecular Neurobiology 25(2):167–189

Garland D, Jones K 1994 Waterbirth, first stage immersion or non-immersion? British Journal of Midwifery 2(3):113–120

Geissbuhler V Eberhard J 2000 Waterbirths: a comparative study. a prospective study on more than 2000 waterbirths. Fetal Diagnosis and Therapy 15:21–300

Gould D 2000 Normal labour: a concept analysis. Journal of Advanced Nursing 31(2):418–427

Haines A & Kimber L 2005 Improving the birthing environment. The Practising Midwife 8(10):18–20

Henley-Einion A 2007 The ecstasy of the spirit: Five Rhythms for healing. British Journal of Midwifery 10(3):20–23

Jones M, Barik S, Mangune H et al 1998 Do birth plans adversely affect the outcome of labour? British Journal of Midwifery 6(1):38–41

Johnson M I 1997 Transcutaneous nerve stimulation in pain management. British Journal of Midwifery 5(7):400–405

Juman Blincoe A 2007 TENS machines and their use in managing labour pain. British Journal of Midwifery 15(8):516–519

Kabeyama K, Miyoshi M 2001 Longitudinal study of the intensity of memorized labour pain. International Journal of Nursing Practice 7:46–53

Kitzinger S 2000 Some cultural perspectives of birth. British Journal of Midwifery 8(12):746–750

Leap N, Anderson T 2004 The role of pain in normal birth and the empowerment of women. In: Downe S (ed.) 2004 Normal childbirth: evidence and debate. Churchill Livingstone, London

Lundgren I, Dahlberg K 2005 Midwives' experience of the encounter with women and their pain during childbirth. In: Wickham S (ed.) Midwifery best practice. Books for Midwives, London, Vol. 3

Mander R 1998 Pain in childbearing and its control. Blackwell Science, London

Martini F H 2001 Fundamentals of anatomy and physiology, 5th edn. Prentice Hall, London

MCWP (Maternity Care Working Party) 2006 Modernising maternity care –A Commissioning Toolkit for England, 2nd edn. The National Childbirth Trust. The Royal College of Midwives. The Royal College of Obstetricians and Gynaecologists.

Melzack R, Wall P D 1965 Pain mechanisms: a new theory. Science 150(3699):971–979

Nolan M 2005 Birth plans – A relic of the past or still a useful tool? In: Wickham S (ed.) Midwifery best practice 2. Books for Midwives, London

Poole D 2007 Use of TENS in pain management: Part 2 How to use TENS. Nursing Times 103(8):28–29

Ransjo-Arvidson A B, Matthieson A S, Lilja G et al 2001 Maternal analgesia during labor disturbs newborn behavior: effects on breastfeeding, temperature and crying. Birth 28 (1):5–11

Ranta P, Joupilla P, Spalding M et al 1994 Parturients' assessment of water blocks, pethidine, nitrous oxide, paracervical and epidural blocks in labour. International Journal of Obstetrics and Anaesthesia 3(4):193–198

RCM (Royal College of Midwives) 2006 Position Statement No. 26 Refocusing the role of the midwife. RCM, London

Robertson A 2003 Watch your language! In: Wickham S (ed.) Midwifery best practice. Books for Midwives, London

Sutton J 2000 Occipito-posterior positioning The Practising Midwife 3(6):20–22

Thorp J A, Hu D H, Albin R M et al 1993 The effect of intrapartum epidural analgesia on nulliparous labour: a randomized, controlled, prospective trial. American Journal of Obstetrics and Gynecology 169(4):851–858

Walsh D 1999 Transcutaneous electrical nerve stimulation. British Journal of Midwifery 7(9):580

Walsh D 2000 Evidence-based care series 1. Birth environment. British Journal of Midwifery 8(5):276–278

Walsh D, El-Nemer A, Downe S 2004 Risk safety and the study of physiological birth. In: Downe S (ed.) Normal childbirth: evidence and debate. Churchill Livingstone, London

FURTHER READING

Downe S 2004 Normal childbirth: evidence and debate. Churchill Livingstone, London

This publication provides an insightful account into how to support women during the birthing process. Chapter 2 on 'The role of pain in normal birth and the empowerment of women', presents some accounts of women's experiences of birth and also proposes many useful strategies and ways of working with pain, to help women during birth. The working with pain paradigm offers very interesting and constructive recommendations and perceptions.

28

The transition and the second stage of labour: physiology and the role of the midwife

Soo Downe

CHAPTER CONTENTS

When labour moves to the phase of active maternal pushing, the whole tempo of activity changes. The change in nature of uterine activity can lead women to express confusion and loss of control. Intense physical effort and exertion is needed as the baby is finally pushed towards its birth. The mother, her supporting companions, and her midwife all require stamina and courage. Excitement and expectation mount as the birth becomes imminent. A positive outcome will depend upon mutual respect and trust between all involved professional groups, and between those groups and the labouring mother and her companions. A mother will never forget a midwife who positively supports her capacity to give birth to her baby. The nature of normality in labour has been subject of debate for a number of years (Anderson 2003, Crawford 1983, Downe 1994, 2004, 2006, 2008, Gould 2000, Montgomery 1958) (See Box 28.1).

The chapter aims to:

- consider the nature of the transitional and second stage of labour
- describe the usual sequence of events during these stages
- summarize signs of transition and of the expulsive phase of labour
- discuss the care of the mother, father, and birth companions
- review the observations which should be carried out at this time.

The nature of the transition and second stage phases of labour

The second stage of labour has traditionally been regarded as the phase between full dilatation of the cervical os, and the birth of the baby. However, most midwives and labouring women are aware of a transitional period between the period of cervical dilatation, and the time when active maternal pushing efforts begin. This is typically characterized by maternal restlessness, discomfort, desire for pain relief, a sense that the process is never-ending, and demands to attendants to end the whole process. Appropriate midwifery care encompasses both knowledge of the usual physiological processes of this phase and of the mechanism of birth, and insight into the needs and choices of each individual labouring woman.

The physiological changes are a continuation of the same forces which occurred in the earlier hours of labour, but activity is accelerated. This acceleration, however, does not occur abruptly. Some women may experience an urge to push before the cervical os is fully dilated, and others may experience a lull before the onset of strong expulsive second stage contractions. This latter phenomenon has been termed the resting phase of the second stage of labour. The formal onset of the second stage of labour is traditionally confirmed with a vaginal examination to check for full dilatation of the cervical os. However, a finding of full cervical dilatation may occur some time after this stage has in fact been reached.

Uterine action

Contractions become stronger and longer but may be less frequent, allowing both mother and fetus regular recovery periods. The membranes often rupture spontaneously towards the end of the first stage or during transition to the second stage. The consequent drainage of liquor allows the hard, round fetal head to be directly applied to the vaginal tissues. This pressure aids distension. Fetal axis pressure increases flexion of the head, resulting in smaller presenting diameters, more rapid progress and less trauma to both mother and fetus. If the mother is upright during this time, these processes are optimized.

The contractions become expulsive as the fetus descends further into the vagina. Pressure from the presenting part stimulates nerve receptors in the pelvic floor. This phenomenon is termed the 'Ferguson reflex'. As a consequence, the woman experiences the need to push. This reflex may initially be controlled to a limited extent but becomes increasingly compulsive, overwhelming and involuntary. The mother's response is to employ her secondary powers of expulsion by contracting her abdominal muscles and diaphragm.

Soft tissue displacement

As the fetal head descends, the soft tissues of the pelvis become displaced. Anteriorly, the bladder is pushed upwards into the abdomen where it is at less risk of injury during fetal descent. This results in the stretching and thinning of the urethra so that its lumen is reduced. Posteriorly, the rectum becomes flattened into the sacral curve and the pressure of the advancing head expels any residual faecal matter. The levator ani muscles dilate, thin out and are displaced laterally, and the perineal body is flattened, stretched and thinned. The fetal head becomes visible at the vulva, advancing with each contraction and receding between contractions until crowning takes place. The head is then born. The shoulders and body follow with the next contraction, accompanied by a gush of amniotic fluid and sometimes of blood. The second stage culminates in the birth of the baby.

Recognition of the commencement of the second stage of labour

Progress from the first to the second stage is not always clinically apparent.

Presumptive evidence

Expulsive uterine contractions

Some women feel a strong desire to push before full dilatation occurs. Traditionally, it has been assumed that an early urge to push will lead to maternal exhaustion and/or cervical oedema or trauma. More recent research indicates that the early pushing urge may in fact be experienced by a significant minority of women, and that, in certain circumstances, early pushing may be physiological (Downe et al 2008, Petersen & Besuner 1997, Roberts & Hanson 2007). It is not clear whether these findings are influenced by factors such as maternal or fetal position, or parity, and there is not enough evidence to date to determine the optimum response to the early pushing urge. The midwife needs to work with each individual woman in the context of each labour to determine the best approach in that specific case.

Rupture of the forewaters

Rupture of the forewaters may occur at any time during labour.

Dilatation and gaping of the anus

Deep engagement of the presenting part may produce this sign during the latter part of the first stage.

Anal cleft line

Some midwives have reported observing this line (also called 'the purple line') as a pigmented mark in the cleft of the buttocks which creeps up the anal cleft as the labour progresses (Hobbs 1998, Wickham 2007). The efficacy of this observation remains to be tested formally.

Appearance of the rhomboid of Michaelis

This is sometimes noted when a woman is in a position where her back is visible. It presents as a dome shaped curve in the lower back, and is held to indicate the posterior displacement of the sacrum and coccyx as the fetal occiput moves into the maternal sacral curve (Sutton & Scott 1996). This seems to lead the labouring woman to arch her back, push her buttocks forward, and throw her arms back to grasp any fixed object she can find. Sutton and Scott (1996) hypothesize that this is a physiological response, since it causes a lengthening and straightening of the Curve of Carus, optimizing the fetal passage through the birth canal.

Upper abdominal pressure and epidural analgesia

It has been observed anecdotally that women who have an epidural *in situ* often have a sense of discomfort under the ribs towards the end of the first stage of labour. This seems to coincide with full cervical dilatation. The efficacy of these observations in predicting the onset of the anatomical second stage of labour remains to be researched.

Show

This is the loss of bloodstained mucus which often accompanies rapid dilatation of the cervical os towards the end of the first stage of labour. It must be distinguished from frank fresh blood loss caused by partial separation of the placenta or a ruptured vasa praevia.

Appearance of the presenting part

Excessive moulding may result in the formation of a large caput succedaneum which can protrude through the cervix prior to full dilatation of the os. Very occasionally, a baby presenting by the vertex may be visible at the perineum at the same time as remaining cervix. This is more common in women of high parity. Similarly a breech presentation may be visible when the cervical os is only 7–8 cm dilated.

Confirmatory evidence

In many midwifery settings, it is held that a vaginal examination must be undertaken to confirm full dilatation of the cervical os. This is both to ensure that a woman is not pushing too early, and to provide a baseline for timing the length of the second stage of labour. However, some maternity settings and some individual midwives do not insist on this unless there are observable maternal and/or fetal signs that the labour is not progressing as anticipated. Enkin et al (2000, p 284) noted that vaginal assessment of cervical dilatation is largely unevaluated. Despite this, regular vaginal examinations are undertaken by most midwives and obstetricians, and expected by many women. Whether the midwife undertakes an examination or not, she should record all the signs she observes and all the measurements she takes, and she should advise and support the labouring woman on the basis of accurate observation and assessment of progress.

Two distinct phases in second stage progress have been recognized in some women. These are the latent phase during which descent and rotation occur, and the active phase with descent and the urge to push.

Phases and duration

The latent phase

In some women, full dilatation of the cervical os is recorded, but the presenting part may not yet have reached the pelvic outlet. She may not experience a strong expulsive urge until the head has descended sufficiently to exert pressure on the rectum and perineal tissues. There is evidence from a study undertaken half a century ago that active pushing during the latent phase does not achieve much, apart from exhausting and discouraging the mother (Benyon 1990). More recent concerns over the impact of epidural analgesia on spontaneous birth have led to an increasing interest in the passive second stage of labour (Simpson & James 2005, NICE 2007). Due to the effect of epidural analgesia on the pelvic floor muscles, there is little benefit in encouraging active pushing until the head has descended and rotated as far as possible if a woman has an effective epidural in situ. Passive descent of the fetus can continue with good midwifery support for the woman until the head is visible at the vulva, or until the mother feels a spontaneous desire to push.

Active phase

Once the fetal head is visible, the woman will usually experience a compulsive urge to push.

Duration of the second stage

There is no good evidence about the absolute time limits of physiological labour (Downe 2004). Mothers and babies who labour for at least twice as long as the traditional limits can do well (Albers 1999). In the presence of regular contractions, maternal and fetal well-being, and progressive descent, considerable variation between women is to be expected. While many maternity units do currently impose limits on the second stage beyond which medical help should be called, these are not based on good evidence (Enkin et al 2000, p 293).

Maternal response to transition and the second stage

Pushing

Traditionally, if the maternal urge to push occurs before confirmation of full dilatation of the cervical os, or the appearance of a visible vertex, the mother is encouraged to avoid active pushing at this stage. This is done to conserve maternal effort and allow the vaginal tissues to stretch passively. Techniques include position change, often to the left lateral, using controlled breathing, inhalation analgesia, or even narcotic or epidural pain relief (Downe et al 2008). However, when mother and baby are well and labour has progressed spontaneously, some midwives have adopted the practice of supporting the overwhelming urge to bear down without confirming full dilatation of the cervical os, while paying close attention to the maternal and fetal condition. As stated above, the optimum response in this situation has not yet been established.

There has been convincing evidence for over a decade that managed active pushing in the second stage of labour accompanied by breath holding (the Valsalva manoeuvre) has adverse consequences (Aldrich et al 1995, Enkin et al 2000, p 290–1, Thomson 1993). Whenever active pushing commences, the woman should be encouraged to follow her own inclinations in relation to expulsive effort. Few women need instruction on how to push unless they are using epidural analgesia (Box 28.2).

Spontaneous pushing efforts usually result in maximum pressure being exerted at the height of a contraction. In turn, this allows the vaginal muscles to become taut and prevents bladder supports and the transverse cervical ligaments from being pushed down in front of the baby's head. It is believed that

> **Box 28.2** Epidural analgesia and spontaneous vaginal birth
>
> Epidural analgesia provides optimal pain relief for women, but its use is associated with an increase in instrumental births (Anim-Somuah et al 2005).
>
> Techniques for reducing the risk of instrumental births in this group have included:
>
> - Minimizing the concentration of local anaesthetic (Turner et al 1988)
> - Letting the block wear off towards the end of labour (Torvaldsen et al 2004)
> - Using oxytocin in the second stage of labour (Saunders et al 1989)
> - Using a device to exert fundal pressure (Cotzias et al 1998)
> - Delaying active pushing between the diagnosis of the onset of full dilatation of the cervix and a fixed point later in the labour (Fraser et al 2000)
> - Using the lateral position in the passive second stage of labour (Downe et al 2004)
> - Using combinations of anaesthetic which allow women to mobilize in labour (COMET Study Group UK 2001).
>
> These techniques have had varying success rates.

this may help to prevent prolapse and urinary incontinence in later life, although this belief has still not been formally tested (Benyon 1990).

Some mothers vocalize loudly as they push. This may aid in coping with the contractions, so women should feel free to express themselves in this way. Reassurance and praise will help to boost confidence, enabling the mother to assert her own control over events. The atmosphere should be calm and the pace unhurried.

Position

If the mother lies flat on her back, vena caval compression is increased, resulting in hypotension. This can lead to reduced placental perfusion and diminished fetal oxygenation (Humphrey et al 1974, Kurz et al 1982). The efficiency of uterine contractions may also be reduced. The semi-recumbent or supported sitting position, with the thighs abducted, is the posture most commonly used in western cultures. While this may afford the midwife good access and a clear view of the perineum, the mother's weight is on her sacrum, which directs the coccyx forwards and reduces the pelvic outlet. In addition, the midwife needs to bend forward and laterally to support the birth, which may lead to injury.

Left lateral position

This position was widely used in the UK in the last century, although it is less common in current practice. The perineum can be clearly viewed and uterine action is effective, but an assistant may be required to support the right thigh, which may not be ergonomic. It provides an alternative for women who find it difficult to abduct their hips. It may also aid fetal rotation, especially in the context of epidural analgesia (Downe et al 2004).

Upright positions; squatting, kneeling, all fours, standing, using a birthing ball. (Figs. 28.1, 28.2)

A review of studies examining upright versus recumbent positions during the second stage of labour

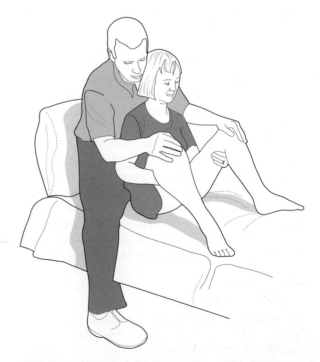

Figure 28.1 Supported sitting position. (After Simkin & Ancheta 2006, with permission from Blackwell Science.)

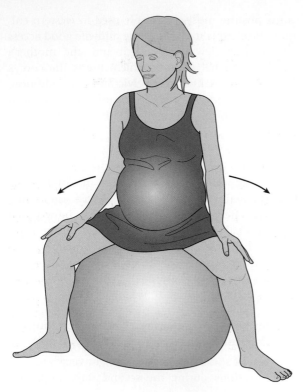

Figure 28.2 Using a birthing ball. (After Simkin & Ancheta 2006, with permission from Blackwell Science.)

showed there were clear advantages for women in adopting an upright position (Gupta et al 2004). These included reduced duration of second stage labour, less assisted deliveries, less episiotomies, reduced severe pain in second stage labour, and fewer abnormal heart rate patterns. However, increased rates of second degree tears and of estimated blood loss >500 mL also occurred. The experimental group included women who used birthing chairs, a technique known to be associated with increased blood loss (Stewart & Spiby 1989, Turner et al 1986). It is not clear if this risk accrues to all upright positions. The 'upright position' group in this review included women who were in supported sitting positions on a bed, and in the lateral position. Data relating to off the bed positions is less easy to locate.

Radiological evidence demonstrates an average increase of 1 cm in the transverse diameter and 2 cm in the anteroposterior diameter of the pelvic outlet when the squatting position is adopted. This produces an average 28% increase in the overall area

of the outlet compare with the supine position (Russell 1969). Some women find the all fours position to be the optimum approach for all or part of their labours, especially in the case of an occipitoposterior position, due to relief of backache (Stremler et al 2005). It can, however, be tiring to maintain for a long period of time. A wide range of other standing and leaning positions can be experimented with to help the mother cope with her labour (Simkin & Ancheta 2006). It is important not to insist on any position as the 'right' one. Positive and dramatic effects on labour progress can be achieved by encouraging the mother to change and adapt her position in response to the way her body feels.

The position the mother may choose to adopt is dictated by several factors:

- The mother's instinctive preference
- The environment should not act as a constraint through lack of privacy or lack of supports such as cushions and chairs. In a hospital setting, it may help to move the labour bed from the middle of the room, and to provide other supports such as cushions and birthing balls, so that the mother can roam from one to another as the labour dictates. Low lighting and music of her choice may help the woman to see the room as a safe and secure place. Minimizing unnecessary intrusion by other members of staff is essential
- The midwife's confidence: A full understanding of the mechanism of labour should enable the midwife to adapt to any position that the woman wishes to adopt, ensuring in the process that the postures adopted by the midwife are protective of her own health (and, specifically, of her back). One way of minimizing this is to refrain from placing the woman in a low supported sitting position with her feet resting on the midwives hip. Minimizing vaginal examinations in labour will also reduce the risk of back injury to the midwife. If the woman has an epidural in situ, it is essential that help is called when the woman needs to be moved, and that ergonomic lifting positions are used.

Maternal and fetal condition

If the mother has had analgesia, or if there is any concern about the well-being of either the woman or her baby then more frequent or continuous monitoring may limit the choices available to her. However, there are often creative solutions to these situations, and good midwifery care involves finding these solutions where possible.

The mechanism of normal labour

As the fetus descends, soft tissue and bony structures exert pressures which lead to descent through the birth canal by a series of movements. Collectively, these movements are called the mechanism of labour. There is a mechanism for every fetal presentation and position which can lead to a vaginal birth. Knowledge and recognition of the normal mechanism enables the midwife to anticipate the next step in the process of descent. Understanding and constant monitoring of these movements can help to ensure that normal progress is recognized, that the woman gives birth safely and positively, or that early assistance can be sought should any unresolvable problems occur. The fetal presentation, position, and size relative to that of the woman will govern the exact mechanism as the fetus responds to external pressures. Principles common to all mechanisms are:

- descent takes place
- whichever part leads and first meets the resistance of the pelvic floor will rotate forwards until it comes under the symphysis pubis
- whatever emerges from the pelvis will pivot around the pubic bone.

It should be noted that, while the mechanism set out below is the most common, it is not an invariant blueprint, but a guide: each labour is unique.

During the mechanism of normal labour, the fetus turns slightly to take advantage of the widest available space in each plane of the pelvis. The widest diameter of the pelvic brim is the transverse: at the pelvic outlet the greatest space lies in the antero-posterior diameter.

At the onset of labour, the most common presentation is the vertex and the most common position either left or right occipitoanterior; therefore it is this mechanism which will be described. In this instance:

- the lie is longitudinal
- the presentation is cephalic

- the position is right or left occipitoanterior
- the attitude is one of good flexion
- the denominator is the occiput
- the presenting part is the posterior part of the anterior parietal bone.

Main movements of the fetus

Descent

Descent of the fetal head into the pelvis often begins before the onset of labour. For a primigravid woman this usually occurs during the latter weeks of pregnancy. In multigravid women muscle tone is often more lax and therefore descent and engagement of the fetal head may not occur until labour actually begins. Throughout the first stage of labour the contraction and retraction of the uterine muscles allow less room in the uterus, exerting pressure on the fetus to descend further. Following rupture of the forewaters and the exertion of maternal effort, progress speeds up.

Flexion

This increases throughout labour. The fetal spine is attached nearer the posterior part of the skull; pressure exerted down the fetal axis will be more forcibly transmitted to the occiput than the sinciput. The effect is to increase flexion which results in smaller presenting diameters which will negotiate the pelvis more easily. At the onset of labour the suboccipito-frontal diameter, which is on average approximately 10 cm, is presenting; with greater flexion the sub-occipitobregmatic diameter, on average approximately 9.5 cm, presents. The occiput becomes the leading part.

Internal rotation of the head

During a contraction, the leading part is pushed downwards onto the pelvic floor. The resistance of this muscular diaphragm brings about rotation. As the contraction fades, the pelvic floor rebounds, causing the occiput to glide forwards. Resistance is therefore an important determinant of rotation (Fig. 28.3). This explains why rotation is often delayed following epidural analgesia which causes relaxation of pelvic floor muscles. The slope of the

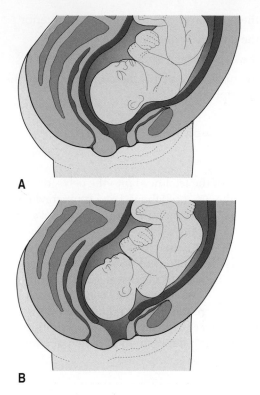

A

B

Figure 28.3 (A) Internal rotation of the head begins. (B) Upon completion, the occiput lies under the symphysis pubis.

pelvic floor determines the direction of rotation. The muscles are hammock-shaped and slope down anteriorly, so whichever part of the fetus first meets the lateral half of this slope will be directed forwards and towards the centre. In a well-flexed vertex presentation the occiput leads, and rotates anteriorly through ⅛ of a circle when it meets the pelvic floor. This causes a slight twist in the neck as the head is no longer in direct alignment with the shoulders. The anteroposterior diameter of the head now lies in the widest (anteroposterior) diameter of the pelvic outlet. The occiput slips beneath the sub-pubic arch and crowning occurs when the head no longer recedes between contractions and the widest transverse diameter (biparietal) is born. If flexion is maintained, the suboccipitobregmatic diameter, usually approximately 9.5 cm, distends the vaginal orifice.

Extension of the head

Once crowning has occurred the fetal head can extend, pivoting on the suboccipital region around the pubic bone. This releases the sinciput, face, and chin, which sweep the perineum, and then are born by a movement of extension (Fig. 28.4).

Restitution

The twist in the neck of the fetus which resulted from internal rotation is now corrected by a slight untwisting movement. The occiput moves ⅛ of a circle towards the side from which it started.

Internal rotation of the shoulders

The shoulders undergo a similar rotation to that of the head to lie in the widest diameter of the pelvic outlet, namely anteroposterior. The anterior shoulder is the first to reach the levator ani muscle and it therefore rotates anteriorly to lie under the symphysis pubis. This movement can be clearly seen as the head turns at the same time (external rotation of the head). It occurs in the same direction as restitution, and the occiput of the fetal head now lies laterally.

Lateral flexion

The shoulders are usually born sequentially. When the mother is in a supported sitting position, the anterior shoulder is usually born first, although it has been noted by midwives who commonly use upright or kneeling positions that the posterior shoulder is commonly seen first. In the former case, the anterior shoulder slips beneath the sub-pubic arch and the posterior shoulder passes over the perineum. In the latter the mechanism is reversed. This enables a smaller diameter to distend the vaginal orifice than if both shoulders were born simultaneously. The remainder of the body is born by lateral flexion as the spine bends sideways through the curved birth canal.

Midwifery care

Care of the parents

The woman and her companions will now realize that the birth of the baby is imminent. They may feel excited and elated but at the same time anxious and frightened by the dramatic change in pace. They will need frequent explanations of events. The midwife's

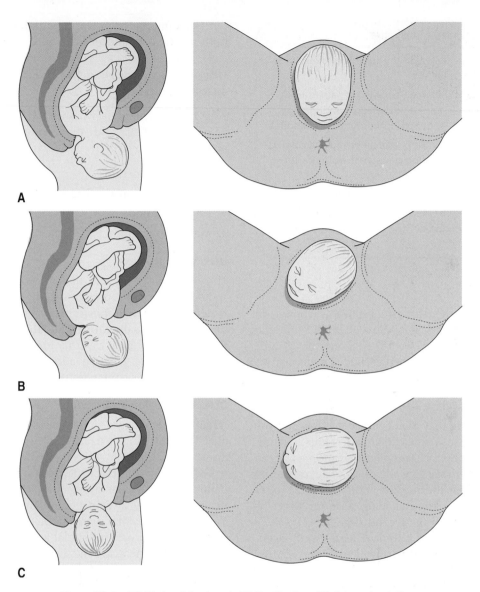

Figure 28.4   (A) Birth of the head. (B) Restitution. (C) External rotation.

calm approach and information about what is happening can ensure the woman stays in control, and is confident. This is critical at the time of transition, when events can result in a sensation of panic. The midwife should praise and congratulate the mother on her hard work, recognizing that she is probably undertaking the most extreme physical activity she will ever encounter. Birth is an intimate act which often takes place in a public setting. The midwife should work hard to ensure that privacy and dignity are maintained (Box 28.3).

Crucially, it is at the time of transition that a maternal request for analgesia may occur, even if she had stated antenatally that she did not want pain relief in labour. Such a request will need to be carefully assessed by the attending midwife. This is especially true when a supportive companion is not present. On the basis of her knowledge of the woman, the midwife may be able to help her over this transient phase with good midwifery support, and without utilizing pharmacological analgesia. The decision for or against pain relief at this stage

Box 28.3 Dilemmas of practice

- The contrast between the current evidence base and actual practices
- The contrast between knowledge gained from experience (empirical knowledge) and that gained from evidence (authoritative knowledge)
- The problem of using guidelines and clinical risk assessments based on population evidence for individual women/babies
- Balancing maternal choice, institutional demands, and midwifery expertise
- Providing optimum care when resources are restricted.

must be made in partnership with the woman. In order to achieve this, it is eminently preferable that the same midwife should support the couple throughout labour (Hodnett et al 2003). Alternatives to pharmacological analgesia include changes in position and scenery, massage and appropriate nutrition. Complementary therapies and optimal fetal positioning may also be offered if the midwife is competent to undertake them. Leg cramp is a common occurrence whichever posture is adopted. It can be relieved by massaging the calf muscle, extending the leg and dorsiflexing the foot. These measures may be crucial in re-energizing a labour which is beginning to flag in the second stage.

The midwife should also have regard to the wellbeing of the woman's partner and other companions as far as possible. Witnessing labour and birth is not easy, especially for the woman's partner. Indeed, recent qualitative research has indicated that birth companions can be profoundly affected by witnessing traumatic birth, and can even exhibit symptoms that appear to be similar to those of post-traumatic stress for years after the birth (White 2007). The midwive's attitude to the labour, to the woman, and to the partner will have a profound effect on the labour, and is likely to have an effect on the family after the birth (El-Nemer et al 2006, Halldorsdottir & Karlsdottir 1996). It is crucial to respect them, and to respect

the meaning that this birth will have for them, both on the day, and in the future.

Observations during the second stage of labour

Four factors determine whether the second stage is continuing safely, and these must be carefully monitored:

1. Uterine contractions
2. Descent, rotation and flexion of the presenting part
3. Fetal condition
4. Maternal condition.

Uterine contractions

The strength, length and frequency of contractions should be assessed continuously by observation of maternal responses, and regularly by uterine palpation. They are usually stronger and longer than during the first stage of labour, with a longer resting phase. The posture and position adopted by the mother may influence the contractions.

Descent, rotation and flexion

Initially, descent may occur slowly, especially in primigravid women, but it usually accelerates during the active phase. It may occur very rapidly in multigravid women. If there is a delay in descent on abdominal palpation, despite regular strong contractions and active maternal pushing, a vaginal examination may be performed with maternal permission. The purpose is to confirm whether or not internal rotation of the head has taken place, to assess the station of the presenting part, and to determine whether a caput succedaneum has formed. If the occiput has rotated anteriorly, the head is well flexed and caput succedaneum is not excessive it is likely that progress will continue. In the absence of good rotation and flexion, and/or a weakening of uterine contractions, change of position, nutrition and hydration, or use of optimal fetal positioning techniques may be helpful (Simkin & Ancheta 2006). Consultation with a more experienced midwife may provide more suggestions to re-orientate the labour. However, if there is evidence that either fetal or maternal condition are compromised, an experienced obstetrician should be consulted.

Fetal condition

If the membranes are ruptured, the liquor amnii is observed to ensure that it is clear. While thin old meconium staining is not always regarded as a sign of fetal compromise, thick fresh meconium is always ominous, and experienced obstetric advice must be sought if this sign appears (Enkin et al 2000, p 268–9, Liu & Harrington 2002).

As the fetus descends, fetal oxygenation may be less efficient owing to either cord or head compression or to reduced perfusion at the placental site. A well-grown healthy baby will not be compromised by this transitory hypoxia. This will tend to produce early decelerations of the fetal heart, with a swift return to the normal baseline after a contraction, and good beat-to-beat variation throughout. While early decelerations are always deemed 'suspicious' in the current National Institute for Health and Clinical Effectiveness (NICE) guidelines (NICE 2001), in practice their occurrence in the active second stage is not usually regarded as pathological in the absence of any other signs of compromise (see Ch 26). The midwife should learn to recognize the normal changes in fetal heart rate patterns during the second stage, so that unwarranted interference is avoided. If the woman is labouring normally, the guideline recommends that a Pinard's stethoscope or other hand held system such as a Sonicaid should be used to monitor the fetal heart. During the second stage, this is usually undertaken immediately after a contraction, with some readings being taken through a contraction if the woman can tolerate this.

Suspicious/pathological changes in the fetal heart

Late decelerations, a lack of return to the normal baseline, a rising baseline, or diminishing beat-to-beat variation are signs of concern. If these are heard for the first time in second stage, they may be due to cord or head compression, which may be helped by a change in position. However, if they persist, experienced obstetric aid must be sought. If the labour is taking place in a unit which is distant from an obstetric unit, an episiotomy may be considered if the birth is imminent, or midwives who are trained and experienced in ventouse birth may consider expediting the birth. Otherwise, with maternal consent, transfer to an obstetric unit should be expedited.

Maternal condition

The midwife's observation includes an appraisal of the mother's ability to cope emotionally as well as an assessment of her physical well-being. Maternal pulse rate is usually recorded half-hourly and blood pressure every few hours, provided that these remain within normal limits. If the woman has an epidural in situ, blood pressure will be monitored more frequently, and continuous electronic fetal monitoring will probably be in use.

Maternal comfort

As a result of her exertions the woman usually feels very hot and sticky and she will find it soothing to have her face and neck sponged with a cool flannel. Her mouth and lips may become very dry. Sips of iced water or other fluids are refreshing and a moisturizing cream can be applied to her lips. Her partner may help with these tasks as a positive contribution to ease her discomfort.

The bladder is vulnerable to damage, due to compression of the bladder base between the pelvic brim and the fetal head. The risk is increased if the bladder is distended. The woman should be encouraged to pass urine at the beginning of the second stage unless she has recently done so.

Preparation for the birth

Once active pushing commences, the midwife should prepare for the birth. There is usually little urgency if the woman is primigravid, but multigravid women may progress very rapidly.

The room in which the birth is to take place should be warm with a spotlight available so that the perineum can be easily observed if necessary. A clean area should be prepared to receive the baby, and waterproof covers provided to protect the bed and floor. Sterile cord clamps, a clean apron, and sterile gloves are placed to hand. In some settings, sterile gowns are also used. An oxytocic agent may be prepared, either for the active management of the third stage if this is acceptable to the woman, or for use during an emergency. A warm cot and clothes should be prepared for the baby. In hospital a heated mattress may be used; at home, a warm (*not* hot) water bottle can be placed in the cot.

Neonatal resuscitation equipment must be thoroughly checked and readily accessible.

The birth of the baby

The midwife's skill and judgement are crucial factors in minimizing maternal trauma and ensuring an optimal birth for both mother and baby. These qualities are refined by experience but certain basic principles should be applied. They are:

- observation of progress
- prevention of infection
- emotional and physical comfort of the mother
- anticipation of normal events, and support for the normal processes of labour
- recognition of abnormal developments, and appropriate response to them.

During the birth, both mother and baby are particularly vulnerable to infection. While there is now evidence that strict antisepsis is unnecessary if the birth is straightforward (Keane & Thornton 1998), meticulous aseptic technique must be observed when preparing sterile equipment such as episiotomy scissors. Surgical gloves should be worn during the birth for the protection of both mother and midwife. Goggles or plain glasses should be available to avoid the risk of ocular contamination with blood or amniotic fluid.

Once she has scrubbed up the midwife prepares her equipment. This includes the following items:

- warm swabbing solution or tap water
- cotton wool and pads
- sterile cord scissors and clamps
- sterile episiotomy scissors.

Birth of the head

Once the birth is imminent, the perineum is usually swabbed, and a clean pad is placed under the woman to absorb any faeces or fluids. If she is not in an upright position a pad is placed over the rectum on the perineum (but not covering the fourchette) and a clean towel is placed on or near the mother for receipt of the baby. Throughout these preparations the midwife observes the progress of the fetus. With each contraction the head descends.

As it does so the superficial muscles of the pelvic floor can be seen to stretch, especially the transverse perineal muscles. The head recedes between contractions, which allows these muscles to thin gradually. The skill of the midwife in ensuring that the active phase is unhurried helps to safeguard the perineum from trauma. She must either watch the advance of the fetal head or control it with light support from her hand, or both. One large study, the HOOP trial, indicted that, compared with guarding the perineum, a hands off technique was associated with slightly more maternal discomfort at 10 days postnatally (McCandlish et al 1998). The hands off technique was also associated with a lower risk of episiotomy, but a higher risk of manual removal of placenta. There is some debate about the generalizability of this trial to all settings and positions in labour. However, account should be taken of these findings in working with individual women. Most midwives place their fingers lightly on the advancing head to monitor descent and prevent very rapid crowning and extension, which are believed to result in perineal laceration. However, firm pressure on the head may be associated with vaginal lacerations. Whatever technique the midwife adopts, it should be based on the assumption that it is the woman who is giving birth to her baby, and the midwife is there to add the minimum physical help necessary at any given time.

Once the head has crowned, the mother can achieve control by gently blowing or 'sighing' out each breath in order to minimize active pushing. Birth of the head in this way may take two or three contractions but may avoid unnecessary maternal trauma (Fig. 28.5).

Once crowned, the head is born by extension as the face appears at the perineum. During the resting phase before the next contraction the midwife may check that the cord is not around the baby's neck. If found, it is usual to slacken it to form a loop through which the shoulders may pass. If the cord is very tightly wound around the neck, it is common practice in the UK to apply two artery forceps approximately 3cm apart and to sever the cord between the two clamps (Jackson et al 2007). In the USA, the so-called 'somersault manoeuvre' is often performed (Fig. 28.6) (Mercer et al 2005, 2007). There has been controversy over early cord

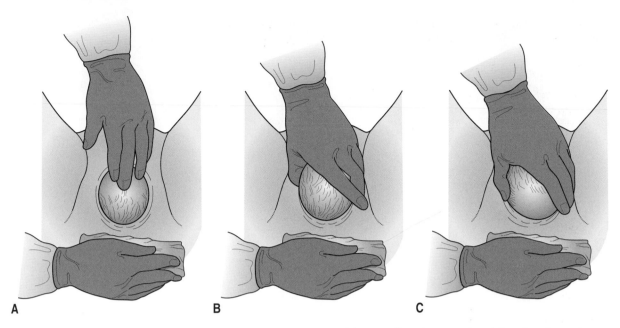

Figure 28.5   Supporting the head. (A) Preventing rapid extension. (B) Controlling the crowning. (C) Easing the perineum to release the face.

cutting for the normal term infant, on the basis that, even if tightly around the neck, the cord is still supplying oxygen. Additionally, the blood volume model proposed by Mercer & Skovgaard (2004) suggests that the loss of blood volume occasioned by clamping and cutting the cord before it stops pulsating may be detrimental to the baby. This hypothesis has been supported by a recent systematic review (Hutton & Hassan 2007). However, these studies have not controlled for the possible adverse effects of a tight nuchal cord.

If the cord is clamped, great care must be taken that maternal tissues are not damaged. Holding a swab over the cord as it is incised will reduce the risk of the attendants being sprayed with blood during the procedure. Once severed, the cord may be unwound from around the neck.

Birth of the shoulders

Restitution and external rotation of the head maximizes the smooth birth of the shoulders and minimizes the risk of perineal laceration. However, it is not uncommon for small babies, or for babies of multiparous women, to be born with the shoulders in the transverse, or even to have a twist in the neck opposite to that expected. While the hands on technique in the HOOP trial included both perineal support and active birth of the trunk and shoulders (McCandlish et al 1998) it is not clear which component of this technique was beneficial for women and babies. If the position is upright, it is more common for the shoulders to be left to birth spontaneously with the help of gravity. During a water birth, it is important not to touch the emerging fetus to avoid stimulating it to gasp underwater. If there is a problem with the birth in this circumstance, the mother should be asked to stand up out of the water before any manoeuvres are attempted.

If the midwife does physically aid the birth of the shoulders and trunk, she should be absolutely sure that restitution has occurred prior to trying to flex the trunk laterally. One shoulder is released at a time to avoid overstretching the perineum. A hand is placed on each side of the baby's head, over the ears, and gentle downward traction is applied (Fig. 28.7). This allows the anterior shoulder to slip beneath the symphysis pubis while the posterior shoulder remains in the vagina. If the third stage is to be

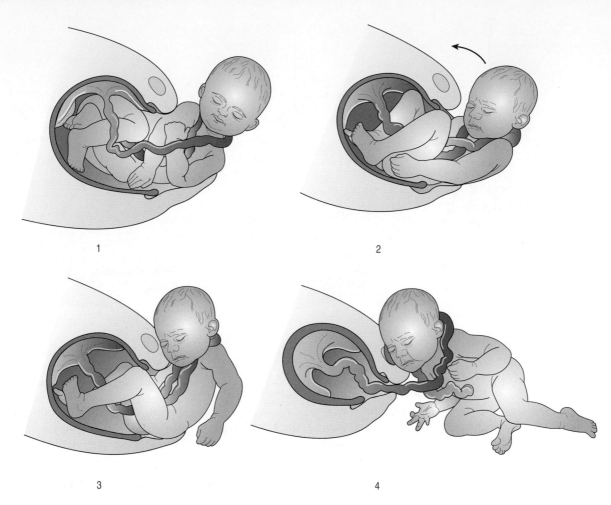

1

2

3

4

Figure 28.6 The somersault manoeuvre. (From Mercer et al 2005.)

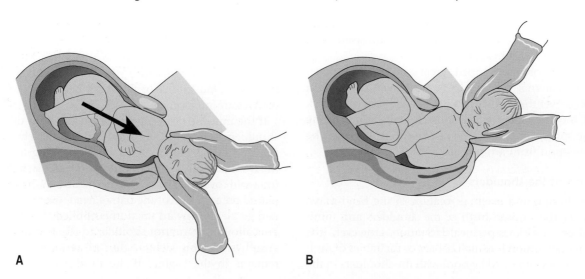

A

B

Figure 28.7 (A) Downward traction releases the anterior shoulder. (B) An upward curve allows the posterior shoulder to escape.

actively managed, the assistant will now give an intramuscular oxytocic drug. When the axillary crease is seen, the head and trunk are guided in an upward curve to allow the posterior shoulder to escape over the perineum. These manoeuvres are reversed if the mother is in a forward facing position such as all fours. The midwife or mother may now grasp the baby around the chest to aid the birth of the trunk and lift the baby towards the mother's abdomen. This allows the mother immediate sighting of her baby and close skin contact, and removes the baby from the gush of liquor which accompanies release of the body. If the midwife does not actively assist, she should be ready to support the head and trunk as the baby emerges. The time of birth is noted.

If this has not already been done, the cord is severed between two cord clamps placed close to the umbilicus at whatever time is considered appropriate, with due attention to the theories around the blood volume model set out above (and see Chs 29 and 39). The cord clamp is applied. The baby is dried and placed in the skin-to-skin position with the mother if she is happy with this (Anderson et al 2003). A warm cover is placed over the baby. Swabbing of the eyes and aspiration of mucus during and immediately following birth are not considered necessary providing the baby's condition is satisfactory. Oral mucus extractors should not be used because of the risks of mucus which is contaminated with a virus such as hepatitis or human immunodeficiency virus (HIV) entering the operator's mouth.

The moment of birth is both joyous and beautiful. The midwife is privileged to share this unique and intimate experience with the parents.

Episiotomy

As the perineum distends, an episiotomy may very occasionally be necessary. This is an incision through the perineal tissues which is designed to enlarge the vulval outlet during birth. As this is a surgical incision it cannot be undertaken unless the mother gives consent. A detailed discussion should take place during pregnancy so that each woman is aware of the indications for and implications of the intervention. She should be assured that its use is selective and discretional. The mother's wishes should be clearly documented and respected.

The risks and benefits of episiotomy have been reviewed (Carroli & Belizan 1999). The rationale for its use is the need to minimize the risk of severe trauma to the vagina and perineum, and to expedite the birth when there is evidence of fetal distress. However, the risks of its use should always be borne in mind. During a normal birth the indications are few and the midwife should adopt a restrictive policy.

The timing of the incision

An episiotomy involves incision of the fourchette, the superficial muscles and skin of the perineum and the posterior vaginal wall. It can therefore successfully speed the birth only when the presenting part is directly applied to these tissues. If the episiotomy is performed too early it will fail to release the presenting part and haemorrhage from cut vessels may ensue. In addition, the levator ani muscles will not have had time to be displaced laterally and may be incised as well. If performed too late there will not be enough time to infiltrate with a local anaesthetic. There is also little reason for superimposing an episiotomy if a tear has already begun.

Types of incision

There are two main directions of incision.

Mediolateral

This begins at the midpoint of the fourchette and is directed at a 45° angle to the midline towards a point midway between the ischial tuberosity and the anus. This line avoids the danger of damage to both the anal sphincter and Bartholin's gland but it is more difficult to repair. This is the incision largely used by midwives in the UK.

Median

This is a midline incision which follows the natural line of insertion of the perineal muscles. It is associated with reduced blood loss but a higher incidence of damage to the anal sphincter. It is the easier to repair and results in less pain and dyspareunia. This incision is favoured in the USA.

Infiltration of the perineum

The perineum should be adequately anaesthetized prior to the incision. Lidocaine (formerly termed lignocaine) is commonly used, 0.5% 10 mL or 1% 5 mL. The advantage of the more concentrated solution is that a smaller volume is needed. Lidocaine takes 3–4 min to take effect and, if possible, two or three contractions should be allowed to occur between infiltration and incision. The timing is not always easy to calculate but it is better to infiltrate and not perform an episiotomy than to incise the perineum without an effective local anaesthetic.

Method of infiltration

The perineum is cleansed with antiseptic solution. Two fingers are inserted into the vagina along the line of the proposed incision in order to protect the fetal head. The needle is inserted beneath the skin for 4–5 cm following the same line (Fig. 28.8). The piston of the syringe should be withdrawn prior to injection to check whether the needle is in a blood vessel. If blood is aspirated, the needle should be repositioned and the procedure repeated until no blood is withdrawn. Lidocaine is continuously injected as the needle is slowly withdrawn. Some practitioners inject the whole amount in one operation. Anaesthesia is, however, more effective if about one-third of the amount is used at first and two further injections are made, one either side of the incision line. The needle must be redirected just before the tip is withdrawn.

The incision

A straight-bladed, blunt-ended pair of Mayo scissors is usually used. The blades should be sharp. Some practitioners prefer to use a scalpel for this reason. Two fingers are inserted into the vagina as before and the open blades are positioned. The incision is best made during a contraction when the tissues are stretched so that there is a clear view of the area and bleeding is less likely to be severe. A single, deliberate cut 4–5 cm long is made at the correct angle. Birth of the head should follow immediately and its advance must be controlled in order to avoid extension of the episiotomy. If there is any delay before the head emerges, pressure should be applied

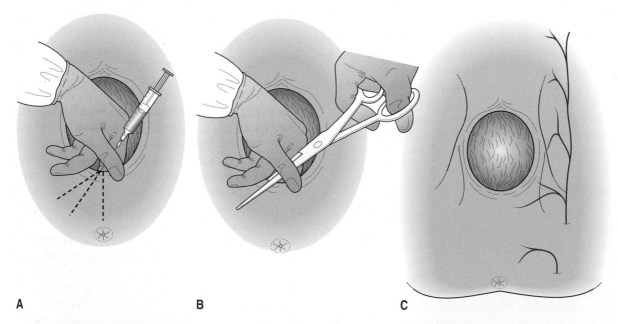

A   B   C

Figure 28.8 (A) Infiltrating the perineum. (B) Performing an episiotomy. (C) Innervation of the vulval area and perineum.

to the episiotomy site between contractions in order to minimize bleeding. Postpartum haemorrhage can occur from an episiotomy site unless bleeding points are compressed.

Perineal repair

Trauma is best repaired as soon as possible after the birth in order to secure haemostasis and before oedema forms. It is also much kinder to the mother to complete this aspect of her care without undue delay and while the tissues are still anaesthetized. Prior to commencement the mother must be made as warm and comfortable as possible. The lithotomy position is usually chosen as it affords a clear view. Other positions may be more appropriate in the home setting. A good, directional light is essential and the operator should be seated comfortably during the procedure.

The appropriate instruments, antiseptic solution, suture materials and local anaesthetic, should be prepared before the mother's legs are placed in the stirrups. This minimizes the time spent in this uncomfortable, undignified position and reduces the risks of complications such as deep vein thrombosis. The midwife scrubs and puts on sterile gown and gloves. The perineum is cleaned with warm antiseptic solution. Blood oozing from the uterus may obscure the field of vision, so a taped vaginal tampon may be inserted into the vault of the vagina. The tape is secured to the drapes by a pair of forceps as a reminder that it is in situ. Both insertion and removal should be recorded. The full extent of the trauma is assessed and explained to the mother. The procedure for repair should also be outlined so that she is aware of what is happening.

Spontaneous trauma may be of the labia anteriorly, the perineum posteriorly or both. A gentle, thorough examination must be carried out to assess the extent of the trauma accurately and to determine whether an experienced obstetrician should carry out the repair, if it is extensive.

Anterior labial tears

It is debatable whether or not these should be sutured. Much depends upon the control of bleeding as the labia are very vascular. A suture may be necessary to secure haemostasis.

Posterior perineal trauma

Spontaneous tears are usually classified in degrees which are related to the anatomical structures which have been traumatized. This classification only serves as a guideline because it is often difficult to identify the structures precisely.

- 1-degree tear involves the fourchette only
- 2-degree tear involves the fourchette and the superficial perineal muscles, namely the bulbocavernosus and the transverse perineal muscles and in some cases the pubococcygeus
- 3-degree tear comprises a partial or complete disruption of the anal sphincter muscles, which may involve either or both the external and internal anal sphincter muscles
- 4-degree tear involves a disruption of the anal sphincter muscles with a breach of the rectal mucosa.

(RCOG 2007)

Third- and fourth-degree tears should be repaired by an experienced obstetrician. A general anaesthetic or effective epidural or spinal anaesthetic is necessary.

Prior to the commencement of repair, infiltration of the wound with local anaesthetic will be required. Lidocaine 1% is used and time must be allowed for it to take effect before repair begins. If an epidural block is in progress, a 'top up' should be given.

The apex of the vaginal incision is identified and the posterior vaginal wall repaired from the apex downwards (Fig. 28.9). A continuous suture affords better haemostasis (Kettle & Johanson 1998). The thread should not be pulled too tightly as oedema will develop during the first 24–48 hrs. Care must be taken to identify other vaginal lacerations which need to be repaired. Deeper interrupted sutures are then inserted to repair the perineal muscles. Good approximation of tissue is important. The subsequent strength of the pelvic floor will depend largely upon adequate repair of this layer. As long as good approximation is obtained, suturing of the perineal skin is unnecessary, and may lead to increased maternal discomfort (Gordon et al 1998, Oboro et al 2003). If skin closure is carried out, a continuous subcuticular suture (Fig. 28.9) results in fewer short-term problems than interrupted transcutaneous suturing techniques (Kettle & Johanson 1998, RCOG 2004).

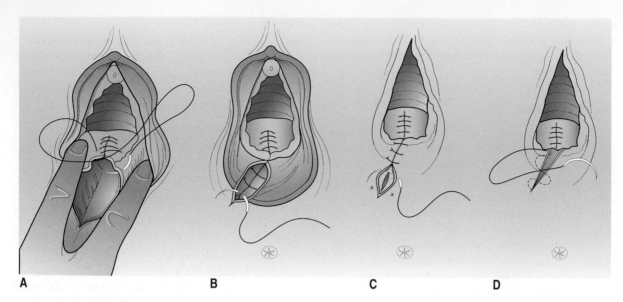

Figure 28.9 Perineal repair. (A) A continuous suture is used to repair the vaginal wall. (B) Three or four interrupted sutures repair the fascia and muscle of the perineum. (C) Interrupted sutures to the skin. (D) Subcuticular skin suture.

Absorbable synthetic polyglycolic acid and rapid-absorption polyglactin 910 sutures are recommended (Kettle & Johanson 1999, RCOG 2004). Repair should begin at the fourchette so that the vaginal opening is properly aligned. When the wound has been closed, any further vulval lacerations should be repaired.

The sutured areas should be inspected in order to confirm haemostasis before the vaginal pack is removed. A vaginal examination is made to ensure that the introitus has not been narrowed. Upon completion, and after warning the mother, a rectal examination is made to ensure that no sutures have penetrated the rectal mucosa. Any such sutures must be removed to prevent fistula formation.

The area is cleaned and a sanitary pad positioned over the vulva and perineum. The mother's legs are then gently and simultaneously removed from lithotomy support and she is made comfortable. The nature of the trauma and repair should be explained to her and information given on whether or not sutures will need to be removed.

Records

It is the responsibility of the midwife assisting the birth to complete the labour record. This should include details of any drugs administered, of the duration and progress of labour, of the reason for performing an episiotomy, and of perineal repair. This information is recorded on the mother's notes and may be duplicated on her domiciliary record as well as in the birth register. Details of the baby's condition including Apgar score are also recorded.

The birth notification must be completed within 36 hrs of the birth (see Ch. 56). This may be undertaken by anyone present at the birth but is usually carried out by the midwife. The notification is sent to the medical officer in the health district in which the baby was born.

New developments such as the All Wales Clinical Pathway for Normal Labour (NHS Wales 2006) provide alternative approaches to record-keeping that may be useful for practitioners in the future. However records are kept, all data in the UK are subject to the Data Protection Act 1998.

Conclusion

The processes of transition and of second stage labour are likely to be very physically and emotionally intense, particularly for the woman, but also for her partner and other birth companions. If maternal

Box 28.4 Diane's birth story

The birth of my first baby should have been one of the happiest days of my life. Instead, I felt I had failed; I was mentally and physically traumatized. Five years on, when I was eventually pregnant again, my fears started creeping back, and I considered having a caesarean section. I was referred to the local caseload midwifery team. When my midwife came to visit, I told her that my first birth had left me traumatized, confused, and scared about everything. This was my big turn around: after talking to her I realized I did not want a caesarean section, and I started to feel confident about giving birth naturally.

The big day arrived. I was over the moon that I had started my labour naturally. After a few hours my midwife came to my house, just to check how everything was going. Eventually, we decided it was time to go to the hospital. When I arrived they organized an epidural for me, which I had discussed, and which was in my birth plan. I was getting excited, knowing I was going to meet my baby soon. My midwife supported me and encouraged me on everything I decided. She was there for me all the time, keeping me focused and positive about my birth. After about 3 hrs, I started pushing hard with contractions. The epidural wore off enough for me turn around on to my knees with my body upright, and I could feel the baby drop down. I gave it my all for two pushes, and out popped the head. I controlled my breathing, pushing slowly, and my beautiful baby girl came out. The midwife brought her through my legs so I could see her and that's when my husband cut her cord, which was memorable and overwhelming for him. I was the happiest person, I had the biggest smile on my face: to me this was a beautiful birth. Thanks to the wonderful midwives – it goes to show that with the right help and guidance you can overcome your fears and anxieties with positive thinking.

Box 28.5 Examples of areas in need of research

- The areas of controversy, as set out in Box 28.1
- The nature of physiological fetal heart patterns in the normal second stage of labour
- Variation and significance of variation in normal fetal heart tones and rhythms as heard with a Pinard's stethoscope
- The mechanisms of labour in upright positions
- The nature of birth in units where no restrictions are imposed as a matter of routine
- Observation of maternal behaviours to assess progress in labour
- The impact of optimal fetal positioning.

Box 28.6 Key points

- The transition and second stage phases of labour are emotionally intense and physically hard
- The majority of labours will progress physiologically
- Maternal behaviour is usually a good indication of progress during this time
- The core midwifery skill is to support the mother in the context of a sound knowledge of the physiology and the mechanisms of this phase of labour
- Support should be unobtrusive
- The woman is the central player
- Clear, comprehensive record keeping is essential
- There are many gaps in the research evidence in this area.

behaviour and instinct are respected, in the context of skilled and watchful waiting, the vast majority of labours will progress physiologically. The skill of the midwife is to support the woman effectively, to guide her when her spirits or the labour are flagging, and to enable her to accomplish her birth safely and in triumph. See Box 28.4, Diane's story. Clear, comprehensive record keeping is essential. While much practice in this area is not based on formal evidence, new observations about normal birth are beginning to be recorded, and these observations will form the basis for future research.

REFERENCES

Albers L L 1999 The duration of labor in healthy women. Journal of Perinatology 19(2):114–119.

Aldrich C J, D'Antona D, Spencer J A et al 1995 The effect of maternal pushing on fetal cerebral oxygenation and blood volume during the second stage of labour. British Journal of Obstetrics and Gynaecology 102(6):448–453

Anderson G 2003 A concept analysis of 'normal birth'. Evidence Based Midwifery 1(2):48–54

Anderson G C, Moore E, Hepworth J, et al 2003 Early skin-to-skin contact for mothers and their healthy newborn infants. Cochrane Database of Systematic Reviews, Issue 2: CD003519

Anim-Somuah M, Smyth R, Howell C 2005 Epidural versus non-epidural or no analgesia in labour. Cochrane Database of Systematic Reviews, Issue 4:CD000331

Benyon C 1990 The normal second stage of labor: a plea for reform in its conduct In: Kitzinger S, Simkin P 1990 (eds) Episiotomy and the second stage of labor, 2nd edn. Pennypress, Seattle (Originally published in 1957 in the Journal of Obstetrics and Gynaecology of the British Empire 64:815–820

Carroli G, Belizan J 1999 Episiotomy for vaginal birth. Cochrane Database of Systematic Reviews, Issue 3: CD000081

COMET (Comparative Obstetric Mobile Trial Study Group) UK 2001 Effect of low-dose mobile versus traditional epidural techniques on mode of delivery: a randomised controlled trial. The Lancet 358:19–23

Cotzias C, Cox J, Osuagwu F et al 1998. Does an inflatable obstetric belt assist in the second stage of labour? British Journal of Obstetrics and Gynaecology 105(Suppl 17):84

Crawford J S 1983 The stages and phases of labour: outworn nomenclature that invites hazard. The Lancet July:271–272

Downe S 1994 How average is normality? British Journal of Midwifery 2(7):303–304

Downe S (ed.) 2008 Normal birth, evidence and debate, 2nd ed. Elsevier, Oxford

Downe S 2004 The concept of normality in the maternity services: application and consequences In: Frith L (ed.). Ethics and midwifery: issues in contemporary practice, 2nd edn Butterworth Heinemann, Oxford

Downe S, Young C, Hall-Moran V, Trent Midwifery Research Group 2008 Multiple midwifery discourses: the case of the early pushing urge. In: Downe S (ed.) Normal birth, evidence and debate. Elsevier, Oxford

Downe S, Gerrett D, Renfrew M J 2004b A prospective randomised trial on the effect of position in the passive second stage of labour on birth outcome in nulliparous women using epidural analgesia. Midwifery 20(2):157–168.

Downe S 2006 Engaging with the concept of unique normality in childbirth. British Journal of Midwifery 14(6):352–356

El-Nemer A, Downe S, Small N 2006' She would help me from the heart': an ethnography of Egyptian women in labour. Social Science and Medicine 62(1):81–92

Enkin M, Keirse M J N C, Neilson J et al 2000 A guide to effective care in pregnancy and childbirth, 3rd edn. Oxford University Press, Oxford

Fraser W D, Marcoux S, Krauss I et al 2000. Multicenter, randomized, controlled trial of delayed pushing for nulliparous women in the second stage of labor with continuous epidural analgesia. American Journal of Obstetrics and Gynecology 182(5):1165–1172

Gordon B, Mackrodt C, Fern E 1998 The Ipswich Childbirth Study: 1. A randomised evaluation of two stage postpartum perineal repair leaving the skin unsutured. British Journal of Obstetrics & Gynaecology 105(4):435–440

Gould D 2000 Normal labour: a concept analysis. Journal of Advanced Nursing 31(2):418–427

Gupta J K, Hofmeyr G J, Smyth R. 2004 Position in the second stage of labour for women without epidural anaesthesia. Cochrane Database of Systematic Reviews, Issue 1: CD002006

Halldorsdottir S, Karlsdottir S I 1996 Empowerment or discouragement: women's experience of caring and uncaring encounters during childbirth. Health Care for Women International 17(4):361–379

Hobbs L 1998. Assessing cervical dilatation without VEs; watching the purple line. The Practising Midwife 1(11):34–35

Hodnett E D, Gates S, Hofmeyr G J et al 2003 Continuous support for women during childbirth. Cochrane Database of Systematic Reviews, Issue 3:CD003766

Humphrey M D, Chang A, Wood E C et al 1974 A decrease in fetal pH during the second stage of labour when conducted in the dorsal position. Journal of Obstetrics and Gynaecology, British Commonwealth 81:600–602

Hutton E K, Hassan E S 2007 Late vs early clamping of the umbilical cord in full-term neonates: systematic review and meta-analysis of controlled trials. Journal of the American Medical Association 297(11):1241–1252

Jackson H, Melvin C, Downe S 2007 Midwives and the fetal nuchal cord: a survey of practices and perceptions. Journal of Midwifery and Womens Health 52:49–55

Keane H E, Thornton J G 1998 A trial of cetrimide/chlorhexidine or tap water for perineal cleaning. British Journal of Midwifery 6(1):34–37

Kettle C, Johanson R B 1998 Continuous versus interrupted sutures for perineal repair. Cochrane Database of Systematic Reviews, Issue 1:CD000947

Kettle C, Johanson R B 1999 Absorbable synthetic versus catgut suture material for perineal repair. Cochrane Database of Systematic Reviews, Issue 4:CD000006

Kurz C S, Schneider H, Hutch R et al 1982 The influence of maternal position on the fetal transcutaneous oxygen pressure. Journal of Perinatal Medicine 10(Suppl 2):74–75

Liu W F, Harrington T 2002 Delivery risk factors for meconium aspiration syndrome American Journal of Perinatology 19(7):367–378

McCandlish R, Bowler U, van Asten H et al 1998 A randomised controlled trial of care of the perineum during second stage of normal labour. British Journal of Obstetrics and Gynaecology 105(12):1262–1272

Mercer J, Skovgaard R Fetal to neonatal transition: first, do no harm. In: Downe S (ed.) Normal birth, evidence and debate. 2004 Elsevier, Oxford

Mercer J, Skovgaard R, Peareara-Eaves J et al 2005 Nuchal cord management and nurse midwifery practice. Journal of Midwifery & Women's Health 50(5):373–379

Mercer J S, Erickson-Owens D A, Graves B et al 2007 Evidence-based practices for the fetal to newborn transition. Journal of Midwifery Women's Health 52(3):262–272

Montgomery T 1958 Physiologic considerations in labor and the puerperium. American Journal of Obstetrics and Gynecology Oct:706

NICE 2001 The use of electronic fetal monitoring. Online. Available: http://www.nice.org.uk

NHS Wales 2006 All Wales Clinical Pathway for Normal Labour. Online. Available: http://www.wales.nhs.uk/sites3/page.cfm?orgid=327&pid=5786 200715 May

NICE 2007 Intrapartum care: management and delivery of care to women in labour. Online. Available: http://www.nice.org.uk

Oboro V O, Tabowei T O, Loto O M et al 2003 A multicentre evaluation of the two-layered repair of postpartum perineal trauma. Journal of Obstetrics and Gynaecology 23(1):5–8

Petersen L, Besuner P 1997 Pushing techniques during labor: issues and controversies. Journal of Obstetric, Gynecologic and Neonatal Nursing 26(6):719–726

RCOG (Royal College of Obstetricians and Gynaecologists) 2004 Materials and methods used in perineal repair: Green top guideline. Online. Available: http://www.rcog.org.uk/resources/Public/pdf/perineal_repair.pdf 2007 24 May 2004

RCOG (Royal College of Obstetricians and Gynaecologists) 2007 The management of third and fourth degree perineal tears. Green-top Guideline No. 29. Online. Available: http://www.rcog.org.uk/index.asp?PageID=532 2007 15 May 2007

Roberts J, Hanson L 2007 Best practices in second stage labor care: maternal bearing down and positioning. Journal of Midwifery and Women's Health 52(3):238–245.

Russell J G B 1969 Moulding of the pelvic outlet. Journal of Obstetrics and Gynaecology 76:817–820

Saunders N J, Spiby H, Gilbert L et al 1989 Oxytocin infusion during second stage of labour in primiparous women using epidural analgesia: a randomised double blind, placebo controlled trial. British Medical Journal 299(6713):1423–1426

Simkin P, Ancheta R 2006 Labor progress handbook, 2nd edn. Blackwell, Oxford

Simpson K R, James D C 2005 Effects of immediate versus delayed pushing during second-stage labor on fetal well-being: a randomized clinical trial. Nurse Researcher 54(3):149–157

Stewart P, Spiby H 1989. A randomized study of the sitting position for delivery using a newly designed obstetric chair. British Journal of Obstetrics and Gynaecology 96(3):327–333

Stremler R, Hodnett E, Petryshen P et al 2005 Randomized controlled trial of hands-and-knees positioning for occipito-posterior position in labor. Birth 32(4):243–251

Sutton J, Scott P 1996 Understanding and teaching optimal fetal positioning, 2nd edn. Birth Concepts, Tauranga

Thomson A M 1993 Pushing techniques in the second stage of labour. Journal of Advanced Nursing 18(2):171–177

Torvaldsen S, Roberts C L, Bell J C et al 2004. Discontinuation of epidural analgesia late in labour for reducing the adverse delivery outcomes associated with epidural analgesia. Cochrane Database of Systematic Reviews, Issue 4: CD004457

Turner M J, Romney M L, Webb J B et al 1986 The birthing chair: an obstetric hazard? Journal of Obstetrics and Gynaecology 6:232–235

Turner M J, Sil J M, Alagesan K et al 1988 Epidural bupivacaine concentration and forceps birth in primiparae. Journal of Obstetrics and Gynecology 9(2):122–125

White G 2007 You cope by breaking down in private: fathers and PTSD following childbirth. British Journal of Midwifery 15(1):39–45

Wickham S 2007 Assessing cervical dilatation without VEs: watching the purple line. Practising Midwife 10(1):26–27

FURTHER READING

Davis E 2004 Heart and hands: a midwife's guide to pregnancy and birth. 4th edn Celestial Arts, Berkeley

This is a manual of midwifery based on the skills and experiences gained by lay midwives working in America. If offers unique tips and insights.

Floyd-Davis R, Sargent C F 1997 Childbirth and authoritative knowledge: cross-cultural perspectives. University of California Press, California

A seminal work, which explores how authority is given to certain kinds of knowledge, and how the knowledge and expertise of women and of less dominant cultures is not privileged, even in the area of childbirth, and even in the face of the evidence.

Leap N, Hunter B 1993 The midwife's tale: an oral history from handywoman to professional midwife. Scarlet Press, London

This is an historical account of trained midwives and laywomen practising in the 1950s. The stories of their experiences and responsibilities while attending women in labour are fascinating. The final chapter offers some accounts of labours from the point of view of women themselves.

Mother friendly campaign. Online. Available: http://www.motherfriendly.org/MFCI/steps.html 22 May 2007

This international campaign is modelled on the baby friendly initiative, and is based on 10 key steps which are believed to promote optimal births for mother and baby.

RCM campaign for normal birth. Online. Available: http://www.rcmnormalbirth.org.uk 22 May 2007

The campaign was set up by the Royal College of Midwives to inspire and support normal birth practice in the midwifery profession. It is a web-based initiative, using real stories and midwives experiences, underpinned with a sound evidence base.

Walsh D 2007 Evidence based care for normal labour and birth. Routledge, London

A clearly written overview of both formal and informal evidence that effectively integrates narrative, evidence, and experiential learning.

29

Physiology and management of the third stage of labour

Sue McDonald

Postpartum haemorrhage (PPH) is still ranked among the top three major causes of maternal death globally (WHO 2007). Although the majority (99%) of deaths reported occur in developing countries, the risk of PPH should not be underestimated for any birth, nor should the potential for the third stage of labour to be the most dangerous stage of labour be underestimated (McDonald et al 2004, WHO 2007). Maternal mortality rates in high resource countries are relatively low when compared to low resource countries, however, maternal morbidity is similar in significance. During this stage, the mother's focus and sense of emotional and physical relief often spontaneously shift from the concentrated exertions of the actual birth to that of exploration and familiarization with her newborn baby. To facilitate a safe and healthy outcome for the mother and her baby, antenatal health as well as intrapartum preparation and postnatal skill, diligence and expertise of the midwife are crucial factors. Research evidence is clearer for some aspects of third stage management than others.

The chapter aims to:

- describe the normal physiological mechanism of placental separation and descent together with factors that facilitate haemostasis
- consider the types and use of uterotonic drugs in third stage management and the relevance of timing of clamping of the umbilical cord
- describe the risk factors most commonly associated with PPH and discuss the current management strategies for both prophylaxis and treatment of it
- discuss the midwife's care of the mother during and immediately after expulsion of the placenta and membranes.

Physiological processes

The third stage is defined as the period from the birth of the baby to complete expulsion of the placenta and membranes, involving the separation, descent and expulsion of the placenta and membranes and control of haemorrhage from the placenta site (Johnson & Taylor 2000). It is an understanding of what has already occurred during pregnancy and labour and the changes that take place that guides the midwife's practice. During the third stage, separation and expulsion of the placenta and membranes occur as the result of mechanical and haemostatic factors. The time at which the placenta actually separates from the uterine wall varies. It may shear off during the final expulsive contractions accompanying the birth of the baby or remain adherent for some considerable time. The third stage usually lasts between 5 and 15 min, but any period up to 1 hr may be considered to be within normal limits.

Separation and descent of the placenta

Mechanical factors

The unique characteristic of uterine muscle lies in its power of retraction. During the second stage of labour, the uterine cavity progressively empties, enabling the retraction process to accelerate. Thus, by the beginning of the third stage, the placental site has already diminished in area by about 75% (Baldock & Dixon 2006). As this occurs, the placenta becomes compressed and the blood in the intervillous spaces is forced back into the spongy layer of the decidua basalis. Retraction of the oblique uterine muscle fibres exerts pressure on the blood vessels so that blood does not drain back into the maternal system. The vessels during this process become tense and congested. With the next contraction the distended veins burst and a small amount of blood seeps in between the thin septa of the spongy layer and the placental surface, stripping it from its attachment (Fig. 29.1). As the surface area for placental attachment reduces, the relatively non-elastic placenta begins to detach from the uterine wall.

Separation usually begins centrally so that a retroplacental clot is formed (Fig. 29.2). This further aids

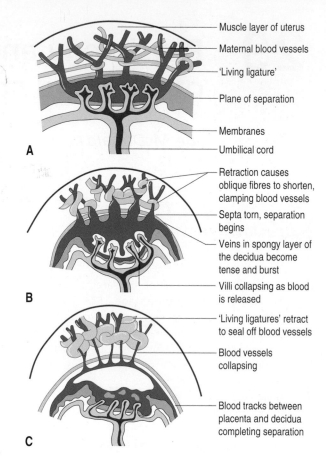

Figure 29.1   The placental site during separation. (A) Uterus and placenta before separation. (B) Separation begins. (C) Separation is almost complete.

separation by exerting pressure at the midpoint of placental attachment so that the increased weight helps to strip the adherent lateral borders and peel the membranes off the uterine wall so that the clot thus formed becomes enclosed in a membranous bag as the placenta descends, fetal surface first. This process of separation (first described by Schultze) is associated with more complete shearing of both placenta and membranes and less fluid blood loss (Fig. 29.3A). Alternatively, the placenta may begin to detach unevenly at one of its lateral borders. The blood escapes so that separation is unaided by the formation of a retroplacental clot. The placenta descends, slipping sideways, maternal surface first. This process (first described by Matthews Duncan in the nineteenth century) takes longer and is associated

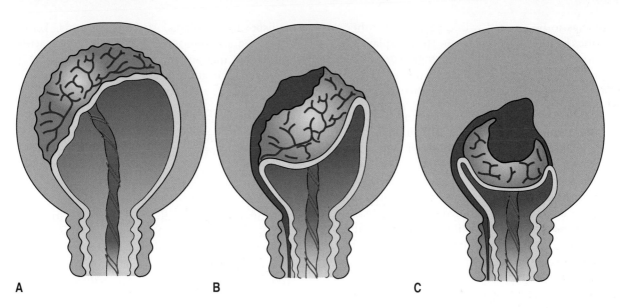

Figure 29.2 The mechanism of placental separation. (A) Uterine wall is partially retracted, but not sufficiently to cause placental separation. (B) Further contraction and retraction thicken the uterine wall, reduce the placental site and aid placental separation. (C) Complete separation and formation of the retroplacental clot. *Note:* The thin lower segment has collapsed like a concertina following the birth of the baby.

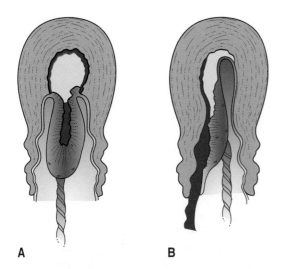

Figure 29.3 Expulsion of the placenta. (A) Schultze method. (B) Matthews Duncan method.

with ragged, incomplete expulsion of the membranes and a higher fluid blood loss (Fig. 29.3B).

Once separation has occurred, the uterus contracts strongly, forcing placenta and membranes to fall into the lower uterine segment (Fig. 29.4) and finally into the vagina.

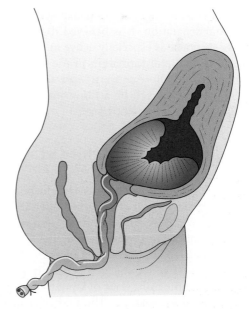

Figure 29.4 Third stage: placenta in lower uterine segment.

Haemostasis

The normal volume of blood flow through the placental site is 500–800 mL/min. At placental separation, this has to be arrested within seconds, as otherwise serious haemorrhage will occur. The interplay of three factors within the normal physiological processes that control bleeding are critical in minimizing blood loss and the serious sequelae of maternal morbidity or mortality, or both, which may result. They are:

1. Retraction of the oblique uterine muscle fibres in the upper uterine segment through which the tortuous blood vessels intertwine – the resultant thickening of the muscles exerts pressure on the torn vessels, acting as clamps, so securing a ligature action. This is shown in Figure 29.1. It is the absence of oblique fibres in the lower uterine segment that explains the greatly increased blood loss usually accompanying placental separation in placenta praevia.

2. The presence of vigorous uterine contraction following separation – this brings the walls into apposition so that further pressure is exerted on the placental site.

3. The achievement of haemostasis – there is a transitory activation of the coagulation and fibrinolytic systems during, and immediately following, placental separation. It is believed that this protective response is especially active at the placental site so that clot formation in the torn vessels is intensified. Following separation, the placental site is rapidly covered by a fibrin mesh utilizing 5–10% of circulating fibrinogen.

Management of the third stage

The midwife's care of the mother should be based on an understanding of the normal physiological processes at work, including having access to as much information as possible about the woman's pregnancy and labour history. Progress of the first and second stages of labour are likely to impact on management of the third stage of labour and should not be reviewed in isolation. The midwife's actions can help to reduce the very real risks of haemorrhage, infection, retained placenta and shock, any of which may increase maternal morbidity and even result in death. A mother's ability to withstand these complications depends, to a large degree, upon her general health and the avoidance of debilitating,

predisposing problems, such as anaemia, ketosis, exhaustion and prolonged hypotonic uterine action. Factors that may influence the risk of haemorrhage are discussed in more detail later.

Uterotonics or uterotonic agents

These are drugs (e.g. Syntometrine, Syntocinon, ergometrine and prostaglandins) that stimulate the smooth muscle of the uterus to contract. They may be administered with crowning of the baby's head, at the time of birth of the anterior shoulder of the baby, after the birth of the baby but prior to placental delivery or following the delivery of the placenta.

Whether women should routinely receive uterotonic drugs, have the umbilical cord clamped or be given assistance with placental delivery has been the subject of a great deal of debate and many research trials. What is of primary importance is that the health professional (whether a midwife, GP or obstetrician) providing clinical care and advice should ensure that, in order to facilitate decision-making by the woman, adequate time for deliberation and questions should be made available, where possible, during the course of her routine antenatal consultations. Information related to the best available research information on the use of uterotonic drugs during the third stage of labour should be offered in an objective manner, which could perhaps be supported with pamphlets that cover topics such as possible management options for the woman in the setting in which she intends to birth, types of uterotonics, explanation of their different applications, risks and benefits, route of administration and timing and method of placental delivery.

Active management

This is a policy whereby prophylactic administration of a uterotonic, as a precautionary measure aimed at reduction in the risk for postpartum haemorrhage, is applied regardless of the assessed obstetric risk status of the woman. An active management policy usually includes the routine administration of a uterotonic agent, either intravenously, intramuscularly or even orally. This is undertaken in conjunction with clamping of the umbilical cord shortly after birth of the baby and delivery of the placenta by the use of controlled cord traction. In situations where women may also be assessed as being at higher risk for PPH (e.g. multiple birth, grande multiparity), a prophylactic infusion of larger doses of uterotonics diluted in intravenous solutions may be administered over several hours following the birth. This would also be considered to be part of an active management policy. Active management in the third stage is the policy of third stage labour management most widely practised throughout the developed world. Like all interventions performed, skill in assisting the delivery of the placenta and membranes is extremely important.

Expectant or physiological management

In expectant management, routine administration of a uterotonic drug is withheld, the umbilical cord is left unclamped until cord pulsation has ceased or the mother requests it to be clamped, or both, and the placenta is expelled by use of gravity and maternal effort. With this approach, therapeutic uterotonic administration would be administered either to stop bleeding once it has occurred or to maintain the uterus in a contracted state when there are indications that excessive bleeding is likely to occur. Emergency use usually indicates an event of uncontrolled haemorrhage. In this situation, it is important for the midwife to be aware of whether, what and how much of a uterotonic agent has already been administered.

No matter what an individual midwife's personal practice experience may be or what the best available research evidence recommends, it is still ultimately the woman's decision as to how she would ideally wish her pregnancy and birth plan to be followed. There may be philosophical, religious or cultural beliefs that influence her decision.

However, it is also fair to suggest that the midwife also has rights and responsibilities. Detailed, accurate, written (contemporaneous wherever possible) documentation is extremely important in all aspects of care, particularly in areas where evidence-based information is relied upon to assess whether due care has been delivered. In the case of third stage management, an example might be: in the circumstance where a woman specifically requests that uterotonic drugs be withheld from routine use in her third stage care, the midwife should clarify the circumstances in which this decision may be reversed. If a uterotonic drug is not to be used, the woman's preference for care must be recorded in her notes antenatally. A record of the discussion may be signed by the woman. It would be prudent for the midwife to notify her clinical manager or the attending medical practitioner of such a request if it is contrary to local guidelines.

In practice, one of the following uterotonic drugs is usually used.

Intravenous ergometrine 0.25 mg

This drug acts within 45 s; therefore it is particularly useful in securing a rapid contraction where hypotonic uterine action results in haemorrhage. If a doctor is not present in such an emergency, a midwife may give the injection. In an overview of the choice of uterotonics for use in the third stage, Prendiville et al (1988a) found that there was no supportive evidence for the continued routine use of intravenous ergometrine, which is associated with an increased risk of retained placenta and this drug is more often used to treat a PPH rather than as a prophylactic drug. If an intravenous cannula is not already *in situ*, any difficulty encountered in locating a vein or sudden movement by the woman may result in failed venepuncture or at least a delay in administration.

Combined ergometrine and oxytocin (a commonly used brand is Syntometrine)

A 1 mL ampoule contains 5 IU of oxytocin and 0.5 mg ergometrine and is administered by i.m. injection. The oxytocin acts within 2½ min, and the ergometrine within 6–7 min (Fig. 29.5). Their combined action results in a rapid uterine contraction enhanced by a stronger, more sustained contraction lasting several hours. It is usually administered as the anterior shoulder of the baby is born, thus stimulating good uterine action at the beginning of the third stage. The use of combined ergometrine/oxytocin or any ergometrine-based drug is associated with side-effects such as elevation of the blood pressure and vomiting (McDonald et al 2004).

Caution

No more than 2 doses of ergometrine 0.5 mg should be given as it can cause headache, nausea and an increase in blood pressure and it is normally contraindicated where there is a history of hypertensive or cardiac disease.

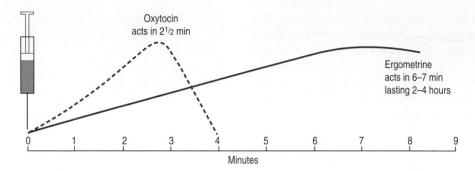

Figure 29.5 The rapid action of oxytocin in comparison with ergometrine.

Oxytocin (a commonly used brand is Syntocinon)

Oxytocin is a synthetic form of the natural oxytocin produced in the posterior pituitary, and is safe to use in a wider context than combined ergometrine/oxytocin agents. It can be administered as an intravenous and or intramuscular injection. However, an intravenous bolus of oxytocin can cause profound, fatal hypotension, especially in the presence of cardiovascular compromise. The recommendation of the CEMD (Lewis & Drife 2001, p 21) is that 'when given as an intravenous bolus the drug should be given slowly in a dose of not more than 5IU'.

Research evidence to date suggests that this is an effective uterotonic choice where routine prophylactic management of the third stage of labour is practised (Choy et al 2002, Khan et al 1995, McDonald et al 1993), more specifically in women who experience a blood loss exceeding 1000 mL. There still, however, does not appear to be an absolute recommendation for practice with regard to choice of uterotonic. This is perhaps partly due to the varied circumstances in which women seek care and clinicians work. It is also perhaps indicative of the need to encompass all the factors that surround the management of labour itself, including induction, use of uterotonics in labour, use of epidurals and tolerance of longer second stages.

Carbetocin originally developed for veterinary use and not widely used for prophylactic use in management of the third stage, is a long-acting synthetic oxytocin analogue which can be administered as a single dose 100 µg injection. This drug has been compared favourably with other injectable oxytocics, such as Syntometrine (oxytocin-ergometrine) and Syntocinon (oxytocin alone) for prevention of PPH (Chaparro et al. 2006, Prendiville & Elbourne 1989, WHO 1990). However, carbetocin still requires refrigeration for stability, so while it provides an alternative uterotonic, there is insufficient evidence as yet regarding its benefit over the drugs that are currently available.

Prostaglandins

The use of prostaglandins for third stage management has up until now been more often associated with the treatment of postpartum haemorrhage than with prophylaxis. This may be partly due to prostaglandin agents being more expensive and associated with side-effects, such as diarrhoea (Chua et al 1995) and cardiovascular complications of increased stroke volume and heart rate (van Selm et al 1995). Prostaglandin administration is most effective when used intramurally (injected directly into the uterine wall) or by intrauterine irrigation (Peyser & Kupfermine 1990). The procedures are time consuming and invasive and the expertise required for undertaking the procedures is unlikely to always be readily available in routine labour management.

In more recent years, a great deal of research time and investment has been invested in seeking alternate ways of implementing strategies to reduce the risk of PPH. Misoprostol (a prostaglandin E1 analogue) was first used to treat gastric ulcers, but when its potential as a uterotonic agent was discovered, optimism regarding its suitability in low resource settings was high. It is cheap, not prone to loss of potency, does not need to be sterile or refrigerated and can be administered vaginally, orally or rectally negating the need for syringes. The Cochrane Library contains several reviews evaluating route and dose of misoprostol compared with either placebo or another uterotonic agent. The largest and most comprehensive trial was conducted by Gülmezoglu et al 2004. The primary endpoint of the study was the number of women reported as having had a PPH >1000 mL. Considering many of the intended settings, which included low resource communities, this seemed unusual as many women in these settings would already be chronically anaemic and would very likely suffer considerable morbidity or even death at a much lower threshold. The difference in the incidence of PPH between the women given 600 mg of misoprostol orally and the women who received other uterotonic agents was 3.6% versus 2.7%. This translated to a >20% difference, which was the tolerance level chosen beyond which it was deemed misoprostol was not as effective. Misoprostol was also found to have unpleasant side-effects, such as severe shivering and higher temperature, both of which were transient but unacceptable to some women. Its use appeared to be no more likely to necessitate manual removal of the placenta. Even though the recommendation was that misoprostol should not replace other uterotonics in settings where they are available, the authors suggest that it may be useful in circumstances where nothing else is available. The transient side-effects associated with misoprostol may not be any more debilitating than the nausea, vomiting (Ng et al 2007) and hypertensive episodes experienced by some women receiving Syntometrine, which remains the most commonly prescribed and administered uterotonic globally.

Clamping of the umbilical cord

This may have been carried out during birth of the baby if the cord was tightly around the neck. However, opinions vary as to the most beneficial time for clamping the cord during the third stage of labour.

Early clamping is normally applied in the first 1–3 min immediately after birth, regardless of whether the cord pulsation has ceased. It has been suggested that this practice may have the following effects:

- It may reduce the volume of blood returning to the fetus by as much as 75–125 mL, especially if clamping occurs within the first minute (van Rheenen & Brabin 2004).

- It may prematurely interrupt the respiratory function of the placenta in maintaining O_2 levels and combating acidosis in the early moments of life. This may be of particular importance in the baby who is slow to breathe.

- It may result in lower neonatal bilirubin levels, although the effect on the incidence of clinical jaundice is unclear (Prendiville & Elbourne 1989).

- It may increase the likelihood of fetomaternal transfusion as a larger volume of blood remains in the placenta. Venous pressure is further increased as retraction continues and may be sufficiently high to rupture surface placental vessels, thus facilitating the transfer of fetal cells into the maternal system; this may be a critical factor where the mother's blood group is Rhesus negative (see Ch. 47).

- It may result in the truncated umbilical vessels containing a quantity of clotted blood, which provides an ideal medium for bacterial growth. Heavier placental weight has also been associated with early cord clamping (Newton et al 1961).

Proponents of late clamping suggest that no action be taken until cord pulsation ceases or the placenta has been completely delivered, thus allowing the physiological processes to take place without intervention. Postulated advantages of late clamping include:

- The route to the low resistance placental circulation remains patent, which provides the newborn with a safety valve for any raised systemic blood pressure. This may be critical when the baby is preterm or asphyxiated, as raised pulmonary and central venous pressures may exacerbate the difficulties in initiating respiration and accompanying circulatory adaptation (Dunn 1985).

- The length of time for the cord to separate postnatally is reduced.

- The transfusion of the full quota of placental blood to the newborn. This may constitute as much as 40% of the circulating volume depending on when the cord is clamped and at what level the baby is held prior to clamping (Yao & Lind 1974); it may therefore be important in maintaining haematocrit levels. The neonatal effects associated with increased placental transfusion include higher mean birth weight and higher neonatal haematocrit accompanied by an increase in the incidence of jaundice (Prendiville et al 1988b). There is growing evidence that delaying cord clamping confers improved iron status in infants up to 6 months post-birth (Chaparro et al 2006, Mercer 2006, Rabe et al 2004).

There is very little evidence concerning how much, if any, of a uterotonic agent the baby receives following birth. In five documented cases of accidental administration of an adult dose of Syntometrine to a newborn infant, no long-term adverse effects were reported (Whitfield & Salfield 1980).

Is the timing of uterotonic administration and cord clamping clinically important in influencing the incidence of PPH?

Background

At the time of birth, the baby is still attached to the mother via the umbilical cord, which is part of the placenta. When the third stage or placental delivery stage is managed actively, an injection of an oxytocic drug is given to the mother at about the same time as the baby's shoulders are born and the umbilical cord is clamped twice. One clamp is placed closer to the baby's navel end. Care should be taken to apply the clamp to the cord end nearer the baby, 3–4 cm clear of the abdominal wall, to avoid pinching the skin or clamping a portion of gut, which, in rare instances, may be in the cord. A greater length of cord is left when umbilical vessels are needed for transfusion, for example in pre-term babies and cases of Rhesus haemolytic disease, and the second clamp is placed closer to the placental end of the cord. The cord between the two clamps is then cut. At this time, the baby may be placed on the mother's abdomen, put to the breast or be more closely examined on a warmed cot if resuscitation is required. Once the placenta is felt to have separated from the wall of the uterus, downward traction may be applied to the remaining length of umbilical cord to assist delivery of the placenta.

Timing of cord clamping is also supposedly routine, but, in practice it varies greatly. Early cord clamping, which is usually part of active management, is in general regarded as clamping of the umbilical cord within 30 s of the birth of the baby. Late cord clamping, a physiological approach, involves clamping of the umbilical cord when cord pulsation has ceased. However, definitions of what constitutes early and late cord clamping vary (Prendiville & Elbourne 1989) and again, in practice, unavoidable factors (e.g. if the cord is around the neck, the number of clinicians in the room, the need for active resuscitation of the infant) can make it difficult to adhere to a particular policy (McDonald 1996). There is no published evidence that this delay is of consequence in term infants (Chaparro et al 2006, McDonald 1996, Mercer 2006, Rabe et al 2004).

Investigations have been undertaken into the advantages and disadvantages of maternal–fetal transfusion and the effect of early or late cord clamping in relation to respiratory distress in the preterm infant (Dunn 1966, Inch 1985, Linderkamp 1982). There is a considerable amount of literature published on timing of cord clamping and associated placental transfusion. Debate continues over the effect of the extra 90–100 mL of blood received by the baby when late cord clamping is practised (Mercer 2006). Recent evidence suggests that the effects of early versus late cord clamping may be different for pre-term and term infants (Rabe et al 2004). Timing of cord clamping appears to be less of an issue in term infants, probably because the normal physiological process of transfer is completed within the first 1–2 min of birth for the majority of these infants (McDonald 1996).

Although active management leads to reduced risk of PPH, it is important to establish which of the components of this package lead to this reduced risk. Given the difficulties of adhering to an active management policy and the preferences of some women for physiological management, it is important to explore practice behaviours to clarify whether it is necessary to continue to promote the policy as it currently stands.

In light of the above information, it may be that whereas there is an obvious advantage to the prophylactic administration of a uterotonic drug, future third stage management policies may be less prescriptive about the necessity to clamp and cut the cord immediately following the birth.

Delivery of the placenta and membranes

Controlled cord traction (CCT). This manoeuvre is believed to reduce blood loss, shorten the third stage of labour and therefore minimize the time during which the mother is at risk from haemorrhage. It is designed to enhance the normal physiological process. Successful results depend upon understanding the principles of placental separation described at the beginning of this chapter.

If CCT is to be used, there are several checks to be made before proceeding:

- that a uterotonic drug has been administered
- that it has been given time to act
- that the uterus is well contracted
- that counter-traction is applied
- that signs of placental separation and descent are present. At the beginning of the third stage, a strong uterine contraction results in the fundus being palpable below the umbilicus (Fig. 29.6). It feels broad as the placenta is still in the upper

segment. As the placenta separates and falls into the lower uterine segment there is a small fresh blood loss, the cord lengthens, and the fundus becomes rounder, smaller and more mobile as it rises in the abdomen above the level of the placenta. There is however debate about whether CCT should be applied before or after the signs of placental separation have been noted.

It is important not to manipulate the uterus in any way as this may precipitate incoordinate action. No further step should be taken until a strong contraction is palpable. If tension is applied to the umbilical cord without this contraction, uterine inversion may occur. This is an acute obstetric emergency with life-threatening implications for the mother (see Ch. 33 Lewis 2007).

When CCT is the preferred method of management, the following sequence of actions is usually undertaken.

Once the uterus is found on palpation to be contracted, one hand is placed above the level of the symphysis pubis with the palm facing towards the umbilicus exerting pressure in an upwards direction. This is counter-traction. The other hand, firmly grasping the cord, applies traction in a downward and

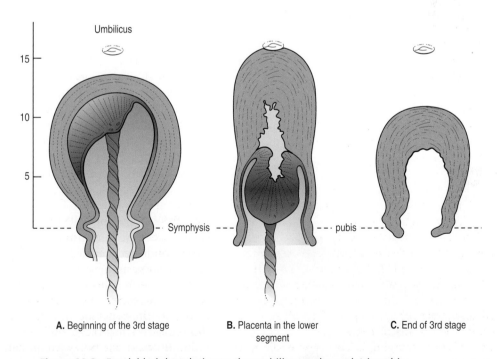

A. Beginning of the 3rd stage   **B.** Placenta in the lower segment   **C.** End of 3rd stage

Figure 29.6 Fundal height relative to the umbilicus and symphysis pubis.

backward direction following the line of the birth canal (Fig. 29.7). Some resistance may be felt but it is important to apply steady tension by pulling the cord firmly and maintaining the pressure. Jerky movements and force should be avoided. The aim is to complete the action as one continuous, smooth, controlled movement. However, it is only possible to exert this tension for a short time as it may be an uncomfortable procedure for the mother and the midwife's hand will tire.

Downward traction on the cord must be released before uterine counter-traction is relaxed as sudden withdrawal of counter-traction while tension is still being applied to the cord may also facilitate uterine inversion. If the manoeuvre is not immediately successful there should be a pause before the uterine contraction is again checked and a further attempt is made. Should the uterus relax, tension is temporarily released until a good contraction is again palpable. Once the placenta is visible it may be cupped in the hands to ease pressure on the friable membranes. A gentle upward and downward movement or twisting action will help to coax out the membranes and increase the chances of delivering them intact. Artery forceps may be applied to gradually ease the membranes out of the vagina. This process should not be hurried; great care should be taken to avoid tearing the membranes.

Expectant management

This management policy allows the physiological changes within the uterus that occur at the time of birth to take their natural course with minimal intervention. The processes of placental separation and expulsion are quite distinct from one another and the signs of separation and descent must be evident before maternal effort can be used to expedite expulsion. If the mother is sitting or squatting at this stage, gravity will aid expulsion.

If good uterine contractions are sustained, maternal effort will usually bring about expulsion. The mother simply pushes as during the second stage of labour. Encouragement is important, as by now she may be exhausted and the contractions will feel weaker and less expulsive than those during the second stage of labour. Providing that fresh blood loss is not excessive, the mother's condition remains stable and her pulse rate normal, there need be no anxiety. This spontaneous process can take from 20 min to 1 hr to complete. It is important that the midwife monitors uterine action by placing a hand lightly on the fundus. She can thus palpate the contraction while checking that relaxation does not result in the uterus filling with blood. Vigilance is crucial as it should be remembered that the longer the placenta remains undelivered, the greater is the risk of bleeding because the uterus cannot contract down fully while the bulk of the placenta is *in situ*. Dombrowski et al (1995) found that the frequency of haemorrhage increased between 10 min and 40 min after the birth of the baby. Patience and confidence are required on the part of the midwife to secure a successful conclusion. A uterotonic agent is usually not administered unless uterine tone is poor.

Early attachment of the baby to the breast may enhance these physiological changes by stimulating the reflex release of oxytocin from the posterior lobe of the pituitary gland, which helps to secure good uterine action.

Evidence for active versus expectant management

There is an increasing amount of appropriate, rigorously conducted research evidence available that strongly suggests that the prophylactic administration of a uterotonic significantly reduces the risk of PPH, results in a lower mean blood loss, fewer blood transfusions are required and there is a reduced need for therapeutic uterotonics (Begley 1990, Khan et al 1997, Prendiville et al 1988a, Rogers et al 1998, Thilaganathan et al 1993). It has

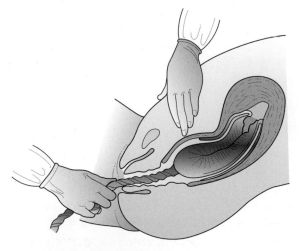

Figure 29.7 Controlled cord traction.

also been highlighted by the wide range of 'risk status' of women included in several studies that it is in fact very difficult to define a group of women who are not at risk for PPH. Taking all the best available evidence into consideration, a systematic review of the literature by Prendiville et al (2002) recommended that all women who birth in circumstances where this option is available should be encouraged to do so. Although the evidence is strongly in favour of prophylactic administration of a uterotonic, there are other aspects of active versus expectant management that may be worth exploring, e.g. prophylactic uterotonic (that is the uterotonic is given as soon as is practicable following the birth of the baby, 2–3 min) administration alone versus active management.

The FIGO/ICM Joint Statement released in November 2006, supports the use of active management by all skilled birth attendants regardless of the setting in which they practise and supplies clear guidelines related to alternative uterotonics and management strategies to be used in the absence of uterotonic drugs.

Not all research has a clearly defined outcome (Sandall & McCandlish 2006). Discussion and practice of management of the third stage of labour also need to take into account that the 'package' of care, whether active or expectant is reliant on the other components of the package being carried out as prescribed. For example, if management is expectant, then the introduction of an oxytocic, cord clamping or pulling on the cord will disrupt the intended sequence of the care process leading to what is often described as a fragmented approach. Once the sequence of the processes is altered, the clinician should commit to completing the process. That is, if the protocol for expectant management is interrupted the clinician should proceed to completing the process with an active management approach. This practice has been shown to significantly reduce the incidence of PPH in a birth centre setting (Patterson 2005).

Position of the woman

The effect of the position adopted by the woman at the time of placental delivery is still largely unclear. It may vary according to the mother's personal preference, the normality of progress and the experience and confidence of the attendant midwife, and may be influenced by the need for the midwife to monitor closely such factors as uterine contraction and blood loss.

Adoption of a dorsal position allows easy palpation of the uterine fundus. However, blood is more likely to pool in the uterus and vagina, thus disguising the true blood loss. Upright, kneeling and all-fours positions may enhance the effect of gravity and increase intra-abdominal pressure, which may in turn hasten the placental delivery process. Palpation of the uterus and/ or use of traction on the umbilical cord are contraindicated in this situation, as there is evidence that these manoeuvres elevate the risk for increased bleeding and retention of the placenta (Sinclair 2004). Blood loss can be more easily observed as fluids will drain out of the vagina. The squatting position has been reported to increase visible blood loss (Gupta & Nikodem 2002). Whichever position is adopted, the use of aids such as wedges, pillows and physical support from her partner will help to ensure the woman's comfort while completion of the third stage is being accomplished. Some women feel cold and shivery at this time, especially if labour has progressed rapidly or has been long and exhausting. This is usually transient and not abnormal.

Asepsis

The need for asepsis is even greater now than in the preceding stages of labour. Laceration and bruising of the cervix, vagina, perineum and vulva provide a route for the entry of micro-organisms. At the placental site, a raw surface provides an ideal medium for infection. Strict attention to the prevention of infection is therefore vital.

Cord blood sampling

This may be required for a variety of conditions:

- when the mother's blood group is Rhesus negative or as a precautionary measure if the mother's Rhesus type is unknown
- when atypical maternal antibodies have been found during an antenatal screening test
- where a haemoglobinopathy is suspected (e.g. sickle cell disease).

The sample should be taken as soon as possible from the fetal surface of the placenta where the blood vessels are congested and easily visible. If the cord has not been clamped prior to placental delivery the fetal vessels will not be congested, but a sample of sufficient volume may still be easily obtained. The appropriate containers should be used for any investigations requested. These may include the baby's blood group, Rhesus type, haemoglobin estimation, serum bilirubin level, Coombs' test or electrophoresis. Maternal blood for Kleihauer testing can be taken upon completion of the third stage.

Completion of the third stage

Once the placenta is delivered, the midwife must first check that the uterus is well contracted and fresh blood loss is minimal. Careful inspection of the perineum and lower vagina is important. A strong light is directed onto the perineum in order to assess trauma accurately prior to instigating repair. This should be carried out as gently as possible as the tissues are often bruised and oedematous. If perineal suturing (see Ch. 28) is required it should be carried out as expediently as possible to prevent unnecessary blood loss, increased risk of oedema at the site of trauma and perhaps unnecessary re-infiltration of additional local anaesthetics.

Blood loss estimation

Blood loss is difficult to measure and is frequently underestimated (Duthie 1990, Prastertcharoensuk et al 2000, WHO 2004). This is an important factor to be considered when assessing blood loss in the immediate postnatal period. The site of the blood loss does not necessarily alter the impact in terms of potential debility for affected women.

Other blood loss studies have been more specifically related to caesarean section. In his paper on blood loss at caesarean section, Brandt (1966) makes a valid point that haemodynamically women can withstand perhaps a 1000–1500 mL blood loss. However, any further blood loss may not be tolerated so readily. Women who undergo elective caesarean section will for the most part have been adequately prepared. Women who undergo emergency caesarean section or vaginal birth who are dehydrated or anaemic may not withstand sudden large volumes of blood loss.

In his study of the importance and difficulties of precise estimation of PPH, Brandt (1967) calculated that 20% of women lose >500 mL of blood after a vaginal birth. It was estimated that 3940 mL of circulating blood volume were required to maintain the central venous pressure at 10 cm of water. Most measurement techniques are not sufficiently sensitive to detect a rapid volume change in the immediate setting when decisions need to be made.

Note. It should also be remembered that any amount of blood loss that causes a physical deterioration such as feeling faint, sudden onset of tachycardia, drop in blood pressure should be immediately investigated.

Examination of placenta and membranes

This should be performed as soon after birth as practicable so that, if there is doubt about their completeness, further action may be taken before the woman leaves the birth room or the midwife prepares to leave the home. A thorough inspection must be carried out in order to make sure that no part of the placenta or membranes has been retained. The membranes are the most difficult to examine as they become torn during delivery and may be ragged. Every attempt should be made to piece them together to give an overall picture of completeness. This is easier to see if the placenta is held by the cord, allowing the membranes to hang. The hole through which the baby was born can then usually be identified and a hand can be spread out inside the membranes to aid inspection (Fig. 29.8). The placenta should then be laid on a flat surface and both placental surfaces minutely examined in a good light. The amnion should be peeled from the chorion right up to the umbilical cord, which allows the chorion to be fully viewed.

Any clots on the maternal surface need to be removed and kept for measuring. Broken fragments of cotyledon must be carefully replaced before an accurate assessment is possible.

The lobes of a complete placenta fit neatly together without any gaps, the edges forming a uniform circle. Blood vessels should not radiate beyond the placental edge. If they do, this denotes

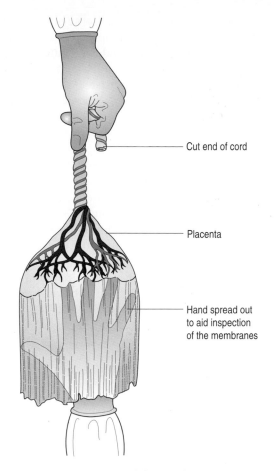

Cut end of cord

Placenta

Hand spread out
to aid inspection
of the membranes

Figure 29.8 Examination of the membranes.

a succenturiate lobe, which has developed separately from the main placenta (see Ch. 11). When such a lobe is visible there is no cause for concern, but if the tissue has been retained the vessels will end abruptly at a hole in the membrane. If there is any suspicion that the placenta or membranes are incomplete, they must be kept for inspection and a doctor informed immediately in case a PPH occurs or there is the possibility that a surgical intervention may be required. Account must be taken of blood that has soaked into linen and swabs as well as measurable fluid loss and clot formation.

Upon completion of the examination, the midwife should return her attention to the mother. The empty uterus should be firmly contracted. If the fundus has risen in the abdomen a blood clot may be present. This should be expelled while the uterus is

in a state of contraction by pressing the fundus gently in a downward and backward direction – with due regard to the risk of inversion and acute discomfort to the woman. Force should never be used.

Immediate care

It is advisable for mother and baby to remain in the midwife's care for at least 1 hr after birth, regardless of the birth setting. Much of this time will be spent in clearing up and completion of records but careful observation of mother and infant is very important. If an epidural cannula is in situ it is usually removed and checked at this time.

Early physiological observations including ensuring a well contracted uterus, assessment of vaginal blood loss and a gentle inspection of the genital tract to inspect for trauma should be undertaken (NICE 2006).

The woman should be encouraged to pass urine because a full bladder may impede uterine contraction. She may not actually feel an urge to do so, especially if she has passed urine immediately prior to giving birth or an effective epidural has been in progress, but she should be asked to try. Uterine contraction and blood loss should be checked on several occasions during this first hour. Once basic procedures to ensure the woman's and baby's safety and comfort have been completed, there is no evidence to suggest that restriction of food or fluids is necessary.

Most women intending to breastfeed will wish to put their babies to the breast during these early moments of contact. This is especially advantageous, as babies are usually very alert at this time and their sucking reflex is particularly strong. There is also evidence to suggest that women who breastfeed soon after birth successfully breastfeed for a longer period of time (Salariya et al 1979). An additional benefit lies in the reflex release of oxytocin from the posterior lobe of the pituitary gland, which stimulates the uterus to contract. This may result in the mother experiencing a sudden fresh blood loss as the uterus empties and she should be pre-warned and reassured that it is a normal response. The desire to feed a newborn baby is a warm, loving and instinctive response. While breastfeeding should be actively encouraged, a formula feed should be available for those who do not wish to breastfeed.

Records

A complete and accurate account of the labour, including the documentation of all drugs, physical examination and observations, is the midwife's responsibility. This should also include details of examination of the placenta, membranes and cord with attention drawn to any abnormalities. The volume of blood loss is particularly important. This record not only provides information that may be critical in the future care of both mother and infant but is a legal document that may be used as evidence of the care given. Signatures are therefore essential, with co-signatories where necessary. Many mothers now carry their own notes related to pregnancy and details of the birth. The completed records are a vital communication link between the midwife responsible for the birth and other caregivers, particularly those who take over care and provide ongoing community support services once the woman returns home.

It is usually the midwife who completes the birth notification form. Timely notification and referral may prevent delay in a woman receiving appropriate assistance should she need it.

Transfer from the birth room

The midwife is responsible for seeing that all observations are made and recorded prior to transfer of mother and baby to the postnatal ward or before the midwife leaves the home following the birth.

The postnatal ward midwife should verify these details prior to transfer of mother and baby. Following a domiciliary birth, the midwife should leave details of a telephone number where she may be contacted should the parents feel any cause for concern.

Complications of the third stage of labour

Postpartum haemorrhage

Primary postpartum haemorrhage is defined as excessive bleeding from the genital tract at any time following the baby's birth up to 24 hrs following the birth (WHO 2000).

PPH is one of the most alarming and serious emergencies a midwife may face and is especially terrifying if it occurs immediately following a straightforward birth. It is always a stressful experience for the woman and any support persons present and may undermine her confidence, influence her attitude to future childbearing and delay her recovery. Although the maternal mortality rate (MMR) in developed countries such as the UK, Australasia, Canada, Japan and USA is quoted as approximately 20/100 000 live births (WHO 2004) the reported MMR for lower resource countries, such as Africa is 830/100 000 live births and Asia 330/100 000 live births with region-specific areas experiencing much higher figures (for example, sub-Saharan Africa best estimates report 920/100 000 live births (WHO 2004). A significant number of the deaths recorded were due to PPH. The midwife is often the first and may be the only professional person present when a haemorrhage occurs, so her prompt, competent action will be crucial in controlling blood loss and reducing the risk of maternal morbidity or even death.

Primary postpartum haemorrhage

Fluid loss is extremely difficult to measure with any degree of accuracy, especially when a mixture of blood and fluid has soaked into the bed linen and spilled onto the floor. It should also be remembered that measurable solidified clots represent only about half the total fluid loss. With these factors in mind, the best yardstick is that any blood loss, however small, that adversely affects the mother's condition constitutes a PPH. Much will therefore depend upon the woman's general well-being. In addition, if the measured loss reaches 500 mL, it must be treated as a PPH, irrespective of maternal condition.

There are several reasons why a PPH may occur, including atonic uterus, retained placenta, trauma and blood coagulation disorder.

Atonic uterus

This is a failure of the myometrium at the placental site to contract and retract and to compress torn blood vessels and control blood loss by a living ligature action. When the placenta is attached, the volume of blood flow at the placental site is approximately 500–800 mL/min. Upon separation, the efficient contraction and retraction of uterine muscle staunch the flow and prevent a haemorrhage, which would otherwise ensue with horrifying speed (Box 29.1).

> **Box 29.1** Causes of atonic uterine action
>
> - Incomplete separation of the placenta
> - Retained cotyledon, placental fragment or membranes
> - Precipitate labour
> - Prolonged labour resulting in uterine inertia
> - Polyhydramnios or multiple pregnancy causing overdistension of uterine muscle
> - Placenta praevia
> - Placental abruption
> - General anaesthesia especially halothane or cyclopropane
> - A full bladder
> - Aetiology unknown.

Incomplete placental separation

If the placenta remains fully adherent to the uterine wall, it is unlikely to cause bleeding. However, once separation has begun, maternal vessels are torn. If placental tissue remains partially embedded in the spongy decidua, efficient contraction and retraction are interrupted.

Retained cotyledon, placental fragment or membranes

These will similarly impede efficient uterine action.

Precipitate labour

When the uterus has contracted vigorously and frequently resulting in a duration of labour that is less than 1 hr, then the muscle may have insufficient opportunity to retract.

Prolonged labour

In a labour where the active phase lasts >12 hrs uterine inertia (sluggishness) may result from muscle exhaustion.

Polyhydramnios or multiple pregnancy

The myometrium becomes excessively stretched and therefore less efficient.

Placenta praevia

The placental site is partly or wholly in the lower segment where the thinner muscle layer contains few oblique fibres: this results in poor control of bleeding.

Placental abruption

Blood may have seeped between the muscle fibres, interfering with effective action. At its most severe this results in a Couvelaire uterus (see Ch. 20).

Induction or augmentation of labour with oxytocin

In some circumstances, the use of oxytocin during labour may result in hyperstimulation of the uterus and cause a precipitate, expulsive birth of the baby. In this instance the uterus may still be responding in a stimulated, but ineffective manner in terms of contracting the empty uterus. In the case of induction or augmentation of a labour, that continues over a prolonged period without establishing efficient uterine contractions, physical and emotional fatigue of the mother, and uterine fatigue or inertia may occur. This inertia inhibits the uterine muscle from providing strong, sustained contraction and retraction of the empty uterus that aids in the prevention of a postpartum haemorrhage occurring.

General anaesthesia

Anaesthetic agents may cause uterine relaxation, in particular the volatile inhalational agents, for example halothane.

Mismanagement of the third stage of labour

'Fundus fiddling' or manipulation of the uterus may precipitate arrhythmic contractions so that the placenta only partially separates and retraction is lost.

A full bladder

If the bladder is full, its proximity to the uterus in the abdomen on completion of the second stage may interfere with uterine action. This also constitutes mismanagement.

Aetiology unknown

A precipitating cause may never be discovered.

There are in addition a number of factors that do not directly cause a PPH, but do increase the likelihood of excessive bleeding (Box 29.2).

Previous history of PPH or retained placenta

There is a risk of recurrence in subsequent pregnancies. A detailed obstetric history taken at the first antenatal visit will ensure that arrangements are made for such a mother to give birth in a consultant unit.

High parity

With each successive pregnancy, fibrous tissue replaces muscle fibres in the uterus; this reduces its contractility and the blood vessels become more difficult to compress. Women who have had five or more births are at increased risk.

Fibroids (fibromyomata)

These are normally benign tumours consisting of muscle and fibrous tissue, which may impede efficient uterine action.

Anaemia

Women who enter labour with reduced haemoglobin concentration (below 10 g/dL) may succumb more quickly to any subsequent blood loss, however small. Anaemia is associated with debility, which is a more direct cause of uterine atony.

HIV/AIDS

Women who have HIV/AIDS are often in a state of severe immunosuppression, which lowers the platelet count to such a degree that even a relatively minor blood loss may cause severe morbidity or death.

Box 29.2 Predisposing factors which might increase the risks of postpartum haemorrhage

- Previous history of postpartum haemorrhage or retained placenta
- High parity resulting in uterine scar tissue
- Presence of fibroids
- Maternal anaemia
- Ketoacidosis
- Multiple pregnancy.

Ketosis

The influence of ketosis upon uterine action is still unclear. Foulkes & Dumoulin (1983) demonstrated that, in a series of 3500 women, 40% had ketonuria at some time during labour. They reported that if labour progressed well, this did not appear to jeopardize either the fetal or maternal condition. However, there was a significant relationship between ketosis and the need for oxytocin augmentation, instrumental delivery and PPH when labour lasted >12 hrs. Correction of ketosis is therefore advisable and can be facilitated by ensuring women have an adequate intake of fluids and light solid nourishment as tolerated throughout labour. There is no evidence to suggest restriction of food or fluids is necessary during the normal course of labour.

Signs of PPH

These may be obvious such as:

- visible bleeding
- maternal collapse.

However, more subtle signs may present, such as:

- pallor
- rising pulse rate
- falling blood pressure
- altered level of consciousness; the mother may become restless or drowsy
- an enlarged uterus as it fills with blood or blood clot; it feels 'boggy' on palpation (i.e. soft and distended and lacking tone); there may be little or no visible loss of blood.

Prophylaxis

By using the above list, it is possible for the midwife to apply some preventive screening in an attempt to identify women who may be at greater risk and to recognize causative factors. During the antenatal period a thorough and accurate history of previous obstetric experiences will identify risk factors such as previous PPH or precipitate labour. Arrangements can then, after careful explanation and in full consultation with the woman, be made for birth to take place in a unit where facilities for dealing with emergencies are available. The early detection and treatment of anaemia will help ensure that women enter labour with a haemoglobin level, ideally, in excess of 10g/dL. The midwife should check that blood tests, if needed, are taken regularly and the results recorded and explained to the woman. If necessary, action can be taken to restore the haemoglobin level before birth. Women more prone to anaemia should be closely monitored, e.g. those with multiple pregnancies.

During labour, good management practices during the first and second stages are important to prevent prolonged labour and ketoacidosis. A mother should not enter the second or third stage with a full bladder. Prophylactic administration of a uterotonic agent is recommended for the third stage, by either intramuscular injection or intravenous infusion. Two units of cross-matched blood should be kept available for any woman known to have a placenta praevia or is known to have pre-disposing risk factors for PPH.

Treatment of PPH

Whatever the stage of labour or crisis that may occur, the midwife should adhere to the underlying principle of always reassuring the woman and her support persons by continually relaying appropriate information and involving them in decision-making.

Three basic principles of care should be applied immediately upon observation of excessive bleeding:

1. Call for medical aid.
2. Stop the bleeding – rub up a contraction – give a uterotonic – empty the uterus.
3. Resuscitate the mother.

Call for medical aid

This is an important initial step so that help is on the way whatever transpires. If the bleeding is brought under control before the doctor arrives, then no action by the doctor will be needed. However, the woman's condition can deteriorate very rapidly, in which case medical assistance will be required urgently. If the mother is at home or in a midwife-led unit, the emergency department of the closest obstetric unit should be contacted and, depending on the policy of the region, an obstetric emergency team summoned or ambulance transfer arranged.

Stop the bleeding

The initial action is always the same, regardless of whether bleeding occurs with the placenta *in situ* or later.

Rub up a contraction

The fundus is first felt gently with the fingertips to assess its consistency. If it is soft and relaxed, the fundus is massaged with a smooth, circular motion, applying no undue pressure. When a contraction occurs, the hand is held still.

Give a uterotonic to sustain the contraction

In many instances, oxytocin 5 units or 10 units, or combined ergometrine/oxytocin 1mL, has already been administered and this may be repeated. Alternatively, ergometrine 0.25–0.5mg may be injected intravenously, which will be effective within 45s. No more than two doses of ergometrine should be given (including any dose of combined ergometrine/oxytocin), as it may cause pulmonary hypertension. Several reports have described the dramatic haemostatic effects of prostaglandins used in cases of uterine atony. Misoprostol or carboprost (Hemabate) are the most common prostaglandin drugs used to increase uterine contractility for the treatment of PPH. However, the side-effects (nausea, vomiting, pyrexia, hypertension, diarrhoea) associated with these drugs can make their use limited (Anderson & Etches 2007).

The baby may be put to the breast to enhance the physiological secretion of oxytocin from the posterior lobe of the pituitary gland, thus stimulating a contraction.

Empty the uterus

Once the midwife is satisfied that it is well contracted, she should ensure that the uterus is emptied. If the placenta is still in the uterus, it should be delivered; if it has been expelled, any clots should be expressed by firm but gentle pressure on the fundus.

Resuscitate the mother

An intravenous infusion should be commenced while peripheral veins are easily negotiated. This will provide a route for an oxytocin infusion or fluid replacement. As an emergency measure, the mother's legs may be lifted up in order to allow blood to drain from them into the central circulation. However, the foot of the bed should not be raised as this encourages pooling of blood in the uterus, which prevents the uterus contracting.

It is usually expedient to catheterize the bladder to ensure a full bladder is not impeding uterine contraction and thus precipitating further bleeding and to minimize trauma should an operative procedure be necessary.

On no account must a woman in a collapsed condition be moved prior to resuscitation and stabilization.

The flow chart (Fig. 29.9) briefly sets out the possible courses of action that may be taken depending upon whether or not bleeding persists. If the above measures are successful in controlling any further loss, administration of oxytocin, 40 units in 1 L of intravenous solution (e.g. Hartmann's or saline) infused slowly over 8–12 hrs, will ensure continued uterine contraction. This will help to minimize the risk of recurrence. Before the infusion is connected, 10 mL of blood should be withdrawn for haemoglobin estimation and for cross-matching compatible blood. If bleeding continues uncontrolled, the choice of further action will depend largely upon whether the placenta remains undelivered.

Placenta delivered

If the uterus is atonic following delivery of the placenta, light fundal pressure may be used to expel residual clots while a contraction is stimulated. If an effective contraction is not maintained, 40 units of Syntocinon in 1 L of intravenous fluid should be started. The placenta and membranes must be re-examined for completeness because retained fragments are often responsible for uterine atony.

Bimanual compression

If bleeding continues, bimanual compression of the uterus may be necessary in order to apply pressure to the placental site. It is desirable for an intravenous infusion to be in progress. The fingers of one hand are inserted into the vagina like a cone; the hand is formed into a fist and placed into the anterior vaginal fornix, the elbow resting on the bed. The other hand is placed behind the uterus abdominally, the fingers pointing towards the cervix. The uterus is brought forwards and compressed between the palm of the hand positioned abdominally and the fist in the vagina (Fig. 29.10). If bleeding persists, a clotting disorder must be excluded before exploration of the vagina and uterus is performed under a general anaesthetic (see also Ch. 55 for aortic compression).

Placenta undelivered

The placenta may be partially or wholly adherent.

Partially adherent

When the uterus is well contracted, an attempt should be made to deliver the placenta by applying CCT. If this is unsuccessful a doctor will be required to remove it manually.

Completely adherent

Bleeding does not usually occur if the placenta is completely adherent. However, the longer the placenta remains *in situ* the greater is the risk of partial separation, which may give rise to profuse haemorrhage.

Retained placenta

This diagnosis is reached when the placenta remains undelivered after a specified period of time (up to 1 hr following the baby's birth). The conventional treatment is to separate the placenta from the uterine wall digitally, effecting a manual removal.

Breaking of the cord

This is not an unusual occurrence during completion of the third stage of labour. Before further action, it is crucial to check that the uterus remains firmly contracted. If the placenta remains adherent, no further action should be taken before a doctor is notified. It is possible that manual removal may be indicated. If the placenta is palpable in the vagina, it is probable that separation has occurred and when the uterus is well contracted then maternal effort may be encouraged (see Expectant management, above). If there is any doubt, the midwife applies fresh sterile gloves before performing a vaginal examination to ascertain whether this is so. As a last resort, if the woman is unable to push effectively then fundal pressure may be used. A uterotonic drug must be given prior to this. Great care is exercised to ensure that placental separation has already occurred and

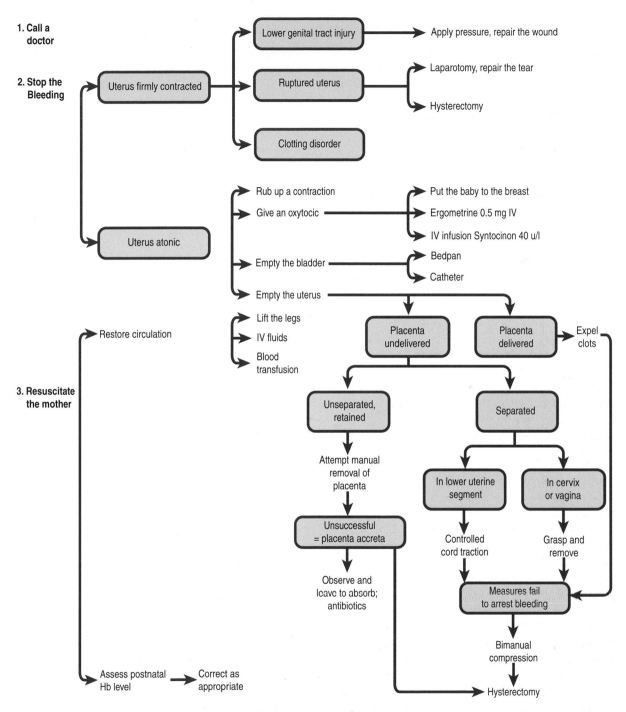

Figure 29.9 Management of primary PPH.

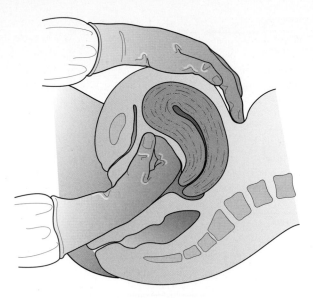

Figure 29.10 Bimanual compression of the uterus.

the uterus is well contracted. The woman should be relaxed as the midwife exerts downward and backward pressure on the firmly contracted fundus. This method can cause considerable pain and distress to the woman and result in the stretching and bruising of supportive uterine ligaments. If it is performed without good uterine contraction, acute inversion may ensue. This is an extremely dangerous procedure in unskilled hands and is not advocated in everyday practice when alternative, safer methods may be employed.

Manual removal of the placenta

This should be carried out by a doctor. An intravenous infusion must first be sited and an effective anaesthetic in progress. The choice of anaesthesia will depend upon the woman's general condition. If an effective epidural anaesthetic is already in progress, a top-up may be given in order to avoid the hazards of general anaesthesia. A spinal anaesthetic offers an alternative but where time is an urgent factor a general anaesthetic will be initiated.

Management

Manual removal is performed with full aseptic precautions and, unless in a dire emergency situation, should not be undertaken prior to adequate analgesia being ensured for the woman. With the left hand,

the umbilical cord is held taut while the right hand is coned and inserted into the vagina and uterus following the direction of the cord. Once the placenta is located the cord is released so that the left hand may be used to support the fundus abdominally, to prevent rupture of the lower uterine segment (Fig. 29.11). The operator will feel for a separated edge of the placenta. The fingers of the right hand are extended and the border of the hand is gently eased between the placenta and the uterine wall, with the palm facing the placenta. The placenta is carefully detached with a sideways slicing movement. When it is completely separated, the left hand rubs up a contraction and expels the right hand with the placenta in its grasp. The placenta should be checked immediately for completeness, so that any further exploration of the uterus may be carried out without delay. A uterotonic drug is given upon completion.

In very exceptional circumstances, when no doctor is available to be called, a midwife would be expected to carry out a manual removal of the placenta. Once she has diagnosed a retained placenta as the cause of PPH, the midwife must act swiftly to reduce the risk of onset of shock and exsanguination. It must be remembered that the risk of inducing shock by performing a manual removal of the placenta is greater when no anaesthetic is given.

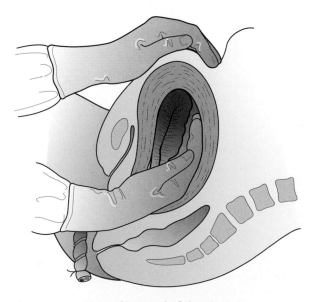

Figure 29.11 Manual removal of the placenta.

In a developed country, the midwife is unlikely to find herself dealing with this situation.

At home

If the placenta is retained following a home birth, emergency obstetric help must be summoned. Under no circumstances should a woman be transferred to hospital until an intravenous infusion is in progress and her condition stabilized.

It is best if the placenta can be delivered without moving the mother but if this is not possible, or if further treatment is needed, she should be transferred to a consultant unit. The baby should accompany her.

Morbid adherence of placenta

Very rarely, the placenta remains morbidly adherent; this is known as placenta accreta. If it is totally adherent, then bleeding is unlikely to occur and it may be left *in situ* to absorb during the puerperium. If, however, only part of the placenta remains embedded then the risks of fatal haemorrhage are high and an emergency hysterectomy may be unavoidable.

Trauma as a cause of haemorrhage

If bleeding occurs despite a well-contracted uterus, it is almost certainly the consequence of trauma to the uterus, vagina, perineum or labia, or a combination of these. Poeschmann et al (1991) cautioned that episiotomy may contribute up to 30% of total blood loss; in their study the severity of blood loss was linked to the length of time that elapsed between incision of the perineum and the commencement of repair. Predictably, the longer the wait the greater is the blood loss.

In order to identify the source of bleeding, the mother is placed in the lithotomy position under a good directional light. An episiotomy wound or tears to the anterior labia, clitoris and perineum often bleed freely. These external injuries are easily identified and torn vessels may be clamped with artery forceps prior to ligation. Internal trauma to the vagina, cervix or uterus more commonly occurs following instrumental or manipulative delivery. A speculum is inserted to enable the cervix and vagina to be clearly visualized and examined. Tissue or artery forceps may be used to apply pressure prior to suturing under general anaesthesia.

If bleeding persists when the uterus is well contracted and no evidence of trauma can be found, uterine rupture must be suspected. Following a laparotomy this is repaired, but if bleeding remains uncontrolled a hysterectomy may become inevitable.

Blood coagulation disorders

As well as the causes already listed above, PPH may be the result of coagulation failure (see Ch. 20). The failure of the blood to clot is such an obvious sign that it can be overlooked in the midst of the frantic activity that accompanies torrential bleeding. It can occur following severe pre-eclampsia, APH, massive PPH, amniotic fluid embolus, intrauterine death or sepsis. Evaluation should include coagulation status and replacing appropriate blood components (Anderson & Etches 2007). Fresh blood is usually the best treatment, as this will contain platelets and the coagulation factors V and VIII. The expert advice of a haematologist will be needed in assessing specific replacement products such as fresh frozen plasma and fibrinogen.

Maternal observation following PPH

Once bleeding is controlled, the total volume lost must be estimated as accurately as possible. Large amounts appear less than they are in reality. Maternal pulse and blood pressure are recorded every 15 min and the temperature taken every 4 hrs. The uterus should be palpated frequently to ensure that it remains well contracted and lochia lost must be observed. Intravenous fluid replacement should be carefully calculated to avoid circulatory overload. Monitoring the central venous pressure (see Ch. 33) will provide an accurate assessment of the volume required, especially if blood loss has been severe. Fluid intake and urinary output are recorded as indicators of renal function. The output should be accurately measured on an hourly basis by the use of a self-retaining urinary catheter.

The woman will, if possible, be transferred to a high dependency care unit if closer monitoring is required, until her condition is stable. All records should be meticulously completed and signed contemporaneously. Continued vigilance will be important for 24–48 hrs. As this woman will need a period of recovery, she will not be suitable for early transfer home.

Secondary postpartum haemorrhage

Secondary postpartum haemorrhage is any abnormal or excessive bleeding from the genital tract occurring between 24 hrs and 12 weeks postnatally. In developed countries, 2% of postnatal women are admitted to hospital with this condition, half of them undergoing uterine surgical evacuation (Alexander et al 2007). It is most likely to occur between 10 and 14 days after birth. Bleeding is usually due to retention of a fragment of the placenta or membranes, or the presence of a large uterine blood clot. Typically occurring during the second week, the lochia is heavier than normal and will have changed from a serous pink or brownish loss to a bright red blood loss. The lochia may also be offensive if infection is a contributory factor. Subinvolution, pyrexia and tachycardia are usually present. As this is an event that is most likely to occur at home, women should be alerted to the possible signs of secondary PPH prior to discharge from midwifery care.

Management

The following steps should be taken:

- call a doctor
- reassure the woman and her support person(s)
- rub up a contraction by massaging the uterus if it is still palpable
- express any clots
- encourage the mother to empty her bladder
- give a uterotonic drug such as ergometrine maleate by the intravenous or intramuscular route
- keep all pads and linen to assess the volume of blood lost
- if bleeding persists, discuss a range of treatment options with the woman and, if appropriate, prepare the woman for theatre.

If the bleeding occurs at home and the woman has telephoned the hospital, midwife or her GP, she should be told to lie down flat until professional assistance arrives (the front door should be left unlocked if the woman is alone). On arrival, the doctor, midwife or paramedic will assess the amount of blood loss and the woman's condition and attempt to arrest the haemorrhage. If the loss is severe or uncontrolled, the nearest emergency obstetric unit will be called and the mother and baby prepared for transfer to hospital. The doctor, midwife or paramedic who attends will start an intravenous infusion and ensure that the mother's condition is stable first.

Careful assessment is usually undertaken prior to the uterus being explored under general anaesthetic. The use of ultrasound as a diagnostic tool is invaluable in minimizing the number of mothers who have operative intervention. If retained products of conception cannot be seen on a scan, the mother may be treated conservatively with antibiotic therapy and oral ergometrine. The haemoglobin should be estimated prior to discharge. If it is below 9 g/dL, options for iron replacement should be discussed with the woman. The severity of the anaemia will assist in determining the most appropriate care, which may be dependent on whether the woman is symptomatic (e.g. feeling faint, dizzy, short of breath). Management may vary from increased intake of iron-rich foods, iron supplements or, in extreme cases, blood transfusion. It is also important to discuss the common symptoms that may be experienced as a result of anaemia following PPH, including extreme tiredness and general malaise. Encourage the woman to seek assistance and stress the importance of making an appointment to see her GP to have her general health and haemoglobin levels checked.

Haematoma formation

PPH may also be concealed as the result of progressive haematoma formation. This may be obvious at such sites as the perineum or lower vagina, but it is more difficult to diagnose if it occurs into the broad ligament or vault of the vagina. A large volume of blood may collect insidiously (up to 1 L). Involution and lochia are usually normal, the main symptom being increasingly severe maternal pain. This is often so acute that the haematoma has to be drained in theatre under a general anaesthetic. Secondary infection is a strong possibility.

Care after a postpartum haemorrhage

Whatever the cause of the haemorrhage, the woman will need the continued support of her midwife until she regains her confidence. Her partner may also be fearful of a recurrence and need much reassurance. If the mother is breast-feeding, lactation may be impaired but this will only be temporary and she should be encouraged to persevere. The midwife is often the first and may be the only professional person present when a haemorrhage occurs, so her prompt, competent action will be crucial in controlling blood loss and reducing the risk of maternal morbidity or even mortality.

Key issues in the management of the third stage of labour are listed in Box 29.3.

Box 29.3 Key issues in the management of the third stage of labour

- Difficulty of implementing well-documented evidence into practice
- Care during the third stage of labour should not be viewed in isolation from what has occurred during the first and second stages of labour
- The global PPH rate has not reduced significantly in the past decade regardless of interventions applied (see Lewis 2007 for UK)
- Possible research: How does delayed childbearing (increased age of women having a first baby), assisted reproductive technology or obesity affect the risk of PPH?

REFERENCES

Alexander J, Thomas P, Sanghera J 2007 Treatments for secondary postpartum haemorrhage. The Cochrane Database of Systematic Reviews, Issue 2:CD002867

Anderson J M, Etches D 2007 Prevention and management of postpartum hemorrhage. American Family Physician 75:875–882

Baldock S, Dixon L 2006 Physiological changes in labour and the postnatal period. In: Pairman S, Pincombe J, Thorogood C et al (eds) Midwifery: preparation for practice. Elsevier, Marrickville, Australia

Begley C M 1990 A comparison of 'active' and 'physiological' management of the third stage of labour. Midwifery 6:3–17

Brandt H A 1966 Blood loss at caesarean section. Journal of Obstetrics and Gynaecology of the British Commonwealth 73:456–459

Brandt H A 1967 Precise estimation of postpartum haemorrhage: difficulties and importance. British Medical Journal 1:398–400

Chaparro C M, Neufeld L M, Alavez G T et al 2006 Effect of timing of umbilical cord clamping on iron status in Mexican infants: A randomised controlled trial. Lancet 367: (9527):1997–2004

Choy C M Y, Lau W C, Tam W H et al 2002 A randomised controlled trial of intramuscular Syntometrine and intravenous oxytocin in the management of the third stage of labour. British Journal of Obstetrics and Gynaecology 109:173–177

Chua S, Shaw S I, Yeoh C L et al 1995 A randomised controlled study of prostaglandin 15 methyl F2 alpha compared with Syntometrine for prophylactic use in the third stage of labour. Journal of Australian and New Zealand Obstetrics and Gynaecology 35:(4):413

Dombrowski M P, Bottoms S F, Saleb A A A et al 1995 Third stage of labour: analysis of duration and clinical practice. American Journal of Obstetrics and Gynecology 172:1279–1284

Dunn P M 1985 Management of childbirth in normal women: the third stage and fetal adaptation. In: Perinatal medicine. Proceedings of the IX European Congress on Perinatal Medicine, Dublin, September 1984. MTP Press, Lancaster, p 47–54

Dunn P M 1966 The placental venous pressure during and after the third stage of labour following early cord ligation. Journal of Obstetrics and Gynaecology of the British Commonwealth 73:747–756

Duthie S J, Ven D, Yung G L K et al 1990 Discrepancy between laboratory determination and visual estimation of blood loss during normal delivery. European Journal of Obstetrics, Gynaecology and Reproductive Biology 38:119–124

FIGO/ICM (International Federation of Gynaecology and Obstetrics/International Confederation of Midwives) Joint Statement 2006 Prevention and treatment of post-partum haemorrhage: New Advances for Low Resource Settings, November

Foulkes J, Dumoulin J G 1983 Ketosis in labour. British Journal of Hospital Medicine 29(6):562–564

Gülmezoglu A M, Forna F, Villar J et al 2004 Prostaglandins for prevention of postpartum hemorrhage. Cochrane Review, Issue 1:CD000494

Gupta J K, Nikodem V C 2002 Position for women during second stage of labour. Cochrane Review, Issue 2:CD002006

Inch S 1985 Management of the third stage of labour – another cascade of intervention. Midwifery 1:114–122

Johnson R, Taylor W 2000. Third stage issues. In: Johnson R (ed.) Skills for midwifery practice Harcourt, London

Khan Q K, John I S, Chan T et al 1995 Abu Dhabi third stage trial: oxytocin versus Syntometrine in the active management of the third stage of labour. European Journal of Obstetrics, Gynaecology and Reproductive Biology 58:147–151

Khan G Q, John I S, Wani S et al 1997 Abstract 56: 'Controlled cord traction' versus 'minimal intervention' techniques in the delivery of the placenta: a randomised controlled trial. American Journal of Obstetrics and Gynecology 177(4):770–774

Lewis G, Drife J (eds) 2001 Why mothers die 1997–1999. The Confidential Enquiries into Maternal Deaths in the United Kingdom. RCOG Press, London, p 21

Lewis, G (ed.) 2007 The Confidential Enquiry into Maternal and Child Health (CEMACH). Saving mothers' lives: reviewing maternal deaths to make motherhood safer 2003–2005. The seventh report on Confidential Enquiries into Maternal Deaths in the United Kingdom. CEMACH, London

Linderkamp O 1982 Placental transfusion: determinants and effects. Clinical Perinatology 9:589–593

McDonald S, Abbott J M, Higgins S P 2004 Prophylactic ergometrine-oxytocin versus oxytocin for the third stage of labour. Cochrane Database of Systematic Reviews, Issue 1:CD000201

McDonald S J, Middleton P 2008 Effect of timing of umbilical cords clamping of term infants on maternal and neonatal outcomes. Cochrane Database of Systematic Reviews 2008 Issue 2 Art no CD 004074

McDonald S J 1996 Timing of interventions in the third stage of labour. In: McDonald S J (ed.) Management in the third stage of labour (Doctoral thesis). Faculty of Medicine, Department of Obstetrics and Gynaecology, University of Western Australia, p 60–81

McDonald S J, Prendiville W J, Blair E 1993 Randomised controlled trial of oxytocin alone versus oxytocin and ergometrine in active management of the third stage of labour. British Medical Journal 307:1167–1171

Mercer J S 2006 Current best evidence: a review of the literature on umbilical cord clamping. In: Wickham S (ed.) Midwifery. Best practice, Vol. 4. Elsevier, London

Newton M, Mosey L M, Egli G E et al 1961 Blood loss during and immediately after delivery. Obstetrics and Gynaecology 17:9–18

Ng P S, Lai C Y, Sahota D S et al 2007 A double-blind randomized controlled trial of oral misoprostol and intramuscular Syntometrine in the management of the third stage of labor. Gynecologic and Obstetric Investigations 63:55–60

NICE (National Institute for Health and Clinical Excellence) 2006 Postnatal care: Routine postnatal care of women and their babies. Online. Available: http://www.nice.org.uk

Patterson D 2005 The views and experiences of childbirth educators providing a breastfeeding intervention during pregnancy. Proceedings of 27th Congress of the International Confederation of Midwives on 'Midwifery: Pathways to Healthy Nations', Brisbane, Australia

Peyser R M, Kupfermine M J 1990 Management of postpartum haemorrhage by uterine irrigation with prostaglandin. American Journal of Obstetrics and Gynecology 162(3):694–696

Poeschmann R P, Docsburg W H, Eskis T K A B A 1991 Randomised comparison of oxytocin, sulprostone and placebo in the management of the third stage of labour. British Journal of Obstetrics and Gynaecology 98:528–530

Prastertcharoensuk W, Swadpanich U, Lumbiganon P 2000 Accuracy of the blood loss estimation in the third stage of labor. International Journal Gynecological Obstetrics 71:9–70

Prendiville W, Elbourne D 1989 Care during the third stage of labour. In: Chalmers I, Enkin M, Keirse M J N C (eds)

Effective care in pregnancy and childbirth. Oxford University Press, Oxford, p 1145–1169

Prendiville W, Elbourne D, Chalmers I 1988a The effects of routine uterotonic administration in the management of the third stage of labour: an overview of the evidence from controlled trials. British Journal of Obstetrics and Gynaecology 95:3–16

Prendiville W J, Elbourne D R, Chalmers I 1988b The Bristol third stage trial: active versus physiological management of the third stage of labour. British Medical Journal 297:1295–1300

Prendiville W J, Elbourne D, McDonald S 2002 Active versus expectant management of the third stage of labour. Cochrane Review, Issue 4:CD001808

Rabe H, Reynolds G, Diaz-Rossello J 2004 Early versus delayed umbilical cord clamping in preterm infants. Cochrane Database of Systematic Reviews, Issue 4:CD003248

Rogers J, Wood J, McCandlish R et al 1998 Active versus expectant management of third stage of labour: the Hinchingbrooke randomised controlled trial. Lancet 351:693–699

Salariya E, Easton P, Cater J 1979 Early and often for best results. Nursing Mirror 148:15–17

Sandall J, McCandlish R 2006 Why Do Research ? In: Page L, McCandlish R (eds) The new midwifery: science and sensitivity in practice, 2nd edn. Churchill Livingstone, Edinburgh, p 251

Sinclair C A 2004 The midwife's handbook. W B Saunders, Missouri

Thilaganathan B, Cutner A, Latimer J et al 1993 Management of the third stage of labour in women at low risk of postpartum haemorrhage. European Journal of Obstetrics and Gynecology and Reproductive Biology 48:19–22

van Rheenen P, Brabin B J 2004 Late umbilical cord clamping as an intervention for reducing iron deficiency anaemia in term infants in developing and industrialized countries: a systematic review. Annals of Tropical Paediatrics 24:3–16

van Selm M, Kanhai H H H, Keiser M I N C 1995 Preventing the recurrence of atonic postpartum haemorrhage: a double-blind trial. Acta Obstetrica et Gynecologica Scandinavica 74:270–274

Whitfield M F, Salfield S A W 1980 Accidental administration of Syntometrine in adult dosage to the newborn. Archives of Disease in Childhood 55:68–70

WHO (World Health Organization) 1990 The prevention and management of postpartum hemorrhage. WHO report of technical working group, No. WHO/MCH/90.7. WHO, Geneva

WHO (World Health Organization) 2000 Managing complications in pregnancy and childbirth: a guide for midwives and doctors, WHO/RHR/00.7. WHO, Geneva

WHO (World Health Organization) 2004 Maternal mortality in 2000: estimates developed by WHO, UNICEF and UNFPA. WHO, Geneva

WHO (World Health Organization) 2007 Maternal mortality in 2005. Estimates developed by WHO, UNICEF, UNFPA, and The World Bank. WHO, Geneva

Yao A C, Lind J 1974 Placental transfusion. American Journal of Diseases of Children 127:128–141

USEFUL WEBSITE

POPPHI 2006: http://www.pphprevention.org

An instructional video on management of the third stage of labour.

30 Prolonged pregnancy and disorders of uterine action

Annie Rimmer

While the decision to intervene in a pregnancy that continues beyond term is based on discussion between the woman and obstetrician, the unique relationship between the woman and midwife is pivotal in enabling the woman to make an informed decision at this time. The midwife continues to play a key role when labour is induced, when there is failure to progress in labour or when labour is prolonged, with or without further complications.

The chapter aims to:

- explore the issues relating to prolonged pregnancy with reference to best evidence and the midwife's role at this time
- outline the indications for the induction of labour and examine the methods used to induce labour
- describe the process where there is failure to progress in labour or labour is prolonged and review the current evidence used to support the management and care in such cases
- describe the serious complication that is obstructed labour and discuss the importance of competent midwifery management and care of women during the antenatal and intrapartum period if such complications are to be avoided
- highlight the significant events in a precipitate labour.

Prolonged pregnancy

Prolonged pregnancy and post-term pregnancy are used synonymously and refer to a specific gestation of the pregnancy and not the fetus or neonate. The term, prolonged pregnancy, will be used in this chapter. Post-maturity refers to a description of the neonate with peeling of the epidermis, long nails, an alert face and loose skin suggestive of recent weight loss (Koklanaris & Tropper 2006). The relationship, if any, between prolonged pregnancy and post-maturity will be explored later in the chapter.

Prolonged pregnancy is associated with increased risk to the fetus and neonate resulting in higher perinatal morbidity and mortality (Briscoe et al 2005, Fok et al 2006, Gülmezoglu et al 2006, RCOG 2001). It is the most common indication given for induction of labour in England accounting for approximately 46% of inductions overall. In 2004–2005, 79% of cases of prolonged pregnancy were induced (Department of Health (DH) 2006). While it is accepted there is evidence of an increase in perinatal mortality and morbidity as the pregnancy goes beyond 41 weeks, this would appear to relate to studies in white women. The racial differences with regards to length of gestation in South Asian and Black women that Balchin et al (2007) highlight must also be considered with regards to a definition of prolonged pregnancy to improve perinatal outcome in these groups.

Definition

The definition of a prolonged pregnancy commonly cited by many authors (Balchin et al 2007, de Miranda et al 2006, Laursen et al 2004) is that taken from WHO (1977) as a pregnancy equal to or more than 42 completed weeks (294 days from the first day of the last menstrual period, LMP). This has become the standard definition of prolonged pregnancy and recognized internationally (Hovi et al 2006, Koklanaris & Tropper 2006, Mogren et al 1999). However, the RCOG in their guideline on induction of labour use a definition of 'those pregnancies continuing past 287 days (41 weeks) from the first day of the last menstrual period' (RCOG 2001, p 15).

The expected date of delivery (EDD) is calculated on the basis of Naegele's rule, the assumption being that the cycle is 28 days and that ovulation occurs on the 14th day (see Ch. 17). It is clear however, that making this assessment based on the LMP is to consider women as a homogenous group with regards to their menstrual cycle. Balchin et al (2007) suggest that defining a pregnancy as prolonged on the basis of the LMP is an 'epidemiological concept' and highlights the racial variations with shorter gestational age in South Asian and Black women. This concept is supported by Laursen et al (2004) who put forward the notion of prolonged pregnancy as 'a normal variation of human gestation'. Only a small proportion of prolonged pregnancies result in babies that are postmature as described above (Hovi et al 2006). We live in a multicultural society and given the perceived risks of prolonged pregnancy, this would appear to highlight the need for further studies in different racial groups to determine a more accurate definition in such groups of women. Accurately defining prolonged pregnancy is important if the woman is to be advised appropriately regarding the possible risks, the options for the birth and to avoid unnecessary intervention in an otherwise 'low risk' pregnancy.

Incidence

The frequency or incidence of prolonged pregnancy is quoted as anything from 5–10% (Briscoe et al 2005, Cardozo et al 1986, Hannah et al 1992, Hovi et al 2006). In 2004–2005 the incidence in England is given as 4% (DH 2006). Based on a definition of 42 weeks, a true incidence of prolonged pregnancy is difficult to assess because in many cases women are induced before reaching that time for specific complications in the pregnancy, for maternal request or because the pregnancy has gone beyond the EDD. Cardozo et al (1986) suggest there might be three sub-groups related to a prolonged pregnancy, which include those where the dates are incorrect, those with a normal prolonged gestation where physiological maturity is achieved after 42 weeks and those with correct dates, are functionally mature but who do not go into labour at term. A number of authors support the use of an early ultrasound scan to date the pregnancy more accurately particularly if there is any uncertainty with LMP in order to reduce the number of pregnancies categorized as prolonged (Balchin 2007, Briscoe et al 2005, Hovi et al 2006,

NICE 2008a). When an early ultrasound scan is used the incidence is reduced from 10% to 3% (Hovi et al 2006).

Associated risks and implication for mother, fetus and baby

The risks with any perceived complication of pregnancy need to be viewed from the perspectives of the mother, the fetus and the neonate with regards to morbidity and mortality. The associated risks for the mother are associated with a large for gestational age or macrosomic infant such as shoulder dystocia, genital tract trauma, postpartum haemorrhage and operative birth. The macrosomic infant is at risk of bony injury, soft tissue trauma, hypoxia, and cerebral haemorrhage. However, in prolonged pregnancy, risk of neonatal morbidity and mortality are more commonly associated with the opposite in terms of growth, i.e. the small for gestational age baby suffering hypoxia, asphyxia, meconium aspiration and stillbirth.

The risks outlined for the fetus and neonate appears to be linked to a reduced liquor volume (oligohydramnios). A number of authors suggest placental insufficiency or placental dysfunction as a contributory factor to fetal problems based on the notion that if the pregnancy is prolonged the placenta is ageing and thus the pregnancy has outgrown placental function (Dasari et al 2007, Hovi et al 2006). Fox (1997) argues that the changes in the placenta over the course of pregnancy are part of a process of maturation and an increase in functional efficiency as opposed to a process of ageing and decrease in functional efficiency. Given that few post-term babies exhibit signs of postmaturity possible changes in placental function might be more appropriately linked to pregnancies where there is evidence of postmaturity in the neonate rather than in prolonged pregnancies *per se* (Koklanaris & Tropper 2006).

In prolonged pregnancy, much of the discussion on the associated risks is focused on fetal and neonatal well-being and the need to reduce perinatal mortality and morbidity with appropriate management. The possible risk to mother, fetus and neonate associated with induction of labour for prolonged pregnancy, particularly where the cervix is unfavourable must also be considered in an otherwise uncomplicated pregnancy.

Predisposing factors

Factors that might predispose a woman to a prolonged pregnancy include nulliparity, previous prolonged pregnancy, male fetus, pre-pregnancy BMI of 25 kg/m^2 or more, anencephaly (Koklanaris & Tropper 2006, Laursen et al 2004, Mogren et al 1999, Neff 2004, Olesen et al 2006). Laursen et al (2004) demonstrate a lower perinatal mortality rate in prolonged pregnancies where the mother has had a previous prolonged pregnancy suggesting a possible genetic influence with a prolonged gestation as a normal variation on human gestation.

Management of prolonged pregnancy

The purpose in determining the most appropriate management is to ensure the optimum outcome for mother and baby. In a prolonged pregnancy where there are any obstetric or medical complications the priority in management should follow the practice for the specific complication. All things being equal the management can follow an active or expectant approach and the decision on which approach to take should be based on the woman and partner receiving the information on the possible benefits and risks of each so that an informed choice can be made. Any management must include an accurate dating of the pregnancy to determine the pregnancy is prolonged for that individual.

The expectant approach involves increased antenatal surveillance including a non-stress test (NST) and ultrasound estimation of amniotic fluid volume (AFV) using either amniotic fluid index (AFI) or maximum vertical pocket (MVP) as the criteria to assess fetal wellbeing (Dasari et al 2007, NICE 2008a). The NST involves a cardiotocograph (CTG) to monitor the fetal heart rate with the expectation of two accelerations of ≥ 15 beats for ≥ 15s above the baseline in a 20-min period. Fetal movements may also be noted on the CTG. Because of difference in the fetal sleep–wake cycle if there are no accelerations seen in that time the CTG is continued for a further 20 min. If no accelerations are seen in the 40-min period (non-reactive trace), or if there are any other irregularities in the CTG the management is reviewed. Measurement of AFV is undertaken to identify cases where there is oligohydramnios because of the association between a reduced liquor volume, intrapartum fetal heart rate decelerations and meconium stained liquor. Other options for monitoring fetal well-being antenatally include a biophysical profile (AFV, fetal breathing movements, fetal movements, fetal tone and NST), contraction stress testing and Doppler velocimetry. There is little or no evidence to support the efficacy of this type of surveillance over those mentioned previously. The suggested frequency of antenatal surveillance is two to three times a week (Hannah et al 1992, Neff 2004, RCOG 2001).

The use of a membrane sweep at 41 weeks' gestation has been seen to significantly increase the spontaneous onset of labour before 42 weeks (de Miranda et al 2006). The purpose of membrane sweeping is to attempt to initiate the onset of labour physiologically, thus avoiding induction for prolonged pregnancy using prostaglandin, ARM and oxytocin. Sweeping of the membranes is designed to separate the membranes from their cervical attachment by introducing the examining fingers into the cervical os and passing them circumferentially around the cervix. The process of detaching the membranes from the decidua results in the release of local prostaglandin that may contribute to the initiation of the onset of labour in some individuals. Massage of the cervix can be used when the cervical os remains closed and this process may also cause release of local prostaglandin. If after an appropriate time labour has not started spontaneously, the process can be repeated. The practice of sweeping the membranes is not associated with any increase in maternal or neonatal infection (NICE 2008a), or pre-labour rupture of membranes (Boulvain et al 2005, Wong et al 2002), although women report more vaginal blood loss and painful contractions in the 24 hrs period following the procedure.

The active approach involves induction of labour (IOL) at 41 or 42 completed weeks (Briscoe et al 2005, Koklanaris & Tropper 2006, Neff 2004, NICE 2008b, RCOG 2001). The RCOG recommend IOL to women with uncomplicated pregnancies beyond 41 weeks, stating that where routine induction is undertaken after 41 weeks, there is evidence of a reduction in perinatal mortality. Heimstad et al (2007) compared IOL at 41 weeks' gestation with expectant management and found no difference between the two groups with regard to neonatal morbidity or mode of birth. Alexander et al (2000) suggest that intervention at 41 weeks' gestation cannot be justified based on a lack of proven benefit and an increased likelihood of intrapartum complications and Menticoglou and Hall (2002) argue that 'ritual induction' at 41 weeks is based on flawed evidence and interferes with a 'normal physiologic situation'.

The midwife's role

The mechanisms leading to the onset of labour remain largely unknown and the possibility of a prolonged pregnancy being a variation on human gestation within normal parameters should be considered. The debate on the management of prolonged pregnancy centres on the disparate evidence with regards to fetal risk and neonatal outcome in terms of perinatal mortality and morbidity and the management is designed to reduce these risks. The potential risks to the mother of a prolonged pregnancy, often relate to complications that arise where the baby is macrosomic. However, the interventions necessary when labour is induced also pose a potential risk to mother, fetus and neonate. The woman and her partner should be fully informed of the risks and benefits of any management to enable her to make an informed choice. While the obstetrician will take the lead in such cases the midwife has a role in facilitating the woman's right to autonomy by ensuring she fully understands the options available to her and in appropriate cases acting as the woman's advocate. See Box 30.1 for a summary of the key points relating to prolonged pregnancy.

Induction of labour

The induction of labour (IOL) rate in the National Health Service (NHS) in England is 20% and this rate has been slowly rising since 1993 (DH 2006) making it an intervention that has become common practice in maternity units within the NHS.

IOL is an intervention to initiate the process of labour by artificial means and is the term used when initiating this process in pregnancies from 24 weeks'

Box 30.1 Key points about prolonged pregnancy

- Accurate EDD determined by LMP and early ultrasound reduces the incidence of pregnancies diagnosed as prolonged
- The length of gestation in some racial groups must also be considered with regard to a definition of prolonged pregnancy in these groups of women to improve perinatal outcomes
- A membrane sweep can be offered from 41 weeks as a means to initiate the onset of spontaneous labour
- Where there is any complication in a pregnancy approaching or beyond term the priority in management should follow the practice for the specific complication
- Where the choice is for expectant management women must be informed that any deviations highlighted in antenatal surveillance will necessitate a review of the management.

Box 30.2 Indications for induction of labour

Maternal

- Prolonged pregnancy: defined as one that exceeds 42 completed weeks or 294 days
- Hypertension, including pre-eclampsia: the decision to induce labour and expedite delivery is influenced by the severity of the woman's symptoms
- Diabetes: the type and severity of diabetes influence the decision to induce. In women with pre-existing diabetes, the risk of perinatal mortality is significantly increased over the national population and the risk of stillbirth has been shown to be five times greater than the general population (RCOG 2001). The risk of fetal macrosomia is increased where diabetic control is poor. IOL is offered prior to 40 weeks' gestation
- Pre-labour rupture of membranes: the longer the interval between membrane rupture and birth of the baby increases the risk of infection to mother and fetus. For the majority of women, spontaneous labour will commence within 24hrs of rupture of membranes but women should be offered the choice of immediate IOL or expectant management (NICE 2008b)
- Maternal request: this may be for psychological or social reasons. Many women who exceed the expected date of delivery ask for labour to be induced and for some women there are compelling reasons for requesting IOL when there is no clinical indication. In such cases it is important the woman is quite clear about the implications of such a decision.

Fetal

- Intrauterine growth restriction: the decision to induce is made when it is felt the fetus will be compromised further if the pregnancy is allowed to continue. The decision to intervene in such cases where the gestation is <34 weeks must be weighed against the very real risk of mortality and significant morbidity in these infants (Thornton et al 2004)
- Macrosomia: to reduce risks associated with possible shoulder dystocia
- Fetal death
- Fetal anomaly not compatible with life.

gestation, which is the legal definition of fetal viability in the UK (RCOG 2001). Where labour is being induced, a full assessment must be made to ensure that any intervention planned will confer more benefit than risk for the mother and her baby. The decision to induce labour should only be made when it is clear that a vaginal birth is the most appropriate mode of delivery in this pregnancy, for that particular woman and her baby (NICE 2008b, RCOG 2001).

Indication for induction of labour

Induction of labour is considered when the maternal or fetal condition suggests that a better outcome will be achieved by intervening in the pregnancy than by allowing it to continue. This most commonly applies to cases where there are deviations from the normal physiological processes of childbirth as a result of maternal problems for example hypertension or diabetes, or fetal problems such as fetal growth restriction or macrosomia. A list of some of the indications for IOL can be seen in Box 30.2. The mother may also request to have labour induced for social reasons (NICE 2008b, RCOG 2001). However, the grounds on which the decision is made to induce labour must be sound enough to support the outcome whatever that outcome might be. There is no guarantee an IOL will result in a vaginal birth.

The list in Box 30.2 is not considered to be definitive or conclusive and there may be other indications where IOL is recommended.

The contraindications for IOL are situations that would preclude a vaginal birth in the best interests of the mother and/or baby (Chamberlain & Zander 1999), such as:

- placenta praevia
- transverse lie or compound presentation
- HIV-positive women not taking highly active antiretroviral therapy (HAART) (RCOG 2004)
- active genital herpes
- cord presentation or cord prolapse
- known cephalopelvic disproportion
- severe acute fetal compromise.

Methods of induction

During pregnancy the cervix must remain strong and unyielding to the pressure of the gravid uterus to retain the fetus until it has reached maturity. For an induction to be successful, the cervix needs to have undergone the changes that will ensure the uterine contractions are effective in the progressive dilatation and effacement of the cervix, descent of the presenting part and the birth of the baby.

The cervix is said to be ripe when it has undergone the changes described in Chs 14 and 25. Assessing the ripeness of the cervix is by means of a scoring system devised by Bishop in 1964 (Bishop's score) that examines four features of the cervix and the relationship of the presenting part to the ischial spines. Each of these five elements is scored between 0 and 3 on vaginal examination (VE). A score of 8 or more equates to a ripe cervix and one that is favourable for the purpose of IOL in that it is more compliant offering less resistance as the contraction and retraction of the myometrium forces the presenting part down. The scoring system has been modified and it is this version that is used in contemporary obstetric practice (Table 30.1). A VE to assess the cervix and the likelihood of successful induction in this way is by nature a subjective examination and as such there

Table 30.1 Modified Bishop's pre-induction pelvic scoring system

Inducibility features	0	1	2	3
Dilatation of cervix (cm)	<1	1–2	2–4	>4
Consistency of cervix	Firm	Firm	Med	Soft
Cervical canal length (cm)	>4	2–4	1–2	<1
Position of cervix	Post	Mid	Ant	–
Station of presenting part (cm above or below ischial spine)	−3	−2	−1,0	+1, +2

will be inter-observer variations. Elghorori et al (2006) undertook a prospective study to compare subjective and objective assessment of the cervix before IOL and found a transvaginal ultrasound assessment of cervical length was superior to the Bishop's score in predicting the success of IOL. Future research in this area of practice will be interesting to follow particularly with regard to preference and acceptability from the woman's perspective.

Prior to any method used to induce labour, it is extremely important for the midwife to carry out an abdominal examination confirming the lie, presentation, descent of presenting part and fetal well-being. All findings are clearly recorded in the woman's maternity records and if there is any doubt or concern in the findings the process should be stopped and the doctor informed (NMC 2004).

Membrane sweep

A membrane sweep after 40 weeks carried out by a doctor or midwife experienced in the practice has been found to reduce the need for further methods to induce labour (Boulvain et al 2005, Chamberlain & Zander 1999). Wong et al (2002) found that while the procedure was safe in that it did not lead to pre-labour rupture of membranes, bleeding or maternal or neonatal infection it did cause significant discomfort and in their study was not found to reduce the need for IOL. NICE (2008b) recommend sweeping of the membranes prior to formal induction procedures at 40+ weeks' gestation or earlier where there are pregnancy complications, if the woman's clinical condition allows for this. However, a review by Boulvain et al (2005) suggests the possible benefits in terms of a reduction in more formal induction methods needs to be weighed against the discomfort of the VE and other adverse effects of bleeding and irregular contractions not leading to labour.

Prostaglandin E2 (PGE$_2$) (Dinoprostone)

Prostaglandins are naturally occurring female hormones present in tissues throughout the body. Prostaglandin E$_2$ and F$_2$ are known to be produced by tissues of the cervix, uterus, decidua and the fetal membranes and to act locally on these structures. Dinoprostone is the active ingredient in Prostin E$_2$ vaginal tablets, gel, and pessaries (BNF 2007). It replicates prostaglandin E$_2$ produced by the uterus in early labour to ripen the cervix and is seen as a more natural method than the use of oxytocin. Prostin E$_2$ placed in the posterior fornix of the vagina (Fig. 30.1) is absorbed by the epithelium of the vagina and cervix leading to relaxation and dilatation of the muscle of the cervix and subsequent contraction of uterine muscle. The use of Prostin prior to the use of oxytocin potentiates the effects of the oxytocic agent (Chamberlain & Zander 1999).

There are a number of preparations of PGE$_2$, which have been found to be clinically equivalent. In a

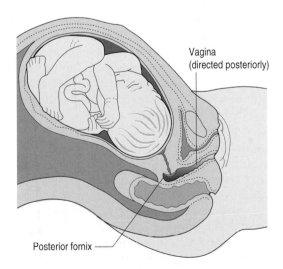

Figure 30.1 Insertion of prostaglandins. The posterior fornix of the vagina is used to insert prostaglandins for ripening or induction of labour. The key point is that when undertaking a vaginal examination to assess the cervix midwives should follow the direction of the vagina which will be directed posteriorly if the woman is semi-recumbent. The uterus is anteverted and anteflexed, creating the posterior fornix. The cervix may appear 'difficult to reach' particularly when unfavourable.

small study by Tomlinson et al (2001) the women receiving the slow release pessary gave a higher satisfaction score with regards to their perception of labour. The slow release preparation would appear to confer more benefit from the woman's perspective with regard to fewer VEs. The cost of PGE$_2$ preparations may vary over time and NICE (2008b) expect cost to be taken into consideration when prescribing a gel, tablet or pessary. It must be remembered that these PGE$_2$ preparations are not bioequivalent.

Following insertion of PGE$_2$, the woman is advised to lie down for 30 min. The fetal heart rate and uterine activity are continuously monitored by CTG to determine fetal well-being. If the trace is found to be reassuring the CTG can be discontinued and intermittent monitoring used. If there are no risk factors such as maternal hypertension, previous caesarean section, fetal growth restriction, etc. the initial process can take place on the antenatal ward with facilities for continuous electronic fetal monitoring (NICE 2008b, RCOG 2001) and appropriate staffing levels. Prior to the administration of the Prostin the midwife should confirm with the midwife in charge of the labour suite that a bed is available in the event there is a need to transfer the woman as a matter of urgency. For the safety of the woman and her baby any decision to proceed with IOL must take cognizance of the current situation on the labour suite because the woman's response to insertion of PGE$_2$ cannot be predicted. If there are any maternal or fetal risk factors in the pregnancy the IOL must take place on the labour suite (NICE 2008b, RCOG 2001).

Where the membranes are intact or ruptured, the recommended initial dose for all women whether it is a first or subsequent pregnancy is PGE$_2$ 3 mg tablet. If the woman has not gone into labour, a further assessment is carried out 6 hrs later and if the cervix remains unfavourable, a further 3 mg tablet is inserted into the posterior fornix the maximum recommended dose of a PGE$_2$ tablet being 6 mg (RCOG 2001). If PGE$_2$ gel is being used, the dosage will depend on parity and Bishop's score. The gel can be given as 1 or 2 mg and the maximum recommended dosage is 4 mg. A review by Kelly et al (2003) suggests that the 'low doses were as effective as higher doses'. However, Selo-Ojeme et al (2007) found that despite having an induction of labour protocol that was said to be in accordance with NICE guidelines a high percentage of units do not comply with these recommendations and exceed the maximum doses particularly when using PGE_2 tablets as opposed to PGE_2 gel. The advice from NICE in cases where the maximum dose has been given but amniotomy is still not possible is for the clinician to use their professional judgement with regard to administering further doses. It is not clear what the legal implications would be if there were complications and the manufacturer's recommendations had been exceeded (Selo-Ojeme et al 2007). There should be a break of no less than 6 hrs from the last PGE_2 to commencement of an oxytocin infusion. Side effects of Prostin include nausea, vomiting and diarrhoea (BNF 2007).

PGE1 (misoprostol) can be given by the oral, sublingual, or vaginal route for IOL but it is not licensed for this purpose in the UK. It is thought the sublingual route might replicate the vaginal route with regards to bioavailability because it avoids first pass effect that occurs when the drug is taken orally. The dosage of tablets currently available is 200 μg and for use in IOL a much smaller dose would need to be available (Shetty et al 2003, Shetty et al 2002). Misoprostol is thought to be more effective and less expensive than PGE_2 and oxytocin for the induction of labour but there are still questions about safety issues with regard to uterine hyperstimulation. More work needs to be done to study the efficacy of these alternative routes.

Risk associated with use of PGE_2

The use of PGE_2 can be unpredictable and may lead to hypertonic uterus, placental abruption, fetal hypoxia, pulmonary or amniotic fluid embolism (Kramer et al 2006). While uterine rupture is rare, occurring between 0.3% and 7% of labours there continues to be debate on the use of prostaglandins in women with a caesarean section scar and the possible effect of the prostaglandin on the fibrous tissue of the scar (Vause et al 1999).

Artificial rupture of membranes

ARM or amniotomy, can be used in an attempt to induce labour if the cervix is favourable and the presenting part is fixed in the pelvis particularly where the woman does not want to use drugs such as PGE_2 or oxytocin. Prior to the procedure an abdominal examination is carried out and if the findings are

satisfactory a VE is done to assess the cervix, confirm the presentation and station and to exclude possible cord presentation or vasa praevia. If these findings are satisfactory, the bag of membranes lying in front of the presenting part (forewaters) is ruptured with the use of an amniohook or similar device to release the amniotic fluid. The fluid is assessed for colour and volume and the midwife or doctor may be able to distinguish other features on the presenting part to identify the position of the fetus. After the procedure, the woman is made comfortable, the fetal heart is auscultated and all findings are recorded in the maternity notes. The longer the interval between ARM and birth increases the risk of the woman developing chorioamnionitis as a result of an ascending infection from the genital tract leading to an increased risk of perinatal mortality (Blackburn 2007). For this reason, if a decision has been made to induce labour for perceived risks it is common practice to start an oxytocin infusion within a few hours if labour has not been established following the ARM. In their review of two trials, Bricker and Luckas (2000) found insufficient evidence on the effects of amniotomy alone for the IOL.

Changes to ripen the cervix are thought to be in response to PGE_2 produced by the amnion and cervix. In pregnancy, the chorion provides a barrier to the amnion and fetus from the vagina and cervix. Prostaglandin dehydrogenase (PGDH) is an enzyme produced by the chorion that breaks down PGE_2. As a result of the actions of this enzyme the changes in the cervix do not take place and pre-term labour is avoided (Smyth et al 2007). Van Meir et al (1997) found that in labouring women the part of the chorion that was in close contact with the cervical os released less of this enzyme allowing the PGE_2 from the amnion to come into contact with the cervix and facilitate ripening of the cervix. The theory is that if an ARM is performed too early the action of the amniotic prostaglandins on the cervix is lost.

Oxytocin

Oxytocin is synthesized in the hypothalamus and then transported to the posterior pituitary gland from where it is episodically released to act on smooth muscle. The number of oxytocin receptors in the myometrium significantly increases by term increasing uterine oxytocin sensitivity (Blackburn 2007).

Table 30.2 Oxytocin dose regimen

Dose of oxytocin	Intravenous fluid (ml normal saline)	Rate (ml/hr)	Rate of oxytocin (mU/min)
30 IU oxytocin	500	1	1
10 IU oxytocin	500	3	1

In its synthetic form oxytocin (Syntocinon) is a powerful uterotonic agent and when used for induction of labour following ARM should be administered by slow intravenous infusion using an infusion pump or syringe driver with non-return valve (BNF 2007, NICE 2001, RCOG 2001). In order to reduce the risk of clinician error, the RCOG (2001) recommend the use of a standardized dilution of oxytocin in 500 mL of normal saline (Table 30.2). There should be an interval of 6 hrs between administration of prostaglandins and commencement of an oxytocin infusion and if the membranes have not previously ruptured an amniotomy should be performed. The dose of oxytocin is titrated against uterine contractions to achieve three to four contractions every 10 min lasting 40 s or more using the lowest possible dose. The contraction rate each 10 min should not exceed this number.

When using an oxytocin infusion, the fetal heart and uterine activity should be monitored using continuous electronic monitoring to ensure the fetus does not become compromised by the induced uterine contractions. The intended outcome is to achieve three to four contractions every 10 min but there is a risk of hyperstimulation and hypertonic uterus leading to fetal compromise. In this event, the infusion should be decreased or discontinued and medical aid summoned. The midwife should also palpate the uterine contractions for their frequency, strength, and duration as well as using electronic monitoring.

Risks associated with use of intravenous oxytocin include:

- uterine hyperstimulation or hypertonus
- fetal hypoxia and asphyxia
- uterine rupture
- fluid retention as a result of the antidiuretic effect of oxytocin
- postpartum haemorrhage
- amniotic fluid embolism (AFE).

The midwife's role when caring for the mother where labour is being induced

The midwife's responsibilities to the mother include care during the antenatal and intrapartum period. Where a decision has been made to induce labour, it is important the midwife ensures the woman and her partner have been fully informed and understand the process and how it might be undertaken. There are a number of ways that labour can be induced and the method will depend on the individual circumstances of each woman. All information should be given in an objective manner to ensure the woman and her partner understand the reason for the induction, any possible consequences or risks of having/not having the procedure as well as any alternatives to the procedure (RCOG 2004). It is important for the woman and her partner to understand that IOL may be delayed if the labour suite is busy, that it might take some time for contractions to be initiated and the possibility that the induction process could be unsuccessful. Time should be allowed for discussion with the midwife or obstetrician and it must be remembered that consent to a treatment can be withdrawn at any time and this decision by the woman should be respected (Dimond 2006). The midwife or doctor should record any discussion that takes place and requests made in the maternity notes.

During the induction process all maternal and fetal observations will be recorded in the maternity notes. Until labour is established and the partogram is commenced, the observation will be recorded in the antenatal section of the notes. Because the layout is not as comprehensive and logical as the partogram it is important the midwife is clear and methodical in her documentation at this time. The frequency and type of monitoring of the mother and fetus will depend on the reason for and method of induction. The midwife is advised to follow the local protocol regarding IOL in each case. It is important when monitoring the well-being of the mother and fetus during the induction process that the midwife understands the possible risks associated with each method of induction so that she can make the necessary observations to recognize any deviations from normal, take whatever action is most appropriate and call medical aid.

Initiation of labour during the induction may be a protracted process and in such cases, the woman may have time to adjust to the changes in her body and be better able to cope with contractions. However, the sudden onset of strong painful contractions occurring every 3–4 min can be quite overwhelming and result in an early request for pain relief. Continuity of care by one midwife in labour is important in developing a rapport with the woman and her partner and in being able to make an assessment of her progress based on physical observations of abdominal examination and VE as well as less tangible observations of body language and behaviour. In this way, a midwife may be better able to advise a woman of her progress to help her in her decision on the type of pain relief. The suggested frequency of VEs will depend on the local policy but it must be remembered that valid consent must be obtained before all such procedures. When a woman is experiencing painful contractions in labour the information about any examinations or procedures that the midwife or doctor may wish to perform should be given between contractions (RCOG 2001).

Alternative approaches to initiating labour

For some women avoidance of any surgical or pharmacological intervention in an otherwise low-risk pregnancy is extremely important and they might seek advice from the midwife on this matter. Alternative approaches include the ingestion of castor oil, nipple stimulation, sexual intercourse, acupuncture and the use of homeopathic methods. The midwife must ensure that any advice given on alternative therapies is in line with the sphere of practice (NMC 2004). In their review, Kelly et al (2001) found there was insufficient research to demonstrate the efficacy of castor oil on cervical ripening or inducing labour.

Stimulation of the breast or more specifically the nipple appears to cause the release of endogenous oxytocin, the effect being to initiate a uterine response. In a review by Kavanagh et al (2005) stimulation of the breast either by massage or nipple stimulation 'appears beneficial in relation to the number of women not in labour after 72 hrs, and reduced postpartum haemorrhage rates'. It appears to be less effective where the cervix is not ripe. Further studies are needed before it can be considered for use in high-risk groups.

Suggesting sexual intercourse as a method of initiating labour to women at or beyond term with uncomplicated pregnancies is based on a number of factors that it is thought might contribute to the induction process; the prostaglandin content in semen, the physical stimulation of the lower segment of the uterus by the act of intercourse, stimulation of the breast during the process of love-making and the release of endogenous oxytocin during maternal orgasm. In the review by Kavanagh et al (2001), the efficacy of sexual intercourse as a method to initiate labour could not be supported.

The review by Smith & Crowther (2004) looking at acupuncture for the induction of labour stated the need for well-designed trials on the subject, but on current evidence the use of acupuncture in the induction of labour had not been fully evaluated for safety and effectiveness. Harper et al (2006) acknowledge the need to conduct further studies in this area.

Caulophyllum is a homeopathic therapy commonly used to initiate labour, however in a review of trials by Smith (2003) there was not enough evidence to recommend homoeopathy as a method of induction.

Failure to progress and prolonged labour

Labour encompasses effective uterine contractions and cervical changes leading to progressive effacement and dilatation of the cervix, rotation of the fetus and descent of the presenting part, the birth of the baby and expulsion of the placenta and membranes and the control of bleeding. For many, this process starts spontaneously and continues that way without the need to intervene. For some however, either in the early or late stages of labour the process slows down and there is 'failure to progress' based on the rate of cervical dilatation/hour or the labour is 'prolonged' when it exceeds the number of hours considered to be normal for a nulliparous or multiparous woman. Dystocia is the term used for a difficult or slow labour and thus includes both failure to progress and prolonged labour (Albers 2001). When dystocia occurs the obstetrician needs to make a decision as to how the situation is best managed from this point onwards with appropriate consideration of all the facts in the context of the individual. Interventions to correct this problem included ARM or oxytocin or a combination of both. The means to augment labour in this way has become common practice in UK with as many as 50% of nulliparae receiving an oxytocin infusion in labour (Hayman 2004). If these means fail an instrumental or operative delivery may be the only course of action depending on the stage of labour reached. The caesarean section rate in England is currently 23% and over half of these are emergencies (DH 2006). Many of these will be for failure to progress or prolonged labour.

The greatest anxiety with prolonged labour is the risk of obstructed labour and uterine rupture and the subsequent maternal and fetal morbidity and mortality associated with that scenario. Other problems when labour is slow to progress or prolonged is the risk of infection with prolonged rupture of membranes, or postpartum haemorrhage as a result of an atonic uterus. It must also be remembered the interventions used to correct a dystocia such as amniotomy, oxytocin infusion, and instrumental or operative delivery are not risk free and therefore any decision to intervene must take account of the full clinical picture. Prolonged labour is not easily defined primarily because there is no consensus as to what constitutes a normal time limit for labour either in the latent or active part of the first stage or the passive or active part of the second stage. The WHO (1994) defines prolonged labour as one that exceeds 18 hrs in primiparous women.

Delay in the latent phase of labour

In the first stage of labour, the latent phase is the period when structural changes occur in the cervix and it becomes softer and shorter (from 3 cm to <0 .5 cm), its position is more central in relation to the presenting part and it dilates to 3 cm (Hayman

2004). The time for this to take place is given as 8–10 hrs based on the original work of Friedman in 1956 (cited El-Hamamy & Arulkumaran 2005, Hayman 2004, Neilson et al 2003,). If progress in this phase of labour is considered to be slow, the emphasis is on conservative management rather than intervention (Hayman 2004). During this time, the woman needs support and encouragement from those caring for her. The contractions may be painful but the perceived result of such painful contractions may be disappointing when hearing the cervix is 3 cm dilated after several hours. Also during this time, making sure there is adequate food and fluid intake not only helps to maintain energy levels but can also bring a sense of normality and comfort. It is important for the woman to rest at this time and not to feel that if she tries to sleep, the contractions will cease. Advice on how to relieve pain might include simple back massage, changes of position, a warm bath or some simple analgesia. Intervention such as an ARM at this stage can interfere with the action of amniotic prostaglandin on the cervix and be counterproductive (Smyth et al 2007).

Delay in the active phase of labour and the use of the partogram

The active phase is the period of time when the cervix dilates from 3 cm to 10 cm with rotation and descent of the presenting part. This part is possibly the most contentious because the expectation is that progress once labour is diagnosed is a cervical dilatation of 1 cm/hr. Albers (2001) suggests a limit of 0.3–0.5 cm/hr might be a more appropriate reflection of the progress of normal labour. The current NICE guideline on intrapartum care (2007) appears to support both perspectives, defining delay in the first stage as progress of <2 cm in 4 hrs in both nulliparous and parous women or slowing in progress in parous women. However, when delay is suspected, the advice is to undertake a VE 2 hrs later at which point progress is defined as more that 1 cm/hr. While the guideline suggests one must also consider descent and rotation of the presenting part, changes in contractions, etc. the emphasis nonetheless seems to remain with the rate of cervical dilatation per hour.

The partogram is a graphical representation of dilatation of the cervix against time with an alert line based on cervical dilatation of 1 cm/hr between 3 cm and 10 cm. When labour is confirmed, the cervical dilatation is plotted on this line. An action line parallel to the alert line is placed 2 or 4 hrs to the right to highlight slow progress and indicate the timing of intervention for failure to progress or prolonged labour. The time frame for the action line varies from unit to unit. The WHO recommends the use of a 4 hrs action line (Lavender et al 2006) and this is supported by NICE (2007). Intervention rates will clearly vary depending on where the action line is placed and these must be considered in the context of improvement to maternal or neonatal outcome. The partogram also provides information on other factors that are critical in making an appropriate assessment where progress is deemed to be deviating from the normal range. These include findings at VE with regard to the presentation, position and station enabling the assessor to determine if there is rotation and descent of the presenting part, and the degree of caput or moulding. Information is also provided from abdominal palpation in terms of the presenting part and fifths palpable to see how this correlates with the VE and the frequency, strength and length of contractions. While such information is helpful it is also very subjective. Continuity of carer over time should reduce the likelihood of inter-observer variations.

The influence of the three 'Ps' (passages, passenger, powers)

Dystocia can be as a result of ineffective uterine contractions, malposition of the fetus leading to a relative or absolute cephalopelvic disproportion (CPD), malpresentation, or any combination of these. These may result in poor progress during the active phase or a cessation of cervical dilatation following a period of normal dilatation (Hayman 2004). An understanding of the role played by the three 'Ps' will help in determining why there is a delay in progress in first or second stage of labour and what action might be taken.

In the developed world, the majority of women have grown up well nourished, fit and healthy and the passages the fetus must negotiate are unlikely to be seriously flawed, excluding possible trauma to the pelvis. However the impact of a full rectum, full bladder and fibroids cannot be ignored in

causing a delay in the progress of labour. A malpresentation, such as shoulder, brow or face (mentoposterior), is one of the causes of poor progress or prolonged labour and this may occur as a result of a problem with the passage (see Ch. 31).

When the fetus is adopting an attitude where the head is deflexed or slightly extended and the occiput is posterior, the presenting diameters are larger and there will be a degree of asynclitism. This inevitably slows progress but does not necessarily mean progress is abnormal. This might be considered a relative cephalopelvic disproportion (CPD) because with effective uterine contractions the fetus might adopt a more flexed attitude; the fetal head is designed to mould and change the dimensions of the presenting part. On some occasions more time is needed to do this safely. Where there is an occipitoposterior position and epidural analgesia, Ferguson's reflex is not effective which results in slowing the progress of labour down at this time. In some cases the head is just (normally) large and any decision to intervene at this point with oxytocin may increase strength and frequency of uterine contractions in such a way as to unduly force this process with inevitable fetal heart rate changes prompting further intervention. El Halta (1998) suggests that rupturing the membranes when the fetus is an occipitoposterior position may result in a sudden descent of the fetal skull resulting in a deep transverse arrest whereby the occipitofrontal diameter (11.5 cm) is caught on the bispinous diameter of the outlet (10–11 cm).

Although the uterus has prepared itself for the metabolic activity of labour, as labour continues the smooth muscle uses up its metabolic reserves and becomes tired. While some ketosis is considered normal in labour, there remains a need for additional supplies of energy if the uterus is to continue contracting effectively. Any change to the strength, length or frequency of contractions will affect progress and is indicative of inefficient uterine action.

When there are concerns about progress in labour, the midwife will inform the obstetrician so that an appropriate assessment can be made to identify the cause and decide on the best course of management. It is important that the woman and her partner are closely involved in any discussions at this time to enable informed consent to be given for any procedures to augment the labour such as artificial rupture of the membranes or an oxytocin infusion if the membranes are ruptured. When a decision has to be made on the next step in managing dystocia it is important that repeat examinations are done by the same person. A full assessment should take place to ensure the decision to augment labour is based on sound and accurate clinical findings.

The midwife's role in caring for a woman in prolonged labour

A prolonged labour leads to increased levels of stress, anxiety and fatigue and increases the risk of infection, postpartum haemorrhage and emergency caesarean section (Svärdby et al 2006). Managing labour should start with appropriate antenatal education. Advice on suitable food and drink to eat in the early stages of labour to maintain energy levels, positions and activities to encourage a forward rotation where there is an occipitoposterior position are just some of the ways that might help to assist the woman in the normal progress of labour.

When the woman and her partner come into hospital, one-to-one care helps to create a sense of trust between the woman, the partner and the midwife but also allows for more accurate assessment over time by the midwife to enable her to suggest non-interventionist ways in which progress can be maintained if appropriate. An upright position might help to facilitate more effective contractions or an alternative position might help to improve pelvic diameters when the position of the baby is posterior. At this stage, it is also important to maintain hydration, to encourage voiding and to suggest non-pharmacological ways to relieve pain. Facilitating her autonomy by keeping the woman and her partner informed of her progress and the choices she has is important in helping her to feel in control and to reduce her anxiety. Raised adrenalin levels as a result of fear, anxiety or pain can impact negatively on uterine activity and slow progress in labour.

Accurate observations in labour are critical in assessing progress. Edmunds (1998, p 13) talks of the importance of the midwife preparing for, expecting and facilitating a normal birth 'while discreetly providing for any contingency necessitating intercession'. Recognition and detection of abnormal progress in labour with appropriate clinical response will improve the outcome of labour for both mother and baby (Neilson et al 2003). An abdominal examination can provide vital information about the labour with regard to the lie, presentation, position and descent of presenting part as well as the length, strength and frequency of contractions whereby any change in the pattern of the contractions can be picked up. When comparing these findings with those from VE a more comprehensive picture of the progress of labour is achieved. On VE the midwife is assessing the presence and degree of moulding of the fetal skull, the presence and position of caput succedaneum in relation to sutures and fontanelles and the dilatation of the cervix noting any thickening and its application to the presenting part. Any changes to the colour of the liquor if the membranes have previously ruptured or to fetal heart rate will give some indication as to how the fetus is coping with the progress of labour.

When the decision to augment labour has been made the woman and her partner will need additional support from the midwife, as the interventions necessary for this process may be very different from the birth they had previously imagined. Psychological as well as physical support is important at this time, as the control of the birth of their baby now appears to be in the hands of a third party and this can lead to very negative feelings of the childbirth experience (Nystedt et al 2005, 2006).

The management of prolonged labour is a collaborative effort involving the woman and her partner, the midwife, obstetrician, and anaesthetist. The normal pattern of observations and care in labour apply and any deviations from normal are reported to the obstetrician. When an ARM has been done to augment labour an appropriate period of grace should be given for effective uterine contractions to resume before commencing an oxytocin infusion. There is no specific regime for the use of oxytocin to augment labour but it is common practice to use that given by the RCOG for the induction of labour (RCOG 2001). The uterus responds with increased sensitivity to the oxytocin infused as the cervix dilates and it may be necessary to reduce the rate as full dilatation is approached to avoid hyperstimulation of the uterus and the concomitant effects on mother and fetus. The timing of how long to continue with augmentation in the first stage of labour will depend on the individual situation and circumstances at that time. An assessment will be made 2–4 hrs after ARM or commencing oxytocin to ascertain the likelihood of a successful vaginal birth. If there is persistent poor progress in the active phase despite optimal contractions of four each 10 min lasting >40 s, and the woman is pain free, well hydrated and with an empty bladder it is unlikely that continuing with an oxytocin infusion will lead to a vaginal birth.

The decision to augment labour in multiparae or in women with prior caesarean section must be made by an experienced obstetrician because of the very real risk of hyperstimulation and uterine rupture. Additional time should be given between ARM and commencing an oxytocin infusion with careful assessment of uterine activity and fetal heart rate. When the obstetrician has excluded absolute CPD a low dose oxytocin infusion may be commenced until optimal contractions are established at which point the infusion may be discontinued (El-Hamamy & Arulkumaran 2005, Hayman 2004).

Delay in the second stage of labour

The second stage of labour can be divided into a passive (pelvic) phase and active (perineal) phase. Delay in this stage of labour may be due to malposition causing failure of the vertex to descend and rotate, ineffective contractions due to a prolonged first stage, large fetus and large vertex, or absence of the desire to push with epidural analgesia. Some of these situations may be rectified with the judicious use of an oxytocin infusion thus avoiding the need for an instrumental or operative delivery.

Time limits in second stage range from 30 min to 2 hrs for multiparae and 1–3 hrs for nulliparae but an understanding of the different phases as the head negotiates the birth canal can avoid the encouragement of premature bearing down efforts, which only serve to tire and demoralize the mother. The variation in time limits takes into consideration the impact of epidural analgesia on the desire to push in the second stage. An imposed time limit is felt by some to be unnecessary if both mother and fetus are doing well (Hayman 2004, Neilson et al 2003).

The active phase when the mother is bearing down is the most critical time. Providing there is obvious progress and mother and fetus are both in good condition intervention may not be necessary. NICE (2007) suggest there is delay if the length of active second stage is 2 hrs in nulliparous women and 1 hr for parous women. When a diagnosis of delay in the second stage has been made the case is referred to the obstetrician for review and assessment. The risk to both mother and fetus if the second stage is allowed to exceed normal time limits must be weighed against the risks of intervening with an instrumental or operative delivery. Where there is any indication that the mother or the fetus is compromised the birth must be expedited as soon as possible.

Obstructed labour

An obstructed labour occurs when despite good uterine contractions there is no advance of the presenting part. Possible causes of obstructed labour include absolute CPD, deep transverse arrest, malpresentation, lower segment fibroids, fetal hydrocephaly and multiple pregnancy with conjoined or locked twins. Because of the high presenting part if the woman goes into labour there may be spontaneous rupture of the membranes and cord prolapse with related risk to the fetus. If the condition is not recognized the mother's uterus will continue to contract to overcome the obstruction. She will become progressively more dehydrated, ketotic, pyrexial, and tachycardic. The fetus will develop a bradycardia because of the relentless contractions. As the uterus continues to contract and retract the upper segment becomes progressively thicker closely enveloping the fetus and the lower segment becomes increasingly thinner. In nulliparous women the contractions may cease for a period before resuming again with increasing strength and frequency with little interval between contractions until the uterus assumes a state of tonic contraction. The difference between upper and lower segment may be seen as a ridge obliquely crossing the abdomen (Bandl's ring). The mother is in severe and unrelenting pain. If VE is possible the presenting part will be high with excessive moulding (Fig. 30.2). The uterus is in

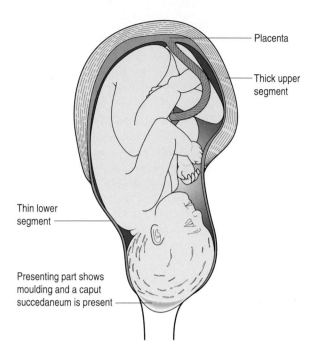

Placenta

Thick upper segment

Thin lower segment

Presenting part shows moulding and a caput succedaneum is present

Figure 30.2 Obstructed labour. The uterus is moulded around the fetus; the thickened upper segment is obvious on abdominal palpation.

imminent danger of rupture and emergency measures must be taken if the situation has been allowed to get this far. Uterine rupture leads to maternal mortality and the tonic contractions and uterine rupture cause hypoxia, asphyxia, and subsequent perinatal mortality (Neilson et al 2003).

If the woman has been discovered in this condition at home, a paramedic ambulance should be called for immediate transfer to hospital. Labour suite should be informed and they in turn will contact the senior obstetrician, anaesthetist, paediatrician, theatre staff, and special care baby unit. While waiting for the ambulance the midwife should cannulate, take blood for urgent cross match, and site an intravenous infusion. The woman's GP can be called if close by to provide additional help and support until the ambulance arrives. Observations of mother and fetus and any actions taken and by whom are recorded in the maternity notes as soon as possible. If the obstruction is discovered in hospital an emergency caesarean section is performed.

Management of obstructed labour is about its prevention in the antenatal and intrapartum period.

The midwife should highlight any predisposing factors antenatally with appropriate referral to the obstetrician so that a decision is made with the woman on the safest mode of birth. During labour skilled abdominal examination will alert the midwife to any malpresentation or failure of the presenting part to advance despite optimal uterine contractions. VE will confirm suspected malpresentation and where the presentation is vertex reveal increasing caput succedaneum or moulding. With a high presenting part in labour cervical dilatation will be extremely slow and there will be little if any application to the presenting part. The obstetrician is informed as soon as possible so that the birth can be expedited. If the labour is becoming obstructed in the first stage an emergency caesarean section will be carried out. If the delay occurs in the second stage as a result of deep transverse arrest the obstetrician may try to deliver the baby vaginally with ventouse but if that fails or is not possible an emergency caesarean is carried out. Despite the very real threat to maternal and perinatal well-being these procedures should only be undertaken with maternal consent.

Precipitate labour

In some women, the uterus is over-efficient and the onset of labour to birth is an hour or less. Much or all of the first stage is not recognized because contractions are not painful and the realization of the birth of the head may be the first indication that labour has actually started.

Such a precipitate birth is not without its problems leading to soft tissue trauma of the maternal genital tract due to sudden stretching and distension as the baby is born. Risks to the baby include: hypoxia as a result of the frequency and strength of the contractions, intracranial haemorrhage from the sudden compression and decompression of the fetal skull as it passes through the birth canal with speed, and possible injury as the head and body deliver rapidly and possibly fall to the floor. The unexpected nature of the event means that the place of birth may be inappropriate and the baby may be further compromised if the importance of maintaining the baby's temperature is not recognized.

The over-efficient uterus may relax after the birth of the baby resulting in retained placenta and/or postpartum haemorrhage. The psychological impact of such a rapid birth must not be underestimated and some women will be in a state of shock after the event.

Precipitate labour will often recur in subsequent pregnancies and the obstetrician may advise induction of labour once term (37 completed weeks) is reached.

The views of midwives and doctors on childbirth are often considered to be diametrically opposite, with midwives looking on childbirth as normal until proved otherwise and obstetricians viewing it as normal retrospectively. El-Hamamy & Arulkumaran (2005) consider every labour a trial of labour. Whatever the perspective taken the primary outcome is the safety of the mother and baby. Childbearing is a time of major life transition and each woman and partner deserve to have a positive birth experience whether labour is spontaneous or induced and the birth is vaginal or by caesarean section. Working together as a team can only help to contribute to that positive birth experience.

REFERENCES

Albers L 2001 Rethinking dystocia: patience please. MIDIRS Midwifery Digest 11(3):351–353

Alexander J M, McIntire D, Leveno K J 2000 Forty weeks and beyond: pregnancy outcomes by week of gestation. Obstetrics and Gynaecology 96(2):291–294

Balchin I, Whittaker C, Patel R et al 2007 Racial variation in the association between gestational age and perinatal mortality: prospective study. British Medical Journal 334:833

Blackburn S 2007 Maternal, fetal, and neonatal physiology: a clinical perspective, 3rd edn. W B Saunders, Philadelphia

BNF 2007 British National Formulary, BNF 53. Online. Available: http://www.bnf.org

Boulvain M, Stan C, Irion O 2005 Membrane sweeping for induction of labour. The Cochrane Database of Systematic Reviews, Issue 1:CD000451

Bricker L, Luckas M 2000 Amniotomy alone for induction of labour. The Cochrane Database of Systematic Reviews, Issue 4:CD002862

Briscoe D, Nguyen H, Mencer M et al 2005 Management of pregnancy beyond 40 weeks' gestation. American Family Physician 71(10):1935–1941

Cardozo L, Fysh J, Pearce J M 1986 Prolonged pregnancy: the management debate. British Medical Journal 293:1059–1063

Chamberlain G, Zander L 1999 ABC of labour care: Induction. British Medical Journal 318(7189):995–998

Dasari P, Niveditta G, Raghavan S 2007 The maximal vertical pocket and amniotic fluid index in predicting fetal distress in prolonged pregnancy. International Journal of Gynaecology and Obstetrics 96(2):89–93

de Miranda E, van der Bom J G, Bonsel G J et al 2006 Membrane sweeping and prevention of post-term pregnancy in low-risk pregnancies: a randomised controlled trial. British Journal of Obstetrics and Gynaecology 113(4A):402–408

DH (Department of Health) 2006 NHS Maternity Statistics, England: 2004–2005 Department of Health, London

Dimond B 2006 Legal aspects of midwifery, 3rd edn. Books for Midwives Press, Hale

Edmunds J 1998 Prolonged labor: past and present. Midwifery Today. Summer:13–14

Elghorori M R M, Hassan I, Dartan W et al 2006 Comparison between subjective and objective assessments of the cervix before induction of labour. Journal of Obstetrics and Gynaecology 26(6):521–526

El Halta V 1998 Preventing prolonged labor. Midwifery Today. Summer:22–27

El-Hamamy E, Arulkumaran S 2005 Poor progress of labour. Current Obstetrics and Gynaecology 15(1):1–8

Fok W Y, Chan L Y, Tsui M H et al 2006 When to induce labour for post-term? A study of induction at 41 weeks versus 42 weeks. European Journal of Obstetrics and Gynaecology and Reproductive Biology 125:206–210

Fox H 1997 Ageing of the placenta. Archives of Diseases in Childhood 77(3):171–175

Gülmezoglu A M, Crowther C A, Middleton P 2006 Induction of labour for improving birth outcomes for women at or beyond term. The Cochrane Database of Systematic Reviews, Issue 4:CD004945

Hannah M E, Hannah W J, Hellman J et al 1992 Induction of labour as compared with serial antenatal monitoring in post-term pregnancy. A randomized controlled trial. The Canadian Multicenter Post-term Pregnancy Trial Group. New England Journal of Medicine 326(24):1587–1592

Harper T C, Coeytaux R R, Chen W et al 2006 A randomized controlled trial of acupuncture for initiation of labour in nulliparous women. Journal of Maternal–Fetal and Neonatal Medicine 19(8):465–470

Hayman R 2004 Poor progress in labour. In: Luesley D M, Baker P N (eds) Obstetrics and gynaecology. An evidence-based text for MRCOG. Arnold, London

Heimstad R, Skogvoll E, Mattsson L A et al 2007 Induction of labour or serial antenatal fetal monitoring in post term pregnancy: a randomised controlled trial. Obstetrics and Gynaecology 109(3):609–617

Hovi M, Raatikainen K, Heiskanen N et al 2006 Obstetric outcome in post-term pregnancies: time for reappraisal in clinical management. Acta Obstetrica et Gynecologica Scandinavica 85(7):805–809

Kavanagh J, Kelly A J, Thomas J 2001 Sexual intercourse for cervical ripening and induction of labour. Cochrane Database of Systematic Reviews, Issue 2:CD003093

Kavanagh J, Kelly A J, Thomas J 2005 Breast stimulation for cervical ripening and induction of labour. Cochrane Database of Systematic Reviews, Issue 3:CD003392

Kelly A J, Kavanagh A J, Thomas J 2001 Castor oil, bath and/or enema for cervical priming and induction of labour. Cochrane Database of Systematic Reviews, Issue 2:CD003099

Kelly A J, Kavanagh J, Thomas J 2003 Vaginal prostaglandin (PGE2 and PGF2a) for induction of labour at term. Cochrane Database of Systematic Reviews, Issue 4:CD003101

Koklanaris N, Tropper P 2006 Post term pregnancy. Female Patient 31(6):14–18

Kramer M S, Rouleau J, Baskett T F et al 2006 Amniotic-fluid embolism and medical induction of labour: a retrospective, population-based cohort study. Lancet 368(954521): 1444–1448

Laursen M, Bille C, Olesen A W, et al 2004 Genetic influence on prolonged gestation: a population-based Danish twin study. American Journal of Obstetrics and Gynaecology 190:489–494

Lavender T, Alfirevic Z, Walkinshaw S 2006 Effect of different partogram action lines on birth outcomes: a randomised controlled trial. Obstetrics and Gynaecology 108:295–302

Menticoglou S M, Hall P F 2002 Routine induction of labour at 41 weeks gestation: nonsensus consensus. British Journal of Obstetrics and Gynaecology 109(5):485–491

Mogren I Stenlund H Hogberg U 1999 Recurrence of prolonged pregnancy. International Journal of Epidemiology 28(2):253–257

Neff M, 2004 ACOG Guidelines on management of post term pregnancy. Obstetrics and Gynaecology 104(3):639–645

Neilson J P, Lavender T, Quenby S et al 2003 Obstructed labour. British Medical Bulletin 67(1):191–204

NICE (National Institute for Health and Clinical Excellence) 2007 Intrapartum care. Care of healthy women and their babies during childbirth National Collaborating Centre for Women's and Children's Health. NICE, London

NICE (National Institute for Clinical Excellence) 2008a Antenatal care: routine care for the healthy pregnant woman National Collaborating Centre for Women's and Children's Health. NICE, London

NICE (National Institute for Clinical Excellence) 2008b Induction of labour. NICE, London

NMC (Nursing and Midwifery Council) 2004 Midwives rules and standards. NMC, London

Nystedt A, Hogberg U, Lundman B 2005 The negative birth experience of prolonged labour: a case-referent study. Journal of Clinical Nursing 14:579–586

Nystedt A, Hogberg U, Lundman B 2006 Some Swedish women's experiences of prolonged labour. Midwifery 22:56–65

Olesen A W, Westergaard J G, Olsen J 2006 Prenatal risk indicators of a prolonged pregnancy. The Danish Birth Cohort 1998–2001. Acta Obstetrica et Gynecologica Scandinavica 85(11):1338–1341

RCOG (Royal College of Obstetricians and Gynaecologists) 2001 Induction of labour. Evidence-based Clinical Guideline No. 9. RCOG, London

RCOG (Royal College of Obstetricians and Gynaecologists) 2004 Management of HIV in pregnancy. Guideline No. 39. Online. Available: http://rcog.org.uk

Selo-Ojeme D, Pisal P, Barigye O et al 2007 Are we complying with NICE guidelines on the use of prostaglandin E2 for induction of labour? A survey of obstetric units in the UK. Journal of Gynaecology and Obstetrics 27(2):144–147

Shetty A, Mackie L, Danielian P et al 2002 Sublingual compared with oral misoprostol in term labour induction: a randomised controlled trial. British Journal of Obstetrics and Gynaecology 109(6):645–650

Shetty A, Livingstone I, Acharya S et al 2003 Oral misoprostol (100 μg) versus vaginal misoprostol (25 μg) in term labour induction: a randomised comparison. Acta Obstetrica et Gynecologica Scandinavica 82(12):1103–1106

Smith C A 2003 Homoeopathy for induction of labour. Cochrane Database of Systematic Reviews, Issue 4:CD003399

Smith C A, Crowther C A 2004 Acupuncture for induction of labour. Cochrane Database of Systematic Reviews, Issue 1:CD002962

Smyth R, Alldred S K, Markham C 2007 Amniotomy for shortening spontaneous labour (Protocol). Cochrane Database of Systematic Reviews, Issue 1:CD006167

Svärdby K, Nordström L, Sellström E 2006 Primiparas with or without oxytocin augmentation: a prospective descriptive study. Journal of Clinical Nursing 16:179–184

Thornton J G, Hornbuckle J, Vail A et al 2004 Infant wellbeing at 2 years of age in the Growth Restriction Intervention Trial (GRIT): multicentred randomised controlled trial. Lancet 364 (9453):513–520

Tomlinson A J, Archer P A, Hobson S 2001 Induction of labour: a comparison of two methods with particular concern to patient acceptability. Journal of Obstetrics and Gynaecology 21(3):239–241

Van Meir C A, Ramirez M M, Matthewset al 1997 Chorionic prostaglandin metabolism is decreased in the lower uterine segment with term labour. Placenta 18:109–114

Vause S, Macintosh M, Glass M R 1999 Evidence based case report: Use of prostaglandins to induce labour in women with a caesarean section scar. British Medical Journal 318:1056–1058

WHO 1977 Recommended definitions, terminology and format for statistical tables related to the perinatal period and use of a new certificate for cause of perinatal deaths: modifications recommended by FIGO. Acta Obstetrica et Gynecologica Scandinavica 56:247–253

WHO 1994 Maternal and Safe Motherhood Programme. World Health Organization partograph in the management of labour. Lancet 343:1399–1404

Wong S F, Hui S K, Choi H et al 2002 Does sweeping of membranes beyond 40 weeks reduce the need for formal induction of labour? British Journal of Obstetrics and Gynaecology 109(6):632–636

Malpositions of the occiput and malpresentations

Terri Coates

Malpositions and malpresentations of the fetus present the midwife with a challenge of recognition and diagnosis both in the antenatal period and during labour.

This chapter aims to:

- outline the causes of these positions and presentations
- discuss the midwife's diagnosis and management
- describe the possible outcomes.

Occipitoposterior positions

Occipitoposterior positions are the most common type of malposition of the occiput and occur in approximately 10% of labours. A persistent occipitoposterior position results from a failure of internal rotation prior to birth. This occurs in 5% of births (Pearl et al 1993).

The vertex is presenting, but the occiput lies in the posterior rather than the anterior part of the pelvis. As a consequence, the fetal head is deflexed and larger diameters of the fetal skull present (Fig. 31.1).

Causes

The direct cause is often unknown, but it may be associated with an abnormally shaped pelvis. In an android pelvis, the forepelvis is narrow and the occiput tends to occupy the roomier hindpelvis. The oval shape of the anthropoid pelvis, with its narrow transverse diameter, favours a direct occipitoposterior position.

Antenatal diagnosis

Abdominal examination

Listen to the mother

The mother may complain of backache and she may feel that her baby's bottom is very high up against her ribs. She may report feeling movements across both sides of her abdomen.

On inspection

There is a saucer-shaped depression at or just below the umbilicus. This depression is created by the 'dip' between the head and the lower limbs of the fetus. The outline created by the high, unengaged head can look like a full bladder (Fig. 31.2).

On palpation

While the breech is easily palpated at the fundus, the back is difficult to palpate as it is well out to the maternal side, sometimes almost adjacent to the maternal spine. Limbs can be felt on both sides of the midline.

The head is usually high, a posterior position being the most common cause of non-engagement in a primigravida at term. This is because the large presenting

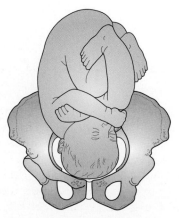

A   Right occipitoposterior position

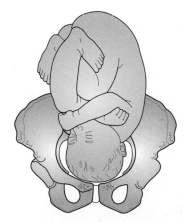

B   Left occipitoposterior position

Figure 31.1   (A) Right occipitoposterior position. (B) Left occipitoposterior position.

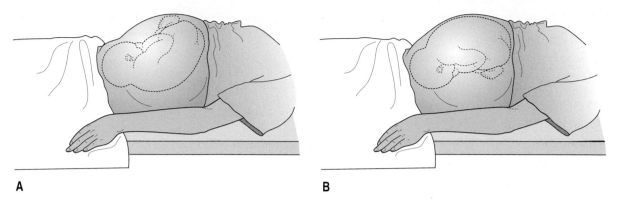

Figure 31.2 Comparison of abdominal contour in (A) posterior and (B) anterior positions of the occiput.

diameter, the occipitofrontal (11.5 cm), is unlikely to enter the pelvic brim until labour begins and flexion occurs. The occiput and sinciput are on the same level (Figs 31.3, 31.4). Flexion allows the engagement of the suboccipitofrontal diameter (10 cm).

The cause of the deflexion is a straightening of the fetal spine against the lumbar curve of the maternal spine. This makes the fetus straighten its neck and adopt a more erect attitude.

On auscultation

The fetal back is not well flexed so the chest is thrust forward, therefore the fetal heart can be heard in the midline. However, the heart may be heard more easily at the flank on the same side as the back.

Antenatal preparation

Anecdotal evidence suggested that active changes of maternal posture would help to achieve an optimal fetal position before labour (El Halta 1998, Sutton

$\frac{5}{5}$	$\frac{4}{5}$	$\frac{3}{5}$
Occiput, sinciput above brim	Sinciput rises	Occiput below brim

Brim

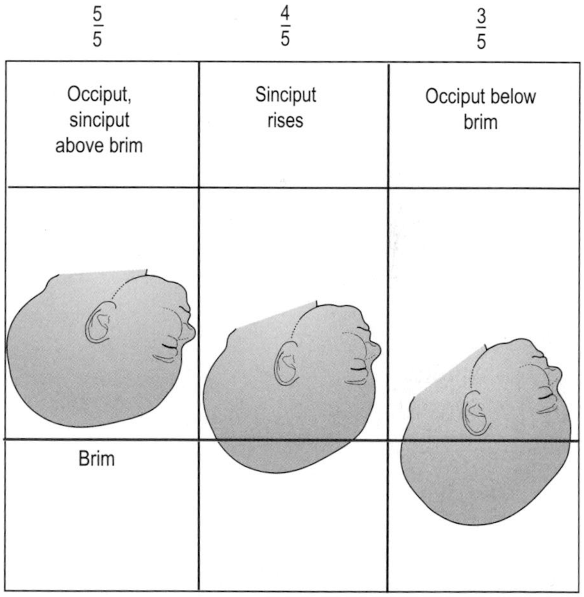

Figure 31.4 Flexion with descent of the head.

1996). Research has shown that the mother adopting a knee–chest position several times a day may achieve temporary rotation of the fetus to an anterior position but only has a short-term effect upon fetal presentation (Kariminia et al 2004). There is insufficient evidence to suggest that mothers adopt the hands and knees posture unless they find it comfortable. Further research is needed to evaluate the effect of adopting a hands and knees posture on the presenting part during labour (Hofmeyr & Kulier 2005).

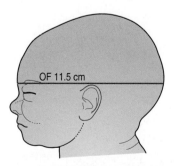

OF 11.5 cm

Figure 31.3 Engaging diameter of a deflexed head: occipitofrontal (OF) 11.5 cm.

Diagnosis during labour

The woman may complain of continuous and severe backache worsening with contractions. However, the absence of backache does not necessarily indicate an anteriorly positioned fetus.

The large and irregularly shaped presenting circumference (Fig. 31.5) does not fit well onto the cervix. Therefore the membranes tend to rupture spontaneously at an early stage of labour and the contractions may be incoordinate. Descent of the head can be slow even with good contractions. The woman may have a strong desire to push early in labour because the occiput is pressing on the rectum.

Vaginal examination

The findings (Fig. 31.6) will depend upon the degree of flexion of the head; locating the anterior fontanelle in the anterior part of the pelvis is diagnostic but this may be difficult if caput succedaneum is present. The direction of the sagittal suture and location of the posterior fontanelle will help to confirm the diagnosis.

Care in labour

Labour with a fetus in an occipitoposterior position can be long and painful. The deflexed head does not fit well onto the cervix and therefore does not produce optimal stimulation for uterine contractions.

First stage of labour

The woman may experience severe and unremitting backache, which is tiring and can be very demoralizing, especially if the progress of labour is slow. Continuous support from the midwife will help the mother and her partner to cope with the labour (Thornton & Lilford 1994) (see Chs 25–27). The midwife can help to provide physical support such as massage and other comfort measures and suggest changes of posture and position. The all-fours position may relieve some discomfort; anecdotal evidence suggests that this position may also aid rotation of the fetal head.

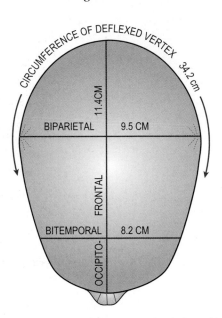

Figure 31.5 Presenting dimensions of a deflexed head.

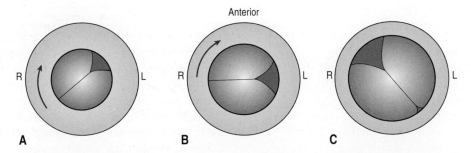

Figure 31.6 Vaginal touch pictures in a right occipitoposterior position. (A) Anterior fontanelle felt to left and anteriorly. Sagittal suture in the right oblique diameter of the pelvis. (B) Anterior fontanelle felt to left and laterally. Sagittal suture in the transverse diameter of the pelvis. (C) Following increased flexion the posterior fontanelle is felt to the right and anteriorly. Sagittal suture in the left oblique diameter of the pelvis. The position is now right occipitoanterior.

Labour may be prolonged and the midwife should do all she can to prevent the mother from becoming dehydrated or ketotic (see Ch. 26).

Incoordinate uterine action or ineffective contractions may need correction with an oxytocin infusion (see Ch. 30).

The woman may experience a strong urge to push long before her cervix has become fully dilated. This is because of the pressure of the occiput on the rectum. However, if the woman pushes at this time, the cervix may become oedematous and this would delay the onset of the second stage of labour. The urge to push may be eased by a change in position and the use of breathing techniques or inhalational analgesia to enhance relaxation. The woman's partner and the midwife can assist throughout labour with massage, physical support and suggestions for alternative methods of pain relief (see Ch. 27). The mother may choose a range of pain control methods throughout her labour depending on the level and intensity of pain that she is experiencing at that time.

Second stage of labour

Full dilatation of the cervix may need to be confirmed by a vaginal examination because moulding and formation of a caput succedaneum may bring the vertex into view while an anterior lip of cervix remains. If the head is not visible at the onset of the second stage, then the midwife could encourage the woman to remain upright (see Ch. 28). This position may shorten the length of the second stage and may reduce the need for operative delivery. In some cases where contractions are weak and ineffective an oxytocin infusion may be commenced to stimulate adequate contractions and achieve advance of the presenting part. As with any labour, the maternal and fetal conditions are closely observed throughout the second stage. The length of the second stage of labour is usually increased when the occiput is posterior, and there is an increased likelihood of operative delivery (Gimovsky & Hennigan 1995, Pearl et al 1993).

Mechanism of right occipitoposterior position (long rotation) (Figs 31.7–31.10)

- The lie is longitudinal
- The attitude of the head is deflexed
- The presentation is vertex
- The position is right occipitoposterior
- The denominator is the occiput
- The presenting part is the middle or anterior area of the left parietal bone
- The occipitofrontal diameter, 11.5 cm, lies in the right oblique diameter of the pelvic brim. The occiput points to the right sacroiliac joint and the sinciput to the left iliopectineal eminence.

Flexion

Descent takes place with increasing flexion. The occiput becomes the leading part.

Internal rotation of the head

The occiput reaches the pelvic floor first and rotates forwards $\frac{3}{8}$ of a circle along the right side of the pelvis to lie under the symphysis pubis. The shoulders follow, turning $\frac{2}{8}$ of a circle from the left to the right oblique diameter.

Crowning

The occiput escapes under the symphysis pubis and the head is crowned.

Extension

The sinciput, face and chin sweep the perineum and the head is born by a movement of extension.

Restitution

In restitution the occiput turns $\frac{1}{8}$ of a circle to the right and the head realigns itself with the shoulders.

Internal rotation of the shoulders

The shoulders enter the pelvis in the right oblique diameter; the anterior shoulder reaches the pelvic floor first and rotates forwards $\frac{1}{8}$ of a circle to lie under the symphysis pubis.

External rotation of the head

At the same time the occiput turns a further $\frac{1}{8}$ of a circle to the right.

Lateral flexion

The anterior shoulder escapes under the symphysis pubis, the posterior shoulder sweeps the perineum and the body is born by a movement of lateral flexion.

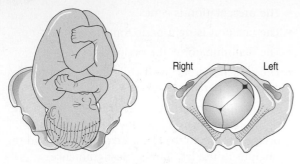

Figure 31.7 Head descending with increased flexion. Sagittal suture in right oblique diameter of the pelvis.

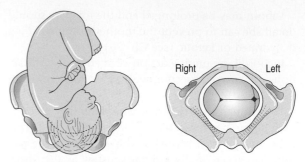

Figure 31.8 Occiput and shoulders have rotated ⅛ of a circle forwards. Sagittal suture in transverse diameter of the pelvis.

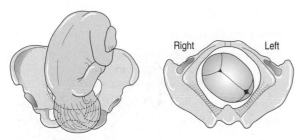

Figure 31.9 Occiput and shoulders have rotated ⅜ of a circle forwards. Sagittal suture in the left oblique diameter of the pelvis. The position is right occipitoanterior.

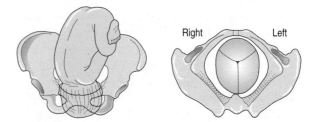

Figure 31.10 Occiput has rotated ⅜ of a circle forwards. Note the twist in the neck. Sagittal suture in the anteroposterior diameter of the pelvis.

Figures 31.7–31.10 Mechanism of labour in right occipitoposterior position.

Possible course and outcomes of labour

As with all labours, complicated or otherwise, the mother should be kept informed of her progress and proposed interventions so that she can make informed choices and give informed consent, ensuring the optimum outcome for herself and her baby.

Long internal rotation

This is the commonest outcome, with good uterine contractions producing flexion and descent of the head so that the occiput rotates forward ⅜ of a circle as described above.

Short internal rotation

The term 'persistent occipitoposterior position' (Figs 31.11, 31.12) indicates that the occiput fails to rotate forwards. Instead the sinciput reaches the pelvic

floor first and rotates forwards. The occiput goes into the hollow of the sacrum. The baby is born facing the pubic bone (face to pubis).

Cause

Failure of flexion. The head descends without increased flexion and the sinciput becomes the leading part. It reaches the pelvic floor first and rotates forwards to lie under the symphysis pubis.

Diagnosis

In the first stage of labour. Signs are those of any posterior position of the occiput, namely a deflexed head and a fetal heart heard in the flank or in the midline. Descent is slow.

In the second stage of labour. Delay is common. On vaginal examination the anterior fontanelle is felt behind the symphysis pubis, but a large caput

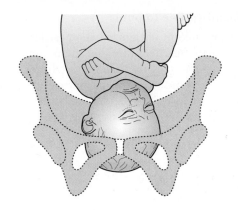

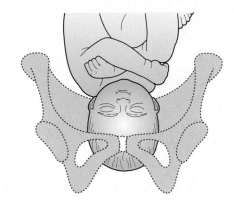

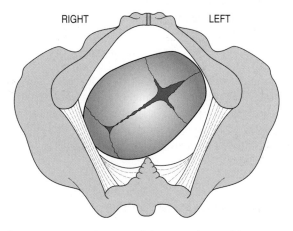

RIGHT   LEFT

Figure 31.11 Persistent occipitoposterior position before rotation of the occiput: position right occipitoposterior.

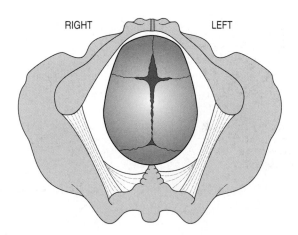

RIGHT   LEFT

Figure 31.12 Persistent occipitoposterior position after short rotation: position direct occipitoposterior.

succedaneum may mask this. If the pinna of the ear is felt pointing towards the mother's sacrum, this indicates a posterior position.

The long occipitofrontal diameter causes considerable dilatation of the anus and gaping of the vagina while the fetal head is barely visible, and the broad biparietal diameter distends the perineum and may cause excessive bulging. As the head advances, the anterior fontanelle can be felt just behind the symphysis pubis; the baby is born facing the pubis. Characteristic upward moulding is present with the caput succedaneum on the anterior part of the parietal bone (Fig. 31.13).

The birth (Figs 31.14–31.17)

The sinciput will first emerge from under the symphysis pubis as far as the root of the nose and the

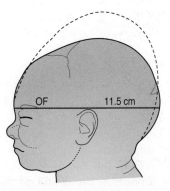

OF   11.5 cm

Figure 31.13 Upward moulding (dotted line) following persistent occipitoposterior position. OF, occipitofrontal.

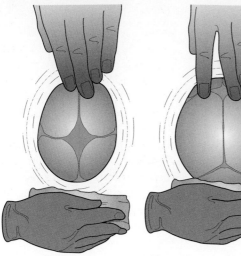

Figure 31.14 Allowing the sinciput to escape as far as the glabella.

Figure 31.15 The occiput sweeps the perineum, sinciput held back to maintain flexion.

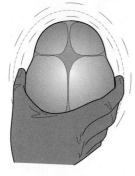

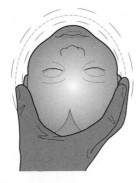

Figure 31.16 Grasping the head to bring the face down from under the symphysis pubis.

Figure 31.17 Extension of the head.

Figures 31.14–31.17 Delivery of head in a persistent occipitoposterior position.

midwife maintains flexion by restraining it from escaping further than the glabella, allowing the occiput to sweep the perineum and be born. She then extends the head by grasping it and bringing the face down from under the symphysis pubis. Perineal trauma is common and the midwife should watch for signs of rupture in the centre of the perineum ('button-hole' tear). An episiotomy may be required, owing to the larger presenting diameters.

Undiagnosed face to pubis

If the signs are not recognized at an earlier stage, the midwife may first be aware that the occiput is posterior when she sees the hairless forehead escaping beneath the pubic arch. She may have been misguidedly extending the head and should therefore now flex it towards the symphysis pubis.

Deep transverse arrest

The head descends with some increase in flexion. The occiput reaches the pelvic floor and begins to rotate forwards. Flexion is not maintained and the occipitofrontal diameter becomes caught at the narrow bispinous diameter of the outlet. Arrest may be due to weak contractions, a straight sacrum or a narrowed outlet.

Diagnosis

The sagittal suture is found in the transverse diameter of the pelvis and both fontanelles are palpable. Neither sinciput nor occiput leads. The head is deep in the pelvic cavity at the level of the ischial spines although the caput may be lower still. There is no advance.

Management

The mother must be kept informed of progress and participate in decisions. Pushing at this time may not resolve the problem; the midwife and the woman's partner can help by encouraging SOS breathing (see Ch. 16). A change of position may help to overcome the urge to bear down.

If an operative delivery is required for the safe delivery of a healthy baby then the mother's informed consent is required. The procedure would be undertaken under local, regional or more rarely general anaesthesia (see Ch. 32). The considerations are the choice of the mother and the condition of the mother and fetus.

Vacuum extraction has been associated with lower incidence of trauma to both the mother and the infant (Pearl et al 1993) (see Ch. 32). The doctor may choose to use forceps to rotate the head to an occipitoanterior position before delivery. Whichever procedure is undertaken, the mother should first be given adequate analgesia or anaesthesia.

Conversion to face or brow presentation

When the head is deflexed at the onset of labour, extension occasionally occurs instead of flexion. If extension is complete then a face presentation results, but if incomplete the head is arrested at the brim, the brow presenting. This is a rare complication of posterior positions, and is more commonly found in multiparous women.

Complications

Apart from prolonged labour with its attendant risks to mother and fetus and the increased likelihood of instrumental delivery, the following complications may occur.

Obstructed labour

This may occur when the head is deflexed or partially extended and becomes impacted in the pelvis (see Ch. 30).

Maternal trauma

Forceps delivery may result in perineal bruising and trauma. Birth of a baby in the persistent occipitoposterior position, particularly if previously undiagnosed, may cause a third-degree tear (Pearl et al 1993).

Neonatal trauma

Neonatal trauma occurring following birth from an occipitoposterior position has been associated with forceps or ventouse delivery. The outcome for a neonate delivered from an occipitoposterior position is comparable with that expected for an infant delivered from an occipitoanterior position.

Cord prolapse

A high head predisposes to early spontaneous rupture of the membranes, which, together with an ill-fitting presenting part, may result in cord prolapse (see Ch. 33).

Cerebral haemorrhage

The unfavourable upward moulding of the fetal skull, found in an occipitoposterior position, can cause intracranial haemorrhage, as a result of the falx cerebri being pulled away from the tentorium cerebelli. The larger presenting diameters also predispose to a greater degree of compression. Cerebral haemorrhage (see Ch. 45) may also result from chronic hypoxia, which may accompany prolonged labour.

Face presentation

When the attitude of the head is one of complete extension, the occiput of the fetus will be in contact with its spine and the face will present. The incidence is about ≤1:500 (Bhal et al 1998) and the majority develop during labour from vertex presentations with the occiput posterior; this is termed *secondary face presentation*. Less commonly, the face presents before labour; this is termed *primary face presentation*. There are six positions in a face presentation (Figs 31.18–31.23); the denominator is the mentum and the presenting diameters are the submentobregmatic (9.5 cm) and the bitemporal (8.2 cm).

Causes

Anterior obliquity of the uterus

The uterus of a multiparous woman with slack abdominal muscles and a pendulous abdomen will lean forward and alter the direction of the uterine axis. This causes the fetal buttocks to lean forwards and the force of the contractions to be directed in a line towards the chin rather than the occiput, resulting in extension of the head.

Contracted pelvis

In the flat pelvis, the head enters in the transverse diameter of the brim and the parietal eminences may be held up in the obstetrical conjugate; the head becomes extended and a face presentation develops. Alternatively, if the head is in the posterior position, vertex presenting, and remains deflexed, the parietal eminences may be caught in the sacrocotyloid dimension, the occiput does not descend, the head becomes extended and face presentation results. This is more likely in the presence of an android pelvis, in which the sacrocotyloid dimension is reduced.

Polyhydramnios

If the vertex is presenting and the membranes rupture spontaneously, the resulting rush of fluid may cause the head to extend as it sinks into the lower uterine segment.

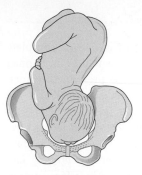

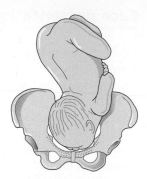

Figures 31.18 Right mentoposterior.

Figure 31.19 Left mentoposterior.

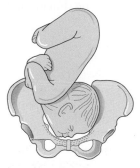

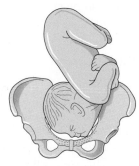

Figure 31.20 Right mentolateral.

Figure 31.21 Left mentolateral.

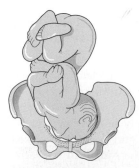

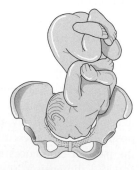

Figure 31.22 Right mentoanterior.

Figure 31.23 Left mentoanterior.

Figures 31.18–31.23 Six positions of face presentation.

Congenital abnormality

Anencephaly can be a fetal cause of a face presentation. In a cephalic presentation, because the vertex is absent the face is thrust forward and presents. More rarely, a tumour of the fetal neck may cause extension of the head.

Antenatal diagnosis

Antenatal diagnosis is rare since face presentation develops during labour in the majority of cases. A cephalic presentation in a known anencephalic fetus may be presumed to be a face presentation.

Intrapartum diagnosis

On abdominal palpation

Face presentation may not be detected, especially if the mentum is anterior. The occiput feels prominent, with a groove between head and back, but it may be mistaken for the sinciput. The limbs may be palpated on the side opposite to the occiput and the fetal heart is best heard through the fetal chest on the same side as the limbs. In a mentoposterior position the fetal heart is difficult to hear because the fetal chest is in contact with the maternal spine (Fig. 31.24).

On vaginal examination

The presenting part is high, soft and irregular. When the cervix is sufficiently dilated, the orbital ridges, eyes, nose and mouth may be felt. Confusion between the mouth and anus could arise, however. The mouth may be open, and the hard gums are diagnostic. The fetus may suck the examining finger.

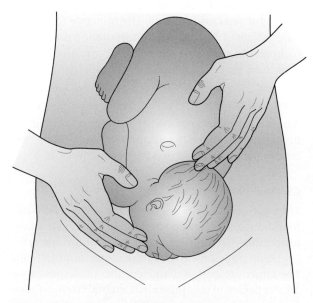

Figure 31.24 Abdominal palpation of the head in a face presentation. Position right mentoposterior.

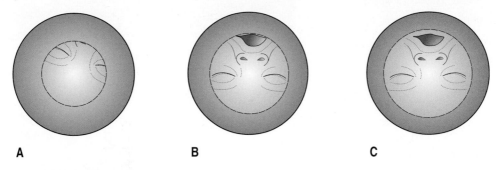

A   B   C

Figure 31.25 Vaginal touch pictures of left mentoanterior position: (A) The mentum is felt to left and anteriorly. Orbital ridges in left oblique diameter of the pelvis. (B) Following increased extension of the head, the mouth can be felt. (C) The face has rotated 1/8 of a circle forwards. Orbital ridges in transverse diameter of the pelvis. Position direct mentoanterior.

As labour progresses the face becomes oedematous, making it more difficult to distinguish from a breech presentation. To determine position the mentum must be located; if it is posterior, the midwife should decide whether it is lower than the sinciput; if so, it will rotate forwards if it can advance. In a left mentoanterior position, the orbital ridges will be in the left oblique diameter of the pelvis (Fig. 31.25). Care must be taken not to injure or infect the eyes with the examining finger.

Mechanism of a left mentoanterior position

- The lie is longitudinal
- The attitude is one of extension of head and neck
- The presentation is face (Fig. 31.26)
- The position is left mentoanterior

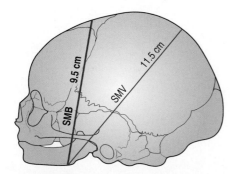

Figure 31.26 Diameters involved in delivery of face presentation. Engaging diameter, sub-mentobregmatic (SMB) 9.5 cm. The sub-mentovertical (SMV) diameter, 11.5 cm, sweeps the perineum.

- The denominator is the mentum
- The presenting part is the left malar bone.

Extension

Descent takes place with increasing extension. The mentum becomes the leading part.

Internal rotation of the head

This occurs when the chin reaches the pelvic floor and rotates forwards ⅛ of a circle. The chin escapes under the symphysis pubis (Fig. 31.27A).

Flexion

This takes place and the sinciput, vertex and occiput sweep the perineum; the head is born (Fig. 31.27B).

Restitution

This occurs when the chin turns ⅛ of a circle to the woman's left.

Internal rotation of the shoulders

The shoulders enter the pelvis in the left oblique diameter and the anterior shoulder reaches the pelvic floor first and rotates forwards ⅛ of a circle along the right side of the pelvis.

External rotation of the head

This occurs simultaneously. The chin moves a further ⅛ of a circle to the left.

Lateral flexion

The anterior shoulder escapes under the symphysis pubis, the posterior shoulder sweeps the perineum and the body is born by a movement of lateral flexion.

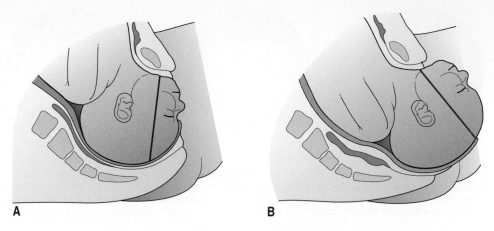

Figure 31.27 Birth of head in mentoanterior position: (A) The chin escapes under symphysis pubis. Sub-mentobregmatic diameter at outlet. (B) The head is born by a movement of flexion.

Possible course and outcomes of labour

The mother should be kept informed of her progress and any proposed intervention throughout labour.

Prolonged labour

Labour is often prolonged because the face is an ill-fitting presenting part and does not therefore stimulate effective uterine contractions. In addition the facial bones do not mould and, in order to enable the mentum to reach the pelvic floor and rotate forwards, the shoulders must enter the pelvic cavity at the same time as the head. The fetal axis pressure is directed to the chin and the head is extended almost at right angles to the spine, increasing the diameters to be accommodated in the pelvis.

Mentoanterior positions

With good uterine contractions, descent and rotation of the head occur (see above) and labour progresses to a spontaneous birth.

Mentoposterior positions

If the head is completely extended, so that the mentum reaches the pelvic floor first, and the contractions are effective, the mentum will rotate forwards and the position becomes anterior.

Persistent mentoposterior position

In this case, the head is incompletely extended and the sinciput reaches the pelvic floor first and rotates forwards ⅛ of a circle, which brings the chin into the hollow of the sacrum (Fig. 31.28). There is no further mechanism. The face becomes impacted because, in order to descend further, both head and chest would have to be accommodated in the pelvis. Whatever emerges anteriorly from the vagina must pivot around the subpubic arch; if the chin is posterior this is impossible because the head can extend no further.

Reversal of face presentation

A face presentation in a persistent mentoposterior position may, in some cases, be manipulated to an occipitoanterior position using bimanual pressure

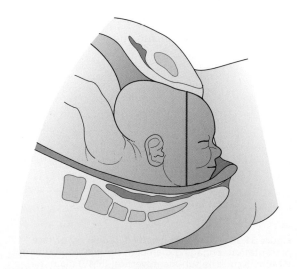

Figure 31.28 Persistent mentoposterior position.

(Gimovsky & Hennigan 1995, Neuman et al 1994). This method was developed to reduce the likelihood of an operative delivery for those women who refused caesarean section. Using a tocolytic drug to relax the uterus, the fetal head is disengaged using upward transvaginal pressure. The fetal head is then flexed with bimanual pressure under ultrasound guidance to achieve an occipitoanterior position.

Management of labour

First stage

Upon diagnosis of a face presentation, the midwife should inform the doctor of this deviation from the normal. Routine observations of maternal and fetal conditions are made as in a normal labour (see Ch. 26). A fetal scalp electrode must not be applied, and care should be taken not to infect or injure the eyes during vaginal examinations.

Immediately following rupture of the membranes, a vaginal examination should be performed to exclude cord prolapse; such an occurrence is more likely because the face is an ill-fitting presenting part. Descent of the head should be observed abdominally, and careful vaginal examination performed every 2–4 hrs to assess cervical dilatation and descent of the head.

In mentoposterior positions the midwife should note whether the mentum is lower than the sinciput, since rotation and descent depend on this. If the head remains high in spite of good contractions, caesarean section is likely. The woman may be prescribed oral ranitidine, 150 mg every 6 hrs throughout labour, if it is considered that an anaesthetic may be necessary.

Birth of the head (Fig. 31.29)

When the face appears at the vulva, extension must be maintained by holding back the sinciput and permitting the mentum to escape under the symphysis pubis before the occiput is allowed to sweep the perineum. In this way, the submentovertical diameter (11.5 cm) instead of the mentovertical diameter (13.5 cm) distends the vaginal orifice. Because the perineum is also distended by the biparietal diameter (9.5 cm), an elective episiotomy may be performed to avoid extensive perineal lacerations.

If the head does not descend in the second stage, the doctor should be informed. In a mentoanterior

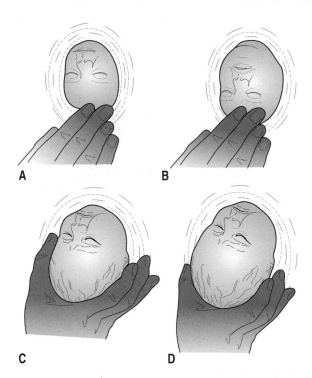

Figure 31.29 Birth of face presentation: (A) The sinciput is held back to increase extension until the chin is born. (B) The chin is born. (C) Flexing the head to bring the occiput over the perineum. (D) Flexion is completed; the head is born.

position it may be possible for the obstetrician to deliver the baby with forceps when rotation is incomplete. If the position remains mentoposterior, the head has become impacted, or there is any suspicion of disproportion, a caesarean section will be necessary.

Complications

Obstructed labour

Because the face, unlike the vertex, does not mould, a minor degree of pelvic contraction may result in obstructed labour (see Ch. 30). In a persistent mentoposterior position the face becomes impacted and caesarean section is necessary.

Cord prolapse

A prolapsed cord is more common when the membranes rupture because the face is an ill-fitting presenting part. The midwife should always perform a

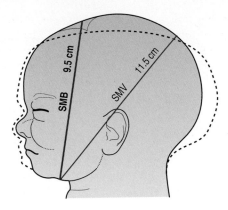

Figure 31.30 Moulding in a face presentation (dotted line). SMB, sub-mentobregmatic; SMV, sub-mentovertical.

vaginal examination when the membranes rupture to rule out cord prolapse (see Ch. 33).

Facial bruising

The baby's face is always bruised and swollen at birth with oedematous eyelids and lips. The head is elongated (Fig. 31.30) and the baby will initially lie with head extended. The midwife should warn the parents in advance of the baby's 'battered' appearance, reassuring them that this is only temporary; the oedema will disappear within 1 or 2 days, and the bruising will usually resolve within a week.

Cerebral haemorrhage

The lack of moulding of the facial bones can lead to intracranial haemorrhage caused by excessive compression of the fetal skull or by rearward compression, in the typical moulding of the fetal skull found in this presentation (Fig. 31.30).

Maternal trauma

Extensive perineal lacerations may occur at birth owing to the large submentovertical and biparietal diameters distending the vagina and perineum. There is an increased incidence of operative delivery, either forceps delivery or caesarean section, both of which increase maternal morbidity.

Brow presentation

In the *brow presentation* the fetal head is partially extended with the frontal bone, which is bounded by the anterior fontanelle and the orbital ridges, lying at the pelvic brim (Fig. 31.31). The presenting diameter of 13.5 cm is the mentovertical (Fig. 31.32), which exceeds all diameters in an average-sized pelvis. This presentation is rare, with an incidence of approximately 1 in 1000 deliveries (Bhal et al 1998).

Causes

These are the same as for a secondary face presentation (see above); during the process of extension from a vertex presentation to a face presentation, the brow will present temporarily and in a few cases this will persist.

Diagnosis

Brow presentation is not usually detected before the onset of labour.

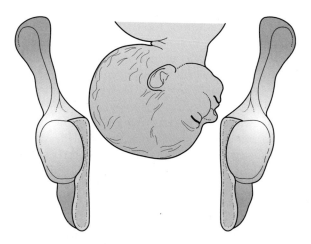

Figure 31.31 Brow presentation.

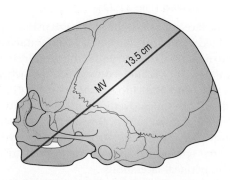

Figure 31.32 Brow presentation. The mentovertical (MV) diameter, 13.5 cm, lies at the pelvic brim.

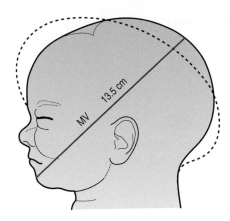

Figure 31.33 Moulding in a brow presentation (dotted line). MV, mentovertical.

On abdominal palpation

The head is high, appears unduly large and does not descend into the pelvis despite good uterine contractions.

On vaginal examination

The presenting part is high and may be difficult to reach. The anterior fontanelle may be felt on one side of the pelvis and the orbital ridges, and possibly the root of the nose, at the other (Fig. 31.33). A large caput succedaneum may mask these landmarks if the woman has been in labour for some hours.

Management

The doctor must be informed immediately this presentation is suspected. This is because vaginal birth is extremely rare and obstructed labour usually results. It is possible that a woman with a large pelvis and a small baby may give birth vaginally. When the brow reaches the pelvic floor the maxilla rotates forwards and the head is born by a mechanism somewhat similar to that of a persistent occipitoposterior position. However, the midwife should never expect such a favourable outcome. The mother should be warned about the possible course of labour and that a vaginal birth is unlikely.

If there is no evidence of fetal compromise, the doctor may allow labour to continue for a short while in case further extension of the head converts the brow presentation to a face presentation. Occasionally spontaneous flexion may occur, resulting in a vertex presentation. If the head fails to descend and the brow presentation persists, a caesarean section is performed, with maternal consent.

Complications

These are the same as in a face presentation, except that obstructed labour requiring caesarean section is the probable rather than a possible outcome.

Breech presentation

A breech presentation is an unusual presentation but it should not be considered abnormal as the fetus lies longitudinally with the buttocks in the lower pole of the uterus. The presenting diameter is the bitrochanteric (10cm) and the denominator the sacrum. This presentation occurs in approximately 3% of pregnancies at term. In mid-trimester the frequency is much higher because the greater proportion of amniotic fluid facilitates free movement of the fetus (Gimovsky & Hennigan 1995). Mothers can be reassured that a normal labour and birth are not excluded just because the presenting part is a breech. Ensuring informed consent the midwife must explain that not all breech babies can or should be born vaginally. The Term Breech Trial (Hannah et al 2000) reported that vaginal birth is more hazardous than caesarean birth for a uncomplicated term breech presentation. However, a 2-year follow-up has shown that there is little difference between outcome comparing mode of delivery (Hannah et al 2004).

Types of breech presentation and position

There are six positions for a breech presentation, illustrated in Figures 31.34–31.39.

Breech with extended legs (frank breech)

The breech presents with the hips flexed and legs extended on the abdomen (Fig. 31.40). Some 70% of breech presentations are of this type and it is particularly common in primigravidae whose good

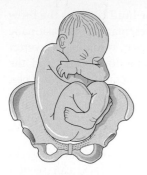

Figure 31.34   Right sacroposterior.

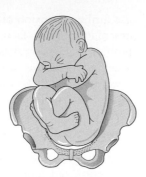

Figure 31.35   Left sacroposterior.

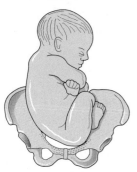

Figure 31.36   Right sacrolateral.

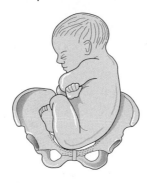

Figure 31.37   Left sacrolateral.

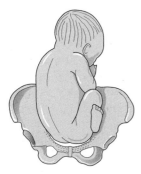

Figure 31.38   Right sacroanterior.

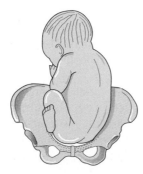

Figure 31.39   Left sacroanterior.

Figures 31.34–31.39   Six positions in breech presentation.

uterine muscle tone inhibits flexion of the legs and free turning of the fetus.

Complete breech

The fetal attitude is one of complete flexion (Fig. 31.41), with hips and knees both flexed and the feet tucked in beside the buttocks.

Footling breech

This is rare. One or both feet present because neither hips nor knees are fully flexed (Fig. 31.42). The feet are lower than the buttocks, which distinguishes it from the complete breech.

Knee presentation

This is very rare. One or both hips are extended, with the knees flexed (Fig. 31.43).

Causes

Often no cause is identified, but the following circumstances favour breech presentation.

Extended legs

Spontaneous cephalic version may be inhibited if the fetus lies with the legs extended, 'splinting' the back.

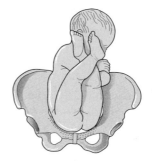

Figure 31.40   Frank breech.

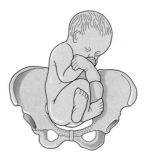

Figure 31.41   Complete breech.

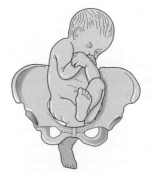

Figure 31.42   Footling presentation.

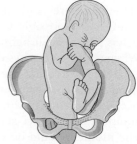

Figure 31.43   Knee presentation.

Figures 31.40–31.43   Types of breech presentation.

Preterm labour

As breech presentation is relatively common before 34 weeks' gestation, it follows that breech presentation is more common in preterm labours.

Multiple pregnancy

Multiple pregnancy limits the space available for each fetus to turn, which may result in one or more fetuses presenting by the breech.

Polyhydramnios

Distension of the uterine cavity by excessive amounts of amniotic fluid may cause the fetus to present by the breech.

Hydrocephaly

The increased size of the fetal head is more readily accommodated in the fundus.

Uterine abnormalities

Distortion of the uterine cavity by a septum or a fibroid may result in a breech presentation.

Placenta praevia

Some authorities believe that this may be a cause of breech presentation but there is some disagreement on this.

Antenatal diagnosis

Abdominal examination

Listen to the mother

She may tell you that she can feel that there is something very hard and uncomfortable under her ribs that makes breathing uncomfortable at times. If her baby's feet are in the lower pole of the uterus she may feel some very hard kicks on her bladder.

Palpation

In primigravidae, diagnosis is more difficult because of their firm abdominal muscles. On palpation the lie is longitudinal with a soft presentation, which is more easily felt using Pawlik's grip (see Fig. 17.7, p 278). The head can usually be felt in the fundus as a round hard mass, which may be made to move independently of the back by balloting it with one or both hands. If the legs are extended, the feet may prevent such nodding. When the breech is anterior and the fetus well flexed, it may be difficult to locate the head but use of the combined grip in which the upper and lower poles are grasped simultaneously may aid diagnosis. The woman may complain of discomfort under her ribs, especially at night, owing to pressure of the head on the diaphragm.

Auscultation

When the breech has not passed through the pelvic brim the fetal heart is heard most clearly above the umbilicus. When the legs are extended the breech descends into the pelvis easily. The fetal heart is then heard at a lower level.

Ultrasound examination

This may be used to demonstrate a breech presentation.

X-ray examination

Although largely superseded by ultrasound, X-ray has the added advantage of allowing pelvimetry to be performed at the same time.

Diagnosis during labour

A previously unsuspected breech presentation may not be diagnosed until the woman is in established labour. If the legs are extended, the breech may feel like a head abdominally, and also on vaginal examination if the cervix is <3 cm dilated and the breech is high.

Abdominal examination

Breech presentation may be diagnosed on admission in labour.

Vaginal examination

The breech feels soft and irregular with no sutures palpable, although occasionally the sacrum may be mistaken for a hard head and the buttocks mistaken for caput succedaneum. The anus may be felt and fresh meconium on the examining finger is usually diagnostic. If the legs are extended (Fig. 31.44) the external genitalia are very evident but it must be

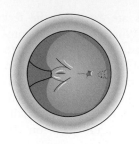
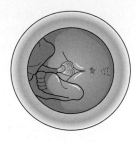

Figure 31.44 No feet felt; the legs are extended.

Figure 31.45 Feet felt; complete breech presentation.

Figures 31.44, 31.45 Vaginal touch pictures of left sacrolateral position.

remembered that these become oedematous. An oedematous vulva may be mistaken for a scrotum.

If a foot is felt (Fig. 31.45), the midwife should differentiate it from the hand. Toes are all the same length, they are shorter than fingers and the big toe cannot be opposed to other toes. The foot is at right angles to the leg, and the heel has no equivalent in the hand.

Presentation may be confirmed by ultrasound scan or X-ray.

Antenatal management

If the midwife suspects or detects a breech presentation at 36 weeks' gestation or later, she should refer the woman to a doctor. The presentation may be confirmed by ultrasound scan or occasionally by abdominal X-ray. There are differing opinions amongst obstetricians as to the management of breech presentation during pregnancy and a decision on management is usually deferred until near term.

External cephalic version

External cephalic version (ECV) is the use of external manipulation on the mother's abdomen to convert a breech to a cephalic presentation. The Royal College of Obstetricians and Gynaecologists (RCOG 1993) recommend that ECV should be offered at term by a practitioner skilled and experienced in the procedure and should be undertaken only in a unit where there are facilities for emergency delivery (CESDI 2000). The success of the procedure depends not only upon the skill and experience of the operator, but also upon the position and engagement of the fetus, liquor volume and maternal parity (Hofmeyr & Hutton 2006).

It has been demonstrated that ECV can reduce the number of babies presenting by the breech at term by two-thirds, and therefore reduce the caesarean section rate for breech presentations (Hofmeyr & Hutton 2006).

According to Zhang et al (1993) turning the fetus from a breech to a cephalic presentation before 37 weeks' gestation does not reduce the incidence of breech birth or rate of caesarean section as it is likely to turn itself back spontaneously but research is in progress (at the time of writing) to test this out. The reasons for attempting ECV and the procedure itself should be explained to the woman so that she can give her informed consent to have ECV performed.

Method

An ultrasound scan is performed to localize the placenta and to confirm the position and presentation of the fetus.

If the procedure is to be performed under tocolysis then a cannula will be sited to allow venous access. A 30 min CTG is performed to establish that the fetus is not compromised at the start of the procedure and maternal blood pressure and pulse are recorded.

The woman is asked to empty her bladder. The midwife then assists the woman into a comfortable supine position. The foot of the bed may be elevated to help free the breech from the pelvic brim. The abdomen is usually dusted with talcum powder to prevent pinching of the mother's skin during the procedure. While ECV may be uncomfortable for the mother it should not be painful. The breech is displaced from the pelvic brim towards an iliac fossa. Simultaneous force is then used as with one hand on each pole the operator makes the fetus perform a forward somersault (Figs 31.46–31.48). If this is not successful then a backward somersault can be attempted. If the fetus does not turn easily, then the procedure is abandoned but may be tried again a few days later.

A CTG is repeated following the procedure.

If the woman is Rhesus negative an injection of anti-D immunoglobulin is given as prophylaxis against iso-immunization caused by any placental separation.

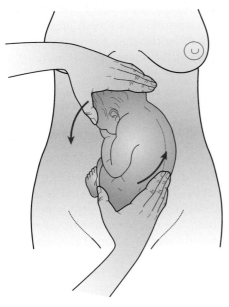

Figure 31.46   The right hand lifts the breech out of the pelvis. The left hand makes the head follow the nose. Flexion of head and back is maintained throughout.

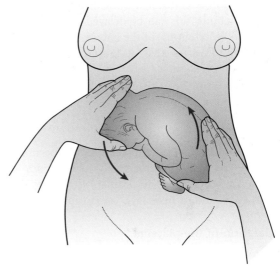

Figure 31.47   Flexion is continued. The left hand brings the head downwards. The right hand pushes the breech upwards.

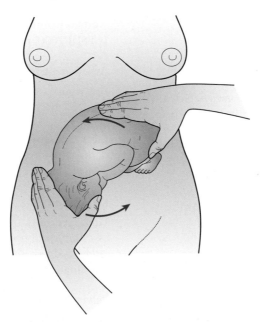

Figure 31.48   Pressure is exerted on head and breech simultaneously until the head is lying at the pelvic brim.

Figures 31.46–31.48   External cephalic version.

If the version is performed immediately prior to the onset of labour, this can be delayed until after birth when the blood group of the baby is known. In this case if anti-D is needed, it must be given within 72 hrs of the version.

Complications

Knotting of the umbilical cord

This should be suspected if bradycardia occurs and persists. The fetus is immediately turned back to a breech presentation. The woman is admitted for observation and, if necessary, caesarean section.

Separation of the placenta

The midwife should ask the woman to report pain or vaginal bleeding during and after the procedure.

Rupture of the membranes

If this occurs the cord may prolapse because neither the head nor the breech is engaged.

Relative contraindications

The presence of a uterine scar was previously thought to be an absolute contraindication to performing an ECV. Evidence, however, suggests that it is a safe and effective procedure used selectively in those women who have previously had a caesarean section (Flamm et al 1991).

Contraindications

These include:

- *pre-eclampsia or hypertension* – because of the increased risk of placental abruption
- multiple pregnancy
- *oligohydramnios* – because too much force has to be applied directly to the fetus and the version is likely to be unsuccessful
- ruptured membranes
- any condition that would require delivery by caesarean section.

Moxibustion for treatment of breech

Moxibustion (see Ch. 50) may be beneficial in reducing the need for ECV. However, there is a need for well-designed randomized controlled trials to evaluate moxibustion for breech presentation which should report on clinically relevant outcomes as well as the safety of the intervention (Cardini et al 2005, Neri et al 2004).

Persistent breech presentation

When external version has been unsuccessful or has not been attempted, then at 37 weeks' gestation a discussion of the available options should take place between the mother and an experienced practitioner (CESDI 2000) and a decision made as to whether to perform an elective caesarean section or to attempt a vaginal birth. The discussion and the plan formulated should be recorded. A planned caesarean section at term reduces the perinatal and neonatal mortality and morbidity but there is an increased risk of maternal morbidity (Hannah et al 2004). A 2-year follow-up did not show any differences in long-term outcomes between planned caesarean or planned vaginal breech births (Hannah et al 2004). 'An increased effort should be made to diagnose presentation at 37 weeks for all women planning to deliver outside an obstetric unit' (CESDI 2000, p 37).

Assessment for vaginal birth

Any doubt as to the capacity of the pelvis to accommodate the fetal head must be resolved before the buttocks are born and the head attempts to enter the pelvic brim. At this point the fetus begins to be deprived of oxygen and a last minute decision to perform caesarean section may be too late.

Fetal size

This, especially in relation to maternal size, can be assessed on abdominal palpation but is more accurately judged in association with an ultrasound examination.

Pelvic capacity

This can be judged on vaginal assessment (see Ch. 17), but it is usual to perform a lateral pelvimetry. This will show the shape of the sacrum and give accurate measurements of the anteroposterior diameters of the pelvic brim, cavity and outlet. No studies have confirmed the value of this procedure in selecting women who are likely to succeed in achieving a vaginal birth of a breech or in improving perinatal outcome (Hannah 1994). In a multigravida, information about the type of birth and the size of previous babies when compared with the size of the present fetus can be helpful.

Mechanism of left sacroanterior position

- The lie is longitudinal
- The attitude is one of complete flexion
- The presentation is breech
- The position is left sacroanterior
- The denominator is the sacrum
- The presenting part is the anterior (left) buttock
- The bitrochanteric diameter, 10 cm, enters the pelvis in the left oblique diameter of the brim
- The sacrum points to the left iliopectineal eminence.

Compaction

Descent takes place with increasing compaction, owing to increased flexion of the limbs.

Internal rotation of the buttocks

The anterior buttock reaches the pelvic floor first and rotates forwards ⅛ of a circle along the right side of the pelvis to lie underneath the symphysis pubis. The bitrochanteric diameter is now in the anteroposterior diameter of the outlet.

Lateral flexion of the body

The anterior buttock escapes under the symphysis pubis, the posterior buttock sweeps the perineum and the buttocks are born by a movement of lateral flexion.

Restitution of the buttocks

The anterior buttock turns slightly to the mother's right side.

Internal rotation of the shoulders

The shoulders enter the pelvis in the same oblique diameter as the buttocks, the left oblique. The anterior shoulder rotates forwards ⅛ of a circle along the right side of the pelvis and escapes under the

symphysis pubis; the posterior shoulder sweeps the perineum and the shoulders are born.

Internal rotation of the head

The head enters the pelvis with the sagittal suture in the transverse diameter of the brim. The occiput rotates forwards along the left side and the suboccipital region (the nape of the neck) impinges on the undersurface of the symphysis pubis.

External rotation of the body

At the same time the body turns so that the back is uppermost.

Birth of the head

The chin, face and sinciput sweep the perineum and the head is born in a flexed attitude.

Management of labour

Vaginal birth should be presented to the woman as the norm for breech presentation (MIDIRS 2007) provided there are no complications or contraindications, and it should be made clear that there is a risk of delivery by caesarean section.

First stage

Basic care during this stage is the same as in normal labour (see Chs 25 and 26) encouraging upright positions a much as possible to aid descent of the presenting part. The breech with extended legs fits the cervix quite well, the complete breech is a less well-fitting presenting part and the membranes tend to rupture early. For this reason there is an increased risk of cord prolapse, and a vaginal examination is performed to exclude this as soon as the membranes rupture. If they do not rupture spontaneously at an early stage, it is considered safer to leave them intact until labour is well established and the breech is at the level of the ischial spines. Meconium-stained liquor is sometimes found owing to compression of the fetal abdomen and is not always a sign of fetal compromise.

Analgesia

An epidural block may be offered to a woman with a breech presentation as it inhibits the urge to push prematurely. However, there is no evidence to suggest that this is indicated. Epidural analgesia has been associated with prolongation of the second stage of labour and has not been associated with any unique advantages for a woman giving birth to a breech at term.

Second stage

Full dilatation of the cervix should always be confirmed by vaginal examination before the woman commences active pushing. This is because in a footling presentation a foot may appear at the vulva when the cervix is only partially dilated; or when the legs are extended, particularly if the fetus is small, the breech may slip through an incompletely dilated cervix. In either case, the head may be trapped by the cervix when the baby is partially born. The woman may like to adopt a supported squat to utilize gravity in the second stage.

If the birth is taking place in hospital it is usual to inform the obstetrician of the onset of the second stage; a paediatrician should be present for the birth and it is usual to inform the anaesthetist also in case a general anaesthetic is required. Active pushing is not commenced until the buttocks are distending the vulva. Failure of the breech to descend onto the perineum in the second stage despite good contractions may indicate a need for caesarean section.

Types of birth

Spontaneous

The birth occurs with little assistance from the attendant.

Assisted breech

The buttocks are born spontaneously, but some assistance is necessary for delivery of extended legs or arms and the head.

Breech extraction

This is a manipulative delivery carried out by an obstetrician and is performed to hasten the birth in an emergency situation such as fetal compromise.

Management of the birth

Breech births can be as normal as any other vaginal birth and a woman who has chosen to birth vaginally needs support from skilled and confident midwives. An explanation is given to the woman so that she can understand the importance of not pushing until full dilatation of her cervix has been confirmed. The midwife should also discuss with the woman beforehand the possibility of the need for other skilled attendants at the birth.

The woman is encouraged to push with the contractions and the buttocks are born spontaneously. If the legs are flexed, the feet disengage at the vulva and the baby is born as far as the umbilicus. A loop of cord is gently pulled down to avoid traction on the umbilicus. Spasm of the cord vessels can be caused by manipulating the cord or by stretching it. If the cord is being nipped behind the pubic bone it should be moved to one side. The midwife should feel for the elbows, which are usually on the chest. If so, the arms will escape with the next contraction. If the arms are not felt, they are extended.

If an obstetrician is assisting the birth the woman may be placed in the lithotomy position when the buttocks are distending the perineum, and the vulva swabbed and draped with sterile towels. The bladder must be empty and it is usually catheterized at this stage. If epidural analgesia is not being used, the perineum is infiltrated with up to 10 mL of 0.5% plain lignocaine prior to an episiotomy being performed. (Pudendal block is sometimes used by a doctor.)

Birth of the shoulders

The uterine contractions and the weight of the body will bring the shoulders down on to the pelvic floor where they will rotate into the anteroposterior diameter of the outlet.

It is helpful to wrap a small towel around the baby's hips, which preserves warmth and improves the grip on the slippery skin. The midwife now grasps the baby by the iliac crests with her thumbs held parallel over his sacrum and tilts the baby towards the maternal sacrum in order to free the anterior shoulder.

When the anterior shoulder has escaped, the buttocks are lifted towards the mother's abdomen to enable the posterior shoulder and arm to pass over the perineum (Fig. 31.49). As the shoulders are born, the head enters the pelvic brim and descends through the pelvis with the sagittal suture in the transverse diameter. The back must remain lateral until this has happened but will afterwards be

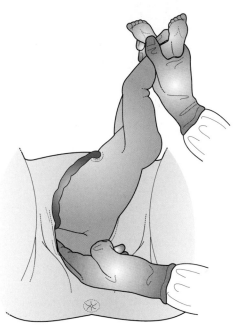

Figure 31.49 Delivery of the posterior shoulder in a breech presentation.

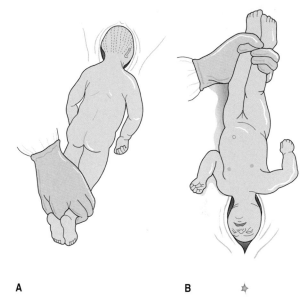

A   B

Figure 31.50 Burns Marshall method of delivering the after-coming head of a breech presentation: (A) The baby is grasped by the feet and held on the stretch. (B) The mouth and nose are free. The vault of the head is delivered slowly.

turned uppermost. If the back is turned upwards too soon, the anteroposterior diameter of the head will enter the anteroposterior diameter of the brim and may become extended. The shoulders may then become impacted at the outlet and the extended head may cause difficulty.

Birth of the head

When the back has been turned the infant is allowed to hang from the vulva without support. The baby's weight brings the head onto the pelvic floor on which the occiput rotates forwards. The sagittal suture is now in the anteroposterior diameter of the outlet. If rotation of the head fails to take place, two fingers should be placed on the malar bones and the head rotated. The baby can be allowed to hang for 1 or 2 min. Gradually the neck elongates, the hair-line appears and the suboccipital region can be felt. Controlled birth of the head is vital to avoid any sudden change in intracranial pressure and subsequent cerebral haemorrhage. There are three methods used.

Forceps delivery. Most breech deliveries are performed by an obstetrician, who will apply forceps to the after-coming head to achieve a controlled birth.

Burns Marshall method can be undertaken once the nape of the neck and hairline are visible. The midwife or doctor stands facing away from the mother and, with the left hand, grasps the baby's ankles from behind with forefinger between the two (Fig. 31.50A). The baby is kept on the stretch with sufficient traction to prevent the neck from bending backwards and being fractured. The suboccipital region, and not the neck, should pivot under the apex of the pubic arch or the spinal cord may be crushed. The feet are taken up through an arc of 180° until the mouth and nose are free at the vulva. The right hand may guard the perineum in order to prevent sudden escape of the head. An assistant may now clear the airway and the baby will breathe. The mother should be asked to take deliberate, regular breaths which allow the vault of the skull to escape gradually, taking 2 or 3 min (Fig. 31.50B).

Mauriceau–Smellie–Veit manoeuvre (jaw flexion and shoulder traction; Fig. 31.51). This is mainly used when there is delay in descent of the head because of extension.

The baby is laid astride the arm with the palm supporting the chest (Fig. 31.51A). One finger is placed

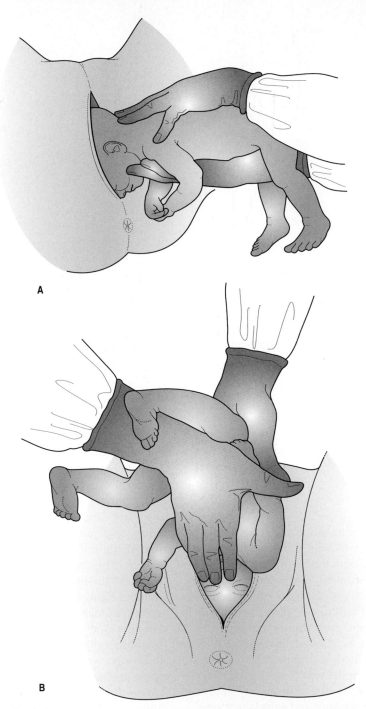

Figure 31.51   Mauriceau–Smellie–Veit manoeuvre for delivering the after-coming head of breech presentation: (A) The hands are in position before the body is lifted. (B) Extraction of the head.

on each malar or cheek bone to flex the head. The middle finger may be used to apply pressure to the chin. Two fingers of the operator's other hand are hooked over the shoulders with the middle finger pushing up the occiput to aid flexion. Suprapubic pressure applied by an assistant may be helpful at this point to increase flexion. Traction is applied to draw the head out of the vagina and, when the sub-occipital region appears, the body is lifted to assist the head to pivot around the symphysis pubis (Fig. 31.51B). The speed of birth of the head must be controlled so that it does not emerge suddenly like a cork popping out of a bottle. Once the face is free, the airways may be cleared and the vault is delivered slowly.

Alternative positions

When the woman has chosen to deliver in an alternative position, it is the upright or supported squat that is the most suitable. The techniques described above will be adapted accordingly and the midwife will observe and encourage the spontaneous mechanism of birth.

Use of uterotonics for third stage

These are withheld until the head is completely born.

Delivery of extended legs

The frank breech descends more rapidly during the first stage of labour. The cervix dilates more quickly and there is a risk of the cord becoming compressed between the legs and the body. Cord prolapse is less likely than in other breech presentations because the frank breech is a better-fitting presenting part. Delay may occur at the outlet because the legs splint the body and impede lateral flexion of the spine.

The baby can be born with legs extended but assistance is usually required. When the popliteal fossae appear at the vulva, two fingers are placed along the length of one thigh with the fingertips in the fossa. The leg is swept to the side of the abdomen (abducting the hip) and the knee is flexed by the pressure on its under surface. As this movement is continued the lower part of the leg will emerge from the vagina (Fig. 31.52). This process should be repeated in order to deliver the second leg. The knee is a hinge joint, which bends in one direction only.

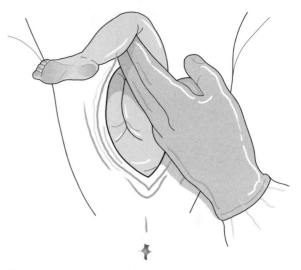

Figure 31.52   Assisting delivery of extended leg by pressure on popliteal fossa.

If the knee is pulled forwards from the abdomen, severe injury to the joint can result.

Delivery of extended arms

Extended arms are diagnosed when the elbows are not felt on the chest after the umbilicus is born. Prompt action must be taken to avoid delay and consequent hypoxia. This may be dealt with by using the Løvset manoeuvre (Figs 31.53, 31.54). This is a combination of rotation and downward traction that may be employed to deliver the arms whatever

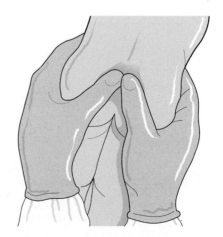

Figure 31.53   Correct grasp for Løvset manoeuvre.

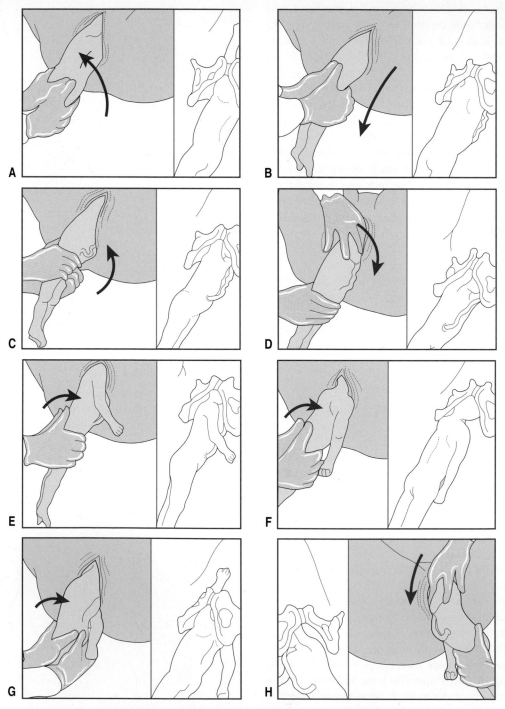

Figure 31.54 Løvset manoeuvre for delivery of extended arms.

position they are in. The direction of rotation must always bring the back uppermost and the arms are delivered from under the pubic arch.

When the umbilicus is born and the shoulders are in the anteroposterior diameter, the baby is grasped by the iliac crests with the thumbs over the sacrum. Downward traction is applied until the axilla is visible.

Maintaining downward traction throughout, the body is rotated through half a circle, 180°, starting by turning the back uppermost. The friction of the posterior arm against the pubic bone as the shoulder becomes anterior sweeps the arm in front of the face. The movement allows the shoulders to enter the pelvis in the transverse diameter.

The arm which is now anterior is delivered. The first two fingers of the hand that is on the same side as the baby's back are used to splint the humerus and draw it down over the chest as the elbow is flexed.

The body is now rotated back in the opposite direction and the second arm delivered in a similar fashion.

Delay in birth of the head

Extended head. If, when the body has been allowed to hang, the neck and hair-line are not visible, it is probable that the head is extended. This may be dealt with by the use of forceps or the Mauriceau–Smellie–Veit manoeuvre. If the head is trapped in an incompletely dilated cervix, an air channel can be created to enable the baby to breathe pending intervention. This is done by inserting two fingers or a Sim's speculum in front of the baby's face and holding the vaginal wall away from the nose. Moisture is mopped away and the airways are cleared. Attempts to release the head from the cervix result in high fetal morbidity and mortality. The McRoberts manoeuvre has been suggested as a method to facilitate the release of the fetal head (Shushan & Younis 1992). The McRoberts manoeuvre requires the woman to lie flat on her back and bring her knees up to her abdomen with hips abducted. This manoeuvre, more commonly used to relieve shoulder dystocia, is described in detail in Ch. 33.

Posterior rotation of the occiput. This malrotation of the head is rare and is usually the result of mismanagement,

for the back should be turned upwards after the shoulders are born.

To assist birth of the head with the occiput posterior, the chin and face are permitted to escape under the symphysis pubis as far as the root of the nose and the baby is then lifted up towards the mother's abdomen to allow the occiput to sweep the perineum.

Complications

Apart from those difficulties already mentioned, other complications can arise, most of which affect the fetus. Many of these can be avoided by allowing only an experienced operator, or a closely supervised learner, to assist the birth.

Impacted breech

Labour becomes obstructed when the fetus is disproportionately large for the size of the maternal pelvis.

Cord prolapse

This is more common in a flexed or footling breech, as these have ill-fitting presenting parts (see Ch. 33).

Birth injury

Superficial tissue damage

The midwife must warn the mother and her partner of the bruising that may be expected during birth. Oedema and bruising of the baby's genitalia may be caused by pressure on the cervix. In a footling breech a prolapsed foot that lies in the vagina or at the vulva for a long time may become very oedematous and discoloured.

If assisting the birth is performed correctly the following are less likely to occur:

Fractures of humerus, clavicle or femur or dislocation of shoulder or hip

These can be caused during manipulation of extended arms or legs.

Erb's palsy

This can be caused when the brachial plexus is damaged. The brachial plexus can be damaged by twisting the baby's neck (see Plate 31).

Trauma to internal organs

A ruptured liver or spleen, may be produced by grasping the abdomen.

Damage to the adrenals

This can be caused by grasping the baby's abdomen, leading to shock caused by adrenaline release.

Spinal cord damage or fracture of the spine

This can be caused by bending the body backwards over the symphysis pubis while assisting birth of the head.

Intracranial haemorrhage

This may be caused by rapid birth of the head, which has had no opportunity to mould. *Hypoxia* may also cause intracranial haemorrhage.

Fetal hypoxia

This may be due to cord prolapse or cord compression or to premature separation of the placenta.

Premature separation of the placenta

Considerable retraction of the uterus takes place while the head is still in the vagina and the placenta begins to separate. Excessive delay in birth of the head may cause severe hypoxia in the fetus.

Maternal trauma

The maternal complications of a breech delivery are the same as found in other operative vaginal deliveries (see Ch. 32).

Shoulder presentation

When the fetus lies with its long axis across the long axis of the uterus (*transverse lie*) the shoulder is most likely to present. Occasionally the lie is oblique but this does not persist as the uterine contractions during labour make it longitudinal or transverse.

Shoulder presentation occurs in approximately 1:300 pregnancies near term. Only 17% of these cases remain as a transverse lie at the onset of labour; the majority are multigravidae (Gimovsky & Hennigan 1995). The head lies on one side of the abdomen, with the breech at a slightly higher level on the other. The fetal back may be anterior or posterior (Figs 31.55, 31.56).

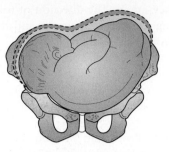

Figure 31.55 Shoulder presentation, dorsoanterior.

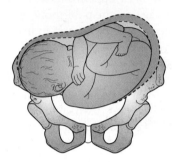

Figure 31.56 Shoulder presentation, dorsoposterior.

Causes

Maternal

Before term, transverse or oblique lie may be transitory, related to maternal position or displacement of the presenting part by an overextended bladder prior to ultrasound examination. Other causes are described below.

Lax abdominal and uterine muscles

This is the most common cause and is found in multigravidae, particularly those of high parity.

Uterine abnormality

A bicornuate or subseptate uterus may result in a transverse lie – as, more rarely, may a cervical or low uterine fibroid.

Contracted pelvis

Rarely, this may prevent the head from entering the pelvic brim.

Fetal

Pre-term pregnancy

The amount of amniotic fluid in relation to the fetus is greater, allowing the fetus more mobility than at term.

Multiple pregnancy

There is a possibility of polyhydramnios but the presence of more than one fetus reduces the room for manoeuvre when amounts of liquor are normal. It is the second twin that more commonly adopts this lie after birth of the first baby.

Polyhydramnios

The distended uterus is globular and the fetus can move freely in the excessive liquor.

Macerated fetus

Lack of muscle tone causes the fetus to slump down into the lower pole of the uterus.

Placenta praevia

This may prevent the head from entering the pelvic brim.

Antenatal diagnosis

On abdominal palpation

The uterus appears broad and the fundal height is less than expected for the period of gestation. On pelvic and fundal palpation, neither head nor breech is felt. The mobile head is found on one side of the abdomen and the breech at a slightly higher level on the other.

Ultrasound

An ultrasound scan may be used to confirm the lie and presentation.

Intrapartum diagnosis

On abdominal palpation

The findings are as above but when the membranes have ruptured the irregular outline of the uterus is more marked. If the uterus is contracting strongly and becomes moulded around the fetus, palpation is very difficult. The pelvis is no longer empty, the shoulder being wedged into it.

On vaginal examination

This should not be performed without first excluding placenta praevia. In early labour, the presenting part may not be felt. The membranes usually rupture early because of the ill-fitting presenting part, with a high risk of cord prolapse.

If the labour has been in progress for some time the shoulder may be felt as a soft irregular mass. It is sometimes possible to palpate the ribs, their characteristic grid-iron pattern being diagnostic (Fig. 31.57). When the shoulder enters the pelvic brim an arm may prolapse; this should be differentiated from a leg. The hand is not at right angles to the arm, the fingers are longer than toes and of unequal length and the thumb can be opposed. No os calcis can be felt and the palm is shorter than the sole. If the arm is flexed, an elbow feels sharper than a knee.

Possible outcome

There is no mechanism for delivery of a shoulder presentation. If this persists in labour, delivery must be by caesarean section to avoid obstructed labour and subsequent uterine rupture (see Ch. 33).

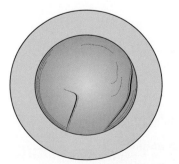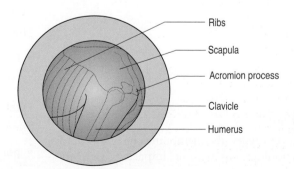

Ribs
Scapula
Acromion process
Clavicle
Humerus

Figure 31.57 Vaginal touch picture of shoulder presentation.

Whenever the midwife detects a transverse lie she must obtain medical assistance.

Management

Antenatal

A cause must be sought before deciding on a course of management. Ultrasound examination can detect placenta praevia or uterine abnormalities, while X-ray pelvimetry will demonstrate a contracted pelvis (see Ch. 8). Any of these causes requires elective caesarean section. Once they have been excluded, ECV may be attempted. If this fails, or if the lie is again transverse at the next antenatal visit, the woman is admitted to hospital while further investigations into the cause are made. She frequently remains there until labour because of the risk of cord prolapse if the membranes rupture.

Intrapartum

If a transverse lie is detected in early labour while the membranes are still intact, the doctor may attempt an ECV, followed, if this is successful, by a controlled rupture of the membranes. (This may be considered before labour in some cases (Hofmeyr & Hutton 2006). If the membranes have already ruptured spontaneously, a vaginal examination must be performed immediately to detect possible cord prolapse.

Immediate caesarean section must be performed:

* if the cord prolapses
* when the membranes are already ruptured
* when ECV is unsuccessful
* when labour has already been in progress for some hours.

Complications

Prolapsed cord

This may occur when the membranes rupture (see Ch. 33).

Prolapsed arm

This may occur when the membranes have ruptured and the shoulder has become impacted. Delivery should be by immediate caesarean section.

Neglected shoulder presentation

The shoulder becomes impacted, having been forced down and wedged into the pelvic brim. The membranes have ruptured spontaneously and if the arm has prolapsed it becomes blue and oedematous. The uterus goes into a state of tonic contraction, the overstretched lower segment is tender to touch and the fetal heartbeat may be absent. All the maternal signs of obstructed labour are present (see Ch. 30) and the outcome, if not treated in time, is a ruptured uterus and a stillbirth.

With adequate supervision both antenatally and during labour this should never occur.

Treatment

An immediate caesarean section is performed under general anaesthetic regardless of whether the fetus is alive or dead, as attempts at manipulative procedures or destructive operations can be dangerous for the mother and may result in uterine rupture.

Unstable lie

The lie is defined as *unstable* when after 36 weeks' gestation, instead of remaining longitudinal, it varies from one examination to another between longitudinal and oblique or transverse.

Causes

Any condition in late pregnancy that increases the mobility of the fetus or prevents the head from entering the pelvic brim may cause this.

Maternal

These include:

* lax uterine muscles in multigravidae
* contracted pelvis.

Fetal

These include:

* polyhydramnios
* placenta praevia.

Management

Antenatal

It may be advisable for the woman to be admitted to hospital to avoid unsupervised onset of labour with a transverse lie. An alternative is for the woman to admit herself to the labour ward as soon as labour commences. The risk associated with the possibility of rupture of membranes and cord prolapse should be emphasized if the mother chooses to remain at home.

Ultrasonography is used to rule out placenta praevia. Attempts will be made to correct the abnormal presentation by ECV. If unsuccessful, caesarean section is considered.

Intrapartum

Many obstetricians induce labour after 38 weeks' gestation, having first ensured that the lie is longitudinal; the induction may be performed by commencing an intravenous infusion of oxytocin to stimulate contractions. A controlled rupture of the membranes is performed so that the head enters the pelvis.

The midwife should ensure that the woman has an empty rectum and bladder before the procedure, as a loaded rectum or full bladder can prevent the presenting part from entering the pelvis. She should palpate the abdomen at frequent intervals to ensure that the lie remains longitudinal and to assess the descent of the head. Labour is regarded as a trial (see Ch. 30).

Complications

If labour commences with the lie other than longitudinal, the complications are the same as for a transverse lie.

Compound presentation

When a hand, or occasionally a foot, lies alongside the head, the presentation is said to be *compound*. This tends to occur with a small fetus or roomy pelvis and seldom is difficulty encountered except in cases where it is associated with a flat pelvis. On rare occasions the head, hand and foot are felt in the vagina – a serious situation that may occur with a dead fetus.

If diagnosed during the first stage of labour, medical aid must be sought. If, during the second stage, the midwife sees a hand presenting alongside the vertex, she could try to hold the hand back.

REFERENCES

Bhal P S, Davies N J, Chung T 1998 A population study of face and brow presentation. Journal of Obstetrics and Gynaecology 18(3):231–235

Cardini F, Lombardo P, Regalia A L 2005 A randomised controlled trial of moxibustion for breech presentation. British Journal of Obstetrics and Gynecology 112(6):743–747

CESDI (Confidential enquiry into stillbirths and deaths in infancy) 2000 7th Annual Report. Maternal and Child Health Research Consortium, London

El Halta 1998 Preventing prolonged labour. Midwifery Today 46:22–27

Flamm B L, Fried M, Lonky N M et al 1991 External cephalic version after previous cesarean section. American Journal of Obstetrics and Gynecology 165(2):370–372

Gimovsky M, Hennigan C 1995 Abnormal fetal presentations. Current Opinion in Obstetrics and Gynecology 7(6): 482–485

Hannah W J 1994 The Canadian consensus on breech management at term. Society of Obstetricians and Gynaecologists of Canada policy statement. Journal of the Society of Obstetricians and Gynaecologists of Canada 16(6): 1839–1848

Hannah M E, Hannah W J, Hewson S A et al 2000 Term Breech Trial Collaborative group. Planned cesarean section versus planned vaginal birth for breech presentation at term: a randomized multicentre trial. Lancet 356(9239):1375–1383

Hannah M E, Whyte H, Hannah W J 2004 Maternal outcomes at 2 years after planned caesarean section versus planned vaginal delivery for breech presentation at term: the international randomized term breech trial. American Journal of Obstetrics and Gynecology 191(3):917–p927

Hofmeyr G J, Hutton E K 2006 External cephalic version for breech presentation before term Cochrane Database of Systematic Reviews, Issue 1

Hofmeyr G J, Kulier R 2005 Hands/knees posture in late pregnancy or labour for fetal malposition (lateral or posterior). Cochrane Database of Systematic Reviews, Issue 2

Kariminia A, Chamberlain M E, Keogh J 2004 Randomised controlled trial of effect of hands and knees posturing on incidence of occiput posterior position at birth. British Medical Journal 328(7438):490–493

MIDIRS 2007 Informed choice for professionals. Number 9 breech presentation – options for care. MIDIRS and The NHS Centre for Reviews and Dissemination, Bristol

Neri I, Airola G, Contu G 2004 Acupuncture plus moxibustion to resolve breech presentation: a randomized controlled study. Journal of Maternal–Fetal and Neonatal Medicine 15(4):247–252

Neuman M, Beller U, Lavie O 1994 Intrapartum bimanual tocolytic-assisted reversal of face presentation: preliminary report. Obstetrics and Gynecology 84(10):146–148

Pearl M L, Roberts J M, Laros R K et al 1993 Vaginal delivery from the persistent occiput posterior position. Influence on maternal and neonatal morbidity. Journal of Reproductive Medicine 38(12):955–961

RCOG (Royal College of Obstetricians and Gynaecologists) 1993 Effective procedures in obstetrics suitable for audit. Medical Audit Unit, RCOG, Manchester, p 2

Shushan A, Younis J S 1992 McRoberts maneuver for the management of the aftercoming head in breech delivery. Gynecologic and Obstetric Investigation 34(3):188–189

Sutton J 1996 Birth: medical emergency or engineering miracle? A midwifery approach to keeping birth normal. MIDIRS Digest 6(2):170–173

Thornton J G, Lilford R J 1994 Active management of labour: current knowledge and research issues. British Medical Journal 309(6951):366–369

Zhang J, Bowes W A, Fortney J A 1993 Efficacy of external cephalic version: a review. Obstetrics and Gynecology 82(2):306–312

FURTHER READING

American College of Obstetricians and Gynecologists 2006 Mode of term singleton breech delivery. Obstetrics and Gynecology 108(1):235–237

This publication suggests that planned vaginal birth of a term singleton breech fetus may be reasonable under hospital-specific protocol guidelines for both eligibility and labour management. It states that the patient's informed consent should be documented.

Ben-Arie A, Kogan S, Schachter M 1995 The impact of external cephalic version on the rate of vaginal and cesarean breech deliveries: a 3-year cumulative experience. European Journal of Obstetrics and Gynecology and Reproductive Biology 63(2):125–129

This paper remains relevant to current practice, an interesting European perspective on the experience of ECV and breech deliveries.

CESDI (Confidential enquiry into stillbirths and deaths in infancy) 2000 7th Annual Report. Maternal and Child Health Research Consortium, London

The 7th CESDI report focuses on breech presentation at the onset of labour. Recommendations for management of breech presentation and training of staff should be read in full.

Chapman K 2000 Aetiology and management of the secondary brow. Journal of Obstetrics and Gynaecology 20:(1)39–44

Six cases of vaginal birth from a brow presentation over a career of 39 years are recorded in this article. Most midwives will never see a brow presentation birth vaginally; this is a fascinating record from a long career.

Gardberg M, Tuppurainen M 1994 Anterior placental location predisposes for occiput posterior presentation near term. Acta Obstetrica et Gynecologica Scandinavica 73(2):151–152

In a series of 325 ultrasound examinations the authors demonstrated an association between an anteriorly situated placenta and OP position after 36 weeks of pregnancy.

Gardberg M, Laakkonen E, Salevaara M 1998 Intrapartum sonography and persistent occiput posterior position: a study of 408 deliveries. Obstetrics and Gynecology 91(5):1746–1749

This study showed that in most cases occipitoposterior position develops through a malrotation and only one-third through absence of rotation from an initially occiput posterior position.

Hofmeyr G J, Impey L W M 2006 The management of breech presentation. Royal College of Obstetricians and Gynaecologists, London

Updated comprehensive obstetric guidelines for the management of breech presentation covering: reducing of the incidence of breech presentation, including external cephalic version; elective caesarean section versus planned vaginal breech delivery at term, including intrapartum management and training needs; and management of the preterm breech and twin breech.

Nassar N, Roberts C L, Raynes-Greenow C H et al 2007 Development and pilot-testing of a decision aid for women with a breech-presenting baby. Midwifery 23(1):38–47

This article highlights the importance of giving women sound information. The decision aid described was an effective and acceptable tool for pregnant women that provided an important adjunct to standard counselling for the management of breech presentation.

Waites B 2003 Breech birth. Free Association Books, London

A clearly written comprehensive guide suitable for professionals and pregnant women

32 Assisted births

Adela Hamilton

CHAPTER CONTENTS

This chapter describes alternative methods of delivery that are used when the mother is unable to give birth without medical or surgical assistance. The role of the midwife will be explored and the importance of providing complete and comprehensive information to the woman will be emphasized.

The chapter aims to:

- identify the midwifery care in relation to preparation for assisted (ventouse/forceps) and caesarean section birth
- describe the role of the midwife in relation to such issues as informed consent and prevention of complications following assisted birth
- consider the various techniques used for assisted (ventouse/forceps) and caesarean section birth, and the skills required by the midwife to improve the experience of this, both for the mother and her partner
- discuss the changing role of the midwife in relation to medical intervention and such issues as the midwife ventouse practitioner and rising caesarean section rates.

Assisting birth

Assisted vaginal birth is a frequently and widely practiced intervention in maternity settings. This accounts for 11% of births in the UK (DH 2004). Stephenson (1992) reports that assisted vaginal delivery may be carried out as frequently as 15% in Australia and Canada. The discrepancy between the reported rates may be due to the variation in the management of birth. Johanson & Menon (1999) say that, in general, maternal outcomes would be improved by lowering instrumental birth rates. Women who use epidural as a form of pain relief are at increased risk of having an instrumental assisted birth (Anim-Somuah et al 2007).

Birth by ventouse

The ventouse is used more commonly than forceps in northern Europe and in Africa. The vacuum extractor is an instrument that applies traction. It can be used as an alternative to forceps. The cup cleaves to the baby's scalp by suction and is used to assist maternal effort.

The use of the ventouse

The ventouse may be used when there is a delay in labour and as with forceps, the ventouse should be applied when the head is engaged and there is no cephalopelvic disproportion. It may be useful in the case of a second twin, when the head remains relatively high. It may be safer and simpler to use the ventouse in this event than forceps.

The ventouse has become more frequently employed by obstetricians due to its apparent increased safety and ease of use, when compared with forceps (Evans & Edelstone 2000). However, evidence shows similar degrees of complications resulting from ventouse births as compared with those where forceps are employed (Johanson et al 1995). Johanson & Menon (1999) conclude that the vacuum extractor is significantly less likely to achieve a successful vaginal delivery than forceps. Nevertheless, it is associated with lower caesarean section rate. Although the ventouse is associated with more cephalohaematoma, other facial and cranial injuries are more common with forceps.

Application of the cup

For successful use of the ventouse, it is essential to determine the whereabouts of the flexion point (Evans & Edelstone 2000). This point lies on the sagittal suture, about 3 cm anterior to the posterior fontanelle and 6 cm posterior to the anterior fontanelle. The cup is positioned over the sagittal suture. If this imperative is not respected, this will not allow flexion of the head and may even cause deflexion of

the head, which may impede the birth. The vacuum within the cup will be achieved more readily in this way. It is important that the midwife has an understanding of this principle, as it is frequently the midwife who is called upon to manage the vacuum.

Soft and rigid vacuum extractor cups

The metal cups used are the Bird variety (Johanson & Menon 1999), or the Malstrom type (Evans & Edelstone 2000) and have a central traction chain and a vacuum conduit. These come in 4, 5 and 6 cm diameters. The preferred new silicone rubber cup is shaped to the contour of the baby's head. This allows the cup to be placed further back on the baby's head to increase flexion, reduce the diameter of the head and facilitate delivery (Fig. 32.1).

The advantage of the new malleable silicone cup is that it effects much less of a 'chignon' on the baby's scalp (Miller & Hanretty 1997). Soft cups have a poorer success rate than metal cups, but are less likely to be associated with scalp trauma. Most of the research shows that the two main outcomes, the occurrence of trauma and the likelihood of vaginal delivery, have been well investigated. However, many studies have not considered other important maternal consequences such as the pain experienced, satisfaction or the mother's anxiety about the baby (Johanson & Menon 1999).

Procedure

The woman is usually in the lithotomy position and the same precautions are observed as for a forceps birth. Local anaesthesia may be used or inhalational analgesia may be sufficient. Pudendal nerve block may be employed or epidural, if already in situ, may be topped up. Episiotomy is not routinely carried out.

The procedure is explained and consent obtained; then adequate analgesia is assured and the bladder is emptied. The fetal heart rate is recorded regularly. The cup of the ventouse is placed as near as possible to, or on, the flexing point of the fetal head. The vacuum in the cup is increased gradually so as to achieve a close application of this to the fetal head. Usually a vacuum of $0.8 \, \text{kg/cm}^2$ is reached, by an increase of $0.2 \, \text{kg/cm}^2$ in stages, or an increase from 0.2 to $0.8 \, \text{kg/cm}^2$ is achieved directly. When the

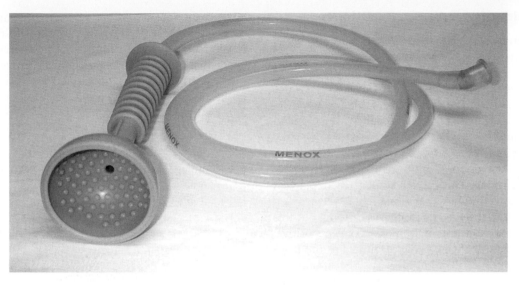

Figure 32.1 The soft cup ventouse.

vacuum is achieved, traction is applied with a contraction, with maternal effort, in an attempt to involve and include the woman in the birth. This traction is done in a downwards and backwards direction, then in a forwards and upwards manner, thus following the curve of Carus. The vacuum is released and the cup then removed at the crowning of the fetal head. The mother can then push the baby for the final part of the birth, thus involving her in this and giving the mother the opportunity to participate. This will result in a more satisfactory experience for the mother and the father.

Precautions in use

These include the following:

- Care should be taken to ensure that no vaginal skin is trapped in the edges of the cup
- Prolonged or excessive traction should not be used.

A useful mnemonic (AAFP 2000) is:

- Ask for help, Address the client, Adequate anaesthesia
- Bladder empty
- Cervix must be completely dilated
- Determine the position of the fetus
- Equipment and extractor ready

- Fontanelle, apply the cup over the sagittal suture [for forceps birth: Forceps ready (lubricate)]
- Gentle traction at right angles to the plane of the cup
- Halt traction and reduce the pressure, repeat the cycle with the next contraction [for forceps birth: Handle elevated]
- Incision, of episiotomy, if necessary
- Jaw is reachable, so, remove the vacuum cup [for forceps birth: remove forceps before head is out to decrease tension].

Complications

As the vacuum actually works by raising an artificial caput succedaneum, it is not logical to then say that caput is a complication of this intervention, as the aim is to form a chignon. However, prolonged traction will increase the likelihood of scalp abrasions, cephalohaematoma or subaponeurotic bleeding (Miller & Hanretty 1997).

Failure of the ventouse may arise in as much as 20% of cases (Drife 1996). This is more likely in the presence of excessive caput, and in the hands of less experienced practitioners. The role of the midwife is to improve the overall efficiency of the manoeuvre, and to support the mother and her partner.

The midwife ventouse practitioner

Some midwives feel that women will be better served by the midwife ventouse practitioner and embrace such innovations, whereas others see it as exceeding the limits of normal midwifery practice (Charles 1999). The fact is that, with the advancement of midwife-led care and the increased demand for less interference in the birth process and also the development of consultant midwives and other resource key persons, midwifery care is changing and developing. There was a similar reaction when midwives commenced suturing, and yet women have been well served by midwives carrying out this activity. The response of women has been positive, with continuity of care being confirmed as the main advantage (Mulholland 1997).

One advantage of the midwife ventouse practitioner role is that women are not traumatized by a change of carer as the midwife is able to provide the panoply of care required by the woman, and this at a very crucial and critical moment. Midwife ventouse practitioners must be well educated and trained before carrying out this procedure. There is more likelihood of the indication being maternal fatigue than for any other reason. Midwives in developing countries and in a few birth centres in the UK are already familiar with this technique.

Birth by forceps

Forceps are most commonly employed to expedite delivery of the fetal head or to protect the fetus or the mother, or both, from trauma and exhaustion. They are also used to assist the delivery of the after-coming head of the breech or to draw the head of the baby up and out of the pelvis at caesarean section birth.

Characteristics of obstetric forceps

Obstetric forceps are composed of two separate blades; a right and a left, and are identified on these as such. The forceps are inserted separately on each side of the head. The forceps are locked together by either an English or a Smellie lock. Rotational forceps have a sliding lock. The blades are spoon shaped (cephalic curve) to accommodate the form of the baby's head and are fenestrated to minimize trauma to the baby's head. In most modern obstetric forceps, the blade is attached to the handle at an angle that corresponds to the pelvic curve. When the blades are correctly positioned the handles will be neatly aligned in the hands of the doctor who applies them.

Classification of obstetric forceps

Forceps operations fall into two categories: low and mid-cavity. Low-cavity forceps are used when the head has reached the pelvic floor and is visible at the vulva. Mid-cavity forceps are used when the head is engaged and the leading part is below the level of the ischial spines. High-cavity forceps are now considered unsafe and a caesarean section will be carried out.

Types of obstetric forceps

Forceps are often described as non-rotational or rotational (Fig. 32.2). Adequate analgesia is required prior to their application to the fetal head.

Wrigley's forceps

These are designed for use when the head is on the perineum. This is a short and light type of forceps, with both pelvic and cephalic curves and an English lock. They are also used for the after-coming head of a breech delivery, or at caesarean section.

Neville-Barnes or Simpson's forceps

These are generally used for a low or mid cavity forceps delivery when the sagittal suture is in the anteroposterior diameter of the cavity/outlet of the pelvis. They have cephalic and pelvic curves and the handles are longer and heavier than those of the Wrigley's. Anderson's and Haig-Ferguson's forceps are also similar in shape and size.

Kielland's forceps

These were originally designed to deliver the fetal head at or above the pelvic brim. They are generally used for the rotation and extraction of the head that is arrested in the deep transverse or in the occipito-posterior position. The blades have little pelvic curve and are for traction. The shallow curve allows safe rotation of the forceps in the vagina. Downward traction encourages rotation of the head. The claw

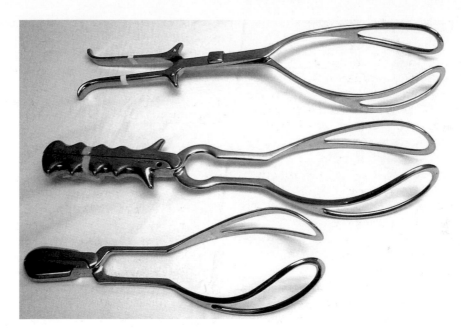

Figure 32.2 Types of forceps. From above: Kielland, Neville-Barnes and Simpson's. Note the difference in cephalic curve. The rotational forceps (Kielland's) have a long shaft and little pelvic curve.

lock allows sliding and corrects asynclitism of the fetal head. These forceps should be used only by an obstetrician skilled in their application and use.

Indications for the use of obstetric forceps

The three main indications for the use of forceps are delay in the second stage of labour, fetal compromise and maternal distress.

Delay in the second stage of labour may be due to:

- insufficient contractions (but this is better corrected by oxytocin infusion)
- epidural analgesia
- malrotation of the head
- maternal fatigue.

Fetal compromise may be due to:

- prematurity
- hypoxia
- intrauterine growth restriction
- a maternal obstetric or medical condition (e.g. pre-eclampsia).

Maternal distress may be caused by:

- hypertension
- cardiac condition
- maternal exhaustion or long labour.

Prerequisites for forceps delivery

(see Mnemonic p. 609)

- *Care of the bladder.* To prevent harm or injury, the bladder must be kept empty
- *Analgesia.* This is generally by epidural or pudendal block plus perineal infiltration of local anaesthetic
- *Information giving and consent.* The couple must be kept informed of the course of events, and must be involved in the decision-making process
- *Paediatrician.* The paediatrician or advanced neonatal practitioner may not be required at birth, but should be kept informed of circumstances
- *Neonatal resuscitation equipment.* This must be checked and prepared in case it becomes necessary.

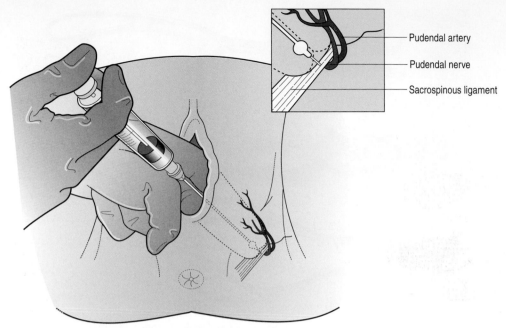

Pudendal artery

Pudendal nerve

Sacrospinous ligament

Figure 32.3 Locating the pudendal nerve.

Pudendal block

This is the infiltration of the area around the pudendal nerve by local anaesthetic. The transvaginal route is used to locate the ischial spine, as the pudendal nerve emerges from vertebrae S2–S4 and crosses this. A particular needle that possesses a ring or guard is employed, called a pudendal block needle. About 10 mL of local anaesthetic, usually 1% lidocaine (lignocaine), is injected into the region just below the ischial spine (Fig. 32.3). Both motor and sensory nerves are affected as both lie in this region. The pudendal nerve supplies the levator ani muscles, also the deep and superficial perineal muscles (Stables & Rankin 2005). It may be used to provide analgesia for the lower vagina and perineum, and is therefore used for forceps and ventouse deliveries. The advantage of this technique is that it does not harm the baby.

Perineal infiltration

A local anaesthetic is used to infiltrate the perineum prior to episiotomy or suturing (see Ch. 28).

Technique

After careful vaginal examination, the presentation and position are identified. There must be no apparent obstruction. The membranes must be ruptured and full dilatation of the cervix must be confirmed. The head must be engaged and there should be no cephalopelvic disproportion. Episiotomy is not routinely carried out but the accoucheur will evaluate whether this accommodates the birth (Figs 32.4–32.7).

Complications

Maternal

Maternal complications include:

- trauma or soft tissue damage, which may occur to the perineum, vagina, or cervix
- haemorrhage from the above
- dysuria or urinary retention, which may result from bruising or oedema to the urethra
- painful perineum
- postnatal morbidity, which is higher in any birth intervention.

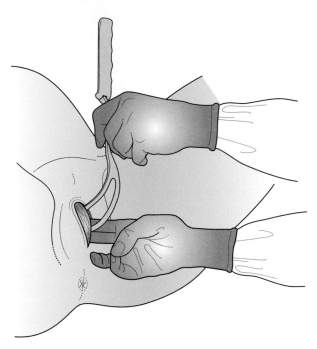

Figure 32.4 Left blade being inserted. The fingers of the right hand guard the vaginal tissue.

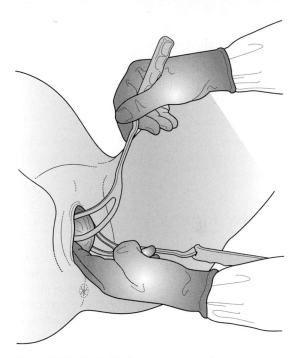

Figure 32.5 Right blade being inserted.

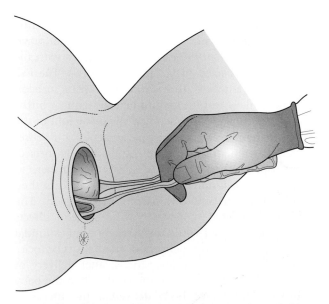

Figure 32.6 Traction of the head is downwards until this point; when the head is low, the direction of pull is outward, towards the operator.

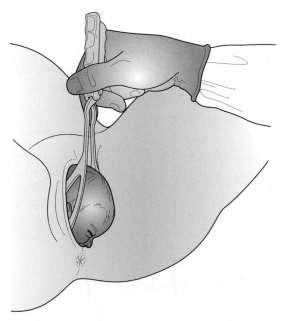

Figure 32.7 As the head crowns it is lifted upwards.

Figures 32.4–32.7 Technique for forceps delivery.

Neonatal

Neonatal complications (see Ch. 45) include:

- marks on the baby's face, which can be caused by the pressure of the forceps, but resolve quite rapidly
- excessive bruising from the forceps
- facial palsy, which may result from pressure from a blade compressing a facial nerve, and is usually temporary.

Symphysiotomy

This is an incision of the fibrocartilage partly through the symphysis pubis and is performed in labour to enlarge the transverse diameter of the pelvis. It is rarely carried out in the UK, but is carried out in countries where the risk of caesarean section is particularly high for the management of cephalopelvic disproportion. A urinary catheter is inserted into the bladder to empty it and to displace the urethra laterally whilst the symphysis is being divided. The fibrocartilage is incised over the centre of the symphysis pubis. A vacuum extractor or forceps may be used to facilitate delivery. Following the operation a bandage is applied around the pelvis to provide support. The catheter may remain in situ for a few days, as oedema is likely.

Caesarean section

Caesarean section is described as being an operative procedure, which is carried out under anaesthesia whereby the fetus, placenta and membranes are delivered through an incision in the abdominal wall and the uterus. This is usually carried out after viability has been reached (i.e. 24 weeks' gestation onwards).

The operative procedure

There are two layers of pelvic peritoneum and the non-gravid uterus is a pelvic organ closely covered by a layer of pelvic peritoneum. As pregnancy advances, the uterus grows up into the abdomen and this peritoneum rises up with the uterus and comes into contact with the abdominal peritoneum. Each of these layers must be incised. The abdominal peritoneum is situated below the abdominal muscle layer.

The anatomical layers are:

- skin
- fat
- rectus sheath
- muscle (rectus abdominis)
- abdominal peritoneum
- pelvic peritoneum
- uterine muscle.

The operation most commonly carried out is the lower uterine segment caesarean section (LSCS). A Pfannenstiel or bikini line incision is usually performed. The lower segment incision is in the less muscular and active part of the uterus and heals better. The main reason for preferring the lower uterine segment technique is the reduced incidence of dehiscence of the uterine scar in subsequent pregnancy. A classical or vertical incision of the uterus may be the only choice in such situations as implantation of the placenta on the lower anterior uterine wall, in the presence of dense adhesions from previous surgery, or in the case of a large fetus with the shoulder impacted in the maternal pelvis. The risk and disadvantage of this is that the uterine incision is more likely to rupture during a subsequent birth.

The abdomen is opened and the loose fold of the peritoneum over the anterior aspect of the lower uterine segment and above the bladder is incised. The operator continues to incise this further, to visualize the fundus of the bladder, which is then pushed down and away from the surgeon. The uterus is incised transversely. The surgeon directs the fetal head out while the assistant applies fundal pressure to help the delivery of the baby. Oxytocics may be given by the anaesthetist after delivery of the baby and clamping of the cord. When the baby and placenta have been delivered, the uterus is sutured. This is usually done in two layers. The peritoneum may then be closed over the uterine wound to exclude it from the peritoneal cavity. The rectus sheath is closed, then the layer of fat and finally the skin is sutured with the surgeon's choice of material; commonly Vicryl, a braided polyglactin preparation, is used for this.

Preparation

Preoperative preparation: an anaesthetic chart/pre-operative assessment, weight and observations of blood pressure, pulse and temperature are undertaken. Gowning and removal of make-up and jewellery (or taping of rings) will be carried out. The woman is visited by the anaesthetist preoperatively, and assessed.

Results of any blood tests that have been requested are obtained and a full blood count is carried out. Blood is grouped and saved. In the case of pre-eclampsia, urea and electrolyte levels will be examined and clotting factors assessed. The woman will have fasted and have taken the prescribed antacid therapy. Attitudes and practices vary regarding pubic shaving.

The woman may prefer to be catheterized in the theatre under epidural, spinal or general anaesthetic, but it may be more private to do this in her room, before entering the operating theatre where others are present.

Positioning of the woman

As the woman will need to lie flat, it is essential that a wedge or cushion is used, or the table is tilted, to direct the weight of the gravid uterus away from the inferior vena cava. Supine hypotensive syndrome is thus avoided.

Caesarean section – some statistics

Internationally, the caesarean section rate is on the increase, with the exception of Norway and Sweden (Chaffer & Royle 2000). The northern European countries have not only the lowest caesarean section rates, but also the lowest perinatal mortality rates.

The results of the National Sentinel Caesarean Section Audit (RCOG 2001) show that caesarean section rates in 2000 were highest in Wales, at 24.2% in 2000 and in Northern Ireland, at 23.9% in 2000–2001. Fear of litigation is thought to be a major contributing factor, but in Canada, where litigation is not widespread, the rates are still rising.

The drive to lower caesarean section rates is economic, but other vital perspectives must be appraised. Chaffer & Royle (2000) state that, by reducing the caesarean section rate by 5%, two to seven maternal deaths could be prevented annually in Britain. The seventh report of the Confidential Enquiries into Maternal Deaths in the UK (Lewis 2007) states that routine use of thromboprophylaxis and antibiotics has reduced deaths from pulmonary embolism and sepsis. However, the report also states that caesarean section is not a risk-free procedure especially in women who are obese.

Women's request for caesarean section

The reasons behind the 'demand' for caesarean section are complex and involved. Accounts of women who have had difficult experiences of childbirth describe knowing something was wrong, and believing they were not listened to. They then go on to request caesarean section for a subsequent birth. Demands therefore stem from previous bad experiences, expressed even as 'nightmare' by some women. There is much evidence to support the fact that very few women actually request caesarean section in the absence of medical indications (Chaffer & Royle 2000, Weaver et al 2001).

Maternal age and caesarean section

There is literature to show that more research is required on obstetrical practices and complications that occur in older women who have had caesarean section, to understand the relationship between these two. It is true that interventions are a consequence of complications (Bell et al 2001), but complications may also result from intervention. The variation in rates of caesarean section between obstetricians and how maternal age affects these requires more consideration.

Other reports show that caesarean section rates rise from teenage years onwards (Marwick & Lynn 2001). These writers state that as findings were particularly uniform, and this from very diverse countries, clinical practice and societal pressures were unlikely to be the cause of the increase in intervention with the increase in maternal age. One paper states that 'concern about complications might be as much of a problem as the complications themselves' (Weaver et al 2001, p 285). The midwife should understand the fears of the childbearing woman, and provide information and support appropriately to disperse these.

Psychological support and the role of the midwife

Choice is an important element in this sequence. One writer makes recommendations following a study on the rise of caesarean section rates, in the attempt to decipher the various reasons why there is such a variation in practice (Chaffer & Royle 2000). Five of the 11 propositions for practice relate to information giving, involvement of the woman in the decision-making process and the provision of consistent advice.

Women expect to be actively involved in their care and the midwife must ensure that recent, valid and relevant information is provided in a straightforward manner for women. This will help women to decide what is best for them, in their circumstances. An informed, confident and competent practitioner will relieve the stress of the situation and help the woman make a decision, supporting her in the midst of her misgivings. The midwife has a pivotal role in giving women clear and unbiased information concerning the choices available (McAleese 2000).

One-to-one care from a support person during labour can influence caesarean section rates (Walker & Golois 2001). It is important that midwives recognize that this is a positive tactic and should value their role and skills. A continual, supportive presence in labour is widely reported as being of considerable benefit. Churchill (1997) states that a friend or partner is appreciated because they are able to act as a mediator on behalf of the woman. They are also able to describe the occurrences and happenings during the operation (Box 32.1, Wendy and Martin's story).

Clarifying the indications for caesarean section

In an effort to try to clarify the precise motive behind women's request for caesarean section, the National Sentinel Caesarean Section Audit (RCOG 2001) formulated the following objectives:

- to determine the frequency of caesarean sections in all maternity units in England and Wales

---

Box 32.1 Wendy and Martin's story

When we came in to have our first baby, we didn't know what to expect (although we had been given lots of information). When you do it for real it's just so different. Things went very quickly. I was quite worried having my epidural. The doctor seemed to take a long time and it was a bit uncomfortable. We got the impression that people thought he was struggling a bit, which doesn't fill you with confidence. Then when they first cut me, I could feel it a bit and got really anxious. Having my husband there all the time helped, and he said a senior doctor was there by then, and he gave me some extra medicine and massaged my head and that was it, I felt much better! We had brought a CD as they said, but we were a bit disappointed that the player was tiny and right down the other end of the room away from my head so that we couldn't hear it. We'd made a special CD, and I had been playing it every night to my baby, so we were used to the sound. Oh well. During the operation we were stuck under a sort of tent, so we couldn't see what was going on. My husband had to really strain to see our baby coming out of me, and no-one asked us if he wanted to cut the cord or anything. But we did feel that everyone was kind to us and looked after us very well. We knew the operation wasn't easy and had taken longer than they thought. We were just so glad that everything went alright in the end, and we have a beautiful healthy son to look after (Fig. 32.8).

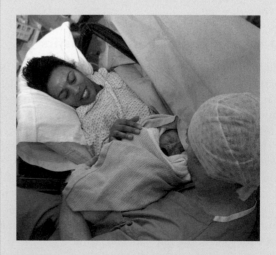

- to determine the factors associated with variations in the rates of caesarean section including maternal request
- to assist in the development of new standards.

The aim of the study was to ascertain the contribution of maternal requests to caesarean section rates and also to interpret the variation of caesarean section rates. There is evidence to support the notion that caesarean section is being used too liberally (Dimond 1999). Many authors state that the number of women who request caesarean section purely for convenience is low (Page 1999, Weaver et al 2001). The same writers observe that, although women are not aware of the morbidity for mother and the baby, they are generally well informed as to the incapacitating consequences of major surgery.

Not all caesarean sections that are non-elective are of an emergency nature. A caesarean section, for example carried out after a few hours of labour when the CTG shows that there may be a degree of fetal compromise present, may be carried out urgently. This will not be an emergency in the strict sense of the word.

Elective caesarean section

This indicates that the decision to carry out the procedure has been taken during the pregnancy, therefore before labour has commenced. If the indication for caesarean section has been a non-recurring one, for example placenta praevia, vaginal birth after caesarean (VBAC) may be attempted. Repeat caesarean section may be indicated in, for example, cephalopelvic disproportion, or on a uterus that has been scarred twice.

Within the umbrella of 'elective' caesarean, there could be merit in re-classification. For example, there are those operations that are truly 'elective' in that they are booked around term at a time convenient for mother and surgeon. The other category includes 'scheduled' caesarean sections when it becomes clear that early delivery is required, but there is no immediate compromise to mother or fetus.

Definite indications

These include:

- cephalopelvic disproportion

- major degree of placenta praevia
- high order multiple pregnancy.

Possible indications

These include:

- breech presentation
- moderate to severe pre-eclampsia
- a medical condition that warrants the exclusion of maternal effort
- diabetes mellitus
- intrauterine growth restriction
- antepartum haemorrhage
- certain fetal abnormalities (e.g. hydrocephalus).

Emergency caesarean section

This is carried out when adverse conditions develop during pregnancy or labour. Standards have been suggested for the maximum time that should elapse from the decision to deliver to the actual time the baby is born. However, this is less straightforward, as in some cases there is a real 'emergency' and everything needs to be in place for immediate delivery of the baby if it is to survive (e.g. cord prolapse with fetal compromise). Then there are other situations where delivery is 'urgent' but more time can be taken to prepare for the operation and proposed actions can be discussed with the parents in a more relaxed manner.

The following are examples of urgent/emergency reasons for caesarean birth:

- antepartum haemorrhage
- cord prolapse
- uterine rupture (dramatic/scar dehiscence)
- cephalopelvic disproportion diagnosed in labour
- fulminating pre-eclampsia
- eclampsia
- failure to progress in the first or second stage of labour
- fetal compromise and birth not imminent.

Vaginal birth after caesarean section

Ziadeh & Sunna (1995) state that widespread adoption of a policy whereby 80% of women with prior caesarean section have a trial of labour could potentially eliminate up to one-third of caesarean sections. Reports state less than a 1% frequency of uterine rupture and no maternal deaths from this cause.

Trial of labour

A trial of labour is carried out whenever there is doubt about the outcome of the labour because of a previous caesarean section. Criteria include:

- after adequate supervision, it is established that the presenting part is capable of flexing adequately to pass through the brim of the pelvis
- all the facilities for assisted birth are readily available
- progress of the labour is sufficient, observed both in the descent of the presenting part and by the dilatation of the cervix
- time limits as to the duration of the trial are set.

Coltart et al (1990) claim that women admitted in active labour have higher vaginal birth rates following caesarean section than those admitted in early labour. Birth weight in previous pregnancies should not exert undue influence on management procedures. Peterson & Saunders (1991) suggest that units allowing longer labours had higher vaginal birth rates following caesarean section. Time limits on the duration of these labours are neither helpful nor reassuring for the woman.

Pare et al (2006) point out that recent arguments about the safety of VBAC have ignored potential downstream consequences of a strategy of multiple elective repeat caesarean sections. These are increased hospital stay, greater risk of placenta praevia and placenta accreta in future pregnancies. They confirmed that for a woman who desires two or more additional children, the risks of multiple caesarean section outweigh the immediate risks of a VBAC attempt. Therefore, for a woman who desires two or more additional children, a VBAC attempt decreases the total number of hysterectomies performed. The decision to carry out an elective caesarean section is complex and the whole clinical picture must be taken into account.

General anaesthesia

Despite the increasing use of regional anaesthesia, general anaesthesia is sometimes required. Regional anaesthesia is incompatible with any maternal coagulation disorder. General anaesthesia can be more rapidly administered, and is of value when speed is important, such as when the fetus is in serious jeopardy (Enkin et al 2000). Women are preoxygenated prior to induction of anaesthesia; that is, they are given oxygen-rich gas mixtures to breathe for several minutes. A muscle relaxant (suxamethonium) is given to allow safe orotracheal intubation; a cuffed tube and cricoid pressure are essential to prevent aspiration of stomach contents. Induction agents include thiopental and propofol. Maternal unconsciousness ensues within seconds. There are minimal side-effects and relatively little negative fetal consequences at the time of birth provided meticulous practices are in place. Regional anaesthesia, however, normally remains the safer option for caesarean birth. Anaesthesia is sustained by inhalational anaesthetic means using Fluothane or Ethrane.

A total of 25 'anaesthetic incidents' were reported in 1998 (CESDI 2000). These fell into three categories, involving:

- serious complications related to giving anaesthetic
- delays with personnel
- delays in the provision of anaesthesia once the anaesthetist was available.

When the midwife recognizes an abnormality she must report it to the appropriate person, giving adequate details, as it is obvious that efficiency and clarity will prevent major incidents from occurring. Speed is essential and the midwife can assist by making sure that optimal care is given and by being an advocate for the mother.

Mendelson's syndrome

This condition was described by Mendelson in 1946 (Stables & Rankin 2005). It is caused if acid gastric contents are inhaled and result in a chemical pneumonitis. This regurgitation may occur during the induction of a general anaesthetic and go unheeded. The acidic gastric contents then damage the alveoli, impairing gaseous exchange. It may become impossible to oxygenate the woman and death may result. The predisposing factors are: the pressure from the gravid uterus when the woman is lying down, the effect of the progesterone relaxing smooth muscle, and the cardiac sphincter of the stomach possibly being relaxed by the effect of the anaesthetic. Analgesics such as pethidine cause significant delay in gastric emptying, thereby exacerbating the above.

Prevention of Mendelson's syndrome

Antacid therapy. Although there are now relatively few cases where general anaesthesia is used for caesarean section, the prevention of Mendelson's syndrome is essential. Prophylactic treatment is given to all women in whom a caesarean is planned or anticipated. A usual regimen is for women having an elective operation to be given two doses of oral ranitidine 150 mg approximately 8 hrs apart, plus 30 mL sodium citrate immediately before transfer to theatre. Women in labour who are thought to have a high risk of caesarean section should have ranitidine 150 mg every 8 hrs. These drugs inhibit the secretion of hydrochloric acid in the stomach.

Cricoid pressure. This is the most important measure in preventing pulmonary aspiration (Enkin et al 2000). The oesophagus is occluded by the use of cricoid pressure. Cricoid pressure is a technique whereby the pressure exerted on the one whole ring of tracheal cartilage, the cricoid cartilage, thus occludes the oesophagus and prevents reflux. Cricoid pressure is maintained by an assistant until the tracheal tube is positioned by the anaesthetist, and the seal of the cuff is verified. The correct use of this manoeuvre is essential in preventing major incidents from occurring (Fig. 32.8).

Difficult or failed intubation

This condition is more likely to occur in pregnant women and particularly with those who have pregnancy-induced hypertension. Laryngeal oedema arises more frequently in these women, therefore anticipation of the disorder is key to its management. If laryngeal oedema is anticipated, a very experienced and well-briefed anaesthetist should carry out the intubation. A well-lubricated stylet or bougie may be used to aid endotracheal intubation. Management of failed intubation is: continued cricoid pressure (but not at the expense of oxygenation) and ventilation by face mask until the effects of suxamethonium and thiopental have worn off (and the woman has regained consciousness and her cough reflex).

Complications

It is suggested that, with the increase in caesarean section rates, there is likely to be a subsequent rise in maternal mortality (Chaffer & Royle 2000, Dimond 1999, Hillan 1995). Morbidity reports reveal that only 9.5% of a sample of women delivered by caesarean section ($n = 619$) had no reported morbidity in the postnatal period (Magill-Cuerden 1996). The evidence suggests that there is also a wide variation in reported morbidity and scanty research on this. Although surgical and anaesthetic techniques have improved, women are still more liable to suffer from complications and to have increased morbidity following caesarean section.

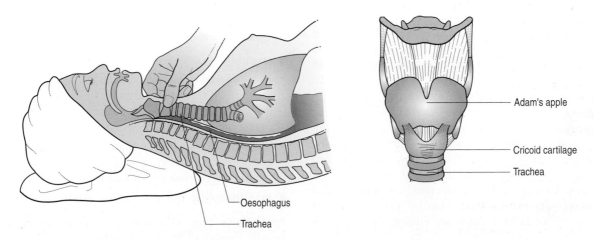

Figure 32.8 Cricoid pressure showing occlusion of the oesophagus by pressure applied to the cricoid cartilage.

Infection

Maternal morbidity following caesarean section has not been studied methodically, but the problem of postoperative infection is considerable (Enkin et al 2000). In one study that considered wound infection (Chaffer & Royle 2000), this was confirmed as being as high as 34%. In the same study, the wound infection rate was even greater, when data covering the first 6 weeks following caesarean section were included. There is now persuasive evidence to indicate that antibiotic prophylaxis markedly reduces the risk of serious postoperative infection such as pelvic abscess, septic shock and septic pelvic vein thrombophlebitis. There is similar evidence to support the fact that women are also safeguarded against endometritis. Protection against wound infection is less sure, but remains considerable (Enkin et al 2000).

Infection is associated with previous rupture of membranes and other factors such as obesity. The prophylactic use of antibiotics was recommended in the 1998 CEMD report (DH 1998) and there is clear evidence showing its benefits, from controlled trials. There is a much greater incidence of infection following emergency caesarean section (Enkin et al 2000, Hillan 1995). The length of stay in hospital prior to operation also influences this incidence. Delaying shaving of the operation site until immediately before operating, ensuring sterilization of all swabs and instruments and a general good sterile and surgical technique would all contribute to a reduction in infection postoperatively.

Urinary tract infection. This was the most consistent of the infectious morbidity described by Hillan's (1995) comprehensive and informative investigation into postoperative morbidity following caesarean section. Urinary tract infection was present in 10.9% of women who had elective and 10.3% of women who had emergency caesarean section. Wound infection rose from 4.1 to 8.3%, intrauterine infection from 1.4 to 6% and chest infection from 0.9 to 5.3%, respectively in elective and emergency caesarean section. Hence the need for attentive and careful observation and care by the midwife of women who have had an emergency caesarean section.

Thromboembolic disorders

These remain the leading direct cause of maternal death, accounting for 41 of the total 132 direct maternal deaths (Lewis 2007). Although there was a small reduction in deaths after caesarean section, further improvements are necessary. Pregnancy and surgery carry increased risks of thromboembolus and the timing of and dose according to body weight of thromboembolic prophylaxis are crucial.

Postoperative care

Immediate care

Observations

The blood pressure, respirations and pulse should be recorded every 15 min in the immediate recovery period. The temperature should be recorded every 2 hrs. The wound must be inspected every 30 min to detect any blood loss. The lochia should also be inspected and drainage should be small initially. Following general anaesthesia the woman is nursed in the left lateral or 'recovery' position until she is fully conscious, since the risks of airway obstruction or regurgitation and silent aspiration of stomach contents are still present.

Analgesia

This is prescribed and is given as required. If the mother intends to breastfeed, the baby should be put to the breast as soon as possible. This can usually be achieved with minimal disturbance to the mother. Postoperative analgesia may be given in a variety of ways:

- an epidural opioid
- rectal analgesia, such as diclofenac (this is contra-indicated if there is continuing bleeding, poor urine output, a history of sensitivity to NSAIDs, or peptic ulcer)
- intramuscular analgesia (though this is never given in conjunction with epidural opioids because of the risk of cumulative effects)
- oral drugs (e.g. dihydrocodeine, paracetamol).

Antiemetics (e.g. cyclizine; prochlorperazine) are usually prescribed by the anaesthetist.

Care following regional block

Following epidural or spinal anaesthesia, the woman may sit up as soon as she wishes, provided her blood pressure is not low. All observations are recorded as described above. Fluids are introduced gradually, followed by a light diet. The intravenous infusion remains in progress for about 12 hrs. Care must be taken to avoid any damage to the legs, which will gradually regain sensation and movement.

As it is possible that an opiate administered via the epidural route may cause some respiratory depression, the woman's respiratory rate must be recorded. This means of pain relief offers the advantage of excellent analgesia without motor block and also seems to give a feeling of well-being. Women are usually able to become mobile very quickly, which reduces the risk of deep venous thrombosis. It is also more conducive to the woman's psychological health.

Ideally, the baby should remain with his mother and they should be transferred to the postnatal ward together once the recovery team says it is safe to do so.

Care in the postnatal ward

On the ward, the blood pressure, temperature respirations and pulse are usually checked every 4 hrs. The intravenous infusion will continue, and the urinary catheter may remain in the bladder until the woman is able to get up to the toilet. The wound and lochia must initially be observed at least hourly. The baby should remain with his mother, and the midwife should offer extra help to ensure that the mother has adequate rest. The mother is encouraged to move her legs and to perform leg and breathing exercises. The physiotherapist will usually teach these and may give chest physiotherapy. Prophylactic low dose heparin and TED antiembolism stockings are often prescribed. The woman is helped to get out of bed as soon as possible following caesarean section, and is encouraged to become fully mobile.

Urinary output must be monitored carefully both before and after removal of the urinary catheter; women may have some difficulty with micturition initially and the bladder may be incompletely emptied. Any haematuria must be reported to the doctor.

Women who have had a general anaesthetic for caesarean section may feel very tired and drowsy for some hours. A woman may complain of a feeling of detachment and unreality and may feel that she does not relate well to the baby. The woman who is concerned should be reassured and be given the opportunity to talk freely.

The mother must be encouraged to rest as much as possible and tactful advice may need to be given to her visitors. If the mother becomes too tired, help is needed with care for the baby. This should preferably take place at the mother's bedside and should include support with breastfeeding. The clip-on cots, which may be attached to the mother's bed can facilitate the handling of baby for the mother (Fig. 32.9).

Some women may have a lingering feeling of failure or disappointment at having had a caesarean section and may value the opportunity to talk this over with the midwife.

Research and the incidence of caesarean section: tackling high and rising caesarean section rates

Low caesarean section rates are associated with low levels of intervention and high levels of psychological support. It is difficult to decipher whether caesarean section rates have been affected by interventions, such as proactive management of labour – that is, artificial rupture of membranes and use of oxytocin – or whether other factors have influenced these. As the protocol of O'Driscoll et al (1993) requires a continuous and supportive presence during labour, this may also have influenced

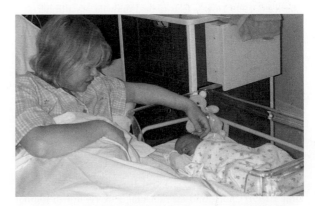

Figure 32.9 Baby in clip-on cot, adjacent to and within easy reach of mother when in bed.

the outcome of the labour and birth; this trial shows an impressive 5% caesarean section rate in Dublin. Other researchers have attempted to interpret these results. Lopez-Zeno et al (1992) did find a significant difference in caesarean section rates between women who were actively managed and those who were not; the actively managed group had much lower caesarean section rates.

The NICE Guidelines (2004) say that the clinical interventions to reduce caesarean section include:

- external cephalic version (ECV) at 36 weeks
- continuous support in labour
- induction of labour for pregnancies beyond 41 weeks
- use of a partogram with a 4 hrs action line in labour
- fetal blood sampling before caesarean section for abnormal cardiotocograph in labour
- support for women who choose vaginal birth after caesarean section.

While there is no accepted optimal rate for caesarean section in the UK, some tertiary units keep their caesarean section rate below 20%. If reductions in the rate are to be achieved, efforts should focus on where there is most potential for reduction: reducing primary caesarean section, particularly in first-time mothers, and increasing rates of VBAC. ECV should be offered to all women with an uncomplicated breech pregnancy at term and vaginal breech birth should be an option for women (MCWP 2006, p 10).

REFERENCES

AAFP (American Academy of Family Physicians) 2000 Advanced life support in obstetrics (ALSO), 4th edn. AAFP, Leawood

Anim-Somuah M, Smyth R, Howell C 2007 Epidural versus non-epidural or no analgesia in labour. The Cochrane Database of Systematic Reviews, Issue 2:CD00031

Bell J S, Campbell D M, Graham W J et al 2001 Do obstetric complications explain high caesarean section among women over 30? British Medical Journal 322:894–895

CESDI (Confidential Enquiry into Stillbirths and Deaths in Infancy) 2000 Seventh annual report, 1 January–31 December 1998. Maternal and Child Health Research Consortium, London, p 1–113

Chaffer D, Royle L 2000 The use of audit to explain the rise in caesarean section. British Journal of Midwifery 8(11):677–684

Charles C 1999 How it feels to be a midwife practitioner. British Journal of Midwifery 7(6):380–382

Churchill H 1997 Caesarean birth experience, practice and history. Books for Midwives Press, Hale

Coltart T, Davies J, Katesmark M 1990 Outcome of second pregnancy after a previous caesarean section. British Journal of Obstetrics and Gynaecology 97:1140–1143

DH (Department of Health) 2004 Statistical Bulletin. Maternity Statistics England 2002–2003. HMSO, London

DH (Department of Health), Welsh Office, Scottish Office Department of Health, Department of Health and Social Services Northern Ireland 1998. Why Mothers Die. Report on Confidential Enquiries into Maternal Deaths in the United Kingdom 1994–1996. Stationery Office, London

Dimond B 1999 Is there a legal right to choose a caesarean? British Journal of Midwifery 7(8):515–518

Drife J 1996 Choice and instrumental delivery. British Journal of Obstetrics and Gynaecology 103:608–611

Enkin M, Keirse M, Neilson J et al 2000 A guide to effective care in pregnancy and childbirth, 3rd edn. Oxford University Press, Oxford

Evans W, Edelstone D I 2000 In: Kean L, Baker P, Edelstone D I (eds) 2000 Best practice in labour ward management. W B Saunders, London

Hillan E M 1995 Postoperative morbidity following caesarean delivery. Journal of Advanced Nursing 22:1035–1042

Johanson R B, Menon V J 1999 Vacuum extraction versus forceps for assisted vaginal delivery. Cochrane Database of Systematic Reviews, Issue 2:CD000224

Johanson R B, Rice C and Doyle M et al 1995 A randomised prospective study comparing vacuum extractor policy with forceps delivery. British Journal of Obstetrics and Gynaecology 100:524–530

Lewis G (ed.) 2007 The Confidential Enquiry into Maternal and Child Health (CEMACH). Saving mothers' lives: reviewing maternal deaths to make motherhood safer 2003–2005. The seventh report on Confidential Enquiries into Maternal Deaths in the United Kingdom. CEMACH, London

Lopez-Zeno J A, Peaceman A M, Adashek J A et al 1992 A controlled trial of a program for the active management of labour. New England Journal of Medicine 326(17):450–454

McAleese S 2000 Caesarean section for maternal choice? Midwifery Matters 84:1–7

Magill-Cuerden J 1996 Intervention in a natural process. Modern Midwife May:4

Marwick J C, Lynn R 2001 High caesarean rates among women over 30. British Medical Journal 323:284

MCWP (Maternity Care Working Party) 2006 Modernising maternity care – A Commissioning Toolkit for England, 2nd edn. The National Childbirth Trust, The Royal College of Midwives, The Royal College of Obstetricians and Gynaecologists, London

Miller A W F, Hanretty K P 1997 Obstetrics illustrated, 5th edn. Churchill Livingstone, London

Mulholland L 1997 Midwife ventouse practitioners. British Journal of Midwifery 5(5):255

NICE (National Centre for Clinical Excellence) National Collaborating Centre for Women's and Children's Health 2004 Caesarean section: clinical guideline. RCOG Press, London.

O'Driscoll K, Meagher D, Boylan P 1993 Active management of labour, 3rd edn. Mosby, London

Page L 1999 Caesarean birth: the kindest cut? British Journal of Midwifery 7(5):296

Pare E, Quinones J, Macones G 2006 Vaginal birth after caesarean section versus elective repeat caesarean section: assessment of maternal downstream health outcomes. British Journal of Obstetrics and Gynaecology 113:75–85

Peterson C M, Saunders N J 1991 Mode of delivery after one caesarean section: audit of current practice in a health region. British Medical Journal 303(6806):818–821

RCOG (Royal College of Obstetricians and Gynaecologists) 2001 Clinical Effectiveness Support Unit. The national sentinel caesarean section audit report. RCOG, London

Stables D, Rankin J 2005 Physiology in childbearing with anatomy and related biosciences, 2nd edn. Elsevier, London

Stephenson P A 1992 International differences in the use of obstetrical inventions. WHO, Copenhagen 112

Walker R, Golois E 2001 Why choose caesarean section? Lancet 357:636–637

Weaver J, Stratham H, Richards M 2001 High rates may be due to perceived potential for complications. British Medical Journal 323:284–285

Ziadeh S M, Sunna E I 1995 Decreased cesarean birth rates and improved perinatal outcome: a seven year study. Birth 22(3):144–147

FURTHER READING

Francome C, Savage W, Churchill H et al 1993 Caesarean birth in Britain. Middlesex University Press, London

A book for health professionals and parents, this presents an international and an historical narration of issues such as causes of, coping with, and policies of British consultants in relation to, caesarean section. Vaginal birth after caesarean section is reviewed.

Kean L, Baker P, Edelstone D 2000 Best practice in labour ward management, 1st ed. W B Saunders, London

This book, written by three obstetricians, is a very useful handbook for students of midwifery and midwives alike. The perspective is research-based and very woman-centred. It contains useful references at the end of each chapter. The whole is focused on care of women on the labour ward, therefore the chapter on Instrumental Delivery and Caesarean Section provides interesting backgrounds on these areas of practice.

33 Midwifery and obstetric emergencies

Terri Coates

The immediate management of the emergencies discussed in this chapter are dependent on the prompt action of the midwife. Recognition of the problem and the instigation of emergency measures may determine the outcome for the mother or the fetus. The midwife should keep calm and try to explain as much as possible to the mother and her partner to ensure her consent and cooperation for procedures that may be needed. All midwifery and medical staff must be updated on the signs and symptoms of critical illness from both obstetric and non-obstetric causes and regular drills should be held to maintain and improve those skills. They should be trained in basic life support to a nationally recognized level and emergency drills for maternal resuscitation should be regularly practised in clinical areas in all maternity units.

The chapter aims to:

- heighten awareness of sudden changes in maternal condition
- describe emergency situations with discussion of possible causes and action to be taken
- consider the rare obstetric conditions of uterine rupture and acute inversion and vasa praevia
- discuss amniotic fluid embolism, in which prompt action is needed to preserve the mother's life
- review the treatment of shock focusing on the conditions of hypovolaemic shock and septic shock, in midwifery practice
- outline the drills for basic resuscitation.

Vasa praevia

The term *vasa praevia* is used when a fetal blood vessel lies over the os, in front of the presenting part. This occurs when fetal vessels from a velamentous insertion of the cord or to a succenturiate lobe (Ch. 11) cross the area of the internal os to the placenta. The fetus is in jeopardy, owing to the risk of rupture of the vessels, which could lead to exsanguination. Good outcome depends on antenatal diagnosis and delivery by caesarean section before the membranes rupture (Oyelese & Smulian 2006).

Vasa praevia may be diagnosed antenatally using ultrasound. Sometimes, vasa praevia will be palpated on vaginal examination when the membranes are still intact. If it is suspected a speculum examination should be made.

Ruptured vasa praevia

When the membranes rupture in a case of vasa praevia, a fetal vessel may also rupture. This leads to exsanguination of the fetus unless birth occurs within minutes.

Diagnosis

Fresh vaginal bleeding, particularly if it commences at the same time as rupture of the membranes, may be due to ruptured vasa praevia. Fetal distress disproportionate to blood loss may be suggestive of vasa praevia.

Management

The midwife should call for urgent medical assistance. The fetal heart rate should be monitored. If the mother is in the first stage of labour and the fetus is still alive, an emergency caesarean section is carried out. If in the second stage of labour, delivery should be expedited and a vaginal birth may be achieved. Caesarean section may be carried out but mode of birth will be dependent on parity and fetal condition.

There is a high fetal mortality associated with this emergency and a paediatrician should therefore be present for the birth. If the baby is born alive, resuscitation, haemoglobin estimation and a blood transfusion will be necessary.

Presentation and prolapse of the umbilical cord (see Box 33.1)

Predisposing factors

These are the same for both presentation and prolapse of the cord. Any situation where the presenting part is neither well applied to the lower uterine segment nor well down in the pelvis may make it possible for a loop of cord to slip down in front of the presenting part. Such situations include:

- high or ill-fitting presenting part
- high parity
- prematurity

Box 33.1 Definitions

Cord presentation

This occurs when the umbilical cord lies in front of the presenting part, with the fetal membranes still intact.

Cord prolapse

The cord lies in front of the presenting part and the fetal membranes are ruptured (see Fig. 33.1).

Occult cord prolapse

This is said to occur when the cord lies alongside, but not in front of, the presenting part.

- malpresentation
- multiple pregnancy
- polyhydramnios.

(Lin 2006, Mesleh et al 1993, Murphy & MacKenzie 1995).

High head

If the membranes rupture spontaneously when the fetal head is high, a loop of cord may be able to pass between the uterine wall and the fetus resulting in its lying in front of the presenting part. As the presenting part descends the cord becomes trapped and occluded.

Multiparity

The presenting part may not be engaged when the membranes rupture and malpresentation is more common.

Prematurity

The size of the fetus in relation to the pelvis and the uterus allows the cord to prolapse. Babies of very low birth weight (<1500g) are particularly vulnerable (Mesleh et al 1993, Lin 2006).

Malpresentation

Cord prolapse is associated with breech presentation, especially complete or footling breech. This relates to the ill-fitting nature of the presenting parts and also the proximity of the umbilicus to the buttocks. In this situation, the degree of compression may be less than with a cephalic presentation, but there is still a danger of asphyxia.

Shoulder and compound presentation and transverse lie carry a high risk of prolapse of the cord, occurring with spontaneous rupture of the membranes.

Face and brow presentations are less common causes of cord prolapse (see Ch. 31).

Multiple pregnancy

Malpresentation, particularly of the second twin, is more common in multiple pregnancy.

Polyhydramnios

The cord is liable to be swept down in a gush of liquor if the membranes rupture spontaneously. Controlled release of liquor during artificial rupture of the membranes is sometimes performed to try to prevent this.

Murphy & MacKenzie (1995) found in 55 cases out of a total 132 that none of the above factors could be attributed as the reason for cord prolapse.

Cord presentation

This is diagnosed on vaginal examination when the cord is felt behind intact membranes. It is, however, rarely detected but may be associated with aberrations in fetal heart monitoring such as decelerations, which occur if the cord becomes compressed.

Management

Under no circumstances should the membranes be ruptured. The midwife should discontinue the vaginal examination, in order to reduce the risk of rupturing the membranes. Medical aid should be summoned. To assess fetal well-being continuous electronic fetal monitoring should be commenced or the fetal heart should be auscultated as continuously as possible. The mother should be helped into a position that will reduce the likelihood of cord compression. Caesarean section is the most likely outcome.

Cord prolapse

Diagnosis

Whenever there are factors present that predispose to cord prolapse (Fig. 33.1), a vaginal examination should be performed immediately on spontaneous rupture of membranes.

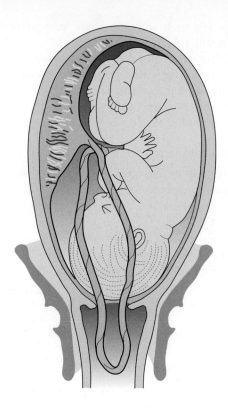

Figure 33.1 Cord prolapse.

Bradycardia, and variable or prolonged decelerations of the fetal heart are associated with cord compression, which may be caused by cord prolapse. The diagnosis of cord prolapse is made when the cord is felt below or beside the presenting part on vaginal examination. The cord may be felt in the vagina or in the cervical os or a loop of cord may be visible at the vulva (Lin 2006).

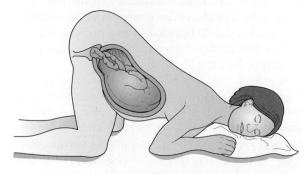

Figure 33.2 Knee–chest position. Pressure on the umbilical cord is relieved as the fetus gravitates towards the fundus.

Immediate action

Where the diagnosis of cord prolapse is made, the time should be noted and the midwife should call for urgent assistance. The midwife should explain her findings and emergency measures that may be needed to the mother and her birth partner.

If an oxytocin infusion is in progress this should be stopped. If the cord lies outside the vagina, then it should be gently replaced to prevent spasm, to maintain temperature and prevent drying. Administering oxygen to the mother by face mask at 4L/min may improve fetal oxygenation.

Relieving pressure on the cord

The risks to the fetus are hypoxia and death as a result of cord compression. The risks are greatest with prematurity and low birth weight (Murphy & MacKenzie 1995). The midwife may need to keep her fingers in the vagina and hold the presenting part off the umbilical cord, especially during a contraction. The mother can be helped to change position to further reduce pressure on the cord. Raising her pelvis and buttocks or adopting the knee–chest position will cause the fetus to gravitate towards the diaphragm (Fig. 33.2). The foot of the bed may also be raised (Trendelenburg position) to relieve compression on the cord. Alternatively, the mother can be helped to lie on her left side, with a wedge or pillow elevating her hips (exaggerated Sims' position) (Fig. 33.3). There is some evidence to suggest that bladder filling may also be an effective technique for managing cord prolapse (Houghton 2006, Katz et al 1988). A self-retaining 16G Foley catheter is used to instil approximately 500–700mL of sterile saline into the bladder. The full bladder can relieve compression of the cord by elevating the presenting part about 2cm above the ischial spines

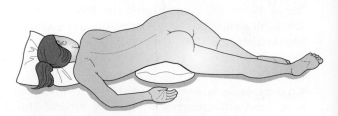

Figure 33.3 Exaggerated Sims' position. Pillows or wedges are used to elevate the woman's buttocks to relieve pressure on the umbilical cord.

until delivery by caesarean section. The bladder would be drained in theatre immediately before delivery.

Birth must be expedited with the greatest possible speed to reduce the mortality and morbidity associated with this condition. Caesarean section is the treatment of choice in those instances where the fetus is still alive and vaginal birth is not imminent.

If cord prolapse is diagnosed in the second stage of labour, with a multiparous mother, the midwife may perform an episiotomy to expedite the birth. Where the presentation is cephalic, assisted birth may be achieved through ventouse or forceps.

If cord prolapse occurs in the community, emergency transfer to hospital is essential. The midwife should carry out the same procedures to relieve the compression on the cord. Consultant unit staff should be informed and be prepared to perform an emergency caesarean section.

Shoulder dystocia

Definition

The term *'shoulder dystocia'* is used in this chapter to describe failure of the shoulders to traverse the pelvis spontaneously after birth of the head (Smeltzer 1986). However, a universally accepted definition of shoulder dystocia has yet to be produced (Roberts 1994).

The anterior shoulder becomes trapped behind or on the symphysis pubis, while the posterior shoulder may be in the hollow of the sacrum or high above the sacral promontory (Fig. 33.4). This is, therefore, a bony dystocia, and traction at this point will further impact the anterior shoulder, impeding attempts at delivery.

Incidence

Shoulder dystocia is not a common emergency: the incidence is reported as varying between 0.37% and 1.1% (Bahar 1996).

Risk factors

Although it would be useful to identify those women at risk from a birth complicated by shoulder dystocia, most risk factors can give only a high index

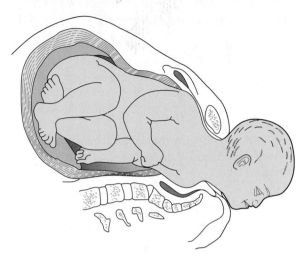

Figure 33.4 Shoulder dystocia.

of suspicion (Al-Najashi et al 1989). Antenatally, these risk factors include post-term pregnancy, high parity, maternal age over 35 and maternal obesity (weight over 90 kg).

Fetal macrosomia (birth weight over 4000 g) has been associated with an increased risk of shoulder dystocia, the incidence increasing as birth weight increases (Delpapa & Mueller-Heubach 1991, Hall 1996). However, ultrasound scanning for prediction of macrosomia to prevent shoulder dystocia has a poor record of success (Combs et al 1993, Hall 1996). If a large baby is suspected then this fact must be communicated clearly to the team caring for the woman in labour (CESDI 1999, p 47).

Maternal diabetes and gestational diabetes have been identified as important risk factors (Athukorala 2007). In diabetic women, a previous birth complicated by shoulder dystocia increases the risk of recurrence to 9.8%; this compares with a risk of recurrence of 0.58% in the general population (Smith et al 1994).

In labour, risk factors that have been consistently linked with shoulder dystocia include oxytocin augmentation, prolonged labour, prolonged second stage of labour and operative deliveries (Al-Najashi et al 1989, Bahar 1996, Benedetti & Gabbe 1978, Keller et al 1991). For a clinically suspected large baby the delivery team must be alert for the possibility of shoulder dystocia (CESDI 1999).

Warning signs and diagnosis

The birth may have been uncomplicated initially, but the head may have advanced slowly and the chin may have had difficulty in sweeping over the perineum. Once the head is born, it may look as if it is trying to return into the vagina, which is caused by reverse traction.

Shoulder dystocia is diagnosed when manoeuvres normally used by the midwife fail to assist the birth (Resnik 1980).

Management (see Box 33.2 for the HELPERR mnemonic)

Upon diagnosing shoulder dystocia, the midwife must summon help immediately. An obstetrician, an anaesthetist and a person proficient in neonatal resuscitation should be called.

Box 33.2 HELPERR mnemonic

Help

Episiotomy need assessed

Legs in McRoberts position

Pressure suprapubically

Enter vagina (internal rotation)

Remove posterior arm

Roll the woman over and try again

(Adapted from the Advanced Life Support in Obstetrics course.)

Shoulder dystocia is a frightening experience for the mother, for her partner and for the midwife. The midwife should keep calm and try to explain as much as possible to the mother to ensure her full cooperation for the manoeuvres that may be needed to complete the birth.

The purpose of all these manoeuvres is to disimpact the shoulders. The principle of using the most simple manoeuvres first should be applied. The midwife will need to make an accurate and detailed record of the type of manoeuvre(s) used and the time taken, the amount of force used and the outcome of each manoeuvre attempted.

Non-invasive procedures

Change in maternal position

Any change in the maternal position may be useful to help release the fetal shoulders as shoulder dystocia is a mechanical obstruction. However, certain manoeuvres have proved useful and are described below. It is anticipated that following the use of one or more of these manoeuvres the midwife should be able to proceed with the birth.

The McRoberts manoeuvre

This manoeuvre involves helping the woman to lie flat and to bring her knees up to her chest as far as possible (Fig. 33.5).

This manoeuvre will rotate the angle of the symphysis pubis superiorly and use the weight of the mother's legs to create gentle pressure on her

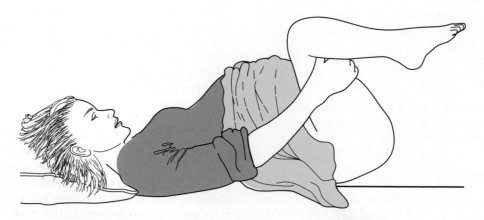

Figure 33.5 The McRoberts manoeuvre position.

abdomen, releasing the impaction of the anterior shoulder (Gonik et al 1983, 1989). It is the manoeuvre associated with the lowest level of morbidity and requires the least force to assist the birth (Bahar 1996, Gross et al 1987, Nocon et al 1993).

Suprapubic pressure

Pressure should be exerted on the side of the fetal back and towards the fetal chest. This manoeuvre may help to adduct the shoulders and push the anterior shoulder away from the symphysis pubis into the larger oblique or transverse diameter (Fig. 33.6).

All fours position

The all-fours position (or Gaskin manoeuvre) is achieved by assisting the mother onto her hands and knees; the act of turning the mother may be the most useful aspect of this manoeuvre (Bruner et al 1998). In shoulder dystocia, the impaction is at the pelvic inlet and the force of gravity will keep the fetus against the anterior aspect of the mother's uterus and pelvis. However, this manoeuvre may be especially helpful if the posterior shoulder is impacted behind the sacral promontory as this position optimizes space available in the sacral curve and may allow the posterior shoulder to be delivered first. In a retrospective study of 82 consecutive cases

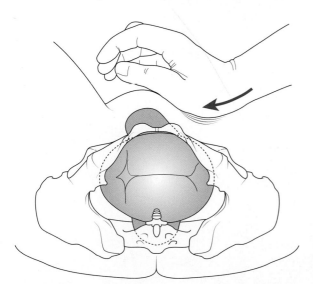

Figure 33.6 Correct application of suprapubic pressure for shoulder dystocia. (After Pauerstein C 1987, with permission.)

of shoulder dystocia and the all fours manoeuvre, 83% of women were delivered with no other manoeuvres required (Bruner et al 1998). Manipulative manoeuvres can be performed while the woman is on all fours but clear verbal communication is needed as eye contact is difficult.

Manipulative procedures

Where non-invasive procedures have not been successful, direct manipulation of the fetus must now be attempted.

Positioning of the mother

The McRoberts position as detailed above can be used, or the mother could be placed in the lithotomy position with her buttocks well over the end of the bed so that there is no restriction on the sacrum. If neither the McRoberts nor lithotomy positions are appropriate, then the all-fours position may prove useful. Any of the following manoeuvres can be undertaken with the mother in one of these positions.

Episiotomy

The problem facing the midwife is an obstruction at the pelvic inlet which is a bony dystocia, not an obstruction caused by soft tissue. Although episiotomy will not help to release the shoulders per se, the midwife should consider the need to perform one (see Ch. 28) to gain access to the fetus without tearing the perineum and vaginal walls.

Rubin's manoeuvre

This manoeuvre (Rubin 1964) requires the midwife to identify the posterior shoulder on vaginal examination, then to push the posterior shoulder in the direction of the fetal chest, thus rotating the anterior shoulder away from the symphysis pubis. By adducting the shoulders this manoeuvre reduces the 12 cm bisacromial diameter (Fig. 33.7).

Woods' manoeuvre

Woods' (1943) manoeuvre requires the midwife to insert her hand into the vagina and identify the fetal chest. Then, by exerting pressure on to the posterior fetal shoulder, rotation is achieved. Although this manoeuvre does abduct the shoulders, it will rotate the shoulders into a more favourable diameter and enable the midwife to complete the birth (Fig. 33.8).

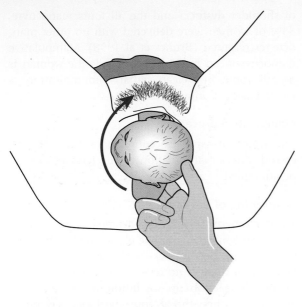

Figure 33.7   The Rubin manoeuvre.

Delivery of the posterior arm

The midwife has to insert her hand into the vagina making use of the space created by the hollow of the sacrum (Fig. 33.9A, B). Then two fingers splint the humerus of the posterior arm (Fig. 33.9C), flex the elbow and sweep the forearm over the chest to deliver the hand (Fig. 33.9D) (O'Leary 1992). If the rest of the birth is not then accomplished, the second arm can be delivered following rotation of the shoulder using either Woods' or Rubin's manoeuvre or by reversing the Løvset manoeuvre (see Ch. 31).

Zavanelli manoeuvre

If the manoeuvres described above have been unsuccessful, the obstetrician may consider the Zavanelli manoeuvre (Sandberg 1985) as a last hope for birth of a live baby.

The Zavanelli manoeuvre requires the reversal of the mechanisms of birth so far and reinsertion of

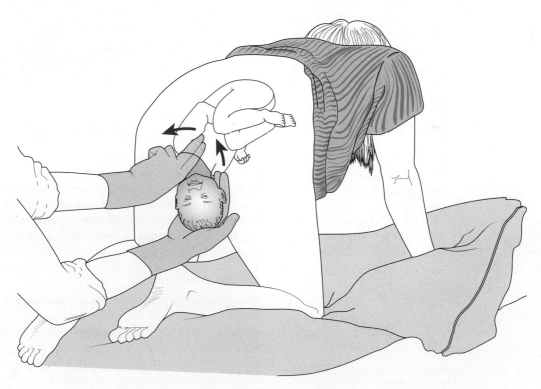

Figure 33.8   The Woods manoeuvre. (After Sweet & Tiran 1996, p 664, with permission.)

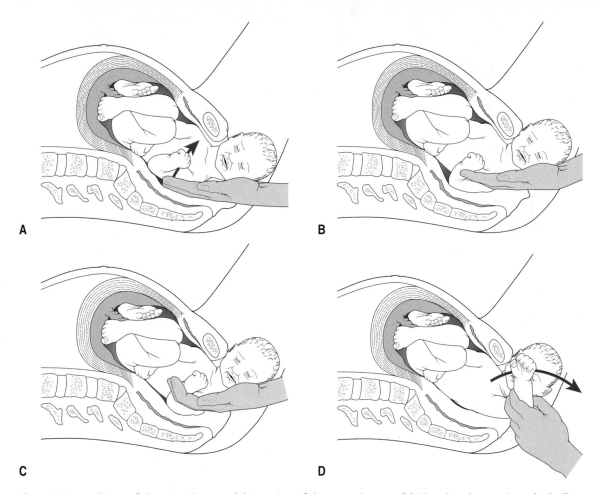

Figure 33.9 Delivery of the posterior arm: (A) Location of the posterior arm. (B) Directing the arm into the hollow of the sacrum. (C) Grasping and splinting the wrist and forearm. (D) Sweeping the arm over the chest and delivering the hand.

the fetal head into the vagina. Delivery is then completed by caesarean section.

Method. The head is returned to its pre-restitution position (Fig. 33.10A). Pressure is then exerted onto the occiput and the head is returned to the vagina (Fig. 33.10B). Prompt delivery by caesarean section is then required.

Symphysiotomy

Symphysiotomy is the surgical separation of the symphysis pubis and is used to enlarge the pelvis to enable the birth. It is usually performed in cases of cephalopelvic disproportion and is used more routinely in the developing world. There are a few

recorded cases where symphysiotomy has been used successfully to relieve shoulder dystocia (Reid & Osuagwu 1999), but the procedure has usually been associated with a high level of maternal morbidity. The rarity of reported cases makes it difficult to assess the technique for the relief of shoulder dystocia.

Outcomes following shoulder dystocia

Maternal

Approximately two-thirds will have a blood loss of >1000 mL from injury associated with the birth (Benedetti & Gabbe 1978). Maternal death from uterine rupture has been reported following the use of

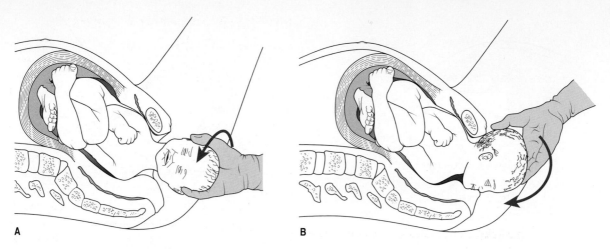

Figure 33.10   The Zavanelli manoeuvre: (A) Head being returned to direct anteroposterior (pre-restitution) position. (B) Head being returned to the vagina. (After Sandberg 1985, with permission.)

fundal pressure (Seigworth 1966) and from haemorrhage during and following the birth (O'Leary 1992).

Fetal

Neonatal asphyxia may occur following shoulder dystocia in 5.7–9.7% of cases and the attending paediatrician must be experienced in neonatal resuscitation (CESDI 1999, Naef & Morrison 1994).

Brachial plexus injury with damage to cervical nerve roots 5 and 6 may result in an Erb's palsy (see also Ch. 45). This is commonly associated with shoulder dystocia when the head and neck have been twisted and pulled (Ubachs et al 1995).

Neonatal morbidity may be as high as 42% following shoulder dystocia. Fetal damage may occur even with excellent management using appropriate obstetric manoeuvres (Naef & Morrison 1994). Shoulder dystocia remains a cause of intrapartum fetal death (CESDI 1999).

The midwife must ensure that she takes opportunities to practise the practical skills needed to complete a birth complicated by shoulder dystocia. Mannequins may help in simulation training and practice drills (Crofts et al 2006).

Rupture of the uterus

Rupture of the uterus is one of the most serious complications in midwifery and obstetrics. It is often fatal for the fetus and may also be responsible for the death of the mother. It remains a significant problem worldwide. With effective antenatal and intrapartum care some cases may be avoided.

Rupture of the uterus is defined as being complete or incomplete:

- *complete rupture* involves a tear in the wall of the uterus with or without expulsion of the fetus
- *incomplete rupture* involves tearing of the uterine wall but not the perimetrium.

Dehiscence of an existing uterine scar may also occur. This involves rupture of the uterine wall but the fetal membranes remain intact. The fetus is retained within the uterus and not expelled into the peritoneal cavity (Cunningham et al 1997).

Causes

Cases of spontaneous rupture of an unscarred uterus in primigravid mothers are reported in the literature (Guirgis & Kettle 1989, Roberts & Trew 1991), but are rare.

Rupture of the uterus can be precipitated in the following circumstances:

- antenatal rupture of the uterus, where there has been a history of previous classical caesarean section
- neglected labour, where there is previous history of caesarean section

- high parity
- use of oxytocin, particularly where the mother is of high parity
- use of prostaglandins to induce labour, in the presence of an existing scar (Lydon-Rochelle et al 2001, Vause & Macintosh 1999)
- obstructed labour: the uterus ruptures owing to excessive thinning of the lower segment
- extension of severe cervical laceration upwards into the lower uterine segment – the result of trauma during an assisted birth (DoH et al 1996)
- trauma, as a result of a blast injury or an accident (Awwad et al 1993, Michiels et al 2007)
- perforation of the non-pregnant uterus can result in rupture of the uterus in a subsequent pregnancy (Howe 1993, Usta et al 2007).

Signs of intrapartum rupture of the uterus

Complete rupture of a previously non-scarred uterus may be accompanied by sudden collapse of the mother, who complains of severe abdominal pain. The maternal pulse rate increases; simultaneously, alterations of the fetal heart may occur, including the presence of variable decelerations (Flannelly et al 1993, Phelan 1990). Three intrapartum fetal deaths associated with ruptured uterus were reported (Acolet 2007). There may be evidence of fresh vaginal bleeding. The uterine contractions may stop and the contour of the abdomen alters. The fetus becomes palpable in the abdomen as the presenting part regresses. The degree and speed of the mother's collapse and shock depend on the extent of the rupture and the blood loss (Box 33.3).

Box 33.3 Signs of rupture of uterus

- Abdominal pain or pain over previous c/s scar
- Abnormalities of the fetal heart rate and pattern
- Vaginal bleeding
- Maternal tachycardia
- Poor progress in labour.

Incomplete rupture of the uterus

Incomplete rupture may have an insidious onset found only after birth or during a caesarean section. This type is more commonly associated with previous caesarean section. Blood loss associated with dehiscence, or incomplete rupture, can be scanty, as the rupture occurs along the fibrous scar tissue which is avascular (O'Connor & Gaughan 1993).

Whenever shock during the third stage of labour is more severe than the type of birth or blood loss warrants, or the mother fails to respond to treatment given, the possibility of incomplete rupture should be considered. Incomplete rupture may also be manifest as a cause of abdominal pain and or postpartum haemorrhage following vaginal birth.

Management

All units should have a protocol for dealing with uterine rupture. An immediate caesarean section is performed in the hope of delivering a live baby. Following the birth of the baby and placenta, the extent of the rupture can be assessed. Choice between the options to perform a hysterectomy or to repair the rupture depends on the extent of the trauma and the mother's condition. Further clinical assessment will include evaluation of the need for blood replacement and management of any shock.

The mother will be unprepared for the events that have occurred and therefore may be totally opposed to hysterectomy. Reports of successful pregnancy following repair of uterine rupture are available (O'Connor & Gaughan 1993).

Rupture of the uterus following previous caesarean section

The risk of uterine rupture is increased for those women who have a uterine scar. Studies cite figures of between 0.3 and 0.7% of labours following a previous caesarean section (Miller et al 1994, Vause & Macintosh 1999). Rates of rupture are lowest following a lower segment caesarean section.

Amniotic fluid embolism

Amniotic fluid embolism (AFE) is rare, unpredictable and unpreventable (Lewis 2007). AFE occurs when amniotic fluid enters the maternal circulation via the uterus or placental site; maternal collapse can be rapidly progressive.

The body responds to AFE in two phases. The initial phase is one of pulmonary vasospasm causing hypoxia, hypotension, pulmonary oedema and cardiovascular collapse. The second phase sees the development of left ventricular failure, with haemorrhage and coagulation disorder and further uncontrollable haemorrhage. Mortality and morbidity are high (Lewis 2007) though early diagnosis may lead to better outcome (Tuffnell 2002) and early transfer to an intensive care unit is associated with decreased morbidity.

Emergency drills for maternal resuscitation should be regularly practised in clinical areas in all maternity units (Lewis 2007).

Predisposing factors

Amniotic fluid embolism can occur at any gestation. It is mostly associated with labour and its immediate aftermath, but cases in early pregnancy and postpartum have been documented (Clark et al 1995).

Chance entry of amniotic fluid into the circulation under pressure may occur through the uterine sinuses of the placental bed (Clark et al 1995).

The barrier between the maternal circulation and the amniotic sac may be breached during periods of raised intra-amniotic pressure, such as termination of pregnancy or during placental abruption. Procedures, such as ARM and insertion of an intra-uterine catheter, have been associated with AFE. Amniotic fluid embolism can also occur during an intrauterine manipulation, such as internal podalic version or during a caesarean section.

It is a condition that is difficult to predict and equally difficult to prevent. Amniotic fluid embolism is associated with a high maternal mortality rate. A total of 17 women died in the years 2003–2005, diagnosis having been confirmed clinically and by post mortem (Lewis 2007).

Clinical signs and symptoms (Box 33.4)

Premonitory signs and symptoms (restlessness, abnormal behaviour, respiratory distress and cyanosis) may occur before collapse (Lewis 2007). There is maternal hypotension and uterine hypertonus. The

---

Box 33.4 Summary of key signs and symptoms of amniotic fluid embolism

- Fetal compromise
- Respiratory
  - Cyanosis
  - Dyspnoea
  - Respiratory arrest
- Cardiovascular
  - Tachycardia
  - Hypotension
  - Pale clammy skin/shivering
  - Cardiac arrest
- Haematological
  - Haemorrhage from placental site
  - Coagulation disorders, DIC
- Neurological
  - Restlessness, panic
  - Convulsions
  - Pain less likely.

---

latter will induce fetal compromise and is in response to uterine hypoxia. Cardiopulmonary arrest follows quickly. Only minutes may elapse before arrest. Blood coagulopathy develops following the initial collapse, if the mother survives.

Emergency action

Any one of the above symptoms is indicative of an acute emergency. As the mother is likely to be in a state of collapse, resuscitation needs to be commenced at once. An emergency team should be called, since the midwife responsible for the care of the mother requires immediate help. If collapse occurs in a community setting, basic life support should be commenced prior to the arrival of emergency services.

Despite improvements in intensive care the outcome of this condition is poor. Specific management for the condition is life support, and high levels of oxygen are required. Mothers who survive are likely to have suffered a degree of neurological impairment (Clark et al 1995).

Complications of amniotic fluid embolism

Disseminated intravascular coagulation (DIC) is likely to occur within 30 min of the initial collapse. In some cases the mother bleeds heavily prior to developing amniotic fluid embolism, which contributes to the severity of her condition. It has also been reported that the amniotic fluid has the ability to suppress the myometrium, resulting in uterine atony.

Acute renal failure is a complication of the excessive blood loss and the prolonged hypovolaemic hypotension. The mother will require continuous assessment of urinary output, using an indwelling catheter. Accurate records of fluid intake and urinary output and urinalysis should be maintained by the midwife. A urinary output of <30 mL/hr should be reported, as should the presence of proteinuria. Prompt transfer to an intensive therapy unit for specialized care improves the outcome in AFE (Lewis 2007). Midwifery support and advice should be continued for the family. The mother should be given the opportunity to talk about emergency treatment when she has recovered sufficiently (Mapp 2005, Mapp & Hudson 2005).

Effect of amniotic fluid embolism on the fetus

Perinatal mortality and morbidity are high where amniotic fluid embolism occurs before the birth of the baby. Delay in the time from initial maternal collapse to delivery needs to be minimal if fetal compromise or death is to be avoided. However, maternal resuscitation may, at that time, be a priority. Box 33.5 is a summary of the key points relating to amniotic fluid embolism.

> **Box 33.5** Summary of key points for amniotic fluid embolism
>
> - Major cause of maternal death worldwide
> - Universal features: maternal shock, dyspnoea and cardiovascular collapse
> - Fetal compromise
> - Can occur at any time, most common immediately after labour
> - Should be suspected in cases of sudden collapse or uncontrollable bleeding.

All cases of suspected or proven amniotic fluid embolism, whether fatal or not, should be reported to the National Amniotic Fluid Embolism Register: UKOSS, National Perinatal Epidemiology Unit, University of Oxford, Old Road Campus, Old Road, Headington, Oxford OX3 7LF.

Acute inversion of the uterus

This is a rare but potentially life-threatening complication of the third stage of labour. It occurs in approximately 1 in 20000 births (Calder 2000). A midwife's awareness of the precipitating factors enables her to take preventive measures to avoid this emergency.

Classification of inversion

Inversion can be classified according to severity as follows:

- *first-degree* – the fundus reaches the internal os
- *second-degree* – the body or corpus of the uterus is inverted to the internal os (Fig. 33.11)

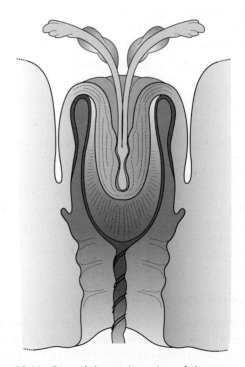

Figure 33.11 Second-degree inversion of the uterus.

- *third-degree* – the uterus, cervix and vagina are inverted and are visible.

It is also classified according to timing of the event:

- *acute inversion* – occurs within the first 24 hrs
- *subacute inversion* – occurs after the first 24 hrs, and within 4 weeks
- *chronic inversion* – occurs after 4 weeks and is rare (Brar et al 1989).

It is the first of these, acute inversion, that the remainder of this section considers.

Causes

Causes of acute inversion are associated with uterine atony and cervical dilatation, and include:

- mismanagement in the third stage of labour, involving excessive cord traction to manage the delivery of the placenta actively
- combining fundal pressure and cord traction to deliver the placenta
- use of fundal pressure while the uterus is atonic, to deliver the placenta
- pathologically adherent placenta
- spontaneous occurrence, of unknown cause
- primiparity
- fetal macrosomia
- short umbilical cord
- sudden emptying of a distended uterus.

(Brar et al 1989, Calder 2000, Platt & Druzin 1981).

Careful management of the third stage of labour is needed to prevent inversion. In active management of the third stage, palpation of the fundus is essential to confirm that contraction has taken place, prior to controlled cord traction.

Warning signs and diagnosis

The major sign of acute inversion is profound shock and usually haemorrhage. The blood loss is within a range of 800–1800 mL (Platt & Druzin 1981, Watson et al 1980).

Inversion of the uterus will cause the woman severe abdominal pain. On palpation of the uterus, the midwife may feel an indentation of the fundus. Where there is a major degree of inversion the uterus may not be palpable abdominally but may be felt upon vaginal examination or in a severe case the uterus may be seen at the vulva.

The pain is thought to be caused by the stretching of the peritoneal nerves and the ovaries being pulled as the fundus inverts. Bleeding may or may not be present, depending on the degree of placental adherence to the uterine wall. The cause of the symptoms may not be readily apparent and diagnosis may be missed if inversion is incomplete.

Management

Immediate action

A swift response is needed to reduce the risks to the mother.

Throughout the events the mother and her partner should be kept informed of what is happening. Assessment of vital signs, including level of consciousness, is of utmost importance.

1. Urgent medical help is summoned.
2. The midwife in attendance should immediately attempt to replace the uterus. If replacement is delayed the uterus can become oedematous and replacement will become increasingly difficult. Replacement may be achieved by pushing the fundus with the palm of the hand, along the direction of the vagina, towards the posterior fornix. The uterus is then lifted towards the umbilicus and returned to position with a steady pressure (Johnson's manoeuvre). If replacement cannot be achieved immediately the foot of the bed can be raised to reduce traction on the uterine ligaments and ovaries (Calder 2000).
3. An intravenous cannula should be inserted, blood should be taken for cross-matching prior to starting an infusion. Analgesia such as morphine may be given to the mother.
4. If the placenta is still attached, it should be left *in situ* as attempts to remove it at this stage may result in uncontrollable haemorrhage.

5. Once the uterus is repositioned, the operator should keep the hand in situ until a firm contraction is palpated. Oxytocics should be given to maintain the contraction (Calder 2000, Cunningham et al 1997).

Medical management

The hydrostatic method of replacement involves the instillation of several litres of warm saline infused through a giving set into the vagina. The pressure of the fluid builds up in the vagina and restores the uterus to the normal position, while the operator seals off the introitus by hand or using a soft ventouse cup.

If the inversion cannot be replaced manually a cervical constriction ring may have developed. Drugs can be given to relax the constriction and facilitate the return of the uterus to its normal position. Surgical correction via a laparotomy may be needed to correct inversion. Full support and explanation of the emergency should be offered to the mother in the postnatal period (Mapp 2005, Mapp & Hudson 2005).

Basic life-support measures

Cardiac arrests are rare in maternity units but they can and do happen and their management is sometimes suboptimal. All medical and midwifery staff should be trained to a nationally recognized level: Basic Life Support, Immediate Life Support or Advanced Life support (BLS, ILS and ALS), as appropriate (Lewis 2007).

Emergency drills for maternal resuscitation should be regularly practised in clinical areas in all maternity units. These drills should include the identification of the equipment required and appropriate methods for ensuring that cardiac arrest teams know the location of the maternity unit and theatres in order to arrive promptly. Specialized courses such as Advanced Life Support in Obstetrics (ALSO) and Managing Obstetric Emergencies and Trauma (MOET) provide additional training for obstetric, midwifery and other staff.

Standards of basic life support have been agreed internationally for health professionals and lay people (Resuscitation Council UK 2005). Basic life support refers to the maintenance of an airway and support for breathing, without any specialist equipment other than possibly a pharyngeal airway. The basic principles are:

A – airway

B – breathing

C – circulation.

1. The level of consciousness is established by shaking the woman's shoulders and enquiring whether she can hear.

2. If there is no response urgent assistance is called for by the most appropriate means.

3. The woman is laid flat on her back removing pillows. A pregnant woman should be further positioned with a left lateral tilt to prevent aortocaval compression.

4. The woman's head should be tilted back and the chin lifted upwards to open the airway (Fig. 33.12). If needed, mucus or vomit should be cleared away.

   – listen for breath sounds

   – look for chest movements.

5. If the midwife is experienced in clinical assessment then she should feel for the presence of a carotid pulse for no more than 10 seconds.

6. The hands are placed palm downwards in the centre of the chest one on top of the other with the fingers interlinked. The heel of the lower hand is

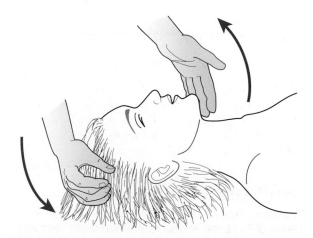

Figure 33.12 The airway is opened by tilting the head backwards and lifting the chin upwards.

positioned in the middle of the sternum. With arms straight, the midwife undertakes chest compressions depressing 4–5 cm. releasing at the same rate as compression. The chest should recoil completely after each compression.

7. The action should be repeated 100 times/min. Interruptions to chest compressions should be minimized.

8. The midwife may need to kneel over the woman or find something to stand on to ensure that she is suitably positioned to carry out resuscitation (Fig. 33.13). The surface under the woman must be firm for the manoeuvre to succeed.

9. After 30 chest compressions the midwife should give two rescue breaths (Fig. 33.12) preferably by bag and mask but mouth-to-mouth if necessary, remembering to pinch the woman's nose to make a seal. Each breath should only last for 1 s. The midwife should ensure that the woman's chest rises with each breath and is seen to fall again.

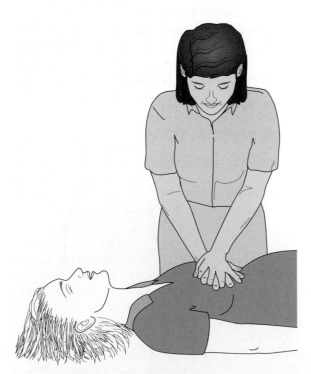

Figure 33.13 Chest compression. The midwife leans well over the patient, with arms straight. Hands are one on top of the other with fingers interlinked. The heel of the hand is used to compress the chest.

Box 33.6 Summary of basic life-support guidelines

1. Shake and shout
2. Call for help
3. Check breathing
4. Check pulse
5. Use 2 breaths to 30 compressions
6. Continue until help arrives.

Chest compression and rescue breathing should be continued until help arrives and until those experienced in resuscitation are able to take over. A ratio of 30 chest compression to two breaths should be maintained (Resuscitation Council UK 2005).

The exact sequences of resuscitation will depend on the training of staff and their experience in assessment of breathing and circulation.

These measures are summarized in Box 33.6.

Shock

Shock is a complex syndrome involving a reduction in blood flow to the tissues that may result in irreversible organ damage and progressive collapse of the circulatory system. If left untreated it will result in death. Shock can be acute but prompt treatment results in recovery, with little detrimental effect on the mother. However, inadequate treatment or failure to initiate effective treatment can result in a chronic condition ending in multisystem organ failure, which may be fatal.

Shock can be classified as follows:

- *hypovolaemic* – the result of a reduction in intravascular volume such as in severe obstetric haemorrhage

- *cardiogenic* – impaired ability of the heart to pump blood. In midwifery it may be seen following a pulmonary embolism or in women with cardiac defects.

- *neurogenic* – results from an insult to the nervous system as in uterine inversion

- *septic or toxic* – occurs with a severe generalized infection.
- *anaphylactic* – may occur as the result of a severe allergy or drug reaction.

This section deals with the principles of hypovolaemic shock and septic shock, either of which may develop as a consequence of childbirth.

Hypovolaemic shock

This is caused by any loss of circulating fluid volume, as in haemorrhage, but may also occur when there is severe vomiting. The body reacts to the loss of circulating fluid in stages as follows:

Initial stage

The reduction in fluid or blood decreases the venous return to the heart. The ventricles of the heart are inadequately filled, causing a reduction in stroke volume and cardiac output. As cardiac output and venous return fall, the blood pressure is reduced. The drop in blood pressure decreases the supply of oxygen to the tissues and cell function is affected.

Compensatory stage

The drop in cardiac output produces a response from the sympathetic nervous system through the activation of receptors in the aorta and carotid arteries. Blood is redistributed to the vital organs. Vessels in the gastrointestinal tract, kidneys, skin and lungs constrict. This response is seen by the skin becoming pale and cool. Peristalsis slows, urinary output is reduced and exchange of gas in the lungs is impaired as blood flow diminishes. The heart rate increases in an attempt to improve cardiac output and blood pressure. The pupils of the eyes dilate. The sweat glands are stimulated and the skin becomes moist and clammy. Adrenaline (epinephrine) is released from the adrenal medulla and aldosterone from the adrenal cortex. Antidiuretic hormone (ADH) is secreted from the posterior lobe of the pituitary. Their combined effect is to cause vasoconstriction, increased cardiac output and a decrease in urinary output. Venous return to the heart will increase but, unless the fluid loss is replaced, will not be sustained.

Progressive stage

This stage leads to multisystem failure. Compensatory mechanisms begin to fail, with vital organs lacking adequate perfusion. Volume depletion causes a further fall in blood pressure and cardiac output. The coronary arteries suffer lack of supply. Peripheral circulation is poor, with weak or absent pulses.

Final, irreversible stage of shock

Multisystem failure and cell destruction are irreparable. Death ensues.

Effect of shock on organs and systems

The human body is able to compensate for loss of up to 10% of blood volume, principally by vasoconstriction. When that loss reaches 20–25%, however, the compensatory mechanisms begin to decline and fail. In pregnancy the plasma volume increases, as does the red cell mass. The increase is not proportionate, but allows a healthy pregnant woman to sustain significant blood loss at birth as the plasma volume is reduced with little disturbance to normal haemodynamics. In a woman who has not had a healthy increase in plasma volume, or has sustained an antepartum haemorrhage, a much lower blood loss is required to have a pathological effect on the body and its systems. Individual organs are affected as below.

Brain

The level of consciousness deteriorates as cerebral blood flow is compromised. The mother will become increasingly unresponsive. She may not respond to verbal stimuli and there is a gradual reduction in the response elicited from painful stimulation.

Lungs

Gas exchange is impaired as the physiological dead space increases within the lungs. Levels of carbon dioxide rise and arterial oxygen levels fall. Ischaemia within the lungs alters the production of surfactant and, as a result of this, the alveoli collapse. Oedema in the lungs, due to increased permeability, exacerbates the existing problem of diffusion of oxygen. Atelectasis, oedema and reduced compliance impair ventilation and gaseous exchange, leading ultimately to respiratory failure. This is known as *adult respiratory distress syndrome* (ARDS).

Kidneys

The renal tubules become ischaemic, owing to the reduction in blood supply. As the kidneys fail, urine output falls to less than 20mL/hr. The body does not excrete waste products such as urea and creatinine, so levels of these in the blood rise.

Gastrointestinal tract

The gut becomes ischaemic and its ability to function as a barrier against infection wanes. Gram-negative bacteria are able to enter the circulation.

Liver

Drug and hormone metabolism ceases, as does the conjugation of bilirubin. Unconjugated bilirubin builds up and jaundice develops. Protection from infection is further reduced as the liver fails to act as a filter. Metabolism of waste products does not occur, so there is a build-up of lactic acid and ammonia in the blood. Death of hepatic cells releases liver enzymes into the circulation.

Management

Urgent resuscitation is needed to prevent the mother's condition deteriorating and causing irreversible damage. Women who decline blood products must have their wishes respected and a treatment plan in case of haemorrhage should be discussed with them before labour (Lewis 2007).

The priorities are to:

1. *Call for help* – Shock is a progressive condition and delay in correcting hypovolaemia can lead ultimately to maternal death.
2. *Maintain the airway* – if the mother is severely collapsed she should be turned on to her side and 40% oxygen administered at a rate of 4–6L/min. If she is unconscious an airway should be inserted.
3. *Replace fluids* – two wide-bore intravenous cannulae should be inserted to enable fluids and drugs to be administered swiftly. Blood should be taken for cross-matching prior to commencing intravenous fluids. A crystalloid solution such as Normal Saline, Hartmann's, or Ringer's lactate is given until the woman's condition has improved. A systematic review of the evidence found that colloids

were not associated with any difference in survival and were more expensive than crystalloids (Alderson et al 2001). Crystalloids are, however, associated with loss of fluid to the tissues, and therefore to maintain the intravascular volume colloids are recommended after 2L of crystalloid have been infused. No more than 1000–1500mL of colloid such as Gelofusine or Haemocel should be given in a 24hrs period. Packed red cells and fresh frozen plasma are infused when the condition of the woman is stable and these are available.

4. *Warmth* – it is important to keep the woman warm, but not overwarmed or warmed too quickly, as this will cause peripheral vasodilatation and result in hypotension.
5. *Arrest haemorrhage* – the source of the bleeding needs to be identified and stopped. Any underlying condition needs to be managed appropriately.

Assessment of clinical condition

An interprofessional team approach to management should be adopted to ensure that the correct level of expertise is available. A clear protocol for the management of shock should be used, with the midwife fully aware of key personnel required. Once the mother's immediate condition is stable, the midwife should continue to assess and record the woman's condition or liaise with staff on the intensive care unit if the woman is transferred.

Hypovolaemic shock in pregnancy will reduce placental perfusion and oxygenation to the fetus. This will result in fetal distress and possibly death. Where maternal shock is caused by antepartum factors, the midwife should determine whether the fetal heart is present, but as swift and aggressive treatment may be required to save the mother's life this should be the first priority.

Detailed observation charts including fluid balance should be accurately maintained. The extent of the mother's illness may require her transfer to a critical care unit.

Observations and clinical signs of deterioration in hypovolaemic shock

1. Assess level of consciousness in association with the Glasgow coma score. This is a reliable,

objective tool for measuring coma, using eye opening, motor response and verbal response. A total of 15 points can be achieved, and one of <12 is cause for concern. Any signs of restlessness or confusion should be noted (Mallett & Dougherty 2000).

2. Assess respiratory status using respiratory rate, depth and pattern, pulse oximetry and blood gases. Humidified oxygen should be used if oxygen therapy is to be maintained for some time.

3. Monitor blood pressure continuously, or at least every 30 min, with note taken of any drop in blood pressure.

4. Monitor cardiac rhythm continuously.

5. Measure urine output hourly, using an indwelling catheter.

6. Assess skin colour, core and peripheral temperature hourly.

7. If a CVP (central venous pressure) line has been sited, haemodynamic measures of pressure in the right atrium are taken to monitor infusion rate and quantities. The fluid balance is maintained accurately (see below).

8. Observe for further bleeding, including lochia, or oozing from a wound or puncture sites.

9. Take blood for haemoglobin and haematocrit to assess the degree of blood loss.

10. The mother is likely to be nursed flat in the acute stages of shock. Clinical assessment will also include review of pressure areas, with positional changes made as necessary to prevent deterioration. A lateral tilt should be maintained to prevent aortacaval compression if a gravid uterus is likely to compress the major vessels.

Box 33.7 is a summary of key points relating to hypovolaemic shock.

Central venous pressure

Central venous pressure (CVP) is the pressure in the right atrium or superior vena cava. It is an indicator of the volume of blood returning to the heart and reflects the competence of the heart as a pump and the peripheral vascular resistance. In the presence of acute peripheral circulatory failure, which accompanies severe

> **Box 33.7** Key points for hypovolaemic shock
>
> - Call for help
> - Gain venous access and insert two wide-bore cannulae
> - Immediate rapid infusion of fluid is needed to correct loss
> - Identify the source of bleeding and control temporarily if necessary
> - Assess for coagulopathy and correct
> - Manage the underlying condition.

shock, the monitoring of CVP aids assessment of blood loss and indicates the fluid replacement required. In such a situation it is extremely dangerous to base an intravenous regimen on guesswork. Hyper- or hypovolaemia, cardiac and renal failure may result.

The normal pressure varies between 5 and 10 cm H_2O. In shock the pressure will be persistently low (i.e. below 5 cm) and may even register a negative reading, indicating hypovolaemia. The correct volume of replacement fluids may then be assessed with greater accuracy.

Method of measuring CVP

A catheter is inserted by a doctor (usually an anaesthetist) into a major vein such as the subclavian or external jugular vein and advanced into the right atrium. The catheter is then connected to a manometer and an intravenous infusion using a three-way tap.

To take a manometer reading, the mother should be lying flat and the base of the manometer should be calibrated to measure 0 cm of water when aligned with the level of the right atrium (Fig. 33.14). This point is level with a mid-axillary line for most people. The three-way tap is opened and filled with intravenous fluid. The fluid will fall and rise with respiratory effort and should be allowed to stabilize before a reading is taken. The highest level the fluid reaches is used for the CVP measurement. Once the reading is completed the tap is returned to the infusion position.

A baseline observation is taken when the CVP catheter is inserted and the position in which the mother was lying is noted. Minor changes in position should be noted, as they may alter the CVP reading.

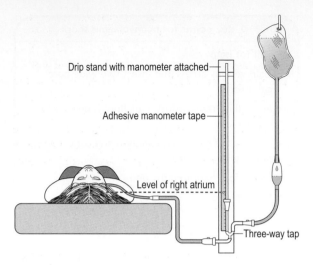

Drip stand with manometer attached

Adhesive manometer tape

Level of right atrium

Three-way tap

Figure 33.14 Monitoring central venous pressure.

Principles of care of CVP lines

1. *Prevention of infection* – insertion of the catheter requires strict asepsis. The site should be inspected regularly for signs of infection and precautions taken to protect against inadvertent contamination during clinical procedures.
2. *Maintaining a closed system* – the mother will bleed profusely if the catheter becomes disconnected, or incur a possible air embolus. Connections in particular should be checked (Mallett & Dougherty 2000).
3. *Maintaining patency of the catheter by preventing clot formation* – positive pressure of the infusion should be maintained.

Additional complications include pneumothorax, hydrothorax, trauma to lung or veins and cardiac arrhythmias during and due to insertion.

Septic shock

This is a distributive form of shock, where an overwhelming infection develops. Certain organisms produce toxins that cause fluid to be lost from the circulation into the tissues. The commonest form of sepsis causing death in childbearing in the UK is reported to be that caused by beta haemolytic *Streptococcus pyrogenes* (Lancefield Group A) (Lewis 2007). This is a Gram-positive organism, responding to intravenous antibiotics, specifically those that are penicillin based. In the general population, infections from Gram-negative organisms such as *Escherichia coli*, *Proteus* or *Pseudomonas pyocyaneus* are predominant, which are common pathogens in the female genital tract.

The placental site is the main point of entry for an infection associated with pregnancy and childbirth. This may occur following prolonged rupture of fetal membranes, obstetric trauma, septic abortion or in the presence of retained placental tissue. A total of 22 women died over 3 years as a result of genital tract sepsis in the last Confidential Enquiry (Lewis 2007). Of these, 18 were counted as *Direct* deaths, one as early pregnancy and three *late* deaths, i.e. >6 weeks postpartum.

Clinical signs

The mother may present with a sudden onset of tachycardia, pyrexia, rigors and tachypnoea. The mother may also exhibit a change in her mental state and gastrointestinal symptoms are common in pelvic sepsis. Signs of shock, including hypotension, develop in septic shock as the condition takes hold.

Haemorrhage may be present. This could be a direct result of events due to childbearing, but it occurs in septic shock because of DIC (Ch. 20).

Management

This is based on preventing further deterioration by restoring circulatory volume and then eradication of the infection. Replacement of fluid volume will restore perfusion of the vital organs. Satisfactory oxygenation is also needed.

Measures are needed to identify the source of infection and to protect against reinfection by maintaining high standards of care in clinical procedures. A full infection screening should be carried out including a high vaginal swab, midstream specimen of urine and blood cultures. Infusion sites and indwelling catheters should be checked for signs of contamination and changed as appropriate. Rigorous treatment with intravenous antibiotics, after blood cultures have been taken, is essential to halt the illness.

Retained products of conception can be detected on ultrasound, and these can then be removed.

In all situations where the mother requires to be transferred for critical or intensive care, relatives should be kept informed of progress. The midwife may be the person with whom the relatives have formed a relationship and therefore is relied on to give information.

Conclusion

The emergency situations included in this chapter are rare, but the actions of the midwife are fundamental to the well-being of mother, baby and also the partner. Awareness of local emergency procedures and knowledge of correct use of any supportive equipment are essential. Midwives in all practice settings should maintain skills that enable them to act in an emergency. The use of multiprofessional workshops to rehearse simulated situations can ensure that all members of the care team know exactly what is required when needed. Midwives should also engage in reviews of practice to ensure that policies and protocols are regularly reviewed to incorporate best practice and current evidence.

REFERENCES

Acolet D ed. 2007 CEMACH Confidential Enquiries into Maternal and Child Health. Perinatal Mortality 2005 England and Wales and Northern Ireland. CEMACH, London. Online. Available: www.cemach.org.uk

Alderson P, Schierhout G, Roberts I et al 2001 Colloids versus crystalloids for fluid resuscitation in critically ill patients (Cochrane review). The Cochrane Library, Issue 3. Update Software, Oxford

Al-Najashi S, Al-Suleiman S A, El-Yahia A et al 1989 Shoulder dystocia – a clinical study of 56 cases. Australian and New Zealand Journal of Obstetrics and Gynaecology 29:129–131

Athukorala C, Crowther C, Wilson K et al 2007 Women with gestational diabetes mellitus in the ACHOIS trial: Risk factors for shoulder dystocia. Australian and New Zealand Journal of Obstetrics and Gynaecology 47:37–41

Awwad J T, Azar G B, Aswad N K et al 1993 Uterine rupture in pregnancy caused by blast injury with fetal survival. Journal of Obstetrics and Gynaecology 13(6):448

Bahar A M 1996 Risk factors and fetal outcome in cases of shoulder dystocia compared with normal deliveries of a similar birthweight. British Journal of Obstetrics and Gynaecology 103:868–872

Benedetti T J, Gabbe S G 1978 Shoulder dystocia: a complication of fetal macrosomia and prolonged second stage of labour with mid pelvic delivery. Obstetrics and Gynecology 52(5):526–529

Brar H S, Greenspoon J S, Platt L D et al 1989 Acute puerperal uterine inversion. New approaches to management. Journal of Reproductive Medicine 34(2):173–177

Bruner J P, Drummond S B, Meenan A L et al 1998 Journal of Reproductive Medicine 43(5): 439–443

Calder A A, 2000 Emergencies in operative obstetrics. Baillière's Clinical Obstetrics and Gynaecology 14(1):43–55

CESDI (Confidential enquires into stillbirths and deaths in infancy) 1999 Sixth annual report. Maternal and Child Health Research Consortium, London

Clark S L, Hankins G D V, Dudley D A et al 1995 Amniotic fluid embolism: an analysis of the national registry. American Journal of Obstetrics and Gynecology 172:1158–1169

Combs C A, Singh N B, Khoury J C 1993 Elective induction versus spontaneous labour after sonographic diagnosis of fetal macrosomia. Obstetrics and Gynecology 81 (4):492–496

Crofts J F, Bartlett C, Ellis D et al 2006 Training for shoulder dystocia. A trial of simulation using low-fidelity and high fidelity mannequins. Obstetrics and Gynecology 108 (6):1477–1485

Cunningham F G, MacDonald P C, Gant N F et al 1997 Williams obstetrics, 20th edn. Prentice Hall, London, p 773

Delpapa E, Mueller-Heubach E 1991 Pregnancy outcome following ultrasound diagnosis of macrosomia. Obstetrics and Gynecology 78(1):340–343

DoH (Department of Health), Welsh Office, Scottish Home and Health Department, Department of Health and Social Services, Northern Ireland 1996 Report on confidential enquiries into maternal deaths in the United Kingdom 1991–1993. HMSO, London

Flannelly G M, Turner M J, Rassmussen M J et al 1993 Rupture of the uterus in Dublin: an update. Journal of Obstetrics and Gynaecology 13:440–443

Gonik B, Allen Stringer C, Held B 1983 An alternate maneuver for management of shoulder dystocia. American Journal of Obstetrics and Gynecology 145:882–883

Gonik B, Allen R, Sorab J 1989 Objective evaluation of the shoulder dystocia phenomenon: effect of maternal pelvic orientation on force reduction. Obstetrics and Gynecology 74(1):44–48

Gross S J, Shime J, Forrine D 1987 Shoulder dystocia: predictors and outcome. A five year review. American Journal of Obstetrics and Gynecology 56(2):334–336

Guirgis R R, Kettle M J 1989 Uterine rupture in a primigravid patient. Journal of Obstetrics and Gynaecology 9(3): 214–215

Hall M 1996 Guessing the weight of the baby. British Journal of Obstetrics and Gynaecology 103:734–736

Houghton G 2006 Bladder filling: an effective technique for managing cord prolapse British Journal of Midwifery 14(2): 88–89

Howe R S 1993 Third trimester uterine rupture following hysteroscopic uterine perforation. Obstetrics and Gynecology 81:827–829

Katz Z, Shoham Z, Lancet M et al 1988 Management of labour with umbilical cord prolapse: a five year study. Obstetrics and Gynaecology 72(2)278–281

Keller J D, Lopez J A, Dooley S L et al 1991 Shoulder dystocia and birth trauma in gestational diabetes: a five year experience. American Journal of Obstetrics and Gynecology 165:928–930

Lewis G (ed.) (2007) The Confidential Enquiry into Maternal and Child Health (CEMACH). Saving mothers' lives: reviewing maternal deaths to make motherhood safer 2003–2005. The seventh report on Confidential Enquiries into Maternal Deaths in the United Kingdom. CEMACH, London

Lin M G 2006 Umbilical cord prolapse. Obstetrical and Gynecological Survey 61(4):269–277

Lydon-Rochelle M, Holt V L, Easterling T R et al 2001 Risk of uterine rupture among women with a prior cesarean delivery. New England Journal of Medicine 345(1):3–8

Mallett J, Dougherty L (eds) 2000 The Royal Marsden NHS Trust manual of clinical nursing procedures, 5th edn. Blackwell Science, Oxford

Mapp T, 2005 Feelings and fears during obstetric emergencies 2. British Journal of Midwifery 13(1):36–40

Mapp T, Hudson K. 2005 Feelings and fears during obstetric emergencies 1. British Journal of Midwifery 13(1):30–35

Mesleh R, Sultan M, Sabagh T et al 1993 Umbilical cord prolapse. Journal of Obstetrics and Gynaecology 13(1):24–28

Michiels I, De Valck C, De Loor J et al 2007 Spontaneous uterine rupture during pregnancy, related to a horse fall 8 weeks earlier. Acta Obstetrica et Gynecologica Scandinavica 86(3):380–381

Miller D A, Diaz F G, Paul R H 1994 Vaginal birth after cesarean: a ten year experience. Obstetrics and Gynecology 84:255–258

Murphy D J, MacKenzie I Z 1995 The mortality and morbidity associated with umbilical cord prolapse. British Journal of Obstetrics and Gynecology 102:826–830

Naef R W, Morrison J C 1994 Guidelines for management of shoulder dystocia. Journal of Perinatology 15(6):435–441

Nocon J J, McKenzie D K, Thomas L J et al 1993 Shoulder dystocia: an analysis of risk and obstetric maneuvers. American Journal of Obstetrics and Gynecology 168(6):1732–1739

O'Connor R A, Gaughan B 1993 Rupture of the gravid uterus and its management. Journal of Obstetrics and Gynaecology 13:29–33

O'Leary J A 1992 Shoulder dystocia and birth injury: prevention and treatment. McGraw-Hill, New York

Oyelese Y, Smulian J C 2006 Placenta previa, placenta accreta, and vasa previa Obstetrics and Gynecology 107(4):927–941

Pauerstein C (ed.) 1987 Clinical obstetrics. Churchill Livingstone, New York

Phelan J P 1990 Uterine rupture. Clinical Obstetrics and Gynecology 33(3):432–437

Platt L D, Druzin M L 1981 Acute puerperal inversion of the uterus. American Journal of Obstetrics and Gynecology 141 (2):187–190

Reid P C, Osuagwu F I 1999 Symphysiotomy in shoulder dystocia. Journal of Obstetrics and Gynaecology 19(6):664–666

Resnik R 1980 Management of shoulder girdle dystocia. Clinical Obstetrics and Gynecology 23(2):559–564

Resuscitation Council UK Resuscitation guidelines 2005. Resuscitation Council (UK) Trading, London

Roberts L 1994 Shoulder dystocia. In: Studd J (ed.) Progress in obstetrics and gynaecology. Churchill Livingstone, Edinburgh, Vol 11, p 201–216

Roberts L, Trew G 1991 Uterine rupture in a primigravida. Journal of Obstetrics and Gynaecology 11(4):261–262

Rubin A 1964 Management of shoulder dystocia. Journal of the American Medical Association 189:835

Sandberg E C 1985 The Zavanelli maneuver: a potentially revolutionary method for the resolution of shoulder dystocia. American Journal of Obstetrics and Gynecology 152:479–487

Seigworth G R 1966 Shoulder dystocia: review of five years experience. Obstetrics and Gynecology 25(6):764–767

Smeltzer J S 1986 Prevention and management of shoulder dystocia. Clinical Obstetrics and Gynecology 29(2):299–308

Smith R B, Lane C, Pearson J F 1994 Shoulder dystocia: what happens at the next delivery? British Journal of Obstetrics and Gynaecology 101:713–715

Sweet B R, Tiran D 1996 Mayes' midwifery. Baillière Tindall, London

Tuffnell D J 2002 Amniotic fluid embolism Maternal morbidity and mortality. RCOG, London

Ubachs J M H, Slooff A C J, Peeters L L H 1995 Obstetric antecedents of surgically treated obstetric brachial plexus injuries. British Journal of Obstetrics and Gynaecology 102:813–817

Usta I M, Hamdi M A, Abu Musa A A et al 2007 Pregnancy outcome in patients with previous uterine rupture. Acta Obstetrica et Gynecologica Scandinavica 86(2):172–176

Vause S, Macintosh M 1999 Use of prostaglandins to induce labour in women with a caesarean scar. British Medical Journal 318:1056–1058

Watson P, Besch N, Bowes W A 1980 Management of acute and subacute puerperal inversion of the uterus. Obstetrics and Gynecology 55(1):12–16

Woods C E 1943 A principle of physics as applied to shoulder delivery. American Journal of Obstetrics and Gynecology 45:796–805

FURTHER READING

Allott H 1994 A grief shared. British Medical Journal 6308:602

A chilling contemporary account of a delivery complicated by shoulder dystocia.

Brook L A, Weindling A M 1995 The paediatric. Clinical focus: shoulder dystocia. Clinical Risk 1(2):55–60

Shoulder dystocia from the paediatrician's perspective; useful descriptions of possible sequelae.

Grady K, Prasad B G R, Howell C. 2003 Cardiopulmonary resuscitation in the non-pregnant and pregnant patient. In: Johanson R, Cox C, Grady K, et al (eds). Managing Obstetric Emergencies and Trauma. RCOG Press, London

An in depth view of obstetric management.

Hofmeyr G J, Mohlala B K F 2001 Hypovolaemic shock – best practice in research. Clinical Obstetrics and Gynaecology 15(4):645–662

This article presents best practice for the management of hypovolaemic shock in childbearing. It revisits the pathophysiology of the condition and examines some of the evidence that informs current practice.

Jevon P, Raby M 2001 Resuscitation in pregnancy. A practical approach. Books for Midwives, Hale

The authors of this book are a resuscitation officer and midwife respectively and they have provided a concise guide that addresses the key issues of resuscitation. The topics covered include those required for effective practice, as well as ethical and professional issues.

Johnstone F D, Myerscough P R 1998 Shoulder dystocia. British Journal of Obstetrics and Gynaecology 105:811–815

Gives clinically useful overview of shoulder dystocia from an obstetric perspective.

RCM (Royal College of Midwives) 2000 Clinical risk management. Shoulder dystocia. RCM Midwives Journal 3(11):348–351

Looks at shoulder dystocia from a risk management perspective with the authority of the RCM.

Resuscitation Council UK, Resuscitation guidelines 2005. Resuscitation Council (UK) Trading, London

This publication provides internationally agreed information and guidance on resuscitation and emergency life support. The website www.resus.org.uk contains a range of information and posters that can be downloaded and publications that can be ordered.

Knight M, Kurinczuk J J, Tuffnell D, 2005 The UK Obstetric Surveillance System for rare disorders of pregnancy. British Journal of Obstetrics and Gynaecology 112(3):263–265

UKOSS. A system set up to study rare disorders of pregnancy. It is has become part of routine midwifery practice to provide information for the UKOSS Surveillance System, which are used to study uncommon disorders of pregnancy.www.npeu.ox.ac.uk/UKOSS

Section 5
The puerperium

SECTION CONTENTS

34 Physiology and care in the puerperium

Sally Marchant

CHAPTER CONTENTS

Current post-birth care in the UK involves midwives, health visitors, general practitioners and others within the primary healthcare network working together on behalf of the new mother, baby and family members (DH 2005, NICE 2006, NMC 2004). The framework for this care differs from that offered to women once they have given birth in most other developed countries where the provision for regular contact with midwives as the main healthcare professionals responsible for post-birth care is less well defined. (Pathology and potential morbidity for the mother is discussed in Chapter 35.)

The chapter aims to:

- explore the role of the midwife in the assessment of women's postpartum health and psychosocial needs
- review the current evidence for the normal parameters of women's health after childbirth
- discuss the current challenges to the provision of postpartum care in the light of women's experiences.

Defining the puerperium and the postnatal period

Following the birth of the baby and expulsion of the placenta, the mother enters a period of physical and psychological recuperation (Buckley 2006). The *puerperium*, starts immediately after delivery of the placenta and membranes and continues for 6 weeks. The overall expectation is that by 6 weeks after the birth all the systems in the woman's body will have recovered from the effects of pregnancy and returned to their non-pregnant state. However, it is only comparatively recently that there has been any professional recognition or substantial interest in the diversity and extent of the morbidity experienced by women in the weeks after childbirth (RCM 2000). Some women continue to experience problems related to childbirth that extend well beyond the 6-week period defined as the puerperium, and the possibility of a longer duration is now accepted alongside the range of initial morbidity (Alexander et al 1997, Ball 1994, Glazener et al 1995, MacArthur et al 1991).

It has been customary to refer to the first weeks after the birth as the *postnatal period*; defined in the UK as a period after the end of labour during which the attendance of a midwife upon a woman and baby is required, being not less than 10 days and for such longer period as the midwife considers necessary (NMC 2004, 2006).

By no longer stating an endpoint in time when midwifery care can still be made available to women, it is to be hoped that offering more flexibility to the provision of midwifery care will in time also make a positive difference to the experiences of women and midwives of this aspect of midwifery care and services (Cattrell et al 2005, Redshaw et al 2007).

Midwives and the management of postpartum care

The provision of midwifery care to women following the birth of their baby aims to encompass aspects of observing and monitoring the health of the new mother and her baby as well as offering support and guidance in breastfeeding and parenting skills. Where the timeframe for attendance from the midwifery services might now be viewed as being more flexible, this could also be seen as an opportunity to extend the midwife's role to include the broader aspects of public and social health and more specialized areas of neonatal care. In addition there is increasing interest in the use of healthcare assistants and other voluntary support networks during this time (NCT 2007, Sewell 2007).

Statutory framework and regulation for the practice of midwifery

The initial framework for hospital postnatal care in the early twentieth century involved a period of prescribed bed rest and compliance with hospital regimens that included vulval swabbing, separation from the baby and routine feeding times. Even where such strict adherence to these practices declined, the approach taken of the 'sickness' model, remained as the framework around which hospital postnatal care operated, and in particular in the undertaking of routine observations which were considered pivotal to the essence of 'good' and viewed therefore as effective care from the point of view of the maternity services (Garcia & Marchant 1996). The current practice where women return home in a few hours after the birth, is now considered both safe and desirable from the viewpoint of most women and most maternity services. However, it is only comparatively recently that the provision of postpartum care has been reviewed with regard to its content, purpose or effectiveness (Garcia & Marchant 1993, Marchant & Garcia 1993, Marsh & Sargent 1991, Twaddle et al 1993); as a result there have been increasing numbers of research studies that challenge the traditional pattern of postpartum care and its overall provision and value (Bick et al 2002, Shaw et al 2006, Walsh 1997, Winter et al 2001, Wray 2006).

The provision of and need for postnatal care

In the UK, it is still usual for a midwife to 'attend' a postpartum woman on a regular, if not daily basis for the first 4–5 days regardless of whether the mother is in hospital or at home (NMC 2004). During the course of this contact, midwifery practice has been to undertake a regular physical examination to assess the new mother's recovery from the birth (Garcia et al 1994, Marsh & Sargent 1991, Murphy-Black 1989). From an international perspective this practice is unusual; it is only comparatively recently that postpartum home visits, and postpartum support programmes, have been initiated in America and Canada (Boulvain et al 2004, Eaton 2001, Evans 1995, Gupton 1995, Peterson et al 2005) and that women in these countries have recognized a need for and their satisfaction with current services (De Clerc 2006). Recent studies have reviewed the use of support workers in the community in the UK (Morrell et al 2000) and the extension of care and support in the community, rather than in the form of direct care. Social intervention in the form of SureStart funding has proved effective in some areas (Wilyman-Bugter & Tucker 2004).

When the extraordinary changes in physiology that occur throughout pregnancy are considered, it should come as no surprise that the period of physiological adjustment and recovery following the end of pregnancy is both complex and closely related to the overall health status of the individual. The intricate relationships between physiological, psychological and sociological factors are all encompassed in the remit of caring for the postnatal woman and her newborn (Ball 1994, MaGuire 2000, Wiggins 2000). A common reference to postnatal services being the 'Cinderella' of the maternity service provision as a whole, has led to repeated reports from women of poor support, disappointment in the services and in some cases evidence of negligence as a result of sub-standard care (Garcia et al 1998, Lewis 2007, Lewis & Drife 2001, 2004, RCM 2000, Redshaw et al 2007).

The framework for assessing resources released from the NHS costs would appear to be based on a measurement of clinical need resulting in the main providers of health services having to make comparisons between postpartum women's needs and other members of the population who are suffering from acute or chronic illnesses (O'Sullivan & Tyler 2007). Therefore, it is not unreasonable to realize that women recovering from what is seen as a positive health event in the birth of a baby does not attract the same level of funding as those with long-term conditions or terminal diseases. However, there has been a growing awareness that there are important aspects around maintaining optimal health of the developing fetus and neonate, that has an overall impact on the nation's health and the costs of sustaining it. It would now appear that there is greater recognition in the UK of the need to allocate resources appropriately to improve services to new mothers and their babies so that postnatal care in the UK is recognized for the corner stone it is with regard to outcomes for the future population (Ladyman 2005, NICE 2006).

Postnatal care in the UK

Brief historical background

The background to the current postpartum observations routinely undertaken by midwives is unclear but it is likely that key observations associated with signs of potential morbidity became part of the routine procedures undertaken by those employed to care for the lying-in woman, her house and family as well as her health (Garcia & Marchant 1996, Reid 2005). With the introduction of the National Health Service in 1948, social changes influenced the duties of the midwife and focused care on assessment of health needs rather than domestic duties. The NHS aimed to provide a cost free service which should have improved care in many areas but after a time, it was clear that women were very dissatisfied with the care they were receiving after the birth of their baby (Garcia et al 1998, RCM 2000, Singh & Newburn 2000), and at the same time, midwives were also questioning the nature, purpose and value of what was being provided (Marchant 1997).

With the focus set on health assessment, it was common for midwifery textbooks on this topic to describe the activities of the midwife with regard to physical examination of the mother and the baby (Silverton 1993,). However, over the past decade there have been increasing moves to view care for postpartum women as a partnership where the woman is encouraged to explore how she is feeling physically and emotionally and to seek the advice and support of the midwife where she needs it (MaGuire 2000, Proctor 1999, RCM 2000). The importance for all postpartum women to have access to, and appropriately receive, postpartum midwifery care has been underpinned by the recent publication of a national guideline defining core care, and what should be provided for the mother and baby in the days and weeks following birth (NICE 2006). This might involve midwives assessing a woman's capability with regard to self-knowledge and communication skills in order to provide the care needed for that woman as an individual. Midwives need to have the appropriate knowledge and skills to determine when to be proactive with regard to undertaking specific observations where these might be required. Therefore the midwife must be totally familiar with the range of normal outcomes following any birth and be able to identify signs of morbidity that require further investigation and discuss the future management of these with the woman. Such a model of care can be challenging to practitioners who lack confidence in their autonomy and decision-making skills (Marchant 2005), or where they feel there is a lack of support, both in hospital and community settings (McCourt & Percival 2000, Ridgers et al 2002).

In the area of postpartum physiology, information has been inconsistent and lacking in what is now considered to be authoritative evidence based on research (Hytten 1995, Marchant et al 1999). Although there has been increased interest in women's health after birth, research in the area of physical morbidity remains relatively sparse. This was demonstrated by the lack of robust evidence that was available to support the NICE guidelines for core postnatal care (Marchant 2006, NICE 2006). The framework adopted by the NICE guidelines, was to set out the initial context of establishing what should be viewed as core care. This is defined as the care that every woman should be offered in order to establish her needs and wishes with regard to her care and that of her newborn infant. This is a philosophical stance which replaces what has become the conventional more didactic approach which approached care needs as being what everyone *would* receive regardless of whether or not they needed it, which is the framework that underpins a routinized approach to the provision of care. This chapter follows a similar framework to that of NICE and aims to assist the practitioner to explore the environment surrounding the woman as a new mother as well as a woman recovering from the physical exertions, and sometimes psychological, trauma, of giving birth. Within this context, any decisions made by the midwife in relation to reassurance of normality or referral for actual or potential morbidity must centre on the circumstances of the individual woman.

Midwifery postpartum visits

Culture and respect

The majority of post-birth care in the UK now occurs in the community setting of the woman or a relative's home. Expectations of women about the nature and purpose of the visits by the midwife may vary according to their cultural backgrounds, from one of welcoming enthusiasm to views that reflect negativity and suspicion. For example, some faiths hold important ceremonies for the baby soon after the birth. This might involve many family members gathering in the home and the visit from the midwife in the middle of these celebrations might not be convenient (McCourt & Percival 2000, Schott & Henley 1996). Other women who have experienced motherhood before and feel the need for only minimal support from the maternity services might consider visits from the midwife as interrupting their day-to-day activities with no real particular benefit to them (Murphy-Black 1989). The concept of postpartum care is one that aims to assist the mother and her baby towards attaining an optimum health status. Where the visit from the midwife can be seen as supportive and useful to the mother and her family, this purpose is more likely to be achieved. The social changes that have occurred over the past 20 or more years will have had an effect on how different members of society view the need for care for new mothers, both from health professionals and from family members. Research that has explored the experiences of women from different ethnic backgrounds have demonstrated very marked inequalities in both the provision of services as well as the actual direct contact with care givers (Hirst & Hewison 2002). In contrast, where the timing of midwifery postpartum care is extended beyond 28 days, there is greater opportunity for midwives to continue midwifery support where this might be appropriate, and this has been welcomed as progress although the focus would appear to be more on social or psychological outcomes, or for breastfeeding support than overt clinical or physical morbidity (Bick et al 2002, Winter et al 2001).

Physiological observations

Regardless of place of birth, the midwife is primarily concerned with the observation of the health of the postpartum mother and the new baby. As such, it has been common practice to have an overall framework upon which to base the assessment of the mother's state of health and for the observations contained within the examination to link with pre-stated categories in the postnatal midwifery records. This formalized approach to the postpartum review might be an appropriate tool to use if there is concern about a woman who is feeling unwell and there is a need for a comprehensive picture of the woman's state of health (see Ch. 35). Where this is not the case such an approach might be less useful from the viewpoint of the needs of a healthy woman who has recently given birth (Gready et al 1997, Redshaw et al 2007, Ridgers 2007). The concern centres on whether, by taking the time to complete a 'top to toe' examination as a thorough review of someone who is generally well, the midwife might ignore or give less attention to what the mother really wants to talk about (Garcia et al 1998, Ridgers 2007) (Box 34.1).

The skill of the midwife's care is to achieve a balance when deciding which observations are appropriate so that she does not fail to detect potential aspects of morbidity. The next part of this chapter identifies areas of physiology that are likely either to cause women the most anxiety or to have the greatest outcome with regard to morbidity. These descriptions relate to observations undertaken for women who have had vaginal births and uncomplicated pregnancies.

The uterus and vaginal fluid loss

After the birth, oxytocin is secreted from the posterior pituitary gland to act upon the uterine muscle and assist separation of the placenta. Following expulsion of the placenta, the uterine cavity collapses inwards; the now opposed walls of the uterus compress the newly exposed placental site and effectively seal the exposed ends of the major blood vessels. The muscle layers of the myometrium are said to simulate the action of ligatures that compress the large sinuses of the blood vessels exposed by placental separation. These occlude the exposed ends of the large blood vessels and contribute further to reducing blood loss. In addition, vasoconstriction in the overall blood supply to the uterus results in the tissues being denied their previous blood supply; de-oxygenation and a state of ischaemia arise. Through the process of autolysis, autodigestion of the ischaemic muscle fibres by proteolytic enzymes occurs resulting in an overall reduction in their size. There is phagocytic action of polymorphs and macrophages in the blood and lymphatic systems upon the waste products of autolysis, which are then excreted via the renal system in the urine. Coagulation takes place through platelet aggregation and the release of thromboplastin and fibrin (Cunningham et al 2005, Hytten 1995).

Box 34.1 Thinking about the parameters that constitute 'postnatal care'

The setting is on a postnatal ward where the midwife is undertaking the daily 'check' on a postpartum mother. This was recorded as part of an observation study into hospital postnatal care (Ridgers 2007):

> '... the woman tells the midwife – "I'm going back to an empty house"
>
> Brief pause, followed by the midwife asking the mother "Have you had your bowels open?"
>
> The woman confirmed this.
>
> Further brief pause. Following which the midwife said to the woman – "it's a lovely time to have a baby." (it is December and Christmas is coming up).

> The midwife opened the bed curtains by the foot of the bed and then left the woman's bed space. As she passed the woman in the adjacent bed, she informed her – "I'll come and see you shortly."
>
> The midwife left the bay. The first woman remained behind the partially opened bed curtains; at no time did she move around or attempt to converse with any of the other women in the bay.
>
> This mother was later heard to confide to a telephone caller:
>
> "This week has been a bit tough ... a bit raw ... it's a bit tricky".'

(Extract from Ridgers 2007 Passing through but needing to be heard; an ethnographic study of women's perspectives of their care on the postnatal ward. Unpublished PhD thesis, Ch. 8.)

What remains of the inner surface of the uterine lining apart from the placental site, regenerates rapidly to produce a covering of epithelium. Partial coverage occurs within 7–10 days after the birth; total coverage is complete by the 21st day (Cunningham et al 2005).

Once the placenta has separated, the circulating levels of oestrogen, progesterone, human chorionic gonadotrophin and human placental lactogen are reduced. This leads to further physiological changes in muscle and connective tissues as well as having a major influence on the secretion of prolactin from the anterior pituitary gland.

Once empty, although the uterus retains its muscular structure, it can be likened to an empty sac. It is therefore important to remember that the uterus, although at this point markedly reduced in size, still retains the potential to be a much larger cavity. This underpins the requirement to undertake immediate and then regular observations of fundal height and the degree of uterine contraction in the first few hours after the birth. Abdominal palpation of the uterus is usually performed soon after placental expulsion to ensure that the physiological processes are beginning to take place. On abdominal palpation, the fundus of the uterus should be located centrally, its position being at the same level or slightly below the umbilicus, and should be in a state of contraction, feeling firm under the palpating hand. The woman may experience some uterine or abdominal discomfort especially where uterotonic drugs have been administered to augment the physiological process (Anderson et al 1998).

Traditionally textbooks have described precise measurements for the size of the uterus at various points in this process. Inconsistencies in these descriptions in the various textbooks cast doubt on the validity of the information overall (Marchant et al 1999). The *process of involution*, however, is essential background knowledge for midwives monitoring the physiological process of the return of the uterus to its non-pregnant state. Research findings would suggest that the information required by both midwives and women is that a well-contracted uterus will gradually reduce in size until it is no longer palpable above the symphysis pubis (Cluett et al 1997, Marchant et al 2000). The rate at which this occurs and the duration of time taken have been demonstrated to be highly individual (Cluett et al 1997) rather than occurring specifically at a daily rate.

Overall, the uterus should not be tender during this process and, although women may be experiencing afterpains, the presence of these should be defined separately from any uterine tenderness. The observations obtained by the midwife about the state of involution of the uterus should be placed into context alongside the colour, amount and duration of the woman's vaginal fluid loss and her general state of health at that time.

Assessment of postpartum uterine involution

There are several aspects to the abdominal palpation of the postpartum uterus that contribute to the observation as a whole. The first is to identify height and location of the fundus (the upper parameter of the uterus). Assessment should then be made of the condition of the uterus with regard to uterine muscle contraction and finally whether palpation of the uterus causes the woman any pain. When all these dimensions are combined, this provides an overall assessment of the state of the uterus and the progress of uterine involution can be described. Findings from such an assessment should clearly record the position of the uterus in relation to the umbilicus or the symphysis pubis, the state of uterine contraction and the presence of any pain during palpation. A suggested approach to how this is undertaken in clinical practice can be found in Box 34.2.

Record-keeping, appropriate use

Clear and accurate records of any observation that has been undertaken are essential tools to competent practice (NMC 2004). Although the usefulness of uterine assessment is not in doubt where this contributes to the confirmation of abnormality, it is questionable whether this assessment when it is carried out routinely (regardless of clinical indication) contributes to the prediction of potential problems associated with involution. Recording of the findings from assessment of uterine involution has been found to be inconsistent between midwives and a wide range of abbreviation and hieroglyphics have been used to describe the involuting uterus (Marchant et al 2000). Such activities are at variance to the professional guidance which states that the record of

Box 34.2 Suggested approach to undertaking postpartum assessment of uterine involution

- Discuss the need for uterine assessment with the woman and obtain her agreement to proceed. She should have emptied her bladder within the previous 30 min

- Ensure privacy and an environment where the woman can lie down on her back with her head supported. Locate a covering to put over her lower body

- The midwife should have clean, warm hands and should help the woman to expose her abdomen; the assessment should not be done through clothing

- The midwife places the lower edge of her hand at the umbilical area and gently palpates inwards towards the spine until the uterine fundus is located

- The fundus is palpated to assess its location and the degree of uterine contraction. Any pain or tenderness should be noted

- Once the midwife has completed the assessment she should help the woman to dress and to sit up

- The midwife should then ask the woman about the colour and amount of her vaginal loss and whether she has passed any clots or is concerned about the loss in any way

- Following the assessment, the woman should be informed about what has been found and any further action that is required, and then a record of the assessment is made in the midwifery notes.

any assessment should be written contemporaneously, clearly and be devoid of abbreviation and ambiguity (NMC 2004).

Postpartum vaginal blood loss

Blood products constitute the major part of the vaginal loss immediately after the birth of the baby and expulsion of the placenta. As involution progresses the vaginal loss reflects this and changes from a predominantly fresh blood loss to one that contains stale blood products, lanugo, vernix and other debris from the unwanted products of the conception. This loss varies from woman to woman, being a lighter or darker colour, but for any woman the shade and density tends to be consistent.

'Lochia' is a Latin word traditionally used to describe the vaginal loss following the birth (Cunningham et al 2005). Medical and midwifery textbooks have described three phases of lochia and have given the duration over which these phases persist. Recent research has explored the relevance of these descriptions for women and raised questions about the use of these descriptions in clinical practice. One study identified that not all women were even aware that they would have a vaginal blood loss after the birth (Marchant et al 1999), but of more importance was the wide variation experienced by women in colour, amount and duration of vaginal loss in the first 12 weeks' postpartum (Marchant et al 1999, Oppenheimer et al 1986, Sherman et al 1999). This suggests that, overall, descriptions of normality ascribed to the traditional descriptions of lochia are outdated and unhelpful to women and midwives in accurately describing a clinical observation. Women also appreciate the use of language that is familiar to them and therefore it is recommended that the description of vaginal loss as 'lochia' should be abandoned and replaced with postpartum 'vaginal blood' or 'fluid' loss.

Plate 14 illustrates the colour of vaginal blood loss reported by women in the first 28 days' postpartum.

Assessment of vaginal blood loss

Most women can clearly identify colour and consistency of vaginal loss if asked and, more importantly, will be able to describe key changes from what has happened previously. Therefore it is of more use to the midwife to ask focused questions about the current vaginal loss: whether this is more or less, lighter or darker than previously and whether the mother has any concerns about it herself. When asking these questions, women should be asked an open question first: 'can you tell me the colour/amount of your vaginal loss today?' rather than asking whether the vaginal loss is brown or red, etc. It is of particular importance to record any clots passed and when these occurred. Clots can be associated with future episodes of excessive or prolonged bleeding postpartum (see Chs 29 and 35).

Assessment that attempts to quantify the amount of loss or the size of clot is problematic. The use of descriptions that are common to both woman and midwife can improve accuracy in these assessments.

Examples are asking the woman to describe the size of the spread of the vaginal loss on a sanitary pad, the frequency of changing the pad because of the saturation level, or comparison of the size of clots to familiar items such as a 50 pence coin or a plum (Marchant et al 1999, 2000).

Perineal pain

Regardless of whether the birth resulted in actual perineal trauma, women are likely to feel bruised around the vaginal and perineal tissues for the first few days after the birth. Women who have undergone any degree of actual perineal injury will experience pain for several days until healing takes place (Albers & Borders 2007, McCandlish et al 1998, Sleep 1995, Steen 2007, Wylie 2002). It has been said that the effects of perineal trauma significantly blight the first experiences of motherhood for many women because of the degree of pain experienced and the effects of this on the activities of daily living (McCandlish et al 1998, Sleep 1995). Long-term psychological and physiological trauma is also evident.

Whose perineum is it?

As with palpation of the uterus, the perineum is not easily viewed by the woman herself and so appropriate midwifery care might involve observing the perineal area to ascertain progress of healing from any trauma (WHO 1999). However, the woman will be well aware of how it feels with regard to degrees of pain and discomfort, or the absence of these. Appropriate care immediately after the birth or where suturing has taken place can help to reduce oedema and bruising (Bick et al 2002, NICE 2006, Sleep 1995, Steen et al 2000, Steen 2007). When the midwife is undertaking the postpartum review it is recommended that, particularly in the first few days after the birth, all women are asked about discomfort in the perineal area regardless of whether there is a record of actual perineal trauma. Clear information and reassurance are helpful where women have poor understanding of what happened and are anxious or embarrassed about urinary, bowel or sexual function in the future.

Where women appear to have no discomfort or anxieties about their perineum, it is not essential for the midwife to examine this area and arguably it is an intrusion on the woman's privacy to do so. The basic principles of morbidity or infection (Cunningham et al 2005) indicate that it is unusual for morbidity to occur without inflammation and pain although these factors are also integral to the healing process (Steen 2007); therefore, although the area might be causing discomfort from the original trauma, where this is unchanged or absent a pathological condition should not be developing. There may be occasions, however, where the midwife might consider that the woman is declining this observation because she is embarrassed or anxious. In such cases, the midwife should use her skills of communication to explore whether there is a clinical need for this observation to be undertaken and, if so, to advise the woman accordingly. For the majority of women, the perineal wound gradually becomes less painful and healing should occur by 7–10 days after the birth.

Advice on what might help perineal pain

Sleep (1995) identified a number of studies aimed at providing evidence of effectiveness in this area. Treatments included the use of salt or Savlon in bathwater, pulsed electromagnetic energy, infra-red heat and ultrasound. None of these trials produced evidence that was persuasive about overall benefit in the area of reducing pain or improving healing. Further enquiry is still needed within the overall aim of giving relief without destabilizing the most suitable environment for healing. However, women may still find soaking in a bath of great comfort to them regardless of any additive, and relief may be derived from the use of a bidet or cool water poured over the area that is tender. Research has supported the use of cool gel pads to reduce pain and these are readily available to purchase at minimal cost as opposed to more expensive medications (Steen et al 2000).

There is also increasing interest and research being undertaken into the use of complementary therapeutic preparations (see Ch. 50).

Vital signs and general health

The following information is based on the premise that the midwife is exploring the health of the postpartum woman from a viewpoint of confirming normality. 'Common sense' although a concept that is very difficult to define is probably a well understood paradigm and taking such an approach is an important part of midwifery care with regard to addressing the issues that are visible before seeking out the less obvious. In this instance, an overall assessment of the woman's physical appearance will add considerably to the management of what will be undertaken prior to continuing any further investigation for either the woman or her baby.

Observations of pulse, temperature, respiration and blood pressure

Making a note of the pulse rate is probably one of the least invasive and most cost-effective observations a midwife can undertake. If undertaken when seated alongside or at the same level as the woman, it can create positive feelings of care while also obtaining valuable clinical information. While observing the pulse rate, particularly if this is done for a full minute, the midwife can also observe a number of related signs of well-being: the respiratory rate, the overall body temperature, any untoward body odour, skin condition and the woman's overall colour and complexion, as well as just listening to what the woman is saying.

It is not necessary to undertake observations of temperature routinely for women who appear to be physically well and who do not complain of any symptoms that could be associated with an infection. However, where the woman complains of feeling unwell with flu-like symptoms, or there are signs of possible infection or information that might be associated with a potential environment for infection, the midwife should undertake and record the temperature. This will enhance the amount of clinical information available where further decisions about potential morbidity may need to be made.

Blood pressure

Following the birth of the baby, a baseline recording of the woman's blood pressure will be made. In the absence of any previous history of morbidity associated with hypertension, it is usual for the blood pressure to return to a normal range within 24 hrs after the birth. Routinely undertaking observations of blood pressure without a clinical reason is therefore not required once a baseline recording has been taken, NICE suggest this should be within six hours of the birth (NICE 2006).

Circulation

The body has to reabsorb a quantity of excess fluid following the birth and for the majority of women this results in passing large quantities of urine, particularly in the first day, as diuresis is increased (Cunningham et al 2005, Hytten 1995). Women may also experience oedema of their ankles and feet and this swelling may be greater than that experienced in pregnancy. These are variations of normal physiological processes and should resolve within the puerperal time scale as the woman's activity levels also increase. Advice should be related to taking reasonable exercise, avoiding long periods of standing, and elevating the feet and legs when sitting where possible. Swollen ankles should be bilateral and not accompanied by pain; the midwife should note particularly if this is present in one calf only as it could indicate pathology associated with a deep vein thrombosis.

Skin and nutrition

Women who have suffered from urticaria of pregnancy or cholestasis of the liver should experience relief once the pregnancy is over. The pace of life once the baby is born might lead to women having a reduced fluid intake or eating a different diet than they had formerly (Tuffery & Scriven 2005). This in turn might affect their skin and overall physiological state. Women should be encouraged to maintain a balanced fluid intake and a diet that has a greater proportion of fresh food in it (DH 2007a, Tuffery & Scriven 2005). This will improve gastrointestinal activity and the absorption of iron and minerals, and reduce the potential for constipation and feelings of fatigue.

Urine and bowel function

For some women, discussions about bladder and bowel functions may be personal and embarrassing. Midwives need to consider that women might either think that problems are 'to be expected' (because they have just had a baby) or that they are unique to them. Women may be unable to tell the midwife about it in case it is either worse than they had dreamed or too trivial to worry someone about. These primarily psychological and sociological barriers can result in women suffering from serious and debilitating urinary or bowel problems for years after the birth (Bishop 2005, MacArthur et al 1991, WHO 1998). Taking again the aspect of the range for normal function after childbirth, women need reassurance that, in the first few days after the birth, minor disorders of urinary and bowel function are common. These may be associated with retention or incontinence of urine or constipation, or both. The skill of midwifery care is to try to explore the possible cause of this and decide whether it will resolve spontaneously or requires further investigation.

Expectations of health

It is reasonable for women to look forward to regaining their body for themselves once the baby is born (Gready et al 1997, MaGuire 2000). However, this is not the immediate outcome for many women and, once again, individual women will have their own expectations about the nature and speed at which they would like this recovery to occur. The role of the midwife at this point is to assist the woman to identify actual symptoms of disorder from the gradual process of reorder and advise what action the woman can do for herself in the way of progressive recovery. Advice for new parents in the matter of recovery from the birth is sparse and often superficial; also women may feel they should know what to do, or have unrealistic expectations of motherhood and their ability to cope with these new experiences (Bartell 2004, Marchant et al 2001, Proctor 1999). This is one area where taking the time to talk about what might seem to the midwife a range of peripheral or even superficial issues that might be worrying the otherwise healthy new mother could be of more benefit that day than a range of routine clinical observations (Redshaw et al 2007).

Exercise and healthy activity versus rest, relaxation and sleep

Increasing the understanding in the general population about the value of different forms of exercise and health has been shown to be of psychological as well a physical benefit (Armstrong & Edwards 2004). Exploring each person's level of activity will encourage advice in relation to appropriate exercise and, by association, nutritional intake and rest or relaxation and sleep. Undertaking regular pelvic floor exercises is of benefit to women's long-term health (see Ch. 16).

Afterpains

It has been traditional to associate afterpains with multiparity and breastfeeding. However, women experience afterpains regardless of whether they have had previous pregnancies and when they are not breastfeeding (Mander 1998, Marchant et al 1999). The description of afterpains in parent education books suggests that they are mildly uncomfortable and more an issue of inconvenience. Women themselves, however, have described the pain as equal to the severity of moderate labour pains (Marchant et al 1999). Management of afterpains is by an appropriate analgesic, where possible taken prior to breastfeeding, as it is the production of the oxytocin in relation to the let-down response that initiates the contraction in the uterus and causes pain. It is helpful to explain the cause of afterpains to women and that they might experience a heavier loss at this time, even to the extent of passing clots. Pain in the uterus that is constant or present on abdominal palpation is unlikely to be associated with afterpains and further enquiry should be made about this. Women might also confuse afterpains with flatus pain, especially after an operative birth or where they are constipated. Identifying and treating the cause is likely to relieve the symptoms or raise concern about a more complex condition that needs further attention.

Future health, future fertility

Advice on managing fertility is within the sphere of practice of the midwife and it is an important aspect of postpartum care (see Ch. 37). Midwives need to be aware of a range of different needs with regard to women's sexuality and should be able to offer sensitive and appropriate advice on contraception where this is needed.

Weighing up the 'evidence'

The midwife should have gained a considerable amount of information during her contact with the mother and baby. The wide range for normality and the individuality within this can make it difficult for the midwife to decide whether an observation is related to morbidity. It is more likely to be the relationship between several observations that raises cause for concern and, where these appear to be more related to abnormality than normality, the midwife has a responsibility to make appropriate referral to a medical practitioner or other appropriate healthcare professional. The midwife's statutory framework (NMC 2004) is different from the overall guidance and frameworks for care provision developed under the auspices of various Departments of Health. This is an important distinction with regard to the professional accountability of the midwife and their obligation as an employee (NMC 2008).

Care and the philosophy of dependence to independence

It has been the presumption in this chapter that women will welcome or even actively seek the help and advice of the midwife once the baby has been born. Within this is also the assumption that the woman will have the capability to do this. There may be various reasons why some women do not seem to be so welcoming of the care offered as others. Women from different cultural backgrounds may have traditions that conflict with the current management of postpartum care (Hirst & Hewison 2002, Ockleford et al 2004), or consider that they already have sufficient skills and experience. Not being able to speak or understand English may also inhibit the woman from seeking advice, or may appear to the midwife as being withdrawn and uncommunicative (Schott & Henley 1996). Aspects of domestic disharmony may also lead the woman to decline visits from an outsider. The midwife may have an important role with regard to referral and support for these women, where the worst outcome has been identified within the statistics for maternal death (Lewis 2007, Lewis & Drife 2001, 2004).

Although a visit to the home might have been planned, there will also be times when women are not at home when the midwife visits. It is important to keep in mind individual circumstances and whether these might have any bearing on a failed visit. For example, people with disabilities such as hearing loss or poor mobility might not hear a doorbell. It is important to make arrangements for contact to be made by alternative means (e.g. using a visual alarm or telephone to alert women of the visit beforehand). A very loud television set can prevent the people inside from hearing a doorbell and, simplest of all, although the doorbell has been rung it is not working and no-one is aware that the midwife is standing on the doorstep. Such events may lead to misunderstandings and a breakdown of communication between women and the caregivers with a risk of deterioration in either the uptake or the provision of future services (Disability, Pregnancy and Parenthood International).

One research study reported how some women who have had previous children did not consider that the midwife or health visitor had much to offer them once they had returned home (Murphy-Black 1989). More recent surveys of postnatal care offer rather more insight into women's needs underpinning the approach that offers recognition of each woman as an individual and not someone with an obstetric label, for example referring to women as 'the section in bed 2' or by the previous number of births 'she's a multip' (Ridgers 2007). The midwife needs to recognize situations where the mother perceives that she has different priorities from those 'routinely' provided by the healthcare services. Recent innovations through the SureStart programmes have identified how services can be appropriately reconfigured to meet the needs of vulnerable groups (Wilyman-Bugter & Tucker 2004). The midwife can then ensure that the woman has access to sufficient information (in a format that she can utilize) and to feel able to make contact with any of the services if she or the baby requires it in the future (Gready et al 1997, McCourt & Percival 2000). Where there are concerns about the safety or protection of the newborn infant, the supervisor of midwives should be informed and advice sought from the local social services (the Safeguarding Children Board).

It is important that those undertaking postpartum care, whether in an active or passive format, are appropriately educated and supported so that they can meet the diverse health needs of the mother and baby over the postnatal period. In addition, recent government policy has re-enforced the urgent need for midwives to work in collaboration with other health and social care professionals during this time, and to incorporate midwifery services into a broader framework of a family network (DH 2005, DH 2007b). The social environment has a marked impact on the overall health outcomes for both mother and baby and the acknowledgement of this has drawn midwifery care into the overall public health arena and long term outcomes for health initiatives (or lack of them) at this time.

REFERENCES

Albers L L, Borders N 2007 Minimizing genital tract trauma and related pain following spontaneous vaginal birth. Journal of Midwifery and Women's Health 52(3):246–253

Alexander J, Garcia J, Marchant S 1997 The BLiPP study – final report for the South and West Research and Development Committee. IHCS, Bournemouth University

Anderson B, Torvin Anderson L, Sørensen T 1998 Methylergometrine during the early puerperium; a prospective randomised double blind study. Acta Obstetrica et Gynecologica Scandinavica 77:54–57

Armstrong K, Edwards H 2004 The effectiveness of a pram-walking exercise programme in reducing depressive symptomatology for postnatal women. International Journal of Nursing Practice 10(4):177–194

Ball J 1994 Reactions to motherhood, 2nd edn. Books for Midwives Press, Hale

Bartell S S 2004 Self-nurturance as a crucial element in mothering. International Journal of Childbirth Education 19(4):8–11

Bick D, MacArthur C, Knowles H et al 2002 Postnatal care: evidence and guidelines for management. Churchill Livingstone, Edinburgh

Bishop M 2005 Improving support for women with incontinence. British Journal of Midwifery 13(9):590

Boulvain M, Perneger T V, Othenin-Girard V et al 2004 Home-based versus hospital-based postnatal care: a randomised trial. British Journal of Obstetrics and Gynaecology 111(8):807–813

Buckley S J 2006 Mother and baby – a good start. In: Wickham S (ed.) Midwifery: best practice, 4. Edinburgh: Elsevier p 201–206

Cattrell R, Lavender T, Wallymahmed A et al 2005 Postnatal care: what matters to midwives. British Journal of Midwifery 13(4):206–213

Cluett E R, Alexander J, Pickering R M 1997 What is the normal pattern of uterine involution? An investigation of post-partum involution measured by the distance between the symphysis pubis and the uterine fundus using a tape measure. Midwifery 13:9–16

Cunningham F G, Leveno K J, Bloom S et al 2005 Williams obstetrics, 22nd edn. McGraw Hill Medical, New York, Ch 5, p 121–150; Ch 30, p 695–710

De Clerc E, Sakal C, Corry M et al 2006 Listening to mothers II Report of the second National US survey of Childbearing Women's Childbearing Experiences. Childbirth Connections, New York, p 45–48, 55–61

DH (Department of Health) 2005 National service framework for children, young people and maternity services. Standard 11. Maternity Services, Department of Health, London

DH (Department of Health) 2007a The pregnancy book. the early weeks: you. Department of Health, London, Ch. 15

DH (Department of Health) 2007b Maternity matters: choice, access and continuity of care in a safe service. DH, London

Disability Pregnancy and Parenthood International. Online. Available: www.dppi.org.uk

Eaton A P 2001 Early postpartum discharge: recommendations from a preliminary report to Congress. Pediatrics 107 (2):400–404

Evans C 1995 Postpartum home care in the United States. Journal of Obstetrics, Gynecology and Neonatal Nursing 24 (2):180–187

Garcia J, Marchant S 1993 Back to normal? Postpartum health and illness. In: Research and the Midwife Conference Proceedings, University of Manchester, Manchester, p 2–9

Garcia J, Marchant S 1996 The potential of postnatal care. In: Kroll D (ed.) Issues in midwifery care for the future. Baillière Tindall, London, p 58–74

Garcia J, Renfrew M, Marchant S 1994 Postnatal home visiting by midwives. Midwifery 10(1):40–43

Garcia J, Redshaw M, Fitzsimmons B et al 1998 First class delivery, a national survey of women's views of maternity care. Audit Commission Publications, Abingdon

Glazener C, Abdalla M, Stroud P et al 1995 Postnatal maternal morbidity: extent, causes, prevention and treatment. British Journal of Obstetrics and Gynaecology 102(4):282–287

Gready M, Buggins E, Newburn M et al 1997 Hearing it like it is: understanding the views of users. British Journal of Midwifery 5(8):496–500

Gupton A 1995 The Canadian perspective on postpartum care. Journal of Obstetrics and Gynecologic and Neonatal Nursing February:173–179

Hirst J, Hewison J 2002 Hospital postnatal care: obtaining the views of Pakistani and indigenous 'white' women. Clinical Effectiveness in Nursing 6(1):10–18

Hytten F 1995 The clinical physiology of the puerperium. Farrand Press, London, Ch 7, p 121–145; Ch 8, p 146–162

Ladyman S 2005 Improving postnatal care for every woman. British Journal of Midwifery 13(2):68, 70

Lewis G, Drife J (eds) 2001 Why mothers die: 1997–1999. The fifth report of the Confidential Enquiries into Maternal Death in the United Kingdom. RCOG Press, London

Lewis G, Drife (eds) 2004 Why mothers die: 2000–2002. The sixth report of the Confidential Enquiries into Maternal Deaths in the United Kingdom. RCOG Press, London

Lewis, G (ed.) 2007 The Confidential Enquiry into Maternal and Child Health (CEMACH). Saving mothers' lives: reviewing maternal deaths to make motherhood safer 2003–2005. The seventh report of the Confidential Enquiries into Maternal Deaths in the United Kingdom. CEMACH, London

MacArthur C, Lewis M, Knox G 1991 Health after childbirth: an investigation of long term health problems beginning after childbirth in 11701 women. HMSO, London

MaGuire M 2000 The transition to parenthood. In: Life after birth: reflections on postnatal care, report of a multi-disciplinary seminar, 3 July 2000. RCM, Cardiff

Mander R 1998 Postnatal pain. In: Pain in childbearing and its control. Blackwell Science, Oxford, p 165–194

Marchant S, Garcia J 1993 The NPEU postnatal care project. Proceedings of the International Confederation of Midwives, 23rd international congress, Vancouver, 9–14 May, p 343–344

Marchant S 1997 Postnatal care and the 'busying, hurrying midwife'. Midwives 110(1319):308

Marchant S, Alexander J, Garcia J et al 1999 Blood loss in the postnatal period – the BLiPP study. A survey of women's experiences of vaginal loss from twenty four hours to three months after childbirth. Midwifery 15:72–81

Marchant S, Alexander J, Garcia J 2000 How does it feel to you? Uterine palpation and lochial loss as guides to postnatal recovery 2 – the BLiPP study (blood loss in the postnatal period). Practising Midwife 3(7):31–33

Marchant S, Alexander J, Garcia J 2001. One small drop in the ocean: blood loss in the postnatal period: the development and pilot testing of information leaflets for women about vaginal loss after childbirth (BLiPP 2). MIDIRS Midwifery Digest 11(Suppl 1):S9–S13

Marchant S, 2005 Developing clinical judgements. In: Raynor M D, Marshall J E, Sullivan A (eds) Decision making in midwifery practice. Churchill Livingstone, Edinburgh, Ch. 7

Marchant S 2006 The postnatal care journey – are we nearly there yet? MIDIRs Midwifery Digest 16(3):295–304

Marsh J, Sargent E 1991 Factors affecting the duration of postnatal visits. Midwifery 7:177–182

McCandlish R, Bowler U, van Asten H et al 1998 A randomised controlled trial of care of the perineum during the second stage of normal labour. British Journal of Obstetrics and Gynaecology 105(12):1262–1272

McCourt C, Percival P 2000 Social support in childbirth. In: Page L (ed.) The new midwifery: science and sensitivity in practice. Churchill Livingstone, Edinburgh, p 245–268

Morrell C J, Spiby H, Stewart P et al 2000 Costs and benefits of community postnatal support workers: randomised controlled trial. British Medical Journal 321:593–598

Murphy-Black T 1989 Postnatal care at home: a descriptive study of mother's needs and the maternity services. University of Edinburgh, Edinburgh

NCT (National Childbirth Trust) 2007 Are you a born leader? New Generation Spring:11

NICE (National Institute for Health and Clinical Excellence) 2006 Routine postnatal care of women and their babies. National Institute for Health and Clinical Excellence, London

NMC (Nursing and Midwifery Council) 2008 The code: standards of conduct, performance and ethics for nurses and midwives. NMC, London

NMC (Nursing and Midwifery Council) 2004 Midwives rules and standards. NMC, London

Ockleford E M, Berryman J C, Hsu R 2004 Postnatal care: what new mothers say. British Journal of Midwifery 12(3):166–171

Oppenheimer L W, Sherrif E, Goodman D S et al 1986 The duration of lochia. British Journal of Obstetrics and Gynaecology 93:754–757

O'Sullivan S, Tyler S 2007 Payment by results: speaking in code. RCM Midwives 10(5):241

Peterson W E, Charles C, DiCenso A et al 2005 The Newcastle satisfaction with nursing scales: a valid measure of maternal satisfaction with inpatient postpartum nursing care. Journal of Advanced Nursing 52(6):672–681

Proctor S 1999 Women's reactions to their experience of maternity care. British Journal of Midwifery 7(8):492–498

RCM (Royal College of Midwives) 2000 Life after birth: reflections on postnatal care, report of a multi-disciplinary seminar, 3 July 2000. RCM, Cardiff

Redshaw M, Rowe R, Hockley C et al 2007 Recorded delivery – a national survey of women's experiences of maternity care in Oxford. National Perinatal Epidemiology Unit, Oxford

Reid L 2005 Midwifery in Scotland: the shaping of postnatal care. British Journal of Midwifery 13(8):492–496

Ridgers I, Marchant S, Alexander J et al 2002 What is happening on the postnatal ward? Non-participant observation. The International Confederation of Midwives. Midwives and women working together for the family of the world. ICM proceedings, CD-ROM, Vienna. ICM, The Hague.

Ridgers I 2007 Passing through but needing to be heard. An ethnographic study of women's perspectives of their care on the postnatal ward. Unpublished PhD thesis. Bournemouth University, Bournemouth

Sewell B 2007 The right kind of help. RCM Midwives 10(2):85

Schott J, Henley A 1996 Culture. In: Schott J, Henley A (eds) Religion and childbearing in a multi-racial society. Butterworth Heinemann, Oxford, p 172–185

Shaw E, Levitt C, Wong S et al 2006 Systematic review of the literature on postpartum care: Effectiveness of postpartum support to improve maternal parenting, mental health, quality of life and physical health. Birth 33(30):210–220

Sherman D, Lurie S, Frenkel E et al 1999 Characteristics of normal lochia. American Journal of Perinatology 16(8):399–402

Silverton L 1993 Postnatal care. In: Silverton L. (ed.) The art and science of midwifery. Prentice Hall, New York, Ch 28

Singh D, Newburn M 2000 Women's experiences of postnatal care. National Childbirth Trust, London

Sleep J 1995 Postnatal perineal care revisited. In: Alexander J, Levy V, Roche C (eds) Aspects of midwifery practice: a research based approach. MacMillan, Chatham, p 132–153

Steen M, Cooper K, Marchant P, et al 2000 A randomised controlled trial to compare the effectiveness of icepacks and Epifoam with cooling maternity gel pads at alleviating perineal trauma. Midwifery 16(1):48–55

Steen M 2007 Perineal tears and episiotomy: how do wounds heal? British Journal of Midwifery 15(5):273–274, 276–280

Tuffery O, Scriven A 2005 Factors influencing antenatal and postnatal diets of primigravid women. Journal of the Royal Society of Health 125(5):227–231

Twaddle S, Liao X, Fyvie H 1993 An evaluation of postnatal care individualised to the needs of the woman. Midwifery 9:154–160

Walsh D 1997 Hospital postnatal care: the end is nigh. British Journal of Midwifery 5(9):516–518

WHO (World Health Organization) 1998 Postpartum care of the mother and newborn. Report of a technical working group. WHO, Geneva

WHO (World Health Organization) 1999 Postpartum care of the mother and newborn: a practical guide. Birth 26(4):255–258

Wiggins M 2000 Psychosocial needs after childbirth. Life after birth: reflections on postnatal care, report of a multi-disciplinary seminar, 3rd July. RCM, Cardiff

Wilyman-Bugter M, Tucker L 2004 Using SureStart to develop an integrated model of postnatal midwifery care. MIDIRS Midwifery Digest 14(3):379–382

Winter H R, MacArthur C, Bick D E et al 2001 Postnatal care and its role in maternal health and well-being. MIDIRS Midwifery Digest 11(Suppl 1):S3–S7

Wray J 2006 Seeking to explore what matters to women about postnatal care. British Journal of Midwifery 14(5):246–254

Wylie L 2002 Postnatal pain. Practising Midwife 5(1):13–15

35

Physical problems and complications in the puerperium

Sally Marchant

This chapter reviews the care of women who either entered the postpartum period having experienced obstetric or medical complications, including those who did not undergo a vaginal birth, or whose postpartum recovery, regardless of the mode of delivery, did not follow a normal pattern.
It includes the care for women with obvious risks for increased postpartum physical morbidity.
(The effects of morbidity related to psychological trauma are covered in Chapter 36.)

The chapter aims to:

- discuss the role of midwifery care in the detection and management of postpartum morbidity
- review best practice in the management of problems associated with trauma and pathology arising from pregnancy and childbirth
- review the role of the midwife where postpartum health is complicated by an instrumental or operative birth.

The need for women-centred and women-led postpartum care

A women-centred approach to care in the postpartum period should assist physical and psychological recovery by being focused on the needs of women as individuals rather than fitting women into a routine care package (DH 2004, MaGuire 2000, NICE 2006). The midwife needs to be familiar with the woman's background and antenatal and labour history when assessing whether or not the woman's progress is following the expected postpartum pattern (DH 2004, Garcia et al 1998, Redshaw et al 2007).

The effects of obstetric or medical complications will be described within the context of the ongoing review by the midwife of the woman's health over the postnatal period. The role of the midwife in these cases is first to identify whether a potentially pathological condition exists and if so, to refer the woman for appropriate investigations and care (NMC 2004). Where the birth involves obstetric or medical complications, a woman's postpartum care is likely to differ from those women whose pregnancy and labour are considered straightforward. However, it must also be considered that some women have a perception of the whole birth experience as traumatic, although to the obstetric or midwifery staff no untoward events occurred (Singh & Newburn 2000).

Maternal mortality and morbidity after the birth

The discovery of penicillin and the provision of a blood transfusion were major contributions to saving women's lives over the past century (Loudon 1986, 1987) and maternal death after childbirth where there has been no preceding antenatal complication is now a rare occurrence in the UK (Lewis 2007).

Thrombosis or thromboembolism continues to be the major cause of direct death but, despite the apparent advances in medication and practice, women still die postpartum as a result of haemorrhage or from sepsis associated with genital tract infection (Lewis 2007). The value of this information is to raise awareness of the degree to which care can contribute to the prevention as well as the detection and management of potentially fatal outcomes.

From research, it became clear that maternal morbidity after childbirth was remarkable in the extensive nature of the problems and the duration of time over which such problems continue to be experienced by women (Bick & MacArthur 1995, Brown & Lumley 1998, Garcia & Marchant 1993, Glazener et al 1995, Glazener & MacArthur 2001, MacArthur et al 1991, Marchant et al 1999, Waterstone et al 2003).

The midwife has a duty to undertake midwifery care for at least the first 28 days postpartum. The activities of the midwife are to support the new mother and her family unit by monitoring her recovery after the birth and to offer her appropriate information and advice as part of the statutory duties of the midwife (NMC 2004).

Immediate untoward events for the mother following the birth of the baby

Immediate (primary) postpartum haemorrhage (PPH) is a potentially life-threatening event which occurs at the point of or within 24 hrs of delivery of the placenta and membranes and presents as a sudden, and excessive vaginal blood loss (see Ch. 29). Secondary, or delayed PPH is where there is excessive or prolonged vaginal loss from 24 hrs after birth and for up to 6 weeks' postpartum (Cunningham et al 2005a). Unlike primary PPH, which includes a defined volume of blood loss (≥ 500 mL) as part of its definition, there is no volume of blood specified for a secondary PPH and management differs according to apparent clinical need (Alexander et al 2002).

Regardless of the timing of any haemorrhage, it is most frequently the placental site that is the source. Alternatively, a cervical or deep vaginal wall tear or trauma to the perineum might be the cause in women who have recently given birth. Retained placental fragments or other products of conception are likely to inhibit the process of involution, or reopen the placental wound. The diagnosis is likely to be determined more by the woman's condition and pattern of events (Hoveyda & MacKenzie 2001, Jansen et al 2005) and is also often complicated by the presence of infection (Cunningham et al 2005b; see Ch. 29).

Maternal collapse within 24 hrs of the birth without overt bleeding

Where no signs of haemorrhage are apparent other causes need to be considered (see Chs 22 and 23). Management of all these conditions requires ensuring the woman is in a safe environment until appropriate treatment can be administered, and meanwhile maintaining the woman's airway, basic circulatory support as needed and providing oxygen. It is important to remember that, regardless of the apparent state of collapse, the woman may still be able to hear and so verbally reassuring the woman (and her partner or relatives if present) is an important aspect of the immediate care.

Postpartum complications and identifying deviations from the normal

Following the birth of their baby, women recount feelings that are, at one level, elation that they have experienced the birth and survived and, at another, the reality of pain or discomfort from a number of unwelcome changes as their bodies recover from pregnancy and labour (Gready et al 1997). Women may experience symptoms that might be early signs of pathological events. These might be presented by the woman as 'minor' concerns, or not actually be in a form that is recognized as abnormal by the woman herself. Where the postpartum visit is

undertaken as a form of review of the woman's physical and psychological health, led by the woman's needs, the midwife is likely to obtain a random collection of information that lacks a specific structure. Women will probably give information about events or symptoms that are the most worrying or most painful to them at that time. At this point the midwife needs to establish whether there are any other signs of possible morbidity and determine whether these might indicate the need for referral. Figure 35.1 suggests a model for linking together key observations that suggest potential risk of, or actual, morbidity.

The central point, as with any personal contact, is the midwife's initial review of the woman's appearance and psychological state. This is underpinned by a review of the woman's vital signs, where any general state of illness is evident. It is suggested that a pragmatic approach be taken with regard to evidence of pyrexia as a mildly raised temperature may be related to normal physiological hormonal responses, for example the increasing production

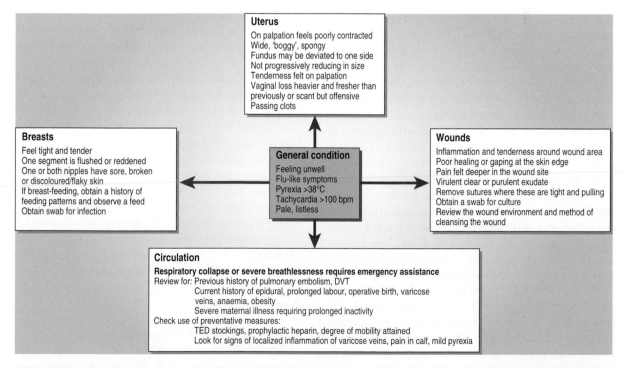

Figure 35.1 Diagrammatic demonstration of the relationship between deviation from normal physiology and potential morbidity.

of breastmilk. However, infection is an important factor in postpartum maternal morbidity and mortality and the midwife should not make an assumption that a mildly raised temperature is part of the normal health parameters (Lewis 2007). The accumulation of a number of clinical signs will assist the midwife in making decisions about the presence or potential for morbidity. Where there is a rise in temperature above 38°C it is usual for this to be considered a deviation from normal and of clinical significance.

The pulse rate and respirations are also significant observations when accumulating clinical evidence. Although there may be no evidence of vaginal haemorrhage for example, a weak and rapid pulse rate (>100 b.p.m.) in conjunction with a woman who is in a state of collapse with signs of shock and a low blood pressure (systolic <90 mmHg) may indicate the formation of a haematoma, where there is an excessive leakage of blood from damaged blood vessels into the surrounding tissues. A rapid pulse rate in an otherwise well woman might suggest that she is anaemic but could also indicate increased thyroid or other dysfunctional hormonal activity.

The midwife needs to be alert to any possible relationship between the observations overall and their potential cause with regard to common illnesses, e.g. that the woman has a common cold, and that the morbidity is associated with or affected by having recently given birth. Where the midwife is in conversation with the woman as part of the postpartum review, if she receives information that suggests the woman has signs deviating from what is expected to be normal, it is important that a range of clinical observations are undertaken to refute or confirm this.

Following an innovative research study into extended midwifery care of women beyond the conventional 10–14-day period, a set of guidelines were compiled to assist midwives make decisions about the need for referral (Bick et al 2002). As part of the NICE (2006) process compiling guidelines for core care, it was recognized that midwives develop skills and processes from their experience to accumulate evidence from their observations and conversations about the overall well-being of the mother and the baby. However, this process was mainly covert and difficult to adapt in any formal way to help less experienced midwives or even explain the course of action to the women themselves

(Marchant 2006, Marchant et al 2003). To clarify the actions necessary, when the NICE guidelines were published, a quick guide was also produced providing a table of the action required for possible signs/symptoms of complications and common health problems in women (NICE 2006, p 22–24).

The uterus and vaginal loss following vaginal birth

It is expected that the midwife will undertake assessment of uterine involution at intervals throughout the period of midwifery care (see Ch. 34). It is recommended that this should always be undertaken where the woman is feeling generally unwell, has abdominal pain, a vaginal loss that is markedly brighter red or heavier than previously, is passing clots or reports her vaginal loss to be offensive (Hoveyda & MacKenzie 2001, Marchant et al 2006).

Where the palpation of the uterus identifies that it is deviated to one side, this might be as a result of a full bladder. Where the midwife has ensured that the woman had emptied her bladder prior to the palpation, the presence of urinary retention must be considered. Catheterization of the bladder in these circumstances is indicated for two reasons: to remove any obstacle that is preventing the process of involution taking place and to provide relief to the bladder itself. If the deviation is not as a result of a full bladder, further investigations need to be undertaken to determine the cause.

Morbidity might be suspected where the uterus fails to follow the expected progressive reduction in size, feels wide or 'boggy' on palpation and is less well contracted than expected. This might be described as subinvolution of the uterus, which can indicate postpartum infection, or the presence of retained products of the placenta or membranes, or both (Howie 1995, Khong & Khong 1993).

Treatment is by antibiotics, oxytocic drugs that act on the uterine muscle, hormonal preparations or evacuation of the uterus (ERPC), usually under a general anaesthetic.

Vulnerability to infection, potential causes and prevention

Infection is the invasion of tissues by pathogenic micro-organisms; the degree to which this results in ill-health relates to their virulence and number. Vulnerability is increased where conditions exist that enable the organism to thrive and reproduce and where there is access to and from entry points in the body. Organisms are transferred between sources and a potential host by hands, air currents and fomites (i.e. agents such as bed linen). Hosts are more vulnerable where they are in a condition of susceptibility because of poor immunity or a pre-existing resistance to the invading organism. The body responds to the invading organisms by forming antibodies, which in turn produce inflammation initiating other physiological changes such as pain and an increase in body temperature.

Acquisition of an infective organism can be *endogenous*, where the organisms are already present in or on the body (e.g. *Streptococcus faecalis* (Lancefield group B), *Clostridium welchii* (both present in the vagina) or *Escherichia coli* (present in the bowel)) or organisms in a dormant state are reactivated (notably tuberculosis bacteria). Other routes are *exogenous*, where the organisms are transferred from other people (or animal) body surfaces or the environment. Other transfer mechanisms include *droplets* – inhalations of respiratory pathogens on liquid particles (e.g. β-haemolytic streptococcus and *Chlamydia trachomatis*), *cross-infection* and *nosocomial* (hospital acquired) transfer from an infected person or place to an uninfected one (e.g. *Staphylococcus aureus*).

The bacteria responsible for the majority of puerperal infection arise from the streptococcal or staphylococcal species. The *Streptococcus* bacterium has a chain-like formation and may be haemolytic or non-haemolytic, and aerobic or anaerobic; the most common species associated with puerperal sepsis is the β-haemolytic *S. pyogenes* (Lancefield group A) although other strains of the streptococcal bacteria have also been identified as the source of serious morbidity (Muller et al 2006). The *Staphylococcus* bacterium has a grape-like structure, of which the most important species is *S. aureus* or *pyogenes*. Staphylococci are the most frequent cause of wound infections; where these bacteria are coagulase positive they form clots on the plasma which can lead to more widely spread systemic morbidity. There is additional concern about their resistance to antibiotics and subsequent management to control spread of the infection. Regardless of the location of care,

postpartum women and healthcare professionals should be aware of how infection can be acquired and should pay particular attention to effective hand-washing techniques, adhere to the accepted practice for aseptic technique when in contact with wound care, including the use of gloves for this, and where there is direct contact with areas in the body where bacteria of potential morbidity are prevalent.

The uterus and vaginal loss following operative delivery

A lower segment caesarean section will have involved cutting of the major abdominal muscles and damage to other soft tissues. Palpation of the abdomen is therefore likely to be very painful for the woman in the first few days after the operation. The woman who has undergone a caesarean section will have a very different level of physical activity from the woman who has had a vaginal birth. It may be some hours after the operation until the woman feels able to sit up or move about at all. Blood and debris will have been slowly released from the uterus during this time and, when the woman begins to move, this will be expelled through the vagina and may appear as a substantial fresh-looking red loss. Following this initial loss, it is usual for the amount of vaginal loss to lessen and for further fresh loss to be minimal. All this can be observed without actually palpating the uterus. For women who have undergone an operative delivery, once 3 or 4 days have elapsed, then abdominal palpation to assess uterine involution can be undertaken by the midwife where this appears to be clinically appropriate. By this time, the uterus or area around the uterus should not be overly painful on palpation.

Where clinically indicated, e.g. where the vaginal bleeding is heavier than expected, the uterine fundus can be gently palpated. If the uterus is not well contracted then medical intervention is needed. Uterine stimulants (uterotonics) are usually prescribed in the form of an intravenous infusion of oxytocin or an intravenous or intramuscular injection of ergometrine (see Ch. 29). If the bleeding continues where such treatment has been commenced, further investigations might include obtaining blood for clotting factors, or the woman might need to return to theatre for further exploration of the uterine cavity. The emergence of ultrasound scans (USS) in the postpartum period has led to some conflicting reports of the state of the normal postpartum uterus and the value of USS in distinguishing potentially pathological conditions (Hertzberg & Bowie 1991). Recent studies appear to support greater use of USS to assist diagnosis and clinical management of problems of uterine sub-involution (Deans & Dietz 2006, Shalev et al 2002).

Wound problems

Perineal problems

It is important that the midwife has an understanding of the effect of trauma as a physiological process and the normal pattern for wound healing (Steen 2007). Pain is a direct result of the assault on the nerve endings in the traumatized tissue and where women have undergone perineal trauma that has required suturing, the most immediate problem that occurs soon after the birth is that the woman complains of severe perineal pain. This might be as a result of the analgesia no longer being effective, of increased oedema in the surrounding tissues or, more seriously, of haematoma formation. Haematoma usually develops deep in the perineal fascia tissues and may not be easily visible to the observer if the perineal tissues are already oedematous and discoloured. The blood contained within such a haematoma can exceed 1000 mL and may significantly affect the overall state of the woman, who can present with signs of acute shock. Treatment is by evacuation of the haematoma and resuturing of the perineal wound, usually under a general anaesthetic.

Perineal pain that is severe and is not caused by a haematoma might arise as a result of oedema, causing the stitches to feel excessively tight. Local application of cold packs can bring relief as they reduce the immediate oedema and continue to provide relief over the first few days following the birth (Steen et al 2006). The use of oral analgesia as well as complementary medicines such as arnica and lavender oil are said to have a beneficial effect, although the effectiveness of such therapies has to date not been confirmed by research findings (Bick et al 2009). Midwives should undertake appropriate training in complementary therapies before advocating their use (see Ch. 50).

Factors that are associated with poor healing include poor diet, obesity, pre-existing medical disorders and negative social conditions such as poor housing, increased stress and smoking (Steen 2007). Where pain in the perineal area occurs at a later stage, or re-occurs, this might be associated with an infection. The skin edges are likely to have a moist, puffy and dull appearance; there may also be an offensive odour and evidence of pus in the wound. A swab should be obtained for microorganism culture and referral made to a GP. Antibiotics might be commenced immediately when there is specific information about any infective agent. Where the perineal tissues appear to be infected, it is important to discuss with the woman about cleaning the area and making an attempt to reduce constant moisture and heat. Women might be advised about using cotton underwear, avoiding tights and trousers and frequently changing sanitary pads. They should also be advised to avoid using perfumed bath additives or talcum powder.

If the perineal area fails to heal, or continues to cause pain once the initial healing process should have occurred, resuturing or refashioning might be advised. Postpartum outcomes were recorded for women who took part in a randomised trial looking at the management of the fetal head at the point of birth (McCandlish et al 1998). A total of 7% of women in the study reported perineal pain 3 months after the birth of their baby. This suggests that quite a substantial proportion of women are left with significant problems long after regular contact with healthcare professionals has ceased. This means it is important to give women information about the timescale by which healing should have occurred so that they can seek appropriate advice earlier rather than later. Women may also need to be encouraged to discuss this with their GP, or be given other support where the vaginal or perineal tissues still cause discomfort within the course of daily activities. Women should be pain free and have been able to resume sexual intercourse without pain by 6 weeks after the birth, although some discomfort might still be present depending on the degree of trauma experienced. Although high levels of sexual morbidity after childbirth have been identified, the approach to discussion and management of this area appears to be problematic (Barrett et al 2000). In giving health advice and support, healthcare professionals are advised to identify an appropriate time, not to make assumptions with regard to sexual activity after childbirth and to be conversant with support agencies relevant to a range of cultural and sexual diversities and associated needs (Barrett et al 2000, Glazener 1997, NICE 2006, RCM 2000).

Caesarean section wounds

It is now common practice for women undergoing an operative birth to have prophylactic antibiotics at the time of the surgery (Smaill & Hofmeyr 2000). This has been demonstrated to significantly reduce the incidence of subsequent wound infection and endometritis. In addition, it is now usual for the wound dressing to be removed after the first 24 hrs, as this also aids healing and reduces infection. Advice needs to be offered to the woman about care of her wound and adequate drying when taking a bath or shower, or for more obese women where abdominal skin folds are present and are likely to create an environment that is constantly warm and moist. For these women, a dry dressing over the suture line might be appropriate.

A wound that is hot, tender and inflamed and is accompanied by a pyrexia is highly suggestive of an infection. Where this is observed, a swab should be obtained for microorganism culture and medical advice should be sought. Haematoma and abscesses can also form underneath the wound and women may identify increased pain around the wound where these are present. Rarely a wound may need to be probed to reduce the pressure and allow infected material to drain, reducing the likelihood of the formation of an abscess. With the hospital stay now being much shorter than previously, these problems increasingly occur after the woman has left hospital.

Circulation

Pulmonary embolism remains a major cause of maternal deaths in the UK and midwives and general practitioners need to be more alert to identify high risk women and the possibility of thromboembolism in puerperal women with leg pain and breathlessness (Lewis 2007). Women who have a *previous* history of pulmonary embolism, a deep vein thrombosis, are obese or who have varicose veins have a higher risk of postpartum problems. Postpartum care of women who have pre-existing or pregnancy-related medical complications relies on prophylactic precautions and should be undertaken for women who undergo surgery and have these pre-existing factors. Thromboembolitic D (TED) stockings should be provided during, or as soon as possible after, the birth and prophylactic heparin prescribed until women attain normal mobility. All women who undergo an epidural anaesthetic, are anaemic, or have a prolonged labour or an operative birth are slightly more at risk of developing complications linked to blood clots. Women with pre-existing problems are at higher risk because of their overall health status and environment of care postpartum. For example, women who undergo a caesarean section as a result of maternal illness are more likely to spend longer in bed, thereby reducing their mobility and increasing their risk of morbidity.

Clinical signs that women might report include the following (from the most common to the most serious). The signs of circulatory problems related to varicose veins are usually localized inflammation or tenderness around the varicose vein, sometimes accompanied by a mild pyrexia. This is superficial thrombophlebitis, which is usually resolved by applying support to the affected area and administering antiinflammatory drugs, where these are not in conflict with other medication being taken or with breastfeeding. Unilateral oedema of an ankle or calf accompanied by stiffness or pain and a positive Homan's sign might indicate a deep vein thrombosis that has the potential to cause a pulmonary embolism. Urgent medical referral must be made to confirm the diagnosis and commence anticoagulant or other appropriate therapy. The most serious outcome is the development of a pulmonary embolism. The first sign might be the sudden onset of breathlessness, which may not be associated with any obvious clinical sign of a blood clot. Women with this condition are likely to become seriously ill and could suffer a respiratory collapse with very little prior warning.

Some degree of oedema of the lower legs and ankles and feet can be viewed as being within normal limits where it is not accompanied by calf pain (especially unilaterally), pyrexia or a raised blood pressure.

Hypertension

Women who have had previous episodes of hypertension in pregnancy may continue to demonstrate this postpartum for several weeks after the birth (Tan & de Swiet 2002). There is still a risk that women who have clinical signs of pregnancy-induced hypertension can develop eclampsia in the hours and days following the birth although this is a relatively rare outcome in the normal population (Atterbury et al 1998, Tan & de Swiet 2002). In addition, some women appear to develop eclampsia postpartum where there has been no previous history of raised blood pressure or proteinuria (Chames et al 2002, Matthys et al 2004). Some degree of monitoring of the blood pressure should be continued for women who were hypertensive antenatally, and postpartum management should proceed on an individual basis (Tan & de Swiet 2002). For these women, the medical advice should determine optimal systolic and diastolic levels, with instructions for treatment with antihypertensive drugs if the blood pressure exceeds these levels. As women can develop postnatal pre-eclampsia without having antenatal problems associated with this, because the symptoms can be fairly non-specific, such as a headache or epigastric pain or vomiting, the woman may delay or fail to contact a healthcare professional for advice, or where they do seek advice, the healthcare professional may not be alert to the possibility of the development of post-partum eclampsia (Chames et al 2002). Failure to detect symptoms at this initial stage may lead to more serious outcomes as the disease develops untreated (Chames et al 2002, Matthys et al 2004, Tan & de Swiet 2002). Therefore, if a postpartum woman presents with signs associated with pre-eclampsia, the midwife should be alert to this possibility and undertake observations of the blood pressure and urine and obtain medical advice.

For women with essential hypertension, the management of their overall medical condition will be reviewed postpartum by their usual caregivers. Undertaking clinical observation of blood pressure for a period after the birth is advisable so that information is available upon which to base the management of this for the woman in the future (Tan & de Swiet 2002).

Headache

This is a common ailment in the general population; concern in relation to postpartum morbidity should therefore centre around the history of the severity, duration and frequency of the headaches, the medication being taken to alleviate them and how effective this is. As this is also associated with hypertension, a recording of the blood pressure should be undertaken to exclude this as a primary factor. In taking the history, if an epidural analgesic was administered, medical advice should be sought. Headaches from a dural tap typically arise once the woman has become mobile after the birth and they are at their most severe when standing, lessening when the woman lies down. They are often accompanied by neck stiffness, vomiting and visual disturbances. These headaches are very debilitating and are best managed by stopping the leakage of cerebral spinal fluid by the insertion of 10–20 mL of blood into the epidural space; this should resolve the clinical symptoms. Where women have returned home after the birth, they would need to return to the hospital to have this procedure.

Headaches might also be precursors of psychological distress and it is important that other issues related to the birth event are explored, taking the time and opportunity to do this in a sensitive manner. Factors that might be overlooked include dehydration, sleep loss and a greater than usual stressful environment (see Ch. 36). However, the midwife should take time to discuss the woman's feelings and offer advice or reassurance about these where possible.

Backache

Many women experience pain or discomfort from backache in pregnancy as a result of separation or diastasis of the abdominal muscles (rectus abdominis diastasis, or RAD, see Ch. 16). Where backache is causing pain that affects the woman's activities of daily living, referral can be made to local physiotherapy services. Pelvic girdle pain experienced in pregnancy should resolve in the weeks after the baby is born but it may continue for a much longer period (Aslan & Fynes 2007).

Urinary problems

Women who have experienced an uncomplicated labour are less likely to experience acute retention of urine following the birth. However, it is still important to monitor urinary function and to ask women about this and the sensations associated with normal bladder control. Management of urine output has been shown to lack consistency and recognition of its potential importance (Zaki et al 2004). For some women a short period of poor bladder control may be present for a few days after the birth, but this should resolve within a week at the most. Women with perineal trauma may have difficulty in deciding whether they have normal urinary control and retention of urine might be detected by the midwife as a result of abdominal palpation of the uterus. Abdominal tenderness in association with other urinary symptoms, for example a poor output, dysuria or offensive urine and a pyrexia or general flu-like symptoms, might indicate a urinary tract infection. Very rarely urinary incontinence might be a result of a urethral fistula following complications from the labour or birth.

Where women have undergone an epidural or spinal anaesthetic, this can have an effect on the neurological sensors that control urine release and flow. This might cause acute retention in some women and be identified within hours of the birth where, as a result of the physiological diuresis, large volumes of urine are produced. In other cases, women may appear to be voiding urine without difficulty but not emptying the bladder each time. They may pass small amounts of urine and be unaware that more urine has remained in the bladder (Lee et al 1999). The main complication of any form of urine retention is that the uterus might be prevented from effective contraction, which leads to increased vaginal blood loss. There is also increased potential for the woman to contract a urine infection with possible kidney involvement and long term effects on bladder function.

It is not uncommon for some women to have a small degree of leakage of urine or retention within the first 2 or 3 days while the tissues recover from the birth, but this should resolve with the practice of postnatal exercise and healing of any localized trauma. Women might feel embarrassed about having urinary problems and midwives may need to consider appropriate ways of encouraging women to talk about any problems so that they can advise women about their future management. Referral to a physiotherapist might be an appropriate first step as pelvic floor exercises and bladder training have been found to improve the outcome significantly in women with long term urinary incontinence (Glazener et al 2001). Specific enquiry about these issues should be made when women attend for their 6-week postnatal examination; further investigations should be made for women who are encountering these problems.

Bowels and constipation

It is the relationship of the regularity of bowel movements to the woman's previous experience that is likely to assist the midwife in determining whether or not there is a problem. The occurrence of haemorrhoids and constipation is not uncommon during pregnancy and is a result of the influence of progesterone on smooth muscle. Additional factors include following an altered diet, a degree of dehydration during labour and concern about further pain from any perineal trauma. A diet that includes soft fibre, increased fluids and the use of prophylactic laxatives that are non-irritant to the bowel can be prescribed to alleviate constipation, the most common and apparently effective of these being lactulose (Eogan et al 2007). Women need advice that any disruption to their normal bowel pattern should resolve within days of the birth, taking into consideration the recovery required by the presence of perineal trauma. They should also be reassured about the effect of a bowel movement on the area that has been sutured as many women may be unnecessarily anxious about the possibility of tearing their perineal stitches. Where women have prolonged difficulty with constipation, anal fissures can result (Corby et al 1997). These are painful and difficult to resolve and therefore advice about bowel management is important in avoiding this situation. Women who have haemorrhoids should also be given advice on following a diet high in fibre and fluids, preferably water and the use of appropriate laxatives to soften the stools as well as topical applications to reduce the oedema and pain.

It is also of concern where women might experience loss of bowel control and whether this is faecal incontinence. It is important to determine the nature of the incontinence and distinguish it from an episode of diarrhoea. It might be helpful to ask whether the woman has taken any laxatives in the previous 24 hrs and explore what food was eaten. Where the problems do not seem to be associated with other factors the woman should first be advised to see her GP. Faecal incontinence is not always associated with a third degree tear and its prevalence is unclear but it is associated with a range of risk factors that include instrumental birth, and primiparity (Guise et al 2007, Thornton & Lubowski 2006). In the last few years, much more attention has been given to it and recent reports suggest that it is more common than was previously thought (Glazener et al 2001, Guise et al 2007, MacArthur et al 1997). The role of the midwife is to facilitate women to talk about these problems by being proactive in asking women about any problems with bowel control. Where women identify any change to their pre-pregnant bowel pattern by the end of the puerperal period, they should be advised to have this reviewed further whether it is constipation or loss of bowel control.

Anaemia

Paterson et al (1994) conducted a study investigating the clinical finding of postpartum anaemia in over 1000 women and the key factors and outcomes related to these findings. While there are now many more studies about treatment and management of postpartum anaemia, including a Cochrane review, no recent study has been identified to date that demonstrates more clearly the relevant issues for women and for midwifery care. The impact of the events of the labour and birth may leave many women looking pale and tired for a day or so afterwards. Where it is evident that a larger than normal blood loss has occurred, it can be valuable to obtain an overall blood profile within which the red blood cell volume and haemoglobin can be assessed so as to provide appropriate treatment to reduce the

effects of the anaemia; these include blood transfusions and iron supplements (Bhandal & Russell 2006, Dodd et al 2004, Paterson et al 1994). The degree to which the haemoglobin level has fallen should determine the appropriate management and this is particularly important in the presence of pre-existing haemoglobinopathies, sickle cell and thalassaemia. Where the haemoglobin level is <9.0 g/dL a blood transfusion might be appropriate, otherwise oral iron and appropriate dietary advice are advocated where the level is <11.0 g/dL. However, where the woman has returned home soon after the birth, the postpartum woman's haemoglobin values might not have been undertaken where there was no history of anaemia prior to labour and the blood loss at birth was not assessed as excessive. If there is no clinical information to hand, the midwife needs to rely on the woman's clinical symptoms; if these include lethargy, tachycardia and breathlessness as well as a clinical picture of pale mucous membranes, it would be prudent to arrange for the blood profile to be reviewed. Some researchers have questioned blood loss estimation after childbirth as well as the timing of blood tests taken to assess the physiological impact of this (Jansen et al 2007, Paterson et al 1994). Therefore the postnatal day when the haemoglobin test was taken might have a clinically significant bearing on the subsequent management.

Breast problems

Regardless of whether women are breastfeeding, they may experience tightening and enlargement of their breasts towards the 3rd or 4th day as hormonal influences encourage the breasts to produce milk (see Ch. 41). For women who are breastfeeding the general advice is to feed the baby and avoid excessive handling of the breasts. Simple analgesics may be required to reduce discomfort. For women who are not breastfeeding, the advice is to ensure that the breasts are well supported but that this is not too constrictive and, again, that taking regular analgesia for 24–48 hrs should reduce the discomfort. Heat and cold applied to the breasts via a shower or a soaking in the bath may temporarily relieve acute discomfort as well as the use of chilled cabbage leaves (Nikodem et al 1993, Roberts et al 1995).

Practical skills for postpartum midwifery care after an operative birth

In the immediate period after an operative birth, the attendant will be closely monitoring recovery from the anaesthetic used for the caesarean section. If the operation was performed under a general anaesthetic, the attendant will observe for signs of cognitive recovery and reorientation as well as taking the usual recording of temperature, pulse, respiration rate and blood pressure. Women who have undergone a spinal anaesthetic will also require monitoring of the level of sensation of their lower body and limbs. Regular observation of vaginal loss, leakage on to wound dressings and fluid loss in any 'redivac' drain system should also be undertaken.

Once the woman has fully recovered from the operation she should be transferred to a ward environment. Midwifery care involves the overall framework of core care (see Ch. 34). Appropriate care is to assess the needs of the individual woman and to formalize this within a stated pattern of care so that she and caregivers have similar and agreed expectations (DH 2004, RCM 2000). Women who have undergone an operative delivery need time to recover from a major physical shock to the systems of the body, for optimal conditions to allow tissue repair to take place as well as psychological adjustment to the events of the birth.

Women who have undergone an operative birth will require assistance with a number of activities they would otherwise have done themselves. In the hospital environment, they will need help to maintain their personal hygiene, to get out of bed and to start to care for their baby. The rate at which each woman will be able to regain control over these areas of activity is *highly individual*. It is strongly suggested that caregivers should not expect all women to have reached a certain level of recovery in line with their 'postnatal day'. Using such a framework to assess the degree to which a woman is recovering from a major operation leads to a tendency to become judgemental. Women may view undergoing a caesarean section or any complication in the birth in different ways depending on their social and cultural background and this might have associations to their ongoing psychological health (Chien et al 2006, McCourt 2006).

It is now common for women to have a much shorter period in hospital after birth; some women might return home 72 hrs after a major operation with very minimal support. Practical advice about the management of their recovery and use of resources at home is also within the remit of midwifery postpartum care. For example; the midwife might suggest that the woman identifies what she will need for herself and the baby and gather this together in one place at the start of the day to reduce the need to go upstairs too often. Alongside this, women can be encouraged to go out with their baby when someone is available to help with all the baby transportation equipment; this will encourage venous return and cardiac output at a level that is beneficial rather than exhausting.

One aspect of current care that can be misunderstood is the need for mobility after surgery. Although women may be supplied with thrombo-embolitic stockings prior to the operation and be prescribed an anticoagulant regimen such as heparin, women need to be encouraged to mobilize as soon as practical after the operation to reduce the risk of circulatory problems. Although women need an explanation that mobility is of benefit soon after the birth, it is also an important part of care to recognize when the woman has reached her limit with regard to physical activity and may need to rest. Regular use of appropriate analgesia should be made available to women where this is required.

Psychological deviation from normal

Psychological distress and psychiatric illness in relation to childbirth are covered in depth in Chapter 36. However, it is relevant to reflect here on the possible importance of the relationship that develops between the woman and the midwife during their contact postpartum. Clearly, such relationships are of greater depth where there has been antenatal contact or a degree of continuity postpartum, or both, and women have commented positively where such continuity has been achieved (Singh & Newburn 2000). This prior knowledge can mean that the midwife might detect or be concerned about a change in the woman's behaviour that has not been noticed by her family. Any initial concerns of the mother or the family should be explored by the midwife making use of open questions and listening skills during the visit in the home or the contact time in the hospital setting (NICE 2007). Behavioural changes may be very subtle, but, however small, they might be of importance in the woman's overall psychological state; it is the balance between the woman's physical condition and her psychological state that might influence an eventual decision to refer for expert advice.

Although the woman and her partner are likely to have an expectation of reduced sleep once the baby is born, the actual experience of this can have very varied effects on individual women. The cause of the lack of sleep or tiredness is what is important – is it being *unable to get to sleep* as a result of anxiety about the future and what is, as yet, unknown? This might include fears about the possibility of a cot death, or a lack of confidence in coping as a mother, or financial or relationship worries. The *opportunity to sleep* might be reduced because the feeding is not yet established or the baby is not in a settled environment and so the mother is constantly disturbed when she tries to sleep. In addition, other people may not be allowing the mother to sleep when the baby does not need her attention. Unravelling these issues can help the midwife and the women to determine what is the underlying cause and whether management of this could improve the situation. As a result of this enquiry, women who come into the category where anxiety prevents them from sleeping when the opportunity arises may benefit from interagency support. Alternatively, where there

is a physiological reason for the tiredness, as a result of anaemia for example, the situation can be managed clinically (Jansen et al 2007). The midwife is an important member of the primary health care team and should operate within an interagency context (see Ch. 36).

Talking after childbirth

The essence of the contact between the woman and the midwife after the birth event is to strive to maintain a framework of support and advice that existed antenatally. Within the current provision of care, it is not always possible to achieve the continuity of carer postnatally and some women will have postnatal home visits from several different midwives possibly previously unknown to them.

Once the birth is over and the woman has returned to her home environment, there may be aspects of the birth that she does not understand or that even distress her to think about. Where appropriate, a midwife undertaking postnatal care in the woman's home might be able to help the woman review and reflect on the birth by talking about it and identifying her concerns and anxieties. Where necessary, the midwife can facilitate referral to the key people involved in order that the woman can discuss the birth or see the notes kept of the birth and clarify any outstanding issues (Allen 1999, Charles & Curtis 1994, NICE 2006). Other forms of support, for instance specific counselling for those with traumatic emotional experiences, might also be appropriate under professional guidance (NICE 2007) (see Ch. 36).

REFERENCES

Allen H 1999 Debriefing for postnatal women: does it help? Professional Care of Mother and Child 9(3):77–79

Alexander J, Thomas P, Sanghera J 2002 Treatments for secondary postpartum haemorrhage. Cochrane Database of Systematic Reviews, Issue 1

Aslan E, Fynes M 2007 Symphysial pelvic dysfunction. Current Opinion in Obstetrics and Gynecology 19 (2):133–139

Atterbury J L, Groome L, Hoff C et al 1998 Clinical presentation of women re-admitted with postpartum severe pre-eclampsia or eclampsia. Journal of Obstetrics, Gynecology and Neonatal Nursing 27(2):134–141

Barrett G, Pendry E, Peacock J et al 2000 Women's sexual health after childbirth. British Journal of Obstetrics and Gynaecology 107(2):186–195

Bick D, MacArthur C 1995 The extent, severity and effect of health problems after childbirth. British Journal of Midwifery 3:27–31

Bick D, MacArthur C, Knowles H et al 2009 Postnatal care: evidence and guidelines for management, 2nd ed. Churchill Livingstone, Edinburgh

Bhandal N, Russell R 2006 Intravenous versus oral iron therapy for postpartum anaemia. British Journal of Obstetrics and Gynaecology 113(11):1248–1252

Brown S, Lumley J 1998 Maternal health after childbirth: results of an Australian population based study. British Journal of Obstetrics and Gynaecology 105:156–161

Chames M C, Livingston J C, Ivester T S et al 2002 Late postpartum eclampsia: a preventable disease? American Journal of Obstetrics and Gynecology 186(6):1174–1177

Charles J, Curtis L 1994 Birth afterthoughts: a listening and information service. British Journal of Midwifery 2(7): 331–334

Chien L Y, Tai C J, Ko Y L et al 2006 Adherence to 'doing-the-month' practices is associated with fewer physical and depressive symptoms among postpartum women. Taiwan Research in Nursing and Health 29(5):374–383

Corby H, Donnelly V S, O'Herlihy C et al 1997 Anal canal pressures are low in women with postpartum anal fissure. British Journal of Surgery 84(1):86–88

Cunningham F G, Leveno K J, Bloom S et al (eds) 2005a Maternal physiology. In: Williams obstetrics, 22nd edn. McGraw Hill Medical, New York, p 121–150, 695–710

Cunningham F G, Leveno K J, Bloom S et al (eds) 2005b Puerperal infection. In: Williams obstetrics, 22nd edn. McGraw Hill Medical, New York, p 710–724

Deans R, Dietz H P 2006 Ultrasound of the post-partum uterus Australian and New Zealand Journal of Obstetrics and Gynaecology 46(4):345–349

DH (Department of Health) 2004 National Service Framework for Children, Young People and Maternity Services, Section 11. Stationery office, London

Dodd J, Dare M R, Middleton P 2004 Treatment for women with postpartum iron deficiency anaemia. The Cochrane Database of Systematic Reviews, Issue 4

Eogan M, Daly L, Behan M et al 2007 Randomised clinical trial of a laxative alone versus a laxative and a bulking agent after primary repair of obstetric anal sphincter injury. British Journal of Obstetrics and Gynaecology 114(6):736–740

Garcia J, Marchant S 1993 Back to normal? Postpartum health and illness. Research and the Midwife Conference Proceedings, 1992, University of Manchester, Manchester, p 2–9

Garcia J, Redshaw M, Fitzsimmons B et al 1998 First class delivery, a national survey of women's views of maternity care. Audit Commission, Abingdon

Glazener C, Abdalla M, Stroud P et al 1995 Postnatal maternal morbidity: extent, causes, prevention and treatment. British Journal of Obstetrics and Gynaecology 102(4):282–287

Glazener C 1997 Sexual function after childbirth: women's experiences, persistent morbidity and lack of professional recognition. British Journal of Obstetrics and Gynaecology 104:330–335

Glazener C, Herbison G P, Wilson C D et al 2001 Conservative management of persistent postnatal urinary and faecal incontinence: a randomised controlled trial. British Medical Journal 323:593–598

Glazener C M A, MacArthur C, 2001 Postnatal morbidity Obstetrician and Gynaecologist 3(4):179–183

Gready M, Buggins E, Newburn M et al 1997 Hearing it like it is: understanding the views of users. British Journal of Midwifery 5(8):496–500

Guise J M, Morris C, Osterweil P et al 2007 Incidence of fecal incontinence after childbirth. Obstetrics and Gynecology 109 (2 Part 1):281–288

Hertzberg B, Bowie J. 1991. Ultrasound of the postpartum uterus. Journal of Ultrasound Medicine 10:451–456.

Howie P W 1995 The puerperium and its complications. In: Whitfield C (ed.) Dewhurst's textbook of obstetrics and gynaecology, 5th edn. Blackwell Science, Oxford, p 421–437

Hoveyda F, MacKenzie I Z 2001 Secondary postpartum haemorrhage: incidence, morbidity and current management. British Journal of Obstetrics and Gynaecology 108(9): 927–930

Jansen A J G, van Rhenen D J, Steegers E A P et al 2005 Postpartum hemorrhage and transfusion of blood and blood components. Obstetrical and Gynecological Survey 60(10):663–671

Jansen A J, Duvekot J J, Hop W C et al 2007 New insights into fatigue and health-related quality of life after delivery. Acta Obstetrica et Gynecologica Scandinavica 86(5):579–584

Khong T Y, Khong T K 1993 Delayed postpartum haemorrhage: a morphologic study of causes and their relation to other pregnancy disorders. Obstetrics and Gynecology 82(1):17–22

Lee S N S, Lee C P, Tang O S F et al 1999 Postpartum urinary retention. International Journal of Gynaecology and Obstetrics 66:287–288

Lewis G (ed.) 2007 The Confidential Enquiry into Maternal and Child Health (CEMACH). Saving mothers' lives: reviewing maternal deaths to make motherhood safer 2003–2005. The seventh report on Confidential Enquiries into Maternal Deaths in the United Kingdom. CEMACH, London

Loudon I 1986 Obstetric care, social class, and maternal mortality. British Medical Journal 293:606–608

Loudon I 1987 Puerperal fever, the streptococcus, and the sulphonamides, 1911–1945. British Medical Journal 295:485–490

MacArthur C, Bick D E, Keighley M 1997 Faecal incontinence after childbirth. British Journal of Obstetrics and Gynaecology 104:46–50

MacArthur C, Lewis M, Knox G 1991 Health after childbirth: an investigation of long term health problems beginning after childbirth in 11701 women. HMSO, London

McCandlish R, Bowler U, van Asten H et al 1998. A randomised controlled trial of care of the perineum during second stage of normal labour. British Journal of Obstetrics and Gynaecology105(2):1262–1272

McCourt C 2006 Becoming a parent. In: Page L A, McCandlish R (eds) The new midwifery: science and sensitivity in practice, 2nd edn. Elsevier, Edinburgh, p 54–56

MaGuire M 2000 The transition to parenthood. In: Life after birth: reflections on postnatal care, report of a multidisciplinary seminar, 3rd July. Royal College of Midwives, London

Marchant S, Alexander J, Garcia J et al 1999 A survey of women's experiences of vaginal loss from 24 hours to three months after childbirth (the BLiPP Study) Midwifery 15(2):72–81

Marchant S, Alexander J, Garcia J 2003 Routine midwifery assessment of postpartum uterine involution. In: Wickham S (ed.) Midwifery best practice. Elsevier, London

Marchant S 2006 The postnatal care journey – are we nearly there yet? MIDIRS Midwifery Digest 16(3):295–304

Marchant S, Alexander J, Thomas P et al 2006 Risk factors for hospital admission related to excessive and/or prolonged postpartum vaginal blood loss after the first 24 h following childbirth. Paediatric and Perinatal Epidemiology 20(5):392–402

Matthys L A, Coppage K H, Lambers D S et al 2004 Delayed postpartum preeclampsia: an experience of 151 cases.

American Journal of Obstetrics and Gynecology 190(5):1464–1466

Muller A E, Oostvogel P M, Steegers E A P et al 2006 Morbidity related to maternal group B streptococcal infections. Acta Obstetrica et Gynecologica Scandinavica 85(9):1027–1037

NICE (National Institute for Health and Excellence) 2006 Routine postnatal care of women and their babies. NICE, London

NICE (National Institute for Health and Excellence) 2007 Antenatal and postnatal mental health: Clinical management and service guidance. NICE, London

Nikodem V C, Danziger D, Gebka N et al 1993 Do cabbage leaves prevent breast engorgement? A randomized, controlled study. Birth 20(2):61–64

NMC (Nursing and Midwifery Council) 2004 Midwives rules and standards. NMC, London

Paterson J, Davis J, Gregory M et al 1994 A study on the effects of low haemoglobin on postnatal women. Midwifery 16: 77–86

RCM (Royal College of Midwives) 2000 Midwifery practice in the postnatal period: recommendations for practice. Davies Communications, London

Redshaw M, Rowe R, Hockley C et al 2007 Recorded delivery: a national survey of women's experience of maternity care. National Perinatal Epidemiology Unit, Oxford

Roberts K L 1995 A comparison of chilled cabbage leaves and chilled gelpaks in reducing breast engorgement. Journal of Human Lactation 11(1):17–20

Shalev J, Royburt M, Fite G et al 2002 Sonographic evaluation of the puerperal uterus: correlation with manual examination. Gynecologic and Obstetric Investigation 53:38–41

Singh D, Newburn M (eds) 2000 Access to maternity information and support: the experiences and needs of women before and after giving birth. National Childbirth Trust, London

Smaill F, Hofmeyr G J 2000 Antibiotic prophylaxis for caesarean section (Cochrane review). The Cochrane Library, Issue 3. Update Software, Oxford

Steen M, Briggs M, King D 2006 Alleviating postnatal perineal trauma: to cool or not to cool? British Journal of Midwifery 14(5):304–306, 308

Steen M 2007 Perineal tears and episiotomy: how do wounds heal? British Journal of Midwifery 15(5):273–274, 276–280

Tan L K, deSwiet M 2002 The management of postpartum hypertension. British Journal of Obstetrics and Gynaecology 109(7):733–736

Thornton M J, Lubowski D Z 2006 Obstetric-induced incontinence: a black hole of preventable morbidity. Australian and New Zealand Journal of Obstetrics and Gynaecology 46(6): 468–473

Waterstone M, Wolfe C, Hooper R et al 2003 Postnatal morbidity after childbirth and severe obstetric morbidity. British Journal of Obstetrics and Gynaecology 110(2):128–133

Zaki M M, Pandit M, Jackson S 2004 National survey for intrapartum and postpartum bladder care: assessing the need for guidelines. British Journal of Obstetrics and Gynaecology 111(8):874–876

36

Perinatal mental health

Maureen D. Raynor   Margaret R. Oates

CHAPTER CONTENTS

Pregnancy and the puerperium are best construed as major life events or in psychological terms – life crises. Having children is associated with an immense increase in individual life changes that are likely to lead to anxiety and chronic stressors. This may be associated with a change of housing. Pregnant women in employment will inevitably take maternity leave and may return to work in a different capacity or even on a part-time basis. Roles and responsibilities alter with changes to the dynamics of family relationships. Having a child places strains on relationships and there is a higher rate of relationship breakdown around this time. Many women find coping with the physiological adaptation to pregnancy, the plethora of antenatal screening tests, issues around choice, control and communication emotionally draining. Therefore, while many women and their partners experience pregnancy and childbirth as a joyous, exciting and life-affirming event, the transition to parenthood is an emotionally charged time bringing common anxieties, a certain degree of loss and periods of self-doubt. This can culminate in pregnancy and postpartum being a fragile time of physical, psychological and social upheavals. Unlike other stressful life events that can precipitate mental illness, childbirth is known to be associated with an increased risk of psychiatric illness. Pregnancy provides a wealth of opportunities for promoting emotional health while preventing and predicting mental illness. It is important for midwives to be able to identify normal reactions to motherhood from the early warning signs of emotional distress or indeed mental illness.

Parts A and B are two distinct but inter-related parts.

The aim of Part A is to explore:

- *The psychological context of pregnancy and the puerperium* by examining the full range of human emotions that may affect women as they adjust to change and make the transition to motherhood. Having an awareness of the multiplicity of psychosocial factors and what constitutes normal emotions, thoughts, feelings, responses and behaviours are key components in enhancing understanding of mental health and illness during pregnancy and the puerperium.

The aim of Part B is to explore:

- *Perinatal psychiatric disorder*, i.e. psychiatric conditions that pre-exist and co-exist with pregnancy or those conditions typically associated with the puerperium. Using a defined nomenclature, emphasis will be placed on recognition, management (including relevant pharmacology and the implications for breastfeeding) and mother–baby relationship. Included are key recommendations from the National Institute for Health and Clinical Excellence (NICE) and the most recent triennial reports on the Confidential Enquiries into Maternal Deaths in the United Kingdom.

Part A   The psychological context of pregnancy and the puerperium

Maureen D. Raynor

Stress/anxiety

Pregnancy and the puerperium are normal life events, yet they are periods in a woman's life when her vulnerability exposes her to a significant amount of anxiety and stress. Stress during pregnancy is both essential and normal for the psychological adjustment of pregnant women. The 'worry work' that women encounter assists in their psychological adaptation to the emotional changes of pregnancy. Conversely, elevated levels of stress hormones and unnecessary anxiety will stretch coping reserves, and could prove crippling. The deleterious effects for both mother and fetus of raised levels of the stress hormone, cortisol, during pregnancy have been reported (Evans et al 2001, Teixeira et al 1999). Even though such studies have raised the profile of antenatal stress factors as a possible precursor to mental illness, they have provided very little insight as to how antenatal stress may be alleviated. As depicted in Figure 36A.1, there are many factors that contribute to unhappiness in women's lives and affect their emotional health and well-being. Understanding the root cause and expression of mental distress in women is complex as the social circumstances into which women live and children are born play a major role in their health and well-being.

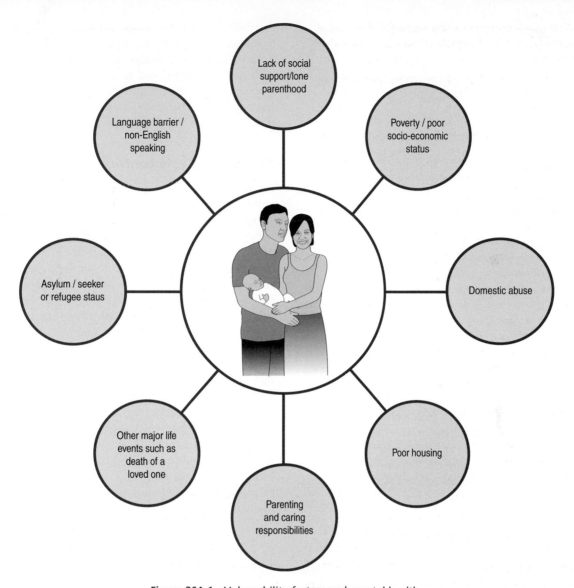

Figure 36A.1 Vulnerability factors and mental health.

Domestic abuse

Domestic abuse as reported by the Home Office for England (Nicholas et al 2005) and CEMACH report 'Saving Mothers' Lives (Lewis 2007) features as a major public health concern. Emotionally and socially, women are affected on many levels as it occurs across society regardless of race, ethnicity, gender, age, wealth and geography. Irion et al (2000) provide some evidence of women in abusive relations and the implications for their emotional well-being. Domestic abuse statistics account for:

- 25% of all violent crimes
- 2 out of 5 murders in England and Wales being committed by partners or ex-partners
- approximately 30% of domestic violence and abuse beginning during pregnancy or after childbirth and escalating during this time

- 1:10 women experiencing some form of sexual abuse including rape but domestic abuse as a whole is 1:4
- pregnancy and the early postnatal period being precursors to domestic abuse.

Antenatal screening for domestic abuse

A firm recommendation is to make routine and sensitive enquiry about domestic abuse during the antenatal period (DH 2006, Lewis 2007). Effective strategies must be in place such as multi-agency support services, to ensure that appropriate help and information is offered to women at an early stage (DH 2004). Domestic abuse causes both physical injury and psychological harm to women and children on a very substantial scale. Furthermore the adverse effects on women's mental health can last for many years (Irion et al 2000). Victims of child sexual abuse can suffer from depression, anxiety, substance abuse, eating disorders, self-harm and suicide. There is a consistent link between domestic abuse and the physical and or sexual abuse of children. This often involves the same male perpetrator, and the majority of these children will witness the violence and abusive behaviour exacted on their mothers. Women who are in abusive relationships are more likely to self-harm, develop eating disorders or other symptoms of mental illness (DH 2003a).

Transition to parenthood

Postnatally, parents may find coping with the demands of a new baby, e.g. infant feeding, financial constraints, the whole process of lifestyle adjustments and role changes, a real strain. For new mothers, this will involve diverse emotional responses ranging from joy and elation to sadness and utter exhaustion. Fatigue, pain and discomfort commonly result once the elation that follows the safe arrival of the baby wears off. Disturbed sleep is inevitable with a new baby. Mothers who are trying to establish breastfeeding, older women, women who are recovering from a caesarean section or those who have had a long and difficult labour/birth, twins or higher multiples, may feel wretched and

constantly weary for months following childbirth. Soreness and pain being experienced from perineal trauma will affect libido, so too will feelings of exhaustion, despair and unhappiness that may be associated with the round-the-clock demands of caring for a new baby. Women may be left feeling bereft and quite miserable after giving birth.

Role change/role conflict

Having a baby, and particularly the transition to parenthood that accompanies the first child, leads to a significant shift in the couple's relationship. Social networks are disrupted, especially those of the mother and the quality and quantity of social support such networks can and do provide. There is a strong possibility that old relationships, particularly with those who are childless or single, may be weakened. However, some relationships are strengthened or even replaced gradually by new contacts established with other parents. The dynamics of relationships with family members are also altered during this process of transition and change. The relationship with the woman's parents for example alters as the daughter becomes a mother herself and her parents develop new roles as grandparents. The competing demands on time of caring for a new baby may lead to role conflict and confusion for parents. Mothers may find that there is little time for them to pursue other activities, which can diminish any opportunity for contact with and support from others (Raynor 2006). Postnatal care is therefore essential to women's emotional well-being and should be a continuation of the care given during pregnancy. Its contribution plays a significant part in the positive adjustment to parenthood, as it assists in the acquisition of confident and well-informed parenting skills (DH 2004).

Communication

Effective communication during pregnancy and the puerperium is essential. Yet poor communication is still the single most common factor that is associated with women's dissatisfaction with their care. A survey by the National Perinatal Epidemiology Unit (NPEU) (Redshaw et al 2007) reports that communication remains a matter of concern within the maternity service. Being provided with adequate information will serve to:

- diminish women's anxiety levels and allay emotional distress
- facilitate choice
- enable women to maintain control over decision-making.

The ideology of motherhood

Motherhood, it is thought, ensures that a woman has fulfilled her biological destiny, confirms a woman's femininity and raises her status in society, but without financial gain (Crittenden 2001, Winson 2003). Instead of feeling elated by motherhood some women experience displeasure, harbour feelings of unhappiness and feel dismayed or even disappointed in their role as new mothers (Grabowska 2003). Many may be afraid to speak out about their feelings in case they are judged a 'bad' or not a 'good enough' mother. Painful emotions may be internalized, magnifying difficulties with coping and sleeping, leading many women to suffer in silence. Distress may then manifest as mothers rage against their impossible situation. Some women may even grieve for the loss of their former lifestyle, career or status. Nicholson (1998) contends that healthcare professionals have defined women's postnatal experience through proposing that well-adjusted, 'normal' and therefore 'good' mothers are those who are happy and fulfilled, but those who are unfulfilled, anxious or distressed are 'ill' and may be perceived as 'bad' mothers. This may lead to feelings of isolation, inadequacy and confusion. The ideology of motherhood is therefore an assumption and a paradox with inherent dichotomies as the woman strives to be 'super mum, super wife, super everything' (Choi et al 2005). Midwives have a pivotal role to play in assisting women and their partners to prepare for the physical, social, emotional and psychological demands of pregnancy, labour, the puerperium and, perhaps more importantly, parenthood (Barlow & Coren 2005).

Social support

During periods of stress, supportive and holistic care from midwives will not only assist in promoting emotional well-being of women, but will also help to ameliorate threatened psychological morbidity in the postnatal period (Hodnett 2000, Oakley et al 1996, Webster et al 2000, Wessely et al 2000). Women who are socially isolated or who have poor socioeconomic circumstances are particularly vulnerable to mental health problems and need additional help and support. This includes women from minority ethnic groups who do not speak English, and often have problems accessing healthcare. Bick et al (2002) provide evidence regarding the psychosocial benefits of midwifery care well beyond the historical boundaries of the traditionally defined postnatal period. The restructuring of postnatal care means there is now a social expectation that midwives will respond flexibly and responsively to women's emotional needs on an individual basis (Brown et al 2002, DH 2004, 2007a,b, NICE 2006). This calls for skilled multidisciplinary and multi-agency collaboration as well as effective team work, taking into account the diversity within teams, for example the Department of Health (DH 2003b) acknowledges the contribution of the maternity support worker in maternity care. Social support is further explored in Part B.

Normal emotional changes during pregnancy, labour and the puerperium

Pregnancy

Since many decisions have to be made it is perfectly normal for women to have periods of self-doubt and crises of confidence. Box 36A.1 outlines the many and varied emotions women may experience during the different trimesters of pregnancy. The reality for many women will encompass fluctuations between ambivalence to positive and negative emotions.

Labour

During labour, midwives must facilitate choice to help women maintain control. Factors that induce stress should be prevented, or at least minimized, as the woman's long-term emotional health may be severely compromised by an adverse birth experience (Lyons 1998, Redshaw et al 2007). Choice and control are important psychological concepts

Box 36A.1 Normal emotional changes during pregnancy

First trimester

- pleasure, excitement, elation
- dismay, disappointment
- ambivalence
- emotional lability (e.g. episodes of weepiness exacerbated by physiological events such as nausea, vomiting and tiredness)
- increased femininity.

Second trimester

- a feeling of well-being especially as physiological effects of tiredness, nausea and vomiting start to abate
- a sense of increased attachment to the fetus; the impact of ultrasound scanning generating images for the prospective parents may intensify the experience
- stress and anxiety about antenatal screening and diagnostic tests
- increased demand for knowledge and information as preparations are now on the way for the birth
- feelings of the need for increasing detachment from work commitments.

Third trimester

- loss of or increased libido
- altered body image
- psychological effects from physiological discomforts such as backache and heartburn
- anxiety about labour (e.g. pain)
- anxiety about fetal abnormality, which may disturb sleep or cause nightmares
- increased vulnerability to major life events such as financial status, moving house, or lack of a supportive partner.

to mental health and well-being. Evidence from Green et al's (1998) prospective study of women's expectations and experiences of childbirth suggests that having choice in pregnancy and childbirth, and a sense of being in control, leads to a more satisfying birth experience. The timely publication of 'Maternity Matters' (DH 2007a) epitomizes a real philosophical shift in maternity care in terms of the guaranteed choices for women. 'Recorded Delivery' (Redshaw et al 2007) identifies key factors related to women's perception of control during labour, these are:

- continuity of care with carer
- one-to-one care in labour
- not being left for long periods
- being involved in decision-making.

Ongoing research to determine the relationship between women's perception of control during childbirth and postnatal outcomes is needed in order to measure factors such as postnatal depression, positive parenting relationships and self-esteem. Common emotional responses during labour are detailed in Box 36A.2.

The puerperium

The puerperium is hailed as the 'fourth trimester' – an emotionally complex transitional phase. By definition, it is the period from birth to 6–8 weeks postpartum, when the woman is readjusting

Box 36A.2 Emotional changes during labour

- Great excitement and anticipation to utter dread
- Fear of the unknown
- Fear of technology, intervention and hospitalization
- Tension, fear and anxiety about pain and the ability to exercise control during labour
- Concerns about the well-being of the baby and ability of the partner to cope
- Fear of death: hospitals may be construed as places of illness, death and dying; the magnitude of such feelings may intensify if the woman experiences life-threatening complications or even an emergency caesarean section
- The process of birth thrusts a lot of private data into the realms of the public, so there could be a fear of lack of privacy or utter embarrassment.

physiologically, socially and psychologically to motherhood. Emotional responses may be just as intense and powerful for experienced as well as for new mothers. The major psychological changes are therefore emotional. The woman's mood appears to be a barometer, reflecting the baby's needs of feeding, sleeping and crying patterns. New mothers tend to be easily upset and oversensitive. A sense of proportion is easily lost, as women may feel overwhelmed and agitated by minor mishaps. The woman might start to regain a sense of proportion and 'normality' between 6 and 12 weeks. Exhaustion is also a major factor of women's emotional state. Perhaps the most important factor in regaining any semblance of normality is the mother's ability to sleep throughout the night. A woman's sexual urges, emotional stability and intellectual acuity may take months, if not longer, to return and for the woman to feel whole again. Normal emotional changes in the puerperium are summarized in Box 36A.3.

Box 36A.3 Normal emotional changes during the puerperium

- Immediately following birth, the woman might experience relief. The woman might convey a cool detachment from events, especially if labour was protracted, complicated and difficult

- Contradictory and conflicting feelings ranging from satisfaction, joy and elation to exhaustion, helplessness, discontentment and disappointment as the early weeks seem to be dominated by the novelty and unpredictability of the new baby

- A feeling of closeness to partner or baby; equally the woman may feel disinterested in the baby

- Early skin-to-skin contact and breastfeed will help to nurture the early stages of relationship building between mother and baby

- Disinterest or being very attentive towards the baby

- Fear of the unknown and sudden realization of overwhelming responsibility

- Exhaustion and increased emotionality

- Pain (e.g. perineal, in nipples)

- Increased vulnerability, indecisiveness (e.g. in feeding); loss of libido, disturbed sleep and anxiety.

Postnatal 'blues'

Childbirth is an emotionally intense experience. Mood changes in the early days postpartum are particularly common. The postnatal 'blues' is a transitory state, experienced by 50–80% of women depending on parity (Harris et al 1994). It has been identified as an antecedent to depression following childbirth (Cooper & Murray 1997, Gregoire 1995). The mean onset typically occurs between day 3 and 4 postpartum, but may last up to 1 week or more, though rarely persisting longer than 48 hrs. The main features are mild and may include:

- a state whereby the woman experiences labile emotions (e.g. tearfulness, despair, irritability to euphoria and laughter)

- the woman might feel overwhelmed by the sudden realization of the relentless responsibility of the baby's 24 hrs dependency and vulnerability.

The actual aetiology is unclear but hormonal influences (e.g. changes in oestrogen, progesterone and prolactin levels) seem to be implicated as the period of increased emotionality appears to coincide with the production of milk in the breasts, as well as the quality of social support. This state of heightened emotionality is self-limiting and will resolve spontaneously, assisted by support from loved ones. The midwife should be vigilant during this time as persistent features could be indicative of depressive illness.

Distress or depression?

Repeated contact with women during pregnancy and puerperium afford a wealth of opportunity to explore feelings, experience and emotions, and for midwives to provide clear explanations to women about the differences between distress – a normal reaction to major life events – and depression – an abnormal reaction to life crises. However, midwives should be mindful of over-reliance on the medical model to describe women's moods as such an approach may serve to pathologize or medicalize normal emotional changes (Nicholson 1998).

Emotional distress associated with traumatic birth events

Understanding the root cause and expression of mental distress associated with pregnancy and childbirth is complex. It is important to recognize the inter-relationship between traumatic life events and women's mental health. What is intended to be one of the happiest days in a woman's life can quickly turn into anguish and distress. Effects of intense pain, use of technological interventions, insensitive and disrespectful care may prove very distressing and frightening. Post-traumatic stress disorder (PTSD) a term most commonly associated with individuals who have suffered the onslaught of war, has emerged in the literature around maternity care (Lyons 1998). Unlike mild to moderate depression in the postpartum period, which seems to have its roots in the biophysical and psychosocial domains, obstetric distress after childbirth appears to be directly linked to the stress, fear and trauma of birth, yet its prevalence is unrecognized (Lyons 1998). Psychological interventions such as 'debriefing' has been suggested to manage immediate symptomatology but there is no reliable evidence that it is a useful intervention in reducing psychological morbidity (Alexandra 1998, Bick et al 2002, Wessely et al 2000). Moreover, clinical guidelines from NICE (2007) have stated that following a traumatic birth, women should not routinely be offered 'single-session formal debriefing focused on the birth'. Instead midwives and other healthcare professionals should support women who wish to talk about their experience and draw on the love and support of family and friends. Neither should midwives overlook the impact of birth on the partner.

Conclusion

A plethora of significant social and health policies and clinical guidelines have resulted in wider consideration being given to the social and psychological context of pregnancy and the puerperium. Midwives need to have knowledge and understanding of how they influence care provision. Box 36A.4 provides a summary of key points.

Box 36A.4 Summary of key points

- In the UK pregnancy and the postnatal period are unparalleled periods when women engage with healthcare and have repeated contact with healthcare professionals
- Women during pregnancy, labour and puerperium are in a state of transition punctuated by heightened emotions and anxiety. Family life and daily routines become disrupted by the arrival of a new baby
- Vulnerability factors such as domestic abuse, poverty and social isolation, can impact on mother/baby relationship with consequences for child development
- Risk identification of vulnerable groups of women antenatally presents a unique opportunity for multidisciplinary and multi-agency collaboration in promoting mental health and well-being.

Part B   Perinatal psychiatric disorder

Margaret R. Oates   Maureen D. Raynor

Introduction

Perinatal psychiatric disorder is now an accepted term used both nationally and internationally. It emphasizes the importance of psychiatric disorder in pregnancy as well as following childbirth. It emphasizes the variety of psychiatric disorders that can occur at this time, not just postnatal depression and the importance of psychiatric disorders that were present before conception, but those that arise during the perinatal period (Box 36B.1).

The emotional well-being of women is of primary importance to midwives. Not only do mental health problems affect obstetric outcomes but also the transition to parenthood and emotional well-being and health problems in the infant. Prior to the report 'Saving Mothers' Lives' (Lewis 2007) psychiatric disorder in pregnancy and the postpartum period was leading cause of maternal morbidity and mortality (Oates 2001, 2004). These reports of the Confidential

> **Box 36B.1** What is perinatal psychiatric disorder?
>
> - Psychiatric disorders which complicate pregnancy, childbirth and the postnatal period
> - Includes not only those illnesses which develop at this time but also pre-existing disorders such as schizophrenia, bipolar illness and depression
> - Care involves consideration of the effects of the illness and its treatment on the developing fetus and infant
> - Care involves multidisciplinary and multi-agency working especially close relationships with Maternity and Children's Services.

Enquiry into Maternal Deaths in the United Kingdom, recommend that midwives routinely ask at early pregnancy assessment about previous mental health problems, their severity and care. These recommendations have also been made by the Royal College of Psychiatrists Council (RCPC 2000), the Women's Mental Health Strategy, (part of the Mental Health NSF DH 1999), the Maternity Standard 11 of the Children, Young Peoples and Maternity NSF (DH 2004), the NICE Guidelines (2007) on the management of antenatal and postnatal mental health and the Clinical Negligence Standards for Trusts. In addition, NICE (2007) recommends that midwives should ask questions on at least two occasions, antenatally and following birth about women's current mental health. Systems should be in place locally to ensure that women with mental health problems and those at risk of developing them receive the appropriate care.

It is therefore essential that all midwives have education and training to be familiar with normal emotional changes, commonplace distress and adjustment reactions as well as the signs and symptoms of more serious illnesses.

Types of psychiatric disorder

The term mental health problem is commonly used to describe all types of emotional difficulties from transient and temporary states of distress, often understandable, to severe and uncommon mental illness. It is also used frequently to describe learning difficulties, substance misuse problems and difficulties coping with the stresses and strains of life. It is therefore too general and too non-specific to be of use to the midwife. The term does not discriminate between severity and need and does not help the midwife distinguish between those conditions which she can manage and those which require specialist attention. For this reason, in this chapter, the term psychiatric disorder is preferred as it can be further categorized and the different types can be described aiding recognition and the planning of care.

Psychiatric disorders are conventionally categorized into:

Serious mental illnesses

These include schizophrenia, other psychotic conditions, bipolar illness and severe (unipolar) depressive illness. Previously, these conditions were called psychotic disorders.

Mild to moderate psychiatric disorders

These were previously known as 'neurotic disorders'. These include non-psychotic mild to moderate depressive illness, mixed anxiety and depression, anxiety disorders including phobic anxiety states, panic disorder, obsessive compulsive disorder and post-traumatic stress disorder.

Adjustment reactions

These would include distressing reactions to life events including death and adversity.

Substance misuse

This includes those who misuse or who are dependent upon alcohol and other drugs of dependency including both prescription and legal/illegal drugs.

Personality disorders

This is a term which should only be used to describe people who have persistent severe problems throughout their adult life in dealing with the stresses and strains of normal life, maintaining satisfactory relationships, controlling their behaviour, foreseeing the consequences of their own actions and which persistently cause distress to themselves and other people.

Learning disability

This is a term used to describe people who have a life time evidence of intellectual and cognitive impairment, developmental delay and consequent learning disabilities. This is usually graded as mild, moderate or severe.

Overall psychiatric disorders are very common in the general population. The General Household Survey (2000), as reported by the Office of National Statistics (ONS 2002), reveals a prevalence of over 20% of these disorders. They are commoner in women than in men with the exception of substance misuse problems. However, the majority of psychiatric disorders in the community are mild to moderate conditions, particularly general anxiety and depression. Mild to moderate depressive illness and anxiety disorders are at least twice as common in women than in men and are particularly common in young women with children under the age of five. The majority of these disorders are managed in primary care and do not require the attention of specialist psychiatric services. Mild to moderate depressive illness and anxiety states respond to psychological treatments. Despite this, perhaps because of shortage of such treatments, prescription of antidepressants is widespread in the community, particularly among women.

Serious mental illnesses are less common. Both schizophrenia and bipolar illness affect approximately 1% of the population. Bipolar illness affects men and women equally. However schizophrenia, particularly the more severe chronic forms is commoner among men. These conditions require the attentions of specialist psychiatric services and require medical treatments as well as psychological care.

Psychiatric services are usually organized separately for adult mental health (serious mental illnesses), substance misuse (drug and alcohol treatment services) and learning disability. There are also, but not relevant to this chapter, separate services for psychiatric disorders in the elderly.

Psychiatric disorder in pregnancy

In general, psychiatric disorder in adults is not associated with a decrease in fertility. Therefore all the previously described psychiatric disorders can and do complicate pregnancy and the postpartum period. The prevalence of psychiatric disorder in young women means that at least 20% of women will have current or previous psychiatric disorder in early pregnancy. An equivalent number will also be taking psychiatric medication at this time. However, it can be seen that only a small number will have a past history of a serious mental illness and an even smaller number will be currently suffering from such an illness. Pregnancy is not protective against a recurrence or relapse of a previous psychiatric disorder particularly if the medication for these disorders is stopped when pregnancy is diagnosed. Women with a previous history of serious illness are at increased risk of a recurrence of that illness following birth. It is for these reasons that it is so important for midwives to enquire into women's current and previous mental health at early pregnancy assessment. Table 36B.1 highlights the incidence of perinatal psychiatric disorders.

Table 36B.1   Incidence of perinatal psychiatric disorders

Psychiatric disorder	(%)
'Depression'	15–30
PND (postnatal depression)	10
Moderate/severe depressive illness	3–5
Referred psychiatry	2
Admitted to hospital	0.4
Admitted psychosis	0.2
Births to schizophrenic mothers	0.2

Types of disorder in pregnancy

Mild–moderate conditions

The incidence (new onset) of psychiatric disorder in pregnancy is mostly accounted for by mild depressive illness, mixed anxiety and depression or anxiety states. These disorders present most commonly in the early weeks of pregnancy, becoming less common as the pregnancy progresses. They are probably predominantly of psychosocial aetiology, and for some women they will represent a recurrence of a previous episode, of depression, anxiety, panic or obsessional disorders. Women may also be vulnerable at this time because of:

- previous fertility problems
- previous obstetric loss
- anxieties about the viability of their pregnancy

- social and relationship problems
- ambivalence towards the pregnancy
- other reasons for personal unhappiness.

In the past, it was often assumed that hyperemesis gravidarum (severe vomiting) was a psychosomatic manifestation of personal unhappiness and psychological disturbance. This condition is less common than in the past and usually resolves by 16 weeks of pregnancy. Psychological factors, anxiety and cognitive misattribution remain a significant factor in some women.

Prognosis and management

Most of the conditions are likely to improve as the pregnancy progresses. Psychological treatments and psychosocial interventions are effective for these conditions and caution needs to be exercised before pharmacological interventions are used during pregnancy, although medication may be necessary for the more severe illnesses.

For others, particularly those who develop a psychiatric illness in the later stages of pregnancy, their conditions are likely to continue and worsen in the postpartum period.

Serious conditions

This term refers to schizophrenia, other psychoses, bipolar illness (manic depressive illness) and severe depressive illness (unipolar depression or endogenous depression).

Incidence

Women are at a lower risk of developing a serious mental illness during pregnancy than at other times in their lives. This is in marked contrast to the elevated risk of suffering from such a condition in the first few months following childbirth (Kendell et al 1987). While these conditions are uncommon, they require urgent and expert treatment particularly as an acute psychosis in pregnancy can pose a risk to the mother and developing infant, both directly because of the disturbed behaviour and indirectly because of the treatments. There is a possibility that such an illness can interfere with proper antenatal care.

Prevalence

While new onset psychosis in pregnancy is relatively rare, the prevalence of these illnesses at the beginning of pregnancy will be the same as at other times. Women suffering from schizophrenia or bipolar illness are as likely to become pregnant as the rest of the general population. This means that approximately 2% of women in pregnancy will either have had such an illness in the past or be currently suffering from one. It is important to realize that these women may range from women who are well and stable, leading normal lives through to those who are disabled, chronically symptomatic and on medication. The management of these women in pregnancy therefore has to be individualized and plans made on a case-by-case basis. Nonetheless, there are three broad groups of women.

The first group includes women who have had a previous episode of bipolar illness or a psychotic episode earlier in their lives. They are usually well, stable not on medication and may not be in contact with psychiatric services. These women, if their last episode of illness was more than 2 years ago, may not be at an increased risk of a recurrence of their condition during pregnancy but face at least a 50% risk of becoming psychotic in the early weeks postpartum. The most important aspect of their management is therefore a proactive management plan for the first few weeks following birth.

The second broad group of women are those who have had a previous and/or recent episode of a serious mental illness, who are relatively well and stable but whose health is being maintained by taking medication. This may be antipsychotic medication or in the case of bipolar illness, a mood stabilizer (lithium or an anticonvulsant). These women are at risk of a relapse of their condition during pregnancy. This risk is particularly high if they stop their medication at the diagnosis of pregnancy. As some of these medications may have an adverse effect on the development of the fetus and yet an acute relapse of the illness also is hazardous, it is important that these women have access to expert advice on the risks and benefits of continuing the treatment or changing it as early as possible in pregnancy.

The third broad category includes women who are chronically mentally ill with complex social needs, persisting symptoms and on medication. These women will usually be in contact with psychiatric services. Midwifery and obstetric care needs to be closely integrated into the case management of these women and there needs to be a close working relationship between maternity, psychiatric and social services.

Ideally all women who have a current or previous history of serious mental illness should have advice and counselling before embarking upon a pregnancy. They should be able to discuss the risk to their mental health of becoming pregnant and becoming a parent as well as the risks to the developing fetus of continuing with their usual medication and perhaps the need to change it. However, in the general population, at least 50% of all pregnancies are unplanned at the point of conception. Midwives should therefore enquire at early pregnancy assessment about the women's previous and current psychiatric history and alert psychiatric services as soon as possible about the pregnancy so that relapses of the psychiatric illness during pregnancy and recurrences postpartum can be avoided wherever possible.

Psychiatric disorder after birth

The majority of postpartum onset psychiatric disorders are affective disorders. However, symptoms other than those due to a disorder of mood are frequently present. Conventionally three postpartum disorders are described:

- the 'blues'
- puerperal psychosis
- postnatal depression.

The 'blues' is a common dysphoric, self-limiting state, occurring in the first week postpartum (see Part A).

Puerperal psychosis

Puerperal psychosis, the most severe form of postpartum affective disorder has been recognized and described since antiquity. It leads to 2/1000 women being admitted to a psychiatric hospital following childbirth, mostly in the first few weeks postpartum. Although a relatively rare condition, there is a marked increase in the risk of suffering from a psychotic illness following childbirth (Kendell et al 1987). It is also remarkably constant across nations and cultures.

Risk factors

Most women who suffer from this condition will have been previously well, without obvious risk factors and the illness comes as a shock to them and their families. However, some women will have suffered from a similar illness following the birth of a previous child, some may have suffered from a non-postpartum bipolar affective disorder from which they have long recovered or they may have a family history of bipolar illness. For others there may be marked psychosocial adversity. It is generally accepted that biological factors (neuroendocrine and genetic) are the most important aetiological factors for this condition. This implies that puerperal psychosis can and does strike without warning, women from all social and occupational backgrounds – those in stable marriages with much wanted babies as well as those living in less fortunate circumstances.

Clinical features

Puerperal psychosis is an acute, early onset condition. The overwhelming majority of cases present in the first 14 days postpartum. They rarely arise within 48hrs following birth and most commonly develop suddenly between day 3 and day 7, at a time when most women will be experiencing the 'blues'. Differential diagnosis between the earliest phase of a developing psychosis and the 'blues' can be difficult. However puerperal psychosis steadily deteriorates over the following 48hrs while the 'blues' tends to resolve spontaneously.

During the first 2–3 days of a developing puerperal psychosis there is a fluctuating rapidly changing, undifferentiated psychotic state. The earliest signs are commonly of perplexity, fear – even terror – and restless agitation associated with insomnia. Other signs include: purposeless activity, uncharacteristic behaviour, disinhibition, irritation and fleeting anger and resistive behaviour.

A woman may have fears for her own and her baby's health and safety, or even about its identity. Even at this early stage, there may be, variably throughout the day, elation and grandiosity, suspiciousness, depression or unspeakable ideas of horror.

Women suffering from puerperal psychosis are among the most profoundly disturbed and distressed found in psychiatric practice (Dean & Kendell 1981). In addition to the familiar symptoms and signs of a manic or depressive psychosis, first-rank symptoms of schizophrenia – particularly primary delusions, delusional mood and delusional perception – are commonplace. Delusional ideas about the identity of loved ones, health professionals and even the baby can occur. Depressive delusions about maternal and infant health are commonplace. The behaviour and motives of others are frequently misinterpreted in a delusional fashion. An effect of perplexity and terror is often found, as are delusions about the passage of time and other bizarre delusions. Women can believe that they are still pregnant or that more than one child has been born or that the baby is older than it is.

Women often seem confused and disorientated. In the very common mixed affective psychosis, along with the familiar pressure of speech and flight of ideas, there is often a mixture of grandiosity, elation and certain conviction alternating with states of fearful tearfulness, guilt and a sense of foreboding. The sufferers are usually restless and agitated, resistive, seeking senselessly to escape and difficult to reassure. However, they are usually calmer in the presence of familiar relatives.

The woman may be unable to attend to her own personal hygiene and nutrition and unable to care for her baby. Her concentration is usually grossly impaired and she is distractible and unable to initiate and complete tasks. Over the next few days her condition deteriorates and the symptoms usually become more clearly those of an acute affective psychosis. Most women will have symptoms and signs suggestive of a depressive psychosis, a significant minority a manic psychosis and very commonly a mixture of both – a mixed affective psychosis.

Relationship with the baby

Some women are so disturbed, distractible and their concentration so impaired that they do not seem to be aware of their recently born baby. Others are preoccupied with the baby, reluctant to let it out of their sight and forever checking on its presence and condition. Although delusional ideas frequently involve the baby and there may be delusional ideas of infant ill health or changed identity, it is rare for women with puerperal psychosis to be overtly hostile to their baby and for their behaviour to be aggressive or punitive. The risk to their baby lies more from an inability to organize and complete tasks and to inappropriate handling and tasks being impaired by their mental state. These problems, directly attributable to the maternal psychosis, tend to resolve as the mother recovers.

Management

Most women with psychotic illness following childbirth will require admission to hospital, which should be to a specialist mother and baby unit, the only setting in which the physical needs of the mother who has recently given birth can be met and where specialist psychiatric nursing is available.

Prognosis

In spite of the severity of puerperal psychosis, they frequently resolve relatively quickly over 2–4 weeks. However, initial recovery is often fragile and relapses are common in the first few weeks. As the psychosis resolves, it is common for all women to pass through a phase of depression and anxiety and preoccupation with their past experiences and the implications of these memories for their future mental health and their role as a mother. Sensitive and expert help is required to assist women through this phase, to help them understand what has happened and to acquire a 'working model' of their illness. The overwhelming majority of women will have completely recovered by 3–6 months postpartum. However, they face at least a 50% risk of a recurrence should they have another child and some may go on to have bipolar illness at other times in their lives (Robertson et al 2005).

Postnatal depressive illness

Approximately 10% of all postnatal women will develop a depressive illness. The studies, from which this figure is derived, are usually community studies using the Edinburgh Postnatal Depression Scale (EPDS) either as a diagnostic tool or as a screen prior to the use of other research tools. Studies using a cut-off point of 14 usually give an incidence of 10%; those using lower scores will give a higher incidence. A score on a screening instrument is not the same as a clinical diagnosis. Nonetheless a score of 14 is said to correlate with a clinical diagnosis of major depression and the lower scores with that of major and minor depression (Elliot 1994). The incidence of women who would meet the diagnostic criteria for moderate to severe depressive illness is lower, probably between 3% and 5% (Cox et al

1993). Depression following childbirth has the same range of severity and subtypes as depression at other times. According to the symptomatology, duration and severity, they may be graded as mild to moderate or severe, and subtypes may have prominent anxiety and obsessional phenomena.

Postnatal depressive illness of all types and severities is therefore relatively common and represents a considerable burden of disability and distress in these women. Although postnatal depressive illness is popularly accepted, with the exception of the most severe forms, it is no more common than during pregnancy or in non-childbearing women of the same age (O'Hara & Swain 1996). However, this does not detract from its importance. Depressive illness of any severity occurring at a time when the expectation is of happiness and fulfillment and when major psychological and social adjustments are being made together with caring for an infant, creates difficulties not found at other times in the human lifespan.

The term 'postnatal depression' (PND) is often used as a generic term for all forms of psychiatric disorder presenting following birth. While in the past, this has undoubtedly been helpful in raising the profile of postpartum psychiatric disorders, improving their recognition and reducing stigma, it has also become problematic. Use of the term in this way can diminish the perceived seriousness of other illnesses, and has led to a 'one size fits all' view of diagnosis and treatments (Oates 2001). The term postnatal depression should only be used for a non-psychotic depressive illness of mild to moderate severity which arises within 3 months of childbirth.

Severe depressive illness

Severe depressive illness with biological features affects at least 3% of all women who have given birth, a seven-fold increase in risk in the first 3 months (Cox et al 1993). Again, the majority of women who suffer from this condition will have been previously well. However, women with a previous history of severe postnatal depressive illness or severe depression at other times or a family history of severe depressive illness or postnatal depression are at increased risk. Psychosocial factors are more important in the aetiology of this condition than in puerperal psychosis, although biological factors play an important role in the most severe illnesses. Nonetheless, severe postnatal depression can affect women from all backgrounds not just those facing social adversity.

Like puerperal psychosis, severe depressive illness is an early onset condition in which the woman commonly does not regain her normal emotional state following birth. However, unlike puerperal psychosis, the onset tends not to be abrupt; rather, the illness develops over the next 2–4 weeks. The more severe illnesses tend to present early, by 4–6 weeks postpartum, but the majority present later, between 8 and 12 weeks postpartum. These later presentations may be missed. This is partly because some of the symptoms may be misattributed to the adjustment to a new baby and partly because the mother may 'put on a brave face' concealing how she feels from others.

Risk factors

A variety of risk factors for postnatal depressive illness have been identified and include those associated with depressive illness at other times. To these can be added ambivalence about the pregnancy, high levels of anxiety during pregnancy and adverse birth experiences, to name but a few. All of these risk factors, though statistically significant are so common as to have little positive predictive value. However a clustering of these risk factors might lead to those caring for the woman to be extra vigilant. Of more use are those risk factors which have a higher positive predictive value. These include a family history of severe affective disorder, a family history of severe postnatal depressive illness, developing a depressive illness in the last trimester of pregnancy and the loss of the previous infant (including stillbirth). There may also be an increased risk in those women who have conceived through IVF.

Clinical features

The familiar symptoms of severe depressive illness are often modified by the context of early maternity and the relative youth of those suffering from the condition:

The *somatic syndrome* of broken sleep and early morning wakening, diurnal variation of mood, loss of appetite and weight, slowing of mental functioning, impaired concentration, extreme tiredness and lack of vitality can easily be misattributed to a crying baby, understandable tiredness and the adjustment to new routines.

The all pervasive *anhedonia or loss of pleasure* in ordinary everyday tasks, the lack of joy and fearfulness for the future may be misattributed by the woman herself to 'not loving the baby' or 'not being a proper mother' and all too easily described as 'bonding problems' by professionals. Anhedonia is a particularly painful symptom at a time when most women would expect to feel overwhelmed with joy and happiness and in turn contributes to feelings of *guilt, incompetence and unworthiness* that are very prominent in postnatal depressive illness. These overvalued ideas can verge on the delusional.

It is also common to find *overvalued morbid beliefs* and fears for the woman's own health and mortality and that of her baby. She may misattribute normal infant behaviour to mean that the baby is suffering or does not like her. A baby that settles in the arms of more experienced people may confirm the mother's belief that she is incompetent. Commonplace problems with establishing breastfeeding may become the subject of morbid rumination.

Some women with severe postnatal depressive illness may be slowed, withdrawn and retreat easily in the face of offers of help, avoid the tasks of motherhood and their relationship with the baby. Others may be agitated, restless and fiercely protective of their infant, resenting the contribution of others.

Anxiety and obsessive compulsive symptoms

Although women with pre-existing anxiety and panic disorder or obsessional compulsive disorder (OCD) frequently experience relapses or recurrences postpartum, it is not known whether there is an increase in incidence of these conditions following birth. Nonetheless, severe anxiety, panic attacks and obsessional phenomena are common following birth. These symptoms may dominate the clinical picture or accompany a postnatal depressive illness. They frequently underpin mental health crises, calls for emergency attention and maternal fears for the infant. Repetitive intrusive, and often deeply repugnant, thoughts of harm coming to loved ones, particularly the infant, are commonplace, often leading to repetitive doubting and checking. The woman may doubt that she is safe as a mother and believe that she is capable of harming her infant. Crescendos of anxiety and panic attacks may result from the baby's crying or being difficult to settle and may lead the mother to be frightened to be alone with her child. This is easily misinterpreted by professionals who may fear that the child is at risk.

Obsessional, vacillating indecisiveness is also common and contributes to an overwhelming sense of being unable to cope with everyday tasks in marked contrast to premorbid levels of competence. While complex obsessive compulsive behavioural rituals are relatively rare, obsessive cleaning, housework and checking are very common. Intrusive obsessional thoughts and the typical catastrophic cognitions associated with panic attacks frequently lead to a fear of insanity and loss of control.

Relationship with the baby

Severe depressive symptomatology, particularly when combined with panic and obsessional phenomena can have a profound effect on the relationship with the baby, in many, but by no means all women. Most women who suffer from severe postnatal depression maintain high standards of physical care for their infants. However, many are frightened of their own feelings and thoughts and few gain any pleasure or joy from their infant. Most affected women feel a deep sense of guilt and incompetence and doubt whether they are caring for their infant properly. Normal infant behaviour is frequently misinterpreted as confirming their poor views of their own abilities. While a fear of harming the baby is commonplace, overt hostility and aggressive behaviour towards the infant is extremely uncommon. It should be remembered that the majority of mothers who harm small babies are not suffering from a serious mental illness. The speedy resolution of maternal illness usually results in a normal mother–infant relationship. However, prolonged chronic depressive illness can interfere with attachment and social and cognitive development in the longer term particularly when combined with social and mental problems (Cooper & Murray 1997).

Management

These conditions need to be speedily identified and treated, preferably by a specialist perinatal mental health team. The value of early contact with professionals who recognize and validate the symptoms and distress, and can re-attribute the overvalued ideas of the mother and instill hope for the future cannot be underestimated. The treatment of the depressive illness is the same as the treatment of depressive illness at other times. The use of antidepressants together with good psychological care should result in an improvement of symptoms within 2 weeks and the resolution of the illness between 6 and 8 weeks.

Prognosis

With treatment, these patients should fully recover. Without, spontaneous resolution may take many months and up to one-third of women can still be ill when their child is 1 year old.

Women who have had a severe depressive (unipolar) illness face a 1:2–1:3 risk of a recurrence of the illness following the birth of subsequent children (Cooper & Murray 1995). They are also at elevated risk from suffering from a depressive illness at other times in their lives. However, the long-term prognosis would appear to be better than when the first episode is in non-childbearing women, both in terms of the frequency of further episodes and in their overall functioning (Robling et al 2000).

Mild postnatal depressive illness

This is the commonest condition following childbirth, affecting up to 10% of all women postpartum. It is in fact no commoner after childbirth than among other non-child bearing women of the same age.

Risk factors

Some women who suffer from this condition will be vulnerable by virtue of previous mental health problems or psychosocial adversity, unsatisfactory marital or other relationships or inadequate social support. Others may be older, educated and married for a long time, perhaps with problems conceiving, previous obstetric loss or high levels of anxiety during pregnancy. Unrealistically high expectations of themselves and motherhood and consequent disappointment are commonplace. Also common are stressful life events such as moving house, family bereavement, a sick baby, experience of special care baby units and other such events that detract from the expected pleasure and harmony of this stage of life.

Clinical features

The condition has an insidious onset in the days and weeks following childbirth but usually presents after the first 3 months postpartum. The symptoms are variable, but the mother is usually tearful, feels that she has difficulty coping and complains of irritability and a lack of satisfaction and pleasure with motherhood. Symptoms of anxiety and a sense of loneliness and isolation and dissatisfaction with the quality of important relationships are common. Affected mothers frequently have good days and bad days and are often better in company and anxious when alone. The full biological (somatic subtype) syndrome of the more severe depressive illness is usually absent. However, difficulty getting to sleep and appetite difficulties, both over-eating and under-eating, are common.

Relationship with the baby

Dissatisfaction with motherhood and a sense of the baby being problematic are often central to this condition, particularly when compounded by difficulty in meeting the needs of older children. Lack of pleasure in the baby, combined with anxiety and irritability, can lead to a vicious circle of a fractious and unsettled baby, misinterpreted by its mother as critical and resentful of her and thus a deteriorating relationship between them. However, it should also be remembered that the direction of causality is not always mother to infant. Some infants are very unsettled in the first few months of their life. A baby who is difficult to feed and cries constantly during the day or is difficult to settle at night can just as often be the cause of a mild postnatal depressive illness as the result of it. Even mild illnesses, particularly when combined with socio-economic deprivation and high levels of social adversity can lead to longer-term problems with mother–infant relationships and subsequent social and cognitive development of the child (Cooper & Murray 1997). A very small minority of sufferers from this condition may experience such marked irritability and even overt hostility towards their baby that the infant is at risk of being injured.

Management

Early detection and treatment is essential for both mother and baby. For the milder cases, a combination of psychological and social support and active listening from a health visitor will suffice. For others, specific psychological treatments, such as cognitive behavioural psychotherapy and interpersonal psychotherapy are as, if not more effective, than antidepressants as outlined in Antenatal and Postnatal Mental Health guidelines (NICE 2007).

Prognosis

With appropriate management, postnatal depression should improve within weeks and recover by the time the infant is 6 months old. However, untreated there may be prolonged morbidity. This, particularly in the presence of continuing social adversity, has been demonstrated to have an adverse effect not only on the mother/infant relationship but also on the later social, emotional and cognitive development of the child.

Breastfeeding

There is no evidence that breastfeeding increases the risk of developing significant depressive illness, nor that its cessation improves depressive illness. Continuing breastfeeding may protect the infant from the effects of maternal depression and improve self-esteem.

Treatment of perinatal psychiatric disorders

The role of the midwife

Midwives need knowledge and understanding of the different management strategies for perinatal psychiatric disorder and of the use of psychiatric drugs in pregnancy and lactation. This knowledge is required because the women themselves may wish for advice, because the midwife may have to alert other professionals, for example general practitioners and psychiatrists to ask for a review of the woman's medication and because in case of serious mental illness, the midwife will be part of a multi-professional team caring for the women.

Midwives should routinely ask all women at booking clinic whether they have had an episode of serious mental illness in the past and whether they are currently in contact with psychiatric services. Those women who have a previous episode of serious mental illness (schizophrenia, other psychoses, bipolar illness and severe [unipolar] depressive illness) should be referred to a psychiatric team during pregnancy even if they have been well for many years. This is because they face at least a 50% risk of becoming ill following birth. The midwife should also urgently inform the psychiatric team if the woman is currently in contact with psychiatric services. The psychiatric team may not be aware that their patient is pregnant. A woman who is taking psychiatric medication at the time when the midwife first sees her should be advised not to abruptly stop her medication. The midwife should urgently seek a review of the woman's medication from the general practitioner, obstetrician or psychiatrist as appropriate. This may result in the woman being advised to reduce, change or undertake a supervised withdrawal of her medication.

There are three components to the management of perinatal psychiatric disorder: psychological treatments and social interventions, pharmacological treatments and the skills, resources and services needed.

Those who are seriously mentally ill will require all three. Those with the mildest illnesses may require only psychological and social interventions which can be carried out in primary care.

Psychological treatments

All illnesses of all severities and indeed those who are not ill but experiencing commonplace episodes of distress and adjustment need good psychological care. This can only be based upon an understanding of the normal emotional and cognitive changes and common concerns of pregnancy and the puerperium. It also requires a familiarity with the symptoms and clinical features of postpartum illnesses.

For most women with mild depressive illness or emotional distress and difficulties adjusting, extra time given by the midwife or health visitor, 'the listening visit', will be effective. For others, particularly those with more persistent states associated with high levels of anxiety, brief cognitive therapy treatments and brief interpersonal psychotherapy are as effective as antidepressants and may confer additional benefits in terms of improving the mother/infant relationships and satisfaction. Similar claims have been made for infant massage and other therapies that focus the mother's attention on enjoying her infant. It is particularly important during pregnancy to use psychological treatments wherever possible and avoid the unnecessary prescription of antidepressants.

Social support

Lack of social support particularly when combined with adversity and life events has long been implicated in the aetiology of mild to moderate depressive illness in young women. Social support not only includes practical assistance and advice but also having an emotional confidante, female friends and people who improve self-esteem. There is evidence that organizations that are underpinned by social support theory, such as HomeStart and Sure Start can have a beneficial effect on maternal and infant well-being and perhaps on mild postnatal depression (Oakley et al 1996).

Pharmacological treatment

In general, psychiatric illnesses occurring during the perinatal period respond to the same treatments as at other times. There are no specific treatments for perinatal psychiatric disorder. Moderate to severe depressive illnesses respond to antidepressants, psychotic illnesses to antipsychotics and mood stabilizers may be needed for those with bipolar illnesses. However, the possibility of adverse consequences on the embryo and developing fetus and via breastmilk on the infant makes the choice and dose of the drug important.

The evidence base for the safety or adverse consequences of psychotropic medication is constantly changing both in the direction of increased concern and reassurance. Any text detailing specific advice is in danger of being quickly out of date and the reader is directed to the regularly updated information published by the National Teratology Information Service (NTIS) – via Toxbase website: http://www.spib.axl.co.uk and to NICE (2007) Guidelines on Antenatal and Postnatal Mental Health.

No matter what the changing evidence is, some general principles apply:

- The absence of evidence of harm is not the same as evidence of safety.
- It may take 20–30 years after the introduction of a drug for its adverse consequences to be fully realized. An example of this is sodium valproate in pregnancy.

- In general there is more evidence on older than on newer drugs although this does not necessarily mean they are safer.
- All psychotropic medication passes across the placenta and into the breastmilk.
- Both the architecture and function of the fetal central nervous system continues to develop throughout pregnancy and in early infancy. Concern should not be confined to the adverse effects in the first 3 months of pregnancy.
- The threshold for prescribing medication in pregnancy and breastfeeding should be high. If there is an alternative, non-pharmacological treatment, of equal efficacy then that should be the treatment of choice.
- Serious mental illness requires robust treatment. In all cases of illness, occurring in a pregnant or breastfeeding mother, the clinician must endeavour to balance the risk of not treating the mother on both mother and baby against the risk to the fetus or infant of treating the mother. The more serious the illness is, the more likely it is that the risks of not treating outweigh the risks of treating.
- The fetus and baby is no less likely to suffer from the side effects of psychotropic medication than an adult. Fetal and infant elimination of psychotropic medication is slower and less than adults and their central nervous systems more sensitive to the effects of these drugs.
- Adverse consequences of medication on the fetus and infant are dose related. If medication is used it should be used in the lowest effective dose and given in divided dosage throughout the day.
- The exposure of the baby to psychotropic medication in breastmilk will depend on the volume of milk, the frequency of feeding, weight and age. A totally breastfed baby under 6 weeks old will receive relatively more psychotropic medication than an older baby who is partially weaned.

Antidepressants

Pregnancy

Tricyclic antidepressants (e.g. imipramine, lofepramine, amitriptyline and dosulepin) have been in use for 40 years. There is no evidence of harmful effects in *pregnancy*. Tricyclic antidepressants are not associated with an increased risk of fetal abnormality, early pregnancy loss or growth restriction when used in later pregnancy. However, newborn babies of mothers who were receiving a therapeutic dose of these antidepressants at the point of birth are at risk of suffering from withdrawal effects (jitteriness, poor feeding and on occasion fits). Consideration should therefore be given to a gradual tapering and reduction of the dose prior to birth.

Breastfeeding

The excretion of tricyclic antidepressants in breast milk is very low. However doxepin should not be used because it has been reported to cause sedation in babies. Any adverse effects in the fully breastfed newborn baby can be minimized by dividing the dose, e.g. 50 mg of imipramine t.d.s.

Selective serotonin reuptake inhibitors (SSRIs) (e.g. fluoxetine, paroxetine, citalopram) have been in use for approximately 15 years and are now the antidepressants most used in the treatment of depressive illness at other times.

There has been some recent concern about the possible adverse effects of certain SSRIs in early pregnancy. The evidence continues to emerge and the risks are therefore difficult to quantify. There may be an increased risk of miscarriage associated with the use of all SSRIs. It is likely that there is an increased risk of cardiac abnormalities related to 1st trimester exposure to SSRIs, particularly ventricular septal defects (VSD) and paroxetine (Seroxat). This has led to both the manufacturer and the drug regulation authorities in the USA and the UK advising against the use of paroxetine in pregnancy. At the moment, this restriction does not apply to fluoxetine (Prozac) and sertraline (Lustral) but it remains to be seen whether this adverse effect is related to all SSRI medications. The NICE (2007) guidelines therefore recommend that tricyclic antidepressants should be the treatment of choice if antidepressants are required during pregnancy. They also recommend that antidepressants should not be used for mild to moderate illness and that psychological treatments should be used wherever possible. However, the withdrawal of SSRI antidepressants in early pregnancy, particularly if the woman has been receiving them for some time is often associated with a withdrawal syndrome or the recurrence of her condition. In such circumstances, consideration should be given to changing the woman to a 'safer' alternative or reducing the dose and supervised withdrawal.

Continued use of SSRI medication during pregnancy has been associated with pre-term birth, reduced crown–rump measurement and lower birth weight. Babies born to mothers receiving SSRI medication at the point of birth are likely to experience withdrawal effects particularly those babies who are preterm. SSRIs, such as citalopram and fluoxetine that have a long half life are also associated with a serotonergic syndrome in the newborn (jitteriness, poor-feeding, hypoglycaemia and sleeplessness). Consideration should therefore be given to reducing and withdrawing this medication before birth.

Breastfeeding. The excretion of SSRIs in breastmilk is higher than that of tricyclic antidepressants. The fully breastfed newborn may be vulnerable to serotonergic side-effects. Those SSRIs with a long half life (fluoxetine and citalopram) should be avoided when breastfeeding the newborn. Venlafaxine and paroxetine are not recommended for use in breastfeeding mothers. However, in older and larger weight infants, particularly those who are partially weaned, other SSRIs particularly sertraline may be less problematic.

Tricyclic antidepressants should be the antidepressant of choice in breastfeeding.

Antipsychotics

There are two groups of antipsychotic medications, the older *'typical'* antipsychotics (e.g. trifluoperazine, haloperidol, chlorpromazine) and the newer *atypical antipsychotics* (for example, risperidone, olanzapine, clozapine).

Typical antipsychotics

Pregnancy

Typical antipsychotics have been in use for 40 years. There is no evidence that their use in early pregnancy is associated with an increased risk of fetal abnormality nor that their continuing use in pregnancy is associated with growth restriction or pre-term birth. However, antipsychotic medication freely passes to the developing fetus and its brain and the dose should be reduced to that which is the minimum for clinical effectiveness. Babies born to mothers receiving relatively high doses of typical antipsychotics may experience a withdrawal syndrome and extra pyramidal symptoms (muscle stiffness, rigidity, jitteriness and poor feeding). Consideration therefore should be given to a reduction of the dose before birth and a possibility of induction at term. Withdrawal of medication at any stage in pregnancy may be associated with a risk of a relapse of the maternal condition.

Breastfeeding

Typical antipsychotics are present in breastmilk, although the amount to which the infant is exposed is likely to be very small. The added benefits of breastfeeding to the infant probably justify the continuation of breastfeeding providing that the dose required is small and divided. Drugs such as procyclidine, given to prevent extra pyramidal side effects, are not recommended.

Atypical antipsychotics

The manufacturers advise against the use of atypical antipsychotics in pregnancy and breastfeeding but this reflects lack of data rather than evidence of harm. The use of olanzapine in pregnancy has been associated with an increased risk of gestational diabetes. Women who become pregnant while taking these newer antipsychotics should be urgently reviewed. In some cases, it may be possible to change their medication to the older type of antipsychotic. In others, because of the substantial risk of relapse of their condition, it may be necessary to continue with their medication. Again this should be reduced to the lowest possible dose and consideration given to a further reduction immediately prior to birth and if necessary, a managed delivery. Clozapine should not be used in pregnancy and breastfeeding because of the risk of blood dyscrasias in the infant.

Mood stabilizers

This is a group of drugs used to treat the manic component of bipolar illness and longterm to prevent relapses of the condition. The drugs used as mood stabilizers are lithium carbonate (Priadel) and various anti-epileptic drugs commonly sodium valproate and carbamazepine but also on occasion lamotrigine.

Pregnancy

Lithium carbonate in pregnancy is associated with a substantial increased risk of developing a rare, serious cardiac condition, Ebstein's anomaly. Although the relative risk is large, the absolute risk is low, 2/1000 exposed pregnancies. However, there is also an increased risk of a range of cardiac abnormalities including milder and less serious conditions. The absolute risk of all types of cardiac abnormality is 10/100 exposed pregnancies. Lithium in early pregnancy is not associated with an increased risk of neural tube abnormalities.

The continued use of lithium throughout pregnancy is associated with an increased risk of fetal hypothyroidism, diabetes insipidus, fetal macrosomia and the floppy baby syndrome (neonatal cyanosis and hypotonia). These risks are difficult to quantify. An additional problem is that the woman will require increasing doses of lithium in later pregnancy to maintain a therapeutic serum level because of the increased maternal clearance of lithium. However, the fetal clearance does not increase. Women receiving lithium in pregnancy therefore require frequent estimations of their serum lithium and close monitoring of their condition. During labour and immediately following birth, physiological diuresis can result in toxic levels of maternal lithium. The woman therefore requires frequent estimations of her serum lithium throughout labour and in the early postpartum days.

Women who are taking lithium carbonate should be advised to carefully plan their pregnancies and to seek medical advice. Abrupt cessation of lithium is associated with a substantial risk of a recurrence of their condition. These women will usually be advised to either slowly withdraw their lithium prior to conception or consider changing to another medication. However, there will be rare occasions when it is necessary to continue lithium throughout pregnancy. Such a pregnancy will need to be managed by an obstetrician working closely with psychiatric services and a fully compliant well informed patient.

Breastfeeding

Lithium should not be used in breastfeeding as it is present in substantial quantities in breastmilk and can result in infant lithium toxicity, hypothyroidism and 'floppy baby' syndrome.

Anticonvulsants

Anticonvulsants have been used as mood stabilizers for 30 years. Carbamazepine was first used in this way, sodium valproate is now increasingly the mood stabilizer of choice and recently the newer anticonvulsants such as lamotrigine and topiramate are being used.

Pregnancy

All anticonvulsants are associated with a doubling of the base-line risk of fetal abnormality if used in the first trimester of pregnancy. A total of 4/100 infants exposed to carbamazepine will have a major congenital malformation. The risk of cleft lip and palate is further increased with exposure to lamotrigine. The risks are highest with sodium valproate, 8/100 exposed pregnancies. The use of folic acid reduces but does not eliminate the risk of neural tube abnormalities. Continued use of anticonvulsants throughout pregnancy is associated with an increased risk of neurodevelopmental problems in the child. This is particularly high with sodium valproate. For this reason, NICE (2007) guidelines advise against the use of sodium valproate in pregnancy. Women receiving these medications should carefully plan their pregnancies with expert advice. They should, wherever possible, either have a supervised withdrawal of their medication or change to a 'safer' alternative. They should also take folic acid. If a woman becomes pregnant while still taking these medications, she should be urgently referred for expert advice and for an early fetal anomaly scan. As all harm is dose related, the woman should be advised wherever possible to reduce her sodium valproate to below 1000 mg daily.

Breastfeeding

The advantages of breastfeeding probably outweigh the risks of taking carbamazepine or sodium valproate during breastfeeding. However, the infant should be monitored for excessive drowsiness and in the case of sodium valproate, rashes. Lamotrigine should not be used in breastfeeding because of the increased risk of severe skin reactions in the infant.

Service provision

There are a number of national recommendations for the needs of women with perinatal psychiatric disorders (Table 36B.2). The distinctive clinical features of the conditions, their physical needs and the professional liaison with maternity services all require specialist skills and knowledge (Oates

Table 36B.2 Perinatal mental health: National Documents (regularly updated)

Royal College of Psychiatrist CR88
SIGN Guidelines – postnatal and puerperal psychosis
CNST 2004
National Screening Committee
NICE guidelines on Antenatal Care
NICE guidelines on Antenatal and Postnatal mental health
NICE guidelines on Postnatal Care: routine postnatal care of women and their babies
Department of Health Reports:
    Children's, young person and maternity NSF. Maternity Standard 11
    Women's mental health into the mainstream
    Responding to domestic abuse
CEMACH 'Why mothers die' triennial reports

1996). The frequency of the serious conditions at locality level makes it difficult for general adult psychiatric services to manage the critical mass of patients required to develop and maintain their experience and skills. It is difficult for maternity services to relate to multiple psychiatric teams. However, at supra-locality (regional) level, the frequency of serious perinatal psychiatric disorder is sufficient to justify the joint commissioning and provision of specialist services. Mothers, who require admission to a psychiatric hospital in the early months postpartum should, unless it is positively contraindicated, be admitted to a mother and baby unit. This is not only humane but also in the best interests of the infant and cost-effective as it shortens inpatient stay and prevents re-admission. There should be specialist perinatal community outreach services available to every maternity service, to deal with psychiatric problems that arise postpartum but also to see women in pregnancy who are at high risk of developing a postnatal illness.

The majority of women suffering from postnatal mental illness will not require to be seen by specialist psychiatric services. However, there is a need for integrated care pathways to ensure that women are effectively identified and managed in primary care and if necessary, referred on to specialist services. There is a need to enhance the skills and competencies of health visitors, midwives, obstetricians and GPs to deal with the less severe illnesses themselves.

Prevention and prophylaxis

Prevention

The National Screening Committee (2001) and NICE guidelines (2007) do not recommend routine screening using the Edinburgh Postnatal Depression Scale and other 'paper and pen' scales in the antenatal period for those at risk of postnatal depression. They also find that there is a lack of evidence to support antenatal interventions to reduce the risk of non-psychotic postnatal illness. In contrast, these and other bodies (DH 2004, Lewis 2007, NICE 2008) all recommend that women should be screened at early pregnancy assessment for a previous or family history of serious mental illness, particularly bipolar illness, because they face at least a 50% risk of recurrence of that condition following birth. Those who undertake early pregnancy assessment will need training to refresh their knowledge of psychiatric disorder.

There is little point in screening for women at high risk of developing severe postnatal illness if systems for the pro-active peripartum management of these conditions are not in place and if appropriate resources are not available. It is recommended that all women who are at high risk of developing a severe postpartum illness by virtue of a previous history are seen by a specialist psychiatric team during the pregnancy and a written management plan placed in the maternity records in late pregnancy and shared with the woman, her partner, her general practitioner, midwife, obstetrician and psychiatrist.

Prophylaxis

If a woman has a previous history of bipolar illness or puerperal psychosis, consideration should be given to starting medication on day one postnatally. For bipolar illness the use of lithium carbonate has been shown to reduce the risk of a recurrence. It is plausible that the use of antipsychotic medication may also reduce the risk of recurrence. However, lithium is not compatible with breastfeeding. Some women will not wish to take medication when they perceive there is 50% chance of them remaining well. They may also place a priority on continuing to breastfeed. Breastfeeding mothers at risk of developing a bipolar or mixed affective illness may take carbamazepine or sodium valproate. The evidence that antidepressants taken prophylactically may prevent the onset of a depressive psychosis is lacking. Antidepressants should be used with great caution in any woman who has bipolar disorder in her personal or family history because of the propensity of antidepressants to trigger a manic illness.

Hormones

There is no evidence that progesterone, natural or synthetic, prevents or treats postnatal depression or puerperal psychosis. Indeed there is evidence to suggest they may cause depression. While there is some evidence that transdermal oestrogens are effective in treating postnatal depression the potential adverse physical effects (Dennis et al 1999) and the known efficacy of antidepressants mean this should not be the treatment of choice.

The most important aspect of preventative management and one that will promote early identification and the avoidance of a life threatening emergency is close surveillance and contact in the early weeks, the period of maximum risk. A specialist community perinatal psychiatric nurse together with the midwife should visit on a daily basis for the first two weeks and remain in close contact for the first six. The local mother and baby unit should be aware of the woman's expected date of birth and systems put in place for direct admission if necessary.

The Confidential Enquiries into Maternal Deaths: psychiatric causes of maternal death

The last three Confidential Enquiries into Maternal Deaths (Oates 2001, 2004, 2007) have found that in those cases reported to the Enquiry, suicide and other psychiatric causes of death were the second leading cause (indirect) of maternal death in the UK between 1997 and 2005. However, in the case of the 2001 and 2004 Reports, if those additional deaths ascertained by the Office of National Statistics Linkage Study are included, then suicide emerges as the leading cause of maternal death (15%). Psychiatric causes contribute 25% of all maternal deaths.

Maternal suicide is commoner than previously thought. Overall, the maternal suicide rate appears to be equivalent to that of the general rate in the female population. Suicide in pregnancy is uncommon. The majority of suicides took place in the year following birth, most in the first 3 months. Not only is the assumption of the 'protective effect of maternity' called into question but also the relative risk of suicide for seriously mentally ill women following childbirth is substantially elevated. An elevated standardized mortality ratio (SMR) of 70 for women with serious mental illness in the postpartum year has previously been reported (Appleby et al 1998) and further confirmed by evidence from the Enquiries with improved case ascertainment.

In contrast to other causes of maternal death, suicide was not associated with socioeconomic deprivation. The majority of suicides were older, married and relatively socially advantaged and seriously ill. A worrying number were health professionals. This underlines the error of merging issues of maternal mental health with those of socioeconomic deprivation.

The majority of the suicides occurred violently by jumping from a height or by hanging. This stands in contrast to the commonest method of suicide among women in general (self-poisoning), and underlines the seriousness of the illness from which the women died.

Half of the suicides had a previous history of admission to a psychiatric hospital. In few cases had this risk been identified at booking and in even fewer had any proactive management been put into place. Had their illnesses been anticipated, a substantial number of these deaths might have been avoided.

Women also died from other consequences of psychiatric disorder. Some of these were due to accidental overdoses of illicit drugs. However, deaths also occurred from physical illness that would not have occurred in the absence of a psychiatric disorder. Some of these were the physical consequences of alcohol or illicit drug misuse, others from side effects of psychotropic medication. However, a worrying number of deaths, some of which took place in a psychiatric unit, were due to physical illness being missed because of the psychiatric disorder or mistak-

Box 36B.2 The 4 main categories of psychiatric deaths emerging from 'Saving Mothers' Lives' (Oates 2007)

- Suicide
- Overdose of drugs abuse
- Medical conditions caused by or mistaken for psychiatric disorder
- Violence and accidents related to psychiatric disorders

Note: New themes are included concerning child protection and termination of pregnancy.

enly attributed to a psychiatric disorder. These findings underline the importance of remembering that physical illness can present as or complicate psychiatric disorder. Suicide is not the only risk associated with perinatal psychiatric disorder. Box 36B.2 identifies the four main categories of psychiatric deaths emerging from 'Saving Mothers' Lives' (Oates 2007).

These findings have major implications for psychiatric and obstetric practice. If psychiatrists discussed with their patients plans for parenthood prior to conception; if obstetricians and midwives detected those at risk of serious mental illness; if psychiatric and maternity professionals communicated freely with each other and worked together; if specialist perinatal mental health services were available for those women who needed them and if all had a greater understanding of perinatal mental illness, then not only would a substantial number of maternal deaths be avoided but also the care and outcome of other mentally ill women would be greatly improved.

Conclusion

The full range of psychiatric disorders can complicate pregnancy and the postpartum year. The incidence of affective disorder, particularly at the most severe end of the spectrum, increases following birth. The familiar signs and symptoms of psychiatric disorder are all present in postpartum disorders as well, but the early maternity context and the dominance of infant care and mother–infant relationships exert a powerful pathoplasty effect on the content, if not the form, of the symptomatology. Early maternity is a time when there is an expectation of joy, pleasure and fulfillment. The presence of psychiatric disorder at this time, however mild, is disproportionately distressing. No matter how ill the woman feels, there is still a baby and often other children to be cared for. She cannot rest and is reminded on a daily basis of her symptoms and disability. Compassionate understanding and skilled care aimed at speedy symptom relief and re-establishing maternal confidence are thus essential.

REFERENCES

Alexandra J 1998 Confusing debriefing and defusing postnatally: the need for clarity of terms, purpose and value. Midwifery 14(2):122–124

Appleby L, Mortenson P B, Faragher E B 1998 Suicide and other causes of mortality after post-partum psychiatric admission. British Journal of Psychiatry 173(9):209–211

Barlow J, Coren E 2005 Parent-training programmes for improving maternal psychosocial health. Cochrane Library of Systematic Reviews, Issue 1

Bick D, MacArthur C, Knowles H et al 2002 Postnatal care: evidence and guidelines for management. Churchill Livingstone, Edinburgh

Brown J, Small R, Faber B et al 2002 Early postnatal discharge from hospital for healthy mothers and term infants. Cochrane Library of Systematic Reviews, Issue 3

Choi P, Henshaw C, Baker S et al 2005 Supermum, superwife, super everything: performing femininity in the transition to motherhood. Journal of reproduction and Infant Psychology 23(2):167–180

Cooper P J, Murray L 1995 The course and recurrence of postnatal depression. British Journal of Psychiatry 166:191-195

Cooper P J, Murray L 1997 Effects of postnatal depression on infant development. Archives of Disease in Childhood 77:97–101

Cox J L, Murray D, Chapman G (1993) A controlled study of the onset, duration and prevalence of postnatal depression. British Journal of Psychiatry 163:27–31

Crittenden A 2001 The price of motherhood: why the most important job in the world is still least valued. Metropolitan books, New York

Dean C, Kendell R E 1981 The symptomatology of puerperal illnesses. British Journal of Psychiatry 139:128–133

DH (Department of Health) 1999 National service framework for mental health: modern standards and service models. DH, London

DH (Department of Health) 2003a Mainstreaming gender and women's mental health. DH, London

DH (Department of Health) 2003b Choosing the best: choice and equity in the NHS. DH, London

DH (Department of Health) 2004 National service framework for children, young people and maternity services, maternity services, Standard 11. DH, London

DH (Department of Health) 2006 Responding to domestic abuse. A handbook for health professionals. DH, London

DH (Department of Health) 2007a Maternity matters: choice, access and continuity of care in a safe service. DH, London

DH (Department of Health) 2007b Our health, our care, our say: one year on. DH, London

Dennis C L, Ross L E, Herxheimer 1999 Oestrogens and progestins for preventing and treating postpartum depression. Cochrane Database of Systematic Reviews, Issue 3: CD001690

Elliot S 1994 Uses and misuses of Edinburgh postnatal depression score in primary care: a comparison of models developed in health visiting. In: Cox J L, Holden J M (eds) Perinatal psychiatry: use and misuse of the Edinburgh postnatal depression scale. Gaskell, London, p 221–228

Evans J, Heron J, Francomb H et al 2001 Cohort study of depressed mood during pregnancy and childbirth. British Medical Journal 323:257–260

Grabowska C 2003 Unhappiness after childbirth. In: Squire C (ed.) The social context of birth. Radcliffe Press, Oxon, Ch 14, p 233–245

Green J M, Coupland V A, Kitzinger J V 1998 Great expectations: a prospective study of women's expectations and experiences of childbirth. Books for Midwives, Hale

Gregoire A 1995 Hormones and postnatal depression. British Journal of Midwifery 3(2):99–104

Harris B, Lovett L, Newcombe R G 1994 Maternity blues and major endocrine changes: Cardiff puerperal mood and hormone study 2. British Medical Journal 308:949–953

Hodnett E D 2000 Support during pregnancy for women at increased risk. Cochrane Database of Pregnancy and Childbirth Module of Systematic Reviews, Issue 2. Update Software, Oxford

Irion O, Boulvain M, Straccia A T et al 2000 Emotional, physical and sexual violence against women before or during pregnancy. British Journal of Obstetrics and Gynaecology 107:1306–1308

Kendell R E, Chalmers J C, Platz C 1987.Epidemiology of puerperal psychoses. British Journal of Psychiatry 150:662–673

Lewis G (ed) 2007 The Confidential Enquiry into Maternal and Child Health (CEMACH). Saving mothers' lives: reviewing maternal deaths to make motherhood safer 2003–2005. The seventh report on Confidential Enquiries into Maternal Deaths in the United Kingdom. CEMACH, London

Lyons S 1998 A prospective study of post-traumatic stress symptoms 1 month following childbirth in a group of 42 first time mothers. Journal of Reproduction and Infant Psychology 16: 91–105

National Screening Committee 2001 A screening for postnatal depression. Department of Health, London

NICE (National Institute for Clinical Excellence) 2003 Antenatal care: routine care for the healthy pregnant women. NICE, London

NICE (National Institute for Health and Clinical Excellence) 2006 Postnatal care: routine postnatal care of women and their babies. NICE, London

NICE (National Institute for Health and Clinical Excellence) 2007 Antenatal and postnatal mental health: clinical management service guidance. NICE, London

NICE (National Institute for Health and Clinical Excellence) 2008 Antenatal care. Routine care for the healthy pregnant woman. NICE, London.

Nicholas S, Povey D, Walker A et al 2005 Crime in England and Wales 2004/2005. Online. Available: www.homeoffice.gov.uk/rds/pdfso5/hosb1105 URL 31 December 2007

Nicholson P 1998 Postnatal depression: psychology, science and the transition to motherhood. Routledge, London

Oakley A, Hickey D, Rajan L et al 1996 Social support in pregnancy – does it have long term effects? Journal of Reproduction and Infant Psychology 14:7–22

Oates M R 1996 Psychiatric Services for women following childbirth. International Review of Psychiatry 8:87–98

Oates M R 2001 Deaths from psychiatric causes. In: Lewis G, Drife J (eds) Why mothers die 1997–1999: The fifth report of the Confidential Enquiries into Maternal Deaths in the United Kingdom. RCOG, London

Oates M R 2004 Deaths from psychiatric causes. In: Lewis G, Drife J (eds) Why mothers die 2000–200: The sixth report of the Confidential Enquiries into Maternal Deaths in the United Kingdom. RCOG, London

Oates M R 2007 Deaths from psychiatric causes. In: Lewis, G (ed.) The Confidential Enquiry into Maternal and Child Health (CEMACH). Saving mothers' lives: reviewing maternal deaths to make motherhood safer 2003–2005. The seventh report on Confidential Enquiries into Maternal Deaths in the United Kingdom. CEMACH, London

O'Hara M W, Swain A M 1996 Rates and risk of postpartum depression – a meta-analysis. International Review of Psychiatry 8:87–98

ONS (Office for National Statistics) 2002 Living in Britain, General Household Survey No 31. Office for National Statistics, London

Raynor M 2006 Pregnancy and the puerperium: the social and psychological context. Psychiatry 5(1):1–4

Redshaw M, Rowe R, Hockley C et al 2007 Recorded delivery: a national survey of women's experience of maternity care 2006. National Perinatal Epidemiology Unit, Oxford

Robertson E, Jones I, Hague S et al 2005 Risk of puerperal and non-puerperal recurrence of illness following bipolar affective puerperal (postpartum) psychosis. British Journal of Psychiatry 186(6):258–259

Robling S A, Paykel E S, Dunn V J et al 2000 Long-term outcome of severe puerperal psychiatric illness: a 23 year follow-up study. Psychological Medicine 30:1263–1271

RCPC (Royal College of Psychiatrists Council) 2000 Perinatal maternal mental health services, Report CR88. Royal College of Psychiatrists Council, London

SIGN (Scottish Intercollegiate Guidelines Network) Postnatal depression and puerperal psychosis. SIGN Publication No. 60. Online. Available: www.sign.ac.uk

Teixeira J M A, Fisk N M, Glover V 1999 Association between anxiety in pregnancy and increased uterine artery resistance index: cohort based study. British Medical Journal 318:153–157

Webster J, Linnane J W J, Dibley L M et al 2000 Measuring social support during pregnancy: can it be simple and meaningful? Birth 27(2):97–103

Wessely S, Rose S, Bisson J 2000 Brief psychological interventions ('debriefing') for treating immediate trauma related symptoms and prevention of post traumatic stress disorder. The Cochrane Library of Systematic Reviews, Issue 3. Update Software, Oxford

Winson N 2003 Transition to motherhood. In: Squire C (ed.) The social context of birth. Radcliffe, Oxon, Ch 9, p 137–151

FURTHER READING

National Institute for Health and Clinical Excellence 2007 Intrapartum care: care of healthy women and their babies during childbirth. NICE, London. Online. Available: www.nice.org.uk

Provides evidence and key recommendations on the psychosocial aspects of care during labour such as support, communication and useful coping strategies.

NHS QIS (NHS Quality Improvement Scotland) 2005 Clinical standards: maternity services. Online.

Available: www.nhshealthquality.org 30 December 2007

Sets out the vision for the maternity services in Scotland.

Royal College of Midwives 2006 Domestic abuse: pregnancy, birth and the puerperium. RCM, London. Online. Available:www.rcm.org.uk/info/docs/Domestic_Abuse_positionstatement.doc

Emphasis placed on the importance of multidisciplinary and multi-agency working.

USEFUL WEBSITES

Birth trauma association:
www.birthtraumaassociation.org.uk

Acknowledges the limited research in the area of PTSD, provides useful literature on the risk factors during pregnancy/childbirth that may lead to emotional trauma and calls for further research.

Fathers direct: www.fathersdirect.com

Provides a useful information centre on research summaries, practical guide and support on fatherhood.

Perinatal illness UK: www.pni-uk.com

A charitable organization that supports women and their families with perinatal mental illness.

37 Contraception and sexual health

Pauline Hudson   Salmon Omokanye

CHAPTER CONTENTS

Contraception is an important part of the lives of many women, with needs varying according to age. For many people throughout the world, control of their own fertility is difficult as they do not have access to contraception. The National Institute for Health and Clinical Excellence UK (NICE) guidelines (2005) describe how important it is for women to make an informed choice about what type of contraceptive method will suit their lifestyle best. Information should be appropriate for people with additional needs, for example people with physical, sensory or cognitive needs and those who do not speak or read English or who have different cultural or religious requirements. In 2004, the government recognized that sexual health services needed to be improved, and in their white paper 'Choosing Health: Making Healthy Choices Easier' (DH 2004) they promised a review of sexual health services followed by investment to meet gaps in local services. This should ensure a full range of contraceptive services become available and that services are modernized.

The chapter aims to:

- provide up-to-date knowledge of all forms of contraception
- emphasize the role of the midwife in providing contraceptive education for women in their care.

The role of the midwife

The midwife has a unique and pivotal role in discussing contraception and sexual health. The Nursing and Midwifery Council (2004) in the UK states that one of the activities of a midwife is 'to provide sound family planning information and advice'. Midwives, who are encouraged to take on a wider public health role, are in a key position to create and use opportunities to enable women to express their needs.

The Royal College of Midwives (2000) feel that the most appropriate time to discuss sexual health, resumption of sexual activity and contraception will, in some respect, be dependent on the individual woman. Issues such as loss of libido, adjustment to motherhood, breastfeeding, discomfort of the perineum, vaginal dryness and body image may influence choice and use of a particular method of contraception. The use of a leaflet from the Family Planning Association (FPA) is helpful; the leaflets are clear to understand in both illustration and language.

The knowledge the midwife has about a client will enable her to appreciate influences such as religion, culture, relationships, lifestyle, age, motivation and socioeconomic status, which all affect the choices she will make. The midwife should be familiar with the contraception and sexual health services available in the area in which she practises and know the system of referral to these specialist services.

For most contraceptive methods discussed in this chapter, the failure rate is given per 100 woman years (HWY). This is the number who would become pregnant if 100 women used the method for 1 year. This rate does not reflect the fact that fertility decreases with age and may be suppressed during lactation, or that the success of a method is partially dependent on motivation, experience of using the method and the teaching received on its use. Unprotected intercourse results in 80–90 pregnancies per HWY. Barrett et al (2000) suggest health professionals assume that women will resume intercourse soon after childbirth and consequently discuss contraception, however, at 6 weeks postnatal as many as 60% of women will not have resumed intercourse. Discussions need to take place well before this time to ensure no unintended pregnancies occur. Some mothers may even appreciate information on contraception in the antenatal period, to give them plenty of time to decide which contraceptive method would be right for them. Partnership working between the new mother and midwife is essential, conversations regarding contraception should take place in a quiet, relaxed setting, with the midwife having up-to-date knowledge on all methods available.

In Britain, all contraception is available free of charge from the National Health Service. This is different in other parts of the world, with a range of charges for contraception.

Hormonal contraceptive methods

The combined hormonal contraceptive pill

The combined oral contraceptive pill (COC or 'the pill') (Fig. 37.1) came as a break-through in 1960 and it has proven to be effective and safe. It is the most popular method of contraception in Europe, used by approximately 25 per cent of sexually active couples in Britain, France and Germany. Around 100 million women rely on the pill worldwide (Guillebaud 2004).

The combined pill contains the synthetic steroid hormones oestrogen and progestogen. All COCs available in the UK contain ethinyl oestradiol, with the exception of Norinyl-l, which contains mestranol. There is a variety of COCs available containing different progestogens. This accounts for subtle differences in their biological effects and provides women with a wide choice. The most commonly used pills in the UK are monophasic pills, which deliver a constant dose of steroids throughout the packet. 'Everyday' pills contain 28 pills in the packet, 21 of which are active monophasic pills while the seven remaining pills contain no hormones.

Also available are biphasic and triphasic pills, in which the dose of steroids administered varies in two or three phases throughout the packet to mimic the natural fluctuations of the hormones during the menstrual cycle. These pills are less commonly used in Britain.

The first generation COC pills contained large doses of oestrogen and were associated with a high risk of deep vein thrombosis. They were replaced in the late 1960s with pills that had low doses of oestrogen and progestogen. They were equally as effective as the earlier pills, much safer and well-tolerated. The progestogens in these second generation pills were norethisterone and levonorgestrel. The third generation pills, which came along in the mid-1980s, contained a variety of new synthetic progestogens, which appeared to have better effects on

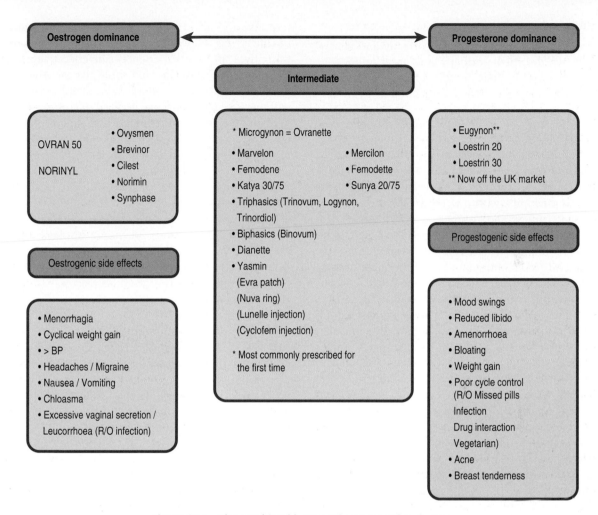

Figure 37.1 The combined hormonal contraceptive choices.

serum lipid profiles. Among these were desogestrel and norgestimate, which were also less androgenic; gestodene, which was the most potent and which achieved the best cycle control and cyproterone acetate, which is anti-androgenic but licensed only as a treatment for acne. Drospirenone has been the most recent addition, included from the late 1990s, with mild antimineralocorticoid activity to counteract oestrogen-induced water retention. It is also anti-androgenic.

Mode of action

COCs work primarily by preventing ovulation. The first seven active pills in a packet inhibit ovulation.

The remaining pills maintain anovulation, according to the Faculty of Family Planning and Reproductive Healthcare (FFPRHC 2006a).

Oestrogen and progestogen suppress follicle stimulating hormone (FSH) and luteinizing hormone (LH) production causing the ovaries to go into a resting state; the ovarian follicles do not mature and ovulation does not normally take place. Progestogen also causes the cervical mucus to thicken, making penetration by spermatozoa difficult. The pill renders the endometrium unreceptive to implantation by the blastocyst. These actions provide additional contraception in the event of breakthrough ovulation occurring.

Failure rate

Provided that the pill is taken correctly and consistently, is absorbed normally and interaction with other medication does not affect its metabolism, its reliability is almost 100% (Guillebaud 2004).

Important considerations

The pill is a reliable contraceptive, which is independent of intercourse and has many advantages. Healthcare providers should manage consultations for contraceptive pills with due regard for the woman's personal context and contraception experience. The woman's ideas, concerns and expectations should be addressed and information should be provided to correct any mistaken notions and perceptions about risks.

Additional benefits of taking the combined oral contraceptive pill, in the short term, are regular, lighter, less painful periods, possible reduction in premenstrual symptoms, protection against pelvic inflammatory disease (PID) – because of the thickened cervical mucus, decreased incidence of ectopic pregnancy and reduced risk of benign breast disease. Taken long term, COC pills offer protection against ovarian and endometrial cancers (International Agency for Research on Cancer 2005) and prevent ovarian cysts and fibroids (Szarewski & Guillebaud 2000).

Use of the COC pill may lead to side-effects such as breast tenderness, nausea, weight increase, depression and loss of libido. These effects often diminish with continued use or may improve with a change of pill. There is a speculative idea that vegetarians have less gut bacteria flora population and consequently less enterohepatic circulation of oestrogen (Guillebaud 2004).

A basic knowledge of the side-effects attributable to the components of the COC pill is helpful when making decisions about changing pills.

Oestrogen dominance in a pill may cause water retention, resulting in breast tension, mild headaches, elevated blood pressure and cyclical weight gain. It may also be responsible for nausea and vomiting, excessive vaginal secretion (leucorrhoea) and skin pigmentation similar to chloasma.

The progestogens may lower mood and libido, provoke acne and seborrhoea and cause mastalgia.

The vast majority of women experience no adverse effects. Every woman is unique in their biological response and also in their perception and tolerance of side-effects. Many women discontinue using contraceptives if they experience side-effects, even if those side-effects seem only subjective or trivial to the providers (Kubba 2005). Most of these women will then use a less effective method of contraception and run the risk of unplanned pregnancy. Women who find any side-effect intolerable should be provided with information about other options and concordance ensured.

The metabolic effects of the COC pill can occasionally result in major side-effects. The risk of venous thromboembolism (VTE) is higher in women with a BMI over 30, heavy smokers, those with a previous history of deep vein thrombosis or a family history of venous thrombosis and those who are immobile. The absolute risk of VTE with COC use remains very small, estimated at 15–25/100 000 woman-years.

The progestogens in third generation COC pills were reported to be associated with an increased risk of venous thromboembolism. A meta-analysis by Kemmeren et al (2001) supported this view. Presenting the risks of VTE for different pills in relative terms may sound alarming, as was the case with the 'pill scare' of 1995. The news media described the risk of VTE as 'double'. The risks of VTE with the COC pill, in absolute terms, recognize the rarity of VTE in women of reproductive age (Table 37.1).

The Committee of Safety of Medicine, UK (2004) concluded that the risks of VTE with all COCs are very small and practically similar. Therefore, any of them may be prescribed first line.

Table 37.1 Risks of venous thromboembolism

	Risk of VTE per 100 000 woman years
Not using COC	5
Using second generation COC containing norethisterone or levonorgestrel	15
Using third generation COC containing desogestrel or gestodene	25
In pregnancy	60

Some women may develop a significantly high blood pressure, which could increase the potential for haemorrhagic stroke and myocardial infarction. Hypertension with blood pressure (BP) between 141/91 mmHg and 159/94 mmHg is considered to be a level of risk, which outweighs the benefits of using the COC. Hypertension with BP of 160/95 mmHg or higher poses an unacceptable health risk with COC use (FFPRHC 2006a).

Cigarette smoking is known to potentiate most of the risks associated with COC pill use such as ischaemic and haemorrhagic stroke and myocardial infarction (Dunn et al 1999).

Following re-analysis of worldwide epidemiological data, women currently using the COC pill are considered to be at a slightly increased risk of developing breast cancer (Collaborative Group on Hormonal Factors in Breast Cancer 1996). Another population-based, case control study found that current COC users appear to have no increased risk compared with those who have never used the COC pill (Marchbanks et al 2002). Any excess risk of breast cancer associated with COC use declines in the first 10 years after discontinuing the pill.

Studies show a small increase in the relative risk of cervical cancer, which is associated with a long duration of use (Beral et al 1999). However, the effects of confounding factors such as sexually transmitted infections (STI), non-use of barrier methods and a high number of sexual partners complicate our understanding of the influence of the COC.

Contraindications to COC pill use are pregnancy, undiagnosed abnormal vaginal bleeding, history of arterial or venous thrombosis (or predisposing factors such as immobility), hypertension, focal migraines, current liver disease, hydatidiform mole (until serum HCG is no longer detectable), smoking (if the woman's age is over 35 years) and BMI over 39.

This is not an exhaustive list. As the pill is not suitable for everyone, women wishing to consider using this form of contraception should have a full history recorded and be fully informed and counselled regarding possible side-effects.

Using the COC pill

When initially commencing the pill, the very first pill is usually taken on the first day of the menstrual period (for postpartum use, see later). Starting on any day up to the 5th day is just as good, provided the first seven pills are taken correctly (Schwarz et al 2002). If a 21-day pill has been prescribed, the contraceptive effect is immediate, provided that the remainder of pills in the packet are taken correctly. If the pill is initially commenced on any day beyond the 5th day of the cycle, additional contraception (such as a condom) should be used, in conjunction with the pill, for the first 7 days. One pill is taken every day for 21 days, then no pills for the next 7 days. Vaginal bleeding usually occurs within the 7-day break, before the next packet of pills is commenced.

When commencing the everyday (ED) COC pill, the active pills are taken first. One pill is taken daily, with care being taken to take the pills in the correct order. Vaginal bleeding will usually occur when the inactive pills are taken, which are usually denoted by a different coloured section on the pill packet. If the pill is forgotten by >12 hrs, the advice given in Figure 37.2 should be followed. If a pill is forgotten from the beginning or end of a packet the pill free interval is lengthened and ovulation may be more likely to occur. If a woman is concerned about a missed or late pill, she can contact the local contraception clinic or GP for reassurance or advice, as emergency contraception may be indicated (see later).

Other factors, which may render the pill less effective, include interaction with other medication, vomiting within 3 hrs of taking a pill and severe diarrhoea. Medications that may hinder the effectiveness of the pill include broad-spectrum antibiotics (such as ampicillin), liver-enzyme-inducing drugs such as rifampicin, some anticonvulsants and some herbal remedies, for example St John's wort.

After absorption, synthetic oestrogen and progestogen are transported to the liver via the portal vein. Liver-enzyme-inducing drugs reduce the efficacy of the pill by increasing the metabolism, and subsequent elimination of oestrogen and progestogen in the bile. Some newer antiepileptics are not enzyme inducers but the COC pill may reduce seizure control with lamotrigine.

Broad-spectrum antibiotics may reduce the gut flora, which free up oestrogen excreted in bile to be reabsorbed. If antibiotics impair the enterohepatic circulation, the oestrogen is disposed of, thereby reducing the amount available in the body for contraception.

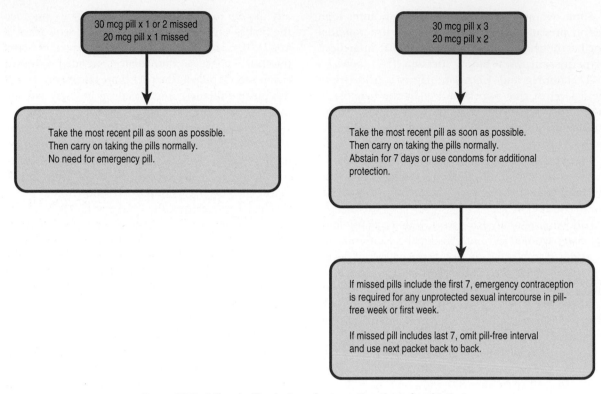

Figure 37.2   Missed pill rule 'two for twenties, three for thirties'.

The advice to be given in cases of an illness with severe vomiting and diarrhoea is to use additional contraception during the illness and for 7 days afterwards. It is important that women are made aware of possible drug interactions and inform their medical practitioner that the COC pill is being taken whenever other medications are prescribed.

Preconception considerations

It is useful to wait for one natural period after stopping the pill before trying to get pregnant as dating the pregnancy can be more accurate and pre-pregnancy care can begin.

Postpartum considerations

The combined oral contraceptive pill reduces milk supply, particularly if lactation is not well established and is therefore not recommended for use in the early months in lactating women. If the mother is bottle-feeding, the COC pill may be commenced 21 days postpartum. This allows the high oestrogen levels of pregnancy to fall before introducing the pill (Guillebaud 2004), thus reducing the risk of thrombo-embolism, but allowing the contraceptive effect to be initiated before ovulation resumes. Women who have experienced pregnancy-induced hypertension may use the combined oral contraceptive pill once their blood pressure has returned to normal levels (Speroff & Darney 2001). Women who have experienced severe pregnancy-induced hypertension with persistent bio-chemical abnormalities are at greater risk of thrombosis and, if no alternative method is acceptable, should delay starting the pill until at least 8 weeks postpartum (Guillebaud 2004).

The COC pill can be commenced immediately following spontaneous abortion or therapeutic termination of pregnancy. Due to the risk of thrombo-embolism, the COC pill should be stopped 4 weeks before major surgery and a progestogen-only method of contraception used; if this is not possible then thromboprophylaxis and compression hosiery are advised. Women who have minor surgery do not need to discontinue the pill.

Further postpartum considerations for discussion with the mother may include whether remembering to take the pill will fit into her current lifestyle and if she can easily access a clinic or surgery.

Research evidence for optimum follow-up intervals is lacking but blood pressure recordings must be reviewed. Common practice is to check the blood pressure at about 10–12 weeks after the initial visit and then at 6-monthly intervals. If this proves difficult for the woman, she may be referred to a domiciliary family planning service, if available, or her health visitor.

The combined hormone injectable (Lunelle)

Lunelle contains 25 mg medroxyprogesterone acetate and 5 mg estradiol cypionate. It is not yet licensed in the UK. It is commenced on the 1st day of a period or within 7 days, and given every 28–33 days. It is very effective and reversible. Side-effects include breakthrough bleeding and weight gain. The efficacy is comparable with perfect use of the COC pill.

The combined hormone patch

The combined hormone patch (EVRA) was licensed in the UK in 2003. One patch is used weekly for 3 weeks followed by 1 week patch-free. It is particularly suitable for women who are unable to tolerate oral medications and those with malabsorption syndrome. It releases 20 µg of ethinyl oestradiol and 150 µg of norelgestromin per 24 hrs. Compliance and cycle control may be improved. The efficacy is comparable with the COC pill. The patch may be worn on most places on the body except the breasts. It is extremely sticky and should stay on during showering or swimming.

The FPA (2005a) suggest it may be used from day 28 in the postnatal period. If the mother is breastfeeding, the patch should not be recommended as it will reduce breastmilk production.

The combined hormone vaginal ring

The combined hormone vaginal ring (NuvaRing) is inserted into the vagina during the first 7 days of the cycle and is used for 3 weeks continuously, followed by 1 week free of its use. It releases 15 µg of ethinyl oestradiol and 120 µg of etonogestrel per 24 hrs. It is not yet licensed in the UK. It seems to be acceptable to many women and well tolerated (Novak et al 2003). Compliance and cycle control were remarkably good in clinical trials (Dieben et al 2002). The efficacy is comparable with the COC pill.

The progestogen-only pills

Progestogen-only pills (POP) were introduced partly to avoid the side-effects of oestrogen in the combined pill, as discussed earlier. They also offer increased choice for women. Currently available in the UK are the older preparations, which contain norethisterone (Noriday, Micronor), etynodiol diacetate (Femulen) and levonorgestrel (Norgeston, Microval) and the new anovulant progestogen-only pills containing desogestrel (Cerazette). All have lower doses of progestogen compared with the COC pill.

Mode of action

The POP exerts its contraceptive effects at different levels. The cervical mucus is viscid, making it impenetrable to spermatozoa; the endometrium is modified to prevent implantation. The older POPs have been shown to suppress ovulation in about 40% of women. The new POP, Cerazette is anovulant and also suppresses FSH and LH consistently.

Drawbacks to the POPs use include menstrual disturbances, encompassing unpredictable and quite often prolonged bleeding, oligomenorrhoea or amenorrhoea. Little is understood about the mechanism of erratic uterine bleeding, which most women experience to some degree. The menstrual disruption is the most common reason for discontinuation of progestogen-only methods. This indicates the need for careful explanation of the drawbacks to potential users.

An increased prevalence of functional ovarian cysts has been demonstrated in women using progestogen-only pills. These may settle with continuation of use and will resolve if the POP is discontinued.

Contraindications to the use of POP are pregnancy, undiagnosed abnormal vaginal bleeding, severe arterial disease and hydatidiform mole (until serum HCG is no longer detectable). The rate of ectopic pregnancy in women using the progestogen-only pill is no higher than in women using no contraception; however, the POP prevents uterine pregnancy more effectively than tubal pregnancy. This is not a problem with the anovulant POP Cerazette.

Antibiotics do not adversely affect progestogen-only methods of contraception but women should be advised to consult the doctor regarding possible interactions if any other medications (especially enzyme inducers such as rifampicin) are prescribed.

Preconception considerations

There is no evidence of a teratogenic effect with the POP.

Postpartum consideration

POP may be started 21 days postpartum for contraception. They have no adverse effect on lactation. Secretion of the hormone in breastmilk and absorption by the neonate is minimal and does not affect the short-term growth and development of infants. The POP can be used immediately following spontaneous or therapeutic termination.

Using the POP

The POP is taken every day; there are no pill-free days and thus tablets are taken throughout periods. If the first tablet is taken on the 1st day of menstruation the contraceptive effect is immediate. If the POP is started on any other day of the cycle then additional contraception, e.g. a condom should be used for the first 7 days.

If a pill is forgotten, the woman has only 3 hrs in which to remember to take it. This is because the effect on cervical mucus is at its maximum between 4 and 22 hrs, and lapses by 27 hrs after the tablet has been taken. For this reason, it is also recommended that the daily tablet be taken about 4 hrs before the usual time of intercourse and at the same time each day. If the woman is over 3 hrs late in taking a tablet, she should continue taking her pills and use additional contraception for the next 7 days. The leeway for the anovulant POP Cerazette is up to 12 hrs.

Following vomiting or severe diarrhoea, additional contraception should be used until 7 days after the illness ceases. Women concerned about missed or late pills should be advised to contact their family planning clinic or GP, as emergency contraception may be indicated (see later). The effects of broad-spectrum antibiotics on the gut flora do not affect the action of the POP.

Failure rate

The effectiveness of the older POP is dependent upon meticulous compliance. Vessey et al (1985) found that the failure rate of this method is clearly related to age, with failure rates ranging from 3/HWY in a population aged 25–29 to only 0.3/HWY in women aged 40 years or over. For women under 25, the failure rate is approximately 4/HWY, suggesting this method is less appropriate for younger women. The new anovulant POP Cerazette has a failure rate of less than 1/HWY.

Long acting reversible contraception

Contraceptives that are used daily or weekly sometimes fail because of non-adherence or incorrect use. The NICE guidelines (2005) recommend giving women wider access to long acting reversible contraceptive (LARC) methods, as a feasible way to reduce unintended pregnancy. Long-acting reversible contraceptive methods, usually referred to as LARC, are considered to be more reliable and cost-effective than other methods.

LARC includes injectable progestogen contraceptives, intrauterine devices, intrauterine hormonal systems and subdermal contraceptive implants. These are all available in the UK but usage is currently low due to inadequate awareness of their availability and access. Most general practitioners and practice nurses do not fit implants and intrauterine methods.

For a long acting method to be initiated, informed choice is crucial because only women who have realistic expectations may tolerate protracted side-effects. The implants and intrauterine systems are expensive, therefore, a reasonable continuation rate is pertinent.

Progestogen injections

The two contraceptive progestogen injections currently available in the UK are depo Provera or depot medroxyprogesterone acetate (DMPA) and Noristerat (norethisterone enanthate). Both methods are given by deep intramuscular injection.

DMPA is the method of choice for many women, not simply those for whom other methods are contraindicated. Over 6 million women use this method worldwide and in some countries it is the most commonly used reversible method. In the UK, <5% of women attending contraception clinics use injectables. The progestogen injections prevent ovulation, thicken cervical mucus and atrophy the endometrium.

Depot medroxyprogesterone acetate

This is the most commonly used injectable and is given in a 150 mg dose at 12-week intervals. It is released slowly from the injection site into the circulation. The failure rate is 0.2/HWY. Prolonged spotting is a common side-effect in the first year but amenorrhoea often prevails in long-term use. Some DMPA users experience other side-effects such as breast discomfort, nausea, vomiting, weight gain, seborrhoea, acne and mood swings. It is now recognized that amenorrhoea for >2 years with DMPA is associated with chronic low serum oestrogen and reduced bone density. All women choosing DMPA should be aware of this information. Teenagers, who may not yet have attained peak bone mass, should preferably use other methods. The peak bone mass is attained around the age of 30 years (Teegarden et al 1995). Women who have been amenorrhoeic for more than 3 years on DMPA may have their bone density checked with dual X-ray absorptiometry (DEXA) scan. It may be reassuring to learn that reduced bone mineral density (BMD) on DMPA does not progress indefinitely but it stabilizes after about 5 years. The BMD returns to normal after discontinuation (Scholes et al 2005).

DMPA offers additional health benefits for women with homozygous sickle cell haemoglobinopathy by reducing haemolytic and bone pain crises (Serjeant 1985).

After discontinuation of DMPA, there may be a delay in the return of fertility for up to 18 months.

Norethisterone enanthate (NET-EN)

Marketed as Noristerat, this is given in a 200 mg dose at 8 week intervals. It is used more commonly in many developing countries. The failure rate for NET-EN is 0.7/HWY. The side-effects are similar to DMPA.

Using injectable progestogens

The initial injection is given within the first 7 days of the menstrual period and the contraceptive effect is immediate. If given at any other time, the practitioner must ensure that there is no likelihood of pregnancy already and advise that additional contraception is used for the next 7 days (WHO 2002).

Specific considerations

This method is irreversible for the time of action; therefore any side-effects may be present until the injection wears off. The efficacy of DMPA is not affected by concurrent use of liver enzyme inducing medications, as hepatic clearance is practically perfect.

Preconception considerations

Injectable progestogen is not recommended as contraception for women who plan to conceive soon.

Postpartum considerations

Injectable progestogen contraceptives can be given prior to day 21 postpartum, thus preventing the earliest ovulation; however, the woman must be warned about the increased risk of bleeding. It can be used by women who are breastfeeding.

Subdermal contraceptive implants

Contraceptive implants have been used internationally for several years. Norplant was used in the UK from 1993 and replaced by Implanon from 1999.

Using implants

Implants are capsules containing progestogen, which are inserted, under local anaesthetic, into the inner aspect of the non-dominant upper arm (Fig. 37.3). The steroid is released into the circulation, producing a change in the cervical mucus which prevents spermatozoa penetration, disturbance of the maturation of the endometrium and suppression of ovulation.

Norplant has six capsules containing levonorgestrel (Norplant 2, also marketed as Jadelle, has two capsules). Norplant and Jadelle are effective for 5 years and still available in some countries. Implanon is a single contraceptive rod containing 68 mg of 3-keto desogestrel (etonogestrel). It should be inserted during the first 7 days of the menstrual cycle and no additional contraceptive cover is required. Ovulation is suppressed within 24 hrs. It is effective for 3 years but can be removed at any time if the

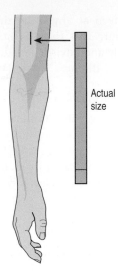

Actual
size

Figure 37.3 Subdermal implant.

woman wishes. After removal, the serum is cleared of etonogestrel within 1 week and fertility is regained promptly.

Failure rate

Norplant has a cumulative failure rate of 0.2/HWY. Implanon has practically zero failure rates if instructions are followed (Guillebaud 2004). Reported implant failures are often due to interaction with enzyme inducing medications used concurrently, unrecognized failure to insert the implant at all and unnoticed pregnancy before the fitting.

Specific considerations

Irregular bleeding is the most common problem for women using this method. Only 20–30% of users become amenorrhoeic. Headache, seborrhoea, acne and mood swings have also been reported as side-effects. Insertion and removal require a minor surgical procedure, with accompanying risks of bleeding and infection. These aspects should be discussed prior to the woman making her decision. Counselling before fitting and during use appears to be the only way to reduce premature discontinuation due to the side-effects.

Preconception considerations

The action of the implant is quickly reversible and ovulation can return within 21 days of removal

(Croxatto & Makarainen 1998). This makes it suitable also for women wishing to 'space' pregnancies.

Postpartum considerations

The implant can be inserted from day 21 postpartum and immediately after miscarriages or induced abortions. No extra contraceptive precautions need to be taken. The implant is safe for women who are breastfeeding.

Intrauterine contraceptive device (IUCD)

These devices are inserted into the uterus, as illustrated in Figure 37.4. They contain copper, which increases contraceptive efficacy. There seems to be an aversion for the use of IUCDs in the UK where only 3% of women use them (Guillebaud 2004). Some myths surrounding the old generation IUCDs perpetuated concerns about efficacy and safety. Service providers need to address these to allay women's fears.

The IUCD is the most popular method in some countries and 156 million women use IUCDs worldwide, of which 60 million are in China.

Mode of action

The IUCD creates an inflammatory response in the endometrium. Leucocytes are capable of destroying spermatozoa and ova. Gamete viability is also impaired by alteration of uterine and tubal fluids. Copper affects endometrial enzymes, glycogen metabolism and oestrogen uptake, thus rendering the endometrium hostile to implantation. Failure rate is 0.4/HWY.

Using the IUCD

A copper IUCD can be inserted up to 5 days following the earliest estimated date of ovulation – that is day 19 in a 28-day cycle. The woman may experience some discomfort during the procedure, which should be performed using aseptic techniques. Depending upon the type of IUCD used, it may be left in place from 5 to 10 years and longer in some instances; e.g. if a woman aged 40 years or over has an IUCD fitted, it may remain in place until 1 year after the menopause, if this occurs after the age of 50. Once *in situ*, the device requires no action of the user and it does not interfere with intercourse.

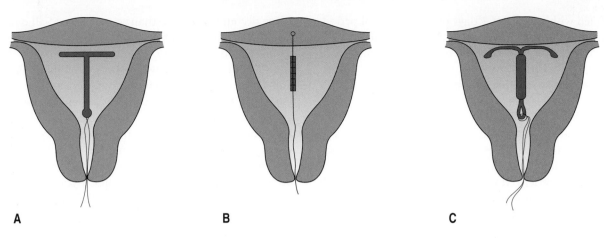

Figure 37.4 Intrauterine contraceptive devices. After insertion through the cervix, the framed devices assume the shape shown; the threads attached to it protrude into the vagina. (A) Copper-carrying device. (B) Frameless copper device. (C) Levonorgestrel-releasing system.

Women are usually taught to feel the threads as reassurance that it remains in place. A follow up in 3–6 weeks is recommended to check for infection, translocation or expulsion. Subsequently, the woman needs a check up only if she has concerns. The traditional routine annual review is no longer recommended (NICE 2005).

Side-effects of using the IUCD include menorrhagia, dysmenorrhoea, bacteria vaginoses and colonization by Actinomycetes-like organisms. When the latter is reported in a routine cervical smear, the woman should be counselled about the options of either changing the IUCD or keeping it and being reviewed periodically to ensure there is no pelvic infection. Removal of the IUCD is easy and painless whenever desired and fertility promptly restored.

The suggestion that IUCDs promote pelvic inflammatory disease (PID) has been refuted; although there is evidence to suggest that asymptomatic sexually transmitted infection (STI) in the cervix may be introduced at the time of insertion of the device. Clinical risk assessment for STI is recommended (WHO 2002). Routine or selective screening for chlamydia and gonorrhoea prior to insertion may prevent pelvic infections, since prompt treatment and contact tracing will be offered. IUCDs are associated with a decreased risk of ectopic pregnancies because of their effectiveness. However, the ratio of ectopic to intrauterine pregnancies is greater among women using IUCDs as, in general, the device prevents more intrauterine pregnancies than ectopic pregnancies. Thus a woman who has an IUCD fitted should be advised to seek early medical advice, should she suspect that she is pregnant.

If uterine pregnancy occurs, there is an increased risk of spontaneous abortion; therefore gentle removal of the device is preferred, to prevent septic miscarriage and premature labour. If removal is not possible it is reassuring to know there is no evidence of teratogenicity.

A newer frameless device, GyneFix (Fig. 37.4B) comprising six copper sleeves crimped onto a polypropylene monofilament thread, is fitted with one end embedded into the fundal myometrium of the uterus. This is associated with lower expulsion rates and less dysmenorrhoea.

Progestogen-releasing intrauterine systems (IUS)

These were developed to overcome some of the problems associated with conventional IUCDs and heavy menstrual bleeding.

The device in current use consists of a small plastic T-shaped frame carrying a Silastic sleeve loaded with 52 mg of levonorgestrel. It is inserted into the uterus and the steroid hormone is released steadily at 20 µg/day. The hormone prevents endometrial proliferation, thickens the cervical mucus and may suppress ovulation in some cycles; the frame, by inducing a sterile inflammatory reaction may also contribute to the contraceptive effect. The system is fitted within the first 7 days of the menstrual period; the contraceptive effect is then immediate. It is licensed for 5 years of use. Failure rate is of 0.2/HWY. A new frameless device containing progestogen has already been developed (Fibroplant- LNG).

Specific considerations

Irregular vaginal bleeding is common initially, and then gradually ceases. The uterine bleeding associated with the IUS is lighter than the menstrual period experienced when using a copper IUCD, with possible amenorrhoea in the long run. The failure rates of both intrauterine methods compare favourably with female sterilization.

Postpartum considerations

The IUS and copper IUCD have no adverse effect on lactation. They can be inserted 4–6 weeks after normal birth and 6–8 weeks after caesarean section (Guillebaud 2004). Following miscarriage or induced abortion, immediate insertion is safe.

Barrier methods of contraception

Barrier methods of contraception prevent the sperm coming into contact with the oocyte. They include male and female condoms, caps and diaphragms. They can be used in conjunction with spermicidal preparations. Barrier methods also offer some protection against cervical cancer (Mindel & Estcourt 2000).

Some of the advantages of using condoms are that they are easily available at many outlets in the UK and using them does not require medical intervention. They offer some protection against sexually transmissible infections and can be used with another method of contraception. This is often called 'double Dutch method'. One of the main disadvantages of using barrier methods of contraception is the possible interruption to intercourse, which may be off-putting for some couples.

It is good practice to ensure that anyone choosing a barrier method is aware of emergency contraception and how to access it, should it be required.

The male condom

Some 44 million couples worldwide use the male condom but with striking geographical differences.

Japan accounts for more than one-quarter of all condom users in the world. By contrast, and despite the massive problem of HIV/AIDS, use of this method of contraception remains low in Africa, the Middle East and Latin America, which together account for an estimated 10% of worldwide use (Guillebaud 2004).

Guillebaud (2004) writes that recent studies show approximately 20% of all couples in the UK use condoms but this may be occasional use or in addition to other methods. There are many varieties of condoms on the market including latex, hypoallergenic and polyurethane. Polyurethane condoms are less sensitive to heat and humidity and not affected by oil-based lubricants (FPA 2005b).

Correct use of condoms is essential. Only condoms with a CE mark should be used and the expiry date should be checked. They should be stored away from extremes of heat, light and damp. Care should be taken when handling the condom to prevent it from tearing. The condom is rolled on to the erect penis before any genital contact is made, this is because it is possible for some sperm to be present in the pre-ejaculate (Guillebaud 2004). About 1 cm of air-free space must be left at the tip of the condom for the ejaculate, otherwise the condom may burst. Some condom designs incorporate a teat end for this purpose. The penis should be withdrawn very soon after ejaculation before it reduces in size and the condom becomes loose. The condom should be held in place during withdrawal of the erect penis so that it does not slip off. The condom should only be used once, and then disposed of in a waste bin. It will not flush down the toilet.

If extra lubrication is required, care must be taken to ensure that the lubrication chosen will not damage the condom. Oil-based lubricants can damage rubber condoms but not polyurethane types. Water-based lubricants are not known to cause damage and are therefore recommended.

The failure rate with condom use is dependent on experience and age of the user and can vary widely between 1 and 10/HWY.

Female condom

This consists of a polyurethane sheath that is inserted into the vagina. The closed inner end is anchored in place by a polyurethane ring, while the outer edge lies flat against the vulva. It is available free from contraception clinics and may be purchased from selected chemists. Great care has to be taken to ensure that the penis is inside the polyurethane sheath and not wrongly positioned between the condom and the vaginal wall.

The efficacy depends on age and experience of the user. The FPA (2005b) state that if it is used correctly it is 95% effective.

Diaphragm

This is a thin rubber dome with a metal circumference to help maintain its shape. It is available in a range of types and sizes and, in the UK, it is individually fitted at contraception clinics and some GP practices. Only approximately 1% of women use this method of contraception in the UK (Guillebaud 2004). It is not used widely in developing countries and Guillebaud (2004) believes this may be due to the fact that it requires medical fitting.

When in place, the rim of the diaphragm should lie closely against the vaginal walls and rest between the posterior fornix and the symphysis pubis. Before insertion, spermicide should be applied. After insertion, the woman has to check that her cervix is covered. In order to preserve spontaneity during intercourse, the diaphragm can be inserted every evening as a matter of routine (Fig. 37.5).

If intercourse occurs >3 hrs after insertion of the diaphragm, then additional spermicide is required.

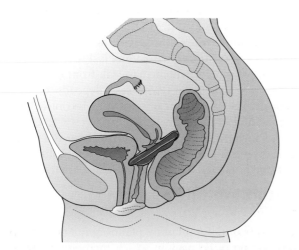

Figure 37.5 The diaphragm in place.

The diaphragm must be left in place for at least 6h after the last intercourse. Once removed the diaphragm should be washed with a mild soap, dried and inspected for damage. A new diaphragm should be fitted annually or following a loss or gain in weight of >3 kg.

The failure rate depends on age and experience of use. The FPA (2004a) quote that it is between 92% and 96% effective if used according to instructions.

In order to feel confident in using this method, the woman must feel comfortable touching her genitalia and have the physical ability to do this. The woman will also need privacy and access to water to clean the diaphragm. Cultural beliefs may affect acceptability of this method (Jogee 2004). The rim of the diaphragm may put pressure on the urethra and bladder base and this could result in cystitis. This could be remedied by a change in size or type of diaphragm.

Postnatal considerations

Following the birth of her baby, the woman should not rely on her previous diaphragm. The size should be reassessed at the 6th postnatal week when the vagina and pelvic floor muscles will have regained some of their tone and any tissue injury sustained from the birth will have healed.

Cervical and vault caps

These cover only the cervix, adhering to it by suction. They are made of rubber and may look smaller in diameter than the diaphragm. They require fitting at a contraception clinic.

Spermicidal creams, aerosols, pessaries

These preparations kill sperm but, as they are not able to penetrate the cervical mucus, they are probably only active in the vagina. Guillebaud (2004) recommends spermicidal creams, aerosols and pessaries are not used without another form of contraception.

The creams or aerosols must be applied immediately before intercourse. Pessaries must be inserted 10 min before intercourse to allow time for them to dissolve. Allergies can occur and couples need to experiment to find the most suitable preparation. Some spermicides are available free from contraception clinics and on prescription or they can be purchased from pharmacies.

Although there is evidence of inactivation of STIs including HIV *in vitro*, Jeffries and Aitken (2000), suggest there is no conclusive evidence that any spermicide will prevent infection *in vivo*. Concern has been expressed about possible teratogenicity if spermicides are used around the time of conception but most studies are reassuring. Guillebaud (2004) states they do not have any detectible teratogenic effect in ordinary use.

Failure rates

General teaching in the UK is that spermicides are not effective when used alone.

Emergency contraception

Emergency contraception is required when contraception was not used before, or during intercourse, used incorrectly or when there is perceived to have been a failure in contraception used, e.g. a condom mishap such as breaking, tearing or coming off. There are two types of emergency contraception.

The emergency hormonal contraception (EHC) is a progestogen preparation with the brand name Levonelle. It is one pill containing 1.5 mg of levonorgestrel, which is available in many countries throughout the world. In the UK it is free from sexual health clinics, walk-in centres, some accident and emergency departments and GP practices. Many Primary Care Trusts provide EHC free of charge through selected pharmacies in an effort to reduce unwanted pregnancies. It can also be purchased over the counter from pharmacies.

The method works by delaying ovulation or preventing implantation of the fertilized oocyte, depending on the stage of ovulation. This method may be contraindicated if there has been more than one episode of unprotected intercourse during the cycle, as the earlier intercourse may already have resulted in a pregnancy. Very careful questioning by the practitioner needs to take place prior to supplying EHC to prevent an unfavourable outcome.

Nausea is uncommon with the progestogen based pill but an additional pill is required if the woman vomits within 3 hrs of taking the medication. The next period may begin earlier or later than expected and the need to use contraception until the next period

should be stressed. If the woman receives the EHC in a contraception clinic in the UK, she is always given an appointment to return to clinic if her period does not arrive on time, or is shorter or lighter than usual. If her period is over 7 days late, a pregnancy test will be offered. Any unusual lower abdominal pain must be investigated as this could be a sign of an ectopic pregnancy.

The failure rate of EHC depends how quickly the emergency contraception is used. If taken within 24 h of intercourse, it will prevent 95% of pregnancies. This gradually decreases to 58% by 72 hrs (FPA 2005c). There are very few contraindications to using this method but anyone administering Levonelle needs to know about any other medication being used by the woman. EHC can be used more than once in each menstrual cycle, but it may disrupt the period pattern.

The copper intrauterine device (IUCD) is the most effective method of emergency contraception, with a failure rate of <1%. Implantation of the fertilized oocyte is avoided if the IUCD is inserted within 5 days of the unprotected intercourse or earliest estimated date of ovulation. This gives the clinician a much longer time range in which to offer emergency contraception. For example in a regular 28-day cycle, the IUCD can be fitted up to day 19 of the cycle. It can then be left in place for use as a regular method of contraception, or removed during the next period.

Coitus interruptus, involves withdrawal of the penis from the vagina prior to ejaculation, and couples should be made aware of emergency contraception. Many euphemisms are used when referring to this, such as 'being careful' or the 'withdrawal method'. Andrews (2006) gives a rate of 90% effectiveness as a contraceptive. Failure is due to the small amount of semen, which may leak from the penis, prior to ejaculation. Its success depends on the man exercising a great amount of self-control and the method is based on trust and honesty.

This method is used widely throughout the world by different cultures. It is the oldest form of contraception and is referred to in the old testament of the Bible.

Natural family planning

The study of natural family planning is a fascinating observation of the way in which the body works to produce the optimum conditions for conception.

According to UK Medical Eligibility Criteria for Contraceptive Use (FFPRHC 2006b), 'Natural Family Planning' includes all the methods of contraception based on the identification of the fertile time in the menstrual cycle. The effectiveness of these methods depends on accurately identifying the fertile time and modifying sexual behaviour. To avoid pregnancy, the couple can either abstain from intercourse or use a barrier method of contraception during the fertile time. Natural methods are attractive to couples that do not wish to use hormonal or mechanical methods of contraception. The success of natural family planning depends on adequate teaching by qualified fertility awareness teachers. Such instruction may be beyond the scope of many midwives but they should be able to provide basic information and appropriate leaflets from the FPA. The midwife can signpost the couple to the local contraception clinic or find local information on natural family planning teachers and available education from the website: www.fertilityuk.com

The method can also be used as a guide to women wishing to become pregnant, by concentrating sexual intercourse on the days they are most fertile. The fertile time lasts around 8–9 days each menstrual cycle. The oocyte lives for up to 24 hrs, the FPA (2005d) suggest that a second oocyte could, occasionally, be released within 24 hrs of the first and that a sperm can live inside a female body for around 7 days. This means that if sexual intercourse takes place 7 days before ovulation a pregnancy could occur.

Fertility awareness

Physiological signs of fertility are:

- cervical secretions (Billings or ovulation method)
- basal body (waking) temperature
- cervical palpation
- calendar calculation.

Cervical secretions

This method monitors the characteristic changes that occur in the cervical mucus throughout the menstrual cycle. Following menstruation there will be dryness at the vaginal entrance. As oestrogen levels rise, the fluid and nutrient content of the secretions increases to facilitate sperm motility. Following menstruation, a sticky white, creamy or opaque secretion is noticed. As ovulation approaches the secretions become wetter, more transparent and slippery with the appearance of raw egg white and capable of considerable stretching between the finger and thumb. The last day of the transparent slippery secretions is called the peak day. This day coincides closely with ovulation. Following ovulation, the hormone progesterone causes the secretions to thicken forming a plug of mucus in the cervical canal, acting as a barrier to sperm. The secretions will then appear sticky and dry until the next menstruation.

When practising this method of contraception, the cervical secretions are observed daily. The fertile time starts when secretions are first noticed following menstruation and ends on the third morning after the peak day. If the secretions are used as a single indicator of fertility, the presence of seminal fluid can make observation difficult. During the preovulatory, relatively infertile dry days it is recommended that intercourse takes place only on alternate dry evenings so that the mucus can be assessed. Intercourse should also be avoided during menstruation as this can mask the first appearance of cervical secretions. Changes in secretions will also be affected by spermicide, vaginal infections and some medications (Guillebaud 2004).

Postpartum considerations

In the first 6 months following the birth, the majority of women who are fully breastfeeding will be able to rely on lactational amenorrhoea (LAM) for contraception. Women who wish to continue using natural methods of contraception should begin observing cervical secretions for the last 2 weeks before the LAM criteria will no longer apply, in order to establish their basic infertile pattern.

Basal body temperature

A woman can calculate her ovulation by recording her temperature immediately on waking each day. If she has been up in the night she must have been resting for at least 3 hrs before recording her temperature. After ovulation, the hormone progesterone produced by the corpus luteum causes the temperature to rise by about 0.2°C and to remain at this higher level until the next menstruation. The infertile phase of the menstrual cycle will begin on the 3rd day after the temperature rise has been observed. Andrews (2006) points out that the temperature can be affected by infection. Therefore care needs to be taken when interpreting temperature charts.

Postpartum considerations

Day-to-day variation is greater at this time, because new mothers are likely to get up more during the night to take care of their baby's needs. Therefore, taking an accurate temperature reading in the morning becomes harder. For this reason, many women prefer to rely on examining cervical secretions, or combine noting secretions with cervical changes at this time.

Cervical palpation

Changes in the cervix throughout the menstrual cycle can be detected by daily palpation by the woman or her partner. After menstruation the cervix is low, easy to reach, feels firm and dry and the os is closed. As ovulation approaches the cervix shortens and sits higher in the vagina, it softens and the os dilates slightly under the influence of oestrogen.

Postpartum considerations

Hormonal changes in pregnancy take around 12 weeks to settle postpartum. The cervix will not revert completely to its pre-pregnant state and the os will always be slightly dilated even in the infertile time.

Calendar calculation (Fig. 37.6)

The calendar method is based on observation of the woman's past menstrual cycles. When starting out using this method, the specialist practitioner and the woman will look at the previous six menstrual cycles (Andrews 2006). The shortest and longest cycles over the previous 6 months are used to identify the likely fertile time. The first fertile day is calculated by subtracting 21 days from the end of the shortest menstrual cycle. In a 28-day cycle, this would be day 7. The last fertile day is calculated by subtracting 11 days from the end of the longest menstrual cycle. In a 28-day cycle, this would be day 17. Cycle length is constantly reassessed and appropriate calculations made. Guillebaud (2004) indicates that

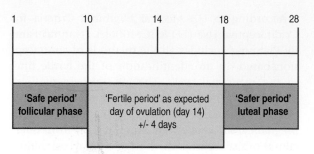

Figure 37.6 Natural family planning: The fertility awareness (rhythm) method. Diagram to illustrate rhythm method of contraception in a 28-day menstrual cycle.

the calendar method is not sufficiently reliable to be recommended as a single indicator of fertility, but is useful when combined with other indicators of fertility. Ovulation usually takes place 14 days before the first day of the next menstrual period. Therefore a woman who has a 28-day period would ovulate on approximately day 14 of her cycle and a woman who had a 30-day cycle would ovulate on approximately day 16 of her cycle.

Postpartum considerations

Calendar calculations must be recalculated once normal periods have begun.

Symptothermal method

This is a combination of temperature charting, observing cervical secretions, calendar calculation and optionally observing cervical palpation, to identify the fertile time. Andrews (2006) also includes in this method the observation of ovulation pain or 'mittelschmerz' and cyclic changes such as breast tenderness. Use of more than one indicator increases the accurate identification of the fertile time. When combining indicators, a couple should avoid intercourse from the first fertile day by calculation, or first change in the cervix until the 3rd day of elevated temperature, provided all elevated temperatures occur after the peak day.

Fertility monitoring device

There are a few different makes of devices on the market now which can be purchased at selected pharmacies. Prices range from £10.99 to £59.99 and they are not available on prescription. It is a hand-held computerized monitor which tests urine sticks. With careful and consistent, use it is between 93% and 97% effective in preventing pregnancy. The device monitors luteinizing hormone and oestrone-3-gluronide, a metabolite of oestradiol, through testing the urine. The 'Persona' monitoring device will detect from the urine test when a woman is fertile and indicate this through a series of lights. A green light indicates that she is in her infertile period and a red light indicates that she is in her fertile period therefore barrier methods must be used if she has sexual intercourse. A yellow light indicates that the database needs more information and a further urine test is required.

Postnatal considerations

The fertility monitor is not recommended as a method of contraception during lactation. The manufacturers recommend that a woman has had two normal menstruations with cycle lengths from 23 to 35 days before using the monitor at the beginning of the third period (Guillebaud 2004).

Lactational amenorrhoea method (LAM)

Before modern forms of contraception, lactation, with its inhibiting action on ovulation, was a major factor in ensuring adequate intervals between births. It is thought that the action of the infant suckling at the breast causes neural inputs to the hypothalamus. This results in the inhibition of gonadotrophin release from the anterior pituitary gland, leading to suppression of ovarian activity. The delay in return of postnatal fertility in lactating mothers varies greatly as it depends on patterns of breastfeeding, which are influenced by local culture and socioeconomic status. The time taken for the return of ovulation is directly related to sucking frequency and duration. The maintenance of night-feeds and the introduction of supplementary feeds also affects the return of ovulation.

Bellfield et al (2006) describe breastfeeding as a very effective method of contraception when used according to the Bellagio Consensus statement. This concludes that there is a 98% protection against pregnancy during the first 6 months following birth if a mother is still amenorrhoeic and fully or almost fully breastfeeding her baby. The mother can be asked if these three rules still apply to confirm LAM remains effective (Fig. 37.7). Mothers who work

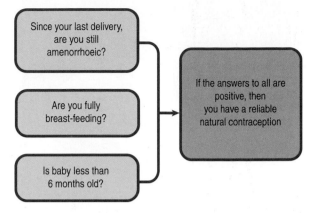

Figure 37.7 Natural contraception: Lactational amenorrhoea method (LAM).

outside the home can still be considered to be nearly fully breastfeeding, provided they stimulate their nipples by expressing breastmilk several times a day.

The LAM is not recommended for use after 6 months following birth, because of the increased likelihood of ovulation. A WHO (1999) multicentre study reported that in the first 6 months after childbirth the pregnancy rate ranged from 0.9% to 1.2% during full breastfeeding.

Male and female sterilization

This is the choice of contraception for many couples once their family is complete. Sterilization should be viewed as permanent, although in a few cases reversal of the operation is requested. Couples requesting sterilization need thorough counselling to ensure that they have considered all eventualities, including possible changes in family circumstances. Although consent of a partner is not necessary, joint counselling of both partners is desirable. The procedure is available on the NHS for both sexes but waiting times vary throughout Britain. There are no alterations to hormone production following sterilization in males or females and some couples find the freedom from fear of pregnancy very liberating.

Female sterilization

An estimated 210 million women worldwide have undergone female sterilization (Fig. 37.8) (Guillebaud 2004). During the procedure, the uterine tube

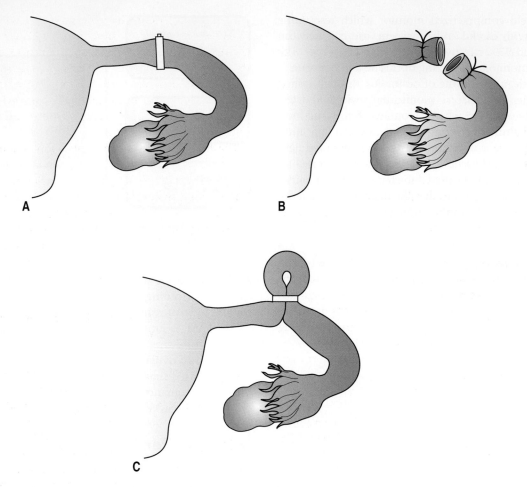

Figure 37.8 Female sterilization.

is occluded using division and ligation, application of clips or rings, diathermy or laser treatment. Modern methods aim to achieve minimal tissue damage with the isthmus section of the uterine tube being chosen as the place to divide the tube as it is of static diameter and this would increase the chance of successful reversal.

The operation is performed under local or general anaesthetic. The procedure can be performed via a laparotomy, minilaparotomy or laparoscopy. It can also be performed vaginally using a hysteroscope. It usually requires a day in hospital.

The effect is immediate, although the woman using the contraceptive pill may be advised to continue to use contraception until the next menstrual period, to prevent ovulation taking place. This is because in the case of failure of the procedure, there may be an increased chance of ectopic pregnancy (Bellfield 2006). Because of this risk, the couple should be advised to seek medical help urgently if they suspect pregnancy following sterilization because of the increased risk of ectopic pregnancy. Following hysteroscopic sterilization (Essure), tubal blockage is confirmed by hysterosalpingography after 3 months.

Postpartum considerations

The woman may experience regret later. This highlights the need for thorough counselling prior to the procedure. FFPRHC (2006b) suggests waiting 6 weeks after the woman has given birth before carrying out the procedure. They also suggest that if sterilization is going to be carried out at the same time as an elective caesarean operation, then 1 week or more should be given for counselling and decision-making before the procedure takes place. Guillebaud (2004) suggests that a waiting period of 12 weeks is desirable to ensure that the couple will have no regrets over the sterilization.

The failure rate for female sterilization is 1 in 200 (FPA 2004b). Reversal of the sterilization is not usually available on the NHS in the UK and can be difficult and expensive to obtain privately.

Male sterilization (vasectomy) (Fig. 37.9)

This procedure involves excision or removal of part of the vas deferens, which is the tube that carries sperm from the testes to the penis. There is a small cut or puncture to the skin of the scrotum. It is easier to access the vas deferens at this point. The tubes are cut and the ends closed by tying them or sealing them with diathermy. The wound on the scrotum will be very small and stitches are not usually required. In the UK, the operation is carried out in an outpatients department or clinic setting. It is usually completed under local anaesthetic and takes around 10–15 min. Men are advised to refrain from excessive physical activity for about 1 week and avoid heavy lifting (Andrews 2006).

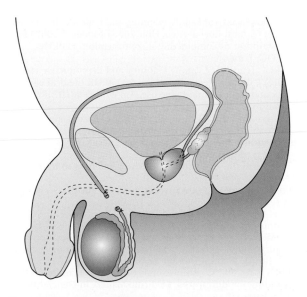

Figure 37.9 Male sterilization (vasectomy).

It may take some time for sperm to be cleared from the vas deferens. Approximately 12 weeks after the operation, the semen must be tested to confirm that it no longer contains sperm and sometimes a second test is necessary to confirm the absence of sperm. Sexual intercourse can take place during this period but contraception must be used until a negative sperm result is confirmed.

The failure rate of male sterilization is 1 in 2000 (FPA 2004b). Careful counselling needs to take place before the procedure is carried out. Reversal of vasectomy is not usually available on the NHS. Even if the reversal is successful in achieving re-anastomosis of the vas, pregnancy may be difficult to achieve because of the development of anti-sperm antibodies in some men. Andrews (2006) quotes a 50% success rate in achieving a pregnancy following successful reversal.

The future of contraception and sexual health services

Development of sexual health and contraception services is now a top priority for the government, as discussed in The National Strategy for Sexual Health and HIV (DH 2002). Primary Care Trusts are now being required to address local priorities in contraception and sexual health, e.g. offering an appointment within 48 hrs at a genito-urinary clinic; prompt referral to abortion services and lowering the teenage pregnancy rate.

In response to the Social Exclusion Unit Report (DH 1999), many PCTs now provide clinics and projects for young people. One of the specific targets of this report was to reduce the teenage pregnancy rate by 50% by 2010. With the development of the Fraser guidelines (Royal College of General Practitioners 2000), it is now possible to give contraceptive advice to young people under 16 years old, provided parental involvement is encouraged and the young person understands the nature of the consequences of treatment. The practitioner should also be of the opinion that, if contraception were withheld, sexual intercourse would still be likely to occur and the young person's physical and mental health could be compromised.

The NICE guidelines (2005) has emphasized the need to promote long-acting reversible contraception.

This requirement will encourage more people to use a form of contraception which does not have to be remembered on a daily basis.

There is a trend in the UK for many women to have their children later in life and to have much smaller families. Throughout the world, people will seek to find new ways to limit their family size as the need to reduce population growth continues (Guillebaud 2004).

Future developments

An extended regimen of combined contraceptive pills for 84 days (e.g. Seasonale) has been confirmed to be safe (Edelman et al 2006) and is presently licensed in many countries. Alternative delivery systems reducing the need for daily pill taking are being explored. Vaginal rings, implants and metered dose transdermal systems (MDTS), frameless intrauterine systems, subcutaneous injections (depo-subQ) and chewable tablets are being developed for progestogens. Research into biodegradable implants (Andrews 2006) and the use of transdermal spray for the delivery of a potent progestogen is ongoing. The Population Council is considering research into proteomics and an immunological approach to contraception (Nass & Strauss 2004). Effective methods for men are still problematic; however long-acting testosterone injections with implanted progestogens may be available in the future (Guillebaud 2004).

REFERENCES

Andrews G (ed.) 2006 Women's sexual health, 3rd edn. Elsevier, Edinburgh

Barrett G, Pendry E, Peacock J et al 2000 Women's sexual health after childbirth. British Journal of Obstetrics and Gynaecology 107(2):186–195

Bellfield T, Carter Y H, Matthews P et al 2006 The handbook of sexual health in primary care. Family Planning Association, London

Beral V, Kay C, Hannaford P, et al 1999 Mortality associated with oral contraceptive use: 25 year follow up of a cohort of 46 000 women from the RCGP's oral contraception study. British Medical Journal 318:96–100

Collaborative Group on Hormonal Factors in Breast Cancer 1996 Breast cancer and hormonal contraceptives: collaborative reanalysis of individual data on 53 297 women with breast cancer and 100 239 women without breast cancer from 54 epidemiological studies. Lancet 347:1713–1727

Committee of Safety of Medicine 2004 Combined oral contraceptives: venous thromboembolism. Current Problems in Pharmacovigilance 30:7

Croxatto H B, Makarainen L 1998 The pharmacodynamics and efficacy of Implanon. An overview of the data. Contraception 58(Suppl):91S–97S

DH (Department of Health) 1999 Teenage pregnancy. Report by the Social Exclusion Unit. The Stationery Office, London

DH (Department of Health) 2002 The National Strategy for Sexual Health and HIV. Implementation of action plan. DoH, London

DH (Department of Health) 2004 Choosing health – making healthier choices easier. DH, London

Dieben T O, Roumen F J, Apter D 2002 Efficacy, cycle control, and user acceptability of a novel combined contraceptive vaginal ring. Obstetrics and Gynecology 100(3):585–593

Dunn N, Thorogood M, Faragher B et al 1999. Oral contraceptives and myocardial infarction: results of the MICA case control study. British Medical Journal 318:1579–1584

Edelman A, Gallo M F, Nichols M D et al 2006 Continuous versus cyclical use of combined oral contraceptive pills: Systematic Cochrane review of randomised control trials. Human Reproduction 21 (3):573–578

FPA (Family Planning Association) (2004a) Leaflet: Your guide to diaphragms and caps

FPA (Family Planning Association) (2004b) Leaflet: Your guide to male and female sterilization

FPA (Family Planning Association) (2005a) Leaflet: Your guide to the contraceptive patch

FPA (Family Planning Association) (2005b) Leaflet: Your guide to male and female condoms

FPA (Family Planning Association) (2005c) Leaflet: Your guide to emergency contraception

FPA (Family Planning Association) (2005d) Leaflet: Your guide to natural family planning

FFPRHC (Faculty of Family Planning and Reproductive Health Care) Clinical Effectiveness Unit 2006a (updated 2007) First prescription of combined oral contraception. FFPRHC, RCOG, London

FFPRHC (Faculty of Family Planning and Reproductive Health Care) Clinical Effectiveness Unit 2006b UK medical eligibility criteria for contraceptive use, 3rd edn. FFPRHC, RCOG, London

Guillebaud J 2004 Contraception: your questions answered, 4th edn. Churchill Livingstone, Edinburgh

International Agency for Research on Cancer (IntARC) 2005 Combined oestrogen-progestogen contraceptives. Monographs on the evaluation of carcinogenic risks to humans No. 91

Jeffries D, Aitken R 2000 Spermicides and virucides. In: Mindel A (ed.) Condoms. BMJ Books, London

Jogee, M 2004 Religions and cultures, 6th edn. R & C Publications, Edinburgh

Kemmeren J, Algra A, Grobbee D 2001 Third generation oral contraceptives and risk of venous thrombosis: a meta-analysis. British Medical Journal 323:131–139

Kubba A A 2005 Combined oral contraceptive choice: understanding the differences. Medicine Matters in General Practice, Issue 101

Marchbanks P A, McDonald J A, Wilson H G et al 2002 Oral contraceptives and risk of breast cancer. New England Journal of Medicine 346:2025–2032

Mindel A, Estcourt C 2000 Condoms for the prevention of sexually transmitted infections. In: Mindel A (ed.) Condoms. BMJ Books, London

Nass S, Strauss J 2004 New frontiers in contraception research: a blue print for action. Washington (DC): Institute of Medicine National Academy Press

NICE (National Institute for Health and Clinical Excellence) 2005 Clinical guideline 30. Department of Health, London

Novak A, de la Logeb C, Abetzc L et al 2003 The combined contraceptive vaginal ring, NuvaRing: An international study of user acceptability. Contraception 67:187–194

Nursing and Midwifery Council 2004 Midwives rules and standards. Nursing & Midwifery Council, London

Royal College of General Practitioners 2000 Confidentiality and young people toolkit. Royal College of General Practitioners and Brook, London

Royal College of Midwives 2000 Midwifery practice in the postnatal period. Royal College of Midwives, London

Scholes D, LaCroix A Z, Ichikawa L E et al 2005 Change in bone mineral density among adolescent women using and discontinuing depot medroxyprogesterone acetate contraception. Archives of Paediatric Adolescent Medicine 159:139–144

Schwarz J L, Creinin M D, Pymar H C, et al 2002 Predicting risk of ovulation in new start oral contraceptive users. Journal of the American College of Obstetricians and Gynaecologists 99:177–182

Serjeant G R 1985 The long acting progestogen-only contraceptive injection: sickle cell disease. Oxford University Press, Oxford, p 287–288

Speroff L, Darney P 2001 A clinical guide for contraception, 3rd edn. Lippincott, Philadelphia

Szarewski A, Guillebaud J 2000 Contraception: a users guide, 3rd edn. Oxford University Press, Oxford

Teegarden D, Proulx W R, Martin R R, Zhao J et al 1995 Peak bone mass in young women. Journal of Bone Mineral Research 10(5):711–715

Vessey M, Lawless M, Yeates D et al 1985 Progestogen-only oral contraception. Findings in a large prospective study with special reference to effectiveness. British Journal of Family Planning 10:117–121

WHO Reproductive Health and Research in Family and Community Health 2002 Selected practice recommendations for contraceptive use. WHO, Geneva

WHO (World Health Organization) 1999 Multicultural study of breast-feeding and lactational amenorrhoea method 111; pregnancy during breast-feeding. Fertility and Sterility 72 (3):431–440

USEFUL ADDRESSES AND WEBSITES

Family Planning Association UK
Scotland: Tel: 0141 576 5088
Northern Ireland: Tel: 028 90 325 488
UK: 0845 310 1334 (open to 6 p.m.)
www.fpa.org.uk
All are open Monday to Friday from 9 a.m.–4.30 p.m.

Brook (putting young people first)
UK: Tel: 0800 0185 023
www.brook.org.uk

Fertility UK
www.fertilityuk.org

Faculty of Family Planning and Reproductive Health Care
www.ffprhc.org.uk

38 Bereavement and loss in maternity care

Rosemary Mander

CHAPTER CONTENTS

This chapter introduces the reader to issues which those working in the maternity area may face in the event of bereavement or loss. It is hoped that it will help the reader to better cope with the situation and, thus, care for those affected. Throughout the chapter, the assumption is made that care is more effective if based on research or, preferably, evidence.

The chapter aims to:

- consider the meaning of bereavement and loss, and their significance in maternity
- discuss forms of loss
- draw on research and evidence to review the care of those affected by the loss.

Introduction

In Western society at the beginning of the twenty-first century, bereavement is inextricably linked with loss through death. In this chapter, to make these concepts more relevant to the midwife, I broaden the focus to include other sources of grief affecting midwifery care. In widening the topic, I reflect the original meaning of 'bereavement', which carries connotations of plundering, robbing, snatching or otherwise removing traumatically and without consent. This meaning may appear to conflict with the other part of my title – 'loss' – also widely used in this context. Such inconsistency is fallacious because, although bereavement may involve 'taking' in a number of ways, the unspoken hopes and expectations invested in the one who is lost remain irretrievable.

In many ways, loss in childbearing is unique. This uniqueness is due to the awful contrast between the sorrow of death and the mystical joy of new life. Additionally, there is the cruel paradox of the 'juxtaposition' of birth and death (Howarth 2001, p 435); we often assume that these events are separated by a lifetime and the experience becomes incomprehensible when they become unified (Bourne 1968). Although any childbearing loss is unique, the uniqueness of both the individual's experience and the phenomenon itself must be contrasted with the frequency with which 'lesser' losses happen during childbearing. Such lesser losses include the parent's loss of their previous independence, the woman's loss of her special relationship with her fetus at birth, or the family's loss of the expectation of a perfect baby when they recognize that the actual baby is all too real.

In this chapter, I focus on the reactions of the woman losing a baby and her care by the midwife. The midwife has a responsibility to draw on her theoretical knowledge, which, as in any care, should be based on the best research evidence. Such knowledge is utilized in skilled care of the woman to facilitate adjustment to these greater and lesser losses. Thus, as well as losing a baby through death, I consider other childbearing-related loss.

Grief and loss

Grief, like death and other fundamentally important matters, is a fact of life. It is something that human beings will invariably meet in some form, sometimes at an early age. In spite of its universality, a woman in a developed country who experiences loss in childbearing may be young enough not to have previously encountered grief due to death. This is another reason for the uniqueness of childbearing loss.

Attachment

Limited understanding of mother–baby attachment, sometimes known as 'bonding', long prevented midwives and others from recognizing the significance of perinatal loss. The strength of the developing relationship between the woman and her fetus emerged in a research project involving bereaved mothers (Kennell et al 1970). This relationship develops with feeling movements and experiencing pregnancy, including investigations, such as ultrasound scans. Ordinarily attachment continues to develop beyond the birth (Bowlby 1997). The development of attachment during pregnancy means, however, that should the relationship not continue it must be ended, just like any parting. Thus, the reality of the mother–baby relationship must be recognized before the loss can be accepted. These processes are crucial to initiating healthy grieving.

Grief

Through grieving we adjust to the more serious as well as the lesser losses that confront us throughout life. Healthy grief means that we can move forward, although probably not directly, from the initial distraught hopelessness. We eventually achieve some degree of resolution, which permits ordinary functioning much of the time; in the process we may even learn something about ourselves and the resources available to us (Vera 2003).

Although grief may be viewed as a state of apathetic passivity, it is better regarded as a time when the bereaved person actively struggles with the emotional tasks facing her; the term 'grief work' describes this struggle (Engel 1961).

The stages of grief through which the person is likely to work have been described in a number of ways, but Kübler-Ross's (1970) account may be useful. These stages (Box 38.1) are not necessarily negotiated in sequence, but individual variations cause the person to move back and forth between them before achieving some degree of resolution (Kastenbaum 1998).

The initial response to any loss comprises a defence mechanism, which protects from the full impact of the news or realization. This reaction comprises shock or denial, which insulates the bereaved person from the unthinkable reality. This initial response allows 'breathing space', during which the person marshals their emotional resources; these facilitate coping with the impending realization.

Denial soon ceases to work and awareness of the reality of loss gradually dawns. Awareness brings powerful emotional reactions, together with their physical manifestations. Feelings of sorrow appear

> **Box 38.1** Stages of grief
>
> - Shock and denial
> - Increasing awareness
>   - Emotions: sorrow – guilt – anger
>   - Searching
>   - Bargaining
> - Realization
>   - Depression
>   - Apathy
>   - Bodily changes
> - Resolution
>   - Equanimity
>   - Anniversary reactions.

but other, less acceptable, emotions may simultaneously overwhelm the bereaved person; such emotions include guilt and dissatisfaction, as well as compulsive searching and, worryingly, anger. Realization dawns in waves as the bereaved person tries coping strategies to 'bargain' with herself to delay accepting reality.

When such fruitless strategies are exhausted, the despair of full realization materializes, bringing apathy and poor concentration as well as bodily changes. At this point in grief, the bereaved person may show anxiety and physical symptoms, typical of depression.

After the loss has eventually been accepted, it becomes integrated into the person's life. As mentioned already, this process is not straightforward and may involve slow progress and many setbacks, featuring oscillation and hesitation. Although the person may never 'get over' the loss, it should eventually be integrated into their life. This ultimate degree of 'resolution' is recognizable in the bereaved person's contemplation with equanimity the strengths, and weaknesses, of the lost relationship.

Significance

Healthy grieving matters. This is because it contributes to the resumption of balance or homeostasis in the life of the bereaved person. Grief crucially helps people recover from the wounds that the greater and lesser losses of life inflict. The hazards of being unable to grieve healthily have long been recognized in emotional terms, but research reveals the association between perinatal loss and the woman's physical illness (Ney et al 1994). This research suggests the woman's need for support, regardless of the nature of the loss or the extent to which it is recognized, or her grief sanctioned, by society.

Culture

I have described a general picture of healthy grieving, and mentioned individual variation, which is common to people of different ethnic backgrounds (Katbamna 2000). It is necessary to emphasize that the manifestations of grief, and the accompanying mourning rituals, vary even more. These variations are influenced by many factors. Cecil (1996) shows the massive differences between ethnic groups in their attitudes towards loss in childbearing. A midwife encounters difficulty accepting the different attitudes to loss in women of cultures other than her own (Mander 2006). Whether midwives are able to work through such feelings, to support women with different attitudes, is uncertain.

Closely bound up with culture, and certainly influencing mourning, is the grieving person's religious orientation or lack thereof. These aspects, however, may be difficult to separate from social class and prevalent societal attitudes.

Despite huge variations in its manifestation, the underlying purpose of mourning is universal. It establishes support for those closely affected, by strengthening links between those remaining. In perinatal loss the midwife initially provides this support. The role of the midwife is to be with the woman when she begins to realize the extent of her loss. The midwife aims to prevent any interference with the woman's healthy initiation of grieving.

Forms of loss

The terms 'loss' and 'bereavement' may be applied to a wide range of experiences, which vary hugely in severity and effects (Despelder & Strickland 2001). We must be careful, however, to avoid making assumptions about the meaning of loss to a particular person. It is difficult, even impossible, for anybody else to understand the significance of a pregnancy or a baby to another person. This is because childbearing carries with it a vast range of profound feelings, which includes unspoken hopes and expectations based on personal and cultural values. We should accept that grief in childbearing, like pain, 'is what the person experiencing it says it is' (McCaffery 1979).

I mention here some situations in which we may encounter grief. Some situations of childbearing grief are not included here and some of the situations listed here do not invariably engender grief.

Perinatal loss

When loss in childbearing is mentioned, loss perinatally comes quickly to mind. This includes stillborn babies and babies dying in the first week.

Attempts have been made to compare the severity of grief of loss at different stages, perhaps to demonstrate that certain women deserve more sympathy. A study investigating this point, however, showed no significant differences in the grief response between mothers losing a baby by miscarriage, stillbirth or neonatal death (Peppers & Knapp 1980). This study emphasizes the crucial role of the developing mother–baby relationship – the understanding of which has facilitated changes in care.

Stillbirth

The mother's long-term recovery from stillbirth was the subject of a retrospective Swedish study. Rådestad and colleagues (1996a) compared the recovery of 380 women who had given birth to a stillborn baby with 379 women who had a healthy child. The 84% response rate shows the mothers' enthusiasm to participate in this study. These researchers found that the mother made a better recovery if she could decide how long to keep her baby with her after the birth and if she could keep mementoes of the birth. The mother whose recovery was more difficult was the one where the birth of the baby was delayed after realization of fetal demise. Clearly, these findings have important implications for midwifery care (see the section on The mother, below). Additionally, the researchers discuss the 'known' stillbirth, when the mother realizes in advance of labour that her baby has died, previously termed 'intrauterine death' or 'IUD'. Alternatively, the loss may be unexpected. While avoiding any comparison of the two mothers' grief, it is understandable that the mother who knows that she is carrying a dead baby bears a particular emotional burden. This burden, compounded by maceration changing the baby's appearance, may impede grieving.

Early neonatal death

Grieving the loss of a baby born alive who dies, may be facilitated by three factors. The first is that the mother will have seen and held her real live baby; giving her a genuine memory of her experience. Second, there is the legal requirement that a baby who dies neonatally must have both their birth and death registered, providing written evidence of the baby having lived. Third is the investment of staff in their care of this dying baby, which increases the likelihood of effective support for the parents (Singg 2003).

Accidental loss in early pregnancy: miscarriage

Early pregnancy loss may be due to a number of pathological processes, such as ectopic pregnancy or spontaneous abortion. The word 'abortion' is avoided in this context, because it carries connotations of deliberate interference, which are unacceptable to a grieving mother. The term 'miscarriage' is preferable, to include all accidental losses. The grief of miscarriage has been ignored in the past, largely owing to its frequency. This has been estimated as 31% of pregnancies (Bansen & Stevens 1992), though the figure may be higher (Oakley et al 1990).

Understanding the woman's experience of miscarriage was sought through a qualitative research project (Bansen & Stevens 1992). Among the 10 mothers whom they interviewed 2–5 months after miscarriage, these researchers identified profound grief; this was associated with anger that their bodies had allowed them to miscarry, and anxiety about future childbearing. Far from being an insignificant event, these mothers were so ill during the miscarriage that they feared for their lives. Although each mother found reassurance in the conception of the pregnancy that was lost, each came to doubt her own fertility. As in other forms of loss, each mother found difficulty in locating support and encountered comments that denigrated the significance of her loss.

It may be necessary to seek the cause of a woman's miscarriage, especially if it happens repeatedly. Although miscarriage has been linked with stressful life events, Nelson and colleagues found no link between psychosocial stress and miscarriage (2003).

The former lack of recognition of miscarriage is now being addressed, and women are encouraged to create their own rituals to assist their grieving. Brin (2004) shows the helpful nature of a religious service, of photographs or of communicating sorrow through writing a poem or letter.

Infertility

The grief associated with involuntary infertility is less focused than that experienced when grieving for a particular person and has been termed 'genetic death' (Crawshaw 1995). In this situation the couple grieve for the hopes and expectations integral to the conception of a baby. Realization of their infertility, and the grief it brings, is aggravated by the widespread assumption that conception is easy. This is sufficiently prevalent for the emphasis, in society generally and healthcare particularly, to be on the prevention of conception. The complex investigations and prolonged treatment for infertility result in emotions comparable with a 'roller-coaster' of hope and despair.

As with any grief, the couple in the infertile relationship grieve differently, engendering tensions. Being told the diagnosis or cause of their infertility resolves some uncertainty about their predicament, but it raises other difficulties. These include the problems of one partner being 'labelled' infertile and, hence, being blamed for the couple's difficulty. A complex spiral of blame and recrimination escalates to damage what is already a vulnerable relationship. Obviously, counselling an infertile couple differs markedly from counselling those bereaved through death.

Relinquishment for adoption

Although long accepted that relinquishment is followed by grief (Sorosky et al 1984) the view still persists that, because relinquishment is voluntary, grief is unlikely (Mander 1995). Each mother in my study was clear that her relinquishment was definitely involuntary and that she had no alternative but to relinquish her baby. These mothers really were 'bereaved' in the original sense (see Introduction, p 727).

The grief of relinquishment is crucially different from grief following death. First, after relinquishment the grief is delayed. This is partly because of the woman's lifestyle at the time and partly because of the secrecy imposed on the woman who does not mother her baby as is usual. Secondly, the grief of relinquishment is unable to be resolved in the short or medium term. This is because, ordinarily, the acceptance of loss is fundamental to resolving grief. After relinquishment, such acceptance is impossible due to the likelihood that the one who was relinquished will make contact when legally able. Being reunited with the relinquished one was fundamentally important to the mothers I interviewed. 'Rosa's' words reflect what many mothers said: 'I'd be delighted if she would turn up on the doorstep'.

Termination of pregnancy (TOP)

Grief associated with termination of an uncomplicated pregnancy is problematic and for this reason it tends not to be included in the research-based literature on grief (Bewley 1993). The experience of grief following TOP for fetal abnormality and of guilt following TOP do, however, tend to be recognized and accepted. In view of the frequency with which TOP happens and the grief engendered, this deserves more attention.

TOP for fetal abnormality (TFA)

The package of investigations that has become known as 'prenatal diagnosis' may ultimately lead to the decision to undergo TFA. Although it may be assumed that the mother's reaction is solely one of relief at avoiding giving birth to a baby with a disability, Iles (1989) suggests several reasons for this mother experiencing conflicting emotions, which impede her grieving:

- the pregnancy is likely to have been wanted
- the TFA is a serious event in both physiological and social terms
- the reason for TFA may arouse guilty feelings
- the recurrence risk may constitute a future threat
- the woman's biological clock will be ticking away
- her failure to achieve a 'normal' outcome may engender guilt.

Interventions have been introduced to facilitate the grieving of the mother who has undergone TFA. These may involve counselling and the creation of memories, as are attempted in other forms of child-bearing loss (see the section on The baby, below). A randomized controlled trial to study the effectiveness of psychotherapeutic counselling in such mothers with no other risk factors was undertaken by Lilford et al (1994). This study suggested that bereavement counselling makes no difference to the difficulty or duration of grieving. Additionally, the researchers concluded that mothers attending for counselling would probably have resolved their grief more satisfactorily than the other group anyway.

TOP for other reasons

The non-recognition of grief associated with TOP may be partly because the mother who has her pregnancy ended may be considered 'undeserving' of the luxury of grief. Further, this may be aggravated by her being blamed for her situation (Hey 1996). Research on the psychological sequelae of TOP has focused on the guilt of having decided to end the pregnancy, as opposed to grief reactions; it may be that this focus is associated with the acrimonious abortion debate in some countries. Thus, the grief and depression, presenting as tearfulness were found to be normal after a termination of pregnancy (Wahlberg 2006). Perhaps these reactions could be prevented by counselling before, as well as after, the TOP.

The baby with a disability

For various reasons a baby may be born with a disability, which may or may not be expected. Disabilities vary hugely in their severity and in their implications for the baby. The mother may have to adjust to the possibility of her baby dying, but many conditions will permit the continuation of a healthy life.

The mother's reaction to the birth of a baby with a disability will involve some grief. This is particularly true if the condition was unexpected, as the mother must grieve for her expected baby before relating to her real baby. The mother may be shocked to find herself thinking that her baby might be better off not surviving (Lewis & Bourne 1989). Although the mother may be reassured that such thoughts are

not unique, she may nevertheless find it difficult to complete her grieving.

If a baby is born with an unexpected disability, the problem of breaking the news emerges. There are no easy answers to how this can be done to avoid trauma, but clear, effective and honest communication is crucial (Farrell et al 2001).

The 'inside baby'

It may be hard to understand that, even in uncomplicated, healthy childbearing, grief may feature. This is because, in spite of obstetric technology, the mother is unable to see her baby before the birth; inevitably the real baby will differ from the one whom she came to love during pregnancy. These differences are likely to be minor, such as hair colour or crying behaviour. Lewis (1979) coined the term 'inside baby' to denote the one she came to love during pregnancy and who was perfect. The 'outside baby' is the real one, for whom she will care and who may have some imperfections, such as having the wrong hair colour. Clearly the mother may have a few moments of regret, during which she grieves the loss of her fantasy 'inside' baby, while at the same time beginning her relationship with her real baby.

The mother's birth experience

A further form of loss, over which the mother may need to grieve, is her loss of her anticipated birth experience. If she was hoping for an uncomplicated birth, even some of the more common interventions may leave her with a sense of failure (Green & Baston 2003). Thus, like the woman grieving her 'inside baby', even though all may appear satisfactory this disappointed mother will have some grief work to complete.

The midwife's experience

The emotional reaction which will be experienced by the midwife may come as a surprise. As a professional person, she may be taken aback by the strength and complexity of her feelings when caring for a bereaved mother. This aspect, while still under-researched, has begun to be opened up to debate (Box 38.2).

Box 38.2 That sad day

This is a summary of feelings and thoughts when I discovered an intrauterine death at 41 weeks' gestation. The woman involved had been admitted for induction and neither of us were prepared for this.

My heart literally sank when on initial palpation her stomach felt cold and then the monitor did not detect the heart beat (I had just used the machine earlier). I knew although it would be difficult that I had to try and prepare her. I stayed later to try and give some continuity of care and support for her and her husband. After the scan confirmed the death I hugged her and her husband and cried with them. After this happened, I had a day off work with a severe migraine caused by stress. I felt very nervous and sick about going back to work, this was compounded when I discovered that the woman had been admitted to Intensive Care and was very ill. However, I did go back to work, visited the woman and sat holding her hand. We talked about her sadness and she said she had been worried about me leaving work late and wondered how I had coped getting home and facing my two children. I couldn't believe that she was concerned about me! She remembered every word I had said to her and praised my honesty. I had told her before the scan that I was sure that the baby had not survived. Two weeks later I attended the funeral in order to seek closure and to demonstrate my sympathy and sadness for the parents.

I have been a midwife for over 12 years and this has NEVER happened to me before, The whole event was very traumatic and upsetting for me. Some colleagues told me not to be upset, cry and/or get involved, but this was ineffective advice. I was so determined that my experience should not be in vain that I wrote this reflective piece. In total I have experienced the loss of over nine friends and relatives including my parents when I was fairly young. However, nothing can prepare someone (even a professional) for discovering that a baby has died and having to prepare the parents for this. Without the love and support of my family, friends and colleagues I would not have coped. As healthcare professionals we should be empathic and display understanding towards our colleagues in similar situations.

As Rosemary Mander (2004b) writes in 'When the professional gets personal':

for professional staff who provide effective care, there is likely to be a personal cost. These are the 'costs of caring', which may be regarded as the negative side of engaging with patients and clients and with one's work.

The whole experience will have a huge effect on my practice in various ways. I will encourage midwives to be honest with the clients. This will ensure that words are carefully chosen and also sensitively put, because they will be clearly remembered in years to come. I will not try to smooth over colleagues' feelings when they are involved in issues like this.

I am also going to liaise with the Local Supervising Authority to look at guidance for other midwives in situations like this. The success of the 'Birth Afterthoughts Service' within the Trust has led me to identify the need for a service for midwives dealing with bereavement and perhaps morbidity as well. Therefore, as a supervisor of midwives I aim to promote separate sessions for midwives – even if the midwife says she is unaffected. This will not be blame-based but will simply allow the members of staff to come to terms with their emotions and feelings by helping them to move on in a positive way.

To summarize, writing about this episode has been a catharsis for me and hopefully my experience will have a positive outcome for other staff who find themselves in the same sad and extremely difficult situation, and therefore benefit the parents as well.

Care

In considering the care that midwives provide in the event of loss, there are difficulties in deciding where to begin. Thus, I have organized this section by focusing first on those who are involved or affected and then on other crucial issues. From this material will emerge the principles of our care in this situation. While recognizing the artificiality of distinguishing care for individuals in this complex situation, this approach may help us to consider the different needs among people affected by a single event.

The baby

It is particularly hard to separate the care of the baby from the care of those who are grieving, because much of our care comprises the creation of memories of the baby, which will facilitate the grieving (Box 38.3).

We may think of the care of the baby beginning before the birth by considering the cot in the labour room (Mander 2006). Although the cot may cause the staff some discomfort, it reminds all concerned of the reality of the baby. If possible, that is if the baby's demise is known, the midwife discusses with the parents prior to the birth the contact which will be made with the baby. This contact may take any of a number of forms, beginning with just a sight of the wrapped baby. Contact with the baby has been said to resolve some of the confusion surrounding the birth. The effects of such care have been called into question, though (Hughes et al 1999).

The midwife faces the quandary of whether, and how much, she will encourage the mother to make contact with her baby, drawing on her knowledge of its beneficial effect on grief (Mander 2006). This quandary is difficult, but midwives tend to be over-cautious in encouraging the mother to make contact with her baby. This was an important finding from a study of 380 mothers who had experienced perinatal loss (Rådestad et al 1996b). These researchers found that one-third of the mothers would have appreciated more encouragement to make contact with their babies.

The mother may choose to have considerable contact with her baby, perhaps keeping the baby with her for some time. During this time, the mother may wish to have her baby baptized which, as well as its religious significance, emphasizes the reality of the baby. This simple act, which may be undertaken by the midwife, additionally presents an opportunity to name the baby. The mother may also during this time have other opportunities to create memories of her experience; these include doing some of the things a mother ordinarily does for a baby, such as bathing and dressing him or her. Whether or not the mother chooses to make contact with her baby immediately, it is usual to collect certain mementoes at the time of the birth, such as a lock of hair, a footprint or photographs. If the mother chooses to make no contact at the birth she may later ask for these mementoes. Taking photographs of a suitable quality may present a challenge to the midwife who is not skilled in using a camera, giving rise to dissatisfaction (Rådestad et al 1996b). Figure 38.1 shows the sensitive way in which a photograph may be used to help create memories of the birth.

In the hope of preventing a future loss, the parents may be advised that the baby should have a post mortem examination. This raises difficult issues for parents, who may consider that their baby has already suffered enough. In the UK, there are guidelines providing information for the parents prior to seeking their consent for the post mortem. These guidelines aim to prevent certain abuses, which have previously caused anguish to some bereaved parents (Dimond 2001, RCP 2000).

The funeral serves a multiplicity of purposes, including a demonstration of general support as well as establishing the reality of the loss. A young woman with no experience of death has difficulty imagining how such a ritual could ever be beneficial.

Box 38.3 Creating memories

- Midwifery activities
  - Information giving
  - Arranging for/taking photographs[a]
  - Cutting a lock of hair[a]
  - Taking a footprint[a]
  - Giving a cot card and/or name-band
- Parental activities
  - Naming baby
  - Seeing baby
  - Holding baby
  - Caring for baby: bathing – dressing
  - Taking photographs
- Other activities
  - Writing in a book of remembrance
  - Service/funeral/burial/cremation
  - Tree planting
  - Writing a letter and/or poem.

[a]Parents' informed consent will be needed.

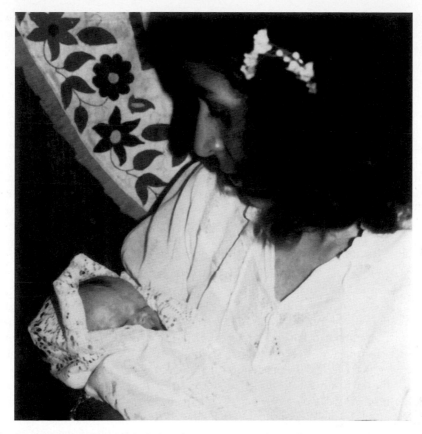

Figure 38.1   Photograph showing a grieving mother cradling her baby, who has been named Baby Shane.

She may be helped, though, by being reminded how cemetery and crematorium staff are sensitive to the need to provide a suitable ceremony and a congenial environment in which the child may subsequently be remembered (Kohner 1995). In some situations, such as early miscarriage, a funeral might not be appropriate. The mother may find that an impromptu service is helpful near the time of her loss or, later, she may create her own memorial by writing a letter to her lost baby or by planting a tree.

The mother

Much of the midwife's care of the grieving mother comprises helping her to make some sense of the incomprehensible experience that has happened to her. As mentioned already, the mother may need help to recognize that she has given birth, even though she no longer has that baby. Integral to this

is assisting her realization that she is a mother, which is achieved through midwifery care.

The mother may start to make sense of her loss by talking about it. Although this sounds simple enough, 'opening up' may present the mother with certain challenges. For example, she may be inexperienced and uncomfortable in talking about such profound feelings. Further, she may have difficulty finding a suitable and willing listener at the precise time when she feels ready. The problem of her finding a listener was identified in a research project showing that senior hospital staff appear too busy, and other staff insufficiently experienced, for her to unburden herself. Family members, who might be able to listen, have their own difficulties to face, making them unreceptive to the mother's needs (Rajan 1994).

In a situation of loss, any of us may feel that our control over our lives is slipping away. Such feelings of losing control are exacerbated when the loss involves a physiological process such as childbearing, which many people achieve successfully and effortlessly. Midwives should be able to help the mother to retain some degree of control. They can do this is by giving her accurate information about the choices open to her and on which she is able to base her decision-making. In this way, the midwife may be able to empower the woman and the two may form a partnership together.

The reality of the grieving mother's control over her care was the subject of Gohlish's research (1985). She interviewed 15 mothers of stillborn babies and asked them to identify the 'nursing' behaviours that they considered most helpful. This study showed the importance to the grieving mother of assuming control over her environment. While the midwife may be keen to share many aspects of control in the form of decision-making with the grieving mother, there are some decisions which are considered unsuitable for the mother to make (Mander 1993). The suitable decisions include the contact that the mother has with her baby; whereas the unsuitable decisions may include the environment in which she is cared for during her hospital stay.

The support offered to the woman was the subject of a systematic review, which found that there is no evidence to indicate the effectiveness of psychological support at this time (Chambers & Chan 2001). A randomized controlled trial by Forrest et al (1982) investigated the effects of support following perinatal loss. The experimental group, comprising 25 bereaved mothers, received ideal supported midwifery care together with counselling; the control group comprised another 25 bereaved mothers who received standard care. Unlike Lilford and colleagues' more psychotherapeutically oriented study (1994), Forrest found that the well-supported and counselled group recovered from their grief more quickly than the control group. Unfortunately, both studies had difficulty retaining contact with the grieving mothers.

The mother may find helpful support in a number of people, who provide support on a more or less formal basis (Forrest et al 1982). Although we may assume that identifying support is easy, research by Rådestad et al (1996b) has shown that, like finding a suitable listener, locating support may be problematic for the mother. These researchers found that for just over one-quarter of bereaved mothers the support lasted for under 1 month; while for just over another quarter the support was non-existent.

Of particular significance to midwives is the contribution of the lay support and self-help groups. My research showed that midwives are happy to recommend that a mother may find a support group, such as the Stillbirth and Neonatal Death Society (SANDS), helpful (Mander 2006). Unfortunately, little is known about their effectiveness or the experiences of those who attend.

If the loss occurs while the woman is in hospital, her transfer home is crucially important, due to the likelihood of other agencies becoming involved in her care. At this point good inter-agency communication ensures that the woman's healthy grieving is not jeopardized. In her large qualitative study, Moulder (1998) identified the quality of the help provided for the grieving mother by community agencies. She found that women experience very different standards of care from the different professionals, such as health visitors, general practitioners, community midwives and a range of counselling personnel. Similarly, the 6-week follow-up presents an opportunity, not only to check the woman's physical recovery, but also to discuss important outstanding issues. These include the couple's emotional recovery from their loss, the post mortem results (if relevant), any questions arising or remaining, as well as plans for the future. The research by Moulder found that this follow-up visit is often handled appropriately sensitively, in a suitable environment, with appropriate personnel present and adequate time to address matters of concern. Unfortunately, for some of the women the appointment was delayed and staff were condescending.

The family

It is the mother who is clearly most intimately involved with, and affected by, a perinatal loss. To a greater or lesser extent those close to her will share her grief. In this context, as well as conventional family members, I would include a range of non-blood and non-marital relationships.

The father

The effect of the loss on the father may previously have been underestimated (Mander 2004a). This is partly because men tend to show their grief differently from women and partly because they are socialized into providing support for their women-folk, possibly at the cost of their own emotional well-being. Further, men are stereotypically unlikely to avail themselves of the therapeutic effects of crying and articulating their sorrow. Men's coping mechanisms may also involve resorting to other less healthy grieving strategies, including returning early to work and using potentially harmful substances such as nicotine or alcohol.

Possibly in association with their different patterns of grieving (Samuelsson et al 2001), the parental relationship is likely to change following perinatal loss. Whether the couple find their relationship strengthened or threatened is unpredictable.

Other family members

Perhaps because they are less closely involved, the grandparents may be disproportionately adversely affected by the loss. This may be due to their inability to protect their children (the bereaved parents) from their painful loss. Inevitably and additionally they will experience their own sense of loss at the threat to the continuity of their family and what it means to them.

The effects of perinatal loss on a sibling may be problematic because of uncertainty about the child's understanding of the event (Hayslip & Hansson 2003). This difficulty is compounded by the parents' limited ability to articulate their pain in a suitable form. The parents may seek to solve these problems by 'protecting' their other child(ren) from the truth. They little know that 'protection' creates a pattern of unhealthy grieving, leaving a family legacy of dysfunctional relationships (Dyregrov 1991).

Whilst midwives tend to assume that the family are the best people to support a grieving mother (Mander 1996), it has been found that family responses may not invariably be healthy or helpful (Kissane & Bloch 1994).

The formal carers

The difficulty that staff face in caring for a grieving mother has been linked with their personal reactions to the loss of a baby (Bourne 1968). This may be part of the reason for the historical neglect of such mothers in particular and this topic in general. Furthermore, the loss of a baby represents all too clearly the failure of the healthcare system, and those who work in it, to give the mother a successful outcome to her pregnancy. The fear of failure in turn engenders a cycle of avoidance, which perpetuates the neglect of the mother.

This vicious cycle has been interrupted so that as the care of the mother has been changed, it is necessary to question whether the care of staff has kept pace (Clarke & Mander 2006). The emotional costs of providing care are now being recognized. Phillips (1996) describes how the devaluation of the emotional component of care is associated with increasing use of the medical model. This devaluation contributes to the increasing recognition of 'burnout'. The remedy has been identified in a midwifery setting to comprise support in the form of development of 'team spirit' (Foster 1996). The need for extra support is particularly important for less experienced staff when providing care for grieving families (Mander 2000). The education of staff for their counselling role is another solution, which is enhanced by supervision for the counsellors. The role of the midwife manager in creating a supportive environment for staff in stressful situations should not be underestimated. The midwife may also be able to locate support in others alongside whom she works, such as the hospital minister or chaplain. Additionally, there are helpful agencies which may be located within or outwith the healthcare system (Stoter 1997).

The involvement of staff in the mother's grief raises some difficult questions. First there is the helpfulness or otherwise of the midwife sharing the bereaved mother's tears. Although some midwives are prepared to cry alongside the mother, others feel that crying is 'unprofessional' and would not be comfortable shedding even a few tears. The midwives in my research said that, generally, crying was not a problem; but any loss of control that impeded their ability to provide care must be avoided at all costs (Mander 2006). Another difficult decision is whether staff should attend the baby's funeral. Some of the midwives I interviewed found this helpful and they had not been uncomfortable attending. In some circumstances, however, this would not apply.

Other aspects of care

Not least because of the possibility of impeding grieving, other aspects of care assume greater importance.

Documentation

Record-keeping in this context becomes even more significant. This is because of the importance of communication in ensuring consistent care, which will facilitate the mother's grieving. Although far from ideal, it may be difficult to avoid this care being provided by a number of personnel. Thus, it is crucial that each midwife should be able to learn from the mother's records about decisions and actions already taken (Horsfall 2001).

The cremation or burial

The documents required for the 'disposal' of the baby differ according to whether the baby was born before or after 24 weeks' gestation (the current legal limit of viability in the UK), according to whether the baby was born alive or not and according to the part of the UK in which the baby was born (see Ch. 56). If the baby was pre-viable, there is no legal requirement for the baby to be buried or cremated. It is, however, essential to ensure that the baby's remains are removed according to the mother's wishes. If she decides not to participate in the removal of the baby's remains, they should still be removed sensitively (RCOG 2006). A book of remembrance in the maternity unit is available to parents to record their names, their baby's details and some thoughts about the baby.

For a baby born after 24 weeks, burial or cremation may be organized by the hospital, with the parents' permission, or by the parents. The local cemetery is likely to have a special plot for babies to be buried individually. This may include the provision of a small tree or rose bush, and a religious or other service may be available. There is also the possibility that the parents may erect a headstone (Mortonhall, Edinburgh City Council, personal communication, 2001).

The statutory documentation is specific to each of the countries of the UK (McDonald 1996). Details of the registration requirements in each of the four countries of the UK are provided on the websites listed in the Useful Addresses at the end of this chapter.

The mother's choices

At the time of the loss of her baby, as well as her grief work, the mother has certain choices. In terms of how the baby's remains should be disposed of, the mother should decide whether she would prefer to arrange this privately or allow the hospital to do it. The mother also needs to decide the extent to which she would like to be involved in organizing the funeral service, the blessing or the memorial ceremony (Kohner 1995). In some hospitals, services of remembrance are arranged on a regular basis, and bereaved parents are able to choose whether to attend. As mentioned above, the mother needs appropriate information in order to make decisions about the funeral and the post mortem.

The death of a mother

A form of loss that fortunately happens even less frequently than the death of a baby is when the mother dies; this is usually known as maternal death. In the UK, the rate of maternal death is approximately 1 in 8771 births (Lewis 2004). This means that in a medium-sized maternity unit a mother is likely to die about once every 3 years.

Although the obstetric and epidemiological aspects of maternal death have been well addressed (Edwards 2004; Lewis 2004; Maclean & Neilson 2002), the personal and emotional aspects have been avoided (Mander 2001a). The English language literature has only addressed a family's experience of loss anecdotally (Dunn 1987). There appears to be, however, no systematic research on the family's experience of loss, or on the life of the motherless baby. Palliative care principles may be appropriately applied to the care of the childbearing woman with or dying from an incurable condition (Mander & Haroldsdottir 2002). The care of this woman and the implications for her baby and the other members of her family are likely to become increasingly important as some women choose to delay childbearing into their more mature years. The care provided for this childbearing woman has not yet been subjected to serious research attention.

However, the experience of the midwife providing care around the time of the death of a mother has begun to be addressed (Mander 2001b). This research shows the dire implications for the midwife of attending a mother who dies, to the extent that the experience assumes the proportions of a disaster. The midwife's desperate need for support may be met by midwifery colleagues who either shared her experience or have been through a similar one. The midwife's family also plays a fundamentally important role in supporting her (Mander 1999).

Conclusion

I have shown in this chapter that, for the midwife's care of the mother grieving a loss in childbearing to be of a suitably high standard, it requires to be research-based knowledge. Although undertaking such research is not easy for any who are involved, it is only by obtaining and using such knowledge that we are able to give this mother and family care of the highest standard. In this way, the midwife facilitates healthy grieving in the mother, having avoided the impediments which interfere with or complicate her grief and prevent its resolution. In this most human of situations, we must remember that 'being nice' is not enough; we need to ensure that our care is based on the strongest evidence available if the woman is eventually to come to terms with her loss.

REFERENCES

Bansen S, Stevens H 1992 Women's experience of miscarriage in early pregnancy. Journal of Nurse Midwifery 37(2):84–90

Bewley C 1993 The midwife's role in pregnancy termination. Nursing Standard 8(12):25–28

Bourne S 1968 The psychological effects of stillbirth on women and their doctors. Journal of the Royal College of General Practitioners 16:103–112

Bowlby J 1997 Attachment and loss, Vol.1 Attachment. Pimlico, London

Brin D J. 2004 The use of rituals in grieving for a miscarriage or stillbirth. Women & Therapy 27(3/4):123–132

Cecil R 1996 The anthropology of pregnancy loss: comparative studies in miscarriage, stillbirth and neonatal death. Berg, Oxford

Chambers H M, Chan F Y 2001 Support for women/families after perinatal death. The Cochrane Database of Systematic Reviews, issue 1. Update Software, Oxford

Clarke J, Mander R 2006 Midwives and loss: the cost of caring. The Practising Midwife 9(4):14–17

Crawshaw M 1995 Offering woman-centred counselling in reproductive medicine. In: Jennings S (ed.) Infertility counselling. Blackwell Science, Oxford, p 38–65

Despelder L A, Strickland A L 2001 Loss. In: Howarth G, Leaman O (eds) Encyclopedia of death and dying. Routledge, London, p 288–290

Dimond B 2001 Alder Hey and the retention and storage of body parts. British Journal of Midwifery 9(3):173–176

Dunn S E 1987 Suddenly, at home. ... Midwives Chronicle 100(1192):132–134

Dyregrov A 1991 Grief in children: a handbook for adults. Kingsley, London

Edwards G 2004 Adverse outcomes in maternity care. Books for midwives, Edinburgh

Engel G C 1961 Is grief a disease? A challenge for medical research. Psychosomatic Medicine 23:18–22

Farrell M, Ryan S, Langrick B 2001 'Breaking bad news' within a paediatric setting: an evaluation report of a collaborative education workshop to support health professionals. Journal of Advanced Nursing 36(6):765–775

Forrest G, Standish E, Baum J 1982 Support after perinatal death: a study of support and counselling after perinatal bereavement. British Medical Journal 285:1475–1479

Foster A 1996 Perinatal bereavement: support for families and midwives. Midwives 109(1303): 218–219

Gohlish M 1985 Stillbirth. Midwife Health Visitor and Community Nurse 21(1):16

Green J M, Baston HA 2003 Feeling in control during labor: concepts, correlates, and consequences. Birth 30(4):235–247

Hayslip B, Hansson R O 2003 Death awareness and adjustment across the life span. In: Bryant C D (ed.) Handbook of death and dying. Sage, Thousand Oaks, Vol 1, Part IV, p 437–447

Hey V 1996 A feminist exploration. In: Hey V, Itzin C, Saunders L et al (eds) Hidden loss: miscarriage and ectopic pregnancy, 2nd edn. The Women's Press, London, p 125–149

Horsfall A 2001 Bereavement: tissues, tea and sympathy are not enough. Royal College of Midwives Journal 4(2):54–57

Howarth G 2001 Stillbirth. In: Howarth G, Leaman O (eds) Encyclopedia of death and dying. Routledge, London, p 434–435

Hughes P M, Turton P, Evans C D 1999 Stillbirth as risk factor for depression and anxiety in the subsequent pregnancy: cohort study. British Medical Journal 318(7200):1721–1724

Iles S 1989 The loss of early pregnancy. In: Oates M R (ed.) Psychological aspects of obstetrics and gynaecology. Baillière Tindall, London, p 769–790

Kastenbaum R (1998) Death, society and human experience, 6th edn. Allyn & Bacon, Boston

Katbamna S 2000 'Race' and childbirth. Open University Press, Buckingham

Kennell J, Slyter H, Klaus M 1970 The mourning response of parents to the death of newborn infant. New England Journal of Medicine 283(7):344–349

Kissane D, Bloch S 1994 Family grief. British Journal of Psychiatry 164:728–740

Kohner N 1995 Pregnancy loss and the death of a baby: guidelines for professionals. SANDS, London

Kübler-Ross E 1970 On death and dying. Tavistock Publications, London

Lewis E 1979 Mourning by the family after a stillbirth or neonatal death. Archives of Disease in Childhood 54:303–306

Lewis E, Bourne S 1989 Perinatal death. In: Oates M (ed.) Psychological aspects of obstetrics and gynaecology. Baillière Tindall, London, p 935–954

Lewis G 2004 Why mothers die 2000–2002 The sixth report of the Confidential Enquiry into Maternal and Child Health. RCOG. London

Lilford R, Stratton P, Godsil S et al 1994 A randomised trial of routine versus selective counselling in perinatal bereavement from congenital disease. British Journal of Obstetrics and Gynaecology 101(4):291–296

Maclean A B, Neilson J P 2002 Maternal morbidity and mortality.RCOG, London

Mander R 1993 Who chooses the choices? Modern Midwife 3(1):23–25

Mander R 1995 The care of the mother grieving a baby relinquished for adoption. Avebury, Aldershot

Mander R 1996 The grieving mother: care in the community? Modern Midwife 6(8):10–13

Mander R 1999 Preliminary report: a study of the midwife's experience of the death of a mother. RCM Midwives Journal 2(11):346–349

Mander R 2000 Perinatal grief: understanding the bereaved and their carers. In: Alexander J, Levy V, Roth C (eds) Midwifery practice: core topics 3. Macmillan, London, p 29–50

Mander R 2001a Death of a mother: taboo and the midwife. Practising Midwife 4(8):23–25

Mander R 2001b The midwife's ultimate paradox: a UK-based study of the death of a mother. Midwifery 17(4):248–259

Mander R 2004a Men and maternity. Routledge, London

Mander R 2004b When the professional gets personal – the midwife's experience of the death of a mother. Evidence Based Midwifery 2(2):40–45

Mander R 2006 Loss and bereavement in childbearing, 2nd edn. Routledge, London

Mander R, Haroldsdottir E 2002 Palliative care and childbearing. European Journal of Palliative Care 9(6):240–242

McCaffery M 1979 Nursing management of the patient with pain. Lippincott, Philadelphia

McDonald M 1996 Loss in pregnancy: guidelines for midwives. Baillière Tindall, London

Moulder C 1998 Understanding pregnancy loss: perspectives and issues in care. Macmillan, London

Nelson D B, Grisso J A, Joffe M M et al 2003 Does stress influence early pregnancy loss? Annals of Epidemiology 13(4):223–229

Ney P, Tak F, Wickett A et al 1994 The effects of pregnancy loss on women's health. Social Science and Medicine 38(9):1193–1200

Oakley A, McPherson A, Roberts H 1990 Miscarriage. Penguin, London

Peppers L, Knapp R. 1980 Maternal reactions to involuntary fetal/infant death. Psychiatry 43:55–59

Phillips S 1996 Labouring the emotions: expanding the remit of nursing work? Journal of Advanced Nursing 24(1):139–143

Rådestad I, Steineck G, Nordin C et al 1996a Psychological complications after stillbirth. British Medical Journal 312(7045):1505–1508

Rådestad I, Nordin C, Steineck G et al 1996b Stillbirth is no longer managed as a non-event: a nationwide study in Sweden. Birth 23(4):209–216

Rajan L 1994 Social isolation and support in pregnancy loss. Health Visitor 67(3):97–101

RCOG 2006 The management of early pregnancy loss. London Royal College of Obstetricians and Gynaecologists, London

RCP 2000 Guidelines for the retention of tissues and organs at post-mortem examination. Royal College of Pathologists, London

Samuelsson M, Rådestad I, Segesten K 2001 A waste of life: fathers' experience of losing a child before birth. Birth 28(2):124–130

Singg S 2003 Parents and the death of a child, Part 7. In: Bryant C D (ed.) Handbook of death and dying. Sage, Thousand Oaks, p 880–888

Sorosky A D, Baran A, Pannor R 1984 The adoption triangle. Anchor, New York

Stoter D J 1997 Staff support in healthcare. Blackwell Science, Oxford

Vera M 2003 Social dimensions of grief, Part 7. In: Bryant C D (ed) Handbook of death and dying. Sage, Thousand Oaks, p 838–846

Wahlberg V 2006 Memories after abortion. Radcliffe, Oxford

FURTHER READING

Field D, HockeyJ, Small N 1997 Death, gender and ethnicity. Routledge, London

The politics of loss.

Dickenson D, Johnson M, Samson Katz J 2000 Death, dying and bereavement, 2nd ed. Sage and The Open University, London

An easily readable examination of a wide range of issues.

Jones A 1996 Psychotherapy following childbirth. British Journal of Midwifery 4(5):239–243

An in-depth exploration of relevant psychoanalytical issues.

Schott J, Henley A 1996 Childbearing losses. British Journal of Midwifery 4(10):522–526

The implications of cultural and religious variations in the context of childbearing loss.

Thompson N 2002 Loss and grief: a guide for human services practitioners. Palgrave, Basingstoke
Very relevant for midwives.

Walter T 1999 On bereavement: the culture of grief. Open University Press, London
Some up-to-date ideas and developments.

USEFUL ADDRESSES AND WEBSITES

Registration and other statutory documentation of a stillborn baby

England & Wales
http://www.gro.gov.uk/gro/content/stillbirths/

Scotland:
http://www.gro-scotland.gov.uk/regscot/registering-a-stillbirth.html

Northern Ireland:
http://www.belfastcity.gov.uk/deaths/stillbirths.asp?menuitem=registering-a-stilldeath

Support groups

The Miscarriage Association
http://www.miscarriageassociation.org.uk/ma2006/index.htm

SANDS (Stillbirth and Neonatal Death Society)
http://www.uk-sands.org/contact.html

CRUSE Bereavement Care
http://www.crusebereavementcare.org.uk/

BLISS – The Premature Baby Charity
http://www.bliss.org.uk/

The Compassionate Friends (UK) Support for bereaved parents and their families.
http://www.tcf.org.uk/

NORCAP – Support for Adults affected by Adoption
http://www.norcap.org.uk/home.asp

Infertility Network UK: Advice Support and Understanding
http://www.infertilitynetworkuk.com/

S.O.F.T.UK – Support Organization for Trisomy 13/18 & Related Disorders.
http://www.soft.org.uk/index.htm

Antenatal Results & Choices (incorporating SATFA)
73 Charlotte Street, London W1P 1LB
Tel: 020 7631 0285

6

Section 6
The newborn baby

SECTION CONTENTS

39 The baby at birth

Philomena Farrell   Norma Sittlington

A newborn baby's survival is dependent on his ability to adapt to an extrauterine environment. This involves adaptations in cardiopulmonary circulation and other physiological adjustments to replace placental function and maintain homeostasis. It is also the commencement of the early parent–baby relationship.

The chapter aims to:

- describe the physiological changes taking place at birth
- discuss the care of the baby during and immediately after birth
- identify factors to be considered when the baby fails to establish respiration at birth and describe the principles of neonatal resuscitation
- consider the early responses of both parents and baby, identifying steps that can be taken to promote good parent–baby relationships.

Introduction

The transition from intrauterine to extrauterine life is a dramatic one and demands considerable and effective physiological alterations by the baby in order to ensure survival. The fetus leaves the uterine environment, which has been completely life sustaining for oxygenation, nutrition, excretion and thermoregulation. The aquatic amniotic sac has permitted movement but freedom to extend the limbs has been limited towards the end of pregnancy as the size of the fetus has increased in relation to the capacity of the uterus. Though the fetus is sensitive to sound, the dim uterine environment has dulled the impact of the noise of the outside world.

Subjected to intermittent diminution of the oxygen supply during uterine contractions, compression followed by decompression of the head and chest, and extension of the limbs, hips and spine during birth, the baby emerges from the mother to encounter light, noises, cool air, gravity and tactile stimuli for the first time. Simultaneously, the baby has to make major adjustments in the respiratory and circulatory systems as well as controlling body temperature. These initial adaptations are crucial to the baby's subsequent well-being and should be understood and facilitated by the midwife at the time of birth.

Respiratory and cardiovascular changes are interdependent and concurrent.

Adaptation to extrauterine life

Onset of respiration

At birth, a baby is transposed from the warm contentment of the uterine environment to the outside world, where the role of independent existence is assumed. The baby must be able to make this sharp transition swiftly, and in order to achieve this, a series of adaptive functions have been developed to accommodate the dramatic change from the intrauterine to extrauterine environment.

Pulmonary adaptation

Until the time of birth, the fetus depends upon maternal blood gas exchange via the maternal lungs and the placenta. Following the sudden removal of the placenta after delivery, very rapid adaptation takes place to ensure continued survival. Prior to birth, the fetus makes breathing movements and the lungs will have matured both biochemically and anatomically to produce surfactant and have adequate numbers of alveoli for gas exchange. Before birth, the fetal lung is full of fluid, which is excreted by the lung itself. During birth, this fluid leaves the alveoli either by being squeezed up the airway and out of the mouth and nose, or by moving across the alveolar walls into the pulmonary lymphatic vessels and into the thoracic duct or to the lung capillaries.

The stimuli of respiration include mild hypercapnia, hypoxia and acidosis, which result from normal labour, due partially to the intermittent cessation of maternal-placental perfusion with contractions. The rhythm of respiration changes from episodic shallow fetal respiration to regular deeper breathing as a result of a combination of chemical and neural stimuli, notably a fall in pH and PaO_2 and a rise in $PaCO_2$. Other stimuli include cold, light, noise, touch and pain. Considerable negative intrathoracic pressure of up to 9.8 kPa (100 cm water) is exerted as the first breath is taken. The pressure exerted to effect inhalation diminishes with each breath taken until only 5 cm water pressure is required to inflate the lungs. This effect is caused by surfactant, which lines the alveoli, lowering the surface tension thus permitting residual air to remain in the alveoli between breaths. Surfactant is a complex of lipoproteins and proteins produced by the alveolar type 2 cells in the lungs, and is primarily concerned with the reduction in surface tension at the alveolar surface, thus reducing the work of breathing (Halliday et al 1998).

Cardiovascular adaptation

Prior to birth, the fetus relies solely on the placenta for all gas exchanges and excretion of metabolic waste. Separated from the placenta at birth, the baby's circulatory system must make major adjustments in order to divert deoxygenated blood to the lungs for re-oxygenation. This involves several mechanisms, which are influenced by the clamping of the umbilical cord and also by the lowered resistance in the pulmonary vascular bed.

During fetal life (see Ch. 12) only approximately 10% of the cardiac output is circulated to the lungs through the pulmonary artery. With the expansion of the lungs and lowered pulmonary vascular resistance, virtually all of the cardiac output is sent to the lungs. Oxygenated blood returning to the heart from the lungs increases the pressure within the left atrium. At almost the same time, pressure in the right atrium is lowered because blood ceases to flow through the cord. As a result, a functional closure of the foramen ovale is achieved. During the first days of life, this closure is reversible; re-opening may occur if pulmonary vascular resistance is high, for example when crying, resulting in transient cyanotic episodes in the baby (Perry 2002). The septa usually fuse within the first year of life, forming the interatrial septum, though in some individuals perfect anatomical closure may never be achieved.

The ductus arteriosus, which is nearly as wide as the aorta, provides a diversionary route to bypass the lungs of the fetus. Contraction of its muscular walls occurs almost immediately after birth. This is thought to occur because of sensitivity of the muscle of the ductus arteriosus to increased oxygen tension and reduction in circulating prostaglandin (Tannenbaum et al 1996). As a result of altered pressure gradients between the aorta and pulmonary artery, a temporary reverse left-to-right shunt through the ductus may persist for a few hours, although there is usually functional closure of the ductus within 8–10 hrs of birth. Intermittent patency has been demonstrated in most healthy infants in the first 3 days of life, but complete closure takes several months. Persistence or reopening of the ductus, with associated cyanosis or cyanotic attacks, may occur if pulmonary vascular resistance is high or hypoxia is present (Linh et al 2007). This is a common problem in pre-term infants with respiratory distress syndrome (see Ch. 44). Persistence of the foramen ovale or ductus arteriosus, or both, may be lifesaving in some forms of congenital heart abnormality (see Ch. 46).

The remaining temporary structures of the fetal circulation – the umbilical vein, ductus venosus and hypogastric arteries – close functionally within a few minutes after birth and constriction of the cord. Anatomical closure by fibrous tissue occurs within

2–3 months, resulting in the formation of the ligamentum teres, ligamentum venosum and the obliterated hypogastric arteries. The proximal portions of the hypogastric arteries persist as the superior vesical arteries.

Thermal adaptation

The baby enters a much cooler atmosphere at birth, with a birthing room temperature of at least 21°C contrasting sharply with an intrauterine temperature of 37.7°C. This causes rapid cooling of the baby as amniotic fluid evaporates from the skin. Each millilitre that evaporates removes 560 calories of heat (Rutter 2005). The baby's large surface area:body mass ratio potentiates heat loss, especially from the head, which comprises 25% of body mass. The subcutaneous fat layer is thin and provides poor insulation, allowing rapid transfer of core heat to the skin, then to the environment, and it also affects blood cooling. In addition to heat loss by evaporation, further heat will be lost by conduction when the baby is in contact with cold surfaces, by radiation to cold objects in the environment, and by convection caused by currents of cool air passing over the surface of the body (Fig. 39.1) (Brueggemeyer 1993, Rutter 2005, Thomas 1994).

The heat-regulating centre in the baby's brain has the capacity to promote heat production in response to stimuli received from thermoreceptors. However,

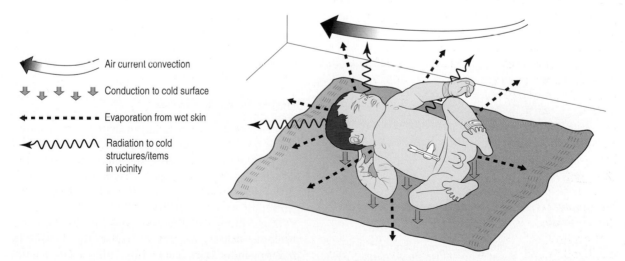

Air current convection

Conduction to cold surface

Evaporation from wet skin

Radiation to cold structures/items in vicinity

Figure 39.1 Modes of heat loss in the neonate.

this is dependent on increased metabolic activity, compromising the baby's ability to control body temperature especially in adverse environmental conditions. The baby has a limited ability to shiver and is unable to increase muscle activity voluntarily in order to generate heat. This means that the baby must depend on his ability to produce heat by metabolism.

The neonate is endowed with brown adipose tissue, which assists in the rapid mobilization of heat resources (namely free fatty acids and glycerol) in times of cold stress. This mechanism is called non-shivering thermogenesis (Sheldon & Korones 2004). Babies derive most of their heat production from the metabolism of brown fat. The term 'brown fat' refers to the reddish-brown colouring of the fat, which is caused by the high degree of vascularization of the tissue. Brown fat is stored in pockets throughout the baby's body. The majority of brown fat is located around the neck, along the line of the spinal column between the scapulae, across the clavicle line and down the sternum (Fig. 39.2). It also surrounds the major thoracic vessels and pads the kidneys (Merkin 2005). The term baby has sufficient brown fat to meet minimum heat needs for 2–4 days after birth, but cold stress results in increased oxygen consumption as the baby strives to maintain sufficient heat for survival. Brown fat uses up to three times as much oxygen as other tissue (Wong 1995), with the undesired effect of diverting oxygen and glucose from vital centres such as the brain and cardiac muscle. In addition, cold stress causes vasoconstriction,

> **Box 39.1** Transient tachypnoea of the newborn
>
> This condition is characterized by rapid respirations of up to 120/min; it is especially common after a caesarian section. The baby may be cyanosed but maintains normal blood gases apart from PaO_2. Little or no recession of the rib cage is evident and there is minimal, if any, grunt on expiration. The respiratory rate may remain elevated for up to 5 days. Treatment consists of oxygen therapy to maintain adequate oxygenation. It is essential that other causes of respiratory distress are excluded, especially infective causes (which mimic this condition) and respiratory distress syndrome (see also Ch. 44).

thus reducing pulmonary perfusion, and respiratory acidosis develops as the pH and PaO_2 of the blood decrease and the $PaCO_2$ increases leading to respiratory distress, exhibited by tachypnoea (Box 39.1), and grunting respirations (see Ch. 44). This, together with the reduction in pulmonary perfusion, may result in the re-opening or maintenance of the right-to-left shunt across the ductus arteriosus. Anaerobic glycolysis (i.e. the metabolism of glucose in the absence of oxygen) results in the production of acid compounding the situation by adding a metabolic acidosis. Protraction of cold stress should therefore be avoided. The peripheral vasoconstrictor mechanisms of the baby are unable to prevent the fall in core body temperature, which occurs within the first few hours after birth. It is important, therefore, for the midwife to ensure that she employs measures to minimize heat loss at birth (Rutter 2005).

Intrauterine hypoxia

Oxygenation of the fetus is dependent on oxygenation of the mother, adequate perfusion of the placental site, placental function, fetoplacental circulation and adequate fetal haemoglobin. Absence or impairment of any of these factors will result in a reduction of oxygen supply to the fetus (Fig. 39.3).

Oxygenation of the mother may be impaired as a result of cardiac or respiratory disease, an eclamptic fit or during induction of general anaesthesia if difficulties arise during intubation. Perfusion of the placental site

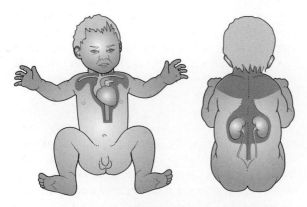

Figure 39.2 Sites of brown fat. (From Brendan Ellis, medical illustrator, Royal Group of Hospitals, Belfast, with permission.)

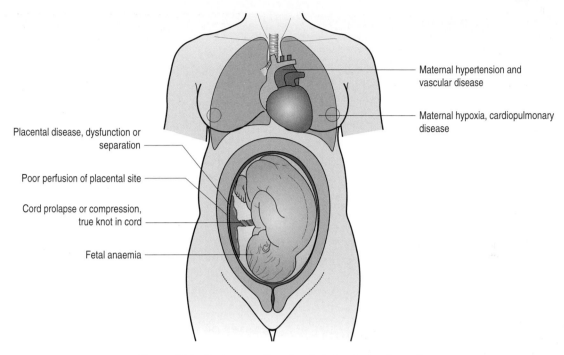

Figure 39.3   Factors predisposing to intrauterine hypoxia.

is dependent on satisfactory blood supply. This may be reduced in the presence of maternal hypertension or if hypotension occurs in response to haemorrhage, shock or aortocaval occlusion. Hypertonic uterine action, when uterine resting tone is elevated, will impede the blood supply to the placental site. This is sometimes due to hyperstimulation of the uterus by oxytocin and necessitates discontinuation of the oxytocic agent to allow the uterus to relax, thus restoring circulation to the placental bed. The umbilical cord transports oxygenated blood to the fetus. If prolapsed or compressed, fetal oxygenation will be reduced. The transport of oxygen within the fetus necessitates the availability of adequate haemoglobin, which may be reduced if Rhesus incompatibility is present. Abnormal fetal cardiac function may also diminish the supply of oxygen to the fetal brain.

The fetus responds to hypoxia by accelerating the heart rate in an effort to maintain supplies of oxygen to the brain. If hypoxia persists, glucose depletion will stimulate anaerobic glycolysis resulting in a metabolic acidosis. Cerebral vessels will dilate and some brain swelling may occur. Peripheral circulation will be reduced. As the fetus becomes acidotic and

cardiac glycogen reserves are depleted, bradycardia develops, the anal sphincter relaxes and the fetus may pass meconium into the liquor. Gasping breathing movements triggered by hypoxia may result in the aspiration of meconium-stained liquor into the lungs, which presents an additional problem after birth.

Auscultation of the fetal heart, use of cardiotocography and observation of meconium staining of the liquor draining from the vagina should alert the midwife to fetal compromise (see Ch. 26). Subsequent fetal blood sampling may confirm a compromised fetus by revealing acidosis. However, Apgar scores do not always correlate with these findings (Fox 1993, Silverman et al 1985).

The length of time during which the fetus or neonate is subjected to hypoxia determines the outcome. It is considered that the human neonate responds to hypoxia in a similar manner to other young mammals (Roberton 2005). This involves an initial response of gasping respirations followed by a period of apnoea lasting 1½ min – primary apnoea – which, if not resolved by intervention techniques, is followed by a further episode of gasping respirations, which

Table 39.1 Degrees of respiratory depression

Mildly depressed	Severely depressed
Heart rate not severely reduced (60–80 b.p.m.)	Slow feeble heart rate (<40 b.p.m.)
Short delay in onset of respiration	No attempt to breathe
Good muscle tone	Poor muscle tone
Responsive to stimuli	Limp, unresponsive to stimuli
Deeply cyanosed	Pale, grey
Apgar score 5–7	**Apgar score <5**
No significant deprivation of oxygen during labour (primary apnoea)	Oxygen lack has been prolonged before or after delivery, circulatory failure is present, baby is shocked (secondary (terminal) apnoea)

Box 39.2 Resuscitation action plan

A: Airway – Open airway

B: Breathing – Inflate lungs and breathe for baby

C: Circulation – Ensure an effective circulation with chest compressions if necessary

D: Drugs – Consider drugs to achieve this if initially unsuccessful

Don't let the baby get cold and observe and record the sequence of events during resuscitation accurately.

(Resuscitation Council (UK) 2006)

and be proficient in the resuscitative measures, to be able to implement emergency care while awaiting medical assistance (Box 39.2).

Causes of respiratory depression

Obstruction of the baby's airway by mucus, blood, liquor or meconium is one of the most common reasons for a baby failing to establish respirations. Depression of the respiratory centre may be due to:

- the effects of drugs administered to the mother, for example narcotic drugs, or diazepam
- cerebral hypoxia during labour or traumatic delivery
- immaturity of the baby, which causes mechanical dysfunction because of underdeveloped lungs, lack of surfactant and a soft pliable thoracic cage
- intranatal pneumonia, which can inhibit successful establishment of respirations and should be considered, especially if the membranes have been ruptured for some time
- severe anaemia, caused by fetomaternal haemorrhage or Rhesus incompatibility, which diminishes the oxygen-carrying capacity of the blood
- major congenital abnormalities, particularly abnormalities of the central nervous system or within the respiratory tract
- a congenital abnormality such as choanal or tracheal atresia (choanal atresia should be suspected when a baby is pink when crying but becomes cyanosed at rest).

accelerate while diminishing in depth until, approximately 8 min after birth, respirations cease completely – secondary (terminal) apnoea. The essential difference between primary and secondary apnoea is the baby's circulatory status. During primary apnoea, the circulation and heart rate are maintained and such babies respond quickly to simple resuscitation measures. In terminal apnoea the circulation is impaired, the heart rate is slow and the baby looks shocked (Table 39.1).

Failure to establish respiration at birth

The first few breaths overcome the surface tension within the lungs, drive any residual fluid from the alveoli into the circulation, and fill the lungs with air. Once the initial opening pressure has been achieved, subsequent breaths need not be so forceful (Hamilton 1999). The majority of babies gasp and establish respirations within 60 s of birth, however if they fail to initiate and sustain respiration at birth, prompt and effective intervention by the midwife is essential.

The principles of resuscitation of the newborn are applicable wherever and whenever apnoea occurs.

The midwife must therefore be aware of the predisposing factors and causes of respiratory depression

Methods of resuscitation

Though the need for resuscitation can be anticipated in many situations, in some instances a baby is born in poor condition without forewarning. It is essential that resuscitation equipment (Box 39.3) is always available and in working order and that personnel in attendance at the birth of a baby are familiar with the equipment, resuscitation techniques and local policies regarding the provision of medical aid.

Box 39.3 Resuscitation equipment

- Resuscitaire with overhead radiant heater (switched on) and light, piped oxygen, manometer, suction and clock timer
- Two straight-bladed infant laryngoscopes, spare batteries and bulbs size 0 and 1
- Neonatal endotracheal tubes 2.0, 2.5, 3.0, and 3.5 mm and connectors
- Neonatal airways sizes 0, 00, 000
- Suction catheters sizes 6, 8 and 10 FG
- Neonatal bag and mask and face masks of assorted sizes (clear, soft masks)
- Magill's forceps
- Endotracheal tube introducer
- Syringes 1 mL, 2 mL, 5 mL and 20 mL and assorted needles
- Drugs
  - Naloxone hydrochloride 1 mL ampoules 400 µg/mL (adult Narcan)
  - Adrenaline (epinephrine) 1:10 000 and 1:1000
  - THAM (tris-hydroxymethyl-amino-methane) 7%
  - Sodium bicarbonate 4.2%
  - Dextrose 10%
  - Vitamin K_1 1 mg ampoules
  - Normal saline 0.9%
- Stethoscope
- Cord clamps
- Warmed dry towels
- Adhesive tape for tube fixation.

In some units resuscitation of babies is undertaken in a specific area, whereas in others each birthing room is equipped to deal with this emergency. Whenever problems are anticipated, such as preterm delivery, instrumental or breech delivery or fetal compromise, it is desirable that a paediatrician, neonatal nurse or midwife experienced in resuscitation techniques is present at the delivery. (In some centres an anaesthetist may be the person responsible for neonatal resuscitation.) At a home birth the midwife is the responsible person.

Aims of resuscitation

- Establish and maintain a clear airway
- Ensure effective circulation
- Correct acidosis
- Prevent hypothermia, hypoglycaemia and haemorrhage.

As soon as the baby is born, the clock timer should be started. The Apgar score is assessed in the normal manner at 1 min and 5 min. In the absence of any respiratory effort, resuscitation measures are commenced. The baby's upper airways should be cleared by gentle suction of the oro- and nasopharynx and the presence of a heartbeat verified. The baby is dried quickly and transferred to a well-lit resuscitaire and placed on a flat, firm surface at a comfortable working height and under a radiant heat source to prevent hypothermia. The baby's shoulders may be elevated on a small towel, which causes slight extension of the head and straightens the trachea (Fig. 39.4). Hyperextension may cause airway obstruction owing to the short neck of the neonate and large, ill-supported tongue.

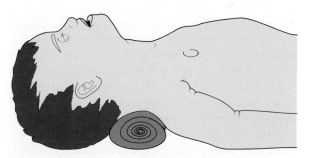

Figure 39.4 Small towel under the neck ('sniffing position').

Airway management

Most babies require no airway clearance at birth; however, if there is obvious respiratory difficulty (absence of chest wall movement) a suction catheter may be used; size 10 FG (8 FG in pre-term babies). It is recommended that the catheter tip should be inserted not further than 5 cm and that each suction attempt should last not longer than 5 s (Resuscitation Council 2005). Even with a soft catheter it is still possible to traumatize the delicate mucosa, especially in the premature baby.

Most babies born through meconium-stained liquor have not inhaled any particulate material into the lower respiratory tract. If they have not done so as a result of a period of anoxic gasping before birth, they will only very rarely do so at birth. There is now good evidence that the long recommended practice of 'prophylactic' suctioning of the oropharynx and nasopharynx of the emerging baby before delivery of the shoulders is of no benefit (Vain et al 2004).

If thick meconium is present and obstructing the airway, suction under direct vision should be performed by passing a laryngoscope and visualizing the larynx (Roberton 2005). Care should be taken to avoid touching the vocal cords as this may induce laryngospasm, apnoea and bradycardia. Thick meconium may need to be aspirated out of the trachea through an endotracheal tube.

Ventilation and oxygenation

If the baby fails to respond to these simple measures, assisted ventilation is necessary. This can be achieved in a variety of ways. Face-mask ventilation is the most commonly used method of inflating the baby's lungs. It is effective and relatively safe in experienced hands. Choose an appropriately sized mask (usually 00 or 0/1) (Fig. 39.5) and position it on the face so that it covers the nose and mouth and ensures a good seal. Use a T Piece with controlled pressure (e.g. Neopuff) or a 500 mL self-inflating bag (Fig. 39.5) (do not use a 250 mL bag as it does not permit sustained inflation) (Hussey et al 2004). Care should be taken not to apply pressure on the soft tissue under the jaw as this may obstruct the airway. To aerate the lungs, deliver five sustained inflations using oxygen or air, or a combination of both, with a pressure of 30 cm H_2O applied for 2–3 s and

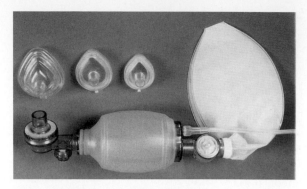

Figure 39.5 Face-mask sizes, self-inflating bag and face mask. (From Medical Photography Department, Royal Group of Hospitals, Belfast, with permission.)

repeated five times, then continue to ventilate at a rate of 40 respirations/min (Drew et al 2000). Insertion of a neonatal airway helps to prevent obstruction by the baby's tongue. Note that overextension of the baby's head causes airway obstruction. A longer inspiration phase improves oxygenation. Higher inflation pressures may be required to produce chest movement. Bag and mask technique and T Piece with controlled pressure therefore require a skilled operator to achieve success (Fig. 39.6). Used correctly these methods can avoid the need for endotracheal intubation.

Endotracheal intubation

If the baby fails to respond to intermittent positive pressure ventilation (IPPV) by bag and mask, or if

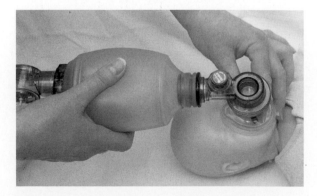

Figure 39.6 Bagging demonstration. (From Medical Photography Department, Royal Group of Hospitals, Belfast, with permission.)

bradycardia is present, an endotracheal tube should be passed without delay. Intubating a baby requires special skill that, once acquired, must be practised to be retained.

Practicalities of intubation

Ensure that all the equipment listed in Box 39.3 is available and in working order. Position the baby on a flat surface, preferably a resuscitaire, and extend the neck into the 'neutral position'. Place a rolled-up towel under the shoulders, which will help maintain proper alignment. Introduce the blade of the laryngoscope over the baby's tongue into the pharynx until the epiglottis is visualized. Elevation of the epiglottis by the tip of the laryngoscope reveals the vocal cords. Any mucus, blood or meconium obstructing the trachea should be cleared by careful suction prior to passing the endotracheal tube a distance of 1.5–2 cm into the trachea (Fig. 39.7). (Pressure on the cricoid cartilage may facilitate visualization of the larynx.) Intubation may be easier if a tracheal introducer made of plastic-covered soft metal wire is used. This will increase the stiffness and curvature of the tube. After the laryngoscope is removed, oxygen is administered by intermittent positive pressure ventilation (IPPV) to the endotracheal tube via the 'Neopuff' or the self inflating bag. A maximum of 30 cm water pressure should be applied, as there is risk of rupture of alveoli or

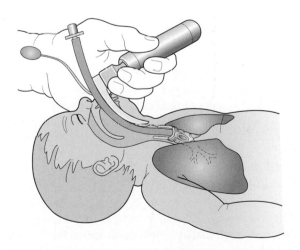

Figure 39.7 Endotracheal intubation. (From Brendan Ellis, medical illustrator, Royal Group of Hospitals, Belfast, with permission.)

tension pneumothorax if higher pressure is applied. The rise and fall of the chest wall should indicate whether the tube is in the trachea. This can be confirmed by auscultation of the chest listening for air entry to be equal on both sides. Distension of the stomach indicates oesophageal intubation necessitating removing and re-siting of the tube.

Mouth-to-face/nose resuscitation

In the absence of a bag and mask, assisted ventilation can be achieved by mouth-to-face resuscitation. With the baby's head in the 'sniffing' position (Fig. 39.4) the operator places his/her mouth over the baby's mouth and nose and, using as much air as he/she can easily keep in their cheeks inflate the babies chest with each breath, at a rate of 20–30 breaths/min, allowing the infant to exhale between breaths (Resuscitation Council 2006). Findings indicate that the nasal route of air entry is more effective than the combined nose and mouth or mouth routes and that neck flexion impedes air entry (Wilson-Davis et al 1997). It may be easier with larger babies to use mouth-to-nose resuscitation (Tonkin et al 1995).

External cardiac massage

Chest compressions should be performed if the heart rate is <60, or between 60 and 100 and falling despite adequate ventilation. The most effective way of achieving this is by encircling the baby's chest with the fingers on the spine and thumbs on the lower third of the sternum (Fig. 39.8) (Milner 1991, Roberton 2005). Research undertaken by Houri et al 1997 concluded that the two thumbs method of chest compression proved haemodynamically more effective. The chest is depressed at a rate of 100–120 times/min, at a ratio of three compressions to one ventilation, and at a depth of 2–3 cm of the baby's chest. (Excessive pressure over the lower end of the sternum may cause rib, lung or liver damage).

Use of drugs for resuscitation

If the baby's response is slow or he remains hypotonic after ventilation is achieved, consideration will be given to the use of drugs. In specialist obstetric

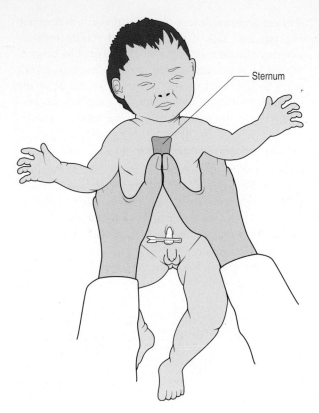

Sternum

Figure 39.8 External cardiac massage.

units, pulse oximetry may be employed to monitor hypoxia (Letko 1996) and blood obtained through the umbilical artery or vein to ascertain biochemical status (Harris et al 1996). Results will enable appropriate administration of resuscitation drugs, as discussed below.

Sodium bicarbonate

This is not recommended for brief periods of cardiopulmonary resuscitation. Once tissues are oxygenated by lung inflation with 100% oxygen and cardiac compression, the acidosis will self-correct unless asphyxia is very severe. If the heart rate is <60, despite effective ventilation, chest compression and two intravenous doses of adrenaline (epinephrine), then sodium bicarbonate 4.2% solution (0.5 mmol/mL), can be administered using 2–4 mL/kg (1–2 mmol/kg) by slow intravenous injection at a rate of 1 mL/min in order to avoid rapid elevation of serum osmolality with the attendant risk of intracranial haemorrhage

(Drew et al 2000). It should not be given prior to ventilation being established. THAM 7% (tris-hydroxymethyl-amino-methane), 0.5 mmol/kg may be used in preference to sodium bicarbonate (Roberton 2005).

Adrenaline (epinephrine)

This is indicated if the heart rate is <60, despite 1 min of effective ventilation and chest compression. An initial dose of 0.1–0.3 mL/kg of 1:10 000 solution (10–30 µg/kg) can be given intravenously; this can be repeated after 3 min for a further two doses. The Royal College of Paediatrics and Child Health (1997) recommends a higher dose of 100 µg/kg i.v. if there is no response to the boluses. It is reasonable to try giving one dose via the endotracheal tube of adrenaline (epinephrine) 0.1 mL/kg of 1:1000 as this sometimes has an immediate effect (Halliday et al 1998).

10% dextrose

Hypoglycaemia is not usually a problem unless resuscitation has been prolonged. A solution of 10% dextrose 3 mL/kg may be given intravenously via the umbilical vein to correct a blood sugar of <2.5 mmol/L.

Volume replacement

On rare occasions, bradycardia will only respond to volume expansion and a bradycardia (as opposed to asystole) that does not respond to chest compressions or drugs is very suggestive of hypovolaemia. Preparation is 0.9% normal saline 10 mL/kg initially via the umbilical vein is given and can be repeated once if necessary (Resuscitation Council 2006).

In rare incidences where the baby has lost blood, e.g. acute feto–maternal transfusion or vasa praevia, replace with emergency 0 Rh neg blood 10 mL/kg.

Naloxone hydrochloride

This is not an emergency drug per se and should be used with caution and only in specific circumstances. It is a powerful anti-opioid drug used to reverse the effects of maternal narcotic drugs given in the preceding 3 hrs. Ventilation should be established prior to its use. It must not be given to apnoeic babies. A dose of up to 100 µg/kg body weight may be administered intramuscularly for prolonged action (Drew et al 2000). As opioid action may persist for some hours, the midwife must be alert for signs of relapse when a repeat dose may be required. *Note*: It should not be administered to babies of narcotic-addicted mothers as this may precipitate acute withdrawal (Zelon et al 1998). Policies relating to dosage and route of administration may vary in different hospitals.

Immediate care of the baby at birth by the attending midwife

Observations during and after resuscitation

Throughout the resuscitation procedure, the baby's response should be monitored and recorded. An accurate written record detailing the resuscitation events is essential, not only because it forms an integral part of the medical and midwifery management of the baby, but also because it can help to protect the practitioner if defence of his/her practice is required. The endotracheal tube may be left in place for a few minutes after the baby starts to breathe spontaneously. Suction may be applied through the endotracheal tube as it is removed. There are some babies who at birth may be somewhat distressed but improve with good resuscitation, and require observations for a few hours before a decision is made whether to admit to a postnatal ward or the neonatal unit. The labour suite is an ideal place for this form of transitional care to take place. A baby whose Apgar score was less than 6 at 5 min, or who was slow to respond to resuscitation, or who requires continued ventilatory assistance, should be transferred to the neonatal unit for a period of observation in order to monitor behaviour and detect early signs of hypoxic ischaemic encephalopathy (HIE) (see Ch. 45).

Explanation about the resuscitation and the need for transfer to hospital (if born at home) or to the neonatal unit must be given to the parents and, if the baby's condition permits, the mother should have the opportunity to see and hold her baby prior to separation. This assists the attachment process described later in this chapter. Babies who respond quickly to resuscitation can be reunited with their parents and remain with them in the labour room until transfer to the postnatal ward is organized.

It can be seen that the midwife's role at the time of birth is one both of privilege and of immense responsibility. Her wish to meet the psychological needs of the parents and the baby must be tempered with the need to accommodate the baby's necessary adaptations at the time of birth and to institute emergency care when required. Continued care of the newborn takes the history of the baby's condition at birth into account and is discussed in Chapter 40.

Assessment of the baby's condition

As soon as the baby has been born, the midwife can proceed with drying the skin, which will help minimize heat loss (Bauer & Versmold 1995). In the vast majority of cases, babies are well and can be handed directly to their parents. Whether a home or hospital birth, the midwife at 1 min and 5 min after the birth will make an assessment of the baby's general condition using the Apgar score (Apgar 1953) (Table 39.2). The assessment at 1 min is important for the further management of resuscitation. However, it has been shown that an assessment at 5 min is more reliable as a predictor of the risk of death during the first 28 days of life, and of the child's neurological state and

Table 39.2 The Apgar score. The score is assessed at 1 min and 5 min after birth. Medical aid should be sought if the score is <7. 'Apgar minus colour' score omits the fifth sign. Medical aid should be sought if the score is <6

Sign	Score		
	0	1	2
Heart rate	Absent	<100 b.p.m.	>100 b.p.m.
Respiratory effort	Absent	Slow, irregular	Good or crying
Muscle tone	Limp	Some flexion of limbs	Active
Reflex response to stimulus	None	Minimal grimace	Cough or sneeze
Colour	Blue, pale	Body pink, extremities blue	Completely pink

risk of major disability at the age of 1 year. The higher the score, the better the outcome for the baby. The Apgar score must be fully documented in the baby's records.

A mnemonic for the Apgar score is:

A: Appearance (i.e. colour)

P: Pulse (i.e. heart rate)

G: Grimace (i.e. response to stimuli)

A: Active (i.e. tone)

R: Respirations (i.e. breathing).

Prevention of heat loss

With the midwife's knowledge of the baby's transitional requirements it is her responsibility to ensure appropriate preparations are made for the birth of the baby. Whether the baby is born at home or in hospital, it is important that the midwife endeavours to provide an ambient temperature in the range 21–25°C. It is accepted that in some remote parts of the world and in emergency situations, this may not be possible. However, within controlled circumstances, provision of an optimal thermal environment is paramount in facilitating a successful transition to extrauterine life. Switching off fans prior to birth helps to minimize heat loss by convection, and closing curtains reduces the radiant heat loss to windows (Karlsson 1996). The baby's temperature can drop by as much as 3–4°C within the first minute (Sinclair 1992, Thomas 1994). After birth, the baby's body and head should be dried immediately thus helping to minimize heat loss by evaporation. It is important to ensure that the wet towel is then removed and the baby wrapped in another dry prewarmed towel. Skin-to-skin contact is an effective method of preventing heat loss, the mother's chest or abdomen is the ideal surface, clean and just at the right temperature. If skin-to-skin is not acceptable the baby should be wrapped or swaddled, a hat put on its head and placed in its mother's arms (WHO 1997). However, considerable heat loss continues by convection, conduction and radiation, particularly from exposed areas of the baby's skin (Karlsson 1996). The midwife's role is to protect and keep the baby warm and she can do this by: keeping the labour room warm, drying the baby at birth, encouraging skin-to-skin, wrapping the baby and encourage breastfeeding (WHO 1997). Pre-term babies in particular can lose heat very rapidly after birth. Research has shown that placing the pre-term baby in a plastic bag up to its neck will prevent heat loss. This method has now been adopted by many labour wards (Knobel & Holditch-Davis 2007).

Clearing the airway

As the baby's head is born, excess mucus may be wiped gently from the mouth. However, care must be taken to avoid touching the nares, as such action may stimulate reflex inhalation of debris in the trachea. Although fetal pulmonary fluid is present in the mouth, most babies will achieve a clear airway unaided. If you are not achieving chest expansion, the airway can be cleared with the aid of a soft suction catheter attached to low pressure (10 cm water) mechanical suction. It is important to aspirate the oropharynx prior to the nasopharynx so that, if the baby gasps as his nasal passages are aspirated, mucus or other material is not drawn down into the respiratory tract. Excess suction can result in vagal stimulation, with laryngospasm and bradycardia.

Stimulation

Rough handling of the baby merely serves to increase shock and is unnecessary. Gentle stimulation by drying the baby and clearing the airway may initiate breathing, but there are a number of different methods that can be used, for example a single finger flick to the sole of the foot, or gentle back rubbing; this will give an indication as to whether tactile stimulation is likely to be effective. Under no circumstances should the method used cause pain or bruising.

Cutting the cord

The umbilical cord is the lifeline of the fetus and of the baby in the first few minutes after birth. Separation of the baby from the placenta is achieved by dividing the umbilical cord between two clamps, which should be applied approximately 8–10 cm from the umbilicus. Application of a gauze swab over the cord while cutting it with scissors will prevent blood spraying the delivery field. The cord should not be cut until it has been clamped securely. Failure to comply with this procedure may result in excessive blood loss from the baby. In some labour suites, it is now common practice for the father of the baby to assist the midwife and cut the umbilical cord. Care of the umbilical cord and stump in the immediate period varies according to social, cultural and geographic factors. The optimal time for umbilical cord clamping after birth remains unknown. Research continues into cord clamping (Mercer et al 2000). In 2007 a controlled trial comparing late versus early cord clamping following birth in infants born at 37 or more weeks' gestation was undertaken and concluded that delaying clamping of the umbilical cord in full-term neonates for a minimum of 2 min following birth is beneficial to the newborn. Although there was an increase in polycythaemia among babies in whom cord clamping was delayed this condition appeared to be benign (Hutton & Hassan 2007).

Some centres advocate delay in cutting until respirations are established and cord pulsation has ceased, thus ensuring that the infant receives a placental transfusion of some 70 mL of blood (Nelle et al 1993). This view is countered by those who maintain that the placental transfusion so acquired may predispose to neonatal jaundice (see Ch. 47). What is agreed is that a term baby at birth can be drawn up on to the mother's abdomen, but raised no higher, and a pre-term baby should be kept at the level of the placenta. This is because, if a pre-term baby is held above the placenta then blood can drain from the baby to the placenta, resulting in anaemia, and if held below can cause the baby to receive a blood transfusion.

Identification of baby

The time of birth and sex of the baby are noted and recorded once the baby has been completely expelled from its mother. It is the practice in many units to apply name-bands to the baby before the cord is cut. Within the baby's own home, unless a twin delivery, identification does not present a problem. However, when babies are born in hospital it is essential that they are readily identifiable from one another. Various methods of indicating identity can be employed, for example name-bands or identity tags. In the UK, two name-bands are applied, each

of which should indicate legibly in indelible pen the family name, sex of the baby, date and time of birth. In some centres, the name-bands are number coded with the baby's case records; in others the number coding corresponds with that of the mother. The amount of information written on the name-bands may vary slightly according to local policy. The mother or father, or both, should verify that the information on the bands or tags is correct prior to these being attached to the baby. The midwife should ensure that the name-bands are fastened securely and are neither too tight, impeding circulation or likely to excoriate the skin, nor too loose, risking loss of the means of identification. Name-bands or tags should remain on the baby until discharged from hospital. The midwives must advise the mother to inform a member of the midwifery or nursing staff if the name-band or tag becomes detached or is removed for any reason. At birth, the midwife will issue the mother with a Personal Child Health Record (Red Book), which will be the main record of their child's health, growth and development. The examination of their baby at birth will be recorded in this and parents will be instructed to bring the book with them when their baby attends for a general practitioner, health visitor, or hospital appointment.

First examination by midwife

Prior to leaving the mother's home, or transferring the baby to the ward, the midwife undertakes a detailed examination of the baby checking for obvious abnormalities, such as spina bifida, imperforate anus, cleft lip or palate, abrasions, fractures or haemorrhage due to trauma. The initial cord clamp is replaced with another method of securing haemostasis by applying a disposable plastic clamp (or a secure ligature) approximately 2–3 cm from the umbilicus and cutting off the redundant cord. The baby's temperature is now recorded. The midwife should ensure that the environmental temperature remains warm, between 21–25°C, as previously discussed. Early transfer of the baby to a postnatal ward has been advocated as a means of minimizing heat loss. The baby should be transferred with its mother, in her arms, to avoid heat loss and to promote mother–baby attachment.

Instillation of eyedrops as prophylaxis against gonococcal infection is not practised in the UK. In other parts of the world, drops or antibiotic ointment may be instilled (Wong 1995). It is suggested that, to be effective, such treatments should be administered within 1 hrs of birth (Tyson 1992). The first bath and other non-urgent procedures may be deferred in order to minimize heat loss. (Further care is discussed in Ch. 40.) All babies should remain with their mother during the first few hours of life, providing both mother and baby are in good condition, as this is the time when parent–baby interactions are initiated and the reality of parenthood begins.

Vitamin K

Depending on local policy, vitamin K, intramuscular or orally may be given as prophylaxis against bleeding disorders (see Ch. 45). Vitamin K is fat soluble; it can only be absorbed from the intestine in the presence of bile salts. The body's capacity to store vitamin K is very low and the half-life of the vitamin-K-dependent coagulation factors is short (Zipursky 1999). Midwives must be aware of and follow their local hospital policy regarding consent and administration of vitamin K (DoH 1998).

Early parent–baby relationships

The safe birth of a healthy baby engenders considerable emotion in most parents and indeed in attendants at the birth. The efforts of the preceding hours are temporarily forgotten as the mother sees her baby for the first time. Characteristically, her first query often relates to the sex of the baby, speedily followed by an anxious enquiry about the baby's state of health: 'is he/she all right?' Reassured on these points, a mother progresses to an examination of her baby, which follows a fairly predictable pattern unless the condition of either the mother or the baby is impaired by the process of labour or by narcotic drugs. Fathers too are involved in this early exploration of the newborn baby. The response of both parents is influenced not only by their prenatal understanding and previous experiences with babies but also by the appearance, behaviour and responses of their baby, who takes an active part in the proceedings (Salariya 1990, Williams 1995). Cultural background may also play a part in parental behaviours at this time (Callister 1995).

The first hour after birth is a time of particular sensitivity for the parents and is a time when the baby has a long period (60%) of 'quiet alert state' (Saigal et al 1981). In this state and while acclimatizing to the outside world, the baby is especially interested in the faces of its mother and father, the sound of their voices, and their smell and touch. Parents can also learn about their baby's natural abilities in this state, in which they can follow the parents' faces or an object, turn to the mother's voice and stop crying when held by the mother or father (Klaus & Klaus 2004).

Regardless of age, parity or marital status, mothers are likely to display a similar behavioural pattern when touching their babies for the first time. This sequence of touching behaviour is enhanced if the baby is naked. The mother begins her examination of her baby by exploring the extremities and head with her fingertips. Thereafter, she caresses her baby's body with her entire hand before gathering her baby in her arms often in the *en face* position where eye-to-eye contact can be established. She talks to her baby with great emotion, looking for positive reinforcement from her partner and other birth attendants (Klaus et al 1975, Sander 1993).

Her emotions at this time may be mixed. She may display great excitement and happiness – laughing, talking or even crying with joy, or she may feel too tired to react positively towards her baby. Factors which may predispose to this latter reaction include prolonged labour, instrumental birth, and baby of the 'wrong' sex or congenital abnormality. Lack of support from partner or parents may influence the behaviour of an unmarried mother and, for some mothers, high parity may dampen their response. Childhood deprivation can inhibit some women from reacting in the anticipated manner.

For some mothers, the sight of an unwashed, wet and sometimes bloody baby is profoundly distasteful and they are not appreciative of skin-to-skin contact with a baby in this condition. A good midwife will ascertain the mother's attitude during pregnancy or early labour. This will allow her to modify her technique in assisting the birth and immediate care of the baby to meet the mother's wishes and so assist the mother to feel comfortable at her first meeting with her baby. Early skin-to-skin contact and breast-feeding are significantly associated with exclusive breastfeeding at discharge and also promote good mother–baby relationships and stimulate lactation (Catlaneo & Buzzetti 2001) (see Ch. 41).

While midwives are providing women-centred care it is important for them to remember to involve the fathers in decision-making and acknowledge their role and needs in one of the most important events in their lifetime (Ratnaike 2007, Tiedje & Darling-Fisher 2003).

Many fathers are surprised at their profound emotional response to the birth of their baby. Sometimes a man's reactions are stronger than those of his partner, who may be rather tired initially. The father feels a sense of deep satisfaction and self-esteem, and is elated and keen to touch and hold his baby and his partner and share his excitement (Barclay & Lupton 1999, Wildman 1995). Intimacy shared between the father and mother at this time is extended to include the baby within an exclusive family group, often oblivious to their surroundings.

Having accomplished the immediate physiological adaptations of respiration and circulation, the baby displays interest in sound, light and nutrition, responding to the mother's voice by moving limbs in synchrony. The response to touch is illustrated in the grasp reflex and in suckling of the breast if offered – or the fist. Newborn babies appear to focus on their mother's face at a distance of 20 cm and respond to movement of bright shiny objects, such as their mother's eyes, by tracking them visually. These responsive behaviours evoke reinforcing responses from parents, thus promoting the interactions essential for survival, which is dependent on good parenting. A slightly darkened birthing room encourages babies to open their eyes widely and look around them, whereas bright lights cause frowning. The midwife's understanding of these responses allows her to create optimal conditions for interaction to occur.

Promotion of parent–baby interaction

The term 'bonding' has been used to describe the establishment of parent–baby relationships in the early neonatal period. The implication of the desirability to feel instant love for one's child can lead to feelings of guilt in some parents who do not identify a strong emotional tie with their baby at birth. It is important to recognize that, as individuals, parents develop a loving relationship with their child at their own pace, some taking longer than others – days, weeks or months. Parents should feel able to express their disappointments as well as their joys without fear of being thought a 'bad' parent (Barclay & Lupton 1999).

A good rapport between the parents and the midwife should enable the development of their love for their baby to progress happily and at its own speed. However, the midwife must be alert to report and document marked negative reactions from either or both parents, as this may be an early sign of future parenting difficulties. Adverse behaviours of note include hostile verbal or non-verbal attitude, lack of supportive interaction between the parents, disinclination to touch or hold their baby, disparaging remarks about the baby or marked disappointment about the sex of the baby.

Involvement of the father in the birth of the baby's body, clamping of the cord and early bathing have been introduced in some centres to help to promote father–baby relationships. The midwife can do much to promote the beginnings of loving relationships by encouraging both parents to handle and examine their baby, by her positive comments, and by undertaking the examination of the baby beside the parents.

Privacy to talk, touch and be alone together with their baby is important for parents and opportunities to do so should be provided whether their baby is born at home or in hospital. The midwife should be sensitive to this often-unexpressed need and leave the family together for some time before progressing with further care of the baby.

The opportunity for this initial intimate family moment is dependent on the baby's condition. A baby whose Apgar score is below 7 requires some form of resuscitation, which may necessitate speedy removal to a special resuscitation area. As parents have entered an entirely new phase of their lives it is essential that they receive a reassuring explanation and adequate information about the need to be separated from their baby, which can be totally unexpected and therefore very frightening.

REFERENCES

Apgar V 1953 A proposal for a new method of evaluation of the newborn infant. Current Research in Anaesthesiology and Analgesics 40:340

Barclay L, Lupton D 1999 The experiences of new fatherhood: a socio-cultural analysis. Journal of Advanced Nursing 29 (4):1013–1020

Bauer K, Versmold H 1995 Prevention of neonatal hypothermia in the delivery room. In: Okken A, Koch J (eds) Thermoregulation of sick and low birth neonates. Springer, Berlin, p 219.

Brueggemeyer A 1993 Neonatal thermoregulation. In: Kenner C, Brueggemeyer A, Gunderson L P (eds) Comprehensive neonatal nursing: a physiologic perspective. W B Saunders, Philadelphia

Callister L C 1995 Cultural meanings of childbirth. Journal of Obstetric, Gynecologic, and Neonatal Nursing 24 (4):327–331

Catlaneo A, Buzzetti P 2001 Effects on rates of breastfeeding in training for the baby friendly hospital initiative. British Medical Journal 323:1358–1362

Department of Health 1998 Vitamin K for babies. PLO/CNO/998/4. DoH, London

Drew D, Jevon P, Ravy M 2000 Resuscitation of the newborn: a practical approach. Butterworth-Heinemann, Oxford

Fox H E 1993 Apgar: A commentary. P&S Medical Review 1 (1):1–3

Halliday H L, McClure B G, Reid M 1998 Handbook of neonatal intensive care, 4th edn. W B Saunders, London.

Hamilton P. 1999 ABC of labour care, care of the newborn in the delivery room. British Medical Journal 318:1403–1406

Harris M, Beckley S L, Garibaldi J M, et al 1996 Umbilical cord blood analysis at the time of delivery. Midwifery 12(3):146–150

Houri P K, Frank L R, Menegazzi J J, et al 1997 A randomized, controlled trial of two-thumbs vs. two finger chest compression in a swine infant model of cardiac arrest. Prehospital Emergency Care 1(2):65–67

Hussey S G, Ryan C A, Murphy B P 2004 Comparison of three manual ventilation devices using an intubated mannequin. Archives of Disease in Childhood Fetal and Neonatal Edition 89:F490–F493

Hutton E K, Hassan E S 2007 Late vs early clamping of the umbilical cord in full-term neonates. Journal of the American Medical Association 297(11):1241–1252

Karlsson H 1996 Skin to skin care: heat balance. Archives of Disease in Childhood 75(2):F130–F132

Klaus P, Klaus M 2004 No separation of mother and baby with unlimited opportunity for breastfeeding. Journal of Perinatal Education 13(2):35–41

Klaus M H, Trause M A, Kennell J H 1975 Does human maternal behaviour after delivery show a characteristic pattern? In: CIBA Foundation Symposium 33, parent–infant interaction. Associated Scientific, Amsterdam

Knobel R, Holditch-Davis D 2007 Thermoregulation and heat loss prevention after birth. Journal of Obstetrics, Gynecology, and Neonatal Nursing 36(3):280–287

Letko M D 1996 Understanding the Apgar score. Journal of Obstetric, Gynecologic, and Neonatal Nursing 25 (4):299–303

Linh G Ly, Hawes J, Whyte H E et al 2007 The hemodynamically significant ductus arteriosus in critically ill full-term neonates. Neonatology 91(4):260–265

Mercer J S, Nelson C C, Skovgaard R L 2000 Umbilical cord clamping: beliefs and practices of American nurse-midwives. Journal of Midwifery and Women's Health 45 (1):58–65

Merkin R J 2005 Growth and distribution of human brown fat. The Anatomical Record 178(3):637–645

Milner A D 1991 Resuscitation of the newborn. Archives of Diseases in Childhood 66(1):66–69.

Nelle M, Zilow E P, Kraus M 1993 The effect of Leboyer delivery on blood viscosity and other hemorheologic parameters in term neonates. American Journal of Obstetrics and Gynecology 169(1):189–193

Perry S E 2002 Nursing care of the newborn. In: Bobak I M, Lowdermilk D L, Jensen M D et al (eds) Maternity nursing, 6th edn. Elsevier Health Sciences, Edinburgh, Ch 18

Puckett R M, Offringa M 2000 The Dutch Cochrane Centre, The Netherlands

Ratnaike D 2007 Father's present or just in the room? Midwives 10(3):106

Resuscitation Council (UK) 2005 Resuscitation guidelines, newborn life support. Online. Available: www.resus.org.uk

Resuscitation Council UK 2006 Newborn Life Support Resuscitation at birth, 2nd edn. TT Litho Printers, Kent.

Roberton N R C 2005 Resuscitation of the newborn. In: Rennie J M (ed.) Roberton's textbook of neonatology, 4th edn. Churchill Livingstone, Edinburgh.

Royal College of Paediatrics and Child Health 1997 Resuscitation of babies at birth. BMJ Publishing, London

Rutter N 2005 Temperature control and disorders. In: Rennie J M (ed.) Roberton's textbook of neonatology, 4th edn. Churchill Livingstone, Edinburgh

Saigal S, Nelson N, Bennett K et al 1981. Observation on the behavioral state of newborn infants during the first hours of life. American Journal of Obstetrics and gynecology 139:715

Sander L W 1993 The earliest relationship: Journal of the American Psychoanalytic Association 41:281–284

Salariya E 1990 Parental-infant attachment. In: Alexander J, Levy V, Roch S (eds) Postnatal care – a research based approach. Macmillan, Basingstoke

Sheldon B, Korones M D 2004 An encapsulated history of thermoregulation in the neonate. NeoReviews 5(3):e78

Silverman F, Suidan J, Wasserman J, et al 1985 The Apgar score: is it enough? Obstetrics and Gynaecology 66:331–336

Sinclair J C 1992 Management of the thermal environment. In: Sinclair J C, Bracken M B (eds) Effective care of the newborn infant. Oxford University Press, Oxford

Tannenbaum J E, Waleh N S, Mauray F, et al 1996 Transforming growth factor-β protein and messenger RND expression is increased in the closing ductus arteriosus. Paediatric Research 39(3):427–434

Thomas K 1994 Thermoregulation in neonates. Neonatal Network 13(2):15–22

Tiedje L B, Darling-Fisher C 2003 Promoting father-friendly healthcare. American Journal of Maternal Child Nursing 28 (6):350–357

Tonkin S L, Davis S L, Gunn T R 1995 Nasal route for infant resuscitation by mothers. Lancet 345(8961):1353–1354

Tyson J E 1992 Immediate care of the newborn infant. In: Sinclair J E, Bracken M B (eds) Effective care of the newborn infant. Oxford University Press, Oxford

Vain N E, Szyld E G, Prudent L M et al 2004 Oropharyngeal and nasopharyngeal suctioning of meconium-stained neonates before delivery of their shoulders: multicentre, randomized controlled trial. Lancet 364;597–602

Wildman J 1995 Is this finally it? New Generation 14(2):5

Williams R P 1995 Family dynamics after childbirth. In: Bobak I M, Lowdermilk D L, Jensen M D (eds) Maternity nursing, 4th edn. CV Mosby, St Louis

Wilson-Davis S L, Tonkin S L, Gunn T R 1997 Air entry in infant resuscitation: oral or nasal routes? Journal of Applied Physiology 82(1):152–155

Wong D L (ed.) 1995 Whaley and Wong's nursing care of infants and children, 5th edn. CV Mosby, St Louis

World Health Organization 1997 Thermal control of the newborn: a practical guide. World Health Organization, WHO/RHT/MSM/97.2 Ch 1, p 5–14

Zelon C, Rubio E, Wasserman E. 1998 Neonatal drug withdrawal. American Academy of Pediatrics 101(6):1079–1088

Zipursky A 1999 Prevention of vitamin K deficiency bleeding in newborns. British Journal of Haematology 104:430–437

FURTHER READING

Beachy P, Deacon J 1993 The core curriculum for neonatal intensive care nursing. W B Saunders, Philadelphia

This book is written for nurses caring for high risk babies. As well as providing information regarding the physiological problems of the sick newborn, it also deals with problems concerning the family, legal and ethical issues.

Bracken M, Sinclair J 1992 Effective care of the newborn infant. Oxford University Press, Oxford

This informative textbook covers all aspects of neonatal conditions with contributions from many neonatal specialists. It should be used as a reference to complement conditions discussed in the chapter.

Brazelton T B and Cramer B 1990 The earliest relationship. Addison Wesley, New York.

This book is a collaboration between a paediatrician and a psychoanalyst and weaves together the fundamentals of new and empirical research in earliest infancy. It is an easy-to-read book which contains a wealth of information and clinical expertise.

Kenner C, Wright Lott J, Flandermeyer A 1998 Comprehensive neonatal nursing: a physiologic perspective, 2nd edn. W B Saunders, Philadelphia

This book provides a comprehensive approach to neonatal care, and is an essential text for those caring for newborn babies and their families.

Rennie J M (ed.) 2005 Textbook of neonatology, 4th edn. Churchill Livingstone, Edinburgh

This is a valuable book for resource material; as well as covering all the conditions that effect the baby it covers topics such as litigation and how the law relates to the baby. It also looks at ethical and moral questions raised because of modern intensive care.

Resuscitation Council (UK) 2006 Newborn life support, 2nd edn. TT Litho Printers, Kent

This informative book covers all aspects of newborn life support, and can be used as a reference source in newborn resuscitation training.

40

The normal baby

Philomena Farrell   Norma Sittlington

The normal neonate continues to adapt to extrauterine life in the first weeks after birth, remaining vulnerable to airway obstruction, hypothermia, hypoglycaemia and infection. This necessitates the provision of an environment that is optimal for physiological needs. The mother takes responsibility for this by continuing to develop and nurture the mother–baby relationship. The father should also play his part and become involved in the care of his baby. It is important for the midwife to remember that after the birth of his baby, a father may display strong emotional feelings towards his child (Ratnaike 2007).

Extrauterine life presents a challenge to the newborn baby. The most important changes – those in the heart and lungs – take place at birth (see Ch. 39); however, continued adaptations are necessary in the first weeks of life as the baby assumes independence from the maternal and placental nurturing which was enjoyed before birth. The baby remains dependent on the mother or other caregiver for nutrition and protection, but is solely responsible for maintaining metabolism and homeostasis among other functions essential for survival.

The chapter aims to:

- describe the external features of the normal newborn baby
- discuss the functioning of the different body systems in relation to their stage of maturity and the changes taking place at birth
- describe the behaviour of the baby during the first weeks of life
- detail the systematic examination of the baby at birth and the subsequent daily examinations
- discuss the care of the baby and the measures employed to ensure security and safety and promotion of normal growth and development
- highlight the role of the midwife in promoting confidence and competence in the parents and encouraging interaction between them and their baby.

General characteristics

Appearance

A normal term baby weighs approximately 3.5 kg, when fully extended measures 50 cm from the crown of the head to the heels, and has on average an occipitofrontal head circumference of 34–35 cm. Most babies are plump and have a prominent abdomen. They lie in an attitude of flexion; with arms extended, their fingers reach upper thigh level.

Physiology

The skin

The skin is the largest organ in the body and is made up of three main layers, the epidermis, the dermis and the underlying subcutaneous fatty tissue. The skin has an important role to play in temperature regulation, it acts as a barrier to infection, balances electrolytes, stores fat and insulates against the cold. It can also give the midwife a guide to the overall well-being of the baby. Vernix caseosa is a white sticky substance, present on the baby's skin at birth. The amount of vernix is variable. It is thought to have a protective function in utero and after birth dries up and flakes off within a few hours.

The midwife must be knowledgeable about the normal parameters of neonatal skin, which differs somewhat from adult skin (Michie 1996).

The skin of a newborn baby is thin, delicate, and easily traumatized by friction, pressure or substances with a different pH. This renders the skin prone to blistering, excoriation and infection. Although sterile at birth, the skin is colonized by micro-organisms within 24 hrs. The skin of babies born at term has a pH of 6.4, which reduces to 4.9 over 3–4 days (Irving 2001). The low pH of the skin surface (pH<5) creates an 'acid mantle', which protects against infection. Baby products along with exposure to urine and faeces could disrupt this delicate protective barrier (Cetta et al 1991).

The best practice based on recent research suggests that the usage of baby products is superfluous to the care of the baby's skin (Trotter 2004) and this is supported by the Postnatal Care Guidelines (NICE 2006).

The umbilical cord's position on the anterior abdominal wall predisposes it to contamination from urine and faeces. Post delivery, the stump is rapidly colonized and necroses and separates by a process of dry gangrene, which usually takes between 7–14 days. The main reasons behind prolonged separation include infection and the use of antiseptics, which reduce the number of normal non-pathogenic flora. Clinical trials continue in relation to best practice in cord care (Janssen et al 2003).

Downy hair, called lanugo, covers the skin and is plentiful over the shoulders, upper arms and thighs. The general colour of the skin depends on the baby's ethnic origin, ranging from pink and white to olive or dark brown. Peripheral cyanosis is common and is usually of no significance. Pigmentation of nipples and genitalia is deeper in babies with darker skins and a linea nigra may be present. Another feature of racial origin is the Mongolian blue spot, which presents as a diffuse bluish-black area usually over the sacral region. Dark-skinned babies become more pigmented in the first weeks of life though the palms of the hands and soles of the feet remain paler than the rest of the body.

A mature baby has many skin creases on the palms of the hands and soles of the feet. The nails are fully formed and adherent to the tips of the fingers, sometimes extending beyond the fingertips. The hair is soft and silky: some babies have virtually no hair, whereas others have a significant amount of straight or curly hair. The eyebrows and eyelashes present a similar variation. The cartilage of the ears is well formed.

Sebaceous glands, though present in the skin, are relatively inactive. Distended glands, milia, may be present over the nose and cheeks. Sweat glands are present but inactive in the first days of life. The vasoconstrictor mechanism is inefficient because the vascular plexuses are underdeveloped. The baby's poor melanin production renders a vulnerability to sunburn.

Sensitivity to touch and pressure, heat and cold, and pain are mediated through the skin.

Temperature regulation

Thermal control in the neonate remains poor for some time. Initial thermal adaptation and modes of heat loss have been described in Chapter 39. Owing to the immaturity of the hypothalamus, temperature regulation is inefficient and the baby remains vulnerable to hypothermia particularly when exposed to cold or draughts, when wet, when unable to move about freely, or when deprived of nutrition. Cold babies are unable to shiver; therefore they attempt to maintain body heat by adopting a flexed fetal posture, increasing their respiratory rate and activity. These activities increase calorie consumption and may result in hypoglycaemia, which in turn will compound the effects of hypothermia, as do hypoxia, acidosis and hyperbilirubinaemia (see Chs 47 and 48).

The baby's normal core temperature is 36.5–37.3°C. A healthy, clothed, term baby will maintain this body temperature satisfactorily, provided the environmental temperature is sustained between 18°C and 21°C, nutrition is adequate and movements are not restricted by tight swaddling. However, like adults, babies are individuals with differing metabolic rates. This makes finite statements of thermoneutral range difficult (Hull et al 1996a, b). Hyperthermia can occur when the baby is exposed to a radiant heat source. Sweating may occur, especially over the forehead, although the neonate's ability to sweat is limited. An unstable temperature may indicate infection.

Respiratory system

At birth, the respiratory system is developmentally incomplete, growth of new alveoli continuing for several years. The lumen of the peripheral airways is narrow, which predisposes to atelectasis. Respiratory secretions are more plentiful than in an adult and the mucous membranes are delicate and sensitive to trauma, the area below the vocal cords being particularly prone to oedema (see also Ch. 39).

The normal baby has a respiratory rate of 40–60 breaths/min, and breathing is diaphragmatic, chest and abdomen rising and falling synchronously. The breathing pattern is erratic. Respirations are shallow and irregular, being interspersed with brief 10–15 s periods of apnoea (Perry 2002). This is known as *periodic breathing*. Apart from the initial profound respiratory efforts at birth, no nasal flaring, sternal or subcostal recession or grunting is present.

The pattern of respiration alters during sleeping and waking states. Babies are obligatory nose breathers and do not convert automatically to mouth breathing when nasal obstruction occurs. Respiratory difficulties can occur because of neurological, metabolic, circulatory or thermoregulatory dysfunction as well as infection, airway obstruction or abnormalities of the respiratory tract itself.

Babies have a lusty cry, which evokes an immediate response from carers. The cry is normally loud and of medium pitch unless neurological damage, infection or hypothermia is present, when it may be high pitched or weak. Transient cyanosis may arise in the first few days when the baby is crying and altered pressure gradients recreate right-to-left shunts within the heart and great vessels. This is of no clinical significance (see Ch. 39).

Cardiovascular system and blood

The changes in the baby's heart at birth have been described in Chapter 39. The heart rate is rapid; 110–160 beats/min (b.p.m.) and fluctuates in accordance with the baby's respiratory function and activity or sleep state. Peripheral circulation is sluggish. This results in mild cyanosis of hands, feet and circumoral areas and in generalized mottling when the skin is exposed. Blood pressure fluctuates according to activity and ranges from 50–55/25–30 mmHg to 80/50 mmHg in the first 10 days of life (Roberton 1996). It is considered that, even at rest, the baby's heart probably functions at full capacity, rendering the baby vulnerable to additional stress (Blackburn 2007).

The total circulating blood volume at birth is 80 mL/kg body weight. However, this may be raised if there is delay in clamping the umbilical cord at birth. The haemoglobin level is high (13–20 g/dL), of which 50–85% is fetal haemoglobin (Blackburn 2007). Conversion from fetal to adult haemoglobin, which commenced in utero, is completed in the first 1–2 years of life. Haemoglobin, red cell count $(5-7 \times 10^{12}/L)$ and haematocrit (55%) levels decrease gradually during the first 2–3 months of life, during which time erythropoiesis is suppressed. The white cell count is high initially $(18.0 \times 10^9/L)$ but decreases rapidly (Perry 2002, Roberton 2005).

Breakdown of excess red blood cells in the liver and spleen predisposes to jaundice in the first week.

Because colonization of the intestine by the bacteria, which synthesize vitamin K, is delayed until feeding is established, vitamin-K-dependent clotting factors II (prothrombin), VII, IX and X are low. This inhibits blood clotting during the first week. Platelet levels equal those of the adult, but there is a reduced capacity for adhesion and aggregation (Blackburn 2007).

Renal system

Though the kidneys are functional in fetal life, their workload is minimal until after birth. They are functionally immature. The glomerular filtration rate is low and tubular reabsorption capabilities are limited. The baby is not able to concentrate or dilute urine very well in response to variations in fluid intake, nor compensate for high or low levels of solutes in the blood. This results in a narrow margin between homeostasis and fluid imbalance (see Ch. 48). The ability to excrete drugs is also limited and the baby's renal function is vulnerable to physiological stress (Blackburn 2007, Perry 2002, Roberton 2005). The first urine is passed at birth or within the first 24 hrs and thereafter with increasing frequency as fluid intake rises. The urine is dilute, straw coloured and odourless. Cloudiness caused by mucus and urates may be present initially until fluid intake increases. Urates may cause pink staining, which is insignificant. As the neonatal pelvis is small, the bladder becomes palpable abdominally when full. It is the midwife's responsibility to observe and record the baby's urinary output.

Gastrointestinal system

The gastrointestinal tract of the neonate is structurally complete, although functionally immature in comparison with that of the adult (Blackburn 2007, Perry 2002, Roberton 2005). The mucous membrane of the mouth is pink and moist. The teeth are buried in the gums and ptyalin secretion is low. Small epithelial pearls are sometimes present at the junction of the hard and soft palates. Sucking pads in the cheeks give them a full appearance. Sucking and swallowing reflexes are coordinated.

The stomach has a small capacity (15–30 mL), which increases rapidly in the first weeks of life. The cardiac sphincter is weak, predisposing to regurgitation or posseting. Gastric acidity, equal to that of the adult within a few hours after birth, diminishes rapidly within the first few days and by the 10th day, the baby is virtually achlorhydric, which increases the risk of infection. Gastric emptying time is normally 2–3 hrs.

In relation to the size of the baby, the intestine is long, containing large numbers of secretory glands and a large surface area for the absorption of nutrients. Enzymes are present, although there is a deficiency of amylase and lipase, which diminishes the baby's ability to digest compound carbohydrates and fat. When food enters the stomach, a gastrocolic reflex results in the opening of the ileocaecal valve. The contents of the ileum pass into the large intestine and rapid peristalsis means that feeding is often accompanied by reflex emptying of the bowel.

The gut is sterile at birth but is colonized within a few hours. Bowel sounds are present within 1 hr of birth. Meconium, present in the large intestine from 16 weeks' gestation, is passed within the first 24 hrs of life and is totally excreted within 48–72 hrs. This first stool is blackish-green in colour, is tenacious and contains bile, fatty acids, mucus and epithelial cells. From the 3rd–5th day the stools undergo a transitional stage and are brownish-yellow in colour. Once feeding is established, yellow faeces are passed. The consistency and frequency of stools reflect the type of feeding. Breastmilk results in loose, bright yellow and inoffensive acid stools. The baby may pass 8–10 stools a day, or pass stools as infrequently as every 2 or 3 days. The stools of the bottle-fed baby are paler in colour, semiformed, less acidic and have a slightly sharp smell (Roberton 2005).

Physiological immaturity of the liver results in low production of glucuronyl transferase for the conjugation of bilirubin. This, together with a high level of red cell breakdown, and stimulation of hepatic blood flow may result in a transient jaundice, which is manifest on the 3rd–5th days (see also Ch. 47). Glycogen stores are rapidly depleted, so early feeding is required to maintain normal blood glucose levels (2.6–4.4 mmol/L). Feeding stimulates liver function and colonization of the gut, which assists in the formation of vitamin K.

Infant-feeding practices are designed to meet the physiological needs and capabilities of the baby and are discussed in Chapter 41.

Immunological adaptations

Neonates demonstrate a marked susceptibility to infections, particularly those gaining entry through the mucosa of the respiratory and gastrointestinal systems. Localization of infection is poor, 'minor' infections having the potential to become generalized very easily.

The baby has some immunoglobulins at birth but the sheltered intrauterine existence limits the need for learned immune responses to specific antigens (Blackburn 2007, Crockett 1995, Perry 2002, Stern 1999). There are three main immunoglobulins, IgG, IgA and IgM, and of these only IgG is small enough to cross the placental barrier. It affords immunity to specific viral infections. At birth, the baby's levels of IgG are equal to or slightly higher than those of the mother. This provides passive immunity during the first few months of life. IgM and IgA do not cross the placental barrier but can be manufactured by the fetus. Levels of IgM at term are 20% those of the adult, taking 2 years to attain adult levels (elevation of IgM levels at birth is suggestive of intrauterine infection). This relatively low level of IgM is thought to render the baby more susceptible to enteric infections. IgA levels are very low and increase slowly, although secretory salivary levels attain adult values within 2 months. IgA protects against infection of the respiratory tract, gastrointestinal tract and eyes. Breastmilk, and especially colostrum, provides the baby with passive immunity in the form of *Lactobacillus bifidus*, lactoferrin, lysozyme and secretory IgA among others (see Ch. 41).

The thymus gland, where lymphocytes are produced, is relatively large at birth and continues to grow until 8 years of age.

Reproductive system: genitalia and breasts

In boys, the testes are descended into the scrotum, which has plentiful rugae; the urethral meatus opens at the tip of the penis and the prepuce is adherent to the glans. In girls born at term, the labia majora normally cover the labia minora; the hymen and clitoris may appear disproportionately large. Spermatogenesis in boys does not occur until puberty, but the total complement of primordial follicles containing primitive ova is present in the ovaries of girls at birth.

In both sexes, withdrawal of maternal oestrogens results in breast engorgement, sometimes accompanied by secretion of 'milk' by the 4th or 5th day. Baby girls may develop pseudomenstruation for the same reason. Both boys and girls have a nodule of breast tissue around the nipple. Midwives should have the knowledge to reassure and explain the physiological nature of these events to the parents.

Skeletomuscular system

The muscles are complete, subsequent growth occurring by hypertrophy rather than by hyperplasia. The long bones are incompletely ossified to facilitate growth at the epiphyses. The bones of the vault of the skull also reveal lack of ossification. This is essential for growth of the brain and facilitating moulding during labour. Moulding is resolved within a few days of birth. The posterior fontanelle closes at 6–8 weeks. The anterior fontanelle remains open until 18 months of age, making assessment of hydration and intracranial pressure possible by palpation of fontanelle tension.

Psychology and perception

Newborn babies at birth are alert and aware of their surroundings and they have long periods (60%) of 'quiet alert state' (Saigal et al 1981). Far from being impassive, they react to stimuli and begin at a very early age to amass information; they are especially interested in the faces of their mother and father, the sound of their voices and their smell and touch (Brazelton & Nugent 1995).

Senses

Vision

Though immature, the structures necessary for vision are present and functional at birth. Babies are sensitive to bright lights, which cause them to frown or blink. They demonstrate a preference for bold black and white patterns and the shape of the human face, focusing at a distance of approximately 15–20 cm. This gives babies the ability to establish eye contact with their mother while being nursed and so enhance the bonding process. They can track a moving object briefly within the first 5 days, and by 2 weeks of age can differentiate their mother's face from that of a stranger. Interest in colour, variety and complexity of patterns develops within the first 2 months of life (Blackburn 2007, Perry 2002, Roberton 2005). The shape of the baby's eyes may reflect racial origin; for instance the epicanthic folds of Oriental babies alter the appearance of the orbital region. No tears are present in the eyes of the newborn, therefore they become infected easily.

Hearing

Newborn babies' eyes turn towards sound. On hearing a high-pitched sound, they first blink or startle and then become agitated, and are comforted by low-pitched sounds. They prefer the sound of the human voice to other sounds and within a few weeks the patterns of adult speech are mimicked by reactive movements. Newborn babies can discriminate between voices, giving preference to their mother's (DeCasper & Fifer 1987). This, too, promotes mother–baby interaction. Neonatal hearing screening is performed on all babies prior to discharge from hospital. The aim of the screening is to identify early and follow-up babies with moderate, severe or profound bilateral permanent hearing impairment (NHS Screening 2006).

Smell and taste

Babies prefer the smell of milk to that of other substances and show a preference for human milk. They prefer the smell of an unwashed breast to that of a washed one (Righard 1995). They turn away from unpleasant smells and show preference for sweet taste, as is demonstrated by vigorous and sustained sucking and a speedy grimacing response to bitter, salty or sour substances (Blackburn 2007).

Touch

Babies are acutely sensitive to touch, enjoying skin-to-skin contact, immersion in water, stroking, cuddling and rocking movements (Blackburn 2007, Perry 2002). A puff of air on the face induces an inspiration or gasp reflex. The grasp reflex enhances the relationship with the mother. Facial coding of pain in babies is expressed by brow bulging, eyelid squeezing, nasolabial furrowing and open-lipped crying (Grunau et al 1998, Rushforth & Levene 1994).

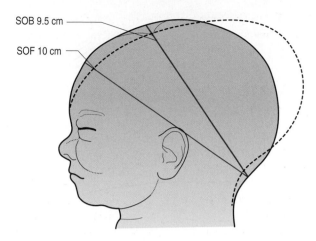

SOB 9.5 cm

SOF 10 cm

Figure 40.1 Type of moulding in a vertex presentation (SOB, suboccipitobregmatic; SOF, suboccipitofrontal).

result of pressure from the cervical os and will disappear spontaneously within 24 hrs. Parents can be reassured that moulding usually resolves within a few days after birth.

The short thick neck of the baby must be examined to exclude the presence of swellings and to ensure that rotation and flexion of the head are possible.

The chest and abdomen

Observation of respiratory movement should reveal that chest and abdominal movements are synchronous. The respirations may still be irregular at this stage. The space between the nipples should be noted; widely spaced nipples being associated with chromosomal abnormality.

The shape of the abdomen should be rounded. The midwife notes any variation, including a scaphoid (boat-shaped) abdomen (which may indicate a malnourished fetus or diaphragmatic hernia, see Ch. 46) or any protrusions, particularly at the base of the umbilical cord.

The artery forceps securing the umbilical cord should be replaced by a plastic disposable clamp, or elastic bands (according to hospital policy) applied approximately 2 cm from the umbilicus. Excess cord is discarded.

Haemostasis of the umbilical cord is vital. A blood loss of 30 mL from a baby is equivalent to almost half a litre of blood from an adult. Prophylactic Vitamin K 1 mg can be given orally or intramuscularly to promote prothrombin formation (Jørgensen et al 1991, Shearer 1995). Midwives must be aware of their local hospital policy regarding consent and administration of Vitamin K (see Ch. 45).

Normally three cord vessels are present. Absence of one of the arteries is occasionally associated with renal anomalies and must be reported to the paediatrician.

The genitalia and anus

The genitalia should be examined carefully. If the sex is uncertain, the paediatrician will initiate investigations. Depending on local policy, the baby's temperature may be taken rectally to detect any excessive cooling and to confirm patency of the anus. This method is less commonly used today. The preferred methods are via the axilla (under the arm), tympanic (ear), or in the groin. The normal baby's skin temperature should range from 36.5°C to 37.3°C.

The limbs and digits

In addition to noting length and movement of the limbs, it is essential that the digits are counted and separated to ensure that webbing is not present. The hands should be opened fully as any accessory digits may be concealed in the clenched fist. The feet are examined for any deformity such as talipes equinovarus, as well as looking for extra digits. The axillae, elbows, groins and popliteal spaces should also be examined for abnormalities. Normal flexion and rotation of the wrist and ankle joints should be confirmed.

The spine

With the baby lying prone, the midwife should inspect and palpate the baby's back. Any swellings, dimples or hairy patches may signify an occult spinal defect. (All abnormalities must be reported to a paediatrician.)

Measurements

The baby's head circumference, length and weight are measured to provide parameters against which future growth can be monitored. The head circumference is measured, encircling it at the occipital protuberance and the supraorbital ridges with a measuring tape. Moulding may reduce this measurement and for this reason, this estimate is sometimes delayed until the 3rd day when the head shape has resumed its normal contours.

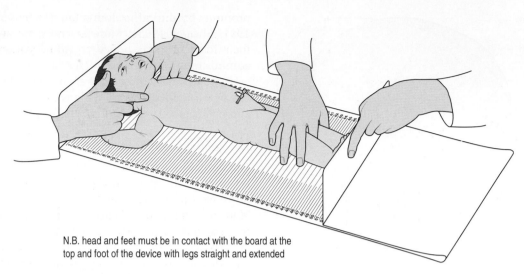

N.B. head and feet must be in contact with the board at the
top and foot of the device with legs straight and extended

Figure 40.2　Calibrated equipment length measurement.

Accurate measurement of the baby's crown–heel length is extremely difficult; this can only be measured accurately using calibrated equipment (Fig.40.2). In circumstances where this is not available, only an approximation of length can be achieved. The midwife should comply with local policy and procedures in this regard.

When the baby is weighed and the identity bands are verified as correct, they are then attached one to the arm and one on the leg, although this may vary according to local hospital policy. The baby is then dressed and wrapped in warm blankets.

Documentation

The midwife records her findings in the baby's case notes, and any abnormalities are brought to the attention of the paediatrician, or GP if a home birth and receiving midwife in the postnatal ward. Midwives must adhere to the guidelines for records and record-keeping (NMC 2007).

Daily examination and care

Each day, the baby should be examined by a midwife, to evaluate progress and identify problems as they arise. The examination is similar to that undertaken at birth but is now concerned with monitoring daily changes with the baby.

In caring for the normal baby, the midwife should ensure that the baby is comfortable, is feeding well and that facilities are available for the parents to help them with the attachment process. It is also important that midwives are aware of the signs of *airway obstruction, infection, jaundice and hypothermia.* They should report any deviation from the normal to the paediatrician.

Prevention of airway obstruction

Babies are obligatory nose breathers; patency can be assessed by watching the baby breathe in a quiet state. If one nostril is blocked, occlusion of the other results in cyanosis with unsuccessful attempts to breathe through the mouth. Bilateral nasal obstruction is of major significance if due to bilateral choanal atresia, which is a major medical emergency. Observe the colour of the baby's skin and mucous membranes. In the normal baby, the lips and mucous membranes are pink and well perfused.

Choking can occur during feeding if coordination is poor, and also following vomiting or regurgitation of mucus or feed. Suction apparatus should be readily available, so that aspiration of the baby's airway can be carried out effectively and quickly in an emergency situation.

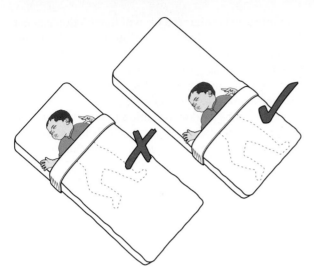

Figure 40.3 'Feet-to-foot' sleeping position.

According to guidelines it is important for a baby to sleep in the supine position (on its back) with the feet at the foot of the cot (Fig. 40.3) (Lerner 1993).

Prevention of infection

The baby's skin is a barrier to infection provided its integrity and pH balance are maintained. Babies should be provided with their own equipment. Adequate linen supplies are essential. This is especially important in hospital. The number of people handling the baby should be restricted. Members of staff who are liable to be a source of infection should not handle babies, and friends and relatives who have colds or sore throats (especially children) should not visit. Parents should be taught the proper technique for hand-washing and instructed that **hand-washing before and after handling babies is essential.** Cross-infection can be a particular problem in hospitals and most hospitals now have a hand sanitizing agent at every bedside. For this reason rooming-in and keeping the baby with the mother is highly recommended. The wearing of gowns for parents when handling babies is not necessary.

A newborn baby usually sleeps for most of the time between feeds but should be alert and responsive when awake. Erratic sleep patterns may prove disconcerting to new parents and they should be reassured by the midwife that this can be normal if the baby looks healthy, is alert and is feeding well. Undue lethargy or irritability may indicate cerebral damage or infection.

Prevention of hypothermia

Overexposure of the baby should be avoided to prevent heat loss. Where possible, the room temperature should be maintained at 18–21°C. In hospital, and where higher ambient temperatures are able to be maintained, the baby should be dressed in a cotton gown or sleep suit and covered by two cellular blankets. An additional blanket underneath the bottom sheet will provide extra warmth for babies who are having difficulty in maintaining a stable body temperature. At home, or in cold environments, extra blankets may be required. Bath water should be warm (36°C) and wet clothing should be changed as soon as possible. It is essential also to avoid overheating (Bacon 1991, Rutter 2005, Thomas 1994). Advice regarding clothing and bedding can only be a guide, as babies have marked individual variations in their metabolic rates (Hull et al 1996a). Parents should be advised to take account of environmental temperature when dressing their baby. Swaddling should be loose enough to permit movement of arms and legs, allowing adjustment to posture in response to the need for a change in temperature (Hull et al 1996b).

Baby cleansing

The timing of the first bath is not critical, although it has been suggested that removal of blood and liquor reduces the risk of transmission of HIV and other organisms to staff (Penny-MacGillivray 1996). Bathing should be deferred until the baby's temperature is above 36.5°C. The temperature of the bath water should be 36°C. The hair is washed and dried carefully at the first bath but need not be washed daily. If the baby has been regurgitating mucus, a thin layer of petroleum jelly may be applied to the cheek to prevent soreness. Petroleum jelly applied to the buttocks will prevent meconium adhering to the skin and causing excoriation.

Daily bathing is not essential but the mother should be given sufficient opportunities to bath her baby in order to increase her confidence. 'Topping and tailing' (cleansing the baby's face, skin flexures and napkin area only) may be carried out once or twice a day. It should be noted that greater heat loss may be incurred during this procedure than when the baby is bathed (Perry 2002).

Cleanliness of the umbilical cord is essential. The umbilical cord base is inspected for redness and the mother is instructed about cord care. Hand-washing is required before and after handling the cord. No specific cord treatment is required, although a wide variety of preparations have been used to promote early separation. However, it should be noted that topical applications could interfere with the normal process of colonization and delay separation. Cleansing with tap water and keeping the cord dry have been shown to promote separation (Barclay et al 1994, Trotter 2003). It is advisable to ensure that the cord is not enclosed within the baby's napkin where contamination by urine or faeces may occur. The cord clamp may be removed on the 3rd day provided the cord is dry and necrosed (WHO 1999). In some Maternity Units, the cord clamp is routinely left in situ because it is thought to help separation due to the added weight (Trotter 2003).

The baby's eyes do not need to be cleansed unless a discharge is present. Sticky eyes are cleaned with sterile water after obtaining a swab for culture and sensitivity testing. The mouth should be clean and moist. Adherent white plaques indicate oral thrush infection. Sucking blisters on the baby's lips may be observed, especially after feeding. These do not require any treatment.

General observation of skin

The skin, between the digits, is inspected for rashes, septic spots, excoriation or abrasions. Skin rashes such as erythema toxicum, a red blotchy rash, are of little significance. Sometimes a harlequin colour change may be noted; this is a very rare but dramatic colour change, with vivid midline demarcation of colour. The baby is red on one side of the trunk and pale on the other side. This is caused by vasomotor instability and is of little importance. However, its appearance is startling and can alarm the mother, so reassurance should be given by the midwife.

Attention should be paid to the washing and drying of skin flexures to prevent excoriation. Promotion of skin integrity is enhanced by avoiding friction against hard fabrics or soiled or wet clothing, and by minimizing the length of time the skin is in contact with irritants, such as gastric contents, urine and stool. Cleansing of the skin should be carried out gently to prevent damage to the epidermis. Skin care preparations should be used with caution to prevent irritation and disturbance of the skin. Research has suggested that the usage of baby products is superfluous to the care of the baby's skin (Trotter 2004). The use of biological powders, fabric softeners and starch should be avoided when laundering babies' clothing (Michie 1996).

All neonates have a transient rise in bilirubin, and some become visibly jaundiced. Babies who become jaundiced in the first 24 hrs of life or who have significant jaundice within 48 hrs need investigation. If a baby remains jaundiced on discharge from hospital, the midwife must contact the community midwife to monitor levels of bilirubin and instruct the parent to report to their GP if the baby's stools become pale or if the urine becomes dark, which may be suggestive of biliary atresia (see Ch. 47).

The fingertips and toes are examined for ragged nails and paronychia. Septic spots must be differentiated from milia, which do not require treatment. Even a few septic spots must be taken seriously. The paediatrician may prescribe topical applications or systemic antibiotics and consider possible isolation of the baby.

In some areas, the baby's temperature is recorded with a low-recording thermometer. This may be taken in the axilla, ear, in the groin or rectally. If the rectal route is used it is essential that the baby's legs and the thermometer are held firmly to prevent sudden movement, which could cause the thermometer to break and perforate the rectum. The midwife should ensure that the bulb of the thermometer is inserted no further than 2.5 cm into the rectum. Concern regarding the risk of injury has led to an increased use of alternative methods of measuring babies' temperatures. This concern must be balanced against the need for an accurate estimate of core temperature when babies are ill (Morley 1992). Midwives should comply with local policy in regard to rectal temperature taking.

Newborn babies' stools are observed for changes in relation to the baby's age and the type of milk ingested (Ch. 41). Non-passage of stools or vomiting helps to identify abnormalities of the gastrointestinal tract, inborn errors of metabolism and infection. Constipation may be alleviated by offering the baby water between feeds. Loose, watery stools may signify sugar intolerance or infection and may cause sore buttocks. Sore buttocks may be treated by exposure to the air, but care must be taken to avoid chilling the baby. The frequency of passing urine and stools in the preceding 24 hrs should be noted and recorded by the midwife.

At feed time, the midwife should observe the baby's eagerness or reluctance to feed and the coordination of sucking and swallowing reflexes, as well as noting the frequency with which the baby demands feeds. During feeding, babies clench their fists, tuck them under the chin and wriggle their toes while grasping their mother's fingers. Eye contact also occurs, which enhances communication between mother and baby. Sucking is interspersed with rest periods. Abnormal feeding behaviour may signify cerebral damage, congenital abnormality or illness. Breast engorgement and pseudomenstruation require no treatment but explanation to the mother is essential. No attempt should be made to express engorged breasts.

If the baby is to be weighed, this is done before dressing, and the result compared with his birth weight. Weight loss is normal in the first few days but more than 10% body weight loss is abnormal and requires investigation. Most babies regain their birth weight in 7–10 days, thereafter gaining weight at a rate of 150–200 g per week.

It is important for the midwife to note responses to handling and noise as she undresses the baby. She can use this time to inspect the identity bands, and have a discussion with the mother about feeding or any other concerns that she may have.

All findings at the daily examination are entered in the baby's records and abnormalities reported to the paediatrician.

Advice to mother

A baby should not be left unattended at any time, especially not on the bed as vigorous activity may result in injury from a fall. When a baby needs transporting from one area to another it should be placed in a cot and not carried in the carer's or parent's arms. The cot design should comply with safety standards and have a tight fitting mattress. Babies do not require a pillow until the age of 2 years and mothers should be advised that placing a pillow behind the baby's head is unsafe. Similarly, polythene bags or sheeting should not be used near a baby and waterproof mattress covers must be tight fitting and enclose the mattress completely to prevent suffocation of the baby by a loose cover.

If safety pins are used to secure the napkin, they should be inserted into the cloth from side-to-side (not vertically) and with one hand protecting the baby's abdomen to avoid penetration of the skin or genitalia. Cotton mittens should be worn to prevent facial scratches.

Advice and information leaflets about safety in the home and reducing the risk of cot death should be given and discussed with parents. Safety in the home should address such issues as use of cat-nets, fireguards, cooker guards, stair gates, pram brakes and car seats. Reducing the risk of cot death concentrates on smoking, back to sleep, feet-to-foot and advice on the importance of seeking early medical advice if the baby becomes unwell.

Discharge examination by the doctor/midwife

All newborn babies should be examined by one of the following: paediatrician, obstetrician, general practitioner, advanced neonatal nurse practitioner or midwife with appropriate training, within the first 72 hrs of life (NICE 2006). Moss et al (1991) believe that a second examination is of little value, apart from a repeat examination of the hips. The mother should be present for the examination. Some of the examination duplicates what has been described above and so only the medical aspects are considered here.

A general appraisal of the baby's colour, overall appearance, muscular activity and response to handling is made throughout the examination.

Head assessment

To start this assessment, the occipital frontal circumference (OFC) is measured using a non-stretchable tape measure. The average OFC in a term baby is

34–38 cm. Next, the size and tension of the anterior fontanelle is checked and suture lines palpated noting cranial moulding, caput succedaneum and cephalhaematoma. Any abnormality detected should be reported to a senior paediatrician and documented in the baby's case notes. Parents should be reassured that moulding, caput and cephalhaematoma usually resolve within a few weeks after birth.

Examination of the face should begin with observing the relationships between all the facial components: eyes, ears, nose and mouth, remembering that unusual facial characteristics may be familial (Boyer Johnson 1996). A general inspection of the eyes for conjunctivitis, cataracts, aniridia and coloboma is carried out before using an ophthalmoscope. The ophthalmoscope is held in the right hand, with the viewing aperture as close as possible to the right eye, and using the right index finger to turn the lens selector dial to the appropriate lens for proper focus (Honeyfield 1996). While positioning the baby's head with the free hand, the illuminating light is aligned along the baby's visual plane, observing for the red reflex and pupil reaction. Parents will need reassurance about common eye trauma such as bruising or oedema of the eyelids and haemorrhage seen around the iris (Boyer Johnson 1996). These can occur after a normal vaginal birth and usually resolve within 1–2 weeks. The ears should be assessed for size, shape and placement; abnormal formation or placement can be associated with chromosomal anomalies and syndromes. The nose should be symmetric and placed vertically in the midline. Its size and shape may be familial (Boyer Johnson 1996).

To examine the mouth a gloved finger should be inserted into the baby's mouth with the fingerpad up, to ensure continuity of the hard and soft palates and to assess suck and gag reflexes. Small white clusters of Epstein's pearls may be seen at the junction of the hard and soft palate and on the gums (Boyer Johnson 1996); these should not be mistaken for the white plaque of oral thrush.

Cardio/respiratory assessment

After inspection of the baby's colour, the next step is to auscultate the heart sounds. It is necessary to have a paediatric stethoscope with a double-headed chest piece; both sides are necessary to listen to the heart. The stethoscope should be placed firmly on bare skin, to assess the heart rate and evaluate cardiac rhythm and regularity (Honeyfield 1996). The practitioner carefully listens to the rhythm of the heart to determine whether there is any irregularity; a note is made of patterns and frequencies of the irregularity, which help identify the type of arrhythmia (Fraser Askin 1996). Murmurs are described as additional heart sounds and must be discussed and reported to a senior paediatrician.

To assess the chest and lungs, the shape of the chest is noted, and the rate and regularity of the respirations. Normal respirations are 40–60/min and relaxed, symmetrical diaphragmatic respirations are normal. Breath sounds can now be assessed using a stethoscope; sounds are louder and coarser in the baby than in the adult. Breath sounds should be assessed for pitch, intensity and duration. The practitioner begins at the top of the chest and moves the stethoscope systematically from side-to-side. Breath sounds in the lower lobes can be assessed adequately only through the baby's back (Fraser Askin 1996). Any irregularities detected must be reported to the paediatrician.

Abdomen

This assessment requires inspection, palpation and auscultation. The practitioner palpates the abdomen with warm hands and observes for pain responses, starting at the groin by placing the index finger just above the groin parallel to the right costal margin and, with a gentle compressing motion, gradually moving the finger upward until the liver edge is felt. The normal liver is smooth and firm with a sharp and well-defined edge, and is felt 1–2 cm below the right costal margin. The spleen is normally not palpable unless infection is present. Next the kidneys and bladder are examined. The bladder when full is easily palpated 1–4 cm above the symphysis pubis, and can be associated with abnormalities if frequently or continuously distended. The kidneys are sometimes difficult to palpate; the left kidney is more easily palpated than the right, unless the descending colon is filled with meconium. The kidney is palpated using a deep smooth firm pressure by placing one hand under the baby's flank and pressing downward with the other. Next, the practitioner auscultates for bowel sounds; using a stethoscope to listen to all four abdominal quadrants, breath sounds are usually heard in the upper abdominal region. Bowel sounds are absent immediately after birth. With crying and sucking, the abdomen begins to fill with air, and bowel sounds become audible within the first 15 min after birth. The sounds have a metallic, tinkling quality and are usually heard every 15–20s. (The above description follows that by Keels Conner 1996.)

Neurological system

The baby's reflex responses are elicited in order to establish normality of the neurological system. These are tested while the baby is in a quiet alert state. Absent or weak responses may indicate immaturity, cerebral damage or abnormality.

In comparison with the other body systems, the nervous system is remarkably immature both anatomically and physiologically at birth. This results in predominantly brain stem and spinal reflex activity with minimal control by the cerebral cortex in the early months, though social interaction occurs early. After birth, brain growth is rapid, requiring constant and adequate supplies of oxygen and glucose. The immaturity of the brain renders it particularly vulnerable to hypoxia, biochemical imbalance, infection and haemorrhage. Temperature instability and uncoordinated muscle movement reflect the incomplete state of brain development and incomplete myelination of nerves.

The baby is equipped with a wide range of reflex activities, the presence of which at varying ages provides an indication of the normality and integrity of the neurological and skeletomuscular systems (Gandy 1999).

Moro reflex

This reflex occurs in response to a sudden stimulus. The baby is held supine, with the trunk and head supported from below. When the head and shoulders are suddenly allowed to fall back, the baby responds by abduction and extension of arms with fingers fanned, and sometimes accompanied by a tremor. The arms then flex and embrace the chest. A similar response may be seen in the legs which, following extension, flex on to the abdomen (Fig. 40.4). The Moro reflex is often accompanied by a cry and may be demonstrated unintentionally when briskly placing a baby in the supine position. Babies do not seem to like this reflex, so it should not be elicited as a routine procedure. The reflex is symmetrical and is present for the first 8 weeks of life. The most common cause of an asymmetric Moro response is a fracture of the humerus or clavicle, or a brachial plexus palsy. Absence of the Moro reflex may indicate brain damage or immaturity. Persistence of the reflex beyond the age of 6 months is suggestive of learning difficulties (Thomas & Harvey 1992).

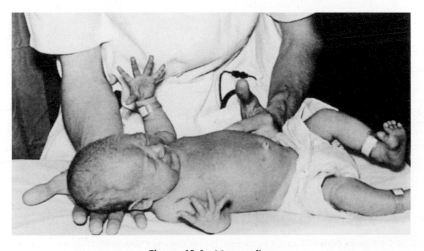

Figure 40.4   Moro reflex.

Rooting reflex

In response to stroking of the cheek or side of the mouth the baby will turn towards the source of stimulus and open the mouth ready to suckle.

Sucking and swallowing reflexes

These are well developed in the normal baby and are coordinated with breathing. This is essential for safe feeding and adequate nutrition.

Gag, cough and sneeze reflexes

These protect the baby from airway obstruction.

Blinking and corneal reflexes

These protect the eyes from trauma.

Grasp reflexes

A palmar grasp is elicited by placing a finger or pencil in the palm of the baby's hand. The finger or pencil is grasped firmly. A similar response can be demonstrated by stroking the base of the toes (plantar grasp).

Walking and stepping reflexes

When supported upright with his feet touching a flat surface, the baby simulates walking. If held with the tibia in contact with the edge of a table, the baby will step up on to the table (limb placement reflex).

Asymmetrical tonic neck reflex

In the supine position the limbs on the side of the body to which the head is turned extend, while those on the opposite side flex. Muscle tone is reflected in the baby's response to passive movements.

Traction response

When pulled upright by the wrists to a sitting position, the head will lag initially (Fig. 40.5) then right itself momentarily before falling forward on to the chest.

Ventral suspension

When held prone, and suspended over the examiner's arm, the baby momentarily holds the head level with the body and flexes the limbs (Fig. 40.6).

These reflexes and responses are self-defence mechanisms, which are designed to attract the mother to her baby and so promote the mother–child attachment.

Examination of hips

It is essential that all babies undergo specific examination to detect developmental dysplasia of the hips (Aronsson et al 1994, Beverley & Nathan 1995). In some centres, the midwife performs this; in others the paediatrician is the person responsible. Care must be taken in order to avoid producing an iatrogenically unstable hip (Beverley & Nathan 1995). The

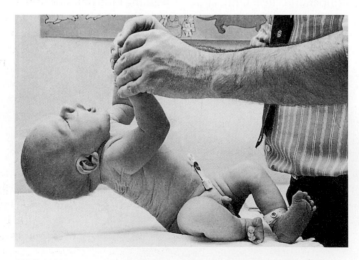

Figure 40.5 Traction response. (From Gandy 1999, with permission.)

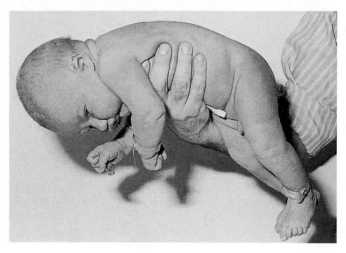

Figure 40.6   Ventral suspension. (From Gandy, 1999, with permission.)

examination should not be undertaken by inexperienced staff. To examine the hips the examiner must place the baby on a firm flat surface at waist height.

Ortolani's test (Fig. 40.7)

The baby's legs are grasped with the flexed knees in the palms of the examiner's hands and the femur splinted between the index and middle fingers and the thumb. Both hips are examined simultaneously. The baby's thighs are flexed on to the abdomen and rotated and abducted through an angle of 70–90° towards the examining surface. *No force should be exerted*. If the hip is dislocated a 'clunk' will be felt as the head of the femur slips into the acetabulum during adduction and the dislocation is reduced.

Barlow's test

With the baby's legs flexed (as above), the head of the femur is held between the examiner's thumb and index finger while the other hand steadies the pelvis. Following the initial movement of flexion and rotation, as the hip is abducted to 70° *gentle pressure* is exerted in a backward and lateral direction. A 'clunk' will be felt as the head of the femur dislocates out of the acetabulum.

In some centres a modified Ortolani/Barlow procedure is followed. This incorporates the essential elements of both of the above manoeuvres (Hall et al 1994). Early referral to a paediatrician is essential if effective treatment for a dislocated, or dislocatable, hip is to be achieved (see Ch. 46).

Circumcision

Although not commonly practised in the UK, in other parts of the world neonatal circumcision may be undertaken while the baby is in hospital. There is little evidence to support this practice as beneficial; rather it is a traditional cultural custom (Gonik & Barrett 1995). It is recommended that appropriate anaesthesia, dorsal penile nerve block is used for this procedure and that postoperative analgesia is also prescribed (Rabinowitz & Hulbert 1995). After care involves the use of a non-adherent dressing, observing for haemorrhage and keeping the area clean and dry.

Blood tests

Certain inborn errors of metabolism and endocrine disorders are detected by means of a blood test, for example the Guthrie test. Blood, obtained from a heel prick made with a stilette on the lateral aspect of the heel to avoid nerves and blood vessels, is dripped on to circles on an absorbent card on to which full details of the baby's identity and history are entered (see Plate 13). This is taken on day 4–6

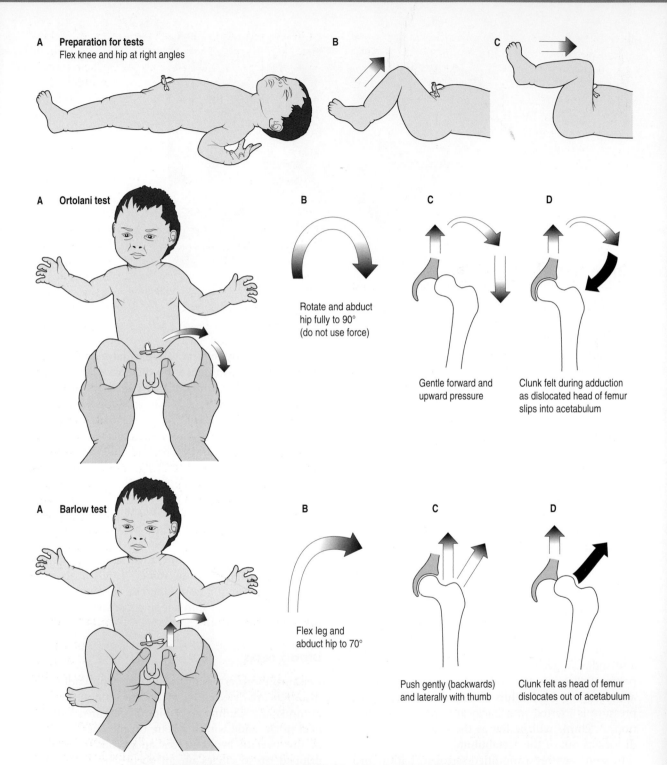

A Preparation for tests
Flex knee and hip at right angles

B

C

A Ortolani test

B
Rotate and abduct
hip fully to 90°
(do not use force)

C
Gentle forward and
upward pressure

D
Clunk felt during adduction
as dislocated head of femur
slips into acetabulum

A Barlow test

B
Flex leg and
abduct hip to 70°

C
Push gently (backwards)
and laterally with thumb

D
Clunk felt as head of femur
dislocates out of acetabulum

Figure 40.7   Examination of the hips. Ortolani's and Barlow's test.

after birth for detection of phenylketonuria, hypothyroidism and cystic fibrosis and if the baby is <35 weeks' gestation, the sample is repeated when the baby reaches 36 weeks. If the baby has received a blood transfusion, the sample cannot be taken until 48hrs post-transfusion and if for any reason the baby or mother is receiving antibiotics, this information should be recorded on the card. Some centres also test routinely for galactosaemia (see Ch. 48.)

The above examination, when completed, must be recorded in the Personal Child Health Record to inform the General Practitioner and Health Visitor.

Child health surveillance

The midwife will hand over care of the mother and baby on the 10th day but may continue to visit until day 28 or to the end of the puerperium to support the mother with, e.g. breastfeeding. Following discharge from the care of the midwife to that of the health visitor, the screening of the baby is continued on a regular basis at the child health clinic.

Vaccination and immunization

While the baby was developing in the uterus it received natural immunity IgG which affords immunity against specific viral infections. A comprehensive immunization programme is in place, which starts when the baby reaches 2 months of age and continues into childhood. Tuberculosis screening is now undertaken at birth and BCG vaccination if applicable will be offered to the baby during the early neonatal period. The date of the immunization, type of vaccine, batch number and injection site, should always be recorded in the baby's record. Consent must be obtained from parents or legal guardian before a baby can receive any vaccinations.

Promoting family relationships

Parent–infant attachment

Positive responses from the baby to his parents reinforce parental attachment and stimulate further interaction. Knowledge of the reflexes, general abilities and sleep and awake states of babies enables the midwife to teach the parents how to take advantage of the occasions when their baby is likely to be most responsive. The resulting interactions continue the process of attachment initiated at birth (see Ch. 39). To help the mother in her new role, it is important to use the baby's name and to speak positively about his/her appearance and activities.

Parents develop their relationship with their babies in individual ways and at their own pace. Some mothers feel somewhat distant from their baby at first; others experience an overwhelming protective urge and intense absorption with their baby (Jowitt 1996). It is important not to overemphasize 'bonding', as this may create non-productive guilt feelings in parents who do not experience instant love for their child and result in negative attitudes towards the baby (Barclay & Lupton 1999, Billings 1995, Rutter 1995).

It is suggested that the parents' relationship with one another is enhanced when the father is encouraged to be involved in discussions, choices and decisions about baby care and to share the responsibility for care. The resultant maternal confidence is reflected in her responsiveness toward her baby, thus promoting the baby's feeling of security (Adams & Cotgrove 1995). The father's reactions to and feelings about his baby should be afforded expression (Heath 1995, McLennan 1995, Ratnaike 2007). Parents may express anxiety about the possible reactions of siblings to the new arrival. A positive attitude on the part of the midwife can do much to allay fears, which are often unfounded (Gullicks & Crase 1993).

Promoting confidence and competence

It is important that the midwife does not let her own maternal feelings 'take over', thus denying the mother opportunity to provide care for her baby. Involvement by the mother and father in the baby's care should be encouraged by the midwife and as the parents gain confidence, they should take over total care of their baby. Teaching the principles and discussing individual care can help to overcome any anxieties the parents may be experiencing.

Promoting communication

The increasing interest in baby massage in recent years capitalizes on the knowledge that the baby is sensitive and responsive to touch (Barnett 2005, Lim 1996). Aromatherapy oils should not be used as the extent of their absorption is unknown. The naked baby is stroked and caressed in a leisurely manner using the fingertips and palms of the hands. Throughout this quiet time together, eye-to-eye contact is promoted by the close proximity of the baby, and the mother (or father) instinctively interacts with the baby's pleasurable responses. This assists in reinforcing the developing emotional relationship.

By applying her knowledge of the physiological and psychological capabilities and potential complications of the newborn, the midwife can ensure that all care is given in a professional manner which will nurture and enhance a happy family relationship.

The foregoing discussions in this chapter have endeavoured to illustrate how the midwife can enhance the parent–baby relationship. Her teaching, support and encouragement of the mother as she learns to provide for her baby's needs is of paramount importance and should culminate in a happy, confident and competent mother being discharged from the midwife's care. The midwife can also do a great deal to encourage a father's interaction with his baby and should take every opportunity to do so. These aspects of midwifery practice are described more fully in Chapters 34 and 36.

REFERENCES

Adams L, Cotgrove A 1995 Promoting secure attachment patterns in infancy and beyond. Professional Care of Mother and Child 5(6):158–160

Aronsson D D, Goldberg M J, Kling T F et al 1994 Developmental dysplasia of the hip. Pediatrics 94(2):201–208

Bacon C J 1991 The thermal environment of sleeping babies and possible dangers of overheating. In: David T J (ed.) Recent advances in paediatrics. Churchill Livingstone, Edinburgh

Barclay L, Lupton D 1999 The experience of new fatherhood: a sociocultural analysis. Journal of Advanced Nursing 29 (4):1013–1020

Barclay L, Harrington A, Conroy R, Royal R et al 1994 A comparative study of neonates' umbilical cord management. Australian Journal of Advanced Nursing 11(3):34–40

Barnett L, 2005 Keep in touch: The importance of touch in infant development. Infant Observation 8(2):115–123

Beverley M, Nathan S 1995 Diagnosing developmental dysplasia of the hip (DDH). Maternal and Child Health 20(4):120,122–124

Billings J R 1995 Bonding theory – tying mothers in knots? A critical review of the application of a theory to nursing. Journal of Clinical Nursing 4(4):207–211

Blackburn S T 2007 Maternal, fetal, and neonatal physiology: a clinical perspective, 3rd edn. Elsevier Science, Edinburgh, Chs 8–15

Boyer Johnson C 1996 Head, eyes, ears, nose, mouth and neck assessment. In: Tappero E P, Honeyfield M E (eds) Physical assessment of the newborn, 2nd edn. NICU INK, California

Brazelton T B 1984 Neonatal behavioural assessment scale, 2nd edn. Spastics International Medical Publications, Blackwell Scientific, London

Brazelton T B, Nugent J K 1995 Neonatal behavioural assessment scale, 3rd edn. Mackeith Press, London.

Cetta F, Lambert GH, Ross SP, 1991 Newborn chemical exposure from over the counter skin-care products. Clinical Pediatrics 30:289–289

Crockett M 1995 Physiology of the neonatal immune system. Journal of Obstetric, Gynecologic and Neonatal Nursing 24(7):627–634

Day M 1995 Babies at risk as maternity units fail to step up security. Nursing Times 91(28):6

DeCasper A, Fifer W 1987 Of human bonding: newborns prefer their mothers' voices. In: Oates J, Sheldon S (eds) Cognitive development in infancy. Lawrence Erlbaum Associates Open University, Hove

Field T 2004 Touch and massage in early childhood development. Johnson&Johnson Paediatric Institute, LLC USA

Fraser Askin D 1996 Chest and lungs assessment. In: Tappero E P, Honeyfield M E (eds) Physical assessment of the newborn, 2nd edn. NICU INK, California

Fry T 1994 Monitoring children's growth: introducing the new child growth standards. Professional Care of Mother and Child 4(8):231–233

Gandy G M 1999 Examination of the neonate including gestational age assessment. In: Roberton N R C Textbook of neonatology, 3rd edn. Churchill Livingstone, Edinburgh, Ch. 17

Gonik B, Barrett K 1995 The persistence of newborn circumcision: an American perspective. British Journal of Obstetrics and Gynaecology 102(12):940–941

Grunau R, Oberlander T, Holsti L et al 1998 Bedside application of the neonatal facial coding system in pain assessment of premature neonates. Pain 76: 277–286

Gullicks J N, Crase S J 1993 Sibling behaviour with a newborn: parents' expectations and observations. Journal of Obstetric, Gynecologic and Neonatal Nursing 22(5):438–444

Hall D, Hill P, Elliman D 1994 The child surveillance handbook, 2nd edn. Radcliffe Medical Press, Oxford

Heath T 1995 New fatherhood. New Generation (June):11

Honeyfield M E 1996 Principles of physical assessment. In: Tappero E P, Honeyfield M E (eds) Physical assessment of the newborn, 2nd edn. NICU INK, California

Hull D, McArthur A J, Pritchard K et al 1996a Metabolic rate of sleeping infants. Archives of Disease in Childhood 75 (4):282–287

Hull D, McArthur A J, Pritchard K et al 1996b Individual variation in sleeping metabolic rates in infants. Archives of Disease in Childhood 75(4):288–291

Irving V 2001 Caring for and protecting the skin of pre-term neonates. Journal of Wound Care 10(7):253–256

Janssen P A, Selwood B L, Dobson S R et al 2003 To Dye or Not to Dye: A randomized clinical trial of a triple dye/alcohol regime versus dry cord care. Paediatrics 111(1):15–20

Jørgensen F S, Felding P, Vinther S et al 1991 Vitamin K to neonates. Per oral versus intramuscular administration. Acta Paediatrica 80:304–307

Jowitt M 1996 Birth and bonding. Midwifery Matters 69 (Summer):3

Keels Conner G 1996 Abdomen assessment. In: Tappero E P, Honeyfield M E (eds) Physical assessment of the newborn, 2nd edn. NICU INK, California

Laurent C 1992 A mother's nightmare. Nursing Times 88(52):18

Lerner H 1993 Sleep position of infants: applying research to practice. Maternal and Child Nursing 18(Sept/Oct):275–277

Lim P, 1996 Baby massage. British Journal of Midwifery (8):439–441

McLennan I 1995 Ian's story. New Generation (June):13

McLintock F 1995 Baby massage. Connections 26(2):4–6

Michie M 1996 A delicate concern: caring for neonatal skin. British Journal of Midwifery 4(3):159–163

Morley C 1992 Measuring infants' temperatures. Midwives Chronicle and Nursing Notes (Feb):26–29

Moss G D, Cartlidge P H T, Speides B D et al 1991 Routine examination in the neonatal period. British Medical Journal 302:878–879

National Health Service Screening 2006 Antenatal and newborn screening programmes. Online. Available: www.screening.nhs.uk

NICE guidelines The postnatal care guidelines (July 2006) National Institute of Clinical Excellence. Online. Available: www.nice.org.uk

Nursing & Midwifery Council 2007 Guidelines for records and record keeping. NMC, London. Online. Available: www.nmc-uk.org/aArticle.aspx?Article ID=1673

Penny-MacGillivray T, 1996 A newborn's first bath: when? Journal of Obstetric, Gynecologic and Neonatal Nursing 25(6):481–487

Perry S E 2002 Nursing care of the newborn. In: Bobak I M, Lowdermilk D L, Jensen M D et al Maternity nursing, 6th edn. Elsevier Health Sciences Edinburgh, p 461–513

Rabinowitz R, Hulbert W C 1995 Newborn circumcision should not be performed without anaesthesia. Birth 22 (1):45–46

Ratnaike D 2007 Fathers present or just in the room? Midwives 10(3):106

Righard L, 1995 How do newborns find their mother's breast? Birth 22(3):174–175

Roberton N R C 2005 Care of the normal term newborn baby. In: Rennie J M (ed.) Roberton's textbook of neonatology, 4th edn. Churchill Livingstone, Edinburgh

Roberton N R C 1996 A manual of normal neonatal care, 3rd edn. Edward Arnold, London

Rushforth J A, Levene M I 1994 Behavioural response to pain in healthy neonates. Archives of Disease in Childhood 70(3): F174–F176

Rutter N 2005 Temperature control and its disorders. In: Rennie J M (ed.) Roberton's textbook of neonatology, 4th edn. Churchill Livingstone, Edinburgh

Rutter M 1995 Clinical implications of attachment concepts: retrospect and prospect. Journal of Child Psychology and Psychiatry 36(4):549–571

Saigal S, Nelson N, Bennett K et al 1981. Observation on the behavioral state of newborn babies during the first hours of life. American Journal of Obstetrics and Gynecology 139:715

Shearer M J 1995 Vitamin K. Lancet 345(8944):229–234

Stern C M 1999 Neonatal immunology. In: Roberton N R C (ed.) Textbook of neonatology, 3rd edn. Churchill Livingstone, Edinburgh, Ch. 43

Thomas K 1994 Thermoregulation in neonates. Neonatal Network 13(2):15–22

Thomas R, Harvey D 1992 Neonatology colour guide, 2nd edn. Churchill Livingstone, Edinburgh

Trotter S, 2003 Management of the umbilical cord – a guide to best care. RCM Midwives Journal 6(7):308–311

Trotter S 2004 Care of the newborn: Proposed new guidelines. British Journal of Midwifery 3:152–157

World Health Organization 1999 Care of the umbilical cord: a review of the evidence. Reproductive Health (technical support). Maternal and Newborn Health/Safe Motherhood. WHO, Geneva

FURTHER READING

Klaus M H, Kennell J H 1996 Bonding: building the foundations of secure attachment and independence. Cedar, London

This book will give the midwife insight into other aspects and studies regarding the parent infant attachment and should be read to compliment the information in this chapter.

Perry S E 2002 The newborn. In: Bobak I M, Lowdermilk D L, Jensen M D (eds) Maternity nursing, 6th edn. Elsevier Health Sciences Edinburgh, Ch. 19

This book will expand on the physiology of the baby's systems at birth, which is discussed in this chapter.

Tappero E P, Honeyfield M E 1996 Physical assessment of the newborn. A comprehensive approach to the art of physical examination, 2nd edn. NICU INK, California

This newborn assessment book is a valuable resource for all midwives involved in the care of the newborn baby. It will also assist the midwife who has extended her role to include the final examination of the newborn baby.

Thomas R, Harvey D 1992 Neonatology colour guide, 2nd edn. Churchill Livingstone, Edinburgh

This is a concise text, clearly integrated with high quality colour clinical photographs; it is an essential resource for midwives involved in the examination of the newborn baby.

41 Infant feeding

Sally Inch

CHAPTER CONTENTS

The establishment of good feeding practices has become even more essential given the recent increase in obesity and allergies in children in the UK. Breastfeeding for the first 6 months of life is the ideal start for babies and midwives have a key role in supporting mothers to breastfeed successfully. For those mothers who are unable to or choose not to breastfeed, the midwife has an equally important role in ensuring families safely and appropriately feed their babies.

This chapter aims to discuss:

- the structure and function of the female breast
- the properties and components of breastmilk
- the role of the midwife, with particular emphasis on ensuring breastfeeding success for both mother and baby
- breastmilk expression
- the different causes of difficulty with breastfeeding
- artificial feeding and the various products available
- human milk banking
- the International code of marketing of breastmilk substitutes
- the Baby Friendly Hospital Initiative

The breast and breastmilk

Anatomy and physiology of the breast
(Fig. 41.1)

The breasts are compound secreting glands, composed of varying proportions of fat, glandular and connective tissue, arranged in lobes. Each lobe is divided into lobules that consist of alveoli and ducts.

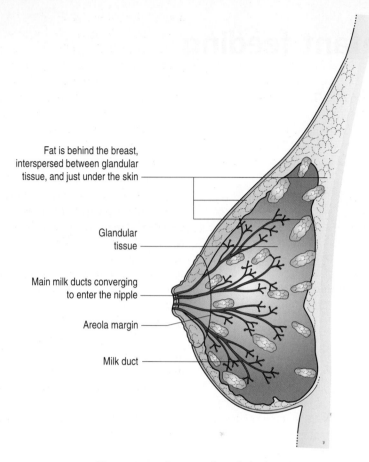

Fat is behind the breast, interspersed between glandular tissue, and just under the skin

Glandular tissue

Main milk ducts converging to enter the nipple

Areola margin

Milk duct

Figure 41.1 Cross-section of the breast.

As there is an intimate and congruous connection between the fat and glandular tissue within the breast (Nickell & Skelton 2005), the relative proportion of fat to glandular tissue is difficult to calculate non-invasively.

However, analysis of 21 non-lactating breasts (surgically removed for carcinoma *in situ*), (Vandeweyer & Hertens 2002) revealed that the percentage weight of fat per total breast varied from 3.6 to 37.6. Mammographic studies of non-lactating breasts have reported breast glandularity decreasing with age (Jamal et al 2004).

Investigations carried out on 25 sections of central breast tissue removed during breast reduction operations (performed on women with an average BMI of 28) found a mean of 61% fat (Cruz-Korchin et al 2002). On average, the central breast area in these

women also contained only 7% glandular tissue and 29% connective tissue.

This finding, that larger breasts contain relatively more fat, is supported by an observational study of 136 patients (with an average BMI of 32), undergoing breast reduction surgery (Nickell & Skelton 2005).

Research on the volumes of 20 complete duct systems ('lobes') in an autopsied breast, found considerable variation in the proportion of breast tissue 'serviced' by each duct; the largest 'lobe' drained 23% of breast volume; half of the breast was drained by three ducts and 75% by the largest six. Conversely, eight small duct systems together accounted for only 1.6% of breast volume (Going & Moffat 2004).

Ultrasound investigations of the *lactating* breasts of 21 subjects (Ramsay et al 2005) have identified nine or so milk ducts per breast (range 4–18), which is fewer than previously believed, and in agreement with investigations conducted by Love and Barsky (2004).

Taneri et al (2006) examined 226 mastectomy specimens and found the mean number of ducts in the nipple duct bundle was 17.5. This is significantly higher than the number reported to open on the nipple surface. They reflected that this discrepancy could be due to duct branching within the nipple or the presence of some ducts which do not reach the nipple surface.

Taken together, the intimate and inseparable relationship between fat and glandular tissue, the uneven distribution of milk glands and the high variability in the number of milk ducts, have implications for those who need breast surgery, particularly breast reduction surgery, since in some cases the loss of only a few ducts may inadvertently compromise a woman's future ability to breastfeed (see Breast surgery, below).

The alveoli contain acini cells, which produce milk and are surrounded by myoepithelial cells, which contract and propel the milk out (Fig. 41.2). Small lactiferous ducts, carrying milk from the alveoli, unite to form larger ducts. Several large ducts (lactiferous tubules) conveying milk from one or more lobe emerge on the surface of the nipple. Myoepithelial cells are oriented longitudinally along the ducts and, under the influence of oxytocin, these smooth muscle cells contract and the tubule becomes shorter

and wider (Ramsay et al 2004, Woolridge 1986). The tubule distends during active milk flow, while the myoepithelial cells are maintained in a state of contraction by circulating oxytocin (2–3 min). The fuller the breast when let down occurs, the greater the degree of ductal distension (Ramsay et al 2004).

The nipple, composed of erectile tissue, is covered with epithelium and contains smooth muscle and elastic fibres, which form a tight sphincter at the end of the teat (as in most mammals; Cross 1977), to prevent unwanted loss of milk from the mammary gland when it is not being suckled.

Surrounding the nipple is an area of pigmented skin called the areola, which contains Montgomery's glands. These produce a sebum-like substance, which acts as a lubricant during pregnancy and throughout breastfeeding. Breasts, nipples and areolae vary considerably in size from one woman to another.

The breast is supplied with blood from the internal and external mammary arteries and branches from the intercostal arteries. The veins are arranged in a circular fashion around the nipple. Lymph drains freely from the two breasts into lymph nodes in the axillae and the mediastinum.

During pregnancy, oestrogens and progesterone induce alveolar and ductal growth as well as stimulating the secretion of colostrum. Other hormones are also involved and they govern a complex sequence of events, which prepare the breast for lactation. Although colostrum is present from the 16th week of pregnancy, the production of milk is held in abeyance until after the birth, when the levels of placental hormones fall. This allows the already high levels of prolactin to initiate milk production. Continued production of prolactin is caused by the baby feeding at the breast, with concentrations highest during night feeds. Prolactin is involved in the suppression of ovulation, and some women may remain anovular until lactation ceases, although for others this effect is not so prolonged (Kennedy et al 1989, Ramos et al 1996) (see Ch. 37).

If breastfeeding (or expressing) has to be delayed for a few days, lactation can still be initiated because prolactin levels remain high, even in the absence of breast use, for at least the first week (Kochenour 1980), although the establishment of lactation will be more secure if breastfeeding or expressing begins as shortly after birth as possible.

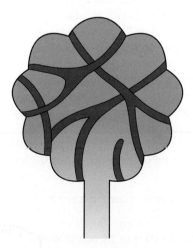

Figure 41.2 Alveoli surrounded by myoepithelial cells, which propel the milk out of the lobule.

Prolactin seems to be much more important to the initiation of lactation than to its continuation. As lactation progresses, the prolactin response to suckling diminishes and milk removal becomes the driving force behind milk production.

This is now known to be due to the presence in secreted milk of a whey protein that is able to inhibit the synthesis of milk constituents (Daly 1993, Prentice et al 1989, Wilde et al 1995).

This protein accumulates in the breast as the milk accumulates and it exerts negative feedback control on the continued production of milk. Removal of this autocrine inhibitory factor, (sometimes referred to as FIL – feedback inhibitor of lactation) by removing the milk, allows milk production to be stepped up again.

It is because this mechanism acts locally (i.e. within the breast) that each breast can function independently of the other. It is also the reason that milk production slows as the baby is gradually weaned from the breast. If necessary, it can be stepped up again if the baby is put back to the breast more often (e.g. because of illness).

Milk is synthesized continuously into the alveolar lumen, where it is stored until milk removal from the breast is initiated. It is only when oxytocin is released, and the myoepithelial cells contract, that milk is made available to the suckling infant.

Milk release is under neuroendocrine control. Tactile stimulation of the breast also stimulates the oxytocin, causing contraction of the myoepithelial cells. This process is known as the 'let-down' or 'milk-ejection' reflex and makes the milk available to the baby. This occurs in discrete pulses throughout the feed and may well trigger the bursts of active feeding.

In the early days of lactation, this reflex is unconditioned. Later, as it becomes a conditioned reflex, the mother may find her breasts responding to the baby's cry (or other circumstances associated with the baby or feeding). In one small study, psychological stress (mental arithmetic or noise) was found to reduce the frequency of the oxytocin pulses, however there was no effect on the amplitude of the pulse. Neither was there any effect on either prolactin levels or the amount of milk the baby received (Ueda et al 1994).

Milk production and the mother

The human mother manages the process of lactation in an entirely different way from her non-primate counterpart. Much of the mis-information to which mothers are subjected derives from extrapolation from veterinary and dairy science (Woolridge 1995). Adequate milk production is largely independent of the mother's nutritional status and body mass index (Prentice et al 1994).

Not only have dietary surveys in developed countries consistently found their calorie intake to be less than the recommended amount (Butte et al 1984, Whitehead et al 1981), but controlled trials conducted in developing countries have demonstrated that giving extra food to mothers, even those who were poorly nourished, did not increase the rate of growth of their babies (Prentice et al 1980, 1983).

It has been suggested that metabolic efficiency is enhanced in lactating women, who are therefore able to conserve energy and 'subsidize' the cost of their milk production (Illingworth et al 1986).

The lactational performance of the human female must become compromised when under-nutrition is sufficiently severe, but it appears that this occurs only in famine or near famine conditions.

As milk production would appear to 'drive' appetite, rather than the reverse, hunger will effectively regulate the calorie intake of a breastfeeding woman, and the practice of encouraging breastfeeding mothers to eat excessively should be abandoned.

Similarly, if healthy breastfeeding women wish to undertake strenuous exercise (from 6 to 8 weeks after birth), or to lose weight (500–1000g/week), they can be assured that neither the quality nor the quantity of their milk will be affected (Dewey et al 1994, Dusdieker et al 1994). Exclusive breastfeeding combined with low fat diet and exercise will result in more effective weight loss than diet and exercise alone (Dewey 1998, Hammer et al 1996).

Milk production is similarly unaffected by fluctuations in the mother's fluid intake. It has been repeatedly demonstrated that neither a significant decrease (e.g. Dearlove & Dearlove 1981) nor a significant increase (e.g. Morse et al 1992) in maternal fluid intake has any effect on milk production or the baby's weight.

Properties and components of breastmilk

Human milk varies in its composition:

- with the time of day (e.g. the fat content is lowest in the morning and highest in the afternoon)

- with the stage of lactation (e.g. the fat and protein content of colostrum is higher than in mature milk)
- in response to maternal nutrition (e.g. although the *total amount* of fat is not influenced by diet, the *type* of fat that appears in the milk will be influenced by what the mother eats)
- because of individual variations.

The most dramatic change in the composition of milk occurs during the course of a feed (Hall 1979). At the beginning of the feed the baby receives a high volume of relatively low fat milk (the *foremilk)*. As the feed progresses, the volume of milk decreases but the proportion of fat in the milk increases, sometimes to as much as five times the initial value (the *hindmilk)* (Jackson et al 1987). The baby's ability to obtain this fat-rich milk is *not* determined by the length of time he spends at the breast, but by the quality of his attachment to the breast. The baby needs to be well attached so that he can use his tongue to maximum effect, stripping the milk from the breast, rather than relying solely on his mother's milk ejection reflex. A poorly attached baby may have difficulty in obtaining enough fat to meet his needs, and may resort to feeding very frequently in order to obtain sufficient calories from low fat feeds. A well-attached baby may, on the other hand, obtain all he needs in a very short time.

The length of the feed, provided that the baby is well attached, is thus determined by the rate of milk transfer from mother to baby. If milk transfer occurs at a high rate, feeds will be relatively short; if it occurs slowly, feeds will be longer (Woolridge et al 1982) (Fig. 41.3). Milk transfer seems to be more efficient in a second lactation than in a first (Ingram et al 2001).

Exclusive breastfeeding for the first 6 months of life

Human milk is species specific. The 54th World Health Assembly, which met in Geneva in May 2001, affirmed the importance of exclusive breastfeeding for 6 months. The new resolution (Agenda Item 13.1, Infant and young child nutrition, A54/45 in para. 2(4).) urged member states to:

support exclusive breastfeeding for six months as a global public health recommendation taking into account the findings of the WHO Expert Technical Consultation on optimal

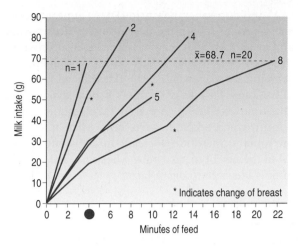

Figure 41.3 Pattern of milk intake at a feed for 20 6-day-old babies. (From Woolridge et al 1982, with permission.)

duration of exclusive breastfeeding and to provide safe and appropriate complementary foods, with continued breastfeeding for up to two years or beyond . . .

(Baby Milk Action 2001.)

It has been known for some time that exclusively breastfed babies who consume enough breastmilk to satisfy their energy needs will easily meet their fluid requirements, even in hot dry climates (Ashraf et al 1993, Sachdev et al 1991).

Extra water will do nothing to speed the resolution of physiological jaundice, should it occur (Carvahlo et al 1981, Nicoll et al 1982). The only consistent effect of giving additional fluids to breastfed infants is to reduce the time for which they are breastfed (Fenstein et al 1986, White et al 1992).

Fats and fatty acids

For the human infant, with his unique and rapidly growing brain, it is the fat and not the protein in human milk that has particular significance.

Some 98% of the lipid in human milk is in the form of *triglycerides*: three fatty acids linked to a single molecule of glycerol. Over 100 fatty acids have so far been identified, about 46% being saturated fat and 54% unsaturated fat. There has been an explosion of interest in recent years in the unsaturated fatty acid content of human milk, particularly in the long chain polyunsaturated variety (LC-PUFAs for short), because of their role in brain growth and myelination. Two of them, arachidonic acid

(AA) and docosahexanoic acid (DHA) appear to play an important role in the development of the retina and visual cortex of the newborn. Fat also provides the baby with >50% of his calorific requirements (Helsing & Savage King 1982). It is utilized very rapidly because *the milk itself* contains the enzyme (bile-salt-stimulated *lipase*) needed for fat digestion, but in a form which becomes active only when it reaches the infant's intestine. Pancreatic lipase is not plentiful in the newborn, so a baby who is not fed human milk is less able to digest fat.

Carbohydrate

The carbohydrate component of human milk is provided chiefly by *lactose*, which provides the baby with about 40% of his calorific requirements. Lactose is converted into galactose and glucose by the action of the enzyme lactase and these sugars provide energy to the rapidly growing brain. Lactose enhances the absorption of calcium and also promotes the growth of lactobacilli, which increase intestinal acidity thus reducing the growth of pathogenic organisms.

Protein

Human milk contains less protein than any other mammalian milk (Akre 1989a) and this accounts in part for its more 'transparent' appearance. Human milk is *whey* dominant (the whey being mainly α-lactalbumin) and forms soft, flocculent curds when acidified in the stomach.

Allergic problems occur less frequently in breastfed babies than in artificially fed babies. This may be because the infant's intestinal mucosa is permeable to proteins before the age of 6–9 months and proteins in cow's milk can act as allergens. In particular, bovine β-lactoglobulin, which has no human milk protein counterpart, is capable of producing antigenic responses in atopic infants (Adler & Warner 1991, Bahna 1987).

Occasionally a baby may react adversely to substances in his mother's milk that come from her diet. However, this is rare and can be resolved by the mother identifying and avoiding the foods that cause the trouble so that she may continue to breastfeed.

Another bovine whey protein, bovine serum albumin, has been implicated as the trigger for the development of insulin-dependent diabetes mellitus (Paronen et al 2000, Vaarala et al 1999).

Vitamins

All the vitamins required for good nutrition and health are supplied in breastmilk, and although the actual amounts vary from mother to mother, none of the normal variations pose any risk to the infant (Worthington-Roberts 1993).

Fat-soluble vitamins

Vitamin A

Vitamin A is present in human milk as *retinol, retinyl esters* and *beta carotene*. Colostrum contains twice the amount present in mature human milk, and it is this that gives colostrum its yellow colour. Bile-salt-stimulated lipase (present in human milk – see fatty acids, above) assists the hydrolysation of the retinyl esters and may account for the rarity of vitamin A deficiency in breastfed babies in affluent societies (Fredrikzon et al 1978).

Vitamin D

Vitamin D plays an essential role in the metabolism of calcium and phosphorus in the body and prevents osteomalacia in adults and rickets in children, and is not strictly a vitamin, but a hormone triggered by ultraviolet light. It is the name given to two fat-soluble compounds, calciferol (vitamin D_2) and cholecalciferol (vitamin D_3). A plentiful supply of 7-dehydrocholesterol, the precursor of vitamin D_3, exists in human skin, and needs only to be activated by sufficient ultraviolet light (<30min of summer sunlight a day) to become fully potent.

For light-skinned babies, exposure to sunlight for 30min/week wearing only a nappy, or 2hrs/week fully clothed but without a hat, will keep vitamin D requirements within the lower limits of the normal range (Specker et al 1985).

However, the latitude and strength of the sunlight is important; research done in the 1970s in Scandinavia and the UK found that photo-conversion of 7-dehydrocholesterol (i.e. sunlight triggering the hormones to do their work) occurred only between March and October, with a maximum in June and July. Those living in regions where exposure to the sun is low have always been at risk for vitamin D deficiency (Garza & Ramussen 2000).

Pregnant women need to ensure that their vitamin D levels are high enough to supply sufficient amounts via the placenta to assure adequate stores in the baby's liver at birth, as the concentration of vitamin D in human milk is low.

It has been suggested (G. Palmer, pers comm) that 9 months is the perfect length for a pregnancy because at some stage the mother should ordinarily have been exposed to adequate sunlight.

In the past, if a baby was born in March the mother's vitamin D levels might be starting to dip by the time of the birth, but the spring sunshine would soon cause the baby's levels to rise. If the baby was born in October he/she might have been well provided for by his mother's (summer) sunlight exposure, but might be at slight risk by March. The introduction of other foods (6 months later) combined with spring sunshine, would raise the baby's levels.

However, in recent years, social mobility, cultural considerations, and concerns over skin cancer from sunlight have increased the risk of vitamin D deficiency by reducing the skin's exposure to sunlight. In the UK, this is of particular concern in women and infants of Asian and Afro-Caribbean ethnic origin (Gregory et al 2000, Leaf 2007).

Maternal vitamin D deficiency during pregnancy has been linked to maternal osteomalacia as well as reduced birthweight, neonatal hypocalcaemia and tetany (Cockburn et al 1980).

Vitamin D is fat soluble, and the principal unfortified dietary source is fish liver oils, with butter, eggs and cheese contributing much smaller amounts. In the UK, only margarine fortification (with 2800–3520 IU/kg of vitamin D) is compulsory. This began in 1940 when dietary sources were in short supply (Kendell & Adams 2002). (In other countries, vitamin D fortification of various other foods is either compulsory or permitted.)

Based on the Expert Group on Vitamins and Minerals (EVM) 2003 report, the Food Standards Agency currently recommends an intake for pregnant women of 10 µg (0.01 mg) (equivalent to 400 IU) of vitamin D each day.

In 2003, the American Academy of Pediatrics published new guidelines on preventing vitamin D deficiency in infants and children, and recommended an intake of 200 IU vitamin D/day, (5 µg) for all infants and children (Gartner & Greer 2003).

In line with these two recommendations, the New UK Healthy Start programme (see below) now provides vitamin D (and A and C) supplements free of charge for all eligible pregnant women and children.

The review of the evidence undertaken and published by NICE in 2008, contains recommendations as follows:

- During the booking appointment at the beginning of pregnancy, midwives should offer *every woman* information and advice on the benefits of taking a vitamin D supplement (10 µg (400 IU) per day) during pregnancy and while breastfeeding.

- They should explain that it will increase both the mother's and her baby's vitamin D stores and reduce the baby's risk of developing rickets.

- Health professionals should take particular care to check that women at greatest risk of deficiency are following advice to take a vitamin D supplement during pregnancy and while breastfeeding. These include women who are obese, have limited skin exposure to sunlight or who are of South-Asian, African, Caribbean or Middle Eastern descent.

- Midwives and health visitors should advise all pregnant and breastfeeding women about the availability of suitable vitamin D supplements such as the Healthy Start vitamin supplements. Women who are not eligible for Healthy Start benefit can obtain the vitamin supplement from their local community pharmacy.

Toxicity

Neither sunlight nor vitamin D consumed from the diet is likely to cause toxicity, unless large amounts of cod liver oil are consumed. It is much more likely to occur from high intakes of vitamin D in supplements, or possibly fortified foods.

Excessive vitamin D intake may lead to hypercalcaemia and hypercalciuria. Vitamin D promotes the absorption of calcium and the resorption of bone; in excess this would result in the deposition of calcium in soft tissues, diffuse demineralization of bones and irreversible renal and cardiovascular toxicity. Patients with sarcoidosis are abnormally sensitive to vitamin D, due to uncontrolled conversion of the vitamin to its active form in the granulomatous tissue.

Although the condition is uncommon, it would be a potential hazard if affected individuals were to take vitamin D in the form of supplements or possibly fortified foods.

In the general population, a daily supplement of 0.025 mg vitamin D (1000 IU) would not be expected to cause adverse effects. This is equivalent to 0.0004 mg/kg per day for a 60 kg adult (EVM 2003).

Vitamin E

Although vitamin E is present in human milk, its role is uncertain. It appears to prevent the oxidization of polyunsaturated fatty acids and may prevent certain types of anaemia to which preterm infants are susceptible.

Vitamin K

Vitamin K (83% of which is present as α-tocopherol), is essential for the synthesis of blood-clotting factors. It is present in human milk and absorbed efficiently. Because it is fat soluble, it is present in greater concentrations in colostrum and in the high fat hindmilk (Kries et al 1987), although the increased volume of milk as lactation progresses means that the infant obtains twice as much vitamin K from mature milk as he does from colostrum (Canfield et al 1991).

It has been suggested that by 2 weeks of age the breastfed baby's gut flora should be synthesizing adequate amounts of vitamin K (Akre 1989b), although others maintain that the diet is the only source of vitamin K in humans (Kries et al 1987).

Babies who are at risk of haemorrhage, such as the pre-term and those delivered precipitately or instrumentally, commonly receive a prophylactic dose, usually by intramuscular injection. Many paediatricians currently consider that all breastfed babies should receive vitamin K soon after birth, although there is little evidence to guide practice. Doubt currently exists as to how much and how often breastfed babies might require additional vitamin K (see Ch. 45). Research undertaken by Greer (1997) has confirmed earlier work suggesting that marked increases in breastmilk concentrations of vitamin K (and corresponding increases in infant blood levels) can be obtained by giving mothers oral vitamin K preparations, although whether this is necessary (since prothrombin times in infants were not altered) is still open to question. Policies in units throughout the UK vary widely, and there is no clear consensus on which babies are at increased risk of bleeding due to vitamin K deficiency (Ansell et al 2001).

Water-soluble vitamins

Unless the mother's diet is seriously deficient, breastmilk will contain adequate levels of all the vitamins. Since most vitamins are fairly widely distributed in foods, a diet significantly deficient in one vitamin will be deficient in others as well. Thus an improved diet will be more beneficial than artificial supplements. With some vitamins, particularly vitamin C, a plateau may be reached where increased maternal intake has no further impact on breastmilk composition.

Minerals and trace elements

Iron

Normal term babies are usually born with a high haemoglobin level (16–22 g/dL), which decreases rapidly after birth. The iron recovered from haemoglobin breakdown is re-utilized. They also have ample iron stores, sufficient for at least 4–6 months. Although the amounts of iron are less than those found in formulae, the bioavailability of iron in breastmilk is very much higher: 70% of the iron in breastmilk is absorbed, whereas only 10% is absorbed from a formula (Saarinen & Siimes 1979). The difference is due to a complex series of interactions that take place within the gut. Babies who are fed fresh cow's milk or a formula may become anaemic because of microhaemorrhages of the bowel.

Zinc

A deficiency of this essential trace mineral may result in failure to thrive and typical skin lesions. Although there is more zinc present in formulae than in human milk, the bioavailability is greater in human milk. Breastfed babies maintain high plasma zinc values compared with formula-fed infants, even when the concentration of zinc is three times that of human milk (Sandstrom et al 1983). Pre-term babies may need zinc supplements.

Calcium

Calcium is more efficiently absorbed from human milk than from breastmilk substitutes because of the higher calcium: phosphorus ratio of human milk. Infant formulas, which are based on cow's milk, inevitably have a higher phosphorus content than human milk, and this has been reported to increase the risk of neonatal tetany (Specker et al 1991).

Other minerals

Human milk has significantly lower levels of calcium, phosphorus, sodium and potassium than formulae. Copper, cobalt and selenium are present at higher levels. The higher bioavailability of these minerals and trace elements ensures that the infant's needs are met while also imposing a lower solute load on the neonatal kidney than do breastmilk substitutes.

Anti-infective factors

Leucocytes

During the first 10 days, there are more white cells/ mL in breastmilk than there are in blood. *Macrophages* and *neutrophils* are among the most common leucocytes in human milk and they surround and destroy harmful bacteria by their phagocytic activity.

Immunoglobulins

Five types of immunoglobulin have been identified in human milk: IgA, IgG, IgE, IgM and IgD. Of these the most important is *IgA*, which appears to be both synthesized and stored in the breast. Although some IgA is absorbed by the infant, much of it is not. Instead it 'paints' the intestinal epithelium and protects the mucosal surfaces against entry of pathogenic bacteria and enteroviruses. It affords protection against *Escherichia coli*, salmonellae, shigellae, streptococci, staphylococci, pneumococci, poliovirus and the rotaviruses.

Lysozyme

Lysozyme kills bacteria by disrupting their cell walls. The concentration of lysozyme increases with prolonged lactation (Hamosh 1998).

Lactoferrin

Lactoferrin binds to enteric iron, thus preventing potentially pathogenic *E. coli* from obtaining the iron they need for survival. It also has antiviral activity (against HIV, CMV and HSV), by interfering with virus absorption or penetration, or both.

Bifidus factor

Bifidus factor in human milk promotes the growth of Gram-positive bacilli in the gut flora, particularly *Lactobacillus bifidus*, which discourages the multiplication of pathogens. (Babies who are fed on cow's-milk-based formulae have more potentially pathogenic bacilli in their gut flora.)

Hormones and growth factors

Epidermal growth factor and *insulin-like growth factor* stimulate the baby's digestive tract to mature more quickly and strengthen the barrier properties of the gastrointestinal epithelium. Once the initially leaky membrane lining the gut matures, it is less likely to allow the passage of large molecules, and becomes less vulnerable to micro organisms. The timing of the first feed also has a significant effect on gut permeability, which drops markedly if the first feed takes place soon after birth.

Management of breastfeeding

Antenatal preparation

Breasts and nipples are altered by pregnancy (see Ch. 14). Increased sebum secretion obviates the need for cream to lubricate the nipple. Women who have inverted and non-protractile (flat) nipples often find that they improve spontaneously during pregnancy (Hytten & Baird 1958). If not, help given with attaching the baby to the breast after birth often results in successful breastfeeding. Neither the wearing of Woolwich shells nor Hoffmann's exercises are of any value (Main Trial Collaborative Group 1994) and should not be recommended, nor should any other un-evaluated commercially available device. Education of the mother is likely to be more use than any physical exercises.

The first feed

The mother should have her baby with her immediately after birth. Early and extended skin contact will ensure the cues that indicate that the baby is ready to feed will not be missed. Early feeding contributes to the success of breastfeeding but the time of the first feed should, to a large extent, depend on the needs of the baby. Some may demonstrate a desire to feed almost as soon as they are born. Other babies may show no interest until they are an hour or so old (Righard & Alade 1990, Widström et al 1987).

The first feed should be supervised by the midwife. If it proceeds without pain and if the baby is allowed to terminate the feed spontaneously, both mother and baby will have been helped to begin the learning process necessary for good breastfeeding in a happy and positive way.

The next feed

All mothers should be offered help with the next feed also. Once the baby is feeding satisfactorily the mother should be told about the cause, and therefore prevention, of sore nipples. She should be urged to seek help if problems do arise. She should be told about the changes that will take place in her breasts during the next few days. Helping mothers to understand that breastfeeding is a learned, not an instinctive, skill will enable them to be patient with themselves and their babies during this time (RCM 2001). Mothers who receive the right help and education at the start will require less support and remedial intervention later.

Positioning the mother

There are two main positions for the mother to adopt while she is breastfeeding. The first is *lying on her side* and this may be appropriate at different times during her lactation (see Plate 5). If she has had a caesarean section, or if her perineum is very painful, this may be the only position she can tolerate in the first few days after birth. It is likely that she will need assistance in placing the baby at the breast in this position, because she will only have one free hand. When feeding from the lower breast it may be helpful if she raises her body slightly by tucking the end of a pillow under her ribs. Once she can do this unaided she may find this a comfortable and convenient position for night feeds, enabling her to get more sleep.

The second position is *sitting up* (see Plate 6). In the early days it is particularly important that the mother's back is upright and at a right angle to her lap.

This is not possible if she is sitting in bed with her legs stretched out in front of her, or if she is sitting in a chair with a deep backward-sloping seat and a sloping back.

Both lying on her side and sitting correctly in a chair (with her back and feet supported) enhance the shape of the breast and also allow ample room in which to manoeuvre the baby.

Positioning the baby

The baby's body should be *turned towards* the mother's body (Fig. 41.4) so that he is coming up to her breast at the same angle as her breast is coming down to him. Thus the more the mother's breast points down, the more on his back he needs to be (Fig. 41.5). (The advice to have the baby *tummy to tummy* may be mistakenly taken to imply that the baby should always

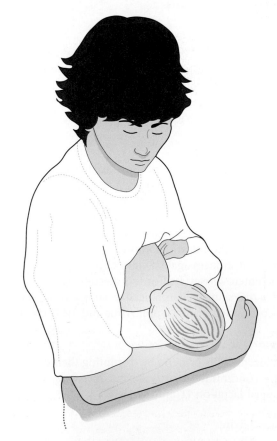

Figure 41.4 Baby turned towards the mother's body. (From an original drawing by Hilary English.)

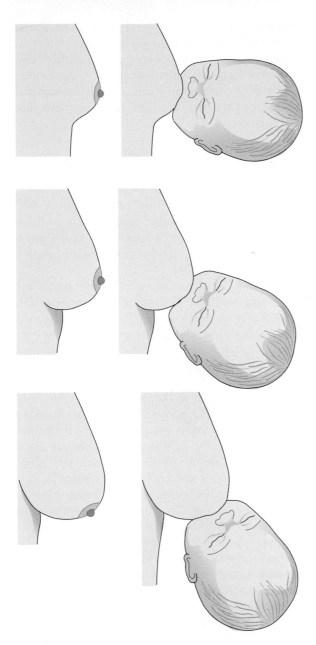

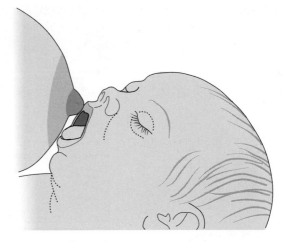

Figure 41.6 The baby's mouth opposite the nipple, the neck slightly extended. (From an original drawing by Jenny Inch.)

Attaching the baby to the breast

The baby should be supported across his shoulders, so that the slight extension of his neck can be maintained. His head may be supported by the extended fingers of the supporting hand (see Plate 7) or on his mother's forearm (see Plate 8). It may be helpful to wrap the baby in a small sheet (Vancouver wrap) so that his hands are by his sides (see Plate 9).

If the baby's mouth is moved gently but persistently against his mother's nipple he will open his mouth wide (see Plate 10). As he gapes (drops his lower jaw and darts his tongue down and forward) he needs to be moved quickly to the breast. The intention is to aim the bottom lip as far away from the base of the nipple as is possible. This allows the baby to draw breast tissue as well the nipple into his mouth with his tongue (see Plate 11). If correctly attached, the baby will have formed a 'teat' from the breast and the nipple (Fig. 41.7) (Woolridge 1986). The nipple should extend almost as far as the junction of the hard and soft palate. Contact with the hard palate triggers the sucking reflex. The baby's lower jaw moves up and down, following the action of the tongue. If the baby is well attached, minimal suction is required to hold the 'teat' within the oral cavity and the tongue can then apply rhythmical cycles of compression and relaxation so that milk is removed from the ducts. Although the mother may be startled by the physical sensation, she should not experience pain.

Figure 41.5 Baby's body in relation to the mother's body, depending on the angle of the breast. (From an original drawing by Hilary English.)

be lying on his side; taking account of the 'angle of the dangle' might be more useful). If the baby's nose is opposite his mother's nipple before he is brought to the breast and his neck is slightly extended, the baby's mouth will be in the correct relationship to the nipple (Fig. 41.6).

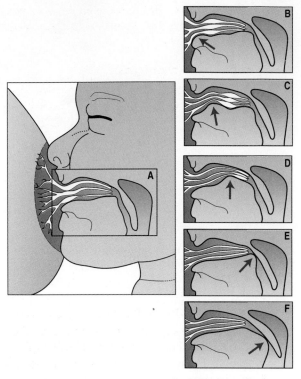

Figure 41.7   The baby has formed a 'teat' from the breast and the nipple, which causes the nipple to extend back as far as the junction of the hard and soft palates. The lactiferous ducts are within the baby's mouth. A generous portion of areola is covered by the bottom lip. (Reproduced from Woolridge 1986, with permission.)

The baby feeds from the breast rather than from the nipple and the mother should guide her baby towards her breast without distorting its shape. The baby's neck should be slightly extended and the chin should be in contact with the breast. If the baby approaches the breast as illustrated in Figure 41.6, a generous portion of areola will be taken in by the lower jaw, but it is positively unhelpful to urge the mother to try to get 'the whole of the areola' in the baby's mouth.

The role of the midwife

The midwife's role during the first few feeds is two-fold. First, she must ensure that the baby is adequately fed at the breast. Second, she must help the mother to develop the necessary skills so that she is able to feed her baby by herself. Women who have not breastfed before, need encouragement and reassurance (*emotional support*), they need to be taught the fundamentals of good attachment so that feeding is pain free (*practical support*) and they need to receive factual information about breastfeeding (*informational support*) in small, manageable chunks.

Some mothers will need more teaching and support than others.

Hands-on help from the midwife

Pragmatically, it may be necessary for the midwife to help attach the baby to the breast for several feeds. In this case, she should think of her own comfort, as well as that of the mother and her baby. She will put less strain on her own back if she kneels (on a foam mat) beside the mother, rather than bending over her (see Plate 12).

She should also consider which hand guides the baby most skillfully. For example, a right-handed midwife who is helping a mother who is lying on her left side will attach the baby to the left breast with her right hand. Instead of asking the mother to turn on her right side (so that she can feed from the right breast), the midwife could raise up the baby on a pillow and attach him to the right breast, again using her right hand. Alternatively, if the mother is sitting up, she could consider placing the baby under the mother's arm on the right side, so that she can again use her right hand. (Some midwives feel more comfortable if they stand behind the mother.)

Once the baby has fed efficiently he is more likely to do so again and it is from this point that the mother can begin to learn how to feed her baby by herself.

If the midwife needs to give hands-on help to the mother, she should also explain what she is doing, and why, so that the mother learns from the encounter. If no explanation is given, or the midwife just attaches the baby and leaves the mother, the mother may have help with every feed and yet still be unable to attach the baby to her breast herself days later.

Feeding behaviour

When the baby first goes to the breast he feeds vigorously, with few pauses. As the feed progresses, pausing occurs more frequently and lasts longer. Pausing is an integral part of the baby's feeding rhythm and should not be interrupted. The midwife should simply encourage the mother to allow the baby to pace the feed. The change in the pattern probably relates to milk flow. The foremilk, which he obtains first, is more generous in quantity but lower in fat than the hindmilk delivered at the end, which is thus higher in calories (Woolridge & Fisher 1988). If the baby receives an excessive quantity of foremilk (owing to either poor attachment or premature breast switching, see below), it may result in increased gut fermentation causing colic, flatus and explosive stools (Woolridge & Fisher 1988).

This is the commonest cause of colic in breastfed babies and is resolved by improving attachment. Simethicone preparations, which are often prescribed for this condition, have been shown to be of no value (Metcalf et al 1994).

Finishing the first breast and finishing a feed

The baby will release the breast when he has had sufficient milk from it. His ability to know this may be controlled either by the calories he has received or by the change in the volume available. The baby *should be offered* the second breast after he has had the opportunity to bring up wind. Sometimes in the early days the baby will not need to feed from the second breast.

The baby should not be deliberately removed from the breast before he releases it spontaneously, unless he is causing pain (in which case he should be reattached, if he is still willing). Taking the baby off the first breast before he has finished may cause two problems. First, the baby is deprived of the high calorie hindmilk; second, if adequate milk removal has not taken place, milk stasis may occur ultimately leading to mastitis or a reduced milk production, or both. Provided that the baby starts each feed on alternate sides, both breasts will be used equally. If the baby does not release the breast or will not settle after a feed, the most likely reason is that he had not been correctly attached to the breast and was therefore unable to remove the milk efficiently.

Other reasons for baby coming off the breast are:

- he may not have been correctly attached
- he may need to let go and pause if the milk flow is very fast
- he may have swallowed air with the generous flow of milk that occurs at the beginning of a feed and need an opportunity to burp.

There is *no justification* for imposing either *one breast per feed* or alternatively *both breasts per feed* as a feeding regimen.

Timing and frequency of feeds

A well, term baby knows better than anyone else how often and for how long he needs to be fed. This is described as baby-led feeding, which is a term preferable to 'demand feeding'.

It is not unusual in the 1st day or so for the baby to feed infrequently, and have 6–8 hrs gaps between good feeds, each of which may be quite long (Inch & Garforth 1989, Waldenström & Swensen 1991). This is normal and provides the mother with the opportunity to sleep if she needs to. As the milk volume increases, the feeds tend to become more frequent and a little shorter. It is unusual for a baby to feed less often than six times in 24 hrs from the 3rd day, and most babies ask for between six and eight feeds per 24 hrs by the time they are 1 week old. Babies who feed infrequently may be consuming less milk than they need, or they may be unwell, or both. Babies who feed very often (10–12 feeds in 24 hrs after the 1st week) may be poorly attached. The feeding technique and the weight should be monitored. However, individual mother–baby pairs develop their own unique pattern of feeding and, provided the baby is thriving and the mother is happy, there is no need to change it.

Volume of the feed

Well-grown term infants are born with good glycogen reserves and high levels of antidiuretic hormone. Consequently they do not need large volumes of milk or colostrum any sooner than these are made available physiologically. In the first 24 hrs, the baby takes an average of 7 mL per feed; in the second 24 hrs, this increases to 14 mL per feed (RCM 2001).

No precise information is available on the actual volume of breastmilk an individual baby requires in order to grow satisfactorily. Previous recommendations (150 mL/kg) were based on the requirements of *artificially fed* babies, and these can therefore be used only as a guideline.

Weight loss and weight gain

Most newborn babies lose some weight during their 1st week of life, and there is a general expectation that the baby will be back to birthweight by 10–14 days.

There is less agreement about how great a weight loss is within the bounds of normal or acceptable. Although the figure of 10% is often cited as the upper limit of normal, there is little evidence to support a figure as high as this. Data from nine studies conducted between 1986 and 1999 suggest a normal range of 3–7%; and more recently, normative data on 435 breastfed babies born in a Scottish 'Baby Friendly' Hospital, reported a median maximum weight loss of 6.6% (Macdonald et al 2003).

Over the first 4 days of life, the stools change from black meconium to the characteristic yellow stool of the baby, fed on breastmilk. A stool that is still 'changing' at 96 hrs of life could indicate that further attention needs to be paid to the way the mother is feeding her baby (see Plate 15).

If the baby is difficult to attach, because he is sleepy or because the breast tissue is inelastic, the same principles ought to apply to this situation as when the baby and mother are separated by virtue of illness or prematurity – namely to teach the mother how to hand express in order to get lactation established. If this is not done, the mother's lactation will be in arrears of her baby's needs when he starts to ask for larger volumes on the 3rd/4th day.

If the mother is still not able to feed effectively as the end of the 1st week approaches, she should make expressing her milk her priority, using either her hands or an effective breast pump, so that her lactation is secured and her baby is fed. Ongoing help with improving breastfeeding will also be needed.

Expressing breastmilk

Although all breastfeeding mothers should know how to hand express milk, *routine* expression of the breasts should not be part of the normal management of lactation, even for mothers who have delivered by caesarean section (Chapman et al 2001).

Provided that no limitation is placed on either feed frequency or duration and the baby is correctly attached, the volume of milk produced will be in step with the requirements of the baby. This will prevent the occurrence of problems (such as engorgement) that would require artificial removal of milk.

The situations where expressing *is* appropriate are:

- where there is concern about the interval between feeds in the early newborn period (expressed colostrum should always be given in preference to formulae to healthy term babies)
- where there are problems in attaching the baby to the breast
- where the baby is separated from the mother, due to prematurity or illness
- where there is concern about the baby's rate of growth, or the mother's milk supply (expressing to top up with the mother's own milk may be necessary in the short term while the cause of the problem is resolved
- later in lactation, when the mother may need to be separated from her baby for periods (occasionally or regularly).

Manual expression of milk

Manual expression has several advantages over mechanical pumping and should be taught to all mothers. It is usually the most efficient method of obtaining colostrum. Some mothers will find hand expressing superior to any breast pump, as illustrated in the new Joint Dept of Health/UNICEF leaflet 'Off to the best start'. There are now a variety of useful teaching aids available; models, videos and leaflets (contact UNICEF-UK Baby Friendly Initiative, see Useful addresses, below).

Expressing with a breast pump

If it is possible and practical, the mother should be able to experiment with a variety of breast pumps, so that she can discover what will suit her best (Auerbach & Walker 1994). Not all pumps work well for all women.

Hand pumps

Manually controlled

Most manually operated pumps are not efficient enough to allow initiation of full lactation but they can be useful when expressing is necessary in established lactation. It is helpful to mothers to explain that the pumps function most efficiently if the vacuum phase is considerably longer than the release phase.

Electrically controlled

Some pumps provide a regular vacuum and release cycle, with variability in the strength of the suction. Some vary the frequency of the cycle as well. Double pumping is possible with most models, and this has repeatedly been shown to be of benefit, either by reducing the time for which the mother needs to pump at each session to obtain the available milk (Groh-Wargo et al 1995, Hill et al 1999), or by increasing the volume of milk obtained, for mothers of both term (Auerbach 1990) and pre-term (Jones et al 2001) babies.

How much and how often?

The mothers of pre-term babies who begin pumping as soon as possible after birth and pump a *minimum* of six times per 24 hrs are more likely to sustain lactation at adequate levels than those who delay pumping or pump less frequently, or both. The earlier the mother is able to express good volumes of milk (per 24 hrs), the better the outlook for continued adequate milk production.

Breast massage (Jones et al 2001) and kangaroo care (Hill et al 1999) have also been positively associated with enhanced milk production.

No time limit should be set for the length of each expressing session. The mother should be guided by the milk flow, not the clock. Expressing should continue until milk flow slows, followed by a short break, and each breast should be expressed twice (either separately (sequential pumping) or together (double pumping)). When milk flow slows for the second time the session should end. Frequent pumping sessions are more likely to have the desired effect than infrequent marathons.

Inadequate milk volume, followed by declining production, are common problems for the mothers of pre-term babies who are expressing their milk. *Prevention*, by the midwife discussing with the mother the importance of early initiation, the appropriate use of the (correct size of) equipment and stressing the importance of the *frequency* (rather than regularity) of expression, is preferable to trying to rescue failing lactation pharmacologically.

Storage of mother's own breastmilk

NICE (2008) advises that expressed milk can be stored for:

- up to 5 days in the main part of a fridge, at 4°C or lower
- up to 2 weeks in the freezer compartment of a fridge
- up to 6 months in a domestic freezer, at minus 18°C or lower.

They also advise that mothers who wish to store expressed breastmilk for <5 days should do so in the fridge, as this preserves its properties more effectively than freezing.

Care of the breasts

Daily washing is all that is necessary for breast hygiene. The normal skin flora are beneficial to the baby. Brassieres may be worn in order to provide comfortable support and are useful if the breasts leak and breast pads (or breast shells) are used.

Breast problems

Sore and damaged nipples

The cause is almost always trauma from the baby's mouth and tongue, which results from incorrect attachment of the baby to the breast. Correcting this will provide immediate relief from pain and will also allow rapid healing to take place. Epithelial growth factor, contained in fresh human milk and saliva, may aid this process.

'Resting' the nipple also enables healing to take place but makes the continuation of lactation much more complicated because it is necessary to express the milk and to use some other means of feeding it to the baby.

Nipple shields should be used with extreme caution, and never before the mother has begun to lactate. They may make feeding less painful, but often they do not. Their use does not enable the mother to learn how to feed her baby correctly, and their longer term use may result in reduced milk transfer from mother to baby. This in turn may result in either mastitis in the mother (reduced milk removal), or slow weight gain or prolonged feeds in the baby (reduced milk transfer), or both. If mothers choose to use them, they should be advised to seek help with learning to attach the baby comfortably without a nipple shield as soon as practicable.

Other causes of soreness

Infection with *Candida albicans* (thrush) can occur, although it is not common during the 1st week. The sudden development of pain when the mother has had a period of trouble-free feeding is suggestive of thrush. The nipple and areola are often inflamed and shiny, and pain typically persists throughout the feed. The baby may show signs of oral or anal thrush. Both mother and baby should receive concurrent fungicidal treatment (such as miconazole, see Ch. 49) and it may take several days for the pain in the nipple to disappear.

Dermatitis

Sensitivity may develop to topical applications such as creams, ointments or sprays (including those used to treat thrush).

Anatomical variations

Long nipples

Long nipples can lead to poor feeding because the baby is able to latch on to the nipple without drawing breast tissue into his mouth.

Short nipples

Short nipples should not cause problems as the baby has to form a teat from both the breast and nipple.

Abnormally large nipples

If the baby is small, his mouth may not be able to get beyond the nipple and onto the breast. Lactation could be initiated by expressing, either by hand or by pump, provided that the nipple fits into the breast cup. As the baby grows and the breast and nipple become more protractile, breastfeeding may become possible.

Inverted and flat nipples

If the nipple is deeply inverted it may be necessary to initiate lactation by expressing and delay attempting to attach the baby to the breast until lactation is established and the breasts have become soft and the breast tissue more protractile.

Problems with breastfeeding

Engorgement

This condition occurs around the 3rd or 4th day postpartum. The breasts are hard (often oedematous), painful and sometimes flushed. The mother may be pyrexial. Engorgement is usually an indication that the baby is not in step with the stage of lactation. Engorgement may occur if feeds are delayed or restricted or if the baby is unable to feed efficiently because he is not correctly attached to the breast.

Management should be aimed at enabling the baby to feed well (Box 41.1). In severe cases the only solution will be the gentle use of a pump. This will reduce the tension in the breast and *will not* cause excessive milk production. The mother's fluid intake should not be restricted, as this has no effect on milk production.

Box 41.1 Babies who are difficult to attach

Inelastic breast tissue, overfull or engorged breasts or deeply inverted nipples may present the baby with more of a challenge.

- If the breast is engorged, pushing away the oedema by gently manipulating the tissue that lies under the areola may be all that is required
- Hand expression, or the use of a breast pump, may relieve fullness to the point where the baby can draw in the inner tissue to create the necessary teat from the breast
- If attachment is still difficult, try asking the mother to lie on her side with the short edge of a pillow under her ribs to raise the breast off the bed. Use your better hand to attach the baby
- If you are not able to attach the baby either, show the mother how to hand express and how to give her colostrum to her baby
- It may also be necessary to show her how to use the electric pump. In the first 24–48 h, the value of the pump is mainly in its effect on the nipple and breast tissue – colostrum is usually best expressed by hand.

When attachment is difficult, the priorities should be to ensure that the baby is adequately fed on his mother's milk, and to work on making the breast tissue more elastic (both of which can be facilitated by hand or electrical expressing). Attaching the baby to the breast directly can come later.

Deep breast pain

In most cases, this responds to improvement in breastfeeding technique and is thus likely to be due to raised intraductal pressure caused by inefficient milk removal. Although it may occur during the feed it typically occurs afterwards, and thus can be distinguished from the sensation of the let-down reflex, which some mothers experience as a fleeting pain. Very rarely, deep breast pain may be the result of ductal thrush infection.

Mastitis

Mastitis means inflammation of the breast. In the majority of cases, it is the result of milk stasis, not infection, although infection may supervene (Thomsen et al 1984). Typically, one or more adjacent segments are inflamed (as a result of milk being forced into the connective tissue of the breast) and appear as a wedge-shaped area of redness and swelling. If milk is also forced back into the bloodstream, the woman's pulse and temperature may rise and in some cases flu-like symptoms, including shivering attacks or rigors, may occur. (The presence or absence of systemic symptoms does not help to distinguish infectious from non-infectious mastitis; WHO 2000.)

Non-infective (acute intramammary) mastitis

Non-infective (acute intramammary) mastitis results from milk stasis. It may occur during the early days as the result of unresolved engorgement or at any time when poor feeding technique results in the milk from one or more segments of the breast not being efficiently removed by the baby. It occurs much more frequently in the breast that is opposite the mother's preferred side for holding her baby (Inch & Fisher 1995). Pressure from fingers or clothing has been blamed for causing the condition, without any supporting evidence. It is extremely important that breastfeeding from the affected breast continues, otherwise milk stasis will increase further and provide ideal conditions for pathogenic bacteria to replicate. An infective condition may then arise which could, if untreated, lead to abscess formation.

Where supervision is available, 12–24 hrs could be allowed to elapse to ascertain whether the mastitis can be resolved by helping the mother to improve her feeding technique and encouraging her to allow the baby to finish the first breast first. If supervision is not available, or if no improvement occurs during that period, antibiotics (e.g. cephalexin, flucloxacillin or erythromycin) should be given prophylactically (RCM 2001, WHO 2000).

Infective mastitis

The main cause of superficial breast infection is damage to the epithelium, which allows bacteria to enter the underlying tissues. The damage usually results from incorrect attachment of the baby to the breast, which has caused trauma to the nipple. The mother therefore urgently needs help to improve her technique, as well as the appropriate antibiotic. Multiplication of bacteria may be enhanced by the use of breast pads or shells. In spite of antibiotic therapy, abscess formation may occur. Infection may also enter the breast via the milk ducts if milk stasis remains unresolved.

Breast abscess

Here a fluctuant swelling develops in a previously inflamed area. Pus may be discharged from the nipple. Simple needle aspiration may be effective, or incision and drainage may be necessary (Dixon 1988). It may not be possible to feed from the affected breast for a few days; however, milk removal should continue and breastfeeding should recommence as soon as practicable because this has been shown to reduce the chances of further abscess formation (WHO 2000). A sinus that drains milk may form, but it is likely to heal in time.

Blocked ducts

Lumpy areas in the breast are not uncommon; the mother is usually feeling distended glandular tissue. If they become very firm and tender (and sometimes flushed) they are often described as 'blocked ducts'. This description carries with it the image of a physical obstruction within the lumen of the duct – like 'a golf ball in a hosepipe'. This is very rarely the cause of the symptoms. It is much more likely to be the case that milk removal has been somewhat uneven (as a consequence of less than optimal attachment) and that the secreted milk is now trying to occupy more space than is actually available – thus distending the alveoli. It may subsequently be forced out into the connective tissue of the breast where it causes inflammation. The inflammatory process then narrows the lumen of the duct by exerting pressure on it from the outside as the tissue swells. A more helpful image might therefore be that of 'compressing the hosepipe'. This is, effectively, mastitis or incipient mastitis. Consequently, the solution is to improve milk removal by improved attachment, and possibly milk expression as well and to treat the accompanying pain and inflammation. Massage, which is often advocated to clear the imagined 'blockage', may make matters worse by forcing more milk into the surrounding tissue.

White spots

Very occasionally, a ductal opening in the tip of the nipple may become obstructed by a white granule or by epithelial overgrowth.

White granules

White granules appear to be caused by the aggregation and fusion of casein micelles to which further materials become added. This hardened lump may obstruct a milk duct as it slowly makes its way down to the nipple, where it may be removed by the baby during a feed, or expressed manually (WHO 2000).

Epithelial overgrowth

Epithelial overgrowth seems to be the more common cause of a physical obstruction. A white blister is evident on the surface of the nipple, and it effectively closes off one of the exit points in the nipple, which leads from one or more milk-producing sections of the breast.

This may also be resolved by the baby feeding. Alternatively, after the baby has fed and the skin is softened, it may be removed with a clean fingernail, a rough flannel, or a sterile needle.

True blockages of this sort tend to recur, but once the woman understands how to deal with them, the progression to mastitis can be avoided.

Feeding difficulties due to the baby

Cleft lip

Provided that the palate is intact, the presence of a cleft in the lip should not interfere with breastfeeding because the vacuum that is necessary to enable the baby to attach to the breast is created between the tongue and the hard palate, not the breast and the lips.

Cleft palate

Because of the cleft, the baby is unable to create a vacuum and thus form a teat out of the breast and nipple. The use of an orthodontic plate is unlikely to help because the baby is unable to feel the breast against the hard palate and this is necessary to elicit the sucking response. There is no reason why the mother should be discouraged from putting the baby to the breast – for comfort, pleasure or food – provided that she is aware of the above and appreciates that it is likely that she will need to give her baby her expressed milk as well.

Many mothers have expressed their milk and used various techniques to feed it to their babies. A device called the Haberman feeder has proved useful. (These are now provided free of charge by CLAPA; see Useful addresses, below). Some mothers have maintained their lactation until the baby has had a surgical repair and have then succeeded in breastfeeding.

Tongue tie

If the baby cannot extend his tongue over his lower gum he is unlikely to be able to draw the breast deeply into his mouth, which he needs to do to feed effectively. Sometimes this is because the tongue is short, and sometimes this is because the frenulum, the whitish strip of tissue that attaches the tongue to the floor of the mouth, is preventing it. As the baby lifts his tongue, the tip becomes heart shaped as the frenulum pulls on it. Previous empirical evidence, which suggested that tongue-tie can interfere with breastfeeding, and of the value of frenotomy (surgical release of the frenulum, which takes a few seconds and is usually bloodless and painless), is now supported by evidence from ultrasound studies (Ramsay 2005) and clinical trials (Dollberg et al 2006, Hogan et al 2005).

The National Institute for Health and Clinical Excellence (NICE 2005) concluded that the division of tongue-tie to help babies with this condition to breastfeed was safe enough and worked well enough for use in the NHS.

Blocked nose

Babies normally breathe through their noses. If there is an obstruction, they have great difficulty with feeding because they have to interrupt the process in order to breathe. A blockage caused by mucus may be relieved with a twist of damp cotton wool, or by instilling drops of normal saline before a feed (Bollag et al 1984).

Down syndrome

Down syndrome babies can be successfully breastfed, although extra help and encouragement may be necessary initially.

Prematurity

Pre-term infants who are sufficiently mature to have developed sucking and swallowing reflexes may successfully breastfeed. Breastfeeding is less tiring than bottle feeding for the pre-term baby (Meier & Cranston-Anderson 1987). If the reflexes are not strongly developed, the baby may tire before the feed is complete and complementary tube feeding may be necessary.

Babies who are too immature to breastfeed may be able to cup feed, as an alternative to being tube-fed (Lang et al 1994). Less mature babies who are unable to suck or swallow at all will be dependent on artificial methods such as tube-feeding and intravenous alimentation.

Illness or surgery

Babies recover quickly following illness or surgery. If they have never been to the breast, or if feeding has been interrupted for a long period, the mother may require skilled help to initiate or re-establish feeding.

Contraindications to breastfeeding

Medications (see Ch. 49)

Breastfeeding may have to be suspended temporarily following the administration of certain drugs or following diagnostic techniques.

Most regions have drug centres where advice may be sought about the safety of drugs for lactating women.

Cancer

If the mother has cancer, the treatment she receives will make it impossible to breastfeed without harming the baby. However, if she wishes to, she could express and discard her milk for the duration of the treatment and resume breastfeeding later. If she has had a mastectomy, she may feed successfully from the other breast. She may also be able to breastfeed following a lumpectomy for cancer. She should seek advice from her surgeon.

Breast surgery

Neither breast reduction nor augmentation are an inevitable contraindication to breastfeeding, but much depends on the techniques used. Where possible, advice should be sought from the surgeon. If the nipple has been displaced, the duct system is not likely to be patent. Nickell & Skelton (2005) recommend that if surgery is proposed for a woman who wishes to breastfeed in the future, it may be possible to alter the surgery to preserve the ductal system.

Ultimately, the only way to determine if the breast will function effectively is to test it out by allowing the baby to go to the breast.

Breast injury

Injuries caused by scalding in childhood may cause such severe scarring that breastfeeding is impossible. Burns or other accidents may also cause serious damage.

One breast only

It is perfectly possible to feed a baby well using just one breast. If the mother has only one functioning breast, she should be reassured that in all women each breast works independently. If the baby is offered only one breast, that breast will make enough milk to feed that one baby. There are documented cases of women feeding two babies with just one breast (Nicolls 1997).

HIV infection

HIV may be transmitted in breastmilk. In developed countries, where artificial feeding is relatively safe, the mother may be advised not to breastfeed if she is HIV-positive (see Ch. 23). In countries where artificial feeding is a significant cause of infant mortality, exclusive breastfeeding may be the safer option (Coovadia et al 2007, Coutsoudis et al 1999).

Cessation of lactation

Suppression of lactation

If a mother chooses not to breastfeed or if she has a late miscarriage or stillbirth, lactation will still begin. The woman may experience discomfort for a day or two, but if unstimulated the breasts will naturally cease to produce milk. Very rarely severe discomfort with engorgement occurs. Expressing small amounts of milk once or twice can afford great relief without interfering with the rapid regression of the condition. The mother will be more comfortable if her breasts are supported but it is doubtful if binding the breasts contributes anything towards suppression.

There is no basis on which to advise the mother to restrict her fluid intake or to seek a prescription for a diuretic, which will be equally ineffective (Hodge 1967).

These measures merely add to the woman's discomfort by making her thirsty. Pharmacological suppression of lactation with dopamine receptor agonists is effective but is not recommended for routine use. Two such drugs, bromocriptine and cabergoline, are currently licensed for this use in the UK, although bromocriptine has now had its USA licence withdrawn.

Discontinuation of breastfeeding

Stopping lactation abruptly once breastfeeding has become established may cause serious problems for the mother. She could develop engorgement or mastitis, or even a breast abscess. She should be encouraged to mimic normal weaning by expressing her breasts but reducing the frequency over several days or possibly weeks. The gradual reduction in the volume of milk removed will result in a corresponding diminution in the production of milk. Eventually she should be encouraged to express only if she feels uncomfortable. Cabergoline might be appropriate following the death of a baby.

Returning to work

If the breastfeeding mother returns to work, her baby will have to be fed in her absence. She may wish her baby to have her own milk at all times and she may express for this purpose.

If the mother finds it difficult to express at work, her baby could receive a formula feed (or 'solid' food if over 6 months) while she is away, but breastfeed at all other times. Returning to work does not mean that breastfeeding has to be terminated.

Weaning from the breast

When the mother or the baby decides to stop breastfeeding, feeds should be tailed off gradually. Breastfeeds may be omitted, one at a time, and spaced further apart. Adding supplementary foods should not begin until about 6 months of age. If the mother is using solid food to give the baby 'tastes' and the experience of different textures before weaning, these should be given after the breastfeed. Solid foods given before the breastfeed (weaning) will result in the baby taking less milk from the breast and thus less will be produced. Allowing the baby to lead the process of weaning (Rapley 2006) may make the transition much easier.

Complementary and supplementary feeds

Complementary feeds (or 'top-ups') are feeds given *after* a breastfeed. Complementary feeds of breastmilk substitutes ('formula milk') should be given as a last resort, not as a quick fix. *Any formula at all* is enough to sensitize susceptible infants (Host 1991).

In Bolling et al's study (2005) 33% of babies born in UK hospitals receive breastmilk substitutes while in hospital. The only demonstrable effect of giving complementary feeds in hospitals is to reduce the overall duration of breastfeeding. The mothers of these babies are three times more likely to have given up breastfeeding by the time their baby is 2 weeks old, in comparison with mothers whose babies have received only breastmilk (White et al 1992).

About 10% of newborns are at risk for hypoglycaemia (see Ch.48), and may thus need a higher intake straight from birth than their mothers are able to provide. Where possible this should be human milk – from a human milk bank.

Babies who are well but sleepy (Box 41.2), jaundiced (see Ch. 47), unsettled (Box 41.3), or difficult to attach (Box 41.1), should, if necessary, be given their mother's own expressed milk in addition to being offered the breast.

If complementary feeds are clinically indicated and the mother is unable to express sufficiently,

---

Box 41.2 'Sleepy' babies

Provided that the baby is otherwise well, which will be determined by checking the baby from time to time, there is no evidence that long intervals between feeds have any adverse affect. As few as three feeds in the first 24 hrs of life is within the normal range.

- The baby could remain in bed with his mother (in accordance with hospital guidelines). His mother will thus be able to respond immediately to her baby's feeding cues

- The baby could be roused at intervals, possibly by changing the nappy, and offered the breast

- The baby could be undressed down to the nappy and placed in skin contact with his mother and offered the breast

- The mother could be shown how to hand express some colostrum, and how to give this to the baby

- It is unnecessary to measure the baby's blood sugar (see Ch. 48).

Box 41.3 If the baby is unsettled

An unsettled baby of any age that is crying again soon after he has been fed may not have been well attached.

- Watch what the mother is doing and, if necessary, guide her or help her directly

- If the attachment is good, then the baby may be reacting to being removed from the closeness of his mother's body. If the mother needs to sleep, suggest that she feed lying down and help her if necessary. Use the cot-side/bed guard to ensure the safety of the baby (as per hospital guidelines for their use)

- The mother might try to express some colostrum/ milk to give to the baby if she is concerned that the baby has not received all that he might from the breast

- Some babies will appear unsettled even if they have fed well at the breast. The baby may be uncomfortable. The act of changing the nappy

may help; so may wrapping the baby comfortably but securely and providing rhythmic motion, such as walking or holding the baby over the shoulder or over the forearm, both of which apply gentle pressure to the baby's abdomen

- Show the mother what you are doing, so that she learns appropriate coping strategies from you

- If *you* give the baby formula or a dummy to 'settle' him, that is what the mother will do when she goes home

- *Do not offer* to remove the baby. Separating mother and baby – particularly removing the baby at night in the mistaken belief that the mother will benefit if she does not wake to breastfeed her baby at night – is strongly correlated with reduced breastfeeding success

- If the mother *asks* you to – and you agree – return the baby to her when he wakes again to be fed.

---

donor milk from a human milk bank could be used. Donors will have been serologically tested for HIV and a negative result received before their milk can be accepted.

If the baby is very young, these additional feeds should be given by oral syringe or cup rather than in a bottle. An oral syringe (or dropper) will reduce wastage and the use of a cup would allow the baby to remain more in control of his intake.

If the problem (such as attachment difficulty) persists, the mother may find it quicker and more efficient to give her expressed milk by bottle. She should be reassured that there is no evidence that the baby will subsequently refuse the breast in these circumstances (Brown et al 1999, Howard et al 2003, Schubiger et al 1997).

Supplementary feeds are feeds given *in place of* a breastfeed. There can be no justification for their use except in extreme circumstances (such as severe illness or unconsciousness) because each breastfeed missed by the baby will interfere with the establishment of lactation and damage the mother's confidence.

Human milk banking

In the late 1970s and early 1980s there were over 60 human milk banks in the UK. Most of them closed in the late 1980s, driven by both the fear of HIV transmission and the rising popularity of pre-term formulae. By the early 1990s there were only six milk banks left in the UK.

Slowly this number has risen, encouraged by research that demonstrated the effectiveness of pasteurization as a means of destroying HIV (Eglin & Wilkinson 1987) and the importance of human milk in the prevention of necrotizing enterocolitis (Lucas & Cole 1990); and aided by the formation, in 1998, of the UK Human Milk Banking Association (UKAMB). Banked human milk is used predominantly for pre-term and sick newborns. Occasionally, if there is sufficient, it is used for term babies whose mothers are temporarily unable to meet their babies' needs with their own (expressed) milk. Mothers who are offered donated milk for their babies should have sufficient

information about the collection and screening of human milk to enable them to make an informed choice whether to accept it or not (Box 41.4).

Feeding the baby – breast or bottle?

Although the majority of women who choose to breastfeed have made this decision very early on, some may not make a final decision until after giving birth. Asking the mother to make a decision antenatally is unhelpful, as it may close the door to further discussion or make her feel that she cannot change her mind, or both.

The subject may be more usefully raised as part of an ongoing discussion in later pregnancy. The midwife should ensure that the mother is aware of the risks of artificial feeding, and knows what the usual practice of the hospital is in relation to skin contact at birth, the management of breastfeeding, rooming-in and so on, so that the woman can make her own preferences known.

Actually seeing a baby being breastfed can strongly influence the decision to breastfeed either positively or negatively, depending on the context (Hoddinott

---

Box 41.4 Donated breastmilk

If you are offering a mother donated human milk for her baby for any reason, she might find the information below helpful in deciding whether to accept it.

- All human milk donors meet the same criteria as blood donors; they are in a low risk group to start with and give consent to an HIV blood test
- All human milk donors sign a form to that effect and all have their blood tested
- Almost all donors are currently feeding their own baby while donating
- No donated milk is used for any baby until the results of the donor's blood test have been received
- All donated milk is collected in sterilized bottles, kept in the fridge and frozen within 24 hrs

- When it arrives, still frozen, at the milk bank, it is thawed, a small sample taken for bacteriological screening and the rest pasteurized
- After pasteurization another small sample is taken (for post-pasteurization bacteriological screening) and the rest refrozen in a holding freezer
- Only when the results of both samples have been received is the milk transferred to the freezer from which it can be used for pre-term and term babies
- Donors are not paid for the milk they donate – it is freely given! Quite often, mothers choose to donate milk because their own babies were themselves helped in this way by the generosity of other mothers.

& Pill 1999). This may be of particular relevance to women for whom theoretical knowledge may have less power than embodied knowledge. It has therefore been suggested that women intending to breastfeed might benefit from an antenatal 'apprenticeship' with a known breastfeeding mother. Peer group support can influence both the initiation and the continuation of breastfeeding (Fairbank et al 2000), and introducing pregnant women to other mothers with young babies, may be helpful.

Time should be taken during the antenatal period to talk briefly about the day-to-day progress and management of early breastfeeding. The woman should be aware that breastfeeding is a learned skill, that it should not hurt and that she may well receive conflicting advice. This does not mean that she will not need to be taught about the major details of management after the baby is born. The midwife's responsibility to the woman is to ensure that her choice is 'fully informed', rather than to persuade her to breastfeed. She will be unable to do this if the midwife withholds information from her.

The nutritional and immunological consequences of not breastfeeding are seen in population studies, and are to do with relative risks. It is not possible to narrow the risk down to the individual. Nevertheless all pregnant women should be made aware that, compared with a fully breastfed baby, a baby who is bottle-fed from birth is:

- five times more likely to be hospitalized with gastroenteritis (within the first 3 months of life)
- five times more likely to suffer from urine infections (within the first 6 months of life)
- twice as likely to suffer from chest infections (within the first 7 years of life)
- twice as likely to suffer from ear infections (within the 1st year of life)
- twice as likely to develop atopic disease where there is a family history
- up to 20 times more likely to develop necrotizing enterocolitis if born prematurely.

Additionally, the pregnant woman should know that she may increase her own risk of pre-menopausal breast cancer, ovarian cancer and osteoporosis if she does not breastfeed (UNICEF and Department of Health 2007).

Artificial feeding

Most breastmilk substitutes (infant formulae) are modified cow's milk. Until the early 1970s, they consisted of crudely modified dried cow's milk with added vitamins. Their high solute loads contributed to infantile hypocalcaemia and to hypernatraemic dehydration.

Currently, the minimum and maximum permitted levels of named ingredients, and named prohibited ingredients, are now laid down by statute in the Infant Formula and Follow-on Formula Regulations 1995. However, considerable variations in composition can (and do) exist within the legally permitted ranges. Over 100 changes a year have been made to commercially available breastmilk substitutes (Messenger 1994).

The two main components used are *skimmed milk* (a by-product of butter manufacture) and *whey* (a by-product of cheese manufacture). Breastmilk substitutes may contain fats from any source, animal or vegetable (except from sesame and cotton seeds), provided that they do not contain >8% transisomers of fatty acids. The fat source may not always be apparent from reading the label: oleo, for example, is beef fat – unacceptable to Hindus and vegetarians; 'oils of vegetable origin' may have come from marine algae. They may also contain, among other things, soya protein, maltodextrin, dried glucose syrup and gelatinized and pre-cooked starch.

Formulae

There are two main types of formula: whey dominant and casein dominant. Both can be used from birth.

Whey-dominant formulae

In these, a small amount of skimmed milk is combined with demineralized whey. The ratio of proteins in the formulae approximates to the ratio of whey to casein found in human milk (60:40). These feeds are more easily digested than the casein-dominant formulae, which will have an effect on gastric emptying times. This leads to feeding patterns that more closely resemble those of breastfed babies.

Casein-dominant formulae

These are also sold as being suitable for use from birth, but they are aimed at mothers whose babies are 'hungrier'. Although the proportions of the macronutrients (fat, carbohydrate, protein, etc.) are the same as is found in whey-dominant formulae, more of the protein present is in the form of casein (20:80). This forms large relatively indigestible curds in the stomach and is intended to make the baby feel full for longer. This will inevitably place even greater metabolic demands on the infant.

Babies intolerant of standard formulae

Predicting which babies will be prone to allergies is an inexact science. It is estimated that the likelihood of a child being predisposed to allergy is about 20–35% if one parent is affected, 40–60% if both parents are affected and 50–70% if both parents have the same allergy (Brostoff & Gamlin 1998, p 261).

Hydrolysate formula

If breastfeeding is not possible, there are (prescription-only) alternatives that carry less risk of allergy than standard formulas – hydrolysates – some of which are designed to *treat* an existing allergy, and some of which are designed for *preventative* use in bottle-fed babies who are at high risk of developing cow's milk protein allergy (Brostoff & Gamlin 1998, p 232). This is reflected in the British National Formulary prescribing guidelines, which require 'proven intolerance' for some hydrolysates, but not for others.

These substances are considerably more expensive than either standard or soya-based formula.

Hydrolysate formula is made of cow's milk, cornstarch and other foods, which is then treated with digestive enzymes so that the milk proteins are partially broken down. This makes them a good deal less allergenic, although they may still cause problems to babies who are highly allergenic.

Whey hydrolysates

These are made from the whey of cow's milk (rather than whole milk) and are thought to be potentially more useful for highly allergenic babies. However, NICE guidance (2008) maintains that there is insufficient evidence to suggest that infant formula based on partially or extensively hydrolysed cow's milk protein helps to prevent allergies.

Amino-acid-based formula, or elemental formula

Amino-acid-based formula, or elemental formula has a completely synthetic protein base, providing the essential and non-essential amino acids, together with fat, maltodextrin, vitamins, minerals and trace elements. (It is very expensive.)

Soya-based formula

Soya-based formula was developed as a response to the emergence of cow's milk protein intolerance in babies fed cow's-milk-based formulae and has been covered by the Infant Formula and Follow-on Formula Regulations since 1995. It was subsequently approved for use (by the Advisory Committee for Borderline Substances) as the sole source of nourishment for young infants and could be purchased without prescription.

However in 2004, The Chief Medical Officer recommended that *soya-based formulas should only be used in exceptional circumstances* to ensure adequate nutrition. For example, they may be given to infants of vegan parents who are not breastfeeding or infants who find alternatives (such as amino acid formulae) unacceptable.

This edict was in response to mounting evidence that soya-based formula's high phytoestrogen content could pose a risk to the long-term reproductive health of infants (Martyn 1999, Minchin 2001), and the advice from the UK's Scientific Advisory Committee on Nutrition (SACN), which questioned the benefit of using any milk protein other than from cows, or any plant protein, including soya (SACN 2003).

Furthermore, many babies who are intolerant of cow's milk are also intolerant of soya. Early soya formula feeding runs the risk of inducing soya protein intolerance in the child and soya protein is much harder to avoid in the weaning diet than dairy products.

Goats' milk formula

In 2006, the European Food Standards Agency concluded that there are insufficient data to establish the suitability of goats' milk protein as a protein source in infant formula. Therefore, since March

2007, infant milks based on goats' milk can no longer be sold in the UK (for further information, see http://www.efsa.eu.int/science/nda/nda_statements/catindex_en.html).

Choosing a breastmilk substitute

Although not always enforced in the past, it is an offence (under UK law) to sell any infant formula as being suitable from birth unless it meets the compositional and other criteria set out in the Infant Formula and Follow-on Formula Regulations 1995. Despite the claims made by formula manufacturers, there is no obvious scientific basis on which to recommend one brand over another.

There is no necessity for the mother to stick to one brand. If she finds that one brand seems to disagree with her baby, she could try switching brands. This has been made easier by the availability of ready-to-feed sachets or cartons, as, with these, mothers can experiment without having to buy large quantities.

Babies with underlying metabolic disorders, such as galactosaemia or phenylketonuria, will need the appropriate, prescribable breastmilk substitute.

Artificial milks are highly processed, factory-produced products. Inevitably, there will be inadvertent errors. Recorded errors in the past include too much or too little of an ingredient, accidental contamination, incorrect labelling and foreign bodies.

Mothers should be advised to inspect the contents of the tin or packet before using it – and if it looks or smells strange, to return it to the place it was purchased.

Preparation of an artificial feed

The introduction of ready-to-feed formula in hospital may have saved staff time, but it reduces the likelihood that the mother who artificially feeds will have been shown how to prepare a bottle feed safely before she goes home (Kaufmann 1999).

All powdered formula feed available in the UK is now reconstituted using one scoopful (provided with the powder) to 30 mL of water. Clear instructions about the volumes of powder and water are also printed on the container.

Many of the major UK manufacturers of formula now produce ready-to-feed cartons which reduces the risk of over or under concentration, but the higher cost of these will preclude universal use.

Another advantage of ready-to-feed formula, is that the contents are sterile prior to opening. Powdered milk, in tins or packets, is not. In response to growing concerns about bacterial contaminants in these powders, the Food Safety Agency (FSA) and Department of Health have changed their recommendations in relation to their reconstitution. Since February 2006, those making up feeds from powder are advised to make each feed just before it is needed, using water that has boiled and cooled to 70°C, adding the powder, allowing the milk to cool and giving the feed straight away. Any remaining milk should be discarded.

An updated leaflet 'Preparing a bottle feed using baby milk powder' is available as a single A4 sheet of instructions (in English). This can be downloaded, free of charge, from the UNICEF UK Baby Friendly website. A similar, companion leaflet 'Sterilization of baby feeding equipment' is also available.

The water supply

It is essential that the water used is free from bacterial contamination and any harmful chemicals. It is generally assumed in the UK that boiled tap water will meet these criteria, but from time to time, this is shown not to be the case. In some areas of the UK, mothers who are artificially feeding their babies have to be provided with a separate supply of water because the tap water is not suitable for babies' consumption.

If bottled water is used, a still, non-mineralized variety suitable for babies must be chosen and it should be boiled as usual. Softened water is usually unsuitable.

Feeding equipment

Concern has been voiced about the nitrosamine content of rubber teats; in some countries mothers have been urged to boil the teat several times with fresh water before using. Silicone teats are now available but, as these have been known to split, the mother should be urged to check for signs of damage in order to ensure that the baby does not swallow any fragments.

It is often easier for the baby to use a simple soft long teat than industry-labelled orthodontic teats (Kassing 2002).

No bottle teat is like a breast. Real-time ultrasound of infants during sucking using different types of teats were measured by researchers (Nowak et al 1994) to determine the percentage lengthening, the percentage lateral compression, and the percentage flattening of the teats. These results were compared with data obtained from studies using breastfed infants. None of the teats lengthened like the human nipple. More recently, Scheel et al (2005) investigated the relative merits of three different types of teats. The rate of milk transfer (mL/min) for the pre-term babies studied was the primary outcome measure. The suction amplitude, and duration of the generated negative intra-oral suction pressure were also measured. No type of teat had any advantage over any other. The mother should feel free to experiment, and use the type of teat that seems to suit her baby.

Feeding bottles should meet the UK standard. This means they will be made of food-grade plastic and have relatively smooth interiors. Crevices and grooves in a bottle may make cleaning difficult. Patterned or decorated bottles may make it less easy to see whether the bottle is clean.

Sterilization of feeding equipment

The effective cleaning of all utensils used should be demonstrated and the method of sterilization discussed. If boiling is to be used, full immersion is essential and the contents of the pan must be boiled for 10min. If cold sterilization using a hypochlorite solution is the method of choice, the utensils must be fully immersed in the solution for the recommended time. The manufacturer's advice should be followed with regard to rinsing items that have been removed from the solution. If the item is to be rinsed, previously boiled water should be used and not water direct from the tap. Both steam and microwave sterilization are now possible, but the mother should check that her equipment can withstand it.

Bottle teats

The size of the hole in the teat causes much anxiety to mothers. It is probably a good idea to have several teats with holes of different sizes so that the mother can experiment as necessary. A useful test for the correct hole size is to turn the bottle upside down; the milk should drip at a rate of about one drop per second.

Feeding the baby with the bottle

Mothers should be warned about the dangers of 'bottle propping', and told that the baby must never be left unattended while feeding from a bottle. They should be told about the need of the baby to relate to a small number of caregivers and that he should not be passed from person to person for feeding.

The baby is 'programmed' to feed from a breast and the mother should use the baby's innate skills when bottle-feeding. The baby's lips should be touched to elicit a gape and the teat should follow the line of the baby's tongue, so that the baby uses the teat effectively. The mother should try to simulate breastfeeding conditions for the baby by holding him close, maintaining eye-to-eye contact and allowing him to determine his intake.

Modern formulae do not, when correctly prepared, cause hypernatraemia, as did the older types. There is therefore no need to give the baby extra water.

The stools and vomit of a formula-fed baby have an unpleasant sour smell. The stools tend to be more formed than those of a breastfed baby and, unlike a breastfed baby, there is a real risk that the artificially fed baby may become constipated.

Healthy Start (and the Welfare Food Scheme)

In 1940 the Welfare Food Scheme was established in the UK. This provided tokens to families on low incomes, which could be exchanged for liquid milk or breastmilk substitutes. This scheme was replaced, in November 2006, by the Health Start Initiative (for more information, see http://www.healthystart.nhs.uk). The new scheme broadened the nutritional base of the scheme to allow fruit and vegetables (as well as liquid milk or breastmilk substitutes previously provided) to be obtained through the exchange of fixed value vouchers at a range of outlets, including local food co-ops and supermarkets.

Those eligible to receive the vouchers include:

- pregnant women and families with children under the age of 4 years who are on:
  - Income Support
  - Income-based Jobseeker's Allowance or
  - Child Tax Credit (but not Working Tax Credit) with an income of $\leq£14495$ a year (in 2008)

- And all pregnant women under the age of 18, whether or not they are receiving benefits.

Those eligible for the vouchers are also entitled to free vitamin supplements for themselves and also for their children from 6 months until their 4th birthday.

Midwives and the International code of marketing of breastmilk substitutes

In 1981, the combined forces of WHO and the United Nations Children's Fund (UNICEF) produced this Code (WHO 1981), which was adopted at the 34th World Health Assembly. The Code has major implications for the work of midwives. Although it is at present a voluntary code in most countries, some countries now have the code enshrined in law.

Recommendations in the code include:

- no advertising or promotion in hospitals, shops or to the general public (this includes posters in hospitals and advertisements in mother-and-baby books)
- no free samples of breastmilk substitutes to be given to mothers
- no free gifts relating to products within the scope of the code to be given to mothers (including discount coupons or special offers)
- no financial or material gifts to be given to health workers for the purpose of promoting products, nor free or subsidized supplies to hospitals or maternity wards

- information provided by manufacturers to health workers should include only scientific and factual material, and should not create or imply a belief that bottle-feeding is equivalent or superior to breastfeeding
- health workers should encourage and protect breastfeeding.

The code does not prevent mothers from bottle-feeding but rather seeks to contribute to safe, adequate nutrition for infants and to promote and protect breastfeeding.

The Baby Friendly Hospital Initiative

The Baby Friendly Hospital Initiative (see: www.babyfriendly.org.uk) is an initiative that was launched worldwide in 1991 (and in the UK in 1994) by WHO and UNICEF to encourage hospitals to promote practices that are supportive of breastfeeding. It was focused around the '10 steps' (Box 41.5), with which all hospitals who wish to achieve 'Baby Friendly' status must comply (WHO 1989). The evidence for the 10 steps is contained in the WHO/UNICEF document of the same name (Vallenas & Savage 1998).

In addition, all 'Baby Friendly Hospitals' will fully implement the International code on the marketing of breastmilk substitutes. Thus if babies are born in a Baby Friendly Hospital, mothers will expect a certain standard of care:

Box 41.5 The 10 steps

1. Have a written breastfeeding policy that is routinely communicated to all healthcare staff
2. Train all healthcare staff in skills necessary to implement this policy
3. Inform all pregnant women about the benefits and management of breastfeeding
4. Help mothers initiate breastfeeding soon after birth
5. Show mothers how to breastfeed and how to maintain lactation even if they should be separated from their infants
6. Give newborn infants no food or drink other than breastmilk, unless medically indicated
7. Practice rooming-in: allow mothers and infants to remain together 24 hrs a day
8. Encourage breastfeeding on demand
9. Give no artificial teats or dummies to breastfeeding infants
10. Foster the establishment of breastfeeding support groups and refer mothers to them on discharge from hospital or clinic.

While they are pregnant they will expect:

- to have a full discussion about caring for and feeding their baby, including the benefits of breastfeeding, so that they have all the facts they need to make an informed choice.

When the baby is born they will expect:

- to be given their baby to hold against their skin straight after he is born, for as long as they want
- that a midwife will offer to help them start breastfeeding as soon as possible after the baby is born
- that their baby will stay with them at all times.

If they decide to breastfeed they will expect:

- a midwife to show them how to hold the baby and how to help him latch on – in order to make sure he gets enough milk and that feeding is not painful
- to be given accurate and consistent advice about how to breastfeed and how to make enough milk for the baby
- that a midwife will offer to show them how to express milk by hand

- to receive information about how to get more support for breastfeeding, should they need it, once they leave hospital
- the baby *not* to be given water or artificial baby milk, unless this is needed for a medical reason.

A mother will expect that the staff will support her even if she decides that she wants to care for her baby differently or if she does not want the information offered. If she decides to bottle-feed, she will expect to be asked if she wants to be shown how to make up a bottle-feed correctly.

The National Institute for Health and Clinical Excellence (NICE 2006) recommended that all maternity care providers should implement an externally evaluated, structured programme that encourages breastfeeding, using the Baby Friendly Initiative as a minimum standard. Acute and Primary Care Trusts are expected to implement NICE guidance and would be required to perform a risk assessment (to be placed on a risk register) if they rejected it. Rejection on the grounds of cost (which has often been cited as a reason for not implementing BFI in the past) is unlikely to be acceptable, as NICE economists have documented the fact that implementation would be cost-effective (see costing Report: http://www.nice.org.uk/download.aspx?o=345136).

REFERENCES

Adler B R, Warner J O 1991 Food intolerance in children. Royal College of General Practitioners members reference book. Camden Publishing, London, p 497–502

Akre J 1989a Infant feeding: the physiological basis. Bulletin of the World Health Organization 67(Suppl 1):25

Akre J 1989b Infant feeding: the physiological basis. Bulletin of the World Health Organization 67(Suppl 1):79

Ansell P, Roman E, Fear N et al 2001 Vitamin K policies and midwifery practice: questionnaire survey. British Medical Journal 322:1148–1152

Ashraf R N, Jalil F, Aperia A et al 1993 Additional water is not needed for healthy babies in a hot climate. Acta Paediatrica 82:1007–1011

Auerbach K G 1990 Sequential and simultaneous breast pumping: a comparison. International Journal of Nursing Studies 27(3): 257–265

Auerbach K G, Walker M 1994 When the mother of a premature infant uses a pump: what every NICU nurse needs to know. Neonatal Network 13(4):23–29

Baby Milk Action 2001 Update. No. 29 (June):3. Online. Available: www.ibfan.org

Bahna S L 1987 Milk allergy in infancy. Annals of Allergy 59:131–136

Bollag U, Albrecht E, Wingert W 1984 Medicated versus saline nose drops in the management of upper respiratory infection. Helvetica Paediatrica Acta 39(4):341–345

Bolling K, Grant C, Hamlyn B et al 2005 Infant Feeding Survey. A survey conducted on behalf of The Information Centre for health and social care and the UK Health Departments by BMRB Social Research. Online. Available: www.ic.nhs.uk/pubs/breastfeed2005

Brostoff J, Gamlin L 1998 The complete guide to allergy and food intolerance. Bloomsbury Publishing, London, p 232, 261

Brown S J, Alexander J, Thomas P 1999 Feeding outcome in breast-fed term babies supplemented by cup or bottle. Midwifery 15:92–96

Butte N F, Garza C, Stuff J E et al 1984 Effect of maternal diet and body composition on lactational performance. American Journal of Clinical Nutrition 39:296–306

Canfield L M, Hopkinson J M, Lima A F et al 1991 Vitamin K in colostrum and mature human milk over the lactation period – a cross sectional study. American Journal of Clinical Nutrition 53(3):730–735

Carvahlo M, Hall M, Harvey D 1981 Effects of water supplementation on physiological jaundice in breast-fed babies. Archives of Disease in Childhood 56:568–569

Chapman D J, Young S, Ferris A M et al 2001 Impact of breast pumping on lactogenesis stage II after caesarean delivery: a randomized clinical trial. Pediatrics 107(6):E94

Cockburn F, Belton N R, Purvis RJ et al 1980 Maternal vitamin D intake and mineral metabolism in mothers and their newborn infants. British Medical Journal 281(6232):11–14

Coovadia H M, Rollins N C, Bland R M et al 2007. Mother-to-child transmission of HIV-1 infection during exclusive breast-feeding in the first 6 months of life: an intervention cohort study. Lancet 369(9567):1107–1116

Coutsoudis A, Pillay K, Spooner E et al 1999 Influence of infant-feeding patterns on early mother-to-child transmission of HIV-1 in Durban, South Africa: a prospective cohort study. South African Vitamin A Study Group. Lancet 354 (9177):471–476

Cross BA 1977 Comparative physiology of milk removal. Symposium of the Zoological Society of London 41:193–210

Cruz-Korchin N, Korchin L, Gonzalez-Keelan C et al 2002 Macromastia: how much of it is fat? Plastic Reconstruction Surgery 109(1): 64–68

Daly S 1993 The short term synthesis and infant regulated removal of milk in lactating women. Experimental Physiology 78:209–220

Dearlove J C, Dearlove B M 1981 Prolactin, fluid balance and lactation. British Journal of Obstetrics and Gynecology 123:845–846

Dewey K G 1998 Effects of maternal caloric restriction and exercise during lactation. Journal of Nutrition 128 (2 Suppl):386S–389S

Dewey K G, Lovelady C A, Nommsen-Rivers L A et al 1994 A randomized study of the effects of aerobic exercise by lactating women on breast-milk volume and composition. New England Journal of Medicine 330(7):449–453

Dixon J M 1988 Repeated aspiration of breast abscess in lactating women. British Medical Journal 297:1517–1518

Dollberg S, Botzer E, Grunis E et al 2006 Immediate nipple pain relief after frenotomy in breast-fed infants with ankyloglossia: a randomized, prospective study. Journal of Pediatric Surgery 41(9):1598–600

Dusdieker L B, Hemingway D L, Stumbo P J 1994 Is milk production impaired by dieting during lactation? American Journal of Clinical Nutrition 59:833–840

Eglin R P, Wilkinson A R 1987 HIV infection and pasteurization of breast milk. Lancet i:1093

EVM (Expert Group on Vitamins and Minerals) 2003 Online. Available: www.food.gov.uk/multimedia/pdfs/evm_d.pdf

Fairbank L, Woolridge M J, Renfrew M J et al 2000 Effective healthcare: promoting the initiation of breast-feeding. NHS Centre for Reviews and Dissemination/University of York, Vol. 6, No. 2, July

Fenstein J, Berkelhamer J, Gruszka M et al 1986 Factors related to early termination of breast-feeding in an urban population. Pediatrics 78(2):210–215

Fredrikzon B, Hernell O, Blackberg L et al 1978 Bile salt-stimulated lipase in human milk: evidence of activity in vivo and of a role in the digestion of milk retinol esters. Pediatric Research 12(11):1048–1052

Gartner LM, Greer F R. 2003 Prevention of rickets and vitamin D deficiency: new guidelines for vitamin D intake. Pediatrics 111(4):908–910

Garza C, Ramussen K M 2000 Pregnancy and Lactation. In: Garrow J S, James W P T, Ralph Alan (eds) Human nutrition and dietetics, 10th edn. Harcourt Medical, Edinburgh, p 437–448

Greer F R 1997 Vitamin K status of lactating mothers and their infants. Acta Paediatrica 88(430):95–103

Going J J, Moffat D F 2004. Escaping from Flatland: clinical and biological aspects of human mammary duct anatomy in three dimensions. Journal of Pathology 203(1):538–544

Gregory J., Great Britain Office for National Statistics Social Survey Division 2000 National diet and nutrition survey young people aged 4–18 years, Vol. 1 Report of the diet and nutrition survey. The Stationery Office, London

Groh-Wargo S, Toth A, Mahoney K et al 1995 The utility of a bilateral breast pumping system for mothers of premature infants. Neonatal Network 14(8):31–36

Hall B 1979 Changing content of human milk and early development of appetite control. Keeping Abreast, April/June:139

Hammer R L, Babcock G, Fisher A G 1996 Low-fat diet and exercise in obese lactating women. Breast-feeding Review 4(1):29–34

Hamosh M 1998 Protective functions of proteins and lipids in human milk. Biology of the Neonate 74:163

Helsing E, Savage King F 1982 Breast-feeding in practice. Oxford University Press, Oxford, p 175

Hill P, Aldag J, Chatterton R 1999 Effect of pumping style on milk production in mothers of non-nursing preterm infants. Journal of Human Lactation 15(3):209–216

Hoddinott P, Pill R 1999 Qualitative study of decisions about infant feeding among women in the East End of London. British Medical Journal 318(7175):30–34

Hodge C 1967 Suppression of lactation by stilboestrol. Lancet ii(7510):286–287

Hogan M, Westcott C, Griffiths M 2005 Randomized, controlled trial of division of tongue-tie in infants with feeding problems. Journal of Paediatrics and Child Health 41(5–6):246–250

Host A 1991 Importance of the first meal on the development of cows' milk allergy and intolerance. Allergy Proceedings 12:227–232

Howard C R, Howard F M, Lanphear B et al 2003 Randomized clinical trial of pacifier use and bottle-feeding or cupfeeding and their effect on breast-feeding. Pediatrics 111(3):511–518

Hytten F E, Baird D 1958 The development of the nipple in pregnancy. Lancet i:1201–1204

Illingworth P J, Jong R T, Howie P W et al 1986 Diminution in energy expenditure during lactation. British Medical Journal 292:437–441

Inch S, Fisher C 1995 Mastitis in lactating women. The Practitioner 239:472–476

Inch S, Garforth S 1989 Establishing and maintaining breast-feeding. In: Chalmers I, Enkin M, Keirse M (eds) Effective care in pregnancy and childbirth. Oxford University Press, Oxford, Ch. 80, p 1364

Infant Formula and Follow-on Formula Regulations 1995. HMSO, London

Ingram J, Woolridge M, Greenwood R 2001 Breast-feeding: it is worth trying with the second baby. Lancet 358 (9286):986–987

Jackson D A, Woolridge M W, Imong S M et al 1987 The automatic sampling shield: a device for sampling suckled breast milk. Early Human Development 15 (5):295–306

Jamal N, Ng KH, McLean D et al 2004 Mammographic breast glandularity in Malaysian women: data derived from radiography. American Journal of Roentgenology 182 (3):713–717

Jones E, Dimmock P, Spencer S A 2001 A randomised controlled trial to compare methods of milk expression after preterm delivery. Archives of Disease in Childhood, Fetal Neonatal 85:F91–F95

Kassing D 2002 Bottle-feeding as a tool to reinforce breastfeeding. Journal of Human Lactation 18(1):56–60

Kaufmann T 1999 Infant feeding: politics vs pragmatism? RCM Midwives Journal 2(8):244

Kendell RE, Adams W 2002 Exposure to sunlight, vitamin D and schizophrenia. Schizophrenia Research 54(3):193–198

Kennedy K I, Rivera R, McNeilly A S 1989 Consensus statement on the use of breast-feeding as a family planning method. Contraception 439:477

Kochenour N K 1980 Lactation suppression. Clinical Obstetrics and Gynecology 23:1052–1059

Kries R V, Shearer M, McCarthy P T et al 1987 Vitamin K1 content of maternal milk: influence of the stage of lactation, lipid composition, and vitamin K1 supplements given to the mother. Pediatric Research 22(5):513–517

Lang S, Lawence C, L'E Orme R 1994 Cup feeding: an alternative method of infant feeding. Archives of Disease in Childhood 71:365–369

Leaf A A 2007 Vitamins for babies and young children: RCPCH Standing Committee on Nutrition. Archives of Disease in Childhood 92(2):160–164

Love S M, Barsky S H. 2004 Anatomy of the nipple and breast ducts revisited. Cancer 101(9):1947–57

Lucas A, Cole T J 1990 Breast milk and neonatal necrotizing enterocolitis. Lancet 336:1519–1523

Macdonald P D, Ross S R, Grant L et al 2003 Neonatal weight loss in breast and formula fed infants. Archives of Disease in Childhood. Fetal and Neonatal Edition 88:F472–F476

Main Trial Collaborative Group 1994 Preparing for breastfeeding: treatment of inverted and non-protractile nipples in pregnancy. Midwifery 10:200–214

Martyn T 1999 Soya in artificial baby milks. Practising Midwife 2(6):17–19

Meier P, Cranston-Anderson J 1987 Responses of small pre-term infants to bottle and breast-feeding. Maternal–Child Nursing Journal 12:97–105

Messenger H 1994 Don't shoot the messenger. Health Visitor 67(5):171

Metcalf I J, Irons T G, Lawrence D S et al 1994 Simethicone in the treatment of infant colic: a randomized placebo-controlled multicentre trial. Pediatrics 94:29–34

Minchin M 2001 Towards safer artificial feeding. Alma publications, Australia, Geelong. Online. Available: almapubs @netlink.com.au

Morse J M, Ewing G, Gamble D et al 1992 The effect of maternal fluid intake on breast milk supply: a pilot study. Canadian Journal of Public Health 83(3):213–216

NICE (National Institute for Health and Clinical Excellence) 2005 IPG149 Division of ankyloglossia (tongue tie) for breastfeeding – information for the public. Online. Available: http://www.nice.org.uk/page.aspx?o=284318

NICE (National Institute for Health and Clinical Excellence) 2006 CG37 Postnatal care: Routine postnatal care of women and their babies – full guideline. NICE, London. Online: Available: http://guidance.nice.org.uk/CG37/guidance/pdf/English

NICE (National Institute for Health and Clinical Excellence) 2008 NICE public health guidance 11. Improving the nutrition of pregnant and breast-feeding mothers and children in low-income households. Online. Available: www.nice.org.uk/guidance/index.jsp?action=byID&o=11943

Nickell W B, Skelton J 2005 Breast fat and fallacies: more than 100 years of anatomical fantasy. Journal of Human Lactation 21(2):126–130

Nicoll A, Ginsburg R, Tripp J 1982 Supplementary feeding and jaundice in newborns. Acta Paediatrica Scandinavica 71:759–761

Nicolls H 1997 Two on to one will go. Midwifery Matters 73:6–7

Nowak A J, Smith W L, Erenberg A 1994 Imaging evaluation of artificial nipples during bottle feeding. Archives of Pediatrics and Adolescent Medicine 148(1):40–42

Paronen J, Knip M, Savilahti E et al. 2000 Effect of cow's milk exposure and maternal type 1 diabetes on cellular and humeral immunization to dietary insulin in infants at genetic risk for type 1 diabetes. Finnish Trial to Reduce IDDM in the Genetically at Risk Study Group. Diabetes 49(10):1657–1665

Prentice A M, Addey C V P, Wilde C J 1989 Evidence for local feed-back control of human milk secretion. Biochemical Society Transactions 17:122, 489–492

Prentice A M, Goldberg G R, Prentice A 1994 Body mass index and lactational performance. European Journal of Clinical Nutrition 48(Suppl 3):S78–S89

Prentice A M, Lunn P G, Watkinson M et al 1983 Dietary supplementation of lactating Gambian women II. Effect on maternal health, nutritional status and biochemistry. Human Nutrition and Clinical Nutrition 37(1):65–74

Prentice A M, Roberts S B, Whitehead R G 1980 Dietary supplementation of Gambian nursing mothers and lactational performance. Lancet ii:886–888

Ramos R, Kennedy K I, Visness C M 1996 Effectiveness of lactational amenorrhoea in prevention of pregnancy in Manila, the Philippines: non-comparative prospective trial. British Medical Journal 313:909–912

Ramsay D 2005 Investigation of the sucking dynamics of the breast-feeding term infant: ultrasound and intraoral vacuum research. Presented at the ILCA conference: Breaking the Barriers to Breast-feeding: Research, Policy and Practice, Chicago, USA.

Ramsay D T, Kent J C, Hartmann R A et al 2005 Anatomy of the lactating human breast redefined with ultrasound imaging. Journal of Anatomy 206(6):525–534

Ramsay D T, Kent J C, Owens R A et al 2004 Ultrasound imaging of milk ejection in the breast of lactating women. Pediatrics 113:361–367

Rapley G 2006 Baby-led weaning. In: Hall Moran V, Dykes F. (eds) Maternal and infant nutrition and nurture: controversies and challenges. Quay Books, London

RCM (Royal College of Midwives) 2001 Successful breast-feeding, 3rd edn. Churchill Livingstone, Edinburgh

Righard L, Alade M O 1990 Effect of delivery room routines on success of first breast-feed. Lancet 336:1105–1107

Saarinen U M, Siimes M A 1979 Iron absorption from breast milk, cow's milk and iron supplemented formula: an opportunistic use of changes in total body iron determined by hemoglobin, ferritin and body weight in 132 infants. Pediatric Research 13:143–147

Sachdev H P S, Krishna J, Puri R K 1991 Water supplementation in exclusively breast-fed infants during the summer in the tropics. Lancet 337:929–933

SACN 2003. Online. Available: www.sacn.gov.uk/pdfs/smcn_03_02.pdf

Sandstrom B, Cederblad A, Lonnerdal B 1983 Zinc absorption from human, cows' milk and infant formula. American Journal of Diseases of Childhood 137:726

Scheel C E, Schanler R J, Lau C. 2005 Does the choice of bottle nipple affect the oral feeding performance of very-low-birth weight (VLBW) infants? Acta Paediatrica 94(9):1266–1272

Schubiger G, Schwartz U, Tonz O 1997 UNICEF/WHO baby-friendly hospital initiative: does the use of bottles and pacifiers in the neonatal nursery prevent successful breast-feeding? European Journal of Paediatrics 156 (11):874–877

Specker B L, Tsang R C, Ho M L et al 1991 Low serum calcium and high para-thyroid hormone levels in neonates fed 'humanized' cows' milk based breast milk substitutes. American Journal of Diseases of Childhood 145:941–945

Specker B L, Valanis B, Hertzberg V R et al 1985 Sunshine exposure and serum 25-hydroxyvitamin D concentrations in exclusively breast-fed infants. Journal of Pediatrics 107 (3):372–376

Taneri F, Kurukahvecioglu O, Akyurek N et al 2006 Micro-anatomy of milk ducts in the nipple. European Surgery Research 38(6):545–549.

Thomsen A C, Espersen M D, Maigaard S 1984 Course and treatment of milk stasis, non-infectious inflammation of the breast, and infectious mastitis in nursing women. American Journal of Obstetrics and Gynecology 149:492–495

Ueda T, Yokoyama Y, Irahara M et al 1994 Influence of psychological stress on suckling-induced pulsatile oxytocin release. Obstetrics and Gynecology 84:259–262

UNICEF and Department of Health 2007. Off to the Best Start. Online. Available: www.breast-feeding.nhs.uk or www.baby-friendly.org.uk/pdfs/otbs_leaflet.pdf

Vaarala O, Knip M, Paronen J et al 1999 Cow's milk formula feeding induces primary immunization to insulin in infants at genetic risk for type 1 diabetes. Diabetes 48(7):1389–1394

Vallenas C, Savage F 1998 Evidence for the ten steps to successful breast-feeding. Division of Child Health and Development. WHO, Geneva

Vandeweyer E, Hertens D 2002. Quantification of glands and fat in breast tissue: an experimental determination. Annals of Anatomy 184(2):181–184.

Waldenström U, Swensen Å 1991 Rooming-in at night in the postpartum ward. Midwifery 7:82–89

White A, Freith S, O'Brien M 1992 Infant feeding 1990. Survey carried out for the Department of Health by the Office of Population Censuses and Surveys. HMSO, London

Whitehead R G, Paul A A, Black A E et al 1981 Recommended dietary amounts of energy for pregnancy or lactation in the UK. In: Torun B, Young V R, Rang W M (eds) Protein energy requirements of developing countries: evaluation of new data. United Nations University, Tokyo, p 259–265

WHO (World Health Organization) 1981 International code of marketing of breast-milk substitutes. WHO, Geneva

WHO (World Health Organization) 2000 Mastitis: causes and management (WHO/RCH/CAH/00.13). Department of Child and Adolescent Health and Development, Geneva

WHO (World Health Organization)/UNICEF 1989 Joint statement – protecting, promoting and supporting breast-feeding. WHO, Geneva

Widström A M, Ransjo-Arvidson A B, Christensson K et al 1987 Gastric suction in healthy newborn infants. Acta Paediatrica Scandinavica 76:566–578

Wilde C J, Addey C V P, Boddy L M et al 1995 Autocrine regulation of milk secretion by a protein in milk. Biochemical Journal 305:51–58

Woolridge M W 1986 The 'anatomy' of sucking. Midwifery 2:164–171

Woolridge M W 1995 Breast-feeding: physiology into practice. In: Davis D P (ed.) Nutrition in child health. Royal College of Physicians, London, p 13–31

Woolridge M W, Baum J D, Drewett R F 1982 Individual patterns of milk intake during breast-feeding. Early Human Development 7:265–272

Woolridge M W, Fisher C 1988 'Overfeeding' and symptoms of malabsorption in the breast-fed baby: a possible artefact of feed management? Lancet ii:382–384

Worthington-Roberts B 1993 Human milk composition and infant growth and development. In: Worthington-Roberts B, Williams S R (eds) Nutrition in pregnancy and lactation, 5th edn. Mosby Year Book, St Louis, p 343

FURTHER READING

Hall Moran V, Dykes F. (eds) 2006 Maternal and infant nutrition and nurture: controversies and challenges. Quay Books, London

This multi-author book uses a sociobiological perspective to examine the complex interaction between political, sociocultural and biological factors in food and health in relation to maternal and infant nutrition.

Inch S, Fisher C 1999 Breast-feeding: into the 21st century. NT clinical monographs, No. 32. Emap Healthcare, London

A concise but wide-ranging review of the importance of breastfeeding, the difficulties facing midwives who want to help breastfeeding women and the ways in which these might be overcome.

Infant Formula and Follow-on Formula Regulations 1995 Stationery Office, London. Online. Available: www.hmso.gov.uk/si/si1995/Uksi_19950077_en_1.htm

This is the UK government's response to the European Directive 1991 (91/321/EEC OJ No. L175, 4.7.91), which sought to persuade all EU countries to adopt the International code of marketing of breastmilk substitutes. It falls short of the code in several important respects, notably in relation to advertising.

Palmer G 1993 The politics of breast-feeding, 2nd edn. Pandora Press, London

This book links biology and politics (sexual, economic and environmental) in an exploration of the consequences of women's changing role in society and the acceleration of the Industrial Revolution, which created the demand for 'artificial milks'.

RCP 2003 Guidelines for the establishment and operation of human milk banks in the UK, 3rd edn. Royal College of Paediatrics and Child Health and United Kingdom Association for Milk Banking, London

Renfrew M, Fisher C, Arms S 2000 Bestfeeding, 2nd edn. Celestial Arts, Berkeley

Taking up where texts addressed primarily to health workers leave off, the authors blend wisdom, experience, idealism and learning to produce a clear, basic breast-feeding guide, addressed primarily to mothers.

WHO/UNICEF International code of marketing of breast milk substitutes 1981. Online. Available: http://www.babymilkaction.org/regs/thecode.html

This was adopted by a resolution (WHA34.22) of the World Health Assembly in 1981. A copy of the code can also be obtained from Baby Milk Action (see Useful addresses, below).

WHO (World Health Organization) 1989 Protecting, promoting and supporting breast-feeding: the special role of maternity services. A joint WHO/UNICEF Statement. WHO, Geneva

This is the document which first set out the 10 steps for successful breastfeeding, which formed the basis of the global Baby Friendly Hospital Initiative, and makes recommendations concerning the structure and function of (maternity) healthcare services. Obtainable also from: Stationery Office, Customer Services, 51 Nine Elms Lane, London SW8 5DR. Tel: (44) 870 600 5522, e-mail: customer.services@theso.co.uk

USEFUL ADDRESSES

National Childbirth Trust breast-feeding
Tel: 0870 444 8708; the enquiry line
Tel: 0870 444 8707

Breast-feeding Network helpline
Tel: 0870 900 8787

Association of Breast-feeding Mothers helpline
Tel: 08444 122 949

La Leche League helpline
Tel: 0207 242 1278

CLAPA (Cleft Lip And Palate Association)
235–237 Finchley Road, London NW3 6LS
Tel: 020 7431 0033

Baby Milk Action
34 Trumpington Street, Cambridge, CB2 1QY
Tel: 01223 464420
www.babymilkaction.org

UNICEF UK Baby Friendly Initiative
Africa House, 64–78 Kingsway, London WC2B 6NB
Tel: 020 7312 7652
www.babyfriendly.org.uk

42 The healthy low birthweight baby

Carole England

It is now generally accepted that healthy babies between 32 and 37 weeks' gestation, with a birthweight of 1.7–2.5 kg, do not need automatic admission to a neonatal intensive care unit (NICU) but instead can be cared for on a postnatal ward, with their mother. There is no doubt that low birthweight (LBW) babies are more vulnerable to illness compared with appropriately grown term babies, and extra monitoring may be a necessary precaution, particularly during the period of adaptation to extrauterine life and the early neonatal period. Caring for healthy LBW babies on a postnatal ward is thought to be advantageous because it removes them from the greater hazard of infection that occurs in neonatal units, prevents separation of mother and baby and finally, eliminates the need for parents to visit the neonatal unit, which is for many, an alien and intimidating environment (Fowlie & McHaffie 2005). There is growing evidence that the majority of these babies remain well, will have minimal or no illness in the neonatal period (Roberton 1999) and can be cared for by midwives as the lead professional. It therefore follows that neonatal nurses will be more able to focus their care on the critically ill, and those babies that are healthy but <1.70 kg, thus utilizing neonatal nurse skills and cot resources to their best effect.

The chapter aims to:

- clarify the terminology and classifications of babies in relation to birthweight and gestational age
- detail the care of pre-term babies and those who are small for their gestational age

- explore the role of the midwife in the provision of holistic care for the mother, her low birthweight baby and her family
- discuss the place and provision of care.

Introduction

Between 6% and 7% of all babies born in the UK weigh <2500g at birth. In 1977, the World Health Organization (WHO 1977a) recommended that babies who weigh <2500g should be called low birthweight (LBW). According to Tucker & McGuire (2005) preterm babies make up two-thirds of LBW babies with the other one-third being small for their gestational age (SGA). Spencer (2003) asserts that 70% of these LBW babies will weigh between 2000 and 2500g. The concepts and categories that surround LBW are complex. The following classification describes the different types of LBW babies seen in practice.

Classification of babies by weight and gestation

Definitions of low birthweight are based upon weight alone and do not consider the gestational age of the baby. Likewise, definitions of gestational age disregard any considerations of birthweight.

Weight

As neonatal technology and care have become more effective, new birthweight categories have been devised to further define babies by birthweight. The low birthweight categories are:

- low birthweight (LBW) babies are those weighing below 2500g at birth
- very low birthweight (VLBW) babies are those weighing below 1500g at birth.
- extremely low birthweight (ELBW) babies are those who weigh below 1000g at birth.

Gestational age

A pre-term baby is one born before completion of the 37th gestational week. Gestational weeks are calculated from the first day of the last menstrual period (LMP) and have no relevance to the baby's weight, length, head circumference, or indeed any other measurement of fetal or neonatal size. As ultrasound scanning has become more accurate, the expected date of delivery (EDD) is sometimes re-calculated at 11–12 weeks, based on the estimation of the fetal crown–rump length. When this data is available, the LMP calculation is disregarded.

Thus, it is the *relationship* between these two separate considerations of weight (for assessment of growth) and gestational age (for assessment of maturity) that is of great importance. This relationship can be plotted on centile charts (Fig. 42.1); these charts visually demonstrate that growth is appropriate, excessive or diminished for gestational age and that the baby is either pre-term, term or post-term. They are based on measurements of fetal growth that have been collected over the last 20 years, from multiple ultrasound measurements, but have limitations. Farrer (2005) believes that to act as a more accurate tool, growth charts should be derived from studies of local populations, because genetically derived growth differences exist between countries, cultures and lifestyles. Tucker & McGuire (2005) also assert that in most of the UK, data on birthweight is collected routinely, but often there is uncertainty and incomplete recording of estimates of gestation.

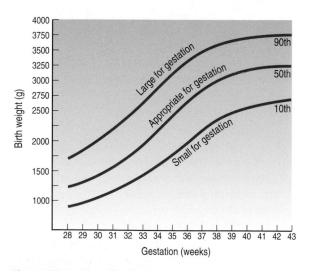

Figure 42.1 A centile chart, showing weight and gestation. (From Simpson 1997, with permission from Baillière Tindall.)

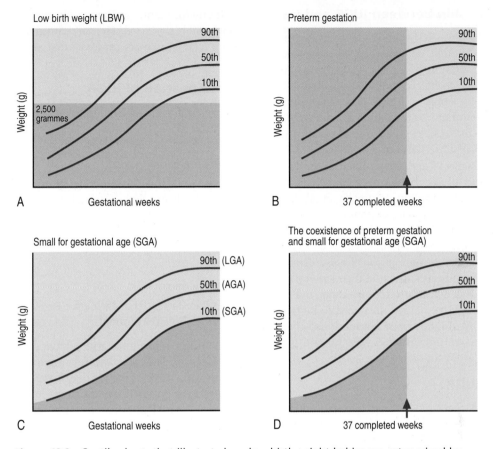

Figure 42.2 Centile charts that illustrate how low birthweight babies are categorized by weight and gestation. (A) Low birthweight. (B) Pre-term gestation. (C) Small for gestational age. (D) Co-existence of pre-term gestation and small for gestational age.

Various types of LBW babies can be described:

1. Babies whose rate of intrauterine growth was normal at the moment of birth: they are small because labour began before the end of the 37th gestational week. These pre-term babies are appropriately grown for their gestational age (AGA).

2. Babies whose rate of intrauterine growth was slowed and who were birthed at or later than term: these term or post-term babies are 'undergrown' for gestational age. They are small for their gestational age (SGA).

3. Babies whose rate of intrauterine growth was slowed and who, in addition, were delivered before term: these pre-term babies are small by virtue of both early birth and impaired intrauterine growth. They are small for gestational age and pre-term babies.

Babies are considered large for their gestational age (LGA) at any weight when they fall above the 90th centile. Therefore, it follows that both term and pre-term babies can be SGA, AGA or LGA (Fig. 42.2).

The small for gestational age (SGA) baby

Expert care of newborn babies requires an understanding of intrauterine growth patterns as they relate to gestational age. A baby's clinical course following birth is largely determined by these factors.

Intrauterine growth restriction rate (IUGR)

Tappero & Honeyfield (2003) define IUGR as a rate of fetal growth that is less than normal for the population and for the growth potential of a specific baby.

The relationship between IUGR and SGA

In the past, the terms IUGR and SGA were used interchangeably. Although related, they are not synonymous. IUGR is a failure of normal fetal growth caused by multiple adverse effects on the fetus, whereas SGA describes a baby whose weight is lower than population norms. SGA babies are defined as having a birth weight below the 10th centile for gestational age, or <2 standard deviations below the mean (the 50th centile) for the gestational age. Thus, all IUGR babies may not be SGA and all SGA babies may not be small as a result of growth restriction (Gomella et al 1999). Indeed, Farrer (2005) contends that at least half of the SGA babies in Britain have no known aetiology. They are proportionately small; their weight, length and head circumference are all on the 3rd centile or below. It is generally accepted that their small parents or grandparents genetically determine their smallness. They are well, healthy babies who need to be treated accordingly and do not need overzealous labeling, which may lead to unwarranted wasteful and potentially harmful interventions (Farrer 2005).

Causes of IUGR

Fetal growth is regulated by maternal, placental and fetal factors and represents a mix of genetic mechanisms and environmental influences through which growth potential is expressed. The mechanisms that appear to limit fetal growth are multifactorial and are presented in Box 42.1.

Classification of IUGR

Factors that influence fetal growth can be intrinsic or extrinsic.

Intrinsic factors

These are factors that operate from *within* the fetus, that arise from chromosomal or genetic abnormalities, or alternatively from infective agents that are transplacental in origin and act by altering the normal process of cell division.

Extrinsic factors

These are factors that influence the fetus through its intrauterine environment.

The clinical appearance and behaviour of the baby at birth can provide relevant information as to the type of growth disruption that may have been sustained and help the midwife to anticipate any future potential problems. There are two types of IUGR clinically recognized.

Box 42.1 Causes of intrauterine growth restriction

Maternal factors

- Pregnancy-induced hypertension, pre-eclampsia
- Chronic hypertension
- Diabetes mellitus
- Undernutrition
- Smoking, alcohol misuse
- Drugs: therapeutic (anticancer drugs) and addictive (narcotic)
- Renal disease, collagen disorders, anaemia
- Irradiation
- Young and elderly mothers
- Poor obstetric history
- Underweight mother/small stature.

Fetal factors

- Multiple gestation
- Chromosomal/genetic abnormality (particularly trisomy conditions), including inborn errors of metabolism, dwarf syndromes
- Intrauterine infection: toxoplasmosis, rubella, cytomegalovirus, herpes simplex (TORCH) and syphilis.

Placental factors

- Abruptio placenta
- Placenta praevia
- Chorioamnionitis
- Abnormal cord insertion
- Single umbilical artery.

Sources: Blackburn (2003), Mupanemunda & Watkinson (2005), Spencer (2003), Tappero & Honeyfield (2003).

Asymmetric growth (sometimes called acute)

Here the fetal weight is reduced out of proportion to the length and head circumference; this is thought to be caused by extrinsic factors such as pregnancy-induced hypertension (Mupanemunda & Watkinson 2005) that adversely affect fetal nutrition during the latter stages of gestation. The head looks disproportionately large compared with the body, but the head circumference is usually within normal parameters and brain growth is usually spared (McGrath et al 2004). The bones are within gestational norms for length and density but the anterior fontanelle may be larger than expected, owing to diminished membranous bone formation. The abdomen looks scaphoid, or sunken owing to shrinkage of the liver and spleen, which surrender their stores of glycogen and red blood cell mass, respectively as the fetus adapts to the adverse conditions of the uterus. Since the ratio of brain mass to liver mass is large, hypoglycaemia is more likely to be seen in such babies. There is decreased subcutaneous fat deposition and the skin is loose, which can give the baby a wizened, old appearance. Vernix caseosa is frequently reduced or absent as a result of diminished skin perfusion and, in the absence of this protective covering, the skin is continuously exposed to amniotic fluid, and its cells will begin to desquamate (shed); thus the skin appears pale, dry and coarse and, if the baby is of a mature gestation, may be stained with meconium. Unless severely affected, these babies appear hyperactive and hungry with a lusty cry (Fig. 42.3).

Symmetric growth (chronic)

Symmetric IUGR is due either to decreased growth potential of the fetus, as a result of congenital infection or chromosomal/genetic defects (intrinsic), or to extrinsic factors that are active early in gestational life (e.g. the effects of maternal smoking, or poor dietary intake), or a combination of intrinsic and extrinsic factors (Mupanemunda & Watkinson 2005). The head circumference, length and weight are all proportionately reduced for gestational age (Gomella et al 1999). These babies are diminutive in size, do not appear wasted, have subcutaneous fat appropriate for their size and their skin is taut. They are generally vigorous and less likely to be hypoglycaemic or polycythaemic, but, because the

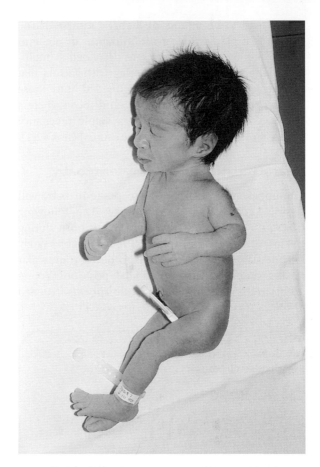

Figure 42.3 Baby with asymmetrical growth restriction. Note the apparently large head compared with the 'undergrown' body.

insult began early with possible interruptions to cell division, they may suffer major congenital abnormalities and can be a source of infection to carers, as a result of transplacental infection.

Symmetric growth (genetically small)

These are small normal babies and should be treated in accordance to their gestational age.

The pre-term baby

This describes a baby born before the end of the 37th gestational week, regardless of birthweight. Most of these babies are appropriately grown and, whereas some are SGA, a small number are LGA (these tend to be infants of diabetic mothers). The factors that play a role in the initiation of pre-term labour are largely unknown, are described as multifactorial and in large part overlay with factors that impair fetal growth. They are divided into those labours that start spontaneously and those where a decision is made to terminate a viable pregnancy before term (referred to as elective causes) (Box 42.2).

Characteristics of the pre-term baby

The appearance at birth of the pre-term baby will depend upon the gestational age. The following description will focus upon the baby born during the last trimester of pregnancy. Pre-term babies rarely become large enough in utero to develop muscular flexion and fully adopt the fetal position (Young 1996) and as a result their posture appears flattened with hips abducted, knees and ankles flexed. Lissauer et al (2006) describe a generally hypotonic baby with a weak and feeble cry. The head is in proportion to the body; the skull bones are soft with large fontanelles and wide sutures. The chest is small and narrow and appears underdeveloped owing to minimal lung expansion during fetal life. The abdomen is prominent because the liver and spleen are large and abdominal muscle tone is poor (Fig. 42.4). The liver is large because it receives a good supply of oxygenated blood via the fetal circulation and is active in the production of red blood

---

Box 42.2 Causes of pre-term labour

Spontaneous causes

- 40% unknown
- Multiple gestation
- Hyperpyrexia as a result of viral or bacterial infection
- Premature rupture of the membranes caused by maternal infection
- Maternal short stature
- Maternal age and parity
- Poor obstetric history; history of pre-term labour
- Cervical incompetence
- Poor social circumstances.

Elective causes

- Pregnancy-induced hypertension, pre-eclampsia, chronic hypertension
- Maternal disease: renal, cardiac
- Placenta praevia, abruptio placenta
- Rhesus incompatibility
- Congenital abnormality
- IUGR.

Sources: Blackburn (2003), Harlow & Spencer (1999), Tucker & McGuire (2005).

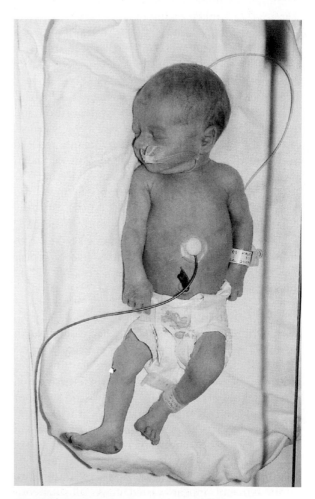

Figure 42.4 Healthy pre-term baby born at 32 weeks' gestation. Note the presence of a nasogastric tube. The thermocouple of the servo skin mode is taped to the baby's upper abdomen.

cells as a result of erythropoiesis. The umbilicus appears low in the abdomen because linear growth is cephalocaudal (it is more apparent nearer to the head than the feet), by virtue of the fetal circulation oxygenation. Subcutaneous fat is laid down from 28 weeks' gestation, therefore its presence and abundance will affect the redness and transparency of the skin. Vernix caseosa is abundant in the last trimester and tends to accumulate at sites of dense lanugo growth (i.e. the face, ears, shoulders and sacral region) and protects the skin from amniotic fluid maceration. The ear pinna is flat with little curve, the eyes bulge and the orbital ridges are prominent. The nipple areola is poorly developed and barely visible. The cord is white, fleshy and glistening. The plantar creases are absent before 36 weeks but soon start to appear as fluid loss occurs through the skin. In girls the labia majora fail to cover the labia minora and in boys the testes descend into the scrotal sac at about the 37th gestational week (Gardner & Johnson 2006).

Management at birth of the healthy LBW baby

Given the unpredictability of the LBW baby and the birth process, the role of the midwife in the birthing room is to prepare adequately the environment, staff and parents for certain eventualities. This takes the form of asking the multiprofessional team (second midwife, paediatrician and neonatal nurse), to be on standby for the birth. The incidence of perinatal asphyxia and congenital abnormality is greater in SGA babies and the baby with a scaphoid abdomen could be physically normal, albeit thin, but alternatively could deteriorate quickly if presenting with a diaphragmatic hernia. Current cot availability in the NICU, transitional care unit (as applicable) and postnatal ward should be known. The labour room ambient temperature should ideally be between 23 and 25°C; the neonatal resuscitaire should be checked and ready for use.

The Apgar score is traditionally scored at 1 and 5 min and acts as a guide in helping staff communicate the resuscitative needs of neonates immediately after birth. Some consider it has limited usefulness in LBW babies because it was originally devised by

Apgar in 1953 for term babies and does not take into account how gestational age, congenital abnormalities or sedation affect the score (Juretschke 2000). Early labeling of the LBW baby is particularly important because separation of mother and baby could happen at any time if the baby's condition becomes unstable. The midwife should cut the cord to leave an extra length, in case access to the umbilical vessels should be necessary at a later time. A detailed but expedient examination of the baby should be conducted by the midwife in the presence of the parents and recorded accordingly. It is particularly important in SGA babies to check that the anal sphincter is patent, which could provide information on the internal integrity of the gastrointestinal system, particularly the oesophagus. This is a good time to allay any parental anxieties about their baby's general appearance, which may be quite different to what they were expecting (Redshaw 1997). Once it is established that the baby appears healthy, the midwife may attempt to normalize the care by emphasizing to the parents the importance of preventing cold stress and suggest skin-to-skin contact for a period of up to 50 min (Philipp & Radford 2006). Lee (2006a) reports that skin-to-skin contact was originally introduced by Klaus & Kennell in the 1970s and later was developed as kangaroo care as an alternative to cot care for LBW babies because of their special physical needs (Klaus & Kennell 1982). The re-introduction of skin-to-skin contact has now been generalized to newborns by the WHO/UNICEF UK Baby Friendly Initiative (1989). The midwife should ensure that the baby is thoroughly dried before skin-to-skin contact is attempted, to prevent evaporative heat losses. This will, according to Sedin (2006) secure the baby's conductive heat transfer gains, and help him to become physically stabilized. Whether the baby will find the breast is open to speculation according to Carfoot et al (2003). Their systematic review based on term infants failed to establish whether skin-to-skin contact had any effect on timing of the first breastfeed or duration of breastfeeding. If the mother chooses not to engage in skin-to-skin contact, the father may wish to do so (Lee 2006a) but if not, the baby can be dressed, wrapped and held by his parents. The baby's axilla temperature should be maintained between 36.4°C and 37°C (Thureen et al 2005).

Assessment of gestational age

It is generally considered essential to obtain an accurate assessment of gestational age, first to anticipate the problems a baby is more likely to develop and secondly to provide valid comparisons with respect to morbidity and mortality statistics (Tappero & Honeyfield 2003). In 1970, Dubowitz et al developed a scoring system for the assessment of gestational age in babies <5 days old, based upon neurological and physical (external) characteristics. The purpose of the assessment, which is still used today, is to confirm the stated gestation, reveal any discrepancies and provide a reliable estimate when uncertainty exists. Despite its usefulness, the accuracy of the assessment is less reliable in babies who have suffered a neurological insult such as birth asphyxia or chronic exposure to drugs. Such babies will obtain a lower score on neurological criteria. Other affected babies are those who have suffered asymmetric IUGR. Their sole creases have extra wrinkles as a result of exposure to amniotic fluid and this feature may confer upon them an enhanced maturity, whereas breast tissue formation, female external genitalia and ear cartilage will give the appearance of less maturity because of diminished amounts of adipose tissue and so they may be underscored on physical assessment, if they are near to term. Hence, gestational age assessments based on physical criteria can be misleading. Mupanemunda & Watkinson (2005) do not totally endorse the Dubowitz scoring system, believing that its margins of error are too wide. They further contend that the handling of LBW babies for the assessment is problematic because it may de-stabilize an otherwise well baby. With the developments of more accurate dating by antenatal ultrasound techniques, it is argued that there is less justification for a full assessment of gestational age in well LBW babies. The exception is applied when the mother deliberately conceals her pregnancy, is unable to communicate or unwilling to divulge requisite information, or is unreliable (e.g. a drug-abusing mother with unfavourable social circumstances). Therefore any assessments that are carried out should be carefully conducted, with the view that no harm should be caused as a result of the process.

Care of the healthy LBW baby

Many of the care issues relevant to the LBW baby apply to both the pre-term and the SGA infant. Where differences do exist, these will receive further consideration. The following areas of focus, although presented separately, do by their nature influence each other and should not be regarded as stand-alone entities.

Principles of thermoregulation

Thermoregulation is the balance between heat production and heat loss and the ideal body temperature should be between 36.5° and 37.3°C. The prevention of cold stress, which may lead to hypothermia which is a body temperature below 36°C, is critical for the intact survival of the LBW baby. Newborn babies are unable to shiver, move very much, or ask for an extra blanket and therefore rely upon physical adaptations that generate heat by raising their basal metabolic rate and utilizing brown fat deposits. Thus, exposure to cool environments can result in multisystem physiological changes, which significantly challenge the baby's health status. As body temperature falls, tissue oxygen consumption rises as the baby attempts to raise its metabolic rate by burning glucose to generate energy and heat. Care measures should aim to provide an environment that supports thermoneutrality. This is otherwise known as the 'neutral thermal environment', a range of ambient temperatures within which the metabolic rate is minimal, the baby is neither gaining or losing heat, oxygen consumption is minimal and the core-to-skin temperature gradient is small (Blackburn 2003).

Thermoregulation and the healthy mature SGA baby

In the neonate, the head accounts for at least one-fifth of the total body surface area and brain heat production is thought to be 55% of total metabolic heat production. Rapid heat loss due to the large head-to-body ratio and large surface area is exaggerated, particularly in the asymmetrically grown SGA baby. Wide sutures and large fontanelles add to the heat-losing tendency. On the plus side, they have increased skin maturity but often depleted stores of subcutaneous fat, which are used for insulation. Their raised basal metabolic rate helps them to produce heat but their high energy demands in the presence of poor glycogen stores and minimal fat deposition can soon lead to hypoglycaemia and then hypothermia. Once the baby is thoroughly dried, a pre-warmed hat will minimize heat loss from the head.

Thermoregulation and the healthy pre-term baby

All pre-term babies are prone to heat loss because their ability to produce heat is compromised by their immaturity, so factors such as their large ratio of surface area to weight, their varying amounts of subcutaneous fat and their ability to mobilize brown fat stores (which have been laid down from 28 weeks) will be affected by their gestational age (Blackburn 2003). During cooling, immaturity of the heat-regulating centres in the hypothalamus and medulla oblongata fail, in different degrees, to recognize and marshall adequately coordinated homeostatic controls. In addition, pre-term babies are often unable to increase their oxygen consumption effectively through normal respiratory function and their calorific intake is often inadequate to meet increasing metabolic requirements (Anderson et al 2006). Furthermore, their open resting postures increase their surface area and along with insensible water losses, these factors render the pre-term baby more susceptible to evaporative heat losses (Sedin 2006). Gestational age and the weight of the baby will influence the type of care initiated. Gardner & Johnson (2006) and Fransson et al (2005) report that skin-to-skin contact is a more effective measure for re-warming cool babies than incubator care. When the baby is not receiving skin-to-skin contact with either parent and the baby is under 2 kg, the warm conditions in an incubator can be achieved either by heating the air to 30–32°C (air mode) or by servo-controlling the baby's body temperature at a desired set point (36°C). In servo mode, a thermocouple is taped to the upper abdomen and the incubator heater maintains the skin at that site at a preset constant (see Fig. 42.4). Within the incubator they are clothed with bedding, in a room temperature of 26°C. Most pre-term babies between 2.0 and 2.5 kg will be cared for in a cot, in a room temperature of 24°C.

Hypoglycaemia

Hypoglycaemia and the healthy LBW baby

The term hypoglycaemia refers to a low blood glucose concentration and in itself is not a medical condition, but a feature of illness or a failure to adapt from the fetal state of continuous transplacental glucose consumption to the extrauterine pattern of intermittent nutrient supply (WHO 1997b). It is more likely to occur in conditions where babies become cold or where the initiation of early feeding (within the first hour) is delayed. Counterregulatory mechanisms (for a more detailed account on hypoglycaemia, see Ch. 48) maintain the blood glucose at safe limits to protect tissue viability; however, it is generally questioned whether LBW babies are able to counter-regulate as effectively as appropriately grown term babies and some caution is recommended (WHO 1997b). The aim of management is to maintain the true blood sugar above the level considered to be the lowest level of normal, which is 2.6 mmol/dL (WHO 1997b). However, this does not mean that every LBW baby should be *routinely* screened. Well LBW babies who show no clinical signs of hypoglycaemia, are demanding and taking nutritive feeds on a regular basis and maintaining their body temperature, do not need screening for hypoglycaemia. The emphasis of care is placed upon the concept of *adequate feeding* and the cornerstone of success is the midwife's ability to assess skillfully whether the baby is feeding sufficiently well to meet energy requirements. Midwives should be guided by their local policies regarding use of reagent strips, but if a baby, despite being fed, presents with clinical signs of hypoglycaemia then a venous sample should be taken by the paediatrician to assess the true blood sugar level, and this should be dispatched to the laboratory for verification purposes. A blood glucose that remains <2.6 mmol/dL, despite the baby's further attempts to feed by breast or colostrum by cup, may warrant transfer to the NICU, because glucose by intravenous bolus may be necessary to correct the metabolic disturbance. In addition, the midwife should consider that there may be some underlying medical condition that may call for more thorough investigation.

Hypoglycaemia and the healthy mature SGA baby

If the SGA baby does not suffer any effects of perinatal asphyxia or develop cold stress, the remaining potential problem is hypoglycaemia. Glycogen storage begins at the beginning of the third trimester and, due to altered placental transport of nutrients during this time, asymmetrically grown babies have reduced glycogen stores in liver and skeletal muscles (Ogata 1999). Their greater brain-to-body mass and a tendency towards polycythaemia increase their energy demands and, since both the brain and the red blood cells are obligatory glucose users, these factors can increase glucose requirements. Mature SGA babies with an asymmetric growth pattern will usually feed within the first 30 min of birth and will demand feeds every 2–3 hrs thereafter, to make up for lost time. Feeding is thought to mature the blunted counterregulatory response, so their susceptibility to hypoglycaemia is relatively short-lived and limited to the first 48 hrs following birth. If the baby is taking formula milk, feeds are usually calculated at 90 mL/kg on the first day, with 30 mL increments/day. Anderson et al (2006) warn however that overfeeding a growth restricted baby has been considered a cause of adult obesity and diabetes.

Hypoglycaemia and the pre-term baby

The pre-term baby may be sleepier, and attempts to take the first feed may reflect gestational age. Total feed requirements (60 mL/kg on the first day, with 30 mL/kg increments/day) may not be taken directly from the breast and supplementary feeds can be given by cup.

Feeding the LBW baby

Both pre-term and SGA babies benefit from human milk because it contains long chain polyunsaturated omega-3 fatty acids, which are thought to be essential for the myelination of neural membranes and for retinal development. Pre-term breastmilk has a higher concentration of lipids, protein, sodium, calcium and immunoglobulins, a low osmolarity, and lipases and enzymes that improve digestion and absorption (Jones & Spencer 1999). The uniqueness of the mother's milk for her own baby cannot be overstated. For any mother to commit to the challenge of breastfeeding her LBW baby, and in particular the pre-term baby, she should be thoroughly prepared both cognitively and emotionally by the midwife, so that her expectations are realistic as she anticipates the likely sequence of events that her baby may take her through (Lang 2002). First, she needs to understand what her baby may be able to achieve related to his development, which is based upon the combined influences of his gestational age at birth and his postnatal age. For a baby to feed for nutritive purposes, the coordination of breathing with suck and swallow reflexes reflect neurobehavioral maturation and organization and is thought to occur between 32 and 36 weeks' gestation (Jones & Spencer 2005, Pinelli & Symington 2001). Pre-term babies are limited in their ability to suck because of their weak musculature and flexor control, which is important for firm lip and jaw closure (Blackburn 2003, Hurst & Meier 2005). Before 32 weeks, they will need to be tube fed on a regular basis, usually on a 3-hourly regimen with preset amounts of breastmilk, hind milk or formula milk based on postnatal age and present weight, to provide the necessary calories for growth, but not at the expense of energy expenditure (King 2005).

It is now common practice for parents to tube feed their own baby. Als & Butler (2006) believe that parents should provide physical support for head, trunk and shoulders as sucking is part of the flexor pattern of development and may be enhanced by giving the baby something to grasp. Jones & Spencer (2005) note that the pre-term head is very heavy for the weak musculature of the neck and would, if not supported, result in considerable head lag, so correct positioning and attachment to the breast can be made much more difficult to achieve (Hurst & Meier 2005). Poor head alignment can result in airway collapse which may lead to apnoea and bradycardia therefore support from the midwife is essential when initiating breastfeeding. Tube feeding has the advantage that the tube can be left in situ during a cup or breastfeed and has been shown to eliminate the need to introduce bottles into a breastfeeding regimen (Philipp & Radford 2006). McGrath (2004) recommends that some of the softer silastic tubes can be left in place for a month or more and this removes the necessity for regular replacement however several problems have been identified with tube feeding. Babies are preferential nose breathers and the presence of a nasogastric tube will inevitably take up part of their available airway. Their prolonged use has been associated with delay in the development of sucking and swallowing reflexes simply because the mouth is bypassed. For these reasons, cup-feeding has been used in addition to tube feeding in order to provide the baby with a positive oral experience, to stimulate saliva and lingual lipases to aid digestion (Lang 2002), and to accelerate the transition from naso/oral gastric feeding to breastfeeding. Oral gastric tubes have been associated with vagal stimulation and have resulted in bradycardia and apnoea. Preference for nasal or oral gastric tubes remains open to debate (McGrath 2004).

Certain behaviours, such as licking and lapping are well established *before* sucking and swallowing (Ritchie 1998) and when babies are given the opportunity, it is not unusual to see them as early as 28 and 29 weeks, licking milk that has been expressed onto the nipple by their mother. Thus, babies between 30 and 32 weeks' gestation can be given expressed breastmilk (EBM) by cup. Lang (2002) makes the point that tongue movement is vital in the efficient stripping of the milk ducts, so cup-feeding can be seen as developmental preparation for breastfeeding. Between 32 and 34 weeks' gestation, cup-feeding can act as the main method of feeding, with the baby taking occasional complete breastfeeds. Cup-feeds tend to last about the same duration it takes to give a feed by bottle. More importantly, however, they utilize little energy, which is a crucial factor in their favour for LBW babies.

A pre-term baby of <35 weeks' gestation can be gently wrapped /swaddled prior to a feed and this is thought to provide reassurance and comfort, not unlike the unique close-fitting tactile stimulation of the uterus. McGrath (2004) argues that this approach supports development of flexion as well as decreasing disorganized behaviours that could detract from feeding success. A pre-term baby may easily tire and the mother can be taught to start the flow of milk by hand expressing, before attaching him to the breast. Long pauses between sucks are to be expected. This burst–pause pattern is a signal of normal development and seems to occur earlier with breastfeeding. The baby may appear to be asleep and a change in position may remind him of the task in hand, but it is thought to be a mistake to force a reluctant baby to feed (Sparshott 1997). If it is obvious that the baby is more interested in sleeping, the mother can complete the feed by tube.

From 35 weeks onwards, cup-feeding can be gradually replaced by complete breastfeeding (Lang 2002). Progress in the feeding method is often dependent upon the pre-term baby, who cues his mother that he is ready to take milk from the breast. In the interim, she must express her milk so that she can maintain her milk supply and provide the milk for cup-feeding as necessary. An unrushed feed can take up to an hour to complete. Any advances on this timeframe should be reviewed in terms of the quality of the baby–nipple attachment (see Ch. 41), maternal milk flow (which may be affected by anxiety or other factors) and the general condition of the baby (e.g. the development of physiological jaundice). Feeding frequency can vary between 6 and 10 feeds/day. The baby should be left to establish his own volume requirements and feeding pattern. The mother should be encouraged to rely upon her own instincts and common sense so that the rhythm of total care she adopts in hospital will thoroughly prepare her for when she goes home (Lang 2002). Often the difference between early and late transfer home is more dependent upon the mother's positive attitude and skill development than the baby's maturity and inherent abilities.

The care environment: promoting health and development of the healthy LBW baby

The importance of providing an appropriate environment for the healthy LBW baby cannot be overstressed and according to Sparshott (1997), the ideal environment should resemble home, which provides a cycle of day and night, regular nourishment, rest, stimulation and loving attention. The midwife's role is to create such an environment, primarily for the physical development of the baby, but at the same time to provide psychological support for the mother and her family. The mother's desire to be involved is seen as an *essential* element in the success of caring for LBW babies in hospital.

The normal sensory requirements of the developing brain depend upon subtle influences, first from the uterus and then from the breast (Reed & Freer 2000). Any disruption to this natural arrangement renders the LBW baby vulnerable to influences in the care environment that can result in poor coordination as a result of delays in the development of different subsystems (autonomic, motor, sensory, etc.). Reid (2000) believes maternal role development depends upon the mother's self-esteem and her perception of mothering. By attempting to adapt the care environment to be more like the intrauterine environment, the midwife can help parents to become aware of their baby's behavioural and autonomic cues and utilize them in organizing care according to their baby's individual tolerance. The ethos of care is for them to listen and learn from their baby, to come to know and see him as an individual, competent for his stage of development and not merely 'a baby born too early', or a dysfunctional term infant. They will be encouraged (but not cajoled) into taking a major role in their baby's emerging developmental agenda, come to understand the situation in which they find themselves, become more able to reset their expectations and thus offer more baby-led support (Lee 2006b, Reed & Freer 2000).

According to McGrath et al (2004) the emerging task of the term newborn baby is increasing alertness, with growing responsiveness to the outside world. By comparison, a pre-term baby is at a stage of development that is more concerned with their internal world. Term babies have stable function of the autonomic and motor systems. Pre-term babies will be at different stages of this development, depending on their gestational age and health status. They will spend more time in rapid eye movement (REM) sleep or drowsy states and have difficulty in achieving deep sleep. They are unable to shut out stimulation that prevents them from sleeping and resting, and sudden noise hazards provoke stress reactions, which can adversely affect respiratory,

cardiovascular and digestive stability. The term baby is able to shut out such stimuli for rest and sleep purposes. The degree to which SGA term babies have been affected by their unique intrauterine experience is difficult to assess in the short term, but hyperactivity is seen as a feature of an adaptive stress reaction. These babies, like their pre-term counterparts, need an environment that supports their level of robustness. Environmental disturbances, excessive or prolonged handling and even activities like feeding may add an extra physiological burden to an already compromised state. Social contact is considered a vital element for the development of parent–child interaction, yet stereotypical notions of social contact that revolve around practical care giving and feeding may not be suitable for some babies and when these activities are clustered together, may draw too heavily on the baby's physical resources. When the baby is over-stimulated and wishes to terminate the interaction, certain cues according to Vergara & Bigsby (2004) are known as coping signals and are recognized as fist clenching, furrowing of the brow, gaze aversion, splayed fingers and yawning. Should the baby wish to initiate or continue an interaction, he tends to demonstrate approach signals such as raised eyebrows, head raising and engagement in different degrees of eye contact with his social partners. The midwife can reassure parents, that by paying attention to their baby's behavioural cues, they can work *with* his capabilities, which is crucial for maintaining his healthy status (Als & Butler 2006).

Handling and touch

Kangaroo care (KC) is used to promote closeness between a baby and mother and involves placing the nappy-clad baby upright between the maternal breasts for skin-to-skin contact (see Plate 20). The LBW baby remains beneath the mother's clothing for varying periods of time that suit the mother. Some mothers may have repeated contacts throughout the day; others may prefer specific periods around which they plan their day's activities. There are no rules or time limitations applied, but contact should be reviewed if there are any clinical signs of neonatal distress. For the benefits of kangaroo care, see Box 42.3.

Box 42.3 Benefits of kangaroo care

- It endorses the notion of togetherness, which is far removed from the threat of separation
- Mothers show thermal synchrony with their babies in a thermoneutral range
- It provides a sense of containment and closeness that is reminiscent of the uterus
- There is an increased reporting of successful lactation because of increased hormonal and sensory stimulation of the mother's milk production
- There is promotion of early tactile, audiovisual and emotional contact for both, and the baby is given the opportunity to further his familiarity with the mother's voice, smell and heartbeat
- It is thought to be influential in the development of strong emotional feelings to the baby
- Mothers are more quickly adapted to the appearance of their babies
- Mothers are more likely to become their baby's advocate
- It is thought to strengthen the mother's confidence in gaining control over her emotions, her competency in mothering skills and her perception of herself as 'a good mother'.

Sources: Jones & Hartmann (2005), Padden & Glen (1997), Sparshott (1997), WHO (1997b).

Noise and light hazards

The time spent in a postnatal ward should be a time of rest and recuperation for both the mother and her LBW baby. Noise should be kept to a minimum. Harrison et al (2004) assert that all extraneous noises should be eliminated from clinical areas such as musical toys and mobiles, harsh clattering footwear, telephones, radios, intercom systems and raised voices. Clinicians should be aware of noise hazards such as the closing of incubator portholes, use of peddle bins, ward doors and general equipment. Ward areas can be carpeted and quiet signs can be posted to remind visitors not to disrupt the peace (Young 1996). In dimmed lighting conditions, pre-term babies are more able to improve their quality of sleep and alert status. Reduced light levels at night will help to promote the development of circadian rhythms and diurnal cycles. Light levels can be adjusted during the day with curtains or blinds to shade windows and protect the room from direct sunlight. Screens to shield adjacent babies from phototherapy lights are essential.

Sleeping position

Hunter (2004) reports that pre-term babies have reduced muscle power and bulk, with flaccid muscle tone, therefore their movements are erratic, weak or flailing. They exert energy to maintain their body position against the pull of gravity. Without support they may, to differing degrees, develop head, shoulder and hip flattening, which in turn can lead to poor mobility. Nesting the more immature pre-term babies into soft bedding, in addition to the use of close flexible boundaries, helps to keep their limbs in midline flexion; however, it is vital that they are nursed in a supine position to prevent asphyxia. Lying the baby in the supine position is thought to be effective in promoting engagement in self-regulatory behaviours such as exploration of the face and mouth, hand and foot clasping, boundary searching, and flexion and extension of the limbs. Pressure on the occiput should over time ensure a more rounded head.

Sudden infant death syndrome (SIDS)

Placing healthy LBW babies to sleep in the prone position has been theoretically eradicated from neonatal practice and Fleming et al (2004) reiterate that all babies should be placed in the supine position and it is incumbent upon health care professionals to accustom the baby and educate the parents in adopting this approach. The midwife needs to explain how the issues apply to individual families and take into consideration the time of year, gestational age and postnatal age when care is transferred to the community midwife. Parental training on

Box 42.4 Benefits and limitations of caring for healthy LBW babies on postnatal wards

Benefits to the mother

- No separation of mother and baby
- No need for mother to visit NICU or father used as an information conduit
- Less acquired nosocomial infections
- Less stressful environment on postnatal ward, therefore more effective communication and understanding of relevant issues and more able to overcome feelings of shock, anxiety and fear of having a LBW baby
- Rooming-in: more social and physical contact with baby
- Greater perceived sense of control; less feelings of failure
- Enhanced sense of role and identity
- Better skill development and related confidence
- Care is more mother–baby focused; more holistic and 'normal'
- The mother feels part of the ward community, not just 'that mother whose baby in on the baby unit'
- More opportunity for support from peers on the ward
- No 'handing over' the baby's care to a more experienced person and then 'taking back' the responsibility
- The transition to home is considered to be easier and more welcomed by the mother.

Limitations that affect the mother

- The mother may not wish to commit to a prolonged and unspecified hospital stay
- The mother may not have any choice but to return home soon after birth (e.g. other caring responsibilities)

- The mother may feel ambivalence toward the birth event and her baby
- The mother may feel that the NICU is the best place for her baby
- The mother may be ill and not able to care for her baby
- There is no option for the mother who wishes after a few days to take her baby home, which may be too early.

Benefits to the organization

- More NICU cots are made available
- Less need to close NICU (a daily concern for some maternity units)
- Less in utero transfers of high risk women to other neonatal units
- More potential for staff development in caring for LBW babies.

Organizational restraints

- Need for designated area in postnatal wards that will require a warm environment (24°C), reduced extraneous noise and subtle lighting conditions
- Longer hospital stay may block bed capacity
- Possible need for a dedicated course to provide extra education for staff
- Lack of consensus on the midwife's role and neonatal care
- Too few midwives, inadequate resourcing, skill-mix issues.

Sources: Bromley (2000), Lee (2006b), Redshaw (1997).

'what to do if my baby stops breathing' is becoming part of a routine preparation for transfer home, although this degree of preparedness can empower some parents but frighten others. The decision to receive training should be the parent's choice (Resuscitation Council 2006).

The prevention of infection

LBW babies, particularly pre-term babies, are especially vulnerable to infections because of the immaturity of their host defence systems (Mupanemunda & Watkinson 1999). (See Chs 43 and 47 for further details.)

The provision of neonatal care: the question of venue and facilities

The decision to transfer a healthy LBW baby to a postnatal ward, a transitional unit or a NICU will depend upon the baby's gestational age and weight. Perhaps more influential will be the availability of facilities and level of staffing that exists at the time. Traditionally, the advantage of a separate transitional care unit has been to divert medium risk babies away from the NICU, and this has been of great value (Bromley 2000), however, some would argue that part of its attraction has been to take healthy LBW babies that otherwise would have been roomed-in with their mothers on postnatal wards. Some offer rooming-in facilities but some are used as an intermediate unit where, in addition to healthy LBW babies, there are convalescing NICU graduates (Farrer 2005), term babies with congenital abnormalities, babies with feeding problems (particularly where tube-feeding is required) and those babies who need antibiotic therapy. Alternatively, transitional care provision can be found on a postnatal ward in a protected area, or transitional care cots can be interspersed randomly throughout the ward. Postnatal ward care is seen as optimal as separation from their babies and lack of contact are reported by mothers as the worst features of having a baby that needs specialist care (Redshaw 1997) but postnatal wards are often busy, noisy places. For women who need hospital postnatal care, midwives need to make the postnatal environment more conducive for rest, relaxation and recuperation (Wray & Davies 2007). Spitzer (2005) believes that mothers are cued by the environment in which they find themselves. If they are less stressed, able to care for their own baby and enjoy being with other postnatal women and being cared for by midwives, these factors may help them to perceive their hospital postnatal experience as a normative life event and better prepare them for when they go home (see Box 42.4 for the benefits and limitations of caring for LBW babies on postnatal wards). Postnatal visiting by the community midwife should continue for as long as necessary to help the family adapt to their new responsibilities (Nursing and Midwifery Council 2004).

REFERENCES

Als H, Butler S 2006 Neurobehavioural development of the pre-term infant. In: Martin R J, Fanaroff A A, Walsh M C (eds) Fanaroff and Martin's neonatal-perinatal medicine. Diseases of the fetus and infant, Vol. 2. Elsevier Mosby, London.

Anderson M S, Wood L L, Keller J et al 2006 Enteral nutrition. In: Merenstein G B, Gardner S L (eds) Handbook of neonatal intensive care. Elsevier Mosby, St Louis.

Blackburn S T 2003 Maternal, fetal and neonatal physiology. A clinical perspective. Saunders, St Louis.

Bromley P 2000 Transitional care: let's think again. Journal of Neonatal Nursing 6:60–64

Carfoot S, Williamson P R, Dickson R 2003 A systematic review of randomized controlled trials evaluating the effect of mother/baby skin to skin care on successful breast-feeding. Midwifery 19:148–155

Dubowitz L M S, Dubowitz V, Golberg C 1970 Clinical assessment of gestational age in the newborn infant. Journal of Paediatrics 77:1–10

Farrer K (2005) Fetal growth, intrauterine growth retardation and small for gestational age babies. In: Rennie J (ed) Roberton's Textbook of neonatology, 4th edn. Churchill Livingstone, London, p 389–398

Fleming P J, Blair P S, Sidebotham P D et al 2004 Investigating sudden unexpected deaths in infancy and childhood and caring for bereaved families: an integrated multiagency approach. British Medical Journal 328: 331–334

Fowlie P W, McHaffie H 2005 Supporting parents in the neonatal unit. In: McGuire W, Fowlie P W (eds) ABC of pre-term birth. Blackwell Publishing, Oxford

Fransson A L, Karlsson H, Nilsson K 2005 Temperature variation in newborn babies: importance of physical contact with the mother. Archives of Disease in Children. Fetal Neonatal Edition 90:F500–F504.

Gardner S L, Johnson J L 2006 Initial nursery care. In: Merenstein G B, Gardner, S L (eds) Handbook of neonatal intensive care. Elsevier Mosby, St Louis.

Gomella T L, Cunningham M D, Eyal F G et al 1999 Neonatology. Appleton & Lange, Stamford

Harrison L L, Lotas M J, Jorgensen K M 2004 Environmental issues. In: Kenner C, McGrath J M (eds) Developmental care of newborns and infants. A guide for health professionals. Mosby Elsevier, St Louis.

Harlow F D, Spencer A D 1999 Obstetrics for the neonatologist. In: Rennie J M, Roberton N R C (eds) Textbook of neonatology. Churchill Livingstone, Edinburgh, p 157–173

Hunter J 2004 Positioning. In: Kenner C, McGrath (eds) Developmental care of newborns and infants. A guide for health professionals. Mosby, St Louis.

Hurst N, Meier P 2005 Breast-feeding the pre-term infant. In: Riordan J (ed) Breast-feeding and human lactation. Jones and Bartlett, London

King C 2005 Nutritional requirements. In: Jones E, King C (eds) Feeding and nutrition in the pre-term infant. Elsevier Churchill Livingstone, London

Klaus M H, Kennell J H 1982 Parent-infant bonding. Mosby, London

Jones E, Hartmann P E 2005 Milk Expression. In: Jones E, King C (eds) Feeding and nutrition in the pre-term infant. Churchill Livingstone, London

Jones L, Spencer A 1999 Successful pre-term breast-feeding. Practising Midwife 2:54–57

Jones E, Spencer S A 2005 How to achieve successful pre-term breast-feeding. Infant 1(4):14–17

Juretschke L J 2000 Apgar scoring: its use and meaning for today's newborn. Neonatal Network 9:17–19

Lang S 2002 Breast-feeding special care babies. Baillière Tindall, London

Lee B 2006a Pre-term birth: a medical miracle with an emotional cost? RSM Forum. Midwives 9:60–62

Lee B 2006b Pre-term birth: a medical miracle with an emotional cost? RSM Forum. Midwives 9:92–94

Lissauer T, Fanaroff A A, Rodriguez R J et al 2006 Neonatology at a glance. Blackwell, London

McGrath J M 2004 Feeding. In: Kenner C, McGrath J M (eds.) Developmental care of newborns and infants. A guide for health care professionals, Mosby, St Louis

McGrath J M, Kenner C, Amspacher K A 2004 Factors that can influence fetal development. In: Kenner C, McGrath J M (eds) Developmental care of newborns and infants. A guide for health professionals. Mosby Elsevier, St Louis

Mupanemunda R H, Watkinson M 1999 Key topics in neonatology. Bios Scientific, Oxford

Mupanemunda R, Watkinson M 2005 Key topics in neonatology. Taylor and Francis, London

Nursing and Midwifery Council 2004 Midwives rules and standards. NMC, London

Ogata E S 1999 Carbohydrate homeostasis. In: Avery G B, Fletcher M A, McDonald M G (eds) Neonatology, physiopathology and management of the newborn. Lippincott, Williams & Wilkins, London, p 699–712

Padden T, Glen S 1997 Maternal experiences of pre-term birth and neonatal care. Journal of Reproductive and Infant Psychology 15:121–139

Philipp B L, Radford A 2006 Baby-friendly: snappy slogan or standard of care? Archives of Disease in Children, 91:145–149

Pinelli K, Symington A, 2001 Non-nutritive sucking for promoting physiologic stability and nutrition in pre-term infants (Cochrane review). In: The Cochrane Library, issue 3. Update Software, Oxford

Redshaw M E 1997 Mothers of babies requiring special care: attitudes and experiences. Journal of Reproductive and Infant Psychology 15:109–120

Reed T, Freer Y 2000 Developmental nursing care. In: Boxwell G (ed) Neonatal intensive care. Routledge, London

Reid T L 2000 Maternal identity in pre-term birth. Journal of Child Health Care 4:23–29

Resuscitation Council UK 2006 Newborn life support resuscitation at birth, 2nd edn. TT Litho Printers, Kent

Ritchie J F 1998 Immature sucking response in premature babies: cup-feeding as a tool in increasing maintenance of breast-feeding. Journal of Neonatal Nursing 14:13–17

Roberton N R C 1999 Fetal growth, intrauterine growth retardation and small for gestational age babies. In: Rennie J M, Roberton N R C(eds) Textbook of neonatology. Churchill Livingstone, London, p 389–398

Sedin G 2006 The thermal environment of the newborn infant. In: Martin R J, Fanaroff A A, Walsh M C. Fanaroff and Martin's neonatal-perinatal medicine. Diseases of the fetus and infant. Vol. 1, Elsevier Mosby, London

Sparshott M 1997 Pain, distress and the newborn baby. Blackwell Science, Oxford

Spencer N 2003 Weighing the evidence – how is birth weight determined? Radcliffe Medical Press, Oxon

Spitzer A R 2005 Care of the family in the neonatal intensive care unit. In: Spitzer A R (ed) Intensive care of the fetus and neonate. Elsevier Mosby, Philadelphia

Tappero E P, Honeyfield M E 2003 Physical assessment of the newborn. A comprehensive approach to the art of physical examination. NICU.INK, Santa Rosa

Thureen P J, Deacon J, Hernandez JA et al 2005 Assessment and care of the well newborn. Elsevier, St Louis

Tucker J, McGuire W 2005 Epidemiology of pre-term birth In: McGuire W, Fowlie P W (eds) ABC of pre-term birth. BMJ Blackwell Publishing, Oxford

Vergara E R, Bigsby R 2004 Developmental and therapeutic interventions in the NICU. Paul Brookes Publishing, London

WHO/UNICEF 1989 Joint statement – protecting, promoting and supporting breast-feeding. World Health Organization, Geneva

WHO 1977a Manual of international statistical classification of diseases, injuries and causes of death. World Health Organization, Geneva, Vol 1

WHO 1997b Hypoglycaemia of the newborn. Review of the literature. World Health Organization, Geneva

Wray J, Davies L 2007 What women want from postnatal care. Midwives 10:131

Young J 1996 Development care of the premature baby. Baillière Tindall, London

FURTHER READING

Lissauer T, Fanaroff A A, Rodriguez R J, Weindling M 2006 Neonatology at a glance. Blackwell, London.

This book provides a concise overview of neonatology with topics confined to one or two pages with colour illustrations and photographs, ideal for the reader who is relatively new to the subject area and needs to have the important points of discussion made clear and free from unnecessary detail.

43 Recognizing the ill baby

Jean E. Bain

CHAPTER CONTENTS

The length of time a mother spends in hospital with her newborn infant is ever decreasing. The focus of this chapter is to aid the midwife in the early detection of diseases which can be used in conjunction with the newborn examination, thus allowing the midwife to distinguish the ill from the well baby.

The chapter aims to:

- assist the midwife in the assessment and identification of the ill neonate
- provide an overview of the potential or presenting problems of the neonate
- consider the needs of the family by the integration of family-centred care in the neonatal unit.

Introduction

The majority of newborn babies are born normal and healthy; they require no intervention after birth except to be dried with a warm towel and then to have skin-to-skin contact with their mothers. However, although the labour and birth may have been straightforward, the baby will still need to be observed at this time to ensure that the respirations are normal, there is good colour, the body temperature is stable and the baby is active and responsive.

The midwife soon becomes familiar with the appearance and behaviour of the well baby, but must also learn the signs and signals caused by illness, some of which may be subtle and non-specific. The labour and birth have an obvious effect on the well-being of the infant, but added to this are the genetic background, the mother's illnesses in pregnancy and any drugs she may have taken or received during that period (Rennie 2005a).

Parents welcome the observation of their newborn as it provides an opportunity for them to discuss any concerns they may have and the midwife can reassure them that their baby is normal and healthy. If the baby is unwell, this needs to be identified quickly and parents need to be made aware of any problem as soon as possible.

Assessment of the infant

Immediately after birth, all infants should be examined for any gross congenital abnormalities or evidence of birth trauma. They should also have their weight and gestational age plotted on a standard growth chart (see Ch. 42).

Classifying infants according to weight and gestation allows the midwife to assess infants who may require specialized care. Infants who are pre-term, small for gestational age (SGA) or large for gestational age (LGA) are at an increased risk of respiratory disease, hypoglycaemia, polycythaemia and disturbed thermoregulation. Later, usually within the next 24 hrs, a more comprehensive, systematic, physical examination should take place.

Decreasing morbidity and mortality are the goal of all those involved with the care of the newborn infant. The early recognition of existing or potential problems is vital if the appropriate treatment is to be initiated as soon as possible.

Maternal health

Any disease in the mother can have an effect on the pregnancy. Some have more specific effects than others do and reviewing the maternal history is an essential starting point in understanding the potential or presenting problems of the neonate. Influencing factors include:

- pregnancy-induced hypertension
- history of epilepsy
- maternal diabetes
- history of substance abuse
- history of sexually transmitted diseases.

Fetal well-being and health in pregnancy

The following are examples of significant questions that a midwife may ask herself as they may have a critical influence on the well-being of the infant:

- was this a twin pregnancy?
- was the baby presenting by the breech?
- is the baby pre-term?
- is the infant SGA?
- was there poor growth in utero?
- was any evidence of congenital abnormality picked up on scanning, such as enlarged heart or bowel obstruction?

Perinatal and birth complications

Labour and birth may also have an effect on the general welfare of the newborn infant. Listed below are important points that can confirm or rule out fetal compromise:

- prolonged rupture of membranes
- abnormal fetal heart rate pattern
- meconium staining
- difficult or rapid birth
- caesarean section and the reason for this.

Over a period of a few hours the newborn baby needs to adapt to living without placental support, and it is during this time that some problems may manifest themselves. The midwife needs to be able to recognize warning signs and initiate prompt action if deterioration of the baby's condition is to be prevented.

Physical assessment

Most of the information the midwife requires for the assessment of a baby's well-being comes from observation. The baby's breathing pattern will alter depending on his level of activity but a respiratory rate consistently above 60 breaths/min is considered as tachypnoea. Much can be learned by observing the baby's resting position. The normal baby will lie with his limbs partially flexed and active. The skin colour should be centrally pink, indicating adequate oxygenation; there should be no rashes or skin lesions. The signs listed in Box 43.1 may indicate an underlying problem.

After the initial observation there should follow a more systematic examination.

The skin

The skin of a neonate varies in its appearance and can often be the cause of unnecessary anxiety in

> **Box 43.1** General assessment warning signs
>
> - Pallor
> - Central cyanosis
> - Jaundice
> - Apnoea lasting longer than 20 s
> - Heart rate <110 or >180 beats/min (taken during spells of inactivity)
> - Respiratory rate <30 or >60 breaths/min
> - Skin temperature (axilla) <36.2°C or >37.2°C
> - Lack of spontaneous movement and responsiveness
> - Abnormal lying position either hypotonic or hypertonic
> - Lack of interest in surroundings.

the mother, midwife and medical staff. It is, however, often the first sign that there may be an underlying problem in the baby.

The presence of meconium on the skin, which is usually seen in the nail beds and around the umbilicus, is frequently associated with infants who have cardiorespiratory problems. More generally, the skin of all babies should be examined for pallor, plethora, cyanosis, jaundice and skin rashes.

Pallor

A pale, mottled baby is an indication of poor peripheral perfusion. At birth, it can be associated with low circulating blood volume or with circulatory adaptation and compensation for perinatal hypoxaemia. The anaemic infant's appearance is usually pale pink, white or, in severe cases where there is vascular collapse, grey. Other presenting signs are tachycardia, tachypnoea and poor capillary refill (to assess capillary refill, press the skin briefly on the forehead or abdomen and observe how long it takes for the colour to return; this should be prompt).

The most likely causes of anaemia in the newborn period are:

- a history in the infant of haemolytic disease of the newborn
- twin-to-twin transfusions in utero (which can cause one infant to be anaemic and the other polycythaemic)

- maternal antepartum or intrapartum haemorrhage.

Pallor can also be observed in infants who are hypothermic or hypoglycaemic. Problems associated with pallor include:

- anaemia and shock
- respiratory disorders
- cardiac anomalies
- sepsis (where poor peripheral perfusion might also be observed).

Plethora

Babies who are beetroot in colour are usually described as plethoric. Their colour may indicate an excess of circulating red blood cells (polycythaemia). This is defined as a venous haematocrit >70%. Newborn infants can become polycythaemic if they are recipients of:

- twin-to-twin transfusion in utero
- a large placental transfusion.

Contributing factors are delayed clamping of umbilical cord, or holding the infant below the level of the placenta, thereby allowing blood to flow into the baby and giving a greater circulating blood volume (sometimes occurring in un-assisted births). Other infants at risk are:

- small for gestational age babies
- infants of diabetic mothers
- those with Down syndrome
- neonatal hypothyroidism
- chromosomal disorders.

Hypoglycaemia is commonly seen in plethoric infants because red blood cells consume glucose. The infant can exhibit a neurological disorder; irritability, jitteriness and convulsions can occur. Other problems that may manifest are:

- apnoea
- respiratory distress
- cardiac failure
- necrotizing enterocolitis.

The diagnosis of polycythaemia is based upon haemoglobin and haematocrit level comparisons with normal values based on gestation. The treatment for symptomatic polycythaemia is to replace red blood cells by means of a partial exchange using a crystalloid solution such as normal saline. Infants who are non-symptomatic should be observed. There is no evidence to support the use of fresh frozen plasma or albumin, both carry a significant risk of transfusion-related sepsis (Roberts 2003).

Cyanosis

Central cyanosis should always be taken very seriously. The mucous membranes are the most reliable indicators of central colour in all babies and if the tongue and mucous membranes appear blue this indicates low oxygen saturation levels in the blood, usually of respiratory or cardiac origin. Episodic central cyanotic attacks may be an indication that the infant is having a convulsion. Peripheral cyanosis of the hands and feet is common during the first 24 hrs of life; after this time it may be a non-specific sign of illness. Central cyanosis always demands urgent attention.

Jaundice

Early onset jaundice (presenting within the first 12 hrs of life) is abnormal and needs investigating. If a jaundiced baby is unduly lethargic, is a poor feeder, vomits or has an unstable body temperature, this may indicate infection and action should be taken to exclude this (see Ch. 47).

Other factors that affect the appearance of the skin

Pre-term infants have thinner skin that is redder in appearance than that of term infants. In post-term infants the skin is often dry and cracked.

The skin is a good indicator of the nutritional status of the infant. The SGA infant may look malnourished and have folds of loose skin over the joints, owing to the lack or loss of subcutaneous fat. This can predispose the infant to problems with hypoglycaemia due to poor glycogen stores in the liver and can also cause problems with hypothermia.

If the infant is dehydrated, the skin looks dry and pale and is often cool to touch. If gently pinched, it will be slow in retracting. Other signs of dehydration are: pallor or mottled skin, sunken fontanelle or eyeball sockets and tachycardia.

Skin rashes

Skin rashes are quite common in newborn babies but most are benign and self-limiting.

Milia

These are white or yellow papules seen over the cheeks, nose and forehead. These invariably disappear spontaneously over the first few weeks of life (Plate 16).

Miliaria

These are clear vesicles on the face, scalp and perineum, caused by retention of sweat in unopened sweat glands. They appear on the chest and around areas where clothes can cause friction. The treatment is to nurse the infant in a cooler environment or to remove excess clothing.

Petechiae or purpura rash

These can occur in neonatal thrombocytopenia, which is a condition of platelet deficiency and usually presents with a petechial rash over the whole of the body. There may also be prolonged bleeding from puncture sites or the umbilicus, or both, and bleeding into the gut. Thrombocytopenia may be found in infants with:

- congenital infections, both viral and bacterial
- maternal idiopathic thrombocytopenia
- drugs (administered to mother or infant)
- severe rhesus haemolytic disease.

Bruising

This can occur extensively following breech extractions, forceps and ventouse deliveries. The bleeding can cause a decrease in circulating blood volume, predisposing the baby to anaemia or, if the bruising is severe, hypotension.

Erythema toxicum

This is a rash that consists of white papules on an erythematous base; it occurs in about 30–70% of infants. This condition is benign and should not be confused with a staphylococcal infection, which will require antibiotics. Diagnosis can be confirmed by examination of a smear of aspirate from a pustule, which will show numerous eosinophils (white cells indicative of an allergic response, rather than infection).

Infectious lesions (see also Ch. 47)

Thrush

This is a fungal infection of the mouth and throat. It is very common in neonates especially if they have been treated with antibiotics. It presents as white patches seen over the tongue and mucous membranes and as a red rash on the perineum.

Herpes simplex virus

If acquired in the neonatal period, is a most serious viral infection. Transmission in utero is rare; the infection usually occurs during birth with the illness presenting after 3 days. Seventy per cent of affected infants will produce a rash, which appears as vesicles or pustules. Mortality depends on severity of the illness and when treatment commenced (Logan 1990) (Plate 24).

Umbilical sepsis

This can be caused by a bacterial infection. Until its separation, the umbilical cord can be a focus for infection by bacteria that colonize the skin of the newborn. If periumbilical redness occurs or a discharge is noted, it may be necessary to commence antibiotic therapy in order to prevent an ascending infection.

Staphylococcal

This commonly presents as a few yellow filled bullae (Plates 25, 26). Severe infections can give rise to **bullous impetigo** which makes the skin look as though it has been scalded. It presents as widespread tender erythema, followed by blisters, which break leaving raw areas of skin. This is particularly noticeable around the napkin area but can also cause umbilical sepsis, breast abscesses, conjunctivitis and, in deep infections, there may also be involvement of the bones and joints.

Respiratory system

Respiratory distress in the newborn can be a presentation of a number of clinical disorders and is the major factor in the morbidity and mortality in the neonatal period.

It is important to observe the baby's breathing when he is at rest and when he is active. The midwife should always start by observing skin colour and then carry out a respiratory inspection, taking into account whether the baby is making either an extra effort or insufficient effort to breathe.

Respiratory inspection

Respirations should be counted by watching the lower chest and abdomen rise and fall for a full minute. The respiration rate should be between 40 and 60 breaths/min but will vary according to the level of activity. Newborn infants are primarily nose breathers and so obstructions of the nares may lead to respiratory distress and cyanosis. *Remember if suction is required at any time; always suction the mouth first and then the nose.* The chest should expand symmetrically. If there is unilateral expansion and breath sounds are diminished on one side, this may indicate that a pneumothorax has occurred. Infants at risk of pneumothorax or other air leaks are:

- pre-term infants with respiratory distress
- term infants with meconium-stained amniotic fluid
- infants who require resuscitation at birth.

Increased work of breathing

If the baby's respiratory rate at rest is above 60 breaths/min, this is described as *tachypnoea*. When observing an infant's respiratory rate the midwife must always take into consideration the environment and the temperature in which the baby is being nursed. Overheating will cause an infant to breathe faster.

Any infant with persistent tachypnoea may be described as having respiratory distress, and the midwife should also observe the quality of the respirations, noting if there is any inspiratory pulling in of the chest wall above and below the sternum, or between the ribs (retraction). If nasal flaring is also present, this may indicate that there has been a delay in the lung fluid clearance (transient tachypnoea of the newborn) or that a more serious respiratory problem is developing (respiratory distress syndrome, meconium aspiration, pneumonia) (Tappero & Honeyfield 2003).

Grunting, heard either with a stethoscope or audibly, is an abnormal expiratory sound. The grunting baby forcibly exhales against a closed glottis in order to prevent the alveoli from collapsing. These infants may require help with their breathing, either by intubation or continuous positive airway pressure ventilation (CPAP) (see also Ch. 44).

Apnoea

Apnoea is defined as a cessation of breathing for 20s or more. It is associated with pallor, bradycardia, cyanosis, oxygen desaturation or a change in the level of consciousness (American Academy 1978). Any baby having apnoeic spells needs to be admitted to a neonatal unit to have his cardiorespiratory system monitored.

The most common cause of apnoea in pre-term babies is pulmonary surfactant deficiency (see Ch. 44) or the immaturity of the central nervous system control mechanism. Other disorders that may produce apnoea in the newborn are:

- hypoxia
- pneumonia
- aspiration
- pneumothorax
- metabolic disorders (e.g. hypoglycaemia, hypocalcaemia, acidosis)
- anaemia
- maternal drugs
- neurological problems (e.g. intracranial haemorrhage, convulsions, developmental disorders of the brain)
- congenital anomalies of the upper airway.

It is very important to remember that apnoea may also be induced by stimulation of the posterior pharynx by suction catheters.

Body temperature

Thermoregulation is a critical physiological function that is closely related to the survival of the infant. It is therefore essential that all those caring for newborn infants are aware of the importance of the thermal environment and understand the need for maintenance of normal body temperature (Merenstein & Gardner 2006).

A neutral thermal environment is defined as the ambient air temperature at which oxygen consumption or heat production is minimal, with body temperature in the normal range (Lissauce & Faranoff 2006).

The normal body temperature range for term infants is 36.5–37.3°C.

Environments that are outside the neutral thermal environment may result in the infant developing hypothermia or hyperthermia. Babies who are too cold or too warm will try and regulate their temperature and this action, especially in the pre-term and SGA infant, can have a detrimental effect (see also Ch. 42).

Note: Intermittent temperature recordings have traditionally been taken using mercury thermometers. Research suggests that this practice is hazardous and should be eradicated (Smith et al 1997).

Hypothermia

Hypothermia is defined as a core temperature below 36°C (Rutter 2005). When the body temperature is below this level the infant is at risk from cold stress. This can cause complications such as increased oxygen consumption, lactic acid production, apnoea, decrease in blood coagulability and, the most commonly seen, hypoglycaemia. In pre-term infants, cold stress may also cause a decrease in surfactant secretion and synthesis.

After birth a baby's body temperature can fall very quickly. The healthy term baby will try to maintain his temperature within the normal range. If, however, he is compromised at birth by any of the following conditions, the added stress of hypothermia can be disastrous:

- severe asphyxia
- extensive resuscitation
- delayed drying at birth
- respiratory distress
- hypoglycaemia
- sepsis – septic infants often have hypothermia rather than hyperthermia
- being pre-term or SGA – these infants have poor glucose stores, decreased subcutaneous tissue and little or no brown fat stores.

When a neonate is exposed to cold he will at first become very restless; then, as his body temperature falls, he adopts a tightly flexed position to try to conserve heat. The sick or pre-term infant will tend to lie supine in a frog-like position with all his surfaces exposed, which maximizes heat loss (Roberton 2002).

Adults can generate heat from shivering, whereas neonates perform non-shivering thermogenesis utilizing their brown fat stores. During brown fat metabolism, oxygen is consumed and this may cause an alteration in the respiratory pattern, usually increasing the rate. Added to this, the baby often looks pale or mottled and may be uninterested in feeding. Hypoglycaemia is a common feature of infants with increased energy expenditure associated with thermoregulation and this can cause the infant to have jittery movements of the limbs, even though he is quiet and often limp.

Hyperthermia

Hyperthermia is defined as a core temperature above 38.0°C (Rutter 2005). The usual cause of hyperthermia is overheating of the environment, but it can also be a clinical sign of sepsis, brain injury or drug therapy. If an infant is too warm, he becomes restless and may have bright red cheeks. Hyperthermia has a similar effect on the body to that of hypothermia and is equally detrimental. An infant will attempt to regulate his temperature by increasing his respiratory rate and this can lead to an increased fluid loss by evaporation through the airways. Other problems caused by hyperthermia are hypernatraemia, jaundice and recurrent apnoea.

Note: Variability in body temperature, either high or low, may be the first and only sign that a baby is unwell.

Cardiovascular system

The normal heart rate of a newborn baby is 110–160 b.p.m., with an average of 130 b.p.m. (Kozier et al 1998). The heart rate varies with respiration in the newborn; however, heart rates persistently outside this range when at rest, may suggest an underlying cardiac problem. Cardiovascular dysfunction should be suspected in infants who commonly present with lethargy and breathlessness during feeding. It is often the baby's mother who first expresses concern: her baby may be slow with his feeds, and she may say he looks pale at times or that he feels very sweaty or has fast or laboured breathing.

It can be very difficult to identify infants with congenital heart disease because the clinical picture of tachycardia, tachypnoea, pallor or cyanosis may be suggestive of a respiratory problem or sepsis.

Problems that occur in neonatal cardiovascular function are usually caused either by congenital defects or by a failure of the transition from fetal to adult circulation. Persistent pulmonary hypertension of the newborn is usually seen in term or post-term infants who have a history of hypoxia or asphyxia at birth. The infants are slow to take their first breath or are difficult to ventilate. Respiratory distress and cyanosis are seen before 12 hrs of age. Hypoxaemia is usually profound and may suggest cyanotic heart disease (see Ch. 46). Risk factors include meconium-stained amniotic fluid, nuchal cord, placental abruption, acute blood loss and maternal sedation.

Congenital heart disease affects just under 1% of newborn infants, many of whom will be asymptomatic in the neonatal period (Fowlie & Forsyth 1995). Infants who appear breathless but have little or no rib recession, are not grunting and have only a moderately raised respiratory rate may have heart disease. Cyanosis can be a prominent feature in some cardiac defects, but not all. Box 43.2 lists signs that may be indicative of congenital heart disease.

Cardiac failure may be rapid in onset; the earlier it presents, the more sinister is the cause. Delays in recognizing and treating heart failure may lead to a rapid deterioration and cardiogenic shock. Cardiac shock may resemble early septicaemia, pneumonia or meningitis (David 1995). The first indication of an underlying cardiac lesion may be the presence of a murmur heard on routine examination. However, a soft localized systolic murmur with no evidence of any symptoms of cardiac disease is usually of no significance.

Central nervous system

Assessment of an infant's neurological status is usually carried out on a baby who is awake but not crying. Abnormal postures, which include neck retraction, frog-like postures, hyperextension or hyperflexion of the limbs, jittery or abnormal involuntary movements and a high-pitched or weak cry, could be indicative of neurological impairment and a need for investigation (Rennie 2005b).

> **Box 43.2** Warning signs suggestive of congenital heart disease
>
> **Presentation**
>
> - Cyanosis (often the cyanosis is out of proportion to the degree of respiratory distress)
> - Persistent tachypnoea
> - Persistent tachycardia at rest
> - Poor feeding: infants may be breathless and sweaty during the feed or after feeding; they may not complete their feeds and subsequently fail to thrive
> - A sudden gain in weight leading to clinical signs of oedema; this is usually noted as the baby having puffy feet or eyelids and, in males, the scrotum being swollen
> - A very loud systolic murmur is invariably significant
> - Evidence of cardiac enlargement on X-ray, persisting beyond 48 hrs of life
> - Enlargement of the liver.

Neurological disorders

Neurological disorders found at or soon after birth may be either prenatal or perinatal in origin. They include:

- congenital abnormalities: hydrocephaly, microcephaly, encephalocele, chromosomal anomalies
- hypoxic-ischaemic cerebral injuries
- birth traumas: skull fractures, spinal cord and brachial plexus injuries, subdural and subarachnoid haemorrhage
- infections passed on to the fetus (toxoplasmosis, rubella, cytomegalovirus (CMV), syphilis).

Neurological disorders that appear in the neonatal period need to be recognized promptly in order to minimize brain damage. These include:

- infection: meningitis, herpes simplex, viral encephalitis
- hypoxia: birth asphyxia, respiratory distress, apnoeic episodes

- metabolic: acidosis, hypoglycaemia, hyponatraemia, hypernatraemia, hypothermia, hypocalcaemia, hypomagnesaemia
- drug withdrawal: narcotics, barbiturates, general anaesthesia
- intracranial haemorrhage or intraventricular haemorrhage (IVH)
- secondary bleeding: intracranial haemorrhage from thrombocytopenia or disseminated intravascular coagulation (DIC).

Cerebral hypoxia and bacterial infections are of prime importance. Prompt diagnosis, investigation and treatment are vital as delay can have a significant impact on neurological development (Rennie 2005a).

Terminology

Terminology that describes abnormal movement in babies is very variable and includes 'fits', 'convulsions', 'seizures', 'twitching', 'jumpy' and 'jittery'. In contrast, a baby with poor muscle tone is described as 'floppy'. It is often very difficult to distinguish a seizure from jitteriness or irritability. The jittery baby has tremors, rapid movement of the extremities or fingers that are stopped when the limb is held or flexed. Jitteriness can be normal but is more often seen in infants who are affected by drug withdrawal or in infants with hypoglycaemia.

Seizures

Seizures in the newborn period can be extremely difficult to diagnose, as they are often very subtle and easily missed (Table 43.1).

The most common causes of seizure activity are:

- asphyxia
- metabolic disturbance
- intracranial or intraventricular haemorrhage
- infection
- malformation or genetic defect.

Hypotonia (floppy infant)

The term *hypotonia* or 'floppy baby' describes the loss of body tension and tone. As a result, the infant adopts an abnormal posture that is noticeable on handling.

Table 43.1 Neonatal seizure chart

Type	Affected infant
Subtle	
Apnoea usually with abnormal eye movements, tonic horizontal deviation, blinking, fluttering eyelids, jerking, drooling, sucking, tonic posturing or unusual movements of the limbs (rowing, peddling or swimming)	Most frequent type and most commonly seen in pre-term infants
Clonic	
Jerking activity. Multifocal or unifocal distinct from jittering	Term infants: hypoxic-ischaemic encephalopathy, or inborn errors of metabolism
Tonic	
Posturing similar to decerebrate posture in adults	Pre-term infants with intraventricular haemorrhage
Myoclonic	
Single or multiple jerks of upper or lower extremities	Possible prediction of myoclonic spasm in early infancy

Adapted from Volpe 2001.

Pre-term infants below 30 weeks' gestation have a resting position that is usually characterized as hypotonic. By 34 weeks, their thighs and hips are flexed and they lie in a frog-like position, usually with their arms extended. At 36–38 weeks' gestation, the resting position of a healthy newborn baby is one of total flexion with immediate recoil. Hypotonia in a term infant is not normal and requires investigation. It is also important to determine whether the hypotonia is associated with weakness or normal power in the infant's limbs. The causes of hypotonia include:

- maternal sedation
- birth asphyxia
- prematurity
- infection
- Down syndrome
- metabolic problems (e.g. hypoglycaemia, hyponatraemia, inborn errors of metabolism)
- neurological problems (e.g. spinal cord injuries (sustained by difficult breech or forceps delivery), myasthenia gravis related to maternal disease, myotonic dystrophy)
- endocrine (e.g. hypothyroidism)
- neuromuscular disorders.

Renal and genitourinary system

Urinary infections in the newborn period are quite common, especially in males. The baby typically presents with lethargy, poor feeding, increasing jaundice and vomiting. Urine that only dribbles out, rather than being passed forcefully, may be an indication of a problem with posterior urethral valves. Urine that is cloudy in appearance or smelly may be an indication of a urinary tract infection.

The genitourinary tract has the highest percentage of anomalies, congenital or genetic, of all the organ systems. Prenatal diagnosis is possible with ultrasound and aids the early assessment and intervention, which is essential if kidney damage is to be prevented. Renal problems may present as a failure to pass urine. The normal infant usually passes urine 4–10 hrs after birth. Normal urine output for a term baby in the first day of life should be 2–4 ml/kg per hour. A urine output of <1 ml/kg per hour (oliguria) in the first few days of life should be investigated (Modi 2005). Urinalysis using reagent strips will give information that may be helpful in diagnosis (Table 43.2).

Common causes of reduced urine output include:

- inadequate fluid intake
- increased fluid loss due to hyperthermia, use of radiant heaters and phototherapy units

Table 43.2 Information obtainable from urinalysis with reagent strips

Test	Significance
Urine pH	Failure to acidify the urine may indicate a dysfunction of the renal tubular system, which plays a primary role in the regulation of bicarbonate concentration
Specific gravity	Indicates urine concentration
Blood	Is suggestive of trauma or inflammation of the genitourinary tract
Protein	May suggest renal disease

- birth asphyxia
- congenital abnormalities
- infection.

Documentation of the passage of urine after birth is important as it provides a record that may help if concerns arise.

Gastrointestinal tract

Some congenital abnormalities of the gastrointestinal tract can now be diagnosed antenatally by ultrasound. Other defects, however, may not be suspected until the infant becomes unwell.

Intestinal obstructions may be caused by atresias, malformations or structural damage anywhere below the stomach. In the newborn period, gastrointestinal disorders often present with vomiting, abdominal distension, a failure to pass stools, or diarrhoea with or without blood in the stools. However, vomiting in the postnatal period can be caused by factors other than gastrointestinal obstructions. The midwife should distinguish between posseting, which occurs with winding and overhandling after feeding, and vomiting due to overfeeding, infection or intestinal abnormalities. Early vomiting may be caused by the infant swallowing meconium or maternal blood at delivery. This can cause a gastritis, which will eventually settle.

All vomit should be checked for the presence of bile or blood. Observe the infant for other signs such as abdominal distension, watery or bloodstained stools and temperature instability.

The normal term baby usually passes about eight stools a day. Breastfed babies' stools are looser and more frequent than those of bottle-fed babies, and the colour varies more and sometimes appears greenish. The infant who has an infection can often display signs of gastrointestinal problems, usually poor feeding, vomiting or diarrhoea, or both. Diarrhoea caused by gastroenteritis is usually very watery and may sometimes resemble urine. The cause is either bacterial or viral. Infants with this condition must be isolated and scrupulous hand washing adhered to (Isaacs & Moxon 2000). Loose stools can also be a feature of infants being treated for hyperbilirubinaemia with phototherapy.

Some of the more commonly seen gastrointestinal problems include: duodenal atresia, malrotation of the gut, volvulus, meconium ileus (see Ch. 46), necrotizing enterocolitis, imperforate anus, rectal fistulas and Hirschsprung's disease.

Necrotising enterocolitis (NEC)

NEC is an acquired disease of the small and large intestine caused by ischaemia of the intestinal mucosa. It occurs more often in pre-term babies, but may also occur in term babies who have been asphyxiated at delivery or babies with polycythaemia and hypothermia (commonly found in SGA babies). NEC may present with vomiting or, if gastric emptying is being monitored, the aspirate is large and bile stained. The abdomen becomes distended (Plate 27), stools are loose and may have blood in them. In the early stages of NEC, the baby can display non-specific signs of temperature instability, unstable glucose levels, lethargy and poor peripheral circulation. As the illness progresses, the baby becomes apnoeic and bradycardic and may need ventilating. (See also Chs 44 and 47.)

Imperforate anus

All babies should be checked at birth for this.

Rectal fistulas

The midwife should look for the presence of meconium in the urine or, in female babies, meconium being passed from the vagina.

Hirschsprung's disease

Hirschsprung's disease should be suspected in term babies with delayed passage of meconium, certainly after the first 24 hrs of life (see Ch. 46). Abdominal distension and vomiting are clinical signs, with the vomit becoming bile stained if meconium is not passed.

Metabolic disorders

Metabolic disorders, such as galactosaemia and phenylketonuria, present in the newborn period with vomiting, weight loss, jaundice and lethargy (see Ch. 48).

Meeting the needs of the ill baby and the family

The baby

Babies who are clearly unwell, distressed or less than 1800g at birth require admission to a neonatal unit (NNU). Early separation of mother and baby is very damaging and should be avoided unless absolutely necessary. Asymptomatic babies above 1800g, irrespective of gestation, should be able to stay with their mother either on a ward, or for infants with minor problems only, in a transitional care unit. Managing these babies can be challenging for midwives as some of them may require tube feeding, monitoring of their blood glucose levels and antibiotic therapy. Drug administration is playing an ever-increasing role in the management of the ill baby. Table 43.3 lists some antibiotic drugs commonly used to treat suspected neonatal sepsis.

Drug administration

Antibiotics are the most common drugs used in NNUs. Premature babies have very little immunity to infections that can be acquired congenitally. Suspected infections are always treated with antibiotics, immediately after blood cultures have been taken. Once the results of the blood cultures are known, antibiotics may be continued or stopped.

Drugs can be given to neonates orally, intramuscularly, intravenously, topically or rectally. The most efficient and effective route to administer drugs to a baby is by the intravenous route; this is because the absorption of drugs via the stomach is dependent on factors in the baby relating to gastric emptying time and gastric and duodenal pH. Intramuscular administration is often a painful route and absorption is

Table 43.3 Commonly used drugs to treat neonatal sepsis

Drug	Some possible neonatal infections	Organism
Acyclovir	Chickenpox, rous sarcoma virus	Virus
Ceftriaxone	Meningitis	Gram −ve cocci
Ceftazidime	Meningitis	Gram −ve cocci
Clarithromycin	Chlamydia	Gram −ve cocci, Gram +ve cocci
Co-amoxiclav	Otis media, lower respiratory infections	Gram −ve cocci, Gram +ve cocci
Flucloxacillin	Skin infections, *Staphylococcus aureus*	Gram −ve cocci
Gentamicin	*Escherichia coli, Klebsiella*	Gram −ve cocci
Metronidazole	Necrotizing enterocolitis	Anaerobes
Penicillin G and V	Group B streptococcus	Gram +ve cocci
Vancomycin	*Staphylococcus epidermidis, Staphylococcus aureus*	Gram +ve cocci

dependent on blood flow to the muscle, which can be compromised in a baby who is poorly perfused.

Whichever route is used, all drugs must be administered safely in accordance with unit/ward/hospital policy and meet the guidelines for administration of medicines (Nursing & Midwifery Council 2007). Many drugs will need to be diluted prior to administration to allow for accurate measurement of the required dose. Unfortunately, mistakes in drug administration are not uncommon, and having two nurses/midwives calculate and check the dose will decrease the risk of an error occurring.

Before administering any drugs to a baby the midwife should always check that it is:

- the right drug
- the right baby
- the right route
- the right dose
- the right time.

Drug calculations

To avoid misinterpretation of doses prescribed, only approved abbreviations should be used.

Before calculating the volume required to give the correct dose, the midwife should write down the strength of the drug in the ampoule or vial; for example, ampoules of gentamicin (paediatric) contain 20 mg of gentamicin diluted in 2 ml of water. If the dose prescribed is 8 mg the calculation is as follows:

> (Dose you require) *times* (the volume of the gentamicin) *divided by* (the amount of gentamicin in the vial) which in this case is: $(8\,mg) \times (2\,ml)/20\,mg = 0.8\,ml$ therefore, *0.8 ml is to be administered to the infant.*
>
> Once you have the answer, ask yourself: *Does it make sense?*

Developmentally focused, family-centred care

For parents, the birth of a baby is a mixture of joy, emotional exhilaration and relief. Most newborn babies are normal and healthy and few parents ever expect or consider the possibility of having a baby that is less than perfect (Cameron 1996). Neither will they have considered the implications of separation if their baby has to be admitted to the NNU. So when a baby requires medical assistance, because of prematurity, illness or congenital malformations, the effect on the parents can be significant and force the family into a crisis that can be as devastating as bereavement. The parents' ability to resolve the crisis will depend on how realistically they perceive their baby's problems.

Separation of mother and baby, even if it is for a short while, may increase the risk of the parents developing parental difficulties, with effects on their pattern of behaviour and general responses towards their baby (Coffman 1992).

The environment of the NNU, however thoughtful the layout and design, is an alarming place to enter, with machinery that bleeps and alarms continuously (Plates 18, 19). Anxiety levels are often high. Midwives, nurses and medical staff have an important part to play to enable parents to feel welcome and equal partners in the care of their baby.

NNUs should be bright, friendly and welcoming. Parents should be encouraged to bring in brightly coloured toys and mobiles for their babies; one or two of these can be placed in the incubator or cot. This is of special importance for longer stay babies to aid their neurological development. In most NNUs, a sitting room, often with kitchen facilities, is provided for parents and children. This is a place of retreat, away from the stresses and strains of busy nurseries. The provision of bedrooms or family rooms, or both, where parents can stay if their baby is critically ill, or sadly if their baby has died, is of crucial importance (see Ch. 38).

If it is known in advance that a baby may require admission to the NNU, parents should be given the opportunity to visit and meet some of the staff. They can be shown the room or area where their baby will be admitted, and a brief explanation of the various items of monitoring equipment may help to alleviate some of their fears about what will happen to their baby after it has been born. Following the delivery and if possible, the parents should be allowed to hold or touch their baby, even if it is for just a few moments, before he is taken to the NNU.

On admission to the NNU, a photograph should be taken. This photograph must be given to the parents as soon as possible, as this will go some way towards reassuring them that their baby is safe and alive (Slade 1988). Parents should be encouraged to visit their baby in the NNU as soon they are able. When discussing the baby with the parents, the midwife should try always to use the name that they have given their child as this establishes the baby's identity and makes the conversation more personalized.

The pre-term infant may require a lengthy stay in the NNU, in which case parenting roles may be difficult to establish owing to the physical condition of the baby who may be on a ventilator, being fed intravenously, or be under phototherapy lights. All of these act as a barrier between the baby and the parents and undermine their confidence. They may look for areas of baby care with which they are familiar, and will often adopt a passive role and concentrate on family routines in order to cope (Redshaw & Harris 1995). It is during this time of crisis, when parents are at their most vulnerable, that they will look to staff to provide information and support. Communication at this time must be on a basic level and backed up with information leaflets in a language they can understand (Taylor 1996).

The most important visual aid for any baby is the human face, especially the talking face, which stimulates both visual and auditory pathways. Parents and siblings should be encouraged to communicate with their baby even if it has to be through the porthole window of the incubator (Gardner & Goldson 2006).

Involving the parents, as partners in care, should be encouraged as soon as the baby's condition and tolerance to handling permits. This early involvement will strengthen their understanding of the baby belonging to them and increase their confidence in their ability to provide care. A supportive environment, in which the parents gain confidence in assuming the role of caregivers, is of fundamental importance to the general well-being of the baby. In order to reinforce the parents' involvement in the care of their baby, it is important to discuss whether the baby is to be breast- or bottle-fed. Midwives and neonatal nurses should encourage mothers to breastfeed their babies, or to express their breastmilk, as it provides a greater protection against infection. Breastfeeding or expressing milk may help the mother feel closer to her baby and may also make her feel that she is contributing to her baby's care in a way that nobody else can.

Minimal handling

Care should be individualized for each baby and not be performed routinely. This requires thoughtful planning to avoid repeatedly disturbing the baby. Questions should be asked about performing unnecessary procedures such as repeated heel stabs. Painful, invasive procedures that are not vital to the individual baby's needs are stress-producing events and should be eliminated. Studies by Sparshott

(1991) and Becker et al (1993) have shown that babies' responses to their environment can be directly linked to their experiences. Increasingly, NNUs are introducing a system of individualized developmental care for pre-term babies aimed at reducing their stress levels. This innovative care programme is based on the studies by Als et al (1994). Day and night cycles should be recognized, lights should be dimmed at nighttime and noise levels, which are often alarmingly high, should be reduced. Remember though that it is essential that ill babies are observed; when monitor alarms are cancelled they need to be reset.

Sibling relationships

Encouraging brothers and sisters to visit their new baby is important. Parents are often anxious about the effect an ill baby may have on the family. However, this may cause anxiety in the siblings and they may feel worried, rejected and left out, causing them to demonstrate behavioural problems.

Discharge home

Effective discharge planning should commence as soon as the baby is admitted to the NNU. Encouraging parents to participate in the care of their baby from the beginning enables them eventually to be the sole caregivers and assume total charge.

Parents should learn how to feed, bathe, dress and generally care for their baby. If the baby has special needs like tube feeding or stoma care, training needs may span several weeks and must be backed up with written information. The parents must feel comfortable about caring for their baby before going home.

REFERENCES

Als H, Lawhon G, Duffy F H 1994 Individualized developmental care for the very low birth weight pre-term infant. Journal of the American Medical Association 272(11):853–858

American Academy of Pediatrics taskforce on prolonged apnea 1978. Prolonged apnea. Pediatrics 61:651–652

Becker P T, Grunwald P C, Moorman J 1993 Effects of developmental care on behavioral organization in very low birth weight infants. Nursing Research 42(4):214–220

Cameron J 1996 Parents as partners in care. British Journal of Midwifery 4(4):218–219

Coffman S 1992 Parent and infant attachment: review of nursing research 1981–1990. Paediatric Nurse 18(4):421–425

David T J 1995. Symptoms of disease in childhood. Blackwell Science, Oxford, p 92–94

Fowlie P, Forsyth J S 1995 Examination of the newborn infant. Modern Midwife 4(12):15–17

Gardner S L, Goldson E 2006 The neonate and the environment: impact on development. In: Merenstein G V, Gardner S L (eds) Handbook of neonatal intensive care, 6th edn. Mosby, St Louis, p 273–349

Isaacs D, Moxon R 2000 Handbook of neonatal infections; a practical guide. W B Saunders, London, p 423–434

Kozier B, Erb G, Blais K et al 1998 Fundamentals of nursing, 5th edn. Addison Wesley, New York

Logan S 1990 Viral infections in pregnancy. In: Chamberlain G L (ed.) Modern ante-natal care of the fetus. Blackwell Scientific, Oxford, p 201–221

Lissauce T, Faranoff A 2006. Neonatology at a glance. Blackwell Science, London

Merenstein G V, Gardner S L 2006 Handbook of neonatal intensive care, 6th edn. C V Mosby, St Louis

Modi N 2005. Fluid and electrolyte balance. In: Rennie J (ed.) Roberton's textbook of neonatology, 4th edn. Churchill Livingstone, Edinburgh, p 335–354

Nursing & Midwifery Council, 2007 Guidelines for the Administration of Medicines, NMC

Redshaw M, Harris A 1995 Maternal perceptions of neonatal care. Acta Paediatrica 84:593–598

Rennie J 2005a Examination of the newborn. In: Rennie (ed.) Roberton's textbook of neonatology, 4th edn. Churchill Livingstone, Edinburgh

Rennie J 2005b Seizures in the newborn, part 2. In: Rennie J (ed.) Roberton's textbook of neonatology, 4th edn. Churchill Livingstone, Edinburgh

Roberts I A G 2003 Hematological problems of the newborn. In: McIntosh N, Helms P, Smyth, R (eds) Forfar and Arneil's, Textbook of Pediatrics, 6th edn. Churchill Livingstone, Edinburgh, p 294–309

Roberton N C R 2002 A manual of neonatal intensive care. Edward Arnold, London

Rutter N 2005. Temperature control and disorders. In: Rennie J (ed.) Roberton's textbook of neonatology, 4th edn. Churchill Livingstone, Edinburgh, p 269–279

Slade P 1988 A psychologist's view of a special care baby unit. Maternal and Child Health 13(8):208–212

Smith S R, Jaffe D M, Skinner M 1997 A case report of metallic mercury injury. Paediatric Emergency Care 13(2):114–116

Sparshott M 1991 This is your baby – a booklet for parents of pre-term infants. Southern Western Regional Health Authority, Plymouth

Tappero E P, Honeyfield M E 2003 Physical assessment of the newborn, 3rd edn. NICU.INK, Santa Rosa, CA 95405–7533V

Taylor B 1996 Parents as partners in care. Paediatric Nursing 8(4):4–7

Volpe J J 2001 Neurology of the newborn, 4th edn. W B Saunders, Philadelphia, p 103–133

FURTHER READING

Kenner C, Wright Lott J 2004 Neonatal nursing handbook, Elsevier Science, St Louis

This book addresses the most common neonatal problems. The illustrations and charts are excellent and aid the reader to a more comprehensive understanding of the clinical situation.

Crawford D, Hickson W 2000 An introduction to neonatal nursing care. Stanley Thornes Ltd, London

An introduction to neonatal nursing care is written in a style that is easily understood by practising midwives, neonatal nurses and students. It covers all aspects of the nursing and medical management of the sick infant.

Lissauce T, Faranoff A 2006 Neonatology at a glance. Blackwell Science, London

This easily understood textbook is a great starting point for midwives and neonatal nurses. It deals with the important aspects of neonatal problems, in a succinct manner, allowing the reader at their own pace to further explore a more in-depth understanding of clinical situations.

44 Respiratory problems

Alison Gibbs

Respiratory compromise in the newborn is a common presentation for a variety of diseases, not all of which may be respiratory in origin. This chapter offers a review of the signs and symptoms of respiratory compromise and an examination of some of the common causes of respiratory distress.

The second part of the chapter describes the typical nursing care for a baby who needs intensive care support for a respiratory disease.

The chapter aims to:

- list the signs of respiratory distress
- describe some of the common neonatal respiratory conditions
- identify the pertinent anatomical features that contribute to neonatal respiratory distress
- discuss neonatal respiratory and cardiovascular support
- define the effects of the environment upon the neonate
- explain the options for maintaining nutrition and hydration
- propose measures to support the parents with a baby in the neonatal unit.

Pathophysiology

Anatomical influences

Neonates are susceptible to respiratory compromise, for a number of reasons.

1. This may be a result of their stage of lung development and contributing lack of maturation in the other body systems. The gestation of the baby at birth has implications for the susceptibility to

disease processes like hyaline membrane disease (HMD), where surfactant production is inhibited. The stages of lung development are, in summary:

- **Embryonic phase.** This lasts until the 5th week of gestation. In this phase the proximal airways develop.
- **Pseudoglandular phase.** This lasts from the 5th to the 16th week of gestation. During this phase there is development of the lower conducting airways, bronchi and large bronchioles.
- **Canalicular phase.** This lasts from the 17th to the 24th week of gestation. It is the period for the development of the gas exchanging bronchioles.
- **Terminal sac phase.** This takes place between the 24th week and the 36th week of gestation. Surfactant production begins with increasing efficiency as the alveolar ducts develop.
- **Alveolar phase.** This is ongoing from the 37th week of gestation until the 8th year of life. During this phase alveoli increase in number and there is maturation of the surfactant production.

2. Neonates experience an increased work of breathing owing to the high compliance of the neonatal lung, resulting from the cartilaginous nature of the rib structure. This flexibility allows for some collapse of the airways with each breath, which would not occur with a rigid rib structure. Subsequently, with each breath, the baby needs to generate larger pressures within the lung to prevent respiratory compromise through airway collapse.

3. Neonates also have a different diaphragmatic muscle structure to adults. The neonatal diaphragm is more susceptible to fatigue owing to the composition and the location of the muscle within the neonatal chest.

4. The size of neonatal airways is smaller, which generates higher resistance to air flow and a smaller area through which perfusion can occur.

5. A final contributing factor is the tendency for pulmonary blood flow to bypass areas of hypoxia, across the alveolar bed, consequently reducing the alveoli perfusion.

Signs of respiratory compromise

Grunting

Grunting is an audible noise heard on expiration. The sound appears when there is partial closure of the glottis as the breath is expired. The baby is attempting to preserve some internal lung pressure and prevent the airways from collapsing completely at the end of the breath.

Retractions

Chest distortions occur due to an increase in the need to create higher inspiratory pressures in a compliant chest. They appear as intercostal, subcostal or sternal recession across the thorax.

Asynchrony

Here the breathing has a 'see-saw' pattern as the abdominal movements and the diaphragm work out of unison. This is a result of increased muscle fatigue and the compliant chest wall.

Tachypnoea

This is a compensatory rise in the respiratory rate initiated from the respiratory centre. It is described as a breathing rate above 60, and aims to remove the hypercarbia and prevent hypoxia.

Nasal flaring

This is an attempt to minimize the effect of the airways resistance by maximizing the diameter of the upper airways. The nares are seen to flare open with each breath.

Apnoea

Apnoea is an absence of breathing for more than 20s. Apnoea occurs as the conclusion of increasing respiratory fatigue in the term baby. The pre-term baby may also experience apnoea of prematurity due to the immature respiratory centre and obstructive apnoea from occluded airways.

Common respiratory problems

Pneumothorax

Seminal research showed that pneumothoraces are known to occur spontaneously in 1% of the newborn population either during or after birth; however, only one-tenth of this 1% will be symptomatic (Steele et al 1971). A pneumothorax at birth is caused by the large pressures generated by the baby's first breaths. These may be in the range of up to 40–80 cm of water. This can lead to alveoli distension and rupture that allows air to leak to a number of sites most notably the potential space between the lung pleura.

Babies receiving any assisted ventilation have an increased susceptibility to a pneumothorax. This could be due to either maldistribution of the ventilated gas in the lungs, high ventilation settings or baby-ventilator breathing interactions.

Term babies may present with symptoms of respiratory distress on the postnatal ward. Although it is difficult to diagnose a pneumothorax in the absence of a chest X-ray, there may be reduced breath sounds on the affected side, displaced heart sounds and a distorted chest/diaphragm movement with respiration and distension of the chest on the affected side. These signs become harder to detect in the baby with bilateral pneumothoraces.

A baby with a suspected pneumothorax needs an immediate paediatric consultation with the view to an emergency procedure. The procedure will be the placement of a chest drain possibly preceded by a needle aspiration. This will drain the air leak and prevent a further accumulation of the air. The placement of a chest drain is a painful procedure and the baby will need some sedation along with nursing on the neonatal unit. Occasionally a pneumothorax can be managed conservatively with observation and breathing oxygen enriched air to aid the reabsorption of the extra-alveolar gas.

Transient tachypnoea of the newborn

The recorded incidence of transient tachypnoea of the newborn (TTN) varies widely; this is partly a result of the variety of recording methods, differences in radiological interpretation and clear diagnostic features. It is frequently seen as a diagnosis of exclusion of other possible respiratory causes. Nevertheless, the chest X-ray may show a streaky appearance with fluid apparent in the horizontal fissure that confirms the diagnosis.

These infants present with respiratory distress normally restricted to tachypnoea alone with rates up to 120 breaths/min. Occasionally supplemental oxygen is required, but during the 24 hrs following birth the condition gradually resolves. The most common predisposing factor for TTN is a caesarean section because the thorax has not been squeezed while the baby descends along the birth canal. This results in lower thoracic pressures after birth. Although these babies tend to require initial care on a neonatal unit, their stay is usually of a short duration with the provision of oxygen and observation.

Infection/pneumonia

A number of infectious disease processes present with signs of respiratory distress in the newborn. All babies presenting with respiratory distress need to be treated for infection until there is proof to the contrary. Wright Lott (2007) notes mortality rates as high as 50% in the developing world and that sepsis rates worldwide range from 0.1% to 0.8%. Pre-term infants have an immature immunological response and hence less resistance to infection.

Pneumonia in the neonate is difficult to diagnose as secretions are difficult to obtain and the radiological appearances can be hard to distinguish. However, pneumonia presenting before 48 hrs of age has normally been acquired either at or before birth whereas presentation after 48 hrs indicates a late onset infection possibly resulting from hospitalization. All infants with infection require antibiotics but their length of stay on a neonatal unit will vary depending upon the nature of the infection, their signs and their antibiotic course. Babies with a mild infection could be cared for in a transitional care setting.

Meconium aspiration syndrome

Greenough & Roberton (1999) report the incidence for meconium aspiration syndrome in one UK hospital as 0.2/1000 live births; however, this incidence is low and other countries, such as the USA, have higher rates of the disease 2–5/1000 (Greenough & Milner 2005). Fetal asphyxia causes the passage of meconium into the liquor. This meconium is unproblematic unless the baby gasps or breathes in amniotic fluid, potentially inhaling meconium simultaneously. Consequently, it is the babies showing signs of fetal hypoxia who develop signs of meconium aspiration syndrome. A baby can develop meconium aspiration syndrome if stimulated to breathe or gasp, either before or after birth, when there is meconium in the airway that could be inhaled. The passage of meconium into the liquor is rarely seen prior to 34 weeks and Matthews & Warshaw (1979) suggest this is due to the immaturity of the pre-term gastrointestinal tract. A significant number of births have meconium-stained liquor but only a few will cause the severe meconium aspiration syndrome, with its associated mortality that is seen in the NNU. In the majority there is a milder disease process that requires initial supportive treatment but quickly resolves over 24–48 hrs.

The initial respiratory distress may be mild, moderate or severe with a gradual deterioration over the first 12–24 hrs in the moderate or severe cases. The baby may present with cyanosis, increased work of breathing and a barrel-shaped chest. This chest appearance occurs as a result of gas being trapped, leading to hyperexpansion of the lung fields. The meconium becomes trapped in the airways and causes a ball-valve effect: although air can enter the lung during inhalation, the meconium then blocks the airway during expiration so that air accumulates behind the blockage. This accumulation can then lead to the rupture of the alveoli and cause the baby to develop a pneumothorax. Where the meconium has contact with the lung tissue a pneumonitis occurs and a fertile site for infection is created. Endogenous surfactant is also broken down in the presence of meconium.

These factors in a previously hypoxic baby combine to produce a severe disease process. The external respiration across the alveoli is inhibited, areas of hypoxic lung are bypassed as blood flow shunts away from them and the pattern of fetal circulation across the arterial duct is difficult to break owing to high pulmonary vascular resistance. These infants will need full intensive care and ventilation to prevent further deterioration. Modalities such as ECMO (extracorporeal membrane oxygenation) have been shown to increase survival by 50% (UK Collaborative ECMO Trial Group 1996) while the use of nitric oxide therapy can further assist these severely compromised infants. A number of the most severely affected will be symptomatic for some months with ongoing residual symptoms during early childhood.

Respiratory distress syndrome

The term respiratory distress syndrome (RDS) is used interchangeably with the diagnosis of HMD in the neonatal culture. The diagnosis of HMD is derived from the presence of hyaline membranes in the airways resulting from the damaged epithelium. The disease occurs as a result of the insufficient production of surfactant and is seen most frequently after a premature birth; however, other disorders like maternal diabetes can also inhibit surfactant production. The 50% of babies born before 30 completed weeks' gestation experience RDS while 1% of all newborn babies may experience RDS (Greenough & Milner 2005).

Surfactant is produced by the type II epithelial cells to reduce the surface tension within the alveoli, preventing their collapse at the end of exhalation. Collapsed alveoli require much greater pressure and exertion to reinflate than do partially collapsed alveoli. The introduction of surfactant therapy into neonatal care has significantly decreased the mortality and morbidity previously seen in RDS. Surfactant consists of several different types of proteins and phospholipids, which also help prevent infection and produce further surfactant.

Pre-term babies are born with a small amount of surfactant but as the time from birth increases, the demands outstrip the supply. This gives a clinical picture of an infant with progressive respiratory distress, in which it may be 4 hrs before there is a significant presentation. The X-ray has a ground-glass appearance across the lung fields, while severe disease is represented by a 'white-out', the greater the density of the 'white out' reflecting the severity of the disease, see e.g. Figure 44.1. The infant has an increasing respiratory distress and work of breathing; it may take 48–72 hrs to reach the peak of the disease without the administration of surfactant. Resolution of the associated inflammation and the hyaline membrane formation may take up to 7 days in the unsupported baby.

Treatment has been revolutionized since the early 1990s with the administration of surfactant directly into the lungs. Surfactant is also used prophylactically when significant disease is anticipated in the most immature babies and is often administered in the birthing room. Mild disease may need oxygen

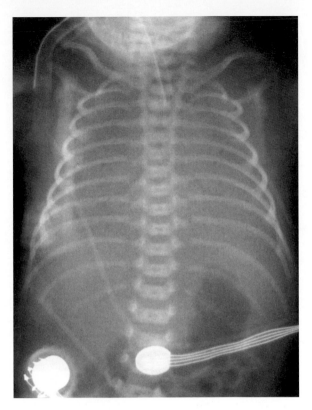

Figure 44.1 X-ray showing lungs of a baby with RDS.

alone but the more severe will need surfactant and ventilatory support. The length of stay on the NNU is dependent upon the severity of the disease and the gestational age of the baby.

A baby may remain in the NNU for a similar number of weeks to the number of weeks he is born pre-term. This allows the midwife to give the parents a ballpark figure to enable them to adjust accordingly, e.g. 'your baby is 16 weeks early so you can anticipate a stay on the NNU for up to about 16 weeks'.

Cardiac disease

Cardiac defects affect 1% of births and can be divided into left-sided and right-sided defects. They account for 30% of congenital defects (Jordan & Scott 1989). Although cardiac disease is not a respiratory disease it presents with respiratory symptoms (see also Ch. 46).

Right-sided lesions

The most frequently seen lesions are transposition of the great arteries, tetralogy of Fallot and pulmonary atresia or stenosis (p. 889). These babies typically present as a 'blue' baby. On examination, there is little to note other than the presence of cyanosis. Their respiratory distress, if present, is mild and consists of tachypnoea alone. These babies will remain cyanotic in the presence of 100% oxygen. An urgent cardiac assessment will need to be sought.

Left-sided lesions

The most frequently occurring left-sided lesions are hypoplastic left heart syndrome and coarctation of the aorta (see p. 891). These frequently present with neonatal heart failure. Initially the baby may appear irritable, lethargic, sweaty and not interested in feeding. The presence of 'effortless' tachypnoea may be seen. This tachypnoea is characterized by the lack of any other sign of respiratory compromise; for example, no grunting is heard and there is no head bobbing and minimal recession. As the heart failure progresses, the infant shows signs of increasing cardiogenic shock and will require full resuscitative measures if left untreated.

When a cardiac condition is suspected a postnatal transfer to a cardiac centre may be necessary for diagnosis and treatment. Parents need clear explanations to enable them to feel supported during this time of anxiety. Prior to departure any resuscitation and stabilization will be managed depending on the advice received from the cardiac centre and the nature of the defect.

Common practice involves the administration of an infusion of prostaglandin to maintain the patency of the arterial duct. The patency of the arterial duct is needed to keep the blood flowing through the heart and around the peripheral circulation. Stabilization may include elective intubation and ventilation of the baby. This assisted mechanical ventilation is commonly provided without oxygen, even if the saturation monitor records saturations in the 80s or 70s, since the additional oxygen may stimulate the arterial duct to close.

Cardiac surgery is complex and some defects require a number of procedures to optimize the baby's future. It is not possible to treat all the different cardiac defects and for some a poor prognosis remains. However, advances are continuously being made in the management of some of the previously fatal defects, e.g. hypoplastic left heart syndrome (Richens 2007).

What to anticipate in the neonatal unit

The anxious and frightened parents will be confronted with a technological environment with an array of buzzers, bleeps, flashing lights and alarms. It is easy to lose sight of the baby behind the technology, as Plate 18 demonstrates. However, all these machines and alarms will have a role to play in the care of the baby. The second part of the chapter explores the environment of the neonatal unit (NNU) and examines some of the technological and therapeutic support available for neonatal intensive care (NIC).

Respiratory care

Babies showing signs of respiratory compromise require a further assessment by a paediatrician or nurse practitioner. This may necessitate an admission to the NNU for continuous supervision and observation of their respiratory status. They require the skills of practitioners who can monitor and assess their critical changes in status and implement the care that is required. To assist in these observations the use of saturation monitors, transcutaneous monitors, arterial catheter readings and blood gas monitoring are used. When satisfactory oxygenation is not being achieved, the baby may need additional oxygen. This can be delivered via nasal cannula, into the incubator or into a headbox, creating an oxygen-enriched micro-environment.

Some babies will need additional ventilatory support to assist the maintenance of an adequate airway or to maximize their respiratory status. Present options for ventilation are mainly pressure controlled although the use of volume controlled strategies is increasing. There is a variety of ventilation styles to choose from. Most frequently these include conventional ventilation (CMV), high frequency oscillation (HFOV) and continuous positive airway pressure (CPAP) and Figure 44.2 shows a neonatal ventilator that offers all three.

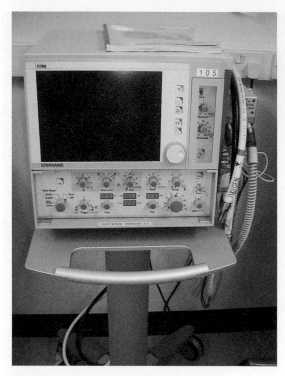

Figure 44.2 Neonatal ventilator.

CMV

Conventional ventilation techniques are increasingly being delivered in ways similar to the natural breathing patterns. During the critical phase of the illness the ventilator may deliver preset rates and pressures only. However, as the baby stabilizes and improves, ventilators are now able to mimic the babies' individual rates, pressures or lung volumes thereby minimizing the associated lung trauma.

CPAP

Nasal continuous positive airway pressure (NCPAP) is used either as a therapy for moderate disease or as weaning tool. Pressure is delivered to the nares and oropharynx which, when transmitted through the bronchial tree, distends the alveoli at the end of respiration preventing their collapse. The aim is to avoid the trauma of an endotracheal tube and the bronchiolar damage from ventilation. Figure 44.3 shows a 'CPAP driver'.

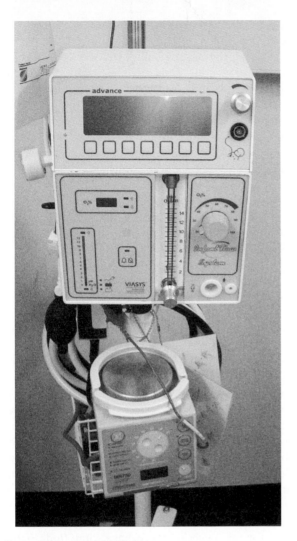

Figure 44.3 Nasal CPAP driver.

Alternative ventilation options

HFOV

This is commonly used for extreme prematurity, as a rescue therapy or in combination with nitric oxide. When babies are being oscillated they are seen to 'vibrate', while some continue to breathe in addition to the ventilation. Pressure is used to reach optimal lung expansion and 'bounce' or oscillations are added to help the distribution of the gases through the lung field. Since Johnson et al (2002) published their study research of conventional ventilation versus HFOV, paediatricians have tended to reserve HFOV for a rescue strategy for the critically ill.

ECMO

This involves the oxygenation of the blood supply outside the body. Large cannulae are inserted to remove and reintroduce the blood to the baby. The procedure uses technology similar to cardiac bypass support for the oxygenation of the blood. During this time the lungs are allowed to rest and heal. This type of ventilation is governed by the availability of the treatment and infant suitability. Generally babies need to be at least 34 gestational weeks, weigh >1.8 kg and be without a bleeding disorder.

NO

Nitric oxide (NO) is a respiratory gas that is inhaled with each ventilation breath. NO works directly upon the pulmonary vessels with minimal effect to the systemic circulation. It has been licensed for use in Europe since 2001 as a pulmonary vasodilator for pulmonary hypertension in babies at 34 weeks' gestation. It has been shown that the use of NO reduces the need for ECMO but the role of inhaled NO for pre-term infants remains unclear awaiting further research (Dewhurst et al 2007).

CNEEP

Continuous nasal end expiratory pressure (CNEEP). This is unsuitable for newly delivered premature babies as the tight fixation around the baby's neck may lead to an increased risk of IVH. However, when this risk has passed, CNEEP works using similar principles to the technology of the iron lung.

These alternative ventilation techniques are available at specialized centres only and may require a postnatal transfer to access. Liquid ventilation is not routinely available in Britain at the time of writing. Box 44.1 shows key points relating to respiratory support.

Box 44.1 Key points – respiratory support

- Respiratory support is frequently provided by conventional ventilation or CPAP
- Other options are available for suitable infants.

Cardiovascular support

Cardiac failure in a neonate is rare and the majority of arrests are respiratory in origin. Nevertheless, neonates may require support to maintain an efficient and effective heart beat. Maintenance of an adequate blood pressure (the mean being equivalent to the gestational age) may need pharmaceutical support too. Continuous observation and supervision of the cardiac parameters will be needed, which can be achieved using either an indwelling catheter or non-invasive monitoring. A bradycardia (a heart rate dropping to below 80) may be a sign of various influences such as a blocked endotracheal tube or sepsis. Normally a respiratory cause is considered first before other explanations are explored.

Occasionally, the transition from a fetal to an adult circulation is compromised and the baby develops persistent pulmonary hypertension (PPHN) of the newborn. This condition has previously been called 'persistent fetal circulation', which describes the tendency of the blood flow to mimic the circulation within the fetus. The compromise may be due to a primary defect in the pulmonary vasculature or secondary to other factors that raise the pulmonary vascular resistance, for example meconium aspiration syndrome. The use of nitric oxide as the vasodilator of choice has replaced other pharmaceutical strategies for PPHN. Box 44.2 gives a key point to note, relating to cardiovascular support.

Nutrition and hydration

The role and benefits of breastmilk are clearly established (see Ch. 41). These benefits are increased further for the pre-term baby, for whom an immature gut can give rise to feeding difficulties. A pre-term baby has little nutritional reserves and will need supplementation soon after birth to meet the continual demand for glucose from the brain. Although the ideal would be to establish oral breastmilk feeding, for a sick neonate this is not possible as the presence of the endotracheal tube, the absence of a suck reflex or critical illness prevents oral feeding.

The majority of such babies will receive a glucose-based intravenous infusion. Meanwhile the practitioner can give milk feeds via a nasogastric, orogastric or nasojejunal tube and increase the volumes as the baby's condition allows. Opinions vary concerning the method of administration and the frequency of these early feedings although there is an increasing trend towards regular bolus feeds rather than continuous feeding with a syringe driver (Grant & Denne 1991, Lucas et al 1986, Newell 1998). Nevertheless sick or immature babies need a cautious introduction to milk, whether expressed breastmilk or formula feeds, as these infants are susceptible to necrotizing enterocolitis (NEC).

When a baby is expected to take more than 4–5 days before full feeding is established, then total parenteral nutrition (TPN) is needed to ensure that all nutritional requirements can be met. TPN is normally administered through a central line, either a longline or umbilical catheter. The strength and irritability of the solution necessitate its delivery into a large vein. Weak TPN solutions can be started on the 1st day of life. TPN typically contains amino acids, fats, carbohydrates, minerals, vitamins and trace elements. All help to prevent the depletion of these essential components, assisting growth and development in the pre-term baby. The strength and composition of the TPN can be built up over a few days as the baby demonstrates its ability to tolerate the solution. Although some babies may need TPN for many weeks, it can have some undesirable side-effects upon the liver, giving rise to a conjugated hyperbilirubinaemia or cholestasis. Prolonged TPN is sometimes needed in very immature babies, infants with gastroschisis and those with NEC.

Necrotizing enterocolitis

NEC is a disease seen in the neonatal population and its causes are multifactorial. Prior to birth the gut mucosa is sterile; consequently during the first few days and weeks of life colonization with the normal bacterial flora must occur. This normal process can be altered by delaying feeding when a baby is unwell or pre-term.

The administration of antibiotics can alter the dominant gut flora, as can formula milk. This can

---

Box 44.2 Key point – cardiovascular support

- Neonates may need additional cardiovascular support through medication.

lead to a proliferation of anaerobes and bacterial invasion into the gut wall. Bacterial infection can also occur following episodes of hypoxia. Variations in blood volume reducing the arterial blood flow through the mesenteric circulation also predispose to NEC, e.g. intrauterine growth restriction. This causes mucosal ischaemia, which when reperfused leads to oedema, haemorrhage, ulceration and necrosis.

The baby may present with mild symptoms of the disease, a painful distended abdomen, blood in the stool and poor food tolerance. However there may be more acute pathology; symptoms may include air within the gut wall, leading to a perforation, hypovolaemic shock and disseminated intravascular coagulation.

Treatment is initially with antibiotics and medical management. However, surgery is needed if there is a perforation or a failure to respond to the medical therapy. The long term problems for those who do recover can be short gut syndrome and gut stenosis (see also Chs 43 and 47). Box 44.3 is a list of key points relating to nutrition.

A safe environment

Neonatal infection

A neonate has an increased susceptibility to infection owing to the immaturity of the neonatal defence mechanisms. These limitations decrease as gestational age lengthens; nevertheless a term baby still has not achieved the immune responses of an adult. Neonates, and pre-term babies especially, experience reduced immunoglobulin protection. Their responses to infection take longer as the organisms are new and not recognized by the memory cells. Consequently there is a delay in response time, as fresh responses are required for each new organism. The complement cascade, a supplementary defence mechanism of plasma proteins, remains inefficient. The phagocytic cells are restricted in their role and the external defences like the skin are immature. Consequently the neonate has a reduced ability to fight infection, whether contracted prior to birth or after.

The uterus is a sterile environment, which cannot be replicated on the neonatal unit. However, strict infection control measures can be exercised e.g. hands are washed by all caregivers and restricted handling by a few individuals. Nursing a baby in an incubator provides a micro-environment that can assist with barrier nursing. However, neonatal infection, whether prenatal or postnatal, continues to contribute to neonatal mortality hence the use of prophylactic antibiotics is widespread throughout developed countries. Box 44.4 gives a key point relating to infection.

Thermoneutral environment

A baby needs the environment to require minimal metabolic activity to maintain temperature stability. Babies born at the extremes of viability have immature skin owing to reduced keratin in the epidermis, hence heat and water is easily lost. This, along with their immature responses to cold stress and no brown adipose tissue before 28 weeks' gestation, makes neonates vulnerable to the effects of a cool environment. Babies for whom an inadequate thermoneutral environment is achieved have an increased mortality and morbidity and hence the diligence given to keeping infants warm.

The use of heated boxes has developed into the use of sophisticated incubators as shown in Figure 44.4. These provide an environment where heat can be controlled and a humidified microclimate can be created for the most immature. Continuous attention to thermoregulation can be made with the use of temperature probes placed upon the skin. Warm delivery rooms are routinely used while the practice of putting pre-term babies into plastic bags immediately after birth has become an effective measure for minimizing heat loss (Bjorklund & Hellstrom-Westas 2000).

Box 44.3 Key points – nutrition

- While nutrition is essential for the neonate, feeding needs to be introduced carefully
- TPN may be given until feeding is established
- NEC remains a serious neonatal disease of the gut.

Box 44.4 Key point – infection

- Neonates have immature defence mechanisms for fighting disease.

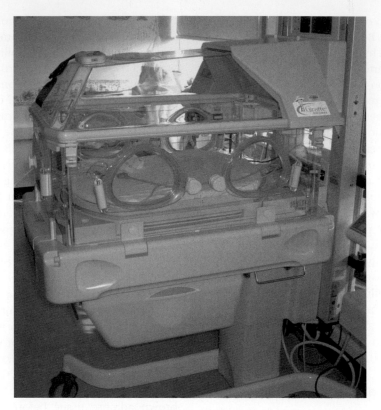

Figure 44.4 Incubator.

A stress-free environment

The neonate experiences a number of stressors within the neonatal environment. Once analgesia and sedation have been administered the baby may still show signs of distress and agitation that can lead to long-term patterns of altered behaviours if left unmanaged.

The use of opiates for pain relief and sedation is routine in neonatal care and recently sucking sucrose has become a non-pharmacological option for pain management (Noerr 2001). The recognition of pain in the neonate has prompted a number of pain assessment tools to aid identification as the behavioural responses may not reflect the severity of the pain. The majority involve some subjectivity and the most preferred tools measure contextual, physiological and behavioural responses; CRIES (Krechel & Bildner 1995), the Neonatal Facial Coding System (Grunau et al 1990) and the Premature Infant Pain Profile (Stevens et al 1996) are frequently used examples.

The pre-term baby can also find other 'routine' stimuli noxious, e.g. the lighting, the noise levels and handling associated with intensive care. Simple comforting measures can be effective for short term use, especially for the non-ventilated baby. These actions include swaddling, nesting, positioning and non-nutritive sucking from a pacifier. These measures can be learnt by the family to aid the attachment process, as some babies demonstrate disorganized behaviours when presented with the usual parental interactions like cuddling and play. Consideration for the environmental stimuli can also be made e.g. by lowering the lighting and minimizing noise levels. Box 44.5 gives a key point relating to stimuli.

Box 44.5 Key point – stimuli

- The environment contains a variety of distressing stimuli for the neonate.

Parents

The importance of attachment for the future relationship between the parents and their baby has been recognized for a number of years now (Klaus & Kennell 1989) and would normally occur as the mother interacts with her baby. Some mothers bond instantaneously, while for others the process occurs more slowly as they meet their baby's needs. When this normal maternal interaction and role is denied, the process of attachment can be delayed and difficult (Bialoskurski et al 1999). McGrath (2007) identifies factors that can influence a family's reactions to a child's hospitalization and lists them as the severity of illness and threat to the baby, previous experiences, familiarity with medical practice and procedures, available support systems, coping strategies, family stresses, cultural or religious beliefs and family communication patterns.

For the majority of parents in the NNU, the question of survival will be paramount. This fear will be intensified with increasing prematurity. The EPICure study data (Costello et al 2000) give the exact data for the outcome of births on the edge of viability. An easily remembered guide suggested by these data is that births at 25 weeks' gestation have a 50% mortality rate, and the surviving babies have a 50% morbidity rate. The survival of their baby is the initial concern for parents, but once there is less of a danger the need for ongoing daily communication should continue as it helps the parents 'feel' for their babies. The mothers rely on this information to help them facilitate an attachment with their baby, since Cox &

Bialoskurski (2001) found that, for 99% of mothers, the information regarding their baby's status was the most important maternal concern during their stay on the NNU.

Some hospital behaviours can become barriers to attachment and nurses and midwives need to be aware of these. Nurses may refer to a baby as 'their baby' for a shift duration, while the baby is actually not theirs but belongs to the family. Exclusion from tasks or reports can reinforce that the baby belongs to the hospital, not the family. The baby's schedule can be controlled by the hospital rather than be family centred, while the family can be treated as guests to their baby rather than partners in care.

The midwife and nursing team can assist the parents to overcome difficulties by improving the quality of their communication, identifying the support structures that are available for parents and by facilitating the parents' easy and frequent access to their baby. The parents should be enabled to develop the skills needed to care for their own baby and be given the information and empowerment to deliver that care, therefore ensuring that the care is family centred, rather than medical and technology focused. Box 44.6 gives a key point relating to parents.

Box 44.6 Key point – parents

- The midwife can augment the parental growth in attachment with effective support and communication.

REFERENCES

Bialoskurski M, Cox C, Hayes J 1999 The nature of attachment in the neonatal intensive care unit. Journal of Perinatal and Neonatal Nursing 13(1):66–77

Bjorklund L J, Hellstrom-Westas L 2000. Reducing heat loss at birth in very pre-term infants. Journal of Pediatrics 137:739–740

Costello K, Hennessy E, Gibson A , et al 2000 The EPICure study: outcomes to discharge from hospital for babies born at the threshold of viability. Pediatrics 106: 659–671

Cox C L, Bialoskurski M 2001 Neonatal intensive care: communication and attachment. British Journal of Nursing 10:668–676

Dewhurst C, Harigopal S, Subhedar N 2007 Recent advances in inhaled nitric oxide therapy in neonates: A review of the evidence. Infant 3(2):69–75

Grant J, Denne S C 1991 Effect of intermittent versus continuous enteral feeding on energy expenditure in premature infants. Journal of Pediatrics 118:928–932

Greenough A, Milner A D 2005 Acute respiratory disease. In: Rennie J M (ed.) Roberton's Textbook of Neonatology, 4th edn. Churchill Livingstone, Edinburgh, p 468–535

Greenough A, Roberton N R C 1999 Acute respiratory distress in the newborn. In: Rennie J M, Roberton N R C (eds) Textbook of neonatology, 3rd edn. Churchill Livingstone, Edinburgh, p 481–607

Grunau R V E, Johnston C C, Craig K D 1990 Pain expression in neonates: Facial action and cry responses to invasive and non-invasive procedures. Pain 42:295–305

Johnson A, Peacock J, Greenough A , et al United Kingdom Oscillation Study Group 2002 High-frequency oscillatory ventilation for the prevention of chronic lung disease of prematurity. New England Journal of Medicine 347 (9):642–663

Jordan S C, Scott O 1989 Heart disease in paediatrics, 3rd edn. Butterworth-Heinemann, Oxford, p 3

Klaus M H, Kennell J H 1989 Parent–infant bonding, 3rd edn. Mosby, St Louis

Krechel S, Bildner J 1995 CRIES: a new neonatal post-operative pain measurement score: initial testing of validity and reliability. Paediatric Anaesthesia 5(1):53–61

Lucas A, Bloom S, Aynsley-Green A 1986 Gut hormones and 'minimal enteral feeding'. Acta Paediatrica Scandinavica 75:719–723

Matthews T G, Warshaw J B 1979 Relevance of the gestational age on distribution of meconium passage in utero. Pediatrics 64:30–31

McGrath J M 2007 Family: essential partner in care. In: Kenner C, Wright-Lott J (eds) Comprehensive neonatal care: an interdisciplinary approach, 4th edn. Saunders, Philadelphia, p 491–509

Newell S 1998 Enteral nutrition. In: Campbell A G M, McIntosh N (eds) Forfar and Arneil's textbook of pediatrics, 5th edn. Churchill Livingstone, New York, p 152–155

Noerr B 2001 Sucrose for neonatal procedural pain. Neonatal Network 20(7):63–67

Richens T 2007 The preoperative management of severe neonatal left ventricular outflow obstruction. Infant 3(1):36–40

Steele R W, Metz J R, Bass J W , et al 1971 Pneumothorax and pneumomediastinum in the newborn. Radiology 98:629–632

Stevens B, Johnston C, Petryshen P , et al 1996 Premature infant pain profile: development and initial validation. Clinical Journal of Pain 12:13–22

UK Collaborative ECMO Trial Group 1996 UK collaborative randomized trial of neonatal extracorporeal membrane oxygenation. Lancet 348:75–82

Wright Lott J 2007 Immune system. In: Kenner C, Wright-Lott J (eds) Comprehensive neonatal care: an interdisciplinary approach, 4th edn. Saunders, Philadelphia, p 203

FURTHER READING

Kenner C, McGrath J (eds) 2004 Developmental care of newborns and infants: a guide for health professionals, Mosby, St Louis

A book with a focus on growth, development and behaviours, including the family role and environmental influences. A book to use alongside the more biomedical science books to facilitate a holistic approach to care.

Merenstein G, Gardner S 2006 Handbook of neonatal intensive care, 6th edn. Mosby, St Louis

A good authority for a combination of pertinent nursing and medical issues. The book covers topics more relevant for holistic management of babies needing intensive care. Although the work is American the balanced approach to all aspects of neonatology ensures the book retains its recommendation as a resource in Britain.

Rennie (ed.) 2005 Roberton's textbook of neonatology, 4th edn. Churchill Livingstone, Edinburgh

A comprehensive coverage of all aspects of neonatology. This book provides an invaluable resource for British neonatologists. It covers an extensive range of medical topics and yet retains an easy to read reference approach.

Rennie J, Roberton N R C 2002 A manual of neonatal intensive care, 4th edn. Arnold, London

A succinct version of their textbook of neonatology for neonatal intensive care. The book provides essential information for the daily management of infants needing extra care. Ideal as a straightforward reference source.

45

Trauma during birth, haemorrhage and convulsions

Claire Greig

CHAPTER CONTENTS

This chapter focuses on complications occurring in specifically vulnerable babies; the midwife's awareness of this vulnerability may prevent such complications. However, if a complication does occur, the midwife must report it to the baby's doctor and may work with that doctor and/or a wider multiprofessional team to diagnose it and implement effective treatment. Parents may be distressed when their baby suffers a complication and the midwife helps them to understand the complication, facilitating their discussions with the multiprofessional team members, and assisting them to care for their baby.

The chapter presents information on:

- trauma during birth to skin and superficial tissues, muscle, nerves and bones
- major types of neonatal haemorrhage due to trauma, disruptions in blood flow, coagulopathies and other causes
- neonatal convulsions
- specific interventions with parents.

Trauma during birth

Despite skilled midwifery and obstetric care in developed, Western societies and a reduction in the incidence, birth trauma still occurs. Efforts continue to reduce the incidence even further.

Trauma during birth includes:

- trauma to skin and superficial tissues
- muscle trauma

- nerve trauma
- fractures.

Trauma to skin and superficial tissues

Skin

Skin damage is often iatrogenic, resulting from forceps blades (Plate 28), vacuum extractor cups, scalp electrodes and scalpels. Poorly applied forceps blades or vacuum extractor cup may result in scalp abrasion (Plate 29), although fewer problems occur with softer vacuum extractor cups. Forceps blades may cause bruising or superficial fat necrosis. Scalp electrodes cause puncture wounds, as do fetal blood sampling techniques. Occasionally, during uterine incision at caesarean section, laceration of the baby's skin may occur.

Superficial fat necrosis is very rare and usually presents between days 1–28 with well-defined areas of induration where pressure was applied (Dudink et al 2003). All other skin injuries should be detected during the midwife's detailed examination of the baby immediately after birth. All trauma should be made known to the parents and reported to the baby's doctor.

Abrasions and lacerations should be kept clean and dry. If there are signs of infection, further medical consultation should be sought by the midwife or parents. Antibiotics may be required. Deeper lacerations may require closure with butterfly strips or sutures. Healing is usually rapid with no residual scarring (Sorantin et al 2006). There is no specific management for fat necrosis that should spontaneously resolve (Dudink et al 2003).

Superficial tissues

Soft tissue trauma involves oedematous swellings and/or bruising. During labour the fetal part overlying the cervical os may be subjected to pressure, a 'girdle of contact', with reduced venous return and resultant congestion and oedema.

Caput succedaneum

With cephalic presentation, there may be a diffuse oedematous swelling under the scalp and above the periosteum, called a caput succedaneum (Fig. 45.1). With an occipitoanterior position, one caput succedaneum may be present. With an occipitoposterior

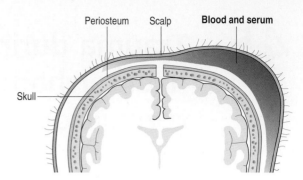

Figure 45.1 Caput succedaneum.

position, a caput succedaneum may form, but if the occiput rotates anteriorly a second caput succedaneum can develop. A second caput succedaneum may also form if, during the second stage of labour, the birth of the head is delayed and the perineum acts as another 'girdle of contact'. A 'false' caput succedaneum can also occur if a vacuum extractor cup is used; because of its distinctive shape, the swelling is known as a 'chignon' (Plate 29).

A caput succedaneum is present at birth, does not usually enlarge, can 'pit' on pressure, can cross a suture line and the oedema may move to the dependent area of the scalp (Furdon & Clark 2001). The baby will usually experience some discomfort and, although care continues as normal, gentle handling is appropriate. Abrasion of a chignon is possible.

The swelling is usually self-limiting, resolving by 36 hrs of life, with no longer-term consequences (Sorantin et al 2006). An abraded chignon usually heals rapidly if the area is kept clean, dry and is not irritated.

Other injuries

The cervical os may restrict venous return when the fetal presentation is not cephalic. When the face presents, it becomes congested and bruised and the eyes and lips become oedematous. In a breech presentation the fetus will develop bruised and oedematous genitalia and buttocks. This type of trauma is apparent at birth. The baby experiences discomfort and pain therefore gentle handling is essential and mild analgesia may be required.

For babies with bruised or oedematous buttocks, maintaining nappy area hygiene is important and needs to be accomplished without inflicting further trauma to the skin. Barrier ointment or cream applications may be required if disposable nappies designed to limit the contact of urine and faecal fluid with the skin are not available. If skin excoriation does occur, the infection risk increases and consultation with a wound care specialist nurse may be required to ensure best skin care practice.

Uncomplicated oedema and bruising usually resolve within days. However, if the baby suffers significant trauma during a vaginal breech birth, resulting serious complications require specific treatment, and take longer to resolve. These complications include excessive haemolysis resulting in hyperbilirubinaemia; excessive blood loss resulting in hypovolaemia, shock, anaemia and disseminated intravascular coagulation (DIC); and damage to muscles resulting in difficulties with micturition and defecation.

Muscle trauma

Injuries to muscle result from tearing or when the blood supply is disrupted.

Torticollis

The most commonly damaged muscle is the sternomastoid muscle. The right and left sternomastoid muscles run from the respective side of the top of the sternum, along the right or left side of the neck and are inserted into the mastoid process of the right or left temporal bone (Tortora & Derrickson 2006). When contracted simultaneously, these muscles allow the head to flex. When contracted separately, each turns the head to the opposite side.

Excessive traction or twisting causing tearing to one of these muscles can occur during the birth of the anterior shoulder of a fetus with a cephalic presentation, or during rotation of the shoulders when the fetus is being born by vaginal breech or caesarean section. A 1–3 cm, apparently painless, hard lump of blood and fibrous tissue is felt on the affected sternomastoid muscle. The muscle length is shortened, therefore the neck is twisted to the affected side: a torticollis or wry neck. If the techniques for assisting at these stages of birth are correctly applied, torticollis is preventable (Butler 2003).

Torticollis management involves carers and parents performing passive muscle-stretching exercises initially under the guidance of a physiotherapist, and actively encouraging the baby to move the neck. The swelling will usually resolve over several weeks to months with minimal sequelae. Occasionally surgical intervention is required if there is no resolution by 1 year. Follow-up to ensure achievement of normal movement is recommended (Butler 2003).

Nerve trauma

The nerves most commonly traumatized are the facial and brachial plexus nerves. Spinal cord injury is very rare and is not discussed here; an excellent explanation is given in Brand (2006).

Facial nerve

The facial nerve runs close to the skin surface and is vulnerable to compression resulting in unilateral facial palsy. Compression may occur in the uterus but is more likely during birth by the maternal sacral promontory or by a mis-applied forceps blade. On the affected side, the baby appears to have no nasolabial fold, the eyelid remains open and the mouth is drawn over to the unaffected side (Plate 30). The baby will drool excessively, may be unable to form an effective seal on the breast or teat, resulting in initial feeding difficulties, and may also have difficulty swallowing (Parker 2006).

There is no specific treatment. If the eyelid remains open, regular instillation of methyl cellulose eye drops lubricate the eyeball. Feeding difficulties are usually overcome by the baby's own adaptation, although alternative feeding positions may help. Spontaneous resolution is usually within 7–10 days; this may extend to months or years if the damage is severe. Cosmetic surgical interventions for the most severely affected babies may be required (Parker 2006).

Brachial plexus

Nerve roots exiting from the spine at the fifth to eighth cervical and the first thoracic vertebrae form a matrix of nerves in the neck and shoulder; the brachial plexus (Tortora & Derrickson 2006). Evans-Jones et al (2003) report a stable incidence of 0.42/ 1000 live births over 40 years for congenital (obstetric) brachial plexus palsy in the United Kingdom (UK) and the Republic of Ireland. Brachial plexus trauma usually results from excessive lateral flexion, rotation or traction of the head and neck during vaginal breech birth or when shoulder dystocia occurs. This force may or may not be excessive or inappropriate (Evans-Jones et al 2003). It is suggested that elective caesarean section for all babies who present breech will prevent such trauma (Dyachenko et al 2006, Evans-Jones et al 2003).

The possible damage ranges from oedema to haemorrhage to tearing of the nerves. There are three main injuries: Erb's palsy, Klumpke's palsy and total brachial plexus palsy. These injuries can be unilateral or bilateral.

Erb's palsy

There is paralysis of the shoulder and arm (not the hand) due to damage to the upper brachial plexus involving the fifth and sixth cervical nerve roots (Parker 2006). The baby's affected arm is inwardly rotated, the elbow extended, the wrist pronated and flexed and the hand partially closed; the 'waiter's tip position'. The arm is limp, although some movement of the fingers and arm is possible (Plate 31).

Klumpke's palsy

The shoulder and upper arm are unaffected but the lower arm, wrist and hand are paralysed resulting in wrist drop and no grasp reflex. This is due to damage to the lower brachial plexus involving the seventh and eighth cervical and the first thoracic nerve roots.

Total brachial plexus palsy

There is complete paralysis of the shoulder, arm and hand, lack of sensation, and circulatory problems due to damage to all brachial plexus nerve roots. If there is bilateral paralysis, spinal injury should be suspected.

All types of brachial plexus trauma will require further investigations such as X-ray and ultrasound scanning (USS) of the clavicle, arm, chest and cervical spine, and assessment of the joints. Passive movements of the joints and limb can be initiated under the direction of a physiotherapist. At 1 month of age, magnetic resonance imaging can offer specific data on nerve damage.

Complete recovery within 6 months is expected for 52% of babies, 2% will have no recovery and 46% will have incomplete recovery (Evans-Jones et al 2003). Erb's palsy tends to resolve more quickly than the other forms. Regular functional follow-up assessments are recommended. Babies with no functional recovery by 6 months may require microsurgical nerve repair (DiTaranto et al 2004, Evans-Jones et al 2003).

Fractures

Fractures are rare but the most commonly affected bones are the clavicle, humerus, femur and those of the skull. With all such fractures, a 'crack' may be heard during the birth.

Clavicle

Clavicular fractures are the second most common type of birth trauma after skin and superficial tissue injury (Parker 2006). Fractures can occur with shoulder dystocia or a vaginal breech birth, or if the baby is macrosomic. The affected clavicle is usually the one that was nearest the maternal symphysis pubis. Brachial plexus and phrenic nerve injuries should be excluded in the affected baby.

Humerus

Midshaft fractures can occur if with shoulder dystocia or during a vaginal breech birth the extended arm is forced down and born.

Femur

Midshaft fractures can occur during vaginal breech birth if the extended legs are forced down and born.

Management of fractures

With most fractures, distortion, deformity, swelling or bruising are usually evident on examination; crepitus may be felt; the baby feels pain and is reluctant to move the affected area. An X-ray examination can usually confirm the diagnosis.

The baby requires careful handling to avoid further pain, and mild analgesia, such as paracetamol may be required (British National Formulary for Children 2005).

Fractures of the clavicle require no specific treatment. To immobilize a fractured humerus, place a pad in the axilla and firmly splint the arm with the elbow bent across the chest with a bandage, ensuring respirations are not embarrassed. Immobilize a fractured femur using a splint and bandage. Traction and plaster casting may be required (Parker 2006). Stable union of a fractured clavicle usually occurs in 7–10 days, while the humerus and femur take 2–3 weeks.

Skull

Although rare, these fractures, linear or depressed, may occur during prolonged or difficult instrumental births. There may be no signs but an overlying cephalhaematoma, or signs of associated complications such as intracranial haemorrhage or neurological disturbances, may suggest a fracture's presence.

X-ray examination can confirm the fracture. An USS may help diagnose associated haemorrhage. Linear fractures usually require no treatment. A depressed skull fracture is a concavity of the bone with no break. External repair using vacuum apparatus is a more recent alternative to the traditional surgical intervention (Sorantin et al 2006). Leakage of CSF through the ear or nose requires antibiotic therapy. Treatment of associated complications is necessary.

Linear skull fractures usually heal quickly with no sequelae. Depressed fractures have a similarly optimistic outcome except if complications occur, when permanent neurological damage is likely (Paige & Carney 2002).

Haemorrhage

Blood volume in the term baby is approximately 80–100 ml/kg and in the pre-term baby 90–105 mL/kg; therefore even a small haemorrhage can be potentially fatal. In this section, haemorrhages are discussed according to their principal cause, or in relation to other factors.

Haemorrhages can be due to:

- trauma
- disruptions in blood flow

or can be related to:

- coagulopathies
- other causes.

Haemorrhage due to trauma

Cephalhaematoma

A cephalhaematoma is an effusion of blood under the periosteum that covers the skull bones (Fig. 45.2).

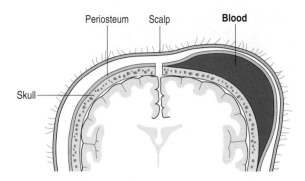

Figure 45.2 Cephalhaematoma.

During a vaginal birth, with friction between the fetal skull and maternal pelvic bones, such as in cephalo-pelvic disproportion or precipitate labour, the periosteum is torn from the bone, causing bleeding underneath. Cephalhaematomas may also occur during vacuum-assisted births. Because the fetal or newborn skull bones are not fused, and as the periosteum is adherent to the edges of the skull bones, a cephalhaematoma is confined to one bone. However, more than one bone may be affected; therefore multiple cephalhaematomas may develop. A double cephalhaematoma is usually bilateral (Fig. 45.3).

A cephalhaematoma is not present at birth; the swelling appears after 12 hrs, grows larger over

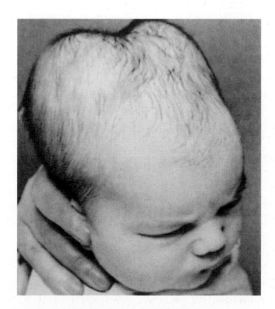

Figure 45.3 Bilateral cephalhaematoma.

subsequent days and can persist for weeks. The swelling is firm, does not pit on pressure, does not cross a suture and is fixed (Furdon & Clark 2001).

No treatment is necessary and the swelling subsides when the blood is reabsorbed. Haemolysis of the extravasated blood may result in hyperbilirubinaemia. A ridge of bone, felt round the periphery of the swelling, is due to the accumulation of osteoblasts.

Subaponeurotic haemorrhage

A subaponeurotic (or subgaleal) haemorrhage is rare. Under the scalp, the epicranial aponeurosis, a sheet of fibrous tissue that covers the cranial vault allowing for muscles to attach to the bone, provides a potential space above the periosteum through which veins travel. Excessive traction on these veins results in haemorrhage, the epicranial aponeurosis is pulled away from the periosteum of the skull bones and swelling is evident (Fig. 45.4). Subaponeurotic haemorrhage may occur with any type of birth but is more often associated with vacuum-assisted births, primiparous women, severe dystocia, occipitolateral or posterior head positions, pre-term babies, precipitate births, macrosomia, coagulopathies and male babies (Sansoucie & Cavaliere 2003).

The swelling is present at birth, increases in size and is a firm, fluctuant mass. The scalp is movable rather than fixed. The swelling can cross sutures and extend into the subcutaneous tissue of neck and eyelids. The baby experiences pain with head movement or handling of the swelling.

Some subaponeurotic haemorrhages are small but there is a risk of excessive haemorrhage and severe shock. This emergency situation requires immediate medical assistance; stabilization and full supportive care, including blood transfusion. Subaponeurotic haemorrhage is associated with a mortality rate of 25% (Sorantin et al 2006).

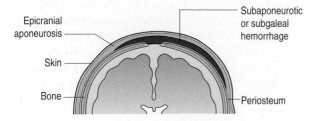

Figure 45.4 Subaponeurotic haemorrhage.

Epicranial aponeurosis

Skin

Bone

Subaponeurotic or subgaleal hemorrhage

Periosteum

With a smaller haemorrhage and in the babies who survive a larger haemorrhage, the blood is reabsorbed and the swelling and bruising resolve over 2–3 weeks. Hyperbilirubinaemia complicates recovery.

Subdural haemorrhage

A sickle-shaped, double fold of dura mater, the falx cerebri, dips into the fissure between the cerebral hemispheres. Attached at right angles to the falx cerebri, between the cerebrum and the cerebellum, is a horseshoe-shaped fold of dura mater; the tentorium cerebelli. In these folds of dura run large venous sinuses draining blood from the brain.

Normally moulding of the skull bones and stretching of the underlying structures during birth are well tolerated. Trauma to the fetal head, such as excessive compression or abnormal stretching, may tear the dura, particularly the tentorium cerebelli, rupturing venous sinuses and resulting in a subdural haemorrhage. Predisposing factors include rapid, abnormal or excessive moulding, such as in precipitate labour or rapid birth, malpositions, malpresentations, cephalopelvic disproportion, or undue compression during forceps manoeuvres (Smith 2006). Subdural haemorrhage may be fatal.

A baby with a small haemorrhage may demonstrate no signs and resolution is spontaneous. Alternatively the haemorrhage may initially be small but if blood continues to leak, the signs develop over several days. As blood accumulates, there is cerebral irritation, cerebral oedema and raised intracranial pressure. The baby is likely to vomit, be non-responsive, and have a bulging anterior fontanelle, abnormal eye movements, apnoea, bradycardia and convulsions. If the subdural haemorrhage is initially large, the baby is likely to be severely asphyxiated and difficult to resuscitate (Smith 2006).

Diagnosis is confirmed by cranial USS. Supportive treatment focuses on replacing blood volume and controlling the consequences of asphyxia and raised intracranial pressure. Subdural taps may be required to drain large collections of blood.

Haemorrhage due to disruptions in blood flow

Subarachnoid haemorrhage

A primary subarachnoid haemorrhage involves bleeding directly into the subarachnoid space. Pre-term babies who suffer hypoxia at birth resulting in disruption of cerebral blood flow, and term babies who suffer traumatic births are vulnerable (Levene et al 2000, Smith 2006). A secondary haemorrhage involves leakage of blood into the subarachnoid space from an intraventricular haemorrhage (Smith 2006).

The affected baby may have generalized convulsions from the second day of life, pre-term babies may have apnoeic episodes, but otherwise the baby appears normal and some babies exhibit no signs. Subarachnoid haemorrhage is difficult to see on USS, although computerized tomography scanning can demonstrate the haemorrhage. If a lumbar puncture is performed, the CSF will be uniformly bloodstained. Management includes replacement of blood volume, and control of the consequences of asphyxia and convulsions. The condition is usually self-limiting.

Post-haemorrhagic hydrocephalus may occur but drainage is not usually required and recovery is usually favourable (Levene et al 2000).

Germinal matrix/intraventricular haemorrhage and intraparenchymal lesions

Germinal matrix/intraventricular haemorrhage (GMH/IVH) and intraparenchymal lesions (IPL) primarily affect babies of <32 weeks' gestation and those weighing <1500g, although term babies can be affected (Rennie & Roberton 2002). The incidence and severity of these haemorrhages/lesions are inversely correlated with gestational age (Smith 2006).

In 1978, Papile et al proposed the following grading system. A grade 1 haemorrhage into the germinal matrix, is a periventricular or subependymal haemorrhage. Extension of the haemorrhage into the lateral ventricle(s), results in an intraventricular haemorrhage (IVH) or grade 2 haemorrhage. The choroid plexus of the lateral ventricles normally produces CSF. If a grade 2 haemorrhage is complicated by blockage to the outflow of CSF, post-haemorrhagic hydrocephalus develops and the ventricles dilate; a grade 3 IVH. A grade 3 haemorrhage may extend into the cerebral tissue, giving rise to a periventricular/parenchymal haemorrhage, known as a grade 4 haemorrhage.

Volpe (1997) proposed that the intraventricular clot in the grade 3 haemorrhage disrupts venous drainage, causing stasis and infarction. Reperfusion of the area caused haemorrhage into the infarcted area and necrotic damage of the white matter. Volpe (1997) reclassified a grade 4 haemorrhage as a complication of a grade 3 IVH, referring to it as a periventricular haemorrhagic infarction (PHI).

More recently, the term 'periventricular' and Papile et al's (1978) grading system have been reconsidered. Improved imaging techniques show that periventricular/parenchymal damage may not always be due to haemorrhage and the lesions vary in size, nature and location. There is still debate about the classification, but Rennie & Roberton (2002) suggest descriptions and the terms GMH/IVH/IPL are now preferred as they indicate the location of the haemorrhage/lesion. An IVH can be with or without ventricular dilatation.

The stage of brain development is a crucial factor in the aetiology of GMH/IVH/IPL. The two lateral ventricles are lined with ependymal tissue. Tissue lying immediately next to the ependyma is the germinal matrix, also known as the subependymal layer. From 8 to 28 weeks' gestation, neuroblasts are produced in the germinal matrix and migrate to the cerebral cortex. During this period, a rich blood supply is provided to the germinal matrix through fragile immature capillaries that lack supporting muscle or collagen fibres. These vessels are particularly vulnerable to increases in cerebral blood flow, rupturing easily causing haemorrhage. After 32 weeks' gestation the germinal matrix becomes less active and by term has almost completely involuted. At the same time the capillaries become more stable; therefore GMH/IVH/IPL in more mature babies are less common than in those <32 weeks' gestation (Kirby 2002, Rennie & Roberton 2002).

In the baby of <32 weeks' gestation, the arterial supply to the area around the lateral ventricles is limited, with arteries forming an end zone or watershed that is relatively poorly supplied with blood. With cerebral blood flow reductions, this area is vulnerable to ischaemic damage, demonstrated as an IPL. The venous drainage from white matter and the deep areas of the brain, including the lateral ventricles, involves a peculiar U-turn route in the area of the germinal matrix. Disruptions to venous flow lead to congestion, with a risk of venous infarctions and ischaemia, demonstrated as an IPL. With reperfusion of these ischaemic areas, there may be haemorrhage, porencephalic cysts may develop and are demonstrated as IPLs (Cullens 2000, Kirby 2002, Rennie & Roberton 2002).

Throughout the perinatal period multiple factors may affect cerebral haemodynamics resulting in GMH/IVH/IPL. Early factors include obstetric haemorrhage, lack of antenatal steroids, birth outside a regional unit, chorioamnionitis, low one minute Apgar score, bruising at birth and low umbilical artery pH. Later risk factors include acidosis, hypotension, hypertension, respiratory distress syndrome (RDS) requiring mechanical ventilation, 'fighting the ventilator', apnoea, rapid volume expansion, rapid administration of sodium bicarbonate or other hyperosmolar solutions, pneumothorax and patent ductus arteriosus (Paige & Carney 2002). Also implicated are excessive handling, exposure to light and noise, lateral flexion of the baby's head and crying.

Approximately 50% of GMHs are small, have a 'silent' onset, and are detectable only on USS. If the haemorrhage is larger or extends, the clinical features may gradually appear and worsen, including apnoeic episodes that become more frequent and severe, bradycardia, pallor, falling packed cell volume, tense anterior fontanelle, metabolic acidosis and convulsions. The baby may be limp or unresponsive. If the haemorrhage is large and sudden in onset, apnoea and circulatory collapse may present (Cullens 2000, Rennie & Roberton 2002).

At-risk babies are screened by 7 days of life for GMH/IVH/IPL using cranial USS. Serial scanning of a lesion may determine any increase, extension or complication.

Care of at-risk babies is focused on prevention (Blackburn 2003). The birth should be in a regional obstetric unit with intensive neonatal facilities. Prenatal maternal steroid administration and postnatal surfactant replacement therapy reduce the incidence of GMH/IVH/IPL. Postnatally, haemodynamic stability is essential, as is prevention of complications. The baby's needs related to respiration and acid–base balance, prevention of hypoxic events, circulation and blood pressure, temperature control, nutrition and elimination, and pain control and comfort must be carefully assessed and meticulously met, with continuing evaluation and appropriate adjustments to care. Mechanical ventilation may be required and endotracheal tube suction should be performed only when necessary. Sophisticated monitoring equipment and the judicious use of analgesic, sedative and inotropic drugs may assist achieving and maintaining stability. If complications develop, such as pneumothorax or patent ductus arteriosus, these should be quickly detected and effectively treated. The baby's developmental needs should be met, particularly in relation to supportive flexed positioning, reduction in bright lighting, a quiet, undisturbed environment and appropriate interaction with parents and others (Blackburn 2003, Paige & Carney 2002, Rennie & Roberton 2002).

Despite preventative measures, babies do develop GMH/IVH/IPL. The outcome depends on the nature of the lesion. The neurological prognosis for babies with a GMH or a small IVH is usually good. An IVH associated with ventricular dilatation may resolve spontaneously with no long-term consequences. However, with a large IVH and ventricular dilatation, the accumulating CSF may require temporary drainage using ventricular taps or external ventricular drainage. Some babies may require permanent CSF drainage via a 'shunt': i.e. a drainage tube surgically inserted into the ventricular system is connected to a one-way valve placed subcutaneously behind the ear. The valve's outflow tube is attached to a catheter allowing drainage of the CSF into a large vein in the neck, or into the peritoneum, where it is reabsorbed and eliminated (Blackburn 2003). The prognosis for these babies is less good. Approximately 50% of babies with a massive IVH die, usually within 48 hrs of the onset and 90% of those who survive develop physical and/or neurological and/or intellectual impairment/s. The prognosis for babies with IPL is variable. If the IPL develops into a porencephalic cyst, hemiplegic cerebral palsy is likely, as is developmental delay. Long-term follow-up is essential and parents need much support (Blackburn 2003, Paige & Carney 2002, Rennie & Roberton 2002).

Periventricular leucomalacia

Although not strictly a haemorrhage, periventricular leucomalacia (PVL) is included because of its association with GMH/IVH/IPL. Between 27 and 30 weeks' gestation, the area of white matter around the lateral ventricles and within the watershed area of the deep cerebral arteries is undergoing considerable development. It is sensitive to any insult that results in reduced cerebral perfusion, such as those associated with GMH/IVH/IPL (Levene et al 2000), and intrauterine infection with or without ruptured membranes (Rennie & Roberton 2002). Reduced perfusion results in areas of ischaemia and degeneration of the nerve fibre tracts, disrupting nerve pathways between areas of the brain and between the brain and spinal cord. This softening and necrosis of tissue is PVL, seen on USS but more clearly with magnetic resonance imaging.

Similar pathogenesis is seen in the older pre-term and term baby, but the lesion occurs in the subcortical region rather than the periventricular region. This is because the watershed moves away from the ventricles to the cortex once the germinal matrix involutes. These lesions are known as subcortical leucomalacia (Levene et al 2000).

Care instituted to reduce the incidence of GMH/IVH/IPL may reduce the incidence of PVL or the severity of the related ischaemic damage. The prognosis is variable. The areas may become cystic, porencephalic cysts, that may regress with little resulting impairment. However bilateral occipital cysts usually result in spastic diplegic cerebral palsy (Rennie & Roberton 2002).

Haemorrhage related to coagulopathies

These haemorrhages occur due to disruption of the baby's blood-clotting abilities.

Vitamin K deficiency bleeding

Vitamin K deficiency bleeding (VKDB) may occur up to 12 months of age, although it more commonly occurs between birth and 8 weeks of life. It was previously known as haemorrhagic disease of the newborn (HDN). Several proteins, factor II (prothrombin), factor VII (proconvertin), factor IX (plasma thromboplastin component), factor X (thrombokinase) and proteins C and S, require vitamin K for their conversion to active clotting factors. A deficiency of vitamin K, as in VKDB, leads to a deficiency of these clotting factors and resultant bleeding.

Vitamin K_1 (phytomenadione) is poorly transferred across the placenta; therefore fetal stores are low. Any stores are quickly depleted after birth and

so, for normal clotting to occur, the baby must receive dietary vitamin K_1, the absorption of which requires fat and bile salts. Vitamin K_2 (menaquinone) is synthesized by bowel flora and may assist in the conversion of proteins to active clotting factors. Because the neonate's bowel is sterile, vitamin K_2 production is restricted until colonization has occurred. Therefore all newborns are deficient in vitamin K and vulnerable to VKDB.

There are three forms of VKDB that were first described by Lane and Hathaway (1985):

- 'early' (0–24 hrs)
- 'classical' (1–7 days)
- 'late' (1–12 months, although the peak onset is before 8 weeks).

Early VKDB is rare, principally affecting babies born to women who, during pregnancy, have taken warfarin, barbiturates, phenytoin, carbamazepine, cephalosporins, or tuberculostatics for treatment of their medical conditions. As these drugs interfere with vitamin K metabolism, avoidance during pregnancy reduces the risk of early VKDB. Taking vitamin K_1 supplements during pregnancy may prevent early VKDB but study results are variable (Moskowitz & Karpatkin 2005).

The babies most susceptible to developing classic VKDB are those with birth trauma, asphyxia, postnatal hypoxia and those who are pre-term, or of low birthweight. They are more likely to spontaneously bleed or have invasive interventions resulting in bleeding that cannot be controlled. Disruptions to the colonization of the bowel due to antibiotic therapy, or lack of or poor enteral feeding, may also result in classic VKDB. Breastfed babies produce bifidobacteria in their bowel that inhibit menaquinone production. Serum menaquinone is naturally low in the newborn breastfed baby, resulting in increased susceptibility to VKDB, although there are doubts as to the role of the menaquinones produced in the bowel, emphasizing the importance of dietary vitamin K_1 (Gasking 1998).

The amount of vitamin K_1 in breastmilk is naturally low, although colostrum and hind milk do contain higher levels than foremilk. The vitamin K_1 in breastmilk is considered insufficient for the exclusively breastfed newborn. Cow's milk has higher concentrations of vitamin K_1 than breastmilk, although the levels are still low. Artificial infant formulae are fortified with vitamin K_1, offering some prophylaxis against VKDB (Manco-Johnson et al 2002).

Late VKDB occurs almost exclusively in breastfed babies. However, babies who have liver disease or a condition that disrupts vitamin K_1's absorption from the bowel, for example cystic fibrosis, may develop late VKDB (Manco-Johnson et al 2002).

The baby may have bruising; or bleeding from the umbilicus, puncture sites, the nose or the scalp; or severe jaundice for >1 week and/or persistent jaundice for >2 weeks. Gastrointestinal bleeding manifests as melaena and haematemesis. In early and late VKDB, there may be extracranial and intracranial bleeding. With severe haemorrhage, circulatory collapse occurs. Late VKDB is associated with higher mortality and morbidity. Blood tests reveal prolonged prothrombin time (PT) and partial thromboplastin time (PTT), with a normal platelet count (Rennie & Roberton 2002).

Babies diagnosed with VKDB require investigation and monitoring to assess their need for treatment. With all forms of VKDB, the baby will require administration of vitamin K_1, 1–2 mg intramuscularly. In severe cases, when coagulation is grossly abnormal and there is severe bleeding, replacement of deficient clotting factors is essential. If circulatory collapse and severe anaemia occur, blood transfusion or exchange transfusion may be required. Affected babies usually require other supportive therapy to assist in their recovery.

As VKDB is a potentially fatal condition, prophylactic administration of vitamin K became the norm. Various types, routes and doses were used, but vitamin K_1 1 mg given intramuscularly within the first hour after birth became the most effective practice, despite some disquiet over such invasive prophylaxis (Soin & Katesmark 1993).

When two case-control studies reported an association between intramuscular vitamin K_1 administration and childhood cancers (Golding et al 1990, 1992), controversy increased. This finding was not confirmed in subsequent case-control studies (Ansell et al 1996, Ekelund et al 1993, Klebanoff et al 1993, McKinney et al 1998, von Kries et al 1996). However, one large retrospective case-control study reported a significant association between the

administration of vitamin K_1 intramuscularly and the development of acute lymphoblastic leukaemia in 1–6 year olds, although not with other cancers (Parker et al 1998).

These studies were limited by their design, with unreliable record keeping of the route and dose of vitamin K_1. The statistical association reported by Golding et al (1990, 1992) and Parker et al (1998) indicates that the children with childhood cancers were more likely to have been given vitamin K_1 intramuscularly at birth, but not that the vitamin K_1 *caused* the cancer. The more recent UK Childhood Cancer Study (Fear et al 2003) showed no causal link with vitamin K_1.

There was a reassessment of vitamin K_1 prophylaxis in the 1990s and a variety of products and regimens emerged. The most recent recommendations offer two prophylactic regimes using vitamin K_1 as Konakion MM Paediatric 2 mg/0.2 mL (Roche 2005). For all pre-term babies, all 'at risk' term babies, and healthy term babies whose parents choose, an intramuscular injection of vitamin K_1 should be administered within one hour of birth to give a transient peak serum concentration, reducing the risk of early VKDB (Puckett & Offringa 2000). Some vitamin K_1 remains within the muscle and acts as a slow release depot, providing prophylaxis for classic and probably also for late VKDB (Hey 2003, Wariyar et al 2000). The dose of vitamin K_1 varies according to the baby's weight and local guidelines should be consulted.

For healthy term babies whose parents decline the single intramuscular injection of vitamin K_1 (phytomenadione), the following oral prophylaxis regimen should be instituted (Roche 2005). Oral vitamin K_1 2.0 mg is given on the first and seventh days of life. If the baby is breastfed, a further dose is required at one month and monthly doses thereafter until solid food and/or milk formula feeding is introduced. This regimen should reduce the risk of all forms of VKDB; however this is dependent on the involvement, motivation and compliance of healthcare professionals and parents. Medical advice should be sought if the baby vomits within 1 hrs of oral administration.

Greer et al (1997) and Bolisetty et al (1998) demonstrated that administration of vitamin K_1 to lactating women increased the levels of vitamin K_1

in the maternal serum and breastmilk. Their babies had higher serum levels of vitamin K_1, giving some VKDB prophylaxis. However, some of these babies were also given intramuscular vitamin K_1, affecting their serum levels of vitamin K_1. Wariyar et al (2000) concluded that while maternal prophylaxis during breastfeeding was a possible alternative to prophylaxis for the baby, it was a more complicated strategy.

All parents should be given the opportunity to discuss vitamin K_1 prophylaxis during pregnancy, understand the specific management of pre-term and 'at risk' babies, and agree on their choice of prophylaxis. They should also understand the signs and treatment of VKDB, especially if their baby has one or more of the risk factors.

Thrombocytopenia

Thrombocytopenia is defined as a platelet count of $<150000/\mu L$ (alternatively described as $150 \times 10^9/L$), and severe thrombocytopenia is a platelet count of $<50000/\mu L$ (Roberts & Murray 2003). It results from a decreased rate of formation of platelets or an increased rate of consumption. In the general neonatal population, thrombocytopenia is rare (Castro et al 2007), however, it develops in up to 35% of preterm and sick babies and in 50% of babies who require intensive care (Chakravorty et al 2005, Roberts & Murray 2003). Babies at risk of developing thrombocytopenia include those who have:

- a severe congenital or acquired infection (e.g. syphilis, cytomegalovirus, rubella, toxoplasmosis, bacterial infection)
- isoimmune thrombocytopenia
- inherited thrombocytopenia

or whose mother:

- has idiopathic thrombocytopenia, purpura, systemic lupus erythematosus or thyrotoxicosis
- takes thiazide diuretics.

Fetal thrombocytopenia, due to congenital infection or an inherited condition, may be monitored during pregnancy to determine the need for maternal immunoglobulin administration and/or prenatal intrauterine platelet transfusions (Roberts & Murray 2003).

Postnatally, early onset thrombocytopenia is mild and due to a lack of platelet production associated with placental insufficiency (Chakravorty et al 2005). Immune thrombocytopenias, asphyxia, disseminated intravascular coagulation and congenital infections also result in early onset cases. Later onset thrombocytopenia is caused by bacterial sepsis and/or necrotizing enterocolitis in 90% of cases and is usually severe (Roberts & Murray 2006). For many babies, multiple causative factors are involved.

A petechial rash appears soon after birth, presenting in a mild case with a few localized petechiae. In a severe case there is widespread and serious haemorrhage from multiple sites. Intracranial haemorrhage may be fatal. Diagnosis is based on history, clinical examination and a reduced platelet count. It is differentiated from other haemorrhagic disorders because coagulation times, fibrin degradation products and red blood cell morphology are normal. Mild early onset cases are usually self-limiting, and require no treatment (Chakravorty et al 2005). In immune-mediated thrombocytopenia, intravenous immunoglobulin administration may help (Levene et al 2000). In severe later onset cases, transfusions of platelet concentrate are required, although the optimum regime is yet to be determined (Chakravorty et al 2005).

Disseminated intravascular coagulation (consumptive coagulopathy)

Disseminated intravascular coagulation (DIC) is an acquired coagulation disorder associated with the release of thromboplastin from damaged tissue, stimulating abnormal coagulation and fibrinolysis with widespread deposition of fibrin in the microcirculation and excessive consumption of clotting factors and platelets. DIC is secondary to primary conditions. Maternal causes include pre-eclampsia, eclampsia and placental abruption. Fetal causes include severe fetal distress, the presence of a dead twin in the uterus and traumatic birth. Neonatal causes include conditions resulting in hypoxia and acidosis, severe infections, hypothermia, hypotension and thrombocytopenia (Baldwin 2001/2002, Chalmers 2004).

As clotting factors and platelets are depleted and fibrinolysis is stimulated, the baby will develop a generalized purpuric rash and bleed from multiple sites. With stimulation of the clotting cascade, multiple microthrombi appear in the circulation. These can occlude vessels, with organ and tissue ischaemia and damage, particularly affecting the kidneys, resulting in haematuria and reduced urine output (Chalmers 2004). The baby becomes anaemic due to haemorrhage and fragmentation of red cells by the fibrin deposits in blood vessels (Baldwin 2001/2002).

The diagnosis is made from clinical signs and laboratory findings that show a low platelet count, low fibrinogen level, distorted and fragmented red blood cells, low haemoglobin and raised fibrin degradation products (FDPs) with a prolonged PT and PTT (Chalmers 2004).

Treatment includes correction of the underlying cause if possible and full supportive care. Control of DIC requires transfusions of fresh frozen plasma, concentrated clotting factors and platelets. Cryoprecipitate is an excellent source of fibrinogen. If there is anaemia, transfusions of whole blood or red cell concentrate are required. Occasionally an exchange transfusion of fresh heparinized blood may be performed, to remove FDPs while replacing the clotting factors. If treatment of the primary disorder and/or replacement of clotting factors is ineffective, the administration of heparin may reduce fibrin deposition (Baldwin 2001/2002).

The prognosis depends on the severity of the primary condition, as well as of the DIC, and the baby's response to treatment.

Haemorrhage related to other causes

Umbilical haemorrhage

This usually occurs as a result of a poorly applied cord ligature. The use of plastic cord clamps has almost eliminated this type of haemorrhage, although it is essential to avoid catching or pulling the clamp. Tampering with partially separated cords before they are ready to separate is discouraged. Umbilical haemorrhage is a potential cause of death. A purse-string suture should be inserted if bleeding continues after 15 or 20 min of manual pressure.

Vaginal bleeding

A small temporary vaginal discharge of blood-stained mucus occurring in the first days of life, pseudomenstruation, is due to the withdrawal of maternal oestrogen. This is a normal expectation but is included here for completeness. Parents need to know that this is a possibility and is self-limiting. Continued or excessive vaginal bleeding warrants further investigation to exclude pathological causes.

Haematemesis and melaena

These signs may present when the baby has swallowed maternal blood during birth, or from cracked nipples during breastfeeding. The diagnosis must be differentiated from VKDB, from other causes of haematemesis that include oesophageal, gastric or duodenal ulceration, and from other causes of melaena, that include necrotizing enterocolitis and anal fissures. These causes need specific and usually urgent treatment.

If the cause is swallowed blood, the condition is self-limiting and requires no specific treatment. If the cause is cracked nipples, appropriate treatment for the mother must be implemented.

Haematuria

Haematuria may be associated with coagulopathies, urinary tract infections and structural abnormalities of the urinary tract. Birth trauma may cause renal contusion and haematuria. Occasionally, after suprapubic aspiration of urine, transient mild haematuria may be observed. Treatment of the primary cause should resolve the haematuria.

Bleeding associated with intravascular access

Some sick or pre-term babies require the insertion of catheters, lines or cannulae into central or peripheral arteries or veins, or both, to provide routes for blood sampling and the infusion of fluids and drugs. However, there is a risk of severe external haemorrhage if there is dislodgement of these from the vessel or accidental disconnection from the sampling or infusion equipment, and of severe haemorrhage if a central vessel is punctured internally.

Skilled technique, close observation and careful handling of babies with intravascular access are imperative to prevent these potentially fatal haemorrhages. If an external haemorrhage does occur, continuous pressure should be applied to the site until natural haemostasis occurs or until haemostatic sutures are inserted. If there is external bleeding from an umbilical vessel, the cord stump should be squeezed between the fingers until haemostasis occurs. A replacement transfusion of whole blood or packed red cells may be required. Internal haemorrhage may require surgical intervention.

Convulsions

A convulsion (seizure/fit) is a sign of neurological disturbance, not a disease, and the occurrence of a convulsion is a medical emergency (Granelli & McGrath 2004). Because the newborn brain is still developing, its function is immature and there is an imbalance between stimulation and inhibition of neural networks, convulsions present quite differently in the neonate and may be more difficult to recognize than those of later infancy, childhood or adulthood. The incidence of convulsions is suggested as 5–8/1000 live births (Levene et al 2000).

Convulsive movement can be differentiated from jitteriness or tremors in that, with the latter two, the movements are rapid, rhythmic, equal, are often stimulated or made worse by disturbance and can be stopped by touching or flexing the affected limb. They are normal in an active, hungry baby and are of no consequence, although their occurrence should be documented. Convulsive movements tend to be slower, less equal, are not necessarily stimulated by disturbance, cannot be stopped by restraint and are always pathological (Granelli & McGrath 2004).

Abnormal, sudden or repetitive movements of any part of the body that are not controlled by repositioning or containment holds require investigation. Levene et al (2000) suggest that the type of movement can help classify the convulsion as subtle, tonic, multifocal clonic, focal clonic or myoclonic. Granelli & McGrath (2004) describe the specific appearance of convulsions as follows.

- *Subtle convulsions* found in term and pre-term babies, include movements such as blinking or fluttering of the eyelids, staring, clonic movements of the chin, horizontal or downward movements of the eyes, sucking, drooling, sticking the tongue out, cycling movements of the legs, and apnoea. These movements should be differentiated from the normal movements associated with rapid eye movement (REM) sleep. Except if there are tonic eye movements, apnoea or chewing movements, there is usually no associated abnormal electroencephalogram (EEG) activity.

- *Focal tonic convulsions* are more common in preterm babies and there is extension or flexion of a limb, asymmetric postures of the body or neck, altered patterns of breathing and maintenance of eye deviations, and abnormal brain electrical activity can be detected on EEG. With *generalized tonic convulsions* the baby sustains a rigid posture that is not usually detected on EEG.

- Term babies demonstrate *clonic convulsions* as *focal or generalized*. In *focal clonic convulsions* there are localized repetitive clonic jerking movements of an extremity, a limb or a localized unilateral muscle group. With *generalized clonic convulsions* there are random jerking movements of the extremities that migrate from limb-to-limb or from side-to-side. Clonic convulsions are usually demonstrated on EEG.

- *Myoclonic convulsions* are the least common and affect term and pre-term babies. They are different from clonic convulsions as they affect flexor muscle groups and the jerking is much faster; they can be focal, multifocal or generalized. *Focal myoclonic convulsions* affect the upper limbs. *Multifocal myoclonic convulsions* affect several areas of the body that jerk asynchronously. These two types of convulsive activity are not usually detected on EEG. With *generalized myoclonic convulsions* there are bilateral jerking movements of the upper and lower limbs that is usually detected on EEG. The jerking movements should not be confused with similar movements in a healthy sleeping baby.

During a convulsion the baby may have tachycardia, hypertension, raised cerebral blood flow and raised intracranial pressure, that predispose to serious complications.

Many conditions cause newborn convulsions and they are classified into central nervous system, metabolic, other and idiopathic causes (Table 45.1).

If a convulsion is suspected, a complete history and physical and laboratory investigations related to the possible cause would be undertaken. An EEG may

Table 45.1 Selected causes of neonatal convulsions

Category	Selected causes
Central nervous system	Intracranial haemorrhage
	Intracerebral haemorrhage
	Hypoxic-ischaemic encephalopathy
	Kernicterus
	Congenital abnormalities
Metabolic	Acquired disorders of metabolism
	Hypo- and hyperglycaemia
	Hypo- and hypercalcaemia
	Hypo- and hypernatraemia
	Inborn errors of metabolism
Other	Hypoxia
	Congenital infections
	Severe postnatally acquired infections
	Neonatal abstinence syndrome
	Hyperthermia
Idiopathic	Unknown

help detect abnormal electrical brain activity and guide treatment (Levene et al 2000). Rennie & Boylan (2007) contend that detection of convulsions and response to anticonvulsants using continuous EEG recordings requires further large-scale study.

Immediate treatment necessitates obtaining assistance from a doctor while ensuring that the baby has a clear airway and adequate ventilation, either spontaneously or mechanically. The baby can be turned to the semiprone position, with the head in a neutral position. Gentle oral and nasal suction may be required to remove any milk or mucus. If the baby is breathing spontaneously but is cyanosed, facial oxygen is given. Active resuscitation may be required. The need for intravenous access should be assessed. Any necessary handling must be gentle and the baby is usually nursed in an incubator to allow for observation and temperature regulation (Granelli & McGrath 2004).

It is important that the nature of the convulsion is documented, noting the type of movement, the areas affected, its length, colour change, change in heart rate, respiratory rate or blood pressure and immediate sequelae.

The aims of care are to treat the primary cause (details of which are not discussed in this chapter), and the pharmacologic control of the convulsions. The latter is controversial due to the potential for damage from the drugs versus the potential damage from the convulsion on the developing brain (Rennie & Boylan 2007). Cochrane reviews suggest that while there is no robust research evidence for the use of any anticonvulsants in neonates, there is consensus for the use of such drugs particularly when the baby experiences prolonged or frequent convulsions (Booth & Evans 2004; Evans & Levene 2001).

If pharmacological treatment is prescribed, the drugs most commonly used are phenobarbital and phenytoin. Newer anticonvulsants such as topiramate and levetiracetam are still being evaluated but may have fewer side-effects (Rennie & Boylan 2007). Anticonvulsant therapy may be discontinued when convulsions cease, preferably before the baby is discharged home (Levene et al 2000). The need for well-conducted randomized controlled trials to determine the most effective treatment remains. The outcome for babies who have convulsions is also controversial and statistics vary. Granelli & McGrath (2004) suggest that the prognosis depends on the cause and type of convulsion, whether it was demonstrated on EEG and whether the tracing became normal following treatment, what type of treatment was used and how long it was before any treatment was successful. Pre-term babies and those babies with congenital malformations of the brain, hypoxic-ischaemic encephalopathy, IVH and IPL, or types of bacterial meningitis tend to have a higher mortality or a poor neurological outcome. Babies with late hypocalcaemia, hyponatraemia, benign familial neonatal seizures or primary subarachnoid haemorrhage are more likely to survive neurologically intact (Paige & Carney 2002). Babies with subtle, generalized tonic and some myoclonic convulsions have a poorer neurological outcome than babies experiencing other types of convulsions. Babies who have short-lived convulsions that respond well to treatment usually have a better outcome than babies who have prolonged and difficult to treat convulsions (Granelli & McGrath 2004).

Parents

The care of parents is more comprehensively discussed elsewhere, and in this section only specific aspects will be summarized. Trauma during birth, haemorrhage and convulsions are unexpected complications and parents may be shocked and anxious, and perhaps find themselves in a crisis situation (Fowlie & McHaffie 2004, McGrath 2003, Seigel et al 2002). However, not all parents experience such feelings and some can adapt quickly to their baby's condition (Carter et al 2005, Greig 2002).

The extent of the midwife's and other professionals' contact with parents will depend on circumstances but the experiences parents have at this time have longer-term implications for them, their response to the situation, their relationships with the multiprofessional teams involved in their care as well as their interaction with and care of their baby. One of the most important aspects of caring for the parents is in relation to communication. All parents are entitled to be given information about their baby's condition, treatment and care in ways that are considered best practice. The 'Right From The Start template' provides an excellent guide (Arnold 2006), and the principles related to the baby, parents and family are summarized as follows:

1. The baby must be valued as a baby:
   - use the baby's name
   - do not predict the future
   - when sharing information, keep the baby with the parents if possible.

2. The parents and family must be respected:
   - facilitate parental support and empowerment
   - acknowledge cultural and religious differences
   - listen to their views and take their concerns seriously
   - give information honestly and sensitively using uncomplicated language
   - ensure understanding and give opportunities for questions
   - facilitate follow-up and provide further information when required.

Parental involvement in their baby's care is essential and the family-centered care/partnership with parents approach should now pervade all midwifery and neonatal settings. Midwives and neonatal nurses have an important role in promoting adaptive coping mechanisms and guiding parents to appropriate resources and support services (Fowlie & McHaffie 2004, McGrath 2003). The premature baby charity BLISS (2005) offers a helpful information guide for parents and their website (www.bliss.org.uk) includes a parent message board. Additional support and information is available from specialized outside agencies and Wilson (2006) suggests that the charity Contact a Family is also a useful resource (www.cafamily.org.uk) in the longer term.

REFERENCES

Ansell P, Bull D, Roman E 1996 Childhood leukaemia and intramuscular vitamin K: findings from a case control study. British Medical Journal 313:204–205

Arnold L 2006 Working with families affected by a disability or health condition from pregnancy to pre-school. A support pack for health professionals. Contact a Family, London. Online. Available: http://www.cafamily.org.uk/Health SupportPack.pdf 15 April 2007.

Baldwin K B 2001/2 Neonatal Disseminated Intravascular Coagulation.Central Lines 17(6):1,2,4–6,10,11

Blackburn S T 2003 Assessment and management of the neurologic system. In: Kenner C, Wright-Lott J (eds) Comprehensive neonatal nursing. A physiologic perspective, 3rd edn. Saunders, Philadelphia, p 624–660

BLISS 2005 Parent Information Guide,3rd edn., BLISS,London

Bolisetty S, Gupta J M, Graham G G et al 1998 Vitamin K in pre-term breast milk with maternal supplementation. Acta Paediatrica 87(9):960–962

Booth D, Evans D J 2004 Anticonvulsants for neonates with seizures.Cochrane Database of Systematic Reviews 3: CD004218

Brand M C 2006 Part 1: Recognizing neonatal spinal cord injury.Advances in Neonatal Care 6(1):15–24

British National Formulary for Children 2005 BMJ Publishing, London

Butler J M 2003 Assessment and management of the musculoskeletal system. In: Kenner C, Wright-Lott J (eds) Comprehensive neonatal nursing. A physiologic perspective, 3rd edn. Saunders, Philadelphia, p 661–672

Carter J D, Mulder R T, Bartram A F et al 2005 Infants in a neonatal intensive care unit: parental response. Archives of Disease in Childhood Fetal and Neonatal 90(2):F109–F113

Castro V, Kroll H, Origa A F et al 2007 A prospective study on the prevalence and risk factors for neonatal thrombocytopenia and platelet alloimmunization among 9332 unselected Brazilian newborns. Transfusion 47(1):59–66

Chakravorty S, Murray N A, Roberts I A 2005 Neonatal thrombocytopenia. Early Human Development 81(1):35–41

Chalmers E A 2004 Neonatal coagulation problems. Archives of Disease in Childhood Fetal and Neonatal 89(6): F475–F478

Cullens V 2000 Brain injury in the premature infant. In: Boxwell G(ed.) Neonatal intensive care nursing. Routledge, London, p 152–163

DiTaranto P, Campagna L, Price A E, et al 2004 Outcomes following nonoperative treatment of brachial plexus birth injuries. Journal of Child Neurology 19(2):87–90

Dudink J, Walther F J, Beekman R P 2003 Subcutaneous fat necrosis of the newborn: hypercalcaemia with hepatic and atrial myocardial calcification. Archives of Disease in Childhood Fetal and Neonatal 88(4):F343–F345

Dyachenko A, Ciampi A, Fahey J et al 2006 Prediction of risk for shoulder dystocia with neonatal injury. American Journal of Obstetrics and Gynaecology 195(6):1544–1549

Ekelund H, Finnström O, Gunnarskog J et al 1993 Administration of vitamin K to newborn infants and childhood cancer. British Medical Journal 307:89–91

Evans D J, Levene M I 2001 Anticonvulsants for preventing mortality and morbidity in full term newborns with perinatal asphyxia. Cochrane Database of Systematic Reviews 2: CD001240

Evans-Jones G, Kay S P J, Weindling A M et al 2003 Congenital brachial palsy: incidence, causes, and outcome in the United Kingdom and Republic of Ireland. Archives of Disease in Childhood Fetal and Neonatal 88(3):F185–F189

Fear N T, Roman E, Ansell P et al 2003 Vitamin K and childhood cancer: a report from the United Kingdom Childhood Cancer Study. British Journal of Cancer 89(7):1228–1231

Fowlie P W, McHaffie H 2004 Supporting parents in the neonatal unit. British Medical Journal 329:1336–1338

Furdon S, Clark D 2001 Differentiating scalp swelling in the newborn. Advances in Neonatal Care 1(1):22–27

Gasking D 1998 Vitamin K: implications for prophylaxis. Journal of Neonatal Nursing 4(1):29–33

Golding J, Patterson M, Kinlen L J 1990 Factors associated with childhood cancer in a national cohort study. British Journal of Cancer 62:304–308

Golding J, Greenwood R, Birmingham K et al 1992 Childhood cancer, intramuscular vitamin K and pethidine given during labour. British Medical Journal 305:341–346

Granelli S L P, McGrath J M 2004 Neonatal Seizures. Diagnosis, pharmacologic interventions, and outcomes. Journal of Perinatal and Neonatal Nursing 18(3):275–287

Greer F R, Marshall S P, Foley A L et al 1997 Improving the vitamin K status of breastfeeding infants with maternal vitamin K supplements. Pediatrics 99(1):88–92

Greig C 2002 Prenatal preparation of parents for neonatal care: A comparative descriptive study. PhD thesis, University of Edinburgh

Hey E 2003 Vitamin K – what, why and when. Archives of Disease in Childhood Fetal and Neonatal 88(2):F80–F83

Kirby C L 2002 Posthemorrhagic hydrocephalus: A complication of intraventricular hemorrhage. Neonatal Network 21 (1):59–68

Klebanoff M A, Read J S, Mills J L et al 1993 The risk of childhood cancer after neonatal exposure to vitamin K. New England Journal of Medicine 329(13):905–908

Lane P A, Hathaway W E 1985 Vitamin K in infancy. Journal of Pediatrics 106:351–359

Levene M I, Tudehope D, Thearle M J 2000 Essentials of neonatal medicine, 3rd edn. Blackwell Science, Oxford

Manco-Johnson M, Rodden D J, Collins, S 2002 Newborn hematology. In: Merenstein G B, Gardner S L (eds) Handbook of neonatal intensive care, 5th edn. Mosby, St Louis, p 419–442

McGrath J M 2003 Family-centered care. In: Kenner C, Wright-Lott J(eds) Comprehensive neonatal nursing. A physiologic perspective, 3rd edn. Saunders, Philadelphia, p 89–107

McKinney P A, Jaszczak E, Findlay E et al 1998 Case-control study of childhood leukaemia and cancer in Scotland: findings for neonatal intramuscular vitamin K. British Medical Journal 316:173–179

Moskowitz N P, Karpatkin M 2005 Coagulation problems in the newborn. Current Paediatrics 15(1):50–56

Paige P L, Carney P R 2002 Neurologic disorders. In: Merenstein G B, Gardner S L (eds) Handbook of neonatal intensive care, 5th edn. Mosby, St Louis, p 644–678

Papile L A, Burnstein J, Burnstein R et al 1978 Incidence and evolution of subependymal and intraventricular hemorrhage: a study of infants with birth weights less than 1500 gm. Journal of Pediatrics 92:529–534

Parker L A 2006 Part 2: Birth trauma: Injuries to the intra-abdominal organs, peripheral nerves, and skeletal system. Advances in Neonatal Care 6(1):7–11

Parker L, Cole M, Craft A W et al 1998 Neonatal vitamin K administration and childhood cancer in the north of England: retrospective case-control study. British Medical Journal 305:341–346

Puckett R M, Offringa M 2000 Prophylactic vitamin K for vitamin K deficiency bleeding in neonates. Cochrane Database of Systematic Reviews 4:CD002776

Rennie J M, Boylan G 2007 Treatment of neonatal seizures. Archives of Disease in Childhood Fetal and Neonatal 92: F148–F150

Rennie J M, Roberton N R C(eds) 2002 A manual of neonatal intensive care, 4th edn. Arnold, London

Roberts I A, Murray N A 2003 Neonatal thrombocytopenia. Archives of Disease in Childhood Fetal and Neonatal 88(5): F359–F364

Roberts I A, Murray N A(2006) Neonatal thrombocytopenia. Current Haematological Reports 5(1):55–63

Roche 2005 How to use Konakion MM Paediatric 2mg/0.2ml (phytomenadione) for the prophylaxis of vitamin K deficiency bleeding (VKDB). Roche, Hertfordshire

Sansoucie D A, Cavaliere, T A 2003 Newborn and infant assessment. In: Kenner C, Wright-Lott J(eds) Comprehensive neonatal nursing. A physiologic perspective, 3rd edn. Saunders, Philadelphia, p 308–347

Seigel R, Gardner, S L, Merenstein G B 2002 Families in crisis: theoretical and practical considerations. In: Merenstein G B, Gardner S L (eds) Handbook of neonatal intensive care, 5th edn., Mosby, St Louis, p 725–753

Smith C 2006 Intracranial haemorrhage in infants. Current Diagnostic Pathology 12(3):184–190

Soin H, Katesmark M 1993 By muscle or mouth. Nursing Times 89(42):32–33

Sorantin E, Brader P, Thimary F 2006 Neonatal trauma. European Journal of Radiology 60(2):199–207

Thomas R, Harvey D 1997 Colour guide: neonatology, 2nd edn. Churchill Livingstone, Edinburgh

Tortora G J, Derrickson B 2006 Principles of anatomy and physiology, 11th edn. John Wiley, Hoboken

Volpe J J 1997 Brain injury in the premature infant. Clinics in Perinatology 24(3):567–587

von Kries R, Gobel U, Hachmeister A et al 1996 Vitamin K and childhood cancer: a population-based case-control study in Lower Saxony, Germany. British Medical Journal 313:199–203

Wariyar U, Hilton S, Pagan J et al 2000 Six years' experience of prophylactic oral vitamin K. Archives of Disease in Childhood Fetal and Neonatal 82:F64–F68

Wilson A K 2006 Contact a family – not just a red book! Infant 2(4):142–145

FURTHER READING

Boxwell G (ed.) 2000 Neonatal intensive care nursing. Routledge, London

This book is primarily written for neonatal nurses and teachers. Student midwives and midwives would benefit from the additional more detailed information about many of the conditions addressed in this chapter. Chapter 2, 7, 8, 9, 17 and 19 are recommended.

Hankins, G D V, Clark S M, Munn M B 2006 Cesarean section on request at 39 week: impact on shoulder dystocia, fetal trauma, neonatal encephalopathy, and intrauterine fetal demise. Seminars in Perinatology 30(5):276–287

Given the controversies about increasing rates, these American authors offer convincing arguments in support of elective caesarean section to prevent complications.

Rennie J M 2005 Roberton's textbook of neonatology, 4th edn. Elsevier, London

A classic British textbook that gives excellent explanations of physiology and discusses the management of neonatal complications, albeit from a mainly medical perspective.

46 Congenital abnormalities

Tom Turner   Judith Simpson

CHAPTER CONTENTS

Anticipating the arrival of a healthy baby is every prospective parent's dream. Sadly for some this dream is shattered when the presence of an abnormality is recognized either prenatally, at birth or in the neonatal period. The incidence of major congenital abnormalities is 2–3% of all births, although this figure is subject to familial, cultural and geographic variations. It is therefore very likely that every practising midwife will at some time in their career be confronted with the challenge of providing appropriate care and support for such babies and their families.

The chapter aims to:

- address issues such as who should tell the parents and how and when they should be told
- describe and explain specific congenital abnormalities
- explore the complementary roles of the midwife and paediatrician in providing care
- consider the psychological impact on staff and the strategies that could be put in place to minimize the accompanying stress.

Communicating the news

It is often the midwife who first notices an abnormality in the baby either during the process of the birth or on routine newborn examination. All abnormalities, identified or suspected, should be notified to medical staff but there is sometimes a difference of opinion as to who should communicate the news to the parents.

There is a very strong argument for suggesting that this should be done by the midwife present at the birth. The midwife–client relationship is, or ought to be, one of mutual trust and respect. Honesty is an implicit tenet of such a relationship. It is well recognized that one of the first questions a mother will ask the midwife after the birth is 'is the baby all right?' For the midwife to be non-committal or economical with the truth is to betray that trust. It is preferable that the midwife tells both parents sensitively but honestly that she has concerns, and shows them any obvious abnormality in the baby.

Where there is doubt in the midwife's mind, for example in cases of suspected chromosomal abnormalities, it could be argued that the issue is less clear cut. Discretion could therefore be exercised in the precise form of words used, but the intention of inviting a second opinion should be made clear to the parents. It is advisable that both the parents and the midwife be present when an experienced paediatrician examines the baby and that the midwife be present during any dialogue between the parents and medical staff so that she is aware of exactly what has been said. She is then in a position to clarify or repeat any points that were not fully understood. Opportunities for follow up consultation with the paediatrician should be offered as and when the parents desire. Patience, tact and understanding are prerequisites for midwives caring for these families.

Some abnormalities are slight and cause no further problems for the parents or child, whereas others are profound and cause the subsequent daily care to be fraught with difficulties. Unlike most others, abnormalities involving the face cannot be disguised or hidden and therefore must rate among the most distressing for parents. This is confirmed by Wirt et al (1992) who claim that congenital defects of the head, face and neck often precipitate a major family crisis. The psychological impact on parents of being told or shown, or both, that their baby has a congenital abnormality is often not dissimilar to the grieving process discussed in Chapter 38. Great sensitivity is required on the part of the midwife when showing the baby to the parents for the first time.

Whatever the abnormality it is essential that families receive accurate, consistent and appropriate information about their baby's condition. Since a comprehensive discussion of every abnormality is clearly not possible, selection has therefore been made of those the midwife is most likely to encounter.

Definition and causes

By definition, a congenital abnormality is any defect in form, structure or function. Identifiable defects can be categorized as follows (Fig. 46.1):

- chromosomal abnormalities
- single gene defects

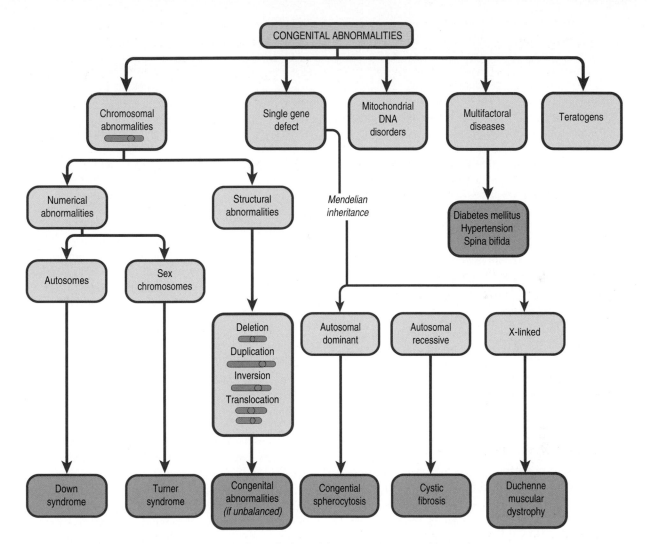

Figure 46.1 Causes of congenital abnormalities. (Adapted from Beattie & Carachi 2005.)

- mitochondrial DNA disorders
- teratogenic causes
- multifactorial causes
- unknown causes.

Chromosomal abnormalities

Box 46.1 provides definitions of terms used in this and subsequent sections.

Every human cell carries a blueprint for reproduction in the form of 44 chromosomes (autosomes) and two sex chromosomes. Each chromosome comprises a number of genes, which are specific sequences of DNA coding for particular proteins. The zygote should have 22 autosomes and one sex chromosome from each parent. Should a fault occur in either the formation of the gametes or following fertilization (see Ch. 10), abnormalities in chromosome number (aneuploidies) or structure (deletions, duplications, inversions, translocations) may occur. Each abnormal chromosomal pattern has a characteristic clinical presentation, the most common of which will be discussed further.

Gene defects (Mendelian inheritance)

Genes are composed of DNA and each is concerned with the transmission of one specific hereditary

Box 46.1 Glossary of terms

Karyotyping	The process of identifying chromosomes by size	Deletion	Breaking off or loss of part of a chromosome
Gamete	Oocyte or spermatozoon	Duplication	Repetition of part of a chromosome
Zygote	Formed by gametes combining at fertilization	Inversion	Rearrangement of part of a chromosome
Meiosis	The type of cell reduction division that occurs in the formation of gametes, in which one of each chromosome pair is 'lost'	Translocation	Transfer of material from one chromosome to another of a different kind. Should this occur during mitosis, the result will be a balanced or reciprocal translocation where the total chromosomal complement is normal. This would be discovered only during karyotyping; there is no clinical manifestation. If, however, translocation happens during meiosis an unbalanced translocation will result in either an excess or deficit of chromosomal material in the gamete formed.
Mitosis	The type of cell division that occurs in somatic cells where each new cell gets a full set of chromosomes		
Aneuploidies	Numerical chromosomal abnormalities		
Non-disjunction	Failure of a chromosome pair to separate during meiosis or paired chromatids during mitosis		
Trisomy	A situation where a particular chromosome is represented three times in the nucleus		

factor. Genetically inherited factors may be dominant or recessive.

A *dominant* gene will produce its effect even if present in only one chromosome of a pair. An autosomal dominant condition can usually be traced through several generations although the severity of clinical expression may vary from generation to generation. Congenital spherocytosis, achondroplasia, osteogenesis imperfecta, adult polycystic kidney disease and Huntington's chorea are examples of dominant conditions.

A *recessive* gene needs to be present in both chromosomes before producing its effect. An individual who is carrying only one abnormal copy of the gene (a heterozygote) is unaffected. Examples of autosomal recessive conditions are cystic fibrosis or phenylketonuria.

Some congenital abnormalities are a consequence of single gene defects. In a dominantly inherited disorder the risk of an affected fetus is 1:2 (50%) for each and every pregnancy. In a recessive disorder, the risk is 1:4 (25%) for each and every pregnancy.

In an X-linked recessive inheritance the condition affects almost exclusively males, although females can be carriers. X-linked recessive inheritance is responsible for conditions such as haemophilia A and B and Duchenne muscular dystrophy. Spontaneous mutations commonly arise in X-linked recessive disorders. When a woman is a carrier of an X-linked condition, there is a 50% chance of each of her sons being affected and an equal chance that each of her daughters will be carriers.

The recent work on the human genome is likely to clarify further some of these disorders and may offer a way into treatment in the future; for example, polycystic kidney disease (see p. 896) arises from a mutation on chromosome 6 and cystic fibrosis is due to a defect on chromosome 7.

Mitochondrial inheritance

Mitochondria are cellular structures responsible for energy production. Mitochondria are always inherited from the mother. Symptoms and signs of mitochondrial disorders can be diverse but tend to occur in tissues which have high energy requirements such as the brain and muscles. Examples are very rare but include lactic acidosis, encephalopathy and stroke-like episodes (MELAS) and myoclonic epilepsy with myopathy (MERFF).

Teratogenic causes

A teratogen is any agent that raises the incidence of congenital abnormality. The list of known and suspected teratogens is continually growing but includes: prescribed drugs (e.g. anticonvulsants, anticoagulants and preparations containing large concentrations of vitamin A such as those prescribed for the treatment of acne), drugs used in substance abuse (e.g. heroin, alcohol and nicotine), environmental factors such as radiation and chemicals (e.g. dioxins, pesticides), infective agents (e.g. rubella, cytomegalovirus) and maternal disease (e.g. diabetes). It should be borne in mind that several factors influence the effect(s) produced by any one teratogen, such as gestational age of the embryo or fetus at the time of exposure, length of exposure and toxicity of the teratogen. Direct cause and effect is sometimes difficult to establish. Accurate recording of all congenital abnormalities on a central register, such as the Scottish Anomaly Register, facilitates the early recognition of new teratogens.

Multifactorial causes

These are due to interactions between specific genes (genetic susceptibility) and environmental influences (teratogens).

Unknown causes

In spite of a growing body of knowledge, the specific cause of the majority of congenital abnormalities remains unspecified and they occur sporadically in families.

The role of preconception advice

Although the midwife may advise on modulation of behaviour or diet during pregnancy, by the time the majority of women present for a booking visit the damage has been done. The burden of prevention therefore lies with dissemination of information and appropriate counselling in preconception clinics. The increasing awareness and availability of preconception advice has helped reduce the incidence of some categories of abnormality, notably those associated with poorly controlled diabetes and neural tube defects. Whyte (1995) cites a 72% decrease in neural tube defects as a result of folic acid supplements being taken prior to conception.

Prenatal screening and diagnosis

Improved prenatal screening and diagnostic techniques (see Ch. 18), have led to increased recognition of abnormality, particularly in early pregnancy. This has resulted in some families making the decision to have their pregnancy terminated, while allowing many others time to adjust and try to come to terms with the news that their baby will be born with a particular problem. One advantage of prenatal diagnosis is that, if necessary, arrangements can be made for the mother to have prenatal transfer to a unit where neonatal surgical or intensive care facilities are available. The disadvantage of transfer is that the mother may then be separated from family, friends and the support of the midwives she knows best. This makes it all the more imperative that the staff in these units are sensitive to the needs of such women.

Chromosomal abnormalities

Trisomy 21 (Down syndrome)

The classic features of what is now known as Down syndrome were first described in 1866 by physician John Down (Fig. 46.2). He recognized a commonly occurring combination of facial features among mentally subnormal individuals. His description included features such as widely set and obliquely slanted eyes, small nose and thick rough tongue. In addition to these, it is now accepted that other signs are evident: a small head with flat occiput, squat broad hands with an incurving little finger, a wide space between the thumb and index finger, a single palmar (simian) crease, Brushfield spots in the eyes, and generalized hypotonia. Not all of these manifestations need be present and any of them can occur alone without implying chromosomal aberration.

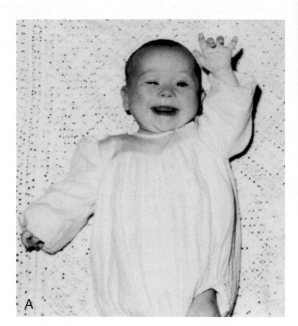
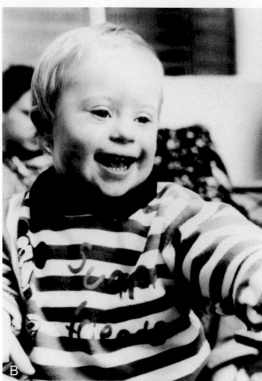

Figure 46.2 (A) Baby with Down syndrome: note slant of eyes and incurving little finger. (B) With good parental involvement and stimulus these infants can reach maximum potential. (Photographs courtesy of Scottish Down's Syndrome Association.)

Babies born with Down syndrome also have a higher incidence of cardiac anomalies, cataracts, hearing loss, leukaemia and hypothyroidism. Intelligence quotient is below average, at 40–80.

Although there may be little doubt in the midwife's mind that a baby has Down syndrome, she should be careful not to make any definitive statements. Family likeness alone may explain some babies' appearance. Parents themselves may voice their suspicions. If they do not, a sensitive but honest approach should be made by either the midwife or paediatrician to alert them to the possibility and to request permission to conduct further investigations. It is inappropriate to transfer the baby to the special care nursery in order to carry out these investigations under the guise of the baby being cold or sleepy. Investigations indicated include chromosome analysis and echocardiography, because of the increased risk of congenital heart disease. Some centres offer rapid diagnosis (see Ch. 18).

Down syndrome arising sporadically as a result of a non-disjunction process occurs in 95% of cases. Unbalanced translocation occurs in 2.5% of cases, usually between chromosomes 14 and 21. Mosaic forms also occur. There is no difference between the types in clinical appearance. Parents who have a baby with Down syndrome, therefore, should be offered genetic counselling to establish the risk of recurrence. The overall incidence of Down syndrome is 1 in 700.

An individual baby's needs will vary depending on whether there are any co-existing abnormalities. Apart from any emotional support the mother may require, the midwife may also offer help with feeding. Problems are likely to be encountered because of the baby's generalized hypotonia. Breastfeeding should be encouraged if the mother had so planned. Providing audiovisual or reading material about Down syndrome for the parents may be helpful, or the address of the local branch of the Down Syndrome Association (see Useful addresses, below).

Trisomy 18 (Edwards syndrome)

This condition is found in about 1 in 5000 births. An extra 18th chromosome is responsible for the characteristic features. The lifespan for these children is short and the majority die during their 1st year. The head is small with a flattened forehead, a receding chin and frequently a cleft palate. The ears are low set and maldeveloped.

The sternum tends to be short, the fingers often overlap each other and the feet have a characteristic rocker-bottom appearance. Malformations of the cardiovascular and gastrointestinal systems are common.

Trisomy 13 (Patau syndrome)

An extra copy of the 13th chromosome leads to multiple abnormalities. These children have a short life. Only 5% live beyond 3 years. Affected infants are small and are microcephalic. Midline facial abnormalities such as cleft lip and palate are common and limb abnormalities are frequently seen. Brain, cardiac and renal abnormalities may coexist with this trisomy.

Turner syndrome (XO)

In this monosomal condition, only one sex chromosome exists: an X. The absent chromosome is indicated by 'O'. The child is a girl with a short, webbed neck, widely spaced nipples and oedematous feet. The genitalia tend to be underdeveloped and the internal reproductive organs do not mature. The condition may not be diagnosed until puberty fails to occur. Congenital cardiac defects may also be found. Mental development is usually normal.

Klinefelter syndrome (XXY)

This is an abnormality affecting boys but it is not normally diagnosed until pubertal changes fail to occur.

Gastrointestinal malformations

Most of the abnormalities affecting this system call for prompt surgical intervention, for example atresias, gastroschisis and exomphalos. With the increasing use of routine ultrasound screening at 18–20 weeks' gestation many are likely to be diagnosed prenatally (Haddock et al 1996). If prenatal diagnosis has been made, the parents will be at least partially prepared. In this event, where possible, the paediatric team of neonatal paediatrician and paediatric surgeon should speak to the parents before birth of the baby to explain the probable sequence of events. Once the baby is born, prior to obtaining their consent for surgery, the paediatric surgeon should have a full discussion with the parents. If the baby's condition allows, the parents should be encouraged to hold the baby and photographs should be taken.

Gastroschisis and exomphalos

Gastroschisis (Fig. 46.3) is a paramedian defect of the abdominal wall with extrusion of bowel that is not covered by peritoneum, thus making it very vulnerable to infection and injury. Surgical closure of

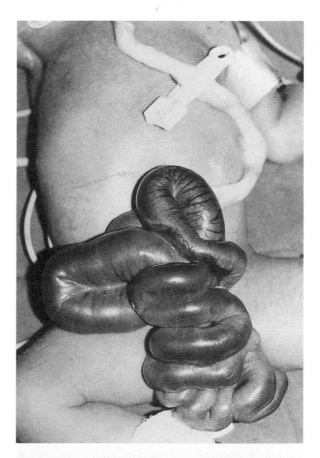

Figure 46.3 Gastroschisis showing prolapsed intestine to the right of umbilical cord. (From Rennie & Roberton 1999, with permission of Churchill Livingstone.)

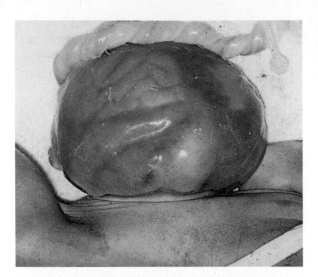

Figure 46.4 Omphalocele defect with bowel visible through sac in the lower part and abnormally lobulated liver in the sac in the upper part. (From Rennie & Roberton 1999, with permission of Churchill Livingstone.)

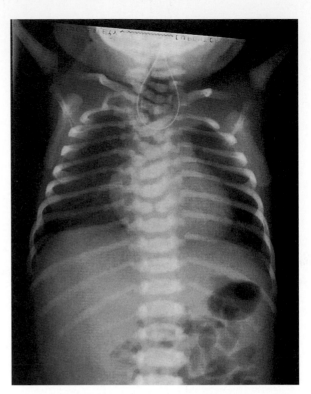

Figure 46.5 Oesophageal atresia. Coiled feeding tube in proximal pouch. Note vertebral and rib abnormalities. Distal gas confirms a tracheo–oesophageal fistula. (From Rennie & Roberton 1999, with permission of Churchill Livingstone.)

the defect is usually possible; the size of the defect will determine whether primary closure is possible or whether a temporary silo made from synthetic materials (e.g. Silastic) is necessary until the abdominal cavity is able to contain all the abdominal organs.

Exomphalos or omphalocele (Fig. 46.4) is a defect in which the bowel or other viscera protrude through the umbilicus. Very often these babies have other abnormalities, for example heart defects, which could be a contraindication to surgery in the immediate neonatal period. Closure of the defect may consequently be delayed as long as 1 or even 2 years.

The immediate management of both the above conditions is to cover the herniated abdominal contents with clean cellophane wrap (e.g. Clingfilm) or warm sterile saline swabs to reduce fluid and heat losses and to give a degree of protection. An orogastric or nasogastric tube should be passed and stomach contents aspirated. Transfer of the baby to a surgical unit is then expedited.

Atresias

Oesophageal atresia

Oesophageal atresia (Fig. 46.5) occurs when there is incomplete canalization of the oesophagus in early intrauterine development. It is commonly associated with tracheo–oesophageal fistula, which connects the trachea to the upper or lower oesophagus, or both. The commonest type of abnormality is where the upper oesophagus terminates in a blind upper pouch and the lower oesophagus connects to the trachea. This abnormality should be suspected in the presence of maternal polyhydramnios and should be screened for after birth in all such affected pregnancies. At birth the baby has copious amounts of mucus coming from the mouth. Early detection is essential. The midwife should attempt to pass a wide orogastric tube but it may travel less than 10–12 cm. Radiography will confirm the diagnosis. The baby must be given no oral fluid but a wide bore oesophageal tube should be passed into the upper pouch and connected to gentle continuous suction apparatus. Usually a double lumen 10 fg (Replogle) tube is used and the baby nursed head up. He should be transferred immediately to a paediatric surgical unit, ensuring that continuous suction is available throughout the transfer. It may be possible to anastomose the blind ends of the oesophagus. If the gap in the oesophagus is too large a series of bouginages can be carried out in an attempt to stretch the ends of the oesophagus, stimulate growth and thereby eventually facilitate repair by end-to-end anastomosis. Alternatively transplant of, for example, a section of colon may be needed at a later date. Rarely, if the repair is delayed, cervical oesophagostomy may be performed to allow drainage of secretions. Meanwhile the baby will need to be fed via a gastrostomy tube. This method of feeding obviously deprives the baby of oral stimuli. Such a baby may be given 'sham' feeds to allow him to taste the milk and to promote sucking, swallowing and normal development of the mandible.

Duodenal atresia

Atresia may occur at any level of the bowel but the duodenum is the most common site. If this has not already been diagnosed in the prenatal period, persistent vomiting within 24–36hrs of birth will be the first feature encountered. The vomit will often contain bile unless the obstruction is proximal to the entrance of the common bile duct. Abdominal distension may not be present and the baby may pass meconium. A characteristic double bubble of gas may be seen on radiological examination (Fig. 46.6). Treatment is by surgical repair. Prognosis is good if the baby is otherwise healthy, but this abnormality is often associated with others; 30% of cases occur in children with Down syndrome.

Rectal atresia and imperforate anus

Careful examination of the perineum is an important aspect of any newborn examination. An imperforate anus should be obvious at birth on examination of the baby, but a rectal atresia might not become apparent until it is noted that the baby has not passed meconium. Occasionally, for the unwary, the passage of meconium through a fistulous connection to the vagina, bladder or urethra may mask an imperforate anus (see Plates 32, 33 & 34). Whatever the anatomical arrangement, all babies should be referred for surgery.

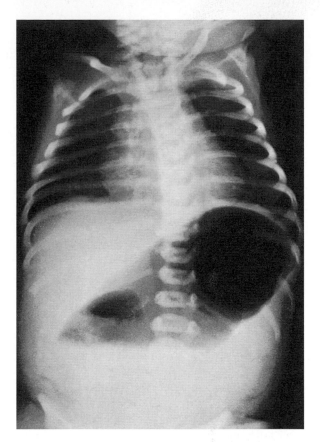

Figure 46.6 Double bubble of duodenal atresia. The stomach is overlapping the duodenum with the second bubble being seen through the stomach. (From Rennie & Roberton 1999, with permission of Churchill Livingstone.)

Should a baby fail to pass meconium in the first 24 hrs, three other possibilities should be considered:

- malrotation/volvulus
- meconium ileus (cystic fibrosis)
- Hirschsprung's disease.

Malrotation/volvulus

This is a developmental abnormality where incomplete rotation of the small bowel has taken place, giving rise to signs of obstruction. There is often bilious vomiting and abdominal distension.

Surgical assessment and correction are necessary. Because of the risks of severe bowel damage secondary to the obstruction of blood flow in the mesentery in unrecognized malrotation, any newborn infant with bile-stained vomiting requires urgent medical assessment.

Meconium ileus (cystic fibrosis)

Some 15% of children with cystic fibrosis present with meconium ileus in the neonatal period. Cystic fibrosis is an autosomal recessive condition affecting 1 in 2500 births. In the past, the majority of cases were not diagnosed until later in infancy or childhood when the child failed to thrive or had repeated chest infections. In meconium ileus the meconium is particularly viscous and causes intestinal obstruction. There is accompanying abdominal distension and bile-stained vomiting. Intravenous fluids and a Gastrografin enema may relieve the obstruction. Definitive diagnosis may be difficult initially, but the presence of a raised immunoreactive trypsin level (IRT) and of markers in the serum using the polymerase chain reaction (PCR) may demonstrate the $\triangle$F508 deletion in both copies of the cystic fibrosis gene on chromosome 7. Histology of any resected bowel may also indicate the likelihood of cystic fibrosis, but a definitive diagnosis is not usually possible until a sweat test has been carried out at 4–6 weeks of age. Treatment of cystic fibrosis is supportive rather than curative and involves administration of pancreatic enzymes and a rigorous programme of chest physiotherapy and antibiotics as indicated by bacteriological evidence.

Hirschsprung's disease

In this disease, which has an incidence of 1 in 5000 births, an aganglionic section of the large bowel is present. This means that peristalsis does not occur and the bowel therefore becomes obstructed. The baby develops abdominal distension and bile-stained vomiting. Definite diagnosis is made by carrying out a rectal biopsy. Resection of the aganglionic segment of bowel is indicated.

Pyloric stenosis

Pyloric stenosis arises from a genetic defect that causes hypertrophy of the muscles of the pyloric sphincter. The characteristic clinical presentation is projectile vomiting usually at around 6 weeks of age, but it may occur earlier and hence is included in this section. There is a gender-related predominance in that it is usually boys who are affected. Surgical repair is effected by pyloromyotomy (Ramstedt's operation), which involves partial splitting of the hypertrophied pyloric muscle along its length.

The remaining abnormalities of the gastrointestinal system, while amenable to surgery, do not usually necessitate immediate action.

Cleft lip and cleft palate

The incidence of cleft lip occurring as a single deformity is 1.3 in 1000. This defect may be unilateral or bilateral. Since it is very often accompanied by cleft palate, both will be considered together.

Clefts in the palate may affect the hard palate, soft palate, or both. Some defects will include alveolar margins and some the uvula. It is recommended that, during the initial examination of the baby, the palate be examined by means of a good light source rather than by digital palpation. The greatest problem for these babies initially is feeding. If the defect is limited to unilateral cleft lip, mothers who had intended to breastfeed should be encouraged to do so. Where there is the additional problem of cleft palate, arranging for the baby to be fitted with an orthodontic plate may facilitate breastfeeding but this obviously does not afford the same stimulus as nipple-to-palate contact.

Middle ear infection is a concomitant risk for babies with cleft palate. Repeated infections of this type could impede hearing and subsequent development of speech. Danner (1992) suggests that breastfeeding be encouraged since passive immunity may protect these babies from the infections to which they are prone. Expressed breastmilk may of course be given. Cup or spoon feeding is an alternative method but for those who wish to bottle feed there is a wide variety of specially shaped teats available to accommodate the different sizes and positions of palate defects. Above all else, an unending supply of patience is required. The midwife should encourage the mother and father to find the most successful technique rather than 'taking over' since this may compound any feelings of guilt or inadequacy the parents may feel. Early referral to the cleft team of paediatric or plastic surgeon and orthodontists should be arranged. These teams may also include specialist nursing staff, speech and language therapists and audiologists.

Corrective surgery will be carried out at some stage but there is some debate as to the most appropriate time to carry out these procedures. Sullivan (1996) examines the arguments for both early and late repair of a cleft lip. He explains that some surgeons advocate effecting closure of the cleft lip within 2 weeks of birth in order to capitalize on the increased tissue-healing properties that are present as a short-lived legacy of intrauterine existence. They also argue that an early repair will be instrumental in encouraging healthy attachment between mother and baby. Advocates of later intervention suggest cleft lip repair at the age of 3–4 months because cleft lip often occurs as a feature of other medical conditions that may not be detected immediately. Surgery in the early neonatal period for such a baby may be too hazardous. Closure of the palate defect is suggested at around the age of 12–15 months. One of the main reasons for this apparently long delay is to allow sufficient growth to take place, which may result in reducing the size of the defect thus increasing the possibility of a more satisfactory repair. Some children have a series of cosmetic operations at some time after the initial repairs are carried out. It is often helpful for the midwife to show families 'before and after' photographs of babies for whom surgery has been a success (Fig. 46.7).

Clearly, although the midwife may offer valuable support in these early days, she is limited in the length of time she has available to help these families. Giving the parents the address of a support group such as the Cleft Lip And Palate Association (CLAPA) is useful (see Useful addresses, below).

Pierre Robin sequence

Pierre Robin sequence is characterized by micrognathia (hypoplasia of the lower jaw), abnormal attachment of muscles controlling the tongue, which allows it to fall backward and occlude the airway, and a central cleft palate. This triad of abnormalities presents a challenge for nursing care. Maintenance of a clear airway is paramount. In order to achieve this, the baby will need to be nursed prone and some may require the insertion of an oral airway. Nasal and nasopharyngeal constant positive airways pressure (CPAP) may be necessary for some time after birth. This is one of the few exceptions to the 'Back to sleep' campaign aimed at reducing cot deaths. Feeding can be problematic. There is a high risk of aspiration occurring. Suction catheter and oxygen equipment should be readily to hand. Some of these babies may be fitted with an orthodontic plate to facilitate feeding. The action of sucking will encourage development of the mandible. Parents will need considerable support during what may for some babies be a protracted period of hospitalization. Discharge will be when the lower jaw has grown sufficiently or when the parents feel comfortable about taking the baby home. Habel et al (1996) suggest that some of these babies can have an earlier transfer

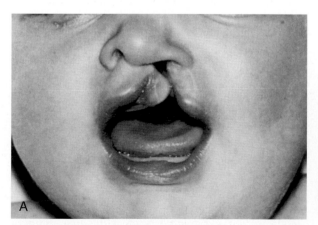
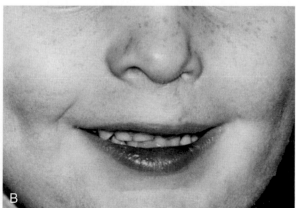

Figure 46.7 (A) Cleft lip and palate. (B) The repaired cleft. (From Raine 1994, with permission of Churchill Livingstone.)

home if a shortened endotracheal tube is in place to ensure a patent nasopharyngeal airway. They recommend replacing the tube every 2 weeks until adequate mandibular development has taken place. Despite this, there remains a small risk of sudden death in these infants.

Abnormalities relating to respiration

Making a successful transition from fetus to neonate includes being able to establish regular respiration. Any abnormality of the respiratory tract or accessory respiratory muscles is likely to hamper this process.

Diaphragmatic hernia

This abnormality consists of a defect in the diaphragm that allows herniation of abdominal contents into the thoracic cavity (Fig. 46.8). The extent

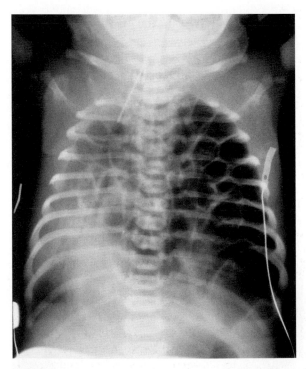

Figure 46.8 Chest radiograph of infant at 1 hr of life, showing left diaphragmatic hernia, displacement of air-filled viscera into the hemithorax and a marked shift of mediastinum and heart. (From Rennie & Roberton 1999, with permission of Churchill Livingstone.)

to which lung development is compromised as a result depends on the size of the defect and the gestational age at which herniation first occurred. The condition is increasingly diagnosed antenatally by ultrasound; where there is prenatal diagnosis, delivery in a specialist unit is advisable. At birth, the condition may be suspected if the baby is cyanosed and unexpected difficulty is experienced in resuscitation. In addition, since the majority of such defects are left sided, heart sounds will be displaced to the right. The abdomen may have a flat or scaphoid appearance. Chest X-ray will confirm the diagnosis. Continuous gastric suction should be commenced. Surgical repair of the defect is necessary, but this is not urgent. It is more important to stabilize the baby's general condition before surgery. It is especially critical to deal with the problem of persistent pulmonary hypertension and right-to-left shunting of blood within the heart. This may necessitate the use of newer ventilation techniques and pharmacological agents such as nitric oxide. Prognosis relates to the degree of pulmonary hypoplasia and reversibility of the pulmonary hypertension. There is also the possibility of co-existent abnormalities such as cardiac defects or skeletal anomalies. The incidence is one in 2000 births.

Choanal atresia

Choanal atresia describes a unilateral or bilateral narrowing of the nasal passage(s) with a web of tissue or bone occluding the nasopharynx (Fig. 46.9). Tachypnoea and dyspnoea are cardinal features, particularly when a bilateral lesion is present. The diagnosis is made relatively easily by noting that the baby mouth breathes and finds feeding impossible without cyanosis. In addition, nasal catheters cannot be passed into the pharynx and if a mirror or cold metal spoon is held under the nose no vapour will collect. A helpful diagnostic aid is that the baby's colour will improve with crying (Bagwell 1993). Maintaining a clear airway is obviously essential and an oral airway may have to be used to affect this. *A unilateral defect may not be noticed until the baby feeds for the first time. The midwife should therefore bear in mind the possibility of this problem if respiratory difficulty and cyanosis occur at this time.* Surgery will be required to remove the obstructing tissue.

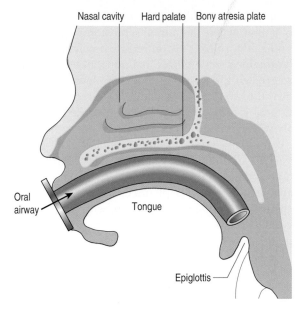

Nasal cavity   Hard palate   Bony atresia plate

Oral airway

Tongue

Epiglottis

Figure 46.9 Choanal atresia. A bony plate blocks the nose. (From Rennie & Roberton 1999, with permission of Churchill Livingstone.)

The incidence is 1 in 8000. Occasionally choanal atresia is associated with other abnormalities such as 'Charge' syndrome, a syndrome in which there are defects found in the eye (coloboma), the heart, the ear, the genitalia, occasionally oesophageal atresia and usually growth retardation.

Laryngeal stridor

This is a noise made by the baby, usually on inspiration and exacerbated by crying. Most commonly the cause is laryngomalacia, which is due to laxity of the laryngeal cartilage. Although it sounds distressing, the baby generally is not at all upset. It is the parents who require comforting and reassurance (often repeatedly). It should be explained to them that the stridor may take some time to resolve, perhaps up to 2 years. If, however, the stridor is accompanied by signs of dyspnoea or feeding problems, further investigations such as bronchoscopy or laryngoscopy would become necessary to rule out a more sinister cause.

Congenital cardiac defects

Babies born with congenital heart defects comprise the second largest group of babies born with abnormalities. Approximately eight in 1000 live-births have some degree of congenital heart disease and about one-third of these babies will be symptomatic in early infancy.

Causes

Approximately 90% of cardiac defects cannot be attributed to a single cause, chromosomal and genetic factors account for 8%, and a further 2% are thought to be caused by teratogens. The critical period of exposure to teratogens in respect of embryological development of cardiac tissue is from the 3rd to the 6th week.

Prenatal detection

An increasing number of cardiac problems are being identified by means of detailed ultrasound scanning (see Ch. 18). However, the detection of many defects is still dependent upon accurate observations and examination during the neonatal period.

Postnatal recognition

Clinically, babies with cardiac anomalies can be divided into two groups: those with central cyanosis and those without, i.e. cyanotic and acyanotic congenital heart disease.

Cardiac defects presenting with cyanosis

Defects included in this group are:

- transposition of the great arteries
- pulmonary atresia
- tetralogy of Fallot
- tricuspid atresia
- total anomalous pulmonary venous drainage
- univentricular/complex heart.

The persistence of central cyanosis (i.e. cyanosis of the lips and mucous membranes), tachypnoea and tachycardia may be the first signs that a cardiac defect is present. If cyanosis is present, administration of oxygen to these babies will be ineffective in improving their colour and oxygen saturation monitoring will show no improvement. Indeed, giving 100% oxygen may encourage closure of the ductus arteriosus, the patency of which, as Paul (1995) remarks, is literally a lifeline for some of these babies. If 100% oxygen therapy does not lead to improvement within 10 min of starting, the midwife should not persist at that concentration without seeking medical advice. Chest X-ray should be carried out to exclude abnormalities of the respiratory tract, respiratory disease and diaphragmatic hernia. The precise nature of the cardiac anomaly will need to be further explored by electrocardiography and echocardiography.

The baby with transposition of the great arteries is worthy of special mention since early detection allows intervention, which will be life saving. This is a condition wherein the aorta arises from the right ventricle and the pulmonary artery from the left ventricle (Fig. 46.10). Consequently, oxygenated blood is circulated back through the lungs and deoxygenated blood back into the systemic circuit. It is apparent therefore that unless there is an opportunity for oxygenated blood to access the systemic circulation, either by means of a patent ductus arteriosus or through accompanying septal defects, such a baby will die. Maintaining the patency of the ductus arteriosus is essential.

Prostaglandin infusion should be commenced to achieve this, but some babies develop apnoea with this treatment and may require ventilatory support.

Arrangements should be made to transfer the baby to a unit where an atrial septostomy (Rashkind) can be performed. This procedure involves enlarging the foramen ovale with a balloon catheter to allow oxygenated blood to cross at atrial level and hence into the systemic circulation. Corrective surgery (arterial switch operation) is then carried out, usually within a few weeks of birth.

Pulmonary atresia usually produces early central cyanosis and responds well to prostaglandin therapy to keep the duct open while surgery (usually a palliative Blalock shunt) is planned.

Tricuspid atresia usually occurs with a ventricular septal defect or an atrial septal defect, or both, allowing mixing of the circulation.

Potentially more distressing for the parents are the defects that do not initially present with marked cyanosis. These babies may for a time be considered to be healthy.

Tetralogy of Fallot (Fig. 46.11) is a good example of this. In this condition there is pulmonary outflow tract obstruction, a ventricular septal defect, right ventricular hypertrophy and an overriding aorta. It seldom presents with cyanosis in the immediate newborn period, but this a may become apparent within a few weeks of birth. Corrective surgery is available.

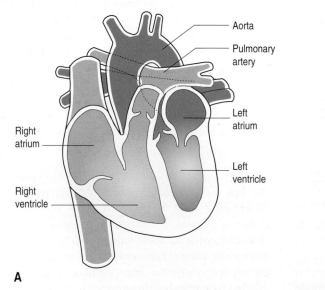 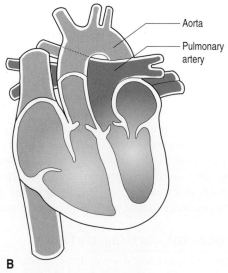

Figure 46.10 Transposition of the great arteries. (A) Normal. (B) Transposition.

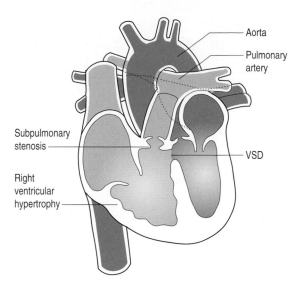

Aorta

Pulmonary artery

Subpulmonary stenosis

VSD

Right ventricular hypertrophy

Figure 46.11 Tetralogy of Fallot. (VSD = ventricular septal defect)

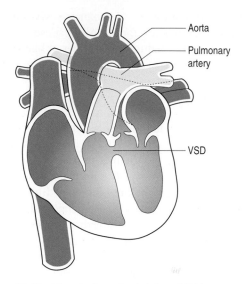

Aorta

Pulmonary artery

VSD

Figure 46.12 Ventricular septal defect (VSD).

'Acyanotic' cardiac defects

Anomalies subsumed under this heading include:

- persistent ductus arteriosus (or arterial duct)
- ventricular or atrial septal defects
- coarctation of the aorta
- aortic stenosis
- hypoplastic left heart syndrome.

Astute midwives may detect in these babies the first subtle signs of cardiac failure, that is tachypnoea, tachycardia and incipient cyanosis, especially following the exertion of crying or feeding. These signs will become more evident, sometimes dramatically so, with the closure of the ductus arteriosus if coarctation of the aorta, hypoplastic left heart syndrome or critical aortic stenosis is present. Detailed examination may disclose heart murmurs and diminution or absence of peripheral pulses. In this event resuscitation with prostaglandin is required to stabilize the baby and allow time for further assessment. While coarctation of the aorta and aortic stenosis are usually amenable to surgical correction, hypoplastic left heart syndrome is still a major surgical challenge with a poor long term outcome. There is a substantial psychological impact on the parents following confirmation of such a diagnosis, which calls for particularly supportive management.

Persistent ductus arteriosus, ventricular septal defects (Fig. 46.12) and atrial septal defects seldom require medical or surgical intervention in early neonatal life, but do require careful follow-up for signs of developing heart failure and may require surgery or interventional cardiology at a later stage.

Changing patterns of postnatal care often mean early transfer home. Ideally each baby should be examined by a competent practitioner before going home. It is important to realize, however, that not all heart murmurs heard at this time are significant. Equally the absence of a murmur at discharge from hospital does not exclude significant heart disease. There is therefore increased responsibility on community midwives to be observant and to communicate effectively with parents. Parents who report any changes in the baby's behaviour such as breathlessness or cyanosis should never be ignored, but rather encouraged to seek medical advice promptly.

Central nervous system abnormalities

Ingestion of folic acid supplements prior to conception and during the early stages of pregnancy has helped prevent such abnormalities. In addition, the ability to recognize these anomalies prenatally (see Ch. 18) has resulted in some parents choosing

selective termination of pregnancies where severe
neural tube defects are found. All of these measures
have combined to reduce the number of babies born
with abnormalities of the central nervous system.

Anencephaly

This major abnormality describes the absence of the
forebrain and vault of the skull. It is a condition that
is incompatible with sustained life but occasionally
such a baby is born alive. The midwife should wrap
the baby carefully before showing him to the
mother. It is recognized that seeing and holding
the baby will facilitate the grieving process. It may
be beneficial for the parents then to see the full
extent of the abnormality, unpleasant though it is.
Seeing the whole baby will help them to accept the
reality of the situation and prevent imagination of
an even more gruesome picture.

Spina bifida

Spina bifida results from failure of fusion of the vertebral column. There is no skin covering the defect,
which allows protrusion of the meninges, hence
the term *meningocele* (Fig. 46.13). The meningeal
membrane may be flat or appear as a membranous
sac, with or without cerebrospinal fluid, but it does
not contain neural tissue. *Meningomyelocele*, on the
other hand, does involve the spinal cord (Figs
46.13, 46.14). This lesion may be enclosed, or the
meningocele may rupture and expose the neural tissue. Meningomyelocele usually gives rise to neural
damage, producing paralysis distal to the defect,
and impaired function of urinary bladder and
bowel. The lumbosacral area is the most common
site for these to present, but they may appear at
any point in the vertebral column. When the defect
is at base of skull level it is known as an *encephalocele*. The added complication here is that the sac
may contain varying amounts of brain tissue. Normal progression of labour may be impeded by a
large lesion of this type.

Immediate management involves covering open
lesions with a non-adherent dressing. Babies with
enclosed lesions should be handled with the utmost
care in an attempt to preserve the integrity of the sac.
This will limit the risk of meningitis occurring.

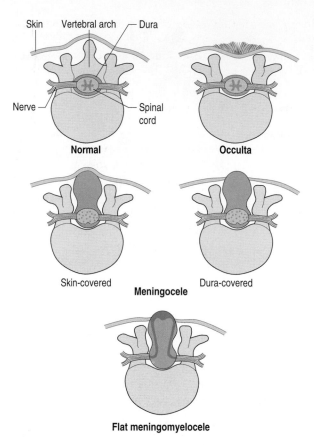

Figure 46.13 Various forms of spina bifida. (After Wallis
& Harvey 1979, with permission of *Nursing Times*.)

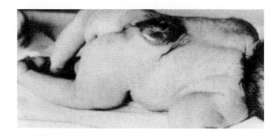

Figure 46.14 Baby with meningomyelocele.

A paediatric surgeon or neurosurgeon should be
contacted. Surgical intervention for myelomeningocele carries a high rate of success of skin closure,
but has no impact on any damage already present
in the cord or more distally. There is usually associated hydrocephalus (see below), which requires
surgical shunting to prevent a rapid increase in the
intracranial pressure. It is seldom necessary to close

the back within 24 hrs of birth. Following examination of the baby, discussion with the parents will allow them to make an informed choice about whether or not they wish their baby to have surgery.

Spina bifida occulta

Spina bifida occulta (see Fig. 46.13) is the most minor type of defect where the vertebra is bifid. There is usually no spinal cord involvement. A tuft of hair or sinus at the base of the spine may be noted on first examination of the baby. Ultrasound investigation will confirm the diagnosis and rule out any associated spinal cord involvement.

Parents who have a baby with a neural tube defect should be offered genetic counselling since the risk of recurrence is one in 25.

Hydrocephalus

This condition arises from a blockage in the circulation and absorption of cerebrospinal fluid, which is produced from the choroid plexuses within the lateral ventricles of the brain. The large lateral ventricles increase in size and eventually compress the surrounding brain tissue. It is a not infrequent accompaniment to the more severe spina bifida lesions because of a structural defect around the area of the foramen magnum known as the Arnold–Chiari malformation. Consequently, hydrocephalus may either be present at birth or develop following surgical closure of a myelomeningocele. In the absence of myelomeningocele, aqueduct stenosis is the commonest cause of hydrocephalus. The risk of cerebral impairment may be minimized by the insertion of a ventriculoperitoneal shunt. As the baby grows, this will need to be replaced. Attendant risks with these devices are that the line blocks and that the shunt is a portal for infection leading to meningitis. The midwife must be alert for the signs of increased intracranial pressure:

- large tense anterior fontanelle
- splayed skull sutures
- inappropriate increase in occipitofrontal circumference
- sun-setting appearance to the eyes
- irritability, or abnormal movements.

Microcephaly

This is where the occipitofrontal circumference is more than two standard deviations below normal for gestational age. The disproportionately small head may be the result of intrauterine infection (e.g. rubella), a feature of fetal alcohol syndrome, or part of a number of defects in some trisomic disorders. Most babies will have learning difficulties with evidence of cerebral palsy and often seizures.

Musculoskeletal deformities

These range from relatively minor anomalies, for example an extra digit, to major deficits such as absence of a limb.

Polydactyly and syndactyly

Careful examination including separation and counting of the baby's fingers and toes during the initial examination is important, otherwise anomalies such as syndactyly (webbing) and polydactyly (extra digits) may go unnoticed.

Syndactyly more commonly affects the hands. It can appear as an independent anomaly or as a feature of a syndrome such as Apert's syndrome; this is a genetically inherited condition in which there is premature fusion of the sutures of the vault of the skull, cleft palate and complete syndactyly of both hands and feet. Whether or not any surgical division needs to be carried out depends on the degree of webbing or fusion.

In *polydactyly* the extra digit(s) may be fully formed or simply extra tissue attached by a pedicle. Even where there is a rudimentary digit without bone involvement, better cosmetic results are obtained if the offending digit is surgically excised and this is mandatory in more complex cases.

Where there is a family history of either of these defects and this is common, the mother will be anxious to examine the baby for herself.

Limb reduction anomalies

Over the years various suggestions have been postulated with regard to the cause(s) of limb reduction anomalies. *Amniotic band syndrome* was the reason most often given for a baby being born with a limb deficit. It was thought that the amnion ruptured, then wrapped itself around a developing limb causing strangulation and necrosis. Although this may account for some instances, it cannot explain all of them. Clustering of cases in certain geographical areas, for example in close proximity to chemical waste plants, has provoked research in an attempt to identify environmental teratogens, as yet to no avail. One possibility being mooted is an iatrogenic cause, namely damage inflicted at the time of chorionic villus sampling (Carr & Lui 1994). They can also occur as part of a syndrome such as the VACTERL spectrum (*v*ertebral anomalies, *a*nal anomalies, *c*ardiac, *t*racheoesophageal, *r*adial aplasia, renal and *l*imb anomalies).

Limb reduction defects, which may be due to failure of formation (arrest of development), comprise a wide range of possibilities. In some either a hand or a foot will be completely missing, whereas in others a normal hand or foot will be present on the end of a shortened limb (longitudinal arrest). Thalidomide has been proven to be teratogenic in this context.

Although, as with any deviation from normal, the parents of a child with a limb defect will grieve for the loss of their perfect child, the child is not ill and will not be upset by the defect. Children usually prove themselves to be most adaptable and able to cope (Fig. 46.15). Specific management plans are often only reached after detailed assessment by an orthopaedic surgeon with a special interest in limb anomalies. For those who require them, different types of prostheses are available and can be fitted as early as 3 months of age. Innovative surgical techniques such as limb lengthening or the transferring of toe(s) to hand to serve as substitute finger(s) are proving successful for some children. Once again one of the most helpful things the midwife can do in these early days of parental adjustment is to offer the address of a support group such as Reach (see Useful addresses, below). This appropriately named support group for parents of children with upper limb deformities has branches throughout the UK.

Talipes

Talipes equinovarus (TEV, club foot) (Plate 17) is the descriptive term for a deformity of the foot where the ankle is bent downwards (plantarflexed) and the front part of the foot is turned inwards (inverted). Talipes

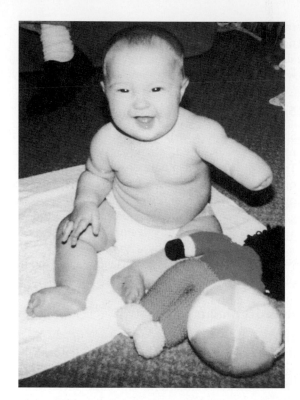

Figure 46.15 A baby with a limb reduction defect quickly learns to adapt. (Photograph courtesy of Reach.)

calcaneovalgus describes the opposite position where the foot is dorsiflexed and everted. It is thought that these deformities are more likely to occur when intrauterine space has been at a premium, for example in multiple pregnancy, macrosomic fetus or oligohydramnios. TEV is also more likely to occur in conjunction with spina bifida deformities. They may be unilateral or bilateral. There is, in some instances, a family history of the defect. Statistically more boys than girls are born with talipes. In the mildest form the foot may easily be turned to the correct position. The midwife should encourage the mother to exercise the baby's foot in this way several times a day. More severe forms will require one or more of manipulation, splinting, or surgical correction. The advice of an orthopaedic surgeon should be sought as soon as possible after birth as early treatment with manipulation or splinting may enhance results. Care should be taken to ensure that, for babies who have splints applied, the strapping is not too tight and that the baby's toes are well perfused.

Developmental hip dysplasia

Congenital hip dysplasia is an abnormality more commonly found where there has been a breech presentation at term, oligohydramnios, a foot deformity or a family history in a first-degree relative. It most often occurs in primigravida pregnancies and there is a higher percentage of girls than boys born with this defect. The left hip is more often affected than the right. The dysplastic hip may present in one of three ways: dislocated, dislocatable or with subluxation of the joint. Prenatal diagnosis by ultrasound is possible; most, however, are diagnosed in the neonatal period. Examination of the hip should be carried out by an experienced practitioner with the baby lying relaxed on a firm surface. It will depend on individual unit policies whether this is an appropriately trained midwife, paediatrician or GP. Repeated examinations by inexperienced people may compound any pre-existing damage to the joint. Either Ortolani's test or Barlow's test is employed (see Ch. 40). Any abnormal findings should be reported and the baby referred for an orthopaedic opinion or ultrasound scan of the hips, or both. Where the diagnosis is confirmed it is usual for the baby to have a splint or harness such as the Pavlik harness (Fig. 46.16) applied, which will keep the hips in a flexed and abducted position of about 60%. The splint should not be removed for napkin changing or bathing. Parents will require additional support in learning how to handle and care for their baby. Particular attention should be paid to skin care and checking for signs of chafing or excoriation.

Achondroplasia

Achondroplasia is an autosomal dominant condition where the baby is generally small with a disproportionately large head and short limbs. Some 80% of cases are new mutations and hence these families may have no anticipation of the disorder unless an antenatal diagnosis has been made. These babies often develop a marked lordosis. Cognitive development is not usually impaired.

Osteogenesis imperfecta

This autosomal dominant disorder of collagen production has at least four forms and leads to unduly brittle bones in the affected fetus and infant. In some types (II–IV) it can cause either lethal multiple fractures of

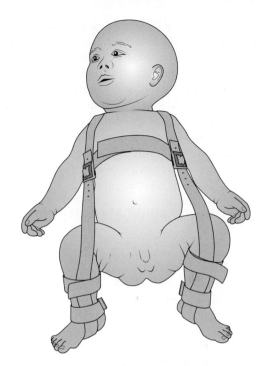

Figure 46.16 Pavlik harness for congenital dislocation of hip. (From Barr 1992, with permission of Churchill Livingstone.)

the skull, ribs and long bones in utero or neonatal long bone fractures. Recognition and genetic counselling are important for future pregnancies.

Abnormalities of the skin

Vascular naevi

These defects in the development of the skin can be divided into two main types, which commonly overlap.

Capillary malformations

These are due to defects in the dermal capillaries. The most commonly observed are 'stork marks'. These are usually found on the nape of the neck. They are generally small and will fade. No treatment is necessary.

Port wine stain

This is a purple-blue capillary malformation affecting the face. It occurs in approximately 1 in 3000 births. It is generally fully formed at birth and does not regress with time. However, laser treatment and the skillful use of cosmetics will help to disguise the problem. The parents, and later the child, may need substantial psychological support.

Should the malformation mimic the distribution of the ophthalmic branch of the trigeminal nerve, further malformations in the eyes (glaucoma), meninges or brain (epilepsy) may be suspected. This is known as the Sturge–Weber syndrome.

Capillary haemangiomata ('strawberry marks')

Capillary haemangiomata are not usually noticeable at birth but appear as red, raised lesions in the first few weeks of life (Plate 35). These common lesions affect up to 10% of the population by the age of 1 year. They are five times more common in girls than boys and are also commoner in preterm infants. They can appear anywhere in the body but cause particular distress to the parents when they appear on the face. However, parents may be reassured that, although the lesion will grow bigger for the first few months it will then regress with associated central pallor (Plate 36) and usually disappears completely by the age of 5–6 years. No treatment is normally required unless the haemangioma is situated in an awkward area where it is likely to be subject to abrasion, such as on the lip, or around the eye where it may interfere with vision. Treatment with steroids or pulsed laser therapy is possible.

Pigmented (melanocytic) naevi

These are brown, sometimes hairy, marks on the skin that vary in size and may be flat or raised. A percentage of this type of birthmark may become malignant. Surgical excision may be recommended to pre-empt this.

It is unlikely that treatment for any of these birthmarks will be carried out in the immediate neonatal period except in the case of larger pigmented naevi. The midwife's responsibilities are therefore to notify appropriate medical staff and offer parents general emotional support.

Genitourinary system

At birth the first indication that there is an abnormality of the renal tract may be finding a single umbilical artery in the umbilical cord, or alternatively recognizing the abnormal facies associated with Potter's syndrome. Attention should be paid at the time of birth to see whether the baby passes urine. If no urine is passed within 24 hrs, the baby is noted to be dribbling urine constantly, or the urine stream seems poor, the paediatrician should be informed. Dribbling of urine is a sign of nerve damage such as occurs with neural tube defects, as previously discussed, whereas a poor urine stream may indicate lower urinary tract obstruction (posterior urethral valve).

Potter syndrome

This collection of features in a series of stillborn infants was first described by Edith Potter, a perinatal pathologist, in 1946. It is due to the compressive effects of longstanding oligohydramnios (from 13–14 weeks' gestation) in renal agenesis or severe hypoplasia.

The baby's face will have a flattened appearance, low set ears, an antimongoloid slant to the eyes, with deep epicanthic folds, and a beaked nose. These babies are usually in poor condition at birth because they have lung hypoplasia. It is a syndrome incompatible with sustained life.

Posterior urethral valve(s)

This is an abnormality affecting boys. The presence of valves in the posterior urethra prevents the normal outflow of urine. As a result the bladder distends, causing back pressure on the ureters and to the kidneys. This will ultimately cause hydronephrosis. Prenatal diagnosis and intervention by intrauterine fetal bladder catheterization is possible. Failing this, early diagnosis in the neonatal period is clearly important but severe renal damage may already have been sustained. Different treatment strategies are possible with surgical procedures featuring prominently.

Polycystic kidneys

It is likely that problems may arise in delivering a baby with polycystic kidneys because of an increase in abdominal girth. On abdominal examination the kidneys will be palpable. Radiological or ultrasound investigations will be carried out to confirm the diagnosis. Unfortunately the prognosis is poor, as renal failure is the likely outcome. The severest forms of polycystic kidney disease are usually linked to an autosomal recessive inheritance, but an autosomal dominant variety also occurs with a less gloomy prognosis.

Hypospadias

Examination of a baby boy may reveal that the urethral meatus opens on to the undersurface of the penis. The meatus can be placed at any point along the length of the penis and in some cases will open onto the perineum. This abnormality often coexists with chordee, in which the penis is short and bent and the foreskin is present only on the dorsal side of the penis. It is anticipated that some babies will require surgery in the neonatal period to 'release' the chordee and enlarge the urethral meatus. It is important that the parents are made aware that circumcision should be deferred until consultation with the paediatric surgeon is completed.

Cryptorchidism

Undescended testes may be unilateral or bilateral and occur in 1–2% of male infants. If on examination of the baby after birth the scrotum is empty, the undescended testes may be found in the inguinal pouch. Sometimes the testis in this position can be manipulated into the scrotal pouch. This augurs well for future normal development. Testes that are found too high in the inguinal canal to manipulate into the scrotum may be malformed. If neither testis is palpable further investigation to exclude endocrine or chromosomal causes is required. In unilateral undescended testis parents should be encouraged to have the baby examined at regular intervals. If descent of the testis has not occurred by the time the child is 2 years old, arrangements for orchidopexy may be made.

Ambiguous genitalia

Ambiguous genitalia describe a situation in which the external appearance is neither definitely male nor female. In this situation it is vital that the midwife is honest and does not assign a gender to the baby. Examination of the baby may reveal any of the following: a small hypoplastic penis, chordee, bifid scrotum, undescended testes (careful examination should be made to detect undescended testes in the inguinal canal) or enlarged clitoris, incompletely separated or poorly differentiated labia. It can be impossible to differentiate by clinical examination alone between male under-virilization and female masculinization and expert clarification is always needed.

Congenital adrenal hyperplasia

One of the commoner reasons for ambiguous genitalia is an autosomal recessive condition called congenital adrenal hyperplasia. In this condition the adrenal gland is stimulated to overproduce androgens because of a deficiency of an enzyme called 21-hydroxylase, which is necessary for normal production of steroid from cholesterol. If aldosterone production is reduced then these babies will rapidly lose salt and may present collapsed and dehydrated. Urea and electrolyte levels, blood glucose and 17-hydroxy progesterone concentrations should be measured and appropriate fluid replacement given. In the process of eliminating or confirming the cause, a 24 hrs urine collection may be requested. It is necessary to ensure that the urine bag is correctly placed to avoid faecal contamination. Placing one end of a catheter or feeding tube in the urine bag and aspirating the contents at regular intervals will help to prevent spillage and the unnecessary trauma to the baby of repeated applications of urine bags. Babies with this condition may require later cosmetic surgery. The condition is not always recognized in boys in the neonatal period.

Intersex

This is where the internal reproductive organs are at variance with the external appearance of the genitalia. Ultrasound examination will help to identify the nature of the internal reproductive organs. True hermaphroditism is extremely rare. The decision of gender attribution is made following chromosomal studies to determine genetic make-up, hormone assays and consideration of the potential for cosmetic surgery.

Clearly, this time of waiting for results of investigations is a time of great concern for parents because they cannot tell relatives and friends the gender of the baby. Delay in naming the baby is an additional pressure. Some parents in this invidious position elect to give the baby a name that would suit either a boy or a girl.

It is, however, more common for a child of truly ambiguous gender to be raised as a girl.

Teratogenic causes

Fetal alcohol syndrome/spectrum

Preconception preparation for pregnancy advice on alcohol intake, if heeded, could dramatically reduce the incidence of this phenomenon. Health promotion objectives and successful outcomes are, however, rarely totally synchronous.

The midwife may be alerted to the possibility of a baby being born with this syndrome prenatally if, in addition to psychosocial markers, clinical intrauterine growth restriction is evident. Postnatally the following characteristics are recognizable: a growth-restricted infant with microcephaly, flat facies, close-set eyes, epicanthic folds, small upturned nose, thin upper lip and low set ears. Most of these features become less pronounced as the child grows. Microcephaly, small stature and learning difficulties remain. The baby may experience acute withdrawal symptoms and require appropriate supportive therapies. The midwife will need to exercise counselling skills to provide much-needed support for the mother. Collaboration with social services is usually called for to ensure that the care options decided are in the best interests of the family.

Establishing such a direct link between a teratogen and such a complex clinical pattern remains the exception rather than the rule although as mentioned earlier accurate recording of all congenital abnormalities on a central register can aid early recognition of potential new teratogens.

Support for the midwife

Caring for a mother whose baby has some major congenital abnormality places extra demands on the midwife. This stress is compounded if the abnormality was not anticipated prior to birth or if the midwife has not previously encountered the particular problem. The exercising of effective counselling and communication skills is invaluable in helping the family to adjust and in facilitating appropriate lines of support. The extra effort expended can be costly in terms not only of time but of the emotional stress the midwife may experience.

It is important that support is available for midwives in these situations (e.g. from her supervisor of midwives). Preparatory courses on grief and bereavement counselling are also of some benefit as many parents with affected babies will experience many of these emotions. Midwives who have acquired experience in this realm should not, however, automatically be targeted as the experts and always be called upon to fulfil this role. Conversely, student midwives ought not to be deliberately shielded from being involved in caring for such families. The provision of quality care for parents who have a child with a congenital abnormality is contingent upon meeting the needs of the carers.

Midwives may also find information available via the internet, however, they should be aware of the dubious quality of some of this information. They should therefore exercise caution in how they utilize it. It might also be wise to caution parents, who often search the internet for further information, of this potential risk.

REFERENCES

Bagwell C E 1993 Surgical lesions of pediatric airways and lungs. In: Koff P B, Eitzman D, Neu J (eds) Neonatal and pediatric respiratory care, 2nd edn. Mosby Year Book, St Louis, Ch 8, p 132

Barr D G D 1992 Disorders of bone. In: Campbell A G M, McIntosh N (eds) Forfar and Arneil's textbook of paediatrics. Churchill Livingstone, Edinburgh, Ch 23, p 1628

Carr A J, Lui D T Y 1994 Chorionic villus sampling. Advantages and disadvantages for prenatal diagnosis. Midwives Chronicle 107(1279):284–287

Danner S C 1992 Breast-feeding the infant with a cleft defect. NAACOGs Clinical Issues in Perinatal and Women's Health Nursing 3(4):634–639

Habel A, Sell D, Mars M 1996 Management of cleft lip and palate. Archives of Disease in Childhood 74(4):360–366

Haddock G, Davis C F, Raine P A M 1996 Gastroschisis in the decade of prenatal diagnosis. European Journal of Paediatric Surgery 6:18–24

Paul K 1995 Recognition, stabilization and early management of infants with critical congenital heart disease presenting in the first days of life. Neonatal Network 14(5):13–25

Raine P 1994 Cleft lip and palate. In: Freeman N V, Burge D M, Griffiths M, Malone P S J (eds) Surgery in the newborn. Churchill Livingstone, Edinburgh, Ch 34, p 375

Sullivan G 1996 Parental bonding in cleft lip and palate repair. Paediatric Nursing 8(1):21–24

Wallis S, Harvey D 1979 Disorders in the newborn 1. Nursing Times 75:1315–1327

Whyte A 1995 Folic acid fortifying the pregnancy message. Health Visitor 68(10):397–398

Wirt S, Algren C L, Arnold S L 1992 Cleft lip and palate: a multidisciplinary approach. Plastic Surgical Nursing 12 (4):140–145

FURTHER READING

Jones K L (ed.) 1997 Smith's recognizable patterns of human malformation, 5th edn. W B Saunders, Philadelphia

This book provides a comprehensive and systematic approach to dysmorphic syndromes.

USEFUL WEBSITES

On-line Mendelian Inheritance in Man (OMIM): www.ncbi.nlm.nih.gov/omim.

This website provides detailed information about clinical features and genetics of all inherited diseases

Contact a family: www.cafamily.org.uk

This website provides information and support for families with disabled children.

Genetic Interest Group (GIG): www.gig.org.uk/members.htm

This is a national alliance of organizations which support children and families affected by genetic disorders.

Association for Spina Bifida and Hydrocephalus (ASBAH): www.asbah.org

Cleft Lip and Palate Association (CLAPA): www.clapa.com

Children's Heart Federation: www.childrens-heart-fed.org.uk

Cystic Fibrosis Research Trust (CF): www.cftrust.org.uk

Down's Syndrome Association: www.downs-syndrome.org.uk

Scottish Down's Syndrome Association (SDSA): www.dsscotland.org.uk

Reach: The Association for Children with Hand or Arm Deficiency: www.reach.org.uk

Support organization for trisomy 13/18 (SOFT): www.soft.org.uk

STEPS (National Association for Children with Lower Limb Abnormalities): www.steps-charity.org.uk

Antenatal Results and Choices (ARC, formerly SAFTA): www.arc-uk.org

Jaundice and infection

Patricia Percival

CHAPTER CONTENTS

Jaundice is a yellow discoloration of skin and sclera caused by raised levels of bilirubin in the blood (hyperbilirubinaemia). Neonatal jaundice is either physiological or pathological. During the first week of life all neonates have a transient rise in serum bilirubin and about 50% of term babies become jaundiced. This physiological jaundice appears about 48 hrs after birth and usually settles within 10–12 days. Pathological jaundice presents earlier, and is persistent or associated with high bilirubin levels. Causes include increased haemolysis, metabolic and endocrine disorders and infection.

Newborn babies are vulnerable to infection. Defence mechanisms are immature and skin thin and easily damaged. Infections may be acquired before, during or soon after birth and, while some are minor, others can be damaging or life-threatening.

The chapter aims to:

- examine the physiological basis of neonatal jaundice and the causes and consequences of pathological jaundice
- emphasize the role of the midwife in preventing Rhesus isoimmunization
- discuss the management of jaundice
- review some neonatal infections acquired before, during and shortly after birth
- discuss the role of the midwife in the prevention, assessment, diagnosis and treatment of infection.

Conjugation of bilirubin

Conjugation changes the end-products of red cell breakdown so they can be excreted in faeces or urine. Understanding this process can increase evidence-based midwifery by increasing knowledge of the importance of such things as early breastfeeding, or early referral for treatment of pathological jaundice.

Ageing, immature or malformed red cells are removed from the circulation and broken down in the reticuloendothelial system (liver, spleen and macrophages). Haemoglobin from these cells is broken down to the by-products of haem, globin and iron.

- *Haem* is converted to biliverdin and then to unconjugated bilirubin
- *Globin* is broken down into *amino acids*, which are used by the body to make proteins
- *Iron* is stored in the body or used for new red cells.

Two main forms of bilirubin are present in the body:

1. *Unconjugated bilirubin* is fat soluble and cannot be excreted easily either in bile or urine. Neonatal jaundice can result from increased levels of this fat soluble bilirubin that cannot be excreted and is instead deposited in fatty tissue.
2. *Conjugated bilirubin* has been made water soluble in the liver and can be excreted in faeces and urine. Neonatal jaundice can also result from increased levels of this water soluble bilirubin if excretion is prevented, e.g. by an obstruction.

Three stages are involved in the process of bilirubin conjugation: transport, conjugation and excretion (Fig. 47.1).

Transport of bilirubin

Unconjugated or fat soluble bilirubin is transported to the liver bound to albumin. If not attached to albumin, this unbound or 'free' bilirubin can be deposited in extravascular fatty and nerve tissues (skin and brain). Skin deposits of unconjugated or fat soluble bilirubin cause jaundice, while brain deposits can cause bilirubin toxicity or *kernicterus* (Box 47.1).

Conjugation

Once in the liver, unconjugated bilirubin is detached from albumin, combined with glucose and *glucuronic acid* and conjugation occurs in the presence of oxygen and the enzyme *Uridine diphosphoglucuronyl transferase* (*UDP-GT*). The conjugated bilirubin is now water soluble and available for excretion.

Excretion

Conjugated bilirubin is excreted via the biliary system into the small intestine where normal bacteria change the conjugated bilirubin into urobilinogen. This is then oxidized into orange-coloured urobilin. Most is excreted in the faeces, with a small amount excreted in urine (Ahlfors & Wennberg 2004, Kaplan et al 2005).

Jaundice

Jaundice is caused by bilirubin deposits in the skin. In term neonates it appears when serum bilirubin concentrations reach 85–120 µmol/L (5–7 mg/dL), with a head to toe progression as levels increase. Babies of full East Asian parentage have a higher bilirubin level and risk of severe jaundice requiring phototherapy, blood transfusion or rehospitalization than Caucasian infants (Setia et al 2002). Babies of African origin have lower levels. Pre-term babies are more likely to develop jaundice (Tyler & McKiernan 2006). Plate 21 shows a Caucasian baby with physiological jaundice who required 24 hrs of fibreoptic phototherapy, and demonstrates the difference in skin tone between the jaundiced baby and her mother.

Physiological jaundice

Neonatal physiological jaundice occurs when unconjugated (fat soluble) bilirubin is deposited in the skin instead of being taken to the liver for processing into conjugated (water soluble) bilirubin that can be excreted in faeces or urine. It is a normal transitional state affecting up to 50% of term and 80% of premature babies who have a *progressive rise* in unconjugated bilirubin levels and jaundice on day 3. Physiological jaundice *never* appears before 24 hrs of life, *usually* fades by 1 week of age and bilirubin levels *never* exceed 200–215 µmol/L (12–13 mg/dL).

Causes

In many newborns, a temporary discrepancy exists between red cell breakdown and their ability to transport, conjugate and excrete the resulting bilirubin. Physiological jaundice results from increased red cell breakdown at a time of newborn immaturity.

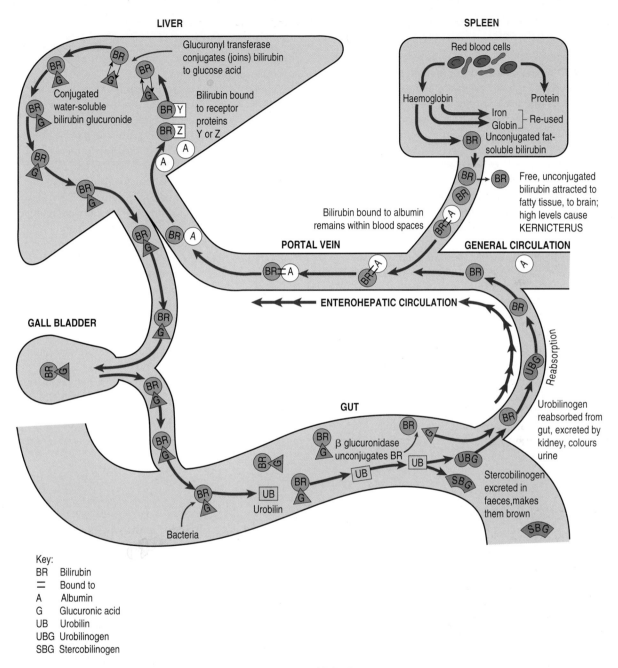

Figure 47.1 Schematic diagram showing the conjugation of bilirubin.

Increased red cell breakdown

Newborn bilirubin production is more than twice that of normal adults per kilogram of weight. In the hypoxic environment of the uterus the fetus relies on haemoglobin F (fetal haemoglobin), which has a greater affinity for oxygen than does haemoglobin A (adult haemoglobin). When the pulmonary system becomes functional at birth, the large red cell

Box 47.1 Kernicterus

Kernicterus (bilirubin toxicity) is an encephalopathy caused by deposits of unconjugated bilirubin in the basal ganglia of the brain. Early signs can be insidious and include lethargy, changes in muscle tone, a high-pitched cry and irritability. These can progress to bilirubin induced neurological dysfunction with muscle hypertonia and possible death. Long-term clinical features can include deafness, blindness, cerebral palsy, developmental delay, learning difficulties and extrapyramidal disturbances such as athetosis, drooling, facial grimace, and chewing and swallowing difficulties (see Shapiro et al 2006).

Kernicterus is usually associated with serum bilirubin levels >340 μmol/L (20 mg/dL), but the critical threshold for long-term morbidity remains unclear. Recent work suggests non-albumin bound or 'free' bilirubin correlates better than total bilirubin concentration with bilirubin toxicity. Important risk factors include hypoxia, acidosis, infection, hypothermia and dehydration, all more likely in pre-term and sick-term infants (these can interfere with albumin- binding capacity). Glucose-6-phosphate dehydrogenase (G-6-PD) deficiency is also important as it increases haemoglobin destruction and produces more unconjugated bilirubin.

Kernicterus rarely occurs in healthy, term breastfed babies. However, it does occur. For example, in one group of six infants with kernicterus Maisels & Newman (1995) identified no cause of hyperbilirubinaemia other than breastfeeding. Watchko (2006) found breastmilk feeding almost uniformly present among late pre-term infants with kernicterus. Inadequate establishment of breastfeeding may play a role in hyperbilirubinaemia in some infants with kernicterus. A small subpopulation of breastfed infants with jaundice may be more susceptible if starved (Bertini et al 2001).

If bilirubin neurotoxicity is suspected, a complete neurodevelopmental examination and diagnostic testing are critical. Treatment of kernicterus is usually aggressive and can include phototherapy, intravenous fluids and exchange transfusion. Ongoing follow-up is essential, including complete neurodevelopmental examinations, repeat MRIs, and behavioural hearing evaluations.

(Ahlfors & Wennberg 2004, Kaplan & Hammerman 2004, Karlsson et al 2006, Maisels & Newman 1995, Newman et al 2000, Shapiro et al 2006, Smitherman et al 2006, Watchko 2006).

mass must be broken down or haemolised, resulting in increased unconjugated bilirubin.

Decreased albumin-binding capacity

Newborns have lower albumin concentrations and decreased albumin-binding capacity (reducing transport of bilirubin to the liver for conjugation). Some drugs also compete for albumin-binding sites. As binding sites on albumin are used, levels of unbound 'free' fat-soluble bilirubin in the blood rise and find tissues with fat affinity (skin and brain).

Enzyme deficiency

Levels of UDP-GT enzyme activity are lower during the first 24 hrs after birth (reducing bilirubin conjugation in the liver). Adult levels are not reached for 6–14 weeks.

Increased enterohepatic reabsorption

This process is increased as the newborn bowel lacks the normal enteric bacteria that break down conjugated bilirubin to urobilinogen (hindering excretion). Newborns also have increased amounts of another enzyme *beta-glucuronidase* which changes conjugated bilirubin back into the unconjugated state (when it is absorbed back into the system). If feeding is delayed then bowel motility is also decreased, further compromising excretion. Babies of East Asian parentage have enhanced enterohepatic circulation of bilirubin, higher peak bilirubin concentrations and more prolonged jaundice (Ahlfors & Wennberg 2004, Bertini et al 2001, Karlsson et al 2006, Setia et al 2002).

Midwifery care and physiological jaundice

Jaundice in newborns is a challenge for midwives as it is important to distinguish between healthy babies with a normal physiological response who need no active treatment, and those who require serum bilirubin testing (see Management of jaundice). For example, a 1-day-old mildly jaundiced baby requires further investigation. Conversely, a 4-day-old moderately jaundiced baby with good urinary output, who wakes regularly and feeds well does not need invasive blood tests.

One effective use of evidence-based practice in managing hyperbilirubinaemia is helping women feed their babies from birth. Early, frequent feeding assists newborns to cope with increased unconjugated bilirubin by promoting factors that deal with this load. Successful breastfeeding supplies glucose to the liver and increases bowel motility and normal bowel flora. In turn, this helps increase albumin-binding capacity, increases enzyme production for conjugation and decreases enterohepatic reabsorption. As well as reducing jaundice, being with women while they learn to breastfeed extends midwives' partnership role with women well beyond the birth.

Midwives can further involve families by making them aware of the importance of excessive sleepiness, reluctance to feed and a decrease in wet nappies. The possible time scale of jaundice in some breastfed babies needs to be explained, and parents asked to report any pale stools and dark urine (these may indicate cholestatic liver disease). In formula-fed babies, prolonged jaundice, persistent pale stools and dark urine are rare, and merit immediate attention. If conjugated hyperbilirubinaemia is present, comprehensive diagnostic investigation is required as early diagnosis is critical for the best outcome (Ratnavel & Ives 2005, Tyler & McKiernan 2006).

In recent years, transcutaneous bilirubinometry (TcB) has reduced the number of blood tests in newborns. In home and hospital settings, midwives can use this method to provide a digital assessment of skin pigmentation with an estimate of plasma bilirubin. However, at high serum bilirubin concentrations Grohmann et al (2006) found all three skin test devices, and one of three non-chemical photometric devices underestimated bilirubin levels. TcB

may also be less accurate in premature babies (Jangaard et al 2006, Nanjundaswamy et al 2005). For routine newborn care, skin testing can be used first. TcB readings above 200 μmol/L (12 mg/dL), and non-chemical photometric readings above 250 μmol/L (15 mg/dL) require standard laboratory testing (Grohmann et al 2006). With phototherapy, TcB is more accurate using a patched skin area (e.g. under the eyeshield) (Jangaard et al 2006, Nanjundaswamy et al 2005).

Exaggerated or prolonged physiological jaundice

In pre-term babies

Physiological jaundice in pre-term babies is characterized by bilirubin levels of 165 μmol/L (10 mg/dL) or greater by day 3 or 4, with peak concentrations on day 5–7 that return to normal over several weeks. Contributing factors include:

- shorter red cell life (increasing production of unconjugated bilirubin)
- hypoxia, acidosis and hypothermia, which can interfere with albumin-binding capacity (decreasing transport to the liver and increasing deposits of 'free' unconjugated bilirubin in the skin and brain)
- delay in the expression of the enzyme UDP-GT (reducing bilirubin conjugation).

Premature infants are at particular risk of bilirubin production-conjugation imbalance. Good midwifery management of any jaundice in pre-term babies is critical as these babies have a higher risk of kernicterus (see Box 47.1) (Ahlfors & Wennberg 2004, Kaplan et al 2005, Karlsson et al 2006, Newman et al 2000, Tyler & McKiernan 2006, Watchko 2006).

In breastfed babies

The exact mechanism of prolonged jaundice in some breastfeeding babies is still unknown. Some researchers have found a significant relationship between breastfeeding and hyperbilirubinaemia or jaundice. For example, in two samples of 51 387 and 1177 healthy term newborns, one of the predictors of hyperbilirubinaemia or jaundice was exclusive breastfeeding (Newman et al 2000). While breastfed neonates in Bertini et al's (2001) study of 2174 babies (at 37 weeks) did not have more hyper-bilirubinaemia, a small group of jaundiced infants were more susceptible to kernicterus if starved. Although rare, kernicterus can occur in healthy, term, breastfed newborns (Maisels & Newman 1995) and breastmilk feeding is almost always present in pre-term infants with kernicterus (Watchko 2006) (see Box 47.1). Some argue a reliable diagnosis of breastmilk jaundice can only be made by excluding pathological causes (Ratnavel & Ives 2005). Stopping breastfeeding is not necessary. Rather, early midwifery help with establishment of breastfeeding is essential (see management).

Pathological jaundice

Pathological jaundice in newborns usually appears within 24 hrs of birth, and is characterized by a *rapid* rise in serum bilirubin. Criteria include:

- jaundice within the first 24 hrs of life
- rapid increase in total serum bilirubin > 85 µmol/L (5 mg/dL) per day
- total serum bilirubin > 200 µmol/L (12 mg/dL)
- conjugated bilirubin > 25–35 µmol/L (1.5–2 mg/dL)
- persistence of clinical jaundice for 7–10 days in term or 2 weeks in pre-term babies.

Causes

The underlying cause of pathological jaundice is any *interference* in bilirubin production, transport, conjugation or excretion (Fig. 47.2). Any disease or disorder that increases bilirubin production or alters transport or metabolism of bilirubin is superimposed upon normal physiological jaundice.

Production

Increased red cell destruction or haemolysis causes increased bilirubin levels. Causes of this increased haemolysis include:

- *blood type/group incompatibility* – including Rhesus (RhD) and ABO incompatibility, anti-E and anti-Kell
- *extravasated blood* – from such causes as cephal-haematoma and bruising

- *sepsis* – can lead to increased haemoglobin breakdown
- *polycythaemia* – too many red cells as in materno-fetal or twin-to-twin transfusion
- *spherocytosis* – fragile red cell membranes
- *haemoglobinopathies* – sickle cell disease and thalassaemia (in babies of African and Mediterranean descent)
- *enzyme deficiencies* – *glucose-6-phosphate dehydrogenase (G6PD)* maintains the integrity of the cell membrane of RBCs. A deficiency results in increased haemolysis (*G6PD* is an X-linked genetic disorder carried by females that can affect male infants of African, Asian and Mediterranean descent).

Transport

Factors that lower blood albumin levels or decrease albumin-binding capacity include:

- hypothermia, acidosis or hypoxia can interfere with albumin-binding capacity
- drugs that compete with bilirubin for albumin-binding sites (e.g. aspirin, sulphonamides and ampicillin).

Conjugation

Immaturity of the neonate's enzyme system interferes with bilirubin conjugation in the liver. Other factors can include:

- dehydration, starvation, hypoxia and sepsis (oxygen and glucose are required for conjugation)
- TORCH infections (toxoplasmosis, others, rubella, cytomegalovirus, herpes)
- other viral infections (e.g. neonatal viral hepatitis)
- other bacterial infections, particularly those caused by *Escherichia coli* (*E. coli*)
- metabolic and endocrine disorders that alter UDP-GT enzyme activity (e.g. Crigler–Najjar disease and Gilbert's syndrome)
- other metabolic disorders such as hypothyroidism and galactosaemia.

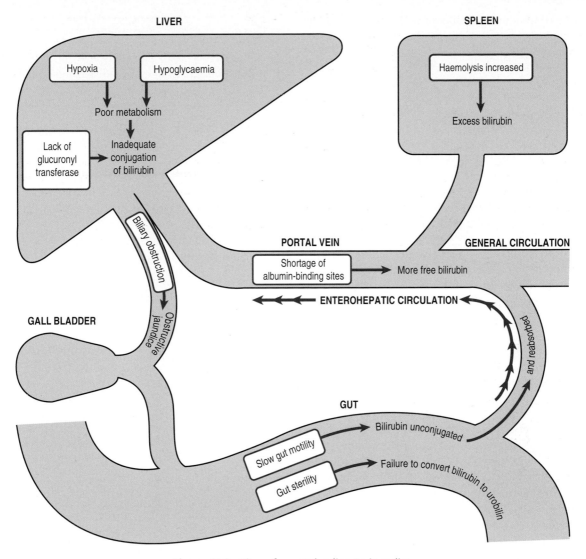

Figure 47.2 Sites of events leading to jaundice.

Excretion

Conditions interfering with bilirubin excretion can include:

- hepatic obstruction caused by congenital anomalies such as extrahepatic biliary atresia
- obstruction by 'bile plugs' from increased bile viscosity (e.g. cystic fibrosis, total parenteral nutrition, haemolytic disorders and dehydration)

- infection, other congenital disorders, and idiopathic neonatal hepatitis, which can also cause an excess of conjugated bilirubin
- saturation of protein carriers needed to excrete conjugated bilirubin into the biliary system.

After processing by the liver, most of the bilirubin is conjugated so babies are at less risk of kernicterus. They may, however, require urgent treatment for other serious conditions (see management) (Ahlfors & Wennberg 2004, Joy et al 2005, Kaplan & Hammerman 2004, Kaplan et al 2005, Karlsson et al 2006, Tyler & McKiernan 2006, Ratnavel & Ives 2005, van Dongen et al 2005).

Haemolytic jaundice

As described above, increased haemoglobin destruction in the fetus or newborn has several causes, for example, Rhesus (RhD) isoimmunization or ABO incompatibility. This increased haemolysis increases bilirubin levels, and causes pathological jaundice. Rhesus (RhD) isoimmunization can occur if blood cells from a Rhesus-positive baby enter a Rhesus-negative mother's bloodstream. Her blood treats the D antigen on positive blood cells as a foreign substance and produces antibodies. While other causes of increased haemolysis are important, this condition is emphasized because of the midwife's critical role in the injection of anti-D immunoglobulin (anti-D Ig). Without this anti-D prophylaxis, RhD isoimmunization can cause severe haemolytic disease of the newborn (HDN) with significant mortality and morbidity (National Institute for Health and Clinical Excellence, NICE 2002).

With the effectiveness of anti-D prophylaxis, antibodies against other blood groups are now more common than anti-D (e.g. anti-A, anti-B and anti-Kell). Although few antibodies to blood group antigens other than those in the Rh system cause such severe HDN, some report mortality and morbidity with antibodies other than anti-D. These include anti-E haemolytic disease of the fetus or newborn (Joy et al 2005), and anti-Kell (van Dongen et al 2005). In this chapter, ABO incompatibility is also emphasized, as it is the most frequent cause of mild to moderate haemolysis in neonates.

RhD incompatibility

RhD incompatibility is commonest among Caucasians, about 15% of whom are Rh-negative, compared with 3–5% of African and about 1% of Asian populations (Bianchi et al 2005). Before the introduction of anti-D Ig in 1969, RhD isoimmunization was a major cause of perinatal mortality and morbidity. In England and Wales, about 500 cases of RhD haemolytic disease of the fetus and newborn still occur each year, resulting

> **Box 47.2** Patterns of Rhesus factor inheritance
>
> DD=homozygous=Rhesus positive blood group
> Dd=heterozygous=Rhesus positive blood group
> dd=Rhesus negative blood group.

in 25 to 30 deaths and 15 children with major permanent developmental problems (NICE 2002).

Patterns of Rhesus factor inheritance

RhD incompatibility can occur when a woman with Rh-negative blood type is pregnant with a Rh-positive fetus (Box 47.2).

With a Rhesus-negative (dd) pregnant women the patterns of Rhesus factor inheritance are as follows:

- If the father is Rhesus-positive blood group (DD homozygous) the baby will always be Rhesus-positive blood group
- If the father is Rhesus-positive blood group (Dd heterozygous) the baby can be Rhesus-positive blood group (Dd), or Rhesus-negative blood group (dd)
- If the father is Rhesus-negative blood group (dd) the baby will always be Rhesus negative-blood group (dd).

Recent improvements in the extraction and amplification of cell-free fetal DNA in maternal plasma can provide a non-invasive diagnosis of fetal Rhesus D genotype (Bianchi et al 2005). In a meta-analysis of 37 publications (3261 samples) of Rh genotyping from maternal peripheral blood, diagnostic accuracy was 94.8% (Geifman-Holtzman et al 2006). In Bristol UK, the International Blood Group Reference Laboratory provides a fetal blood group genotyping service for RhD isoimmunized pregnant women with heterozygous partners (Finning et al 2004). In the UK, antenatal anti-D Ig prophylaxis is currently given to all Rh-negative pregnant women. Ongoing technique improvements may increase accuracy of testing and enable large-scale, risk-free fetal RhD genotyping using maternal blood (Geifman-Holtzman et al 2006). Such future developments may allow anti-D Ig to be restricted to Rh-positive pregnancies (Finning et al 2004).

Causes of RhD isoimmunization

The placenta usually acts as a barrier to fetal blood entering the maternal circulation (Fig. 47.3). However,

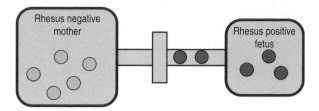

Figure 47.3 Normal placenta with no communication between maternal and fetal blood.

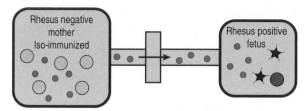

Figure 47.6 In a subsequent pregnancy maternal Rhesus antibodies cross the placenta, resulting in haemolytic disease of the newborn.

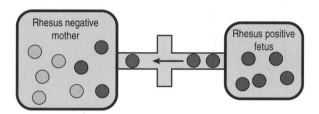

Figure 47.4 Fetal cells enter maternal circulation through 'break' in 'placental barrier', e.g. at placental separation.

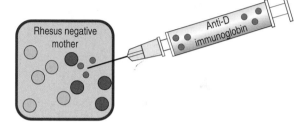

Figure 47.7 Anti-D immunoglobulin administered within 72 hrs of birth or other sensitizing event.

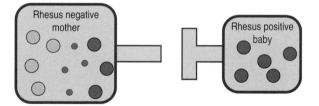

Figure 47.5 Maternal production of Rhesus antibodies following introduction of Rhesus positive blood.

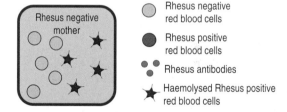

Figure 47.8 Anti-D immunoglobulin has destroyed fetal Rhesus positive red cells and prevented isoimmunization.

Figures 47.3–47.8 Rhesus isoimmunization and its prevention.

during pregnancy or birth, fetomaternal haemorrhage (FMH) can occur, when small amounts of fetal Rh-positive blood cross the placenta and enter the Rh-negative mothers blood (Fig. 47.4). The woman's immune system produces anti-D antibodies (Fig. 47.5). In subsequent pregnancies these maternal antibodies can cross the placenta and destroy the red cells of any Rh-positive fetus (Fig. 47.6).

RhD isoimmunization can result from any procedure or incident where positive blood leaks across the placenta, or from any other transfusion of Rh-positive blood (e.g. blood or platelet transfusion or drug use). Haemolytic disease of the fetus and newborn caused

by RhD isoimmunization can occur during the first pregnancy. However, in most cases sensitization during the first pregnancy or birth leads to extensive destruction of fetal red blood cells during subsequent pregnancies (Bianchi et al 2005, Finning et al 2004, Geifman-Holtzman et al 2006, NICE 2002).

Prevention of RhD isoimmunization

Most cases of RhD isoimmunization can be prevented by injecting anti-D Ig within 72 hrs of birth or any other sensitizing event (Fig. 47.7). Anti-D Ig is a human plasma-based product that is used to prevent women producing anti-D antibodies. Anti-D Ig is of value to women with non-sensitized Rh-negative blood who have a baby with Rh-positive blood type. It is *not* used when anti-D antibodies are already present in maternal blood. As well, Anti-D Ig does not protect against the development of other antibodies that cause haemolytic disease of the newborn.

Routine antenatal prophylaxis

In the UK since 2002 (and some other countries), routine antenatal anti-D prophylaxis at 28 and 34 weeks' gestation is recommended for all non-sensitized Rh-negative women (NICE 2002). With postnatal anti-D Ig prophylaxis, about 1.5% of Rh-negative women still develop anti-D antibodies following a first Rh-positive pregnancy. A meta-analysis (Allaby et al 1999) and Cochrane review (Crowther & Keirse 1999) suggest the antenatal sensitization rate is further reduced by routine antenatal prophylaxis.

Antenatal prophylaxis following sensitizing events

The most recent available evidence suggests anti-D Ig prophylaxis should be given to all non-sensitized Rh-negative women within 72 hrs of the following:

- spontaneous miscarriage before 12 weeks requiring surgical intervention
- any threatened, complete, incomplete or missed abortion *after* 12 weeks of pregnancy
- termination of pregnancy by surgical or medical methods regardless of gestational age
- ectopic pregnancy
- amniocentesis, cordocentesis, chorionic villus sampling, fetal blood sampling or other invasive intrauterine procedure such as shunt insertion
- external cephalic version of the fetus
- fetal death in utero or stillbirth
- abdominal trauma and antepartum haemorrhage
- any other instance of inadvertent transfusion of Rh-positive red blood cells (e.g. transfusion of Rh-positive blood or platelets or drug use).

Postnatal prophylaxis

A systematic review of six eligible trials of over 10 000 women found when given within 72 hrs of birth (and other antenatal sensitizing events), anti-D Ig lowered the incidence of Rh isoimmunization 6 months after birth and in a subsequent pregnancy, regardless of the ABO status of the mother and baby (Crowther & Middleton 2001).

Administration of anti-D Ig

As previously outlined, Anti-D Ig destroys any fetal cells in the mother's blood (Fig. 47.8) before her immune system produces antibodies. Anti-D Ig should *not* be given to women who are RhD-sensitized, as they have already developed antibodies. The process is as follows:

1. During pregnancy blood is grouped for ABO and Rh type, and women who are Rh-negative are screened for Rh antibodies (indirect Coombs' test). A negative test shows an *absence* of antibodies or sensitization.
2. Blood is re-tested at 28 weeks of pregnancy. In countries where antenatal prophylaxis is routine (at 28 and 34 weeks' gestation), the first injection of anti-D Ig is given just after this blood sample.
3. Where a policy of routine antenatal anti-D Ig prophylaxis is *not* in place, blood is re-tested for antibodies at 34 weeks of pregnancy.
4. When anti-D Ig prophylaxis is given at 28 weeks, blood is not retested at 34 weeks as it is difficult to distinguish passive anti-D Ig from immune anti-D. The second routine injection is given at 34 weeks.
5. Following the birth, cord blood is tested for confirmation of Rh type, ABO blood group, haemoglobin and serum bilirubin levels and the presence of maternal antibodies on fetal red cells (direct Coombs' test). Again, a negative test indicates an absence of antibodies or sensitization. However, 20% of Rh-positive babies born to mothers given two doses of antenatal anti-D Ig have a *positive* direct Coombs' test from passive anti-D Ig (Maayan-Metzger et al 2001). The postnatal dose of anti-D Ig *is still given* if passive anti-D Ig is present.
6. A Kleihauer acid elution test is carried out on an anticoagulated maternal blood sample as soon as possible, and within 2 hrs after the birth. This test detects fetal haemoglobin and estimates the number of fetal cells in a sample of maternal blood (see below).
7. Anti-D Ig must always be given as soon as possible, and within 72 hrs of any sensitizing event

and the birth. Some protection may occur when given within 9–10 days (RCOG 2002). Anti-D Ig is injected into the deltoid muscle from which absorption is optimal. Absorption may be delayed if the gluteal region is used (Maayan-Metzger et al 2001, RCOG 2002).

Dose of anti-D Ig

The dose of anti-D Ig, and the requirement for a test to identify the size of FMH, varies in different countries, as does the need for a follow up screening test (e.g. Kleihauer or flow cytometry) (RCOG 2002). Research evidence on the optimal dose of anti-D Ig is still limited (Crowther & Middleton 2001). The best available evidence suggests an intramuscular dose of 500 IU of anti-D Ig will suppress the immunization that could occur following a FMH of 4–5 mL of RhD positive red cells. Most women have a FMH of less than 4 mL at the birth (cited in RCOG 2002).

In the UK, the following doses of anti-D Ig are recommended:

- 500 IU of anti-D Ig at 28 and 34 weeks' gestation for women in their first pregnancy (see NICE 2002)
- 250 IU following sensitizing events *up to* 20 weeks' gestation
- at least 500 IU following sensitizing events *after* 20 weeks' gestation
- at least 500 IU for all non-sensitized Rh-negative woman following the birth of a Rh-positive infant
- larger doses for caesarean birth, twin pregnancies, manual removal of the placenta, stillbirths and intrauterine deaths, unexplained hydrops fetalis and third trimester abdominal trauma (dose calculated on 500 IU of anti-D Ig suppressing immunization from 4 mL of RhD-positive red blood cells)
- larger doses for any other instance of inadvertent maternal transfusion of Rh-positive red blood cells
- *An insufficient dose of anti-D Ig can result in RhD isoimmunization.* In the UK, (and some other countries) a Kleihauer screening test or flow cytometry (when available) is recommended within 2 hrs to quantify FMH, and assess the need for additional anti-D Ig (see RCOG 2002).

RhD isoimmunization can also result from not following established protocols, particularly during pregnancy. For example:

- not administering anti-D Ig appropriately, or women not attending for bleeding in pregnancy
- not administering anti-D Ig for abdominal trauma
- using an inadequate dose of anti-D Ig following antepartum haemorrhage after 20 weeks
- not managing miscarriages and medical terminations of pregnancy
- not managing sensitizing events after 20 weeks' gestation according to guidelines
- interpreting a 'negative' Kleihauer test result as a reason not to give anti-D immunoglobin
- postnatal omissions in women who have recently received antenatal treatment with anti-D Ig.

Ethical and legal issues

A number of ethical, moral, legal and safety issues surround anti-D Ig, a human plasma-based product (see NICE 2002, RCOG 2002). Women have the right to refuse anti-D Ig treatment. To give informed consent, they need to know the possible consequences of treatment versus non-treatment. In the UK because of the hypothetical risk of transmitting new variant Creutzfeldt–Jakob disease, anti-D Ig use from UK residents has been discontinued. Anti-D Ig is now obtained from paid donors in and outside the EC. Midwives also have rights with respect to anti-D Ig, which they usually administer, in particular, involvement in policy decisions affecting anti-D Ig protocols. To assist midwives in their discussion with families, anti-D Ig information and resources are available, e.g. from NICE 2002. In all countries, midwives need to be aware of the content of consumer information leaflets available nationally and locally.

Management of RhD isoimmunization

Effects of RhD isoimmunization

Destruction of fetal RBCs results in fewer mature and more immature red cells. The fetus becomes anaemic, less oxygen reaches fetal tissue, and oedema and congestive cardiac failure can develop. Increased bilirubin levels also increase the risk of neurological damage from bilirubin deposits in the brain. Lesser degrees of red cell destruction result in haemolytic anaemia, while extensive haemolysis can cause hydrops fetalis and fetal death. Mortality rates are higher for those with hydrops fetalis (van Kamp et al 2005). Early referral to specialist care for women with RhD antibodies is essential. While early specialist care influences fetal outcome (Craparo et al 2005, Ghi et al 2004, van Kamp et al 2005), ongoing midwifery information and support remain important.

Antenatal monitoring and treatment of RhD isoimmunization

Treatment aims to reduce the effects of haemolysis. Intensive fetal monitoring is usually required, and often a high level of intervention throughout the pregnancy. Monitoring and treatment can include:

1. In early pregnancy maternal blood is grouped for Rh type, and women who are Rh-negative are screened for RhD antibodies (indirect Coombs' test). A positive test indicates the *presence* of antibodies or sensitization.

2. Maternal blood is re-tested frequently to monitor any increase in antibody titres. Even with low anti-D levels, sudden and unexpected rises in serum anti-D levels can result in hydrops fetalis.

3. Red blood cells obtained by chorionic villus sampling can be Rh-phenotyped as early as 9–11 weeks' gestation.

4. If antibody titres remain stable, ongoing monitoring is continued.

5. If antibody titres increased, for many years amniocentesis and cordocentesis were used to diagnose fetal anaemia. More recently, Doppler ultrasonography of the middle cerebral artery peak systolic velocity is used for non-invasive diagnosis of fetal anaemia. This procedure is as sensitive as amniocentesis in predicting anaemia and bilirubin breakdown products, has less associated risk, and can safely replace invasive testing in the management of RhD-isoimmunized pregnancies (Joy et al 2005, Mari et al 2005, Oepkes et al 2006, van Dongen et al 2005).

6. Intravenous immunoglobulin (IVIG) blocks fetal red cell destruction, reducing maternal antibody levels and may be used to maintain the fetus until intrauterine fetal transfusion can be performed (see below).

7. Intrauterine intravascular transfusion can be used to treat fetal anaemia until the fetus is capable of survival outside the uterus (Craparo et al 2005, van Kamp et al 2005).

8. Some clinicians recommend antenatal phenobarbital to enhance fetal hepatic maturity and reduce the need for neonatal exchange transfusion. In a Cochrane Review, Thomas et al (2007) concluded this treatment in RhD isoimmunized pregnant women has not been evaluated in randomized controlled trials.

9. Detailed fetal neuroimaging using multiplanar sonography and/or magnetic resonance imaging may be used to assess brain anatomy in fetuses with severe anaemia (Ghi et al 2004).

10. The ongoing severity of the haemolysis and the condition of the fetus will influence the duration of the pregnancy. If early birth of the baby needs to be considered, this would be discussed with parents.

Postnatal treatment of RhD isoimmunization

Management aims to:

- prevent further haemolysis
- reduce bilirubin levels
- remove maternal RhD antibodies from the baby's circulation
- combat anaemia.

Treatment depends upon the baby's condition. Careful monitoring but less aggressive management may be adequate with mild to moderate haemolytic anaemia and hyperbilirubinaemia. Severely affected babies often require admission to intensive care units. Babies with hydrops fetalis are pale, have oedema and ascites and may be stillborn. In some cases phototherapy can be effective but exchange transfusion is often required, and packed cell transfusion may be needed to increase haemoglobin levels. Babies are at risk of ongoing haemolytic anaemia. Early work with IVIG treatment suggests it can be effective at blocking ongoing haemolysis in babies, who then require shorter duration of phototherapy and less exchange transfusions. In their Cochrane Review Alcock & Liley (2002) recommended further clinical research before routine use of intravenous immunoglobulin for the treatment of iso-immune haemolytic jaundice.

ABO incompatibility

ABO isoimmunization usually occurs when the mother is blood group O and the baby is group A, or less often group B. Type O women are 5.5 times more likely to have sensitization than type A or B as the latter have a protein or antigen not present in type O blood. Individuals with type O blood develop antibodies throughout life from exposure to antigens in food, Gram-negative bacteria or blood transfusion, and by the first pregnancy may already have high serum anti-A and anti-B antibody titres. Some women produce IgG antibodies that can cross the placenta and attach to fetal red cells and destroy them (see effects of RhD isoimmunization). ABO incompatibility is also thought to protect the fetus from Rh incompatibility as the mother's anti-A and anti-B antibodies destroy any fetal cells that leak into the maternal circulation (David et al 2004). Although first and subsequent babies are at risk, destruction is usually much less severe than with Rh incompatibility. In most cases haemolysis is fairly mild but in subsequent pregnancies can become more severe. ABO erythroblastosis can, rarely, cause severe fetal anaemia and hydrops.

Antibody titres are monitored throughout the pregnancy, but a high level of antenatal intervention is not usually required. Postnatal management depends on the severity of haemolysis and, as with RhD isoimmunization, aims to prevent further haemolysis, reduce bilirubin levels and combat anaemia. After the birth, cord blood can be tested to confirm blood type, check haemoglobin and serum bilirubin levels and identify maternal antibodies on fetal red cells (direct Coombs' test). If antibodies are present, the baby is monitored for jaundice. As with other causes of haemolysis, if infants require phototherapy it is usually commenced at a lower serum bilirubin level (140–165 μmol/L or 8–10 mg/dL). In rare cases, babies with high serum bilirubin level require exchange transfusion. IVIG administration to newborns with significant hyperbilirubinemia due to

ABO haemolytic disease (with a positive direct Coomb's test) has reduced the need for exchange transfusion (Miqdad et al 2004).

Management of jaundice

For more than 50% of term and 80% of pre-term infants, jaundice is a normal physiological response. However, others are at risk of kernicterus and 1 in 500 newborn babies have liver disease. Good management protocols include careful, individual assessment of each case and a range of therapeutic and diagnostic options.

In countries such as the UK, Australia, New Zealand and many European countries, midwives have an important role in diagnosing and treating jaundice. During the first weeks of the baby's life, midwives can identify at risk newborns, make follow-up visits when women are discharged from hospital or birth at home, arrange home phototherapy and inform and teach parents. This is particularly so in the UK, with midwives encouraged to extend their public health role and work with women for up to 6 weeks after the birth. This includes responsibility for referrals and communication with other agencies.

Most jaundice beyond 2 weeks of age in healthy term infants is associated with breastfeeding and is benign. However, it can also result from haematological, hepatobiliary, metabolic, endocrine, infectious and genetic disorders, all associated with significant morbidity. If conjugated hyperbilirubinaemia is present, comprehensive diagnostic investigation is required to ensure early diagnosis (Ratnavel & Ives 2005). Prolonged jaundice in premature infants is a frequent clinical problem. Sick, premature infants can develop cholestasis from parenteral nutrition, delayed enteral nutrition, sepsis, hypoxia and umbilical lines. They are at risk of serious liver disease, including extrahepatic biliary atresia (Tyler & McKiernan 2006).

Assessment and diagnosis

Two initial diagnostic questions are:

1. Does the jaundice result from the physiological breakdown of bilirubin or the presence of another underlying factor?
2. Is the baby at risk of kernicterus (bilirubin toxicity)?

Individual risk factors

Individual midwifery assessment includes identifying particular risk factors for jaundice. These include any disease or disorder that increases bilirubin production, or alters the transport or excretion of bilirubin (see above and Fig. 47.2). For example:

- birth trauma or evident bruising (increased production of unconjugated bilirubin)
- delayed feeding or meconium passage (decreased enzymes, albumin-binding capacity and increased enterohepatic reabsorption)
- pre-term and therefore at greater risk (increased hepatic immaturity)
- family history of significant haemolytic disease, jaundiced siblings or an ethnic predisposition to jaundice or inherited disease (increased unconjugated bilirubin)
- timing of jaundice, for example, within the first 24 hrs (suggesting haemolysis)
- prolonged jaundice (possible underlying serious disease such as hypothyroidism or obstructive jaundice).

Physical assessment

This includes observation of:

- extent of changes in skin and scleral colour
- head to toe progression of jaundice
- other clinical signs such as lethargy and decreased eagerness to feed
- dark urine or light stools
- dehydration, starvation, hypothermia, acidosis or hypoxia
- vomiting, irritability or high-pitched cry.

Laboratory investigations

These may include:

- transcutaneous bilirubinometry and nonchemical photometric estimates
- serum bilirubin to determine levels and if bilirubin is unconjugated or conjugated
- direct Coomb's test to detect presence of maternal antibodies on fetal RBCs
- indirect Coomb's test to detect the presence of maternal antibodies in serum
- reticulocyte count – elevated by haemolysis as new RBCs are produced
- ABO blood group and Rh type for possible incompatibility
- haemoglobin/haematocrit estimation to assess anaemia
- peripheral blood smear – red cell structure for abnormal cells
- white cell count to detect infection
- serum samples for specific immunoglobulins for the TORCH infections
- glucose-6-phosphate dehydrogenase (G6PD) assay
- urine for substances such as galactose.

Treatment strategies

These include phototherapy, exchange transfusion and in some cases drug treatments.

Phototherapy

Indications for phototherapy

Commencement is based on serum bilirubin levels and the individual condition of each baby, particularly when jaundice occurs within the first 12–24 hrs:

- for pre-term infants <1500 g – between 85 and 140 µmol/L (5 and 8 mg/dL)
- for pre-term infants >1500 g, sick infants and those with haemolysis – between 140 and 165 µmol/L (8 and 10 mg/dL)
- for healthy term infants jaundiced after 48 hrs – between 280 and 365 µmol/L (17 and 22 mg/dL).

Consideration of the above individual factors, and serum bilirubin levels <215 µmol/L (13 mg/dL) are usual before stopping phototherapy. Although bilirubin levels can rise following phototherapy, healthy term babies do not require testing to identify this rebound effect. Rebound to clinically significant levels is more likely with prematurity, a positive direct Coombs test, and in those treated before 72 hrs (Kaplan et al 2006).

Types of phototherapy

Phototherapy reduces levels of unconjugated bilirubin in the blood and decreases the likelihood of neurotoxicity or kernicterus. The skin surface is exposed to high intensity light, which converts fat-soluble unconjugated bilirubin into water-soluble bilirubin that can be excreted in bile and urine. Commercially available phototherapy systems include those delivering light via fluorescent bulbs, halogen quartz lamps, light-emitting diodes and fibreoptic mattresses (Stokowski 2006).

1. *Conventional phototherapy systems* – these use high intensity light from conventional white and more recently blue, blue-green, and turquoise fluorescent phototherapy lamps. Some report no difference in duration and total serum bilirubin decrease with blue, blue-green or conventional phototherapy (Seidman et al 2003). Others found a turquoise fluorescent lamp more effective than a blue fluorescent lamp (Ebbesen et al 2003). In one study, low-cost white reflecting curtains hung around a standard phototherapy unit increased the effectiveness of phototherapy without increased adverse effects (Djokomuljanto et al 2006). The baby is placed about 45–60 cm from the light with the entire skin exposed and eyes protected. Recent research found no significant difference in TSB level when babies wore disposable nappies in posturally supported positions, or were naked without postural support (Pritchard et al 2004).

2. *Fibreoptic light systems* – these use a woven fibreoptic pad that delivers high intensity light with no ultraviolet or infrared irradiation. The tungsten-halogen lamp of fibreoptic phototherapy has a broad emission through the blue and green phototherapy group, mainly in the green spectrum. The device can be placed around the baby, under the clothing, again with the entire skin exposed to light. Ramagnoli et al (2006) found fibreoptic phototherapy as effective as conventional phototherapy. In very pre-term infants, combined phototherapy achieved shorter duration of treatment and significant reduction in exchange transfusion. Unlike conventional phototherapy, fibreoptic phototherapy does not cause a significant increase in skin temperature (Pezzati et al 2002) and eye protection is not required.

These systems may also be more comfortable for babies and allow easier accessibility and handling for parents.

Side-effects of phototherapy

Side-effects of conventional white and blue fluorescent phototherapy can include:

- hyperthermia, increased fluid loss and dehydration
- damage to the retina from the high intensity light
- lethargy or irritability, decreased eagerness to feed, loose stools
- skin rashes and skin burns
- alterations in a baby's state and neurobehavioural organization
- isolation and lack of usual sensory experiences, including visual deprivation
- a decrease in calcium levels leading to hypocalcaemia
- low platelet counts and increased red cell osmotic fragility
- bronze baby syndrome, riboflavin deficiency and DNA damage.

Midwifery care and phototherapy

Midwives and family are usually responsible for infant care either in hospital or at home. Phototherapy may be intermittent or continuous (interrupted only for essential care). In a UK study, fibreoptic home treatment was successful with 22 full term, well babies. No babies required re-admission, and all families preferred home treatment (Walls et al 2004). With both systems, *but particularly with conventional phototherapy*, babies need to be monitored:

- *Temperature.* The infant is maintained in a warm thermoneutral environment and observed for hypo- or hyperthermia.
- *Eyes.* Eye shields or patches must cover the eyes without occluding the nose, and not be too tight or cause eye discharge or weeping.
- *Skin.* Skin is cleaned with warm water and observed for rashes, dryness and excoriation.

- *Hydration.* Fluid intake and output are monitored and demand feeding is continued. Extra fluids may be needed for ill or dehydrated babies.

- *Neurobehavioural status.* This includes sleep and wake states, feeding behaviours, responsiveness, response to stress and interaction with parents and other carers.

- *Calcium levels.* In neonates, hypocalcaemia is defined as a total serum of <1.7 µmol/L (7 mg/dL). Symptoms include jitteriness, irritability, rash, loose stools, fever, dehydration and convulsions.

- *Bilirubin levels.* The reduction in bilirubin levels appears to be greatest in the first 24 hrs of phototherapy and bilirubin levels are usually estimated daily.

- *Parent support.* In most cases, parents will be caring for their infant and need adequate information and support to help them in this role. To give informed consent, parents must know the side-effects of phototherapy and the possible risks of not treating their baby.

Exchange transfusion

Excess bilirubin is removed from the baby during a blood exchange transfusion. With HDN, sensitized erythrocytes are replaced with blood compatible with both the mother's and the infant's serum. In recent years, cord blood screening and advances in phototherapy have reduced exchange transfusion for infants with many haemolytic and enzyme deficiency diseases. Except with very premature babies and Rh incompatibility, exchange transfusion may only be used when phototherapy has failed, or there is a risk of kernicterus.

As with phototherapy, exchange transfusion is considered at a lower serum bilirubin level with haemolysis, in smaller, sick or pre-term babies, and jaundice during the first 12–24 hrs:

- 255 µmol/L (15 mg/dL) for pre-term babies <1500 g

- 300–400 µmol/L (17–23 mg/dL) for sick and pre-term babies >1500 g, and those with haemolysis

- 400–500 µmol/L (23–29 mg/dL) for healthy term babies.

In most cases exchange transfusion is carried out in a neonatal intensive care unit (refer to individual hospital protocol). A Cochrane review (Thayyil & Milligan 2006) found insufficient evidence to support a change from double to single volume exchange transfusion for severe jaundice in newborns. Complications can result from the procedure and from blood products. Babies with other medical problems are more likely to have severe complications such as hypocalcaemia, thrombocytopenia and a higher death rate. Necrotizing enterocolitis also increases with exchange transfusions (see Chs 43 and 44).

Drug treatments

Metalloporphyrins are being used experimentally to reduce levels of unconjugated bilirubin in neonates. In a Cochrane Review, Suresh et al (2003) concluded routine treatment of neonatal unconjugated hyperbilirubinaemia with a metalloporphyrin cannot be recommended at present. While treatment may decrease phototherapy and hospitalization, no evidence supported or refuted a decrease in neonatal kernicterus, long-term neurodevelopmental impairment, or increased cutaneous photosensitivity.

Neonatal infection

Modes of acquiring infection

Babies may acquire infections through the placenta (transplacental infection), from amniotic fluid as they traverse the birth canal, or after birth from sources such as carers' hands, contaminated objects or droplet infection.

Vulnerability to infection

Newborns are more immunodeficient and prone to infection than older children and adults, as full immunocompetence requires innate (natural) and acquired immune responses. Pre-term babies are more vulnerable as placental transfer of IgG mainly occurs after 32 weeks' gestation. Cytokines in maternal and fetal tissues influence physical immunity of the fetus and neonate. They play a leading role in the perinatal period, with their inter-regulation critical for normal function and maturation of neonatal immunity.

Innate immunity

Babies initially depend on natural or innate immunity that does not require previous exposure to microorganisms and is a first line of defence against infection. This includes intact skin, mucous membranes, gastric acid and digestive enzymes. However, newborn skin is more easily damaged and the bowel is not immediately colonized with normal protective flora (Hale 2007).

Acquired immunity

This antigen specific immunity develops and improves from ongoing exposure to a pathogen or organism. The newborn has some maternal immune protection, but immunoglobulins are deficient. Maternal exposure and transfer of IgG across the placenta provides passive protection during the first months of life, while breastfeeding confers increased immune protection. During the early weeks the baby also has deficiencies in the quantity and the quality of neutrophils.

Of particular importance for midwives is the increasing evidence base supporting vaginal birth and breastfeeding in the functioning and maturation of neonatal host defences. Vaginal birth promotes the production of various cytokines and their receptors, with significantly higher levels when compared to elective caesarean section (Malamitsi-Puchner et al 2005, Nesin & Cunningham-Rundles 2000). Breastfeeding increases the baby's immune protection through the transmission of secretory IgA in breastmilk (see Ch. 41).

Management of infection

The midwife's role in the management of fetal and neonatal infection includes prevention, diagnosis and treatment of infection in mother, baby and midwife. Meeting these individual needs may involve high levels of collaboration with other professionals and agencies.

Prevention of infection in the mother

Before, during and after pregnancy, good midwifery practice involves evidence-based prevention that informs each woman of potential sources of infection that may harm her or her child. For example, informing women of such things as the importance of avoiding high risk foods, countries or areas with a high prevalence of some infections and contact with individuals with infectious diseases (see below).

Prevention or treatment of infection in the mother during pregnancy can often prevent or reduce short and long term sequelae in her child (see Ch. 23). In the UK, Group B streptococcus (GBS) is the most frequent cause of serious neonatal bacterial sepsis. In high-risk pregnancies, early-onset neonatal GBS infection can be reduced with antibiotics during birth (Law et al 2005). Similarly, antibiotic use for pre-term rupture of membranes is associated with reduced neonatal morbidity (Kenyon et al 2003).

Prevention of infection in the newborn

A safe environment is of central importance, particularly in hospital where babies are at risk of cross-infection. Careful, frequent hand washing with soap or alcohol remains the most important method of preventing infection. In busy situations cleansing with an alcohol-based hand-rub solution may be the most practical means of improving staff compliance, while wearing gloves further reduces contamination. In their Cochrane Review, Gould et al (2007) recommended research to assess short and longer-term strategies to improve hand hygiene compliance, and determine if this reduced rates of infection. Other midwifery strategies to reduce infection in all environments include:

- encouraging and assisting with breastfeeding to increase immune protection
- maintaining skin integrity and pH balance to increase immune function, and avoiding irritation or trauma of the baby's skin and mucous membranes
- discouraging visitors with infections, or exposure to a communicable disease
- early diagnosis and treatment of infection
- always using individual equipment for each baby
- isolating infected babies when absolutely essential
- in hospital, having the baby rooming in with the mother
- adequate spacing of cots if babies are in a hospital nursery
- ongoing education to ensure infection control practice is evidence-based.

For asymptomatic term neonates of mothers with risk factors for neonatal infection, insufficient evidence exists to guide clinical practice on prophylactic versus selective antibiotic treatment. Ungerer et al (2004) identified the need for a large randomized controlled trial to compare the effects of prophylactic versus selective antibiotics on infant morbidity, mortality and costs.

Prevention of infection in the midwife

This is an important midwifery practice issue, as all health professionals are at risk of exposure to blood-borne infection. Universal precautions are based on the *routine* use of techniques that reduce exposure to blood, other body fluids and tissue that may contain bloodborne pathogens, and *every* client is considered a possible source of infection. In England, the Department of Health (DH) (1998) recommended the following precautions to avoid exposure to body fluids:

- wearing gloves, masks, goggles, gowns and protective footwear if there is any risk of exposure to body fluids (e.g. blood)
- covering all skin lesions
- changing gloves between patients and washing hands when gloves are changed
- disinfecting all blood splashes and spillage
- safe disposal of sharp instruments and waste
- appropriate vaccination, e.g. against hepatitis B.

Diagnosis of infection

In newborns, early signs of infection may be subtle and difficult to distinguish from other problems. The mother or midwife may simply feel the baby is 'off colour' (see Ch. 43). Newborn risk factors include a maternal history of prolonged rupture of membranes, pyrexia during birth, chorioamnionitis, and offensive amniotic fluid.

Physical assessment may include observation of:

- temperature instability
- lethargy or poor feeding, dehydration, starvation
- acidosis or hypoxia
- bradycardia or tachycardia, and any apnoea
- reduced urine output and any vomiting
- central nervous system signs.

Laboratory investigations may include:

- amniotic fluid, placental tissue and cord blood for specific organisms
- a complete blood cell count
- specimens of urine and meconium for specific organisms
- swabs from the nose, throat, umbilicus, skin rashes, pustules or vesicles for specific organisms
- MRI, CT scans, ultrasound and chest X-rays
- comprehensive neurodevelopmental examination
- lumbar puncture for examination of CSF.

Treatment of infection

The overall aim is to reduce the risk of septicaemia and life-threatening septic shock in this vulnerable group. Good management includes:

1. caring for the baby in a warm thermoneutral environment and observing for temperature instability
2. good hydration and the correction of electrolyte imbalance, with demand feeding if possible and intravenous fluids as required
3. maintaining skin integrity to increase thermoregulation and prevent excessive fluid loss
4. prompt systemic antibiotic or other drug therapy and local treatment of infection
5. ongoing monitoring of neurobehavioural status
6. reducing separation of mother and baby, particularly in neonatal intensive care units
7. encouraging breastfeeding, or expressing, and informing women of the value of breastmilk in fighting infection
8. providing evidence-based information, support and reassurance to parents.

Infections acquired before or during birth

Infections may be acquired through the placenta, from amniotic fluid, or the birth canal. For management of sexually transmissible and reproductive tract infections, see Ch. 23. Other infections are discussed in this chapter, emphasizing those where midwives have a critical preventive role. Viral infections such as rubella and varicella (chickenpox) can be a major cause of fetal morbidity and mortality, as can the parasite toxoplasmosis. *Candida albicans*, a yeast fungus, as well as causing infant thrush, can also result in systemic candidiasis and death in very pre-term infants.

Rubella

For most immunocompetent children and adults (including pregnant women), the rubella virus causes a mild, insignificant illness spread by droplet infection. Maternal rubella is now rare in many countries with rubella vaccination programmes (Robinson et al 2006). Congenital rubella syndrome (CRS) remains a major cause of developmental anomalies including blindness and deafness (Banatvala & Brown 2004).

Incidence and effects during pregnancy

In most industrialized countries the measles, mumps and rubella (MMR) vaccine has reduced rubella incidence and with it CRS, although in recent years in the UK and some other countries, vaccination rates have declined due to concerns about the vaccine (see prevention). Countries without routine MMR programmes report rates similar to those of industrialized countries before vaccination (Banatvala & Brown 2004). With primary rubella infection during the first 12 weeks of pregnancy maternal-fetal transmission rates are as high as 85%. Intrauterine infection is unlikely when the mother's rash appears before, or within 11 days after the last menstrual period, and with proven infection later than the 16th week, the risk of severe fetal sequelae is less (Enders et al 1988).

First trimester infection can result in spontaneous abortion and in surviving babies a number of serious and permanent consequences. These include cataracts, sensorineural deafness, congenital heart defects, microcephaly, meningoencephalitis, dermal erythropoiesis, thrombocytopenia and significant developmental delay (Banatvala & Brown 2004, Bedford & Tookey 2006).

Diagnosis and treatment

Diagnosis of congenital rubella may include:

- maternal history of a rash or contact with rubella
- laboratory differentiation of rubella from other infections (e.g. measles, parvovirus B19, and human herpesvirus 6)

- serological screening for rubella-specific IgG and IgM antibodies
- cordocentesis for rubella IgM antibody in umbilical cord blood
- detection of viral ribonucleic acid in chorionic villi, amniotic fluid, or fetal blood
- ongoing ultrasonography of the fetus and neonate for eye and cardiac anomalies
- specific antibody detection in cord blood at birth
- isolation of the rubella virus from the throat, urine and CSF of the neonate
- detection of rubella-specific IgG and IgM salivary antibody responses in oral fluid
- ongoing surveillance during early childhood (Banatvala & Brown 2004, Degani 2006, Robinson et al 2006).

Most women with first trimester infection require a great deal of information and support, and some may request termination of pregnancy. Following the birth, management is symptomatic, emphasizing support for parents, and referrals to ensure best outcomes for babies. Infants with CRS are highly infectious and should be isolated from other infants and pregnant women (but not their own mothers). Long-term follow up is essential, as some problems may not become apparent until babies are older.

Prevention

In the UK, a number of factors may contribute to CRS:

- maternal rubella re-infection
- missed opportunities for immunization at school, or after the birth
- immigration from countries without routine, or with recent rubella vaccination programmes
- overseas travel during early pregnancy
- increasing numbers of CRS cases in some European countries, together with poor MMR uptake
- declining measles-mumps-rubella vaccination due to MMR vaccine concerns (Banatvala & Brown 2004, Bedford & Tookey 2006, Robinson et al 2006, Sathanandan et al 2005, Wright & Polack 2006).

Midwives need to emphasize the importance of avoiding contact with rubella during pregnancy, as reinfection has been reported despite previous vaccination. As part of their extended public health role, midwives can encourage vaccination for seronegative women before and after, (but *not* during pregnancy), and also discuss the importance of vaccinating their child. Strategies targeting all children, and offering vaccine to susceptible schoolgirls or women before pregnancy offer the best protection against CRS. Those working with pregnant women may also be offered rubella vaccination.

Midwives and other health professionals can also use evidence-based medicine to offer immunization and health education to groups with low rates. For example, in the UK, women in urban areas have the lowest rates of MMR cover (particularly inner city areas). They may also have the highest levels of deprivation (Wright & Polack 2006). Those born outside the UK, e.g. African- and Asian-born women are more susceptible to a rubella outbreak (Bedford & Tookey 2006). Similarly, in Sydney, Australia, country of birth was a strong predictor of immunity, with 65% non-immune Asian-born women compared with 13% Australian-born. Other significant risk factors for non-immunity were maternal age >35 years and nulliparity (Sathanandan et al 2005).

Also essential are evidence-based programmes (e.g. by midwives and health visitors) to address concerns about perceived adverse effects of measles-mumps-rubella vaccine. Often related to higher levels of education, these concerns include associations between MMR vaccine, autism, and Crohn's disease (Banatvala & Brown 2004, Wright & Polack 2006). In their Cochrane Review, Demicheli et al (2005) found MMR unlikely to be associated with Crohn's disease, ulcerative colitis, autism or aseptic meningitis. However, overall in the 31 reviewed studies MMR was associated with irritability, febrile convulsions, benign thrombocytopenic purpura, parotitis, joint and limb complaints and aseptic meningitis (mumps). The authors commented on the inadequacy of design and reporting of safety outcomes in MMR vaccine studies, and on the absence of studies on the effectiveness of MMR that fulfilled Cochrane inclusion criteria (see Ch. 51 for further discussion on immunization).

Varicella zoster

Varicella zoster virus (VZV) is a highly contagious DNA virus of the herpes family that causes varicella (chickenpox). Transmitted by respiratory droplets and contact with vesicle fluid, it has an incubation period of 10–20 days and is infectious for 48 hrs before the rash appears until vesicles crust over. After primary infection the virus remains dormant in sensory nerve root ganglia, with any recurrent infection resulting in herpes zoster or shingles (Heininger & Seward 2006). Primary infection during pregnancy can result in serious outcomes (Meyberg-Solomayer et al 2006).

Incidence and effects during pregnancy

Up to 90% of women born in countries such as the UK have had chickenpox before pregnancy, and are seropositive for VZV immunoglobulin G (IgG) antibodies. However, many tropical and subtropical areas have lower rates of chickenpox during childhood, leaving women at increased risk for primary infection during pregnancy (Pinot de Moira et al 2006). In adults chickenpox can also be more severe and may be complicated by pneumonia, hepatitis and encephalitis. A UK confidential enquiry reported 7 maternal deaths associated with varicella infection during pregnancy between 1985 and 1997 (cited in Heuchan & Isaacs 2001).

Fetal effects vary with gestation at the time of maternal infection.

1. During the first 20 weeks of pregnancy the baby has about a 2% risk of fetal varicella syndrome (FVS). Symptoms can include skin lesions and scarring, eye problems, such as chorioretinitis and cataracts, and skeletal anomalies, in particular limb hypoplasia. Severe neurological problems may include encephalitis, microcephaly and significant developmental delay. About 30% of babies born with skin lesions die in the first months of life.

2. From 20 weeks' gestation up to almost the time of birth, infection can result in milder forms of neonatal varicella that do not result in negative sequelae for the neonate. The child may have shingles during the first few years of life.

3. Maternal infection after 36 weeks, and particularly in the week before the birth (when cord blood VZV IgG is low) to 2 days after, can result in infection rates of up to 50%. About 25% of those infected will develop neonatal clinical varicella. Newborns are also at risk of contracting varicella from mothers or siblings in the postnatal period. Most affected babies will develop a vesicular rash and about 30% will die. Other complications of neonatal varicella include clinical sepsis, pneumonia, pyoderma and hepatitis.

Diagnosis and treatment

Diagnosis of FVS can include a recent history of maternal chickenpox, polymerase chain reaction (PCR) to identify the specific infectious agent, VZV DNA detection in amniotic fluid, and prenatal ultrasound. Continuing improvements in ultrasonography are valuable in confirming the effects of FVS e.g. limb contractures and deformities, cerebral anomalies, borderline ventriculomegaly, intracerebral, intrahepatic and myocardial calcifications, articular effusions, and intrauterine growth retardation (Degani 2006, Meyberg-Solomayer et al 2006).

Most pregnant women with chickenpox will need a great deal of information and support. Women infected during the first 20 weeks may request termination of pregnancy. Although mother and baby should be isolated from others, they should always be kept together. Varicella zoster immune globulin (VZIG) can be offered to seronegative pregnant women who are exposed to chickenpox, within 72 hrs of contact, and always within 10 days. With parental permission, VZIG should also be given to a baby whose mother develops chickenpox between 7 days before and 28 days after the birth, or whose siblings at home have chickenpox (if the mother is seronegative). Informed consent is essential as VZIG is a human blood product (Heuchan & Isaacs 2001, Murguia-de-Sierra et al 2005).

Although no clinical trials could be found to confirm that antiviral chemotherapy prevents CVS, the antiviral drug acyclovir may reduce the mortality and risk of severe disease in some groups, particularly if VZIG is not available. These include pregnant women with severe complications, and newborns if they are unwell or have added risk factors such as prematurity or corticosteroid therapy (Hayakawa et al 2003, Sauerbrei & Wutzler 2000).

Prevention

At the present time, and particularly in the UK, health education remains the most effective midwifery preventive strategy. As with rubella, midwives need to emphasize the importance of avoiding contact with chickenpox during pregnancy. Antenatal screening is only cost effective as part of a screening and vaccination programme or for groups of women who are at increased risk. Varicella childhood immunization programmes are available in some countries, e.g. the USA, Australia, Uruguay, Germany, Taiwan, and Canada (Heininger & Seward 2006).

As part of their extended public health role, and *where varicella vaccine is readily available*, midwives can encourage vaccination for seronegative women before and after, (but *not* during pregnancy until safety is proven) and also discuss the importance of vaccinating their child. Where varicella vaccine is readily available, midwives and other health professionals can also offer immunization and health education to groups at increased risk. These include women who have emigrated from tropical countries which have lower childhood chickenpox rates, such as Bangladesh (Pinot de Moira et al 2006).

Using a cohort model, Pinot de Moira et al (2006) assessed costs and benefits of screening and vaccination. For susceptible women, verbal plus serological screening would cost less for both UK- and Bangladesh-born women. Universal screening costs more, but was more effective and could be cost-effective in younger immigrant women.

Toxoplasmosis

Toxoplasmosis is caused by *Toxoplasma gondii (T. gondii)*, a protozoan parasite infecting up to a third of the world's population. It is found in uncooked meat and cat and dog faeces. Primary infection can be asymptomatic, or characterized by malaise, lymphadenopathy and ocular disease. Primary infection during pregnancy can cause severe damage to the fetus (Montoya & Liesenfeld 2004). Childhood acquired infection also causes half of toxoplasma ocular disease in UK and Irish children (Gilbert et al 2006).

Incidence and effects during pregnancy

A survey of 1897 pregnant women in Kent, UK, identified a seroprevalence rate of 9.1%. A higher seroprevalence was associated with living in a rural location or in Europe as a child (not UK), feeding a dog raw meat and increased age. This 9.1% toxoplasma immune status leaves 90% at risk of primary infection during pregnancy. However, toxoplasma prevalence in the UK has declined since the 1960s (Nash et al 2005). Increasing gestational age at seroconversion increases the risk of mother-to-child transmission (Systematic Review on Congenital Toxoplasmosis, SYROCOT 2007).

Risks for the infected fetus can include intrauterine death, low birthweight, enlarged liver and spleen, jaundice and anaemia, intracranial calcifications, hydrocephalus and retinochoroidal and macular lesions. Infected neonates may be asymptomatic at birth, but can develop retinal and neurological disease. Those with subclinical disease at birth can develop seizures, cognitive and motor problems and reduced cognitive function over time (Gilbert et al 2006, Schmidt et al 2006, SYROCOT 2007). For example, in one group of 38 children with confirmed toxoplasma infection, 58% had congenital infection. Of these, 9% were stillborn, while 32% of the live births had intracranial abnormalities and/or developmental delay, and 45% had retinochoroiditis with no other abnormalities. Of the 42% of children infected after birth, all had retinochoroiditis (Gilbert et al 2006).

Diagnosis and treatment

Diagnosis can be made by direct detection of the parasite, or serological techniques. Antenatally, a *T. gondii* polymerase chain reaction (PCR) and ultrasound can be used.

Sonographic findings can often enable diagnosis of specific congenital syndromes with serial scanning as conditions change (Degani 2006). Postnatally, *T. gondii* IgM antibodies may be detected from eluate on the infant's PKU Guthrie filter paper card (Montoya & Liesenfeld 2004, Schmidt et al 2006).

The effectiveness of antenatal treatment in reducing the congenital transmission of *T. gondii* is not proven. A meta-analysis of 1438 treated mothers (26 cohorts) also found no evidence that antenatal treatment significantly reduced the risk of clinical symptoms (SYROCOT 2007). Infants with congenital toxoplasmosis are usually treated with pyrimethamine, sulfadiazine and folinic acid for an extended period (Montoya & Liesenfeld 2004, Schmidt et al 2006).

Prevention

Midwives have an essential role in prevention, as health education can result in a 92% reduction in pregnancy seroconversion. Breugelmans et al (2004) found the most effective strategy was a leaflet explaining toxoplasmosis and how to avoid the condition during pregnancy, with this information reinforced in antenatal classes. In the UK, the Toxoplasmosis Trust (1998) educates health professionals and the public (a handbook for midwives is available from the trust). Appropriate information includes advising women about washing kitchen surfaces following contact with uncooked meats, stringent hand washing and avoiding cat and dog faeces.

Of relevance for midwives is an ongoing knowledge of countries with high rates of toxoplasmosis, e.g. France and Brazil, where women may travel. Primary prevention strategies also need to address the toxoplasma ocular disease acquired after birth by UK and Irish children (Gilbert et al 2006).

Maternal serologic screening for toxoplasmosis during pregnancy is offered in some countries. However, controversy exists about primary and secondary prevention (see Montoya & Liesenfeld 2004). Some suggest the current UK policy of not offering prenatal or neonatal screening is supported by the absence of evidence of effective antenatal treatment (Gilbert et al 2006, SYROCOT 2007). The latter reviewers recommended a large randomized clinical trial to identify potential benefits of prenatal treatment.

Candida

Candida is a Gram-positive yeast fungus with a number of strains (see Ch. 23). *C. albicans* is responsible for most fungal infections, including thrush in infants. Infection can affect the mouth (oral candidiasis), skin (cutaneous candidiasis) and other organs (systemic candidiasis).

Oral candidiasis

Thrush presents as white patches on the baby's gums, palate and tongue. It can be acquired during birth and from caregivers' hands or feeding equipment. Raw areas (removed by sucking) on the edge of the infant tongue can assist diagnosis. Risk factors for infant thrush include bottle use during the first 2 weeks, the presence of siblings (Morrill et al 2005), and antibiotic exposure (Dinsmoor et al 2005). Breastfeeding women may also have infected breasts, with flaky or shiny skin of the nipple/areola, sore, red nipples and persistent burning, itching or stabbing pain in the breasts (see Ch. 41). Risk factors for maternal thrush include bottle use in the first 2 weeks after the birth, pregnancy duration of >40 weeks (Morrill et al 2005), and intrapartum antibiotic use (Dinsmoor et al 2005). In a further study of 100 healthy breastfeeding mothers, thrush was best predicted by three or more simultaneous signs or symptoms, or by flaky or shiny skin of the nipple/areola, together or in combination with breast pain (Francis-Morrill et al 2004).

Accurate midwifery diagnosis and treatment of thrush is important for continued breastfeeding. Morrill et al (2005), found 43% of women with thrush 2 weeks after the birth were breastfeeding at 9 weeks, compared with 69% of women with a negative diagnosis. Nystatin is possibly the most effective and least expensive treatment: oral for the baby and topical breast application for the mother (see Wiener 2006 for differential diagnosis and treatment options).

Cutaneous candidiasis

Cutaneous candidiasis presents as a moist papular or vesicular skin rash, usually in the region of the axillae, neck, perineum or umbilicus. Cutaneous fungal infections are found in healthy full-term newborns as well as those who are premature or immunocompromised. Usually benign, recognition and treatment is important in preventing adverse outcomes (Smolinski et al 2005). Management includes keeping the area dry and applying topical nystatin. In pre-term babies the thin cutaneous barrier may contribute to the early onset of systemic *Candida* infection. Antifungal prophylaxis may be used to prevent systemic *Candida* colonization, e.g. oral nystatin or fluconazole.

Disseminated candidiasis

Systemic colonization with *Candida* is associated with such factors as low birth weight, low gestational age, exposure to third-generation cephalosporins, endotracheal intubation, longer stays in the NICU, bacterial sepsis, and colonization of central venous catheter or endotracheal tube (Manzoni et al 2006). Prompt management is essential as the condition can be life threatening, with a high death rate in very low birth weight infants. Complications can include meningitis, endocarditis, pyelonephritis, pneumonia and osteomyelitis. Fluconazole prophylaxis decreases the risk of neonatal candidiasis (Manzoni et al 2006). Treatment may include oral nystatin, fluconazole and amphotericin B. Newer antifungal agents, including voriconazole and caspofungin show promise in treating potentially fatal neonatal fungal infections (Smolinski et al 2005). Clerihew & McGuire (2004), in their Cochrane Review, emphasized the need for a large randomized controlled trial to compare amphotericin B with newer antifungal preparations.

Ophthalmia neonatorum

Ophthalmia neonatorum is a notifiable condition, defined in England as any purulent eye discharge within 21 days of birth, and in Scotland as eye inflammation within 21 days of birth accompanied by a discharge. The condition is usually acquired during vaginal birth. A swab must be taken for culture and sensitivity testing, with immediate medical referral. Differential diagnosis of the organism is essential as chlamydial and gonococcal infections can cause conjunctival scarring, corneal infiltration, blindness and systemic spread (see Ch. 23). Other causes of inflammation must also be excluded. Treatment includes local cleaning and care of the eyes with normal saline, and appropriate drug therapy for the baby and mother if required.

Some infections acquired after birth

After the birth the most common routes for neonatal infection are the umbilicus, broken skin, the respiratory tract and those that result from invasive procedures and devices. Infections acquired after birth are also discussed in Chapters 43 and 44.

Meningitis

Neonatal meningitis is an inflammation of the membranes lining the brain and spinal column caused by such organisms as group B streptococci (GBS), *E. coli*, *Listeria monocytogenes*, and less often *Candida* and herpes. In the UK, neonatal meningitis is most often caused by GBS (Law et al 2005). In Australia and New Zealand, the incidence of GBS early onset neonatal bacterial meningitis decreased significantly between 1993 and 2002, while the incidence of *Escherichia coli* meningitis remained the same (May et al 2005).

Very early signs may be non-specific, followed by those of meningeal irritation and raised intracranial pressure such as crying, irritability, bulging fontanelle, increasing lethargy, tremors, twitching, severe vomiting, diminished muscle tone and alterations in consciousness. Babies may also present with hemiparesis, horizontal deviation and decreased pupillary reaction of the eye, decreased retinal reflex and an abnormal Moro reflex.

Early diagnosis and treatment are critical to prevent collapse and death. Diagnosis may be confirmed by examination of cerebrospinal fluid (CSF). Very ill babies require intensive care, intravenous fluids and antibiotic therapy. Although acute phase mortality has declined in recent years, long-term neurological complications still occur in many surviving infants. For example, in one group aged 5 years, 23% had a serious disability, with isolation of bacteria from CSF the best single predictor (de Louvois et al 2005). For such infants, long-term comprehensive developmental assessment is essential, including audiometry and vision testing.

Eye infections

Mild eye infections are common in babies and can be treated with routine eye care and antibiotics if required. Other more serious conditions must be excluded, such as ophthalmia neonatorum (see above), trauma, foreign bodies, congenital glaucoma and nasolacrimal duct obstruction.

Skin infections

Newborn skin lesions include septic spots or pustules, either as solitary lesions or clustered in the umbilical and buttock areas. For well babies with limited pustules, regular cleaning with an antiseptic solution is adequate. Antibiotic therapy may be required for more extensive pustules (see Ch. 43). Neonatal fungal skin infections can range from benign conditions such as congenital candidiasis and neonatal cephalic pustulosis to serious infections in very low birthweight or immunocompromised neonates (Smolinski et al 2005).

Respiratory infections

These may be minor (nasopharyngitis and rhinitis) or more severe such as pneumonia (see Chs 43 and 44).

Gastrointestinal tract infections

In newborns these can include gastroenteritis or the more severe NEC. Causative organisms for gastroenteritis include rotavirus, *Salmonella*, *Shigella* and a pathogenic strain of *E. coli*. The secretory IgA in breastmilk offers important protection against these organisms, particularly rotavirus. Treatment depends on the severity of symptoms. With nausea and vomiting, correction of fluid and electrolyte imbalance is urgent to avoid dehydration (see Ch. 43).

Umbilical infection

Signs can include localized inflammation and an offensive discharge. In their Cochrane Review of 10 studies, Zupan et al (2004) found keeping the cord clean was as effective and safe as using antiseptics or antibiotics. Although antiseptics prolonged cord separation time, they also reduced the mother's concerns. Untreated infection can spread to the liver via the umbilical vein and cause hepatitis and septicaemia. Treatment can include regular cleaning, antibiotic powder and antibiotic therapy (see Ch. 43).

Urinary tract infections

Urinary tract infections can result from bacteria such as *E. coli*, or less often from a congenital anomaly that obstructs urine flow. The signs are usually those of an early non-specific infection, and diagnosis is usually confirmed through laboratory evaluation of a urine sample (see Ch. 43).

REFERENCES

Ahlfors C E, Wennberg R P 2004 Bilirubin-albumin binding and neonatal jaundice. Seminars in Perinatology 28(5):334–339

Alcock G S, Liley H 2002 Immunoglobulin infusion for iso-immune haemolytic jaundice in neonates (Cochrane Review). The Cochrane Library, issue 3. Online. Available: http://www3.interscience.wiley.com/cgi-bin/home

Allaby M, Forman K, Touch S et al 1999 The use of routine anti-D prophylaxis antenatally to Rhesus negative women. Trent Institute for Health Services Research, Universities of Leicester, Nottingham and Sheffield, ref 99/04

Banatvala J E, Brown D W G 2004 Rubella. Lancet 363 (9415):1127–1137

Bedford H, Tookey P 2006 Rubella and the MMR vaccine. Nursing Times 102(5):55–57

Bertini G, Dani C, Tronchin M et al 2001 Is breast-feeding really favoring early neonatal jaundice. Pediatrics 107(3):E41

Bianchi D W, Avent N D, Costa J M et al 2005 Noninvasive prenatal diagnosis of fetal rhesus D. Ready for prime(r) time. Obstetrics and Gynecology 106(4):841–844

Breugelmans M, Naessens A, Foulon W 2004 Prevention of toxoplasmosis during pregnancy – an epidemiologic survey over 22 consecutive years. Journal of Perinatal Medicine 32 (3):211–214

Clerihew L, McGuire W 2004 Systemic antifungal drugs for invasive fungal infection in pre-term Infants (Cochrane Review). The Cochrane Library, issue 1. Online. Available: http://www3.interscience.wiley.com/cgi-bin/home

Craparo F J, Bonati F, Gementi P et al 2005 The effects of serial intravascular transfusions in ascitic/hydropic RhD-alloim-munized fetuses. Ultrasound in Obstetrics and Gynecology 25(2):144–148

Crowther C, Middleton P 2001 Anti-D administration after childbirth for preventing Rhesus alloimmunization. The Cochrane Library, issue 3. Online. Available: http://www3. interscience.wiley.com/cgi-bin/home

Crowther C A, Keirse M J N C 1999 Anti-D administration during pregnancy for preventing Rhesus alloimmunization (Cochrane review). The Cochrane Library, issue 2. Online. Available: http://www3.interscience.wiley.com/cgi-bin/home

David M, Smidt J, Frank C K et al 2004 Risk factors for fetal-to-maternal transfusion in Rh D-negative women – results of a prospective study on 942 pregnant women. Journal of Perinatal Medicine 32(3):254–257

Degani S 2006 Sonographic findings in fetal viral infections: a systematic review. Obstetrical and Gynecological Survey 61 (5):329–336

de Louvois J, Halket S, Harvey D 2005 Neonatal meningitis in England and Wales: sequelae at 5 years of age – European Journal of Pediatrics 164(12):730–734.

Demicheli V, Jefferson T, Rivetti A et al 2005 Vaccines for measles, mumps and rubella in children (Cochrane Review). The Cochrane Library, issue 4. Online. Available: http://www3.interscience.wiley.com/cgi-bin/home

Dinsmoor M J, Viloria R, Lief L et al 2005 Use of intrapartum antibiotics and the incidence of postnatal maternal and neonatal yeast infections. Obstetrics and Gynecology 106 (1):19–22

Djokomuljanto S, Quah B S, Surini Y et al 2006 Efficacy of phototherapy for neonatal jaundice is increased by the use of low-cost white reflecting curtains. Archives of Disease in Childhood: Fetal and Neonatal Edition 91(6): F439–F442

DH (Department of Health) 1998 Guidance for clinical health care workers: protection against infection with blood-borne viruses. Recommendations of the Expert Advisory Group on AIDS and the Advisory Group on Hepatitis. DH, London

Ebbesen F, Agati G, Pratesi R 2003 Phototherapy with turquoise versus blue light. Archives of Disease in Childhood: Fetal and Neonatal Edition 88(5):F430–F431

Enders G, Pacher U N, Miller E et al 1988 Outcome of confirmed periconceptional maternal rubella. Lancet 1 (8600):1445–1446

Finning K, Martin P, Daniels G 2004 A clinical service in the UK to predict fetal Rh (Rhesus) D blood group using free fetal DNA in maternal plasma. Annals of the New York Academy of Sciences 1022:119–123

Francis-Morrill J, Heinig M J, Pappagianis D et al 2004 Diagnostic value of signs and symptoms of mammary candidosis among lactating women. Journal of Human Lactation 20 (3):288–295

Geifman-Holtzman O, Grotegut C A, Gaughan J P 2006 Diagnostic accuracy of noninvasive fetal Rh genotyping from maternal blood – a meta-analysis. American Journal of Obstetrics and Gynecology 195(4):1163–1173

Ghi T, Brondelli L, Simonazzi G et al 2004 Sonographic demonstration of brain injury in fetuses with severe red blood cell alloimmunization undergoing intrauterine transfusions. Ultrasound in Obstetrics and Gynecology 23 (5):428–431

Gilbert R, Tan H K, Cliffe S et al 2006 Symptomatic toxoplasma infection due to congenital and postnatally acquired infection. Archives of Disease in Childhood 91 (6):495–498

Gould D J, Chudleigh J H, Moralejo D et al 2007 Interventions to improve hand hygiene compliance in patient care (Cochrane Review). The Cochrane Library, issue 2. Online. Available: http://www3.interscience.wiley.com/cgi-bin/home

Grohmann K, Roser M, Rolinski B et al 2006 Bilirubin measurement for neonates: comparison of 9 frequently used methods. Pediatrics 117(4):1174–1183

Hale R 2007 Protecting neonates' delicate skin. British Journal of Midwifery 15(4):231–232, 234–235

Hayakawa M, Kimura H, Ohshiro M et al 2003 Varicella exposure in a neonatal medical centre: successful prophylaxis with oral acyclovir. Journal of Hospital Infection 54 (3):212–215

Heininger U, Seward J F 2006 Varicella. Lancet 368 (9544):1306–1307

Heuchan A M, Isaacs D 2001 The management of varicella-zoster virus exposure and infection in pregnancy and the newborn period. Medical Journal of Australia 174 (6):288–292

Jangaard K A, Curtis H, Goldbloom R B 2006 Estimation of bilirubin using BiliChek, a transcutaneous bilirubin measurement device: effects of gestational age and use of phototherapy. Paediatrics and Child Health 11(2):79–83

Joy S D, Rossi K Q, Krugh D et al 2005 Management of pregnancies complicated by anti-E alloimmunization. Obstetrics and Gynecology 105(1):24–28

Kaplan M, Hammerman C 2004 6 Glucose-6-phosphate dehydrogenase deficiency: a hidden risk for kernicterus – Seminars in Perinatology 28(5):356–364

Kaplan M, Kaplan E, Hammerman C et al 2006 Post-phototherapy neonatal bilirubin rebound: a potential cause of significant hyperbilirubinaemia. Archives of Disease in Childhood 91(1):31–34

Kaplan M, Muraca M, Vreman H J et al 2005 Neonatal bilirubin production-conjugation imbalance: effect of glucose-6-phosphate dehydrogenase deficiency and borderline prematurity. Archives of Disease in Childhood: Fetal and Neonatal Edition 90(2):F123–F127

Karlsson M, Blennow M, Nemeth A et al 2006 Dynamics of hepatic enzyme activity following birth asphyxia. Acta Paediatrica 95(11):1405–1411

Kenyon S, Boulvain M, Neilson J 2003 Antibiotics for pre-term rupture of membranes (Cochrane Review). The Cochrane Library, issue 2. Online. Available: http://www3.interscience.wiley.com/cgi-bin/home

Law M R, Palomaki G, Alfirevic Z et al 2005 The prevention of neonatal group B streptococcal disease: a report by a working group of the Medical Screening Society. Journal of Medical Screening 12(2):60–68

Maayan-Metzger A, Schwartz T, Sulkes J et al 2001 Maternal anti-D prophylaxis during pregnancy does not cause neonatal haemolysis. Archives of Disease in Childhood: Fetal and Neonatal Edition 84(1):F60–F62

Maisels M J, Newman T B 1995 Kernicterus in otherwise healthy, breast-fed term newborns. Pediatrics 96(4):730–733

Malamitsi-Puchner A, Protonotariou E, Boutsikou T et al 2005 The influence of the mode of delivery on circulating cytokine concentrations in the perinatal period. Early Human Development 81(4):387–392

Manzoni P, Farina D, Leonessa M L et al 2006 Risk factors for progression to invasive fungal infection in pre-term neonates with fungal colonization. Pediatrics 118(6):2359–2364

Mari G, Zimmermann R, Moise K J et al 2005 Correlation between middle cerebral artery peak systolic velocity and fetal hemoglobin after 2 previous intrauterine transfusions. American Journal of Obstetrics and Gynecology 193 (3):1117–1120

May M, Daley A J, Donath S et al 2005 Early onset neonatal meningitis in Australia and New Zealand, 1992–2002. Archives of Disease in Childhood 90(4):F324–F327

Meyberg-Solomayer G C, Fehm T, Muller-Hansen I et al 2006 Prenatal ultrasound diagnosis, follow-up, and outcome of congenital varicella syndrome. Fetal Diagnosis and Therapy 21(3):296–301

Miqdad A M, Abdelbasit O B, Shaheed M M et al 2004 Intravenous immunoglobulin G (IVIG) therapy for significant hyperbilirubinemia in ABO hemolytic disease of the newborn. Journal of Maternal-Fetal and Neonatal Medicine 16 (3):163–166

Montoya J G, Liesenfeld O 2004 Toxoplasmosis. Lancet 363 (9425):1962

Morrill J F, Heinig M J, Pappagianis D et al 2005 Risk factors for mammary candidosis among lactating women. Journal of Obstetric, Gynecologic and Neonatal Nursing 34 (1):37–45

Murguia-de-Sierra T, Villa-Guillen M, Villaneuva-Garcia D et al 2005 Varicella zoster virus antibody titers after intravenous zoster immune globulin in neonates, and the safety of this preparation. Acta Paediatrica 94(6):790–793

Nanjundaswamy S, Petrova A, Mehta R et al 2005 Transcutaneous bilirubinometry in pre-term infants receiving phototherapy. American Journal of Perinatology 22(3):127–131

Nash J Q, Chissel S, Jones J et al 2005 Risk factors for toxoplasmosis in pregnant women in Kent, United Kingdom. Epidemiology and Infection 133(3):475–483

Nesin M, Cunningham-Rundles S 2000 Cytokines and neonates. American Journal of Perinatology 17(8):393–404

Newman T B, Xiong B, Gonzales V M et al 2000 Prediction and prevention of extreme neonatal hyperbilirubinemia in a mature health maintenance organization. Archives of Pediatrics and Adolescent Medicine 15(11):1140–1147

NICE (National Institute for Health and Clinical Excellence) 2002 Guidance on the use of routine antenatal anti-D prophylaxis for RhD-negative women. Technology appraisal guidance no 41 (TA41). NICE, London. Online. Available: www./nice.org.uk

Oepkes D, Seaward G, Vandenbussche F P H A et al 2006 Doppler ultrasonography versus amniocentesis to predict fetal anemia. New England Journal of Medicine 355 (2):156–164

Pezzati M, Fusi F, Dani C et al 2002 Changes in skin temperature of hyperbilirubinemic newborns under phototherapy: conventional versus fiberoptic device. American Journal of Perinatology 19(8):439–443

Pinot de Moira A, Edmunds W J, Breuer J 2006 The cost-effectiveness of antenatal varicella screening with post-partum vaccination of susceptibles. Vaccine 24(9):1298–1307

Pritchard M A, Beller E M, Norton B 2004 Skin exposure during conventional phototherapy in pre-term infants: a randomized controlled trial. Journal of Paediatrics and Child Health 40(5/6):270–274

Ramagnoli C, Zecca E, Papacci P et al 2006 Which phototherapy system is most effective in lowering serum bilirubin in very pre-term infants? Fetal Diagnosis and Therapy 21 (2):204–220

Ratnavel N, Ives N K 2005 Investigation of prolonged neonatal jaundice. Current Paediatrics 15(2):85–91

RCOG (Royal College of Obstetricians and Gynaecologists) 2002 Use of anti-D immunoglobulin for Rh prophylaxis. Online. Available: www.rcog.org.uk

Robinson J L, Lee B E, Preiksaitis J K et al 2006 Prevention of congenital rubella syndrome--what makes sense in 2006? Epidemiologic Reviews 28:81–87

Sathanandan D, Gupta L, Liu B et al 2005 Factors associated with low immunity to rubella infection on antenatal screening. Australian and New Zealand Journal of Obstetrics and Gynaecology 45(5):435–438

Sauerbrei A, Wutzler P 2000 The congenital varicella syndrome. Journal of Perinatology 20(8):548–554

Schmidt D R, Hogh B, Andersen O et al 2006 The national neonatal screening programme for congenital toxoplasmosis in Denmark: results from the initial four years, 1999–2002. Archives of Disease in Childhood 91(8):661–665

Seidman D S, Moise J, Ergaz Z et al March 2003 A prospective randomized controlled study of phototherapy using blue and blue-green light-emitting devices, and conventional halogen-quartz phototherapy. Journal of Perinatology 23(2):123–127

Setia S, Villaveces A, Dhillon P et al 2002 Neonatal jaundice in Asian, white, and mixed-race infants. Archives of Pediatrics and Adolescent Medicine 156(3):276–279

Shapiro S M, Bhutani V K, Johnson L 2006 Hyperbilirubinemia and kernicterus. Clinics in Perinatology 33(2):387–410

Smitherman H, Stark A R, Bhutani V K 2006 Early recognition of neonatal hyperbilirubinemia and its emergent management. Seminars in Fetal and Neonatal Medicine 11 (3):214–224

Smolinski K N, Shah S S, Honig P J et al 2005 Neonatal cutaneous fungal infections. Current Opinion in Pediatrics 17(4):486–493

Stokowski L A 2006 Fundamentals of phototherapy for neonatal jaundice. Advances in Neonatal Care 6(6):303–312

Suresh G K, Martin C L, Soll R F 2003 Metalloporphyrins for treatment of unconjugated hyperbilirubinemia in neonates (Cochrane Review). The Cochrane Library, issue 1. Online. Available: http://www3.interscience.wiley.com/cgi-bin/home

SYROCOT (Systematic Review on Congenital Toxoplasmosis) Study Group 2007 Effectiveness of prenatal treatment for congenital toxoplasmosis: a meta-analysis of individual patients' data. Lancet 369(9556):115–122

Thayyil S, Milligan D W A 2006 Single versus double volume exchange transfusion in jaundiced newborn infants (Cochrane Review). The Cochrane Library, issue 4. Online. Available: http://www3.interscience.wiley.com/cgi-bin/home

Thomas J T, Muller P, Wilkinson C 2007 Antenatal phenobarbital for reducing neonatal jaundice after red cell isoimmunization (Cochrane Review). The Cochrane Library, issue 2. Online. Available: http://www3.interscience.wiley.com/cgi-bin/home

Toxoplasmosis Trust 1998 Toxoplasmosis survey reveals ignorance and misconceptions: daisy chain campaign aims to end an avoidable tragedy. Toxoplasmosis Trust London, 18 March

Tyler W, McKiernan P J 2006 Prolonged jaundice in the pre-term infant – what to do, when and why. Current Paediatrics 16(1):43–50

Ungerer R L S, Lincetto O, McGuire W et al 2004 Prophylactic versus selective antibiotics for term newborn infants of mothers with risk factors for neonatal infection (Cochrane Review). The Cochrane Library, issue 4. Online. Available: http://www3.interscience.wiley.com/cgi-bin/home

van Dongen H, Klumper F J C M, Sikkel E et al 2005 Non-invasive tests to predict fetal anemia in Kell-alloimmunized pregnancies. Ultrasound in Obstetrics and Gynecology 25 (4):341–345

van Kamp I L, Klumper F J C M, Oepkes D et al 2005 Complications of intrauterine intravascular transfusion for fetal anemia due to maternal red-cell alloimmunization. American Journal of Obstetrics and Gynecology 192 (1):165–170

Walls M, Wright A, Fowlie P et al 2004 Home phototherapy: a feasible, safe and acceptable practice. Journal of Neonatal Nursing 10(3):92–94

Watchko J F 2006 Hyperbilirubinemia and bilirubin toxicity in the late pre-term infant. Clinics in Perinatology 33 (4):839–852

Wiener S 2006 Diagnosis and management of candida of the nipple and breast. Journal of Midwifery and Women's Health 51(2):125–128

Wright J A, Polack C 2006 Understanding variation in measles-mumps-rubella immunization coverage – a population-based study. European Journal of Public Health 16 (2):137–142

Zupan J, Garner P, Omari A A 2004 Topical umbilical cord care at birth (Cochrane Review). The Cochrane Library, issue 3. Online. Available: http://www3.interscience.wiley.com/cgi-bin/home

48 Metabolic and endocrine disorders and drug withdrawal

Stephen P. Wardle

CHAPTER CONTENTS

The chapter aims to:

- describe the normal mechanisms of control and abnormalities that can occur in electrolyte, fluid and glucose balance in the newborn infant. The emphasis is placed on the normal infant although obviously many of these problems are more common in growth restricted or pre-term infants
- describe the presentation, detection, and management of inherited specific metabolic abnormalities most of which are rare
- describe the presentation and management of abnormalities of hormonal control in the newborn
- describe the effects of fetal exposure to drugs and the effects of this on the newborn, its treatment and prognosis.

Metabolic disturbances in the newborn

Many metabolic abnormalities can occur in the newborn particularly in pre-term or growth restricted infants; by far the most common problem is hypoglycaemia. Some other common problems are also highlighted here.

Glucose homeostasis

In utero the healthy fetus has a constant supply of glucose via the placenta. Following birth, this supply of nutrient ceases and there is a fall in glucose concentration (Srinivasan et al 1986). However at the same time, endocrine changes (decrease in insulin and a surge of catecholamines and release of glucagon) result in an increase in glycogenolysis (breakdown of glycogen stores to provide glucose), gluconeogenesis (glucose production from the liver), ketogenesis (producing ketones, an alternative fuel) and lipolysis (release of fatty acids from adipose) bringing about an increase in glucose and other metabolic fuel. Problems arise in the newborn when either there is a lack of glycogen stores to mobilize (pre-term and growth restricted infants) or excessive insulin production (infants of diabetic mothers) or when infants are sick and have poor supply of energy and increased requirements.

Low glucose concentrations are a potential problem in the newborn infant because if there is a lack of fuel or nutrient available for the brain, cerebral dysfunction and potentially brain injury may occur. The problem for those caring for newborn infants is not only to identify infants who are at risk and treat them appropriately but also to avoid excessive treatment and investigation in infants who are normal and where intervention is not required.

Hypoglycaemia
Definition of hypoglycaemia

The definition of hypoglycaemia is controversial and many different definitions can be found in the literature (Koh et al 1988a). The problem is that defining a specific level of blood glucose is unhelpful because an infant's ability to compensate and use alternative fuels may be as important as the specific glucose concentration. However, pragmatically a specific level is helpful for management purposes. The consensus appears to favour a cut-off value in the newborn of 2.6 mmol/L although the evidence for the use of this level is not strong. This figure comes mainly from two studies (Koh et al 1988b, Lucas et al 1988). Koh et al demonstrated abnormal sensory-evoked brain stem potentials in a small number of term infants. This did not occur in any infants where the blood glucose was above 2.6 mmol/L whether or not symptoms were present (Koh 1988b). In addition, and perhaps more importantly, in a retrospective study of pre-term infants the neurological outcome was less good if the blood glucose concentration had been <2.6 mmol/L on

≥5 days during the neonatal period (Lucas et al 1988). These studies suggest that levels of blood glucose concentration above 2.6 mmol/L are likely to be safe but they do not take into account infants' ability to compensate for low glucose concentrations. Lower values may be safe in some infants.

Symptoms of hypoglycaemia

Any infant who has symptomatic hypoglycaemia has a glucose concentration that is too low and this should be treated whatever the exact glucose level. The symptoms of hypoglycaemia are lethargy, poor feeding, seizures and decreased consciousness level. Jitteriness is commonly ascribed to hypoglycaemia but is a common symptom in the newborn and alone should not be used as an indication for measuring blood glucose concentration.

Normal term infants

It is likely that healthy term infants are able to tolerate low blood glucose concentrations using compensatory mechanisms and use alternative fuels such as ketone bodies, lactate or fatty acids (Hawdon et al 1992). These infants may have blood glucose concentrations as low as 2.0 mmol/L without any ill effects because, if responding normally, they are likely to have increased ketone body concentrations so that fuel is available for the brain (Hawdon et al 1992). Term infants who are breastfed are a group who are particularly likely to have low blood glucose concentrations probably because of the low energy content of breastmilk in the first few postnatal days. However these infants have higher ketone body concentrations to compensate (Hawdon et al 1992) and they are unlikely therefore to suffer any ill effects. Unfortunately however, routine measurements of ketone body concentrations are not readily available and when glucose measurements are made in these infants it becomes difficult for practitioners to resist giving treatment that may involve supplementary formula feeding or even intravenous dextrose at the expense of breastfeeding. This should obviously be avoided unless there are other clinical indications for intervention.

Because of their ability to compensate, clinically well appropriately grown full term infants who are feeding do not require monitoring of their glucose concentration. Doing so would result in many infants being inappropriately treated.

Infants at risk of neurological sequelae of hypoglycaemia

Infants where monitoring and treatment should be considered are those in whom counter-regulation may be impaired for some reason. These groups of infants are:

- Pre-term infants (<37 weeks)
- Growth restricted infants (<3rd centile for gestation)

    Pre-term and growth restricted infants have lower glycogen stores and cannot therefore mobilize glucose as rapidly during the immediate postnatal period. In addition they also have immature hormone and enzyme responses and are less likely to be enterally fed at an early stage.

- Infants of diabetic mothers

    These infants frequently have low blood glucose concentrations because of an excess of insulin. This is produced by the fetal pancreatic gland as a result of stimulation by increased maternal glucose concentrations. This excess of insulin also acts as a growth factor and brings about excessive fat and glycogen deposition. This is why these infants have a characteristic appearance and are relatively macrosomic (see Plate 22; note macrosomic appearance with increased adiposity).

    A study published in 2005 by the Confidential Enquiry into Maternal and Child Health (CEMACH 2005) demonstrated that practice across the UK varies with regard to the management of infants of diabetics and many infants appear to be inappropriately admitted to neonatal intensive care units. This should be avoided where possible but it requires the ability to monitor these infants on routine postnatal wards.

- Sick term infants, e.g. septic or following perinatal hypoxia-ischaemia

    In sick infants following perinatal hypoxia-ischaemia or sepsis there may also be low substrate stores but there are frequently feeding difficulties that add to the problem.

- Infants with inborn-errors of metabolism.

Diagnosis, prevention and management of hypoglycaemia

Term infants who are admitted to the postnatal ward and are feeding should not have measurements of blood glucose unless they are symptomatic. In particular breastfeeding advice and intervention should not be based on blood glucose concentrations.

Infants at risk of neurological complications of hypoglycaemia can be easily identified from the above categories and the following infants should be monitored:

- infants <37 weeks' gestation
- and/or <2.5 kg
- infants of diabetic mothers
- infants with sepsis or following perinatal hypoxia.

Prevention is important in these infants and they should therefore have:

- adequate temperature control – keep warm
- early feeding (within 1 hr of birth) with 100 mL/kg per day if formula feeding
- frequent feeding (≤3-hourly)
- blood glucose check immediately before the second feed and then 4–6-hourly.

There is no advantage to checking the blood glucose concentration earlier than this as long as there are no symptoms as it is likely to be low and the appropriate treatment at that stage is to feed the baby. If there are symptoms the glucose should be checked and treatment given immediately. Breastfed infants are particularly difficult in this situation as it is important to avoid supplemental feeding with formula to promote successful breastfeeding but the risks associated with significant hypoglycaemia in at risk infants out-weigh this advantage.

If the blood glucose concentration is <2.6 mmol/L then feed should be given at an increased volume and decreased frequency (2-hourly or even hourly). This may require supplementary feeding with formula milk in infants who are breastfed and/or nasogastric tube (NGT) feeding. Breastmilk can also be expressed to give via an NGT.

If the blood glucose concentration remains low despite these measures and there is an adequate feed volume intake then intravenous treatment with dextrose is required. It is important in this situation that enteral feeding is continued as feeding contains much more energy than 10% glucose and it promotes ketone body production and metabolic adaptation.

If the blood glucose concentration is >2.6 mmol/L before the second and the third feed than glucose monitoring can be discontinued but feeding should continue at 3-hourly intervals.

In infants where enteral feeding is contraindicated for some reason then i.v. 10% dextrose at least 60 mL/kg per day should commence.

Hyperglycaemia

Hyperglycaemia is much less of a clinical problem than hypoglycaemia and occurs predominantly in pre-term and severely growth restricted infants. It is also seen in term infants in response to stress especially following perinatal hypoxia-ischaemia, surgery or drugs (especially corticosteroids). In general no treatment is required.

In pre-term infants it is usually a transient phenomenon related to the infants immature glucoregulation or inability to deal with excessive glucose intakes. In general, treatment is not required unless there is significant loss of glucose in the urine that may cause an osmotic diuresis. If treatment is required the rate of glucose infusion can be decreased but there may be some advantages in this situation of giving an intravenous insulin infusion. This allows glucose input to continue and sufficient calories to continue to be given and may result in better weight gain (Collins et al 1991).

Electrolyte imbalances in the newborn

Postnatal weight loss, fluid and electrolyte changes

In the first few days after birth all babies lose weight due to a loss of extracellular fluid. This diuresis and loss of weight is associated with cardiopulmonary adaptation; it occurs rapidly in healthy babies but may be delayed in those with respiratory distress syndrome. As extracellular fluid is lost there is a net loss of both water and sodium over these first few days after birth, although the infant's serum sodium should remain within the normal range. The normal infant should lose up to 10% of its birth weight. This weight loss is physiological and should be expected.

Sodium

Sodium is normally excreted via the kidney, controlled by the renin–angiotensin system. This control mechanism is functional in the pre-term infant but loss of sodium may occur in pre-term infants because of renal tubule unresponsiveness. Term breastmilk has relatively little sodium (<1 mmol/kg per day) showing that the normal newborn can preserve sodium via the kidney in order to maintain growth. Normal sodium requirements are 1–2 mmol/kg per day in term infants and 3–4 mmol/kg per day in pre-term infants.

Changes in serum sodium reflect changes in sodium and water balance. In order to assess changes in sodium concentration it is important to know an infant's weight: hypernatraemia in the presence of a loss of weight suggests dehydration whereas when there is weight gain it is due to fluid and sodium overload. Hyponatraemia in the presence of weight gain represents fluid overload whereas a low sodium with inappropriate weight loss represents sodium depletion. The normal serum sodium concentration is 133–146 mmol/L (Green & Keffler 1999).

Hyponatraemia

Hyponatraemia is either due to fluid overload or sodium depletion. The latter may be due to inadequate intake or excessive losses.

Fluid overload

In the first few days after birth this is the commonest cause of a low sodium concentration. It is commonly seen in infants receiving intravenous (i.v.) fluids or in infants with oliguric renal failure.

Causes:

- excessive i.v. fluid administration (to mother or infant)
- oliguric renal failure
- drugs, e.g. indomethacin given to pre-term infants.

Appropriate treatment is to limit the fluid intake whilst maintaining normal sodium intake with appropriate intravenous fluids.

Sodium depletion

This is commonest in pre-term infants after the first few days after birth due to renal losses but is also common in term infants on diuretics (usually for cardiac failure).

Causes:

- renal loss in pre-term infants. This is treated by increasing sodium intake to cope with the losses. Some pre-term infants may require a very large daily intake of i.v. sodium with their i.v. fluids when losses are high
- loss into the bowel due to ileus (intestinal obstruction, sepsis or prematurity) or severe vomiting
- drugs, e.g. diuretics
- adrenocortical failure. This is rare but may be due to congenital adrenal hyperplasia or hypoplasia or adrenal haemorrhage in a sick infant.

Hypernatraemia

Increased sodium concentration is almost always due to water depletion and loss of extracellular fluid but can also rarely be due to an excessive sodium intake. These causes can again be easily differentiated by weighing an infant to assess the change since birth.

Water depletion

This is rare in term babies but does occur occasionally in infants with an inadequate intake of breast-milk. It is more common in pre-term infants.

Causes:

- transepidermal water loss in pre-term infants. This occurs particularly in infants <28 weeks' gestation and can be prevented by adequate environmental humidity and regular weighing to gauge fluid loss to predict fluid requirements
- excessive urine output in pre-term infants during recovery from respiratory distress syndrome
- high rates of fluid loss during vomiting, diarrhoea or bowel obstruction
- inadequate lactation.

For the midwife this is perhaps the most important cause of hypernatraemia. The incidence has been estimated as 2.5/10 000 live births and it typically occurs in term infants of breastfeeding primiparous mothers (Oddie et al 2001). It can be associated with significant morbidity and even mortality (Edmondson et al 1997), however, it can be prevented with sufficient assistance and supervision of feeding. Babies typically present at 5–9 days of age with lethargy and poor feeding. They have lost >15% of their birthweight and are usually significantly jaundiced. The serum sodium concentration can be between 150 and 200 mmol/L.

In general many infants are not weighed during this period. Mothers who are breastfeeding can be discouraged by the fact that their infant has lost weight despite a good technique and this can serve to undermine breastfeeding no matter how carefully the physiology of the phenomenon is explained. Additionally (particularly in primiparous mothers) lactogenesis is only just becoming established between 48 and 72 hrs. Thus the volume of milk transferred to the infant is still rising sharply between 72 and 96 hrs of age. However, weighing babies during this period can be very useful when a baby is unwell or if there are concerns about intake and fluid and electrolyte balance. It has been suggested that routine weighing of infants may be useful to prevent dehydration and hypernatraemia in breastfed infants with referral to hospital if weight loss exceeds 10% (van Dommelen et al 2007).

The infant's fluid deficit can be calculated from the loss in weight and this is then replaced by gradual rehydration over 24–48 hrs. Feeding can continue but i.v. treatment is often required with normal saline and dextrose. Assistance with lactation can then be given to continue to promote breastfeeding.

Excessive sodium intake

In general this is rare in term infants although may be seen in sick pre-term infants due to excessive bicarbonate and other sodium-containing fluids.

Causes:

- incorrect fluid prescription
- excessive administration of sodium bicarbonate
- incorrectly formulated powdered feeds.
- Münchausen's syndrome by proxy – intentional administration of salt to an infant.

Potassium

Potassium is the major intracellular cation. A low serum concentration therefore implies significant potassium depletion. Abnormalities in serum potassium concentration are important because they can cause significant arrhythmias. Potassium concentrations can be severely affected by measurement technique and any haemolysis of the blood sample especially from capillary sampling is likely to lead to a falsely high value.

Hyperkalaemia

Causes:

- acidosis
- acute renal failure
- congenital adrenal hyperplasia.

Treatment is to remove all potassium supplements from i.v. fluids, and to consider giving calcium resonium rectally, calcium gluconate i.v., sodium bicarbonate to increase pH and i.v. glucose and insulin. In general these measures will only be required where there is a serum potassium that is very high (>8 mmol/L) and/or evidence of an abnormal ECG or arrhythmias.

Hypokalaemia

Causes:

- inadequate intake of potassium
- bowel losses (vomiting or diarrhoea)
- diuretic therapy
- hyperaldosteronism.

Hypokalaemia is treated by adding potassium to i.v. infusion fluids or orally. The normal daily requirement of potassium is 2 mmol/kg per day.

Calcium

Calcium metabolism is closely linked to phosphate metabolism and these are very important minerals in relation to bone development. This is of particular importance in pre-term infants as they need much higher concentrations of phosphate and calcium. These are given as intravenous supplements, by supplementing breastmilk with fortifier (Lucas et al 1996) or by giving specific pre-term milk formulae rather than term formula.

High serum calcium concentrations are unusual but there are rare but important causes of low serum calcium. The normal serum concentration is 2.2–2.7 mmol/L but this must be interpreted with the serum albumin concentration as serum calcium is bound to albumin therefore a low albumin concentration will lead to a falsely low serum value.

Calcium concentrations fall within 18–24 hrs of birth as the infant's supply of placental calcium ceases but accretion into bone continues. In the past, hypocalcaemia during the first week after birth used to be caused by giving unmodified cow's milk. This has a high phosphate concentration and a relatively low calcium concentration that depressed the serum calcium concentration and caused seizures. This is now rare with modern formula feeds.

Hypocalcaemia can cause seizures, tremors, jitteriness, lethargy, poor feeding and vomiting. Severe symptoms can be treated by i.v. replacement of calcium. Longer-term management depends on the cause.

Hypocalcaemia can be caused by:

- prematurity
- significant hypoxia-ischaemia
- renal failure
- hypoparathyroidism including DiGeorge syndrome (see later)
- maternal diabetes mellitus.

Inborn errors of metabolism in the newborn

Background/Incidence

Inborn errors of metabolism (IEM) are rare inherited disorders occurring in approximately 1 in 5000 births. They result mainly from enzyme deficiencies in metabolic pathways leading to an accumulation of substrate, leading to toxicity. In utero, the placenta provides an effective dialysis system for most disorders, removing toxic metabolites. Most affected babies are therefore initially born in good condition with normal birth weight. A high index of suspicion is needed when evaluating an acutely ill neonate, as many disorders are treatable and early diagnosis and institution of therapy can reduce morbidity. It has been estimated that 20% of infants presenting with sepsis in the absence of risk factors have an inborn error of metabolism.

Patient group

The mode of inheritance is usually autosomal recessive, therefore family history is crucial and the following features should be sought:

- affected sibling
- previous stillbirth/neonatal death
- parental consanguinity
- symptoms associated with feeding, fasting or a surgical procedure
- improvement when feeds stopped and relapse on restarting.

Clinical examination however is usually normal. The features below may be seen in isolation with many diagnoses, however multiple features indicate that an underlying IEM should be seriously considered:

- septicaemia
- hypoglycaemia
- metabolic acidosis
- convulsions
- coma
- cataracts
- cardiomegaly
- jaundice/liver disease
- severe hypotonia
- unusual body odour
- dysmorphic features
- abnormal hair
- hydrops fetalis
- diarrhoea.

Diagnosis

The following tests are a basic first step in investigation:

- full blood count
- septic screen
- creatinine, urea and electrolytes (including chloride)

- liver enzymes
- blood gas
- blood glucose and lactate concentration
- urine reducing substances
- urine ketones (dipstick)
- plasma ammonia concentration
- coagulation tests.

Many other investigations may be necessary and useful but in general investigations need to be discussed with a consultant biochemist or paediatrician with an interest in metabolic disorders.

Principles of emergency management are to reduce load on affected pathways by removing toxic metabolites and stimulating residual enzyme activity. Hypoglycaemia is corrected, adequate ventilatory support and hydration are maintained, convulsions are treated and significant metabolic acidosis is treated with i.v. sodium bicarbonate, and electrolyte abnormalities are corrected. In general antibiotics are frequently given as infection may have precipitated metabolic decompensation and occasionally dialysis may also be required (Wraith and Walker 1996).

Phenylketonuria

Phenylketonuria (PKU) is important, first because it is a treatable cause of brain injury and second it is possible to successfully screen for it during the first week of life in order to identify affected individuals and treat them appropriately to produce a favourable outcome.

PKU is an autosomal recessive disorder that has an incidence of approximately 1 in 10 000 in the UK. Babies with PKU are born in good condition but begin to be affected by their condition during the first few weeks/months after birth. Untreated it leads to severe mental retardation (IQ<30). However, if it is identified early (within the first 3 weeks), it can be treated by a diet specifically restricted in phenylalanine. The common type is caused by the absence of or reduction in an enzyme in the liver that converts phenylalanine to tyrosine (phenylalanine hydroxylase). This leads to a build up of phenylpyruvic acid that is toxic to the brain.

PKU is particularly suitable for mass screening because there is a simple widely available diagnostic test and because treatment is effective. Midwives collect the blood sample for PKU screening in the UK between days 5–8 after birth. It is commonly collected on the Guthrie Card along with a sample for screening for congenital hypothyroidism (see later). The level of phenylalanine is analysed and babies with increased levels need to be prescribed a low phenylalanine diet and have further assessment to determine whether they are affected by the 'classic' type or other variants.

If it is treated early the prognosis for PKU is good and normal intelligence can result. In females, a return to the low phenylalanine diet is essential prior to conception and during pregnancy. This is because fetal brain injury may result from exposure to high concentrations of phenylalanine and its metabolites in the mother.

Galactosaemia

Galactosaemia is a disorder of carbohydrate metabolism that is autosomal recessive in inheritance and has an incidence of 1 in 60 000. It is caused by an absence or severe deficiency of the enzyme galactose-1-phosphate uridyltransferase (often referred to as Gal-I-P UT). This enzyme is important for converting galactose to glucose and since milk's main sugar lactose is a disaccharide containing glucose and galactose, infants with this condition rapidly become affected when fed either human breastmilk or cow's milk formulae. The metabolite that builds up and is harmful is galactose-1-phosphate.

The clinical signs and symptoms of the disorder are those of liver failure and renal impairment. They tend to present with vomiting, hypoglycaemia, jaundice, bleeding, acidosis, failure to gain weight and hypotonia during the first few days after birth. Another important clinical feature sometimes present is cataracts. Affected babies may also present with septicaemia (particularly E. coli) due to damage to intestinal mucosa by high levels of galactose in the gut. Galactosaemia is an important differential diagnosis to consider when dealing with an infant with unresponsive hypoglycaemia and prolonged or severe jaundice.

Infants with galactosaemia will have galactose but not glucose in their urine. The diagnosis therefore can be made by looking for urine-reducing substances (i.e. galactose) using a Clinitest, whereas a urine test for glucose will be negative. Confirmation of the diagnosis is by assay of the enzyme level (Gal-I-P UT) within red blood cells.

Treatment is with a lactose free milk formula and this must be commenced as soon as the diagnosis is suspected. This results in a rapid correction of the abnormalities. However cataracts and mild brain injury have occurred even when galactosaemic infants have been fed lactose-free milk from birth.

Screening for this disorder is possible but many infants will have presented before the screening test is available and there is little evidence to suggest that diagnosis at or soon after birth gives a better long-term outlook than diagnosis by rapid screening of the symptomatic neonate.

Endocrine disorders in the newborn

Endocrine problems in the newborn are relatively rare but may be serious, even life threatening but are nearly always treatable so identification and diagnosis is important. Disorders of blood glucose homeostasis have already been described so this section will concentrate on other endocrine abnormalities that may present in the newborn.

Thyroid disorders

The thyroid gland produces hormones that have an effect on the metabolic rate in most tissues. They are also essential for normal neurological development. Thyroid stimulating hormone (TSH) is produced by the anterior pituitary gland and this stimulates production of T3 and T4 by the thyroid gland with a feedback mechanism to the anterior pituitary.

Hypothyroidism

The incidence of hypothyroidism in the newborn is 1 in 3500. There are several possible causes for hypothyroidism in the newborn including abnormalities in gland formation (thyroid dysgenesis), defects in hormone synthesis (dyshormonogenesis) and rarely secondary pituitary causes. The latter causes a decrease or lack of TSH, whereas primary (thyroid) causes result in very high TSH values. The presentation is however the same although this has implications for screening.

Infants with hypothyroidism tend to be large, postmature and have a large posterior fontanelle. They have coarse features and often have an umbilical hernia. These features are often missed, however, and this is why screening for this disorder is so important. Untreated infants develop impaired motor development with growth failure, a low IQ, impaired hearing and language problems. With treatment the physical signs of hypothyroidism do not appear but the intellectual and neurological prognosis is poor unless treatment is started within the first few weeks of life but this should always occur when infants are detected by screening.

Screening

Screening for hypothyroidism involves measuring TSH on a blood spot taken along with the screening test for PKU at 5–8 days of age. This method detects almost all cases, however, it cannot detect cases caused by secondary (pituitary) hypothyroidism that will have a low TSH. This condition is however much less common with an incidence of 1 in 60–100 000 (Fisher et al 1979).

Hyperthyroidism

Graves disease is an autoimmune disorder that causes hyperthyroidism. Neonatal hyperthyroidism occurs relatively rarely but is possible when the mother has or has had Graves disease. It occurs not because of neonatal autoantibodies but as a result of the transfer of maternal thyroid stimulating immunoglobulins. These are autoantibodies that are produced and act in the same way as TSH. This can occur when a mother has active, inactive or treated Graves disease (Teng et al 1980). Thyrotoxicosis in the fetus can lead to pre-term labour, low birth weight, stillbirth and fetal death but only a small percentage of infants of mothers with Graves disease become symptomatic

In the neonate the symptoms are irritability, jitteriness, tachycardia, prominent eyes, sweating, excessive appetite and weight loss. These symptoms may be present immediately after birth or presentation may be delayed for as long as 4–6 weeks (Skuza et al 1996). Infants therefore need to be observed for this period and treatment will be required with antithyroid medication if there are symptoms.

Adrenal disorders

The adrenal glands are vital for normal function of many systems within the body. They are divided into a medulla and a cortex. The medulla produces catecholamines these help to maintain blood pressure and are produced at times of stress. Abnormalities of function of the adrenal medulla are not described in the newborn. The adrenal cortex produces three groups of hormones: glucocorticoids, mineralocorticoids and sex hormones that have distinct functions. Glucocorticoids regulate the general metabolism of carbohydrates, proteins and fats on a long-term basis. They have a particular role in modifying the metabolism in times of stress. Mineralocorticoids regulate sodium, potassium and water balance. The sex hormones are responsible for normal development of the genitalia and reproductive organs. Abnormalities in function of the glands represent the functions of these different groups of hormones.

Adrenocortical insufficiency

This is caused by congenital hypoplasia, adrenal haemorrhage, enzyme defects or can be secondary to pituitary problems. It generally presents with symptomatic hypoglycaemia, poor feeding, vomiting, poor weight gain and even prolonged jaundice. Infants may have hyponatraemia, hypoglycaemia, hyperkalaemia and acidosis. Treatment is by i.v. therapy with glucose and electrolytes replacement of corticosteroid and mineralocorticoid hormones is then required.

Adrenocortical hyperfunction

This may occur in the form of congenital adrenal hyperplasia (CAH). This is the name given to a group of inherited disorders that are due to deficiency of enzymes responsible for hormone production within the adrenal. The most common enzyme deficiency results in an excess of androgenic hormones but a deficiency of glucocorticoid and mineralocorticoids often also occurs. These disorders can cause abnormalities in the formation of the genitalia leading to ambiguous genitalia (virilization of females or inadequate virilization of males), and symptoms of adrenal insufficiency (vomiting, diarrhoea, vascular collapse, hypoglycaemia, hyponatraemia, hyperkalaemia) (see Fig. 48.1).

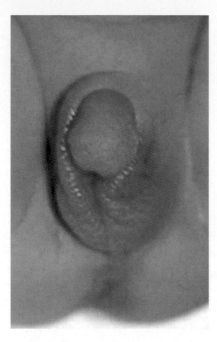

Figure 48.1 Female infant with ambiguous genitalia due to congenital adrenal hyperplasia.

The classification of disorders of sexual differentiation has been revised in recent years. For more information see the consensus statement by Hughes et al (2006).

It is important to make a prompt diagnosis. The genetic sex must be determined (chromosome analysis) and it is important not to assign a sex until the diagnosis has been established. The biochemical diagnosis is made by analysing urine and plasma for steroid hormone metabolites. Treatment is as for adrenocortical insufficiency by replacement of glucocorticoid and mineralocorticoid hormones. Virilized girls may also require surgical intervention to correct the genital abnormalities.

Pituitary disorders

Pituitary insufficiency is rare in the newborn. It may occur in association with other abnormalities, particularly midline developmental defects. Presentation is with signs of glucocorticoid deficiency (hypoglycaemia), prolonged jaundice or signs of hypothyroidism. Growth hormone deficiency generally causes hypoglycaemia but no other signs in the newborn. When it is recognized treatment is with replacement of the missing hormones.

Parathyroid disorders

The parathyroid glands are responsible for control of calcium metabolism but abnormalities of the parathyroids are rare causes of hypo- or hypercalcaemia in the newborn. When hypoparathyroidism does occur it may be familial or may occur in association with deletions of chromosome 22 (22q11 deletion or DiGeorge syndrome). The symptoms associated with hypocalcaemia are detailed above.

Effects of maternal drug abuse/ use during pregnancy on the newborn

The incidence of drug use within the population has a large geographical variation. As a result the incidence of drug withdrawal symptoms amongst infants also has a markedly varying incidence. Inner city areas are more likely to be affected but even within cities large variation is seen in the incidence of problems.

Opiates and other drugs cross the placenta and the fetus during pregnancy is likely to be exposed to the same peaks and troughs of drug exposure that the mother is. Withdrawal may be manifested before birth. The increased incidence of fetal distress may be related in part to drug withdrawal during labour but the effects of drugs and withdrawal on the fetus and newborn are obviously related to the timing of drug doses.

Infants born to mothers who have used illicit drugs during pregnancy are at risk of withdrawal symptoms but there are many other problems associated with these pregnancies and infants that must be considered as well as the obvious problem of withdrawal symptoms. Other problems that are more common in these pregnancies are:

- obstetric complications of pregnancy including placental abruption, fetal growth restriction, fetal distress during labour, stillbirth etc.
- poor attendance for antenatal care
- non-disclosure of information regarding drugs taken during pregnancy
- risk of infectious disease (hepatitis B, hepatitis C and HIV)

- social problems such as poor housing, chaotic lifestyle, care of other children etc.
- poor attendance for neonatal follow-up.

Attendance for antenatal care and supervision during pregnancy may be improved by speciality midwifery support and community liaison. It is important to identify these women during pregnancy in order to try to prevent some of the above problems and offer appropriate support. Identification during pregnancy also allows screening for infectious diseases and this is particularly important for hepatitis B and HIV where treatments are available to decrease the chance of the newborn being affected.

Symptoms

Many drugs have been reported to cause problems of withdrawal in the newborn. The most common seen in the UK are opiates in the form of heroin and methadone but barbiturates, benzodiazepines cocaine and amphetamines are also frequently seen. Multidrug use is common and usually leads to prolonged difficult withdrawal. Each drug has a different half-life and this leads to different patterns of withdrawal symptoms. In general methadone produces symptoms for longer periods than heroin (Herzlinger et al 1977) but benzodiazepines may also contribute to this (Sutton & Hinderliter 1990).

The symptoms most frequently seen are jitteriness, irritability and constant high-pitched crying. Infants often fail to settle between feeds and are hyperactive. When feeds are offered they often feed voraciously although some infants have poor sucking. Vomiting is common. Diarrhoea and an irritant nappy rash are also often seen. Sneezing and yawning are also symptoms and episodes of high temperature in the absence of infection. In rare circumstances infants may also have seizures.

Several scoring systems have been developed to help to guide when to give pharmacological treatment (Finnegan et al 1975). These scoring systems aim to make the assessment more objective, however, most of the symptoms and their severity are difficult to quantify. Infants assessed for signs of drug withdrawal by a scoring system are less likely to be inappropriately treated and may have a shorter hospital stay. It is important not to over-treat infants with drugs as the long-term effects of treatment are not clear and treatment may

then be difficult to withdraw but also treatment in many maternity hospitals means admitting the infant to the neonatal unit and therefore moving the baby away from the mother. On the other hand infants who are withdrawing appear to be in discomfort that we obviously want to relieve and the long-term effects of withdrawal symptoms are also unclear. Personally I find that the most useful symptom is whether infants settle and sleep between feeding. If they do then pharmacological treatment may be unnecessary.

Treatment

Treatment can be divided into general care given to these infants and pharmacological treatment. It is important, if at all possible, to keep the infant with his/her mother. Bonding with and care of these infants by their mother is vital to encourage. The mother is likely to be feeling upset and guilty because of the infant's symptoms and there are frequently already social problems involved with these families. Involving parents in the care of the infant is difficult when he/she provides little positive behavioural return for their effort. Breastfeeding can be encouraged as long as there is no evidence of HIV or on-going drug use that precludes this (cocaine, heroin). This includes methadone although some recommend limiting this to mothers who are taking a dose which is <20 mg/day (Committee on Drugs, American Academy of Pediatrics 1989).

A quiet environment with reduced light and noise is helpful in keeping stimuli to a minimum. Swaddling is useful and feeds may need to be given frequently. These infants often will take large volumes of milk which is acceptable as long as vomiting is not a problem. Rocking or cradling are also useful adjuncts.

Pharmacological treatment

Several different treatments have been recommended in the past. Previously, the four drugs recommended for use were paregoric (a mixture of alcohol and opiate), phenobarbitone, diazepam and chlorpromazine (Committee on Drugs, American Academy of Pediatrics 1983). A number of randomized trials have been performed attempting to assess the use of various drugs in the treatment of neonatal abstinence syndrome (NAS) (Theis et al 1997). It seems logical to treat opiate withdrawal with opiates and now the two most commonly used treatments are oral methadone and oral morphine. These appear to control withdrawal seizures much more effectively (Rivers 1999). They can be given in increasing doses if necessary until symptoms are controlled and then the dose gradually reduced. A possible dosing regimen for oral morphine is shown below:

- initially 0.04 mg/kg morphine sulphate oral 4-hourly
- then 0.03 mg/kg morphine sulphate oral 4-hourly
- then 0.02 mg/kg morphine sulphate oral 4-hourly
- then 0.01 mg/kg morphine sulphate oral 4-hourly.

The dose is reduced every 24 hrs if the baby is feeding well and settling better between feeds. If the feeding and settling does not improve or profuse watery stools and profuse vomiting continue other treatment needs to be considered. Other medication may sometimes be useful, e.g. clonazepam for benzodiazepine use or chloral hydrate as a general sedative.

Cocaine

Cocaine deserves special mention because its effects on the newborn are different. It is a larger problem in the USA than in the UK but the incidence of its use during pregnancy is unknown. It is only present in maternal urine for 24 hrs after exposure therefore detection is difficult (Zuckerman et al 1989). It can produce significant withdrawal symptoms but these are often less severe and less troublesome than with other drugs but it is associated with many other harmful effects on the fetus (Fulroth et al 1989). These include significant fetal growth restriction, brain injury due to haemorrhage or infarction (Hadeed & Siegel 1989), abnormalities of brain development, limb reduction defects and gut atresias. A correlation between cocaine exposure, small head size and developmental scores has been reported (Chasnoff et al 1992).

Discharge and long-term effects

Discharge must be planned with the involvement of other support agencies. This may involve a planning meeting involving all agencies involved in the care of the mother and baby.

Although it seems intuitive that exposure to drugs in utero would cause neurodevelopmental impairment this is not borne out by carefully controlled studies (Lifschitz et al 1985). This implies that impairment in intellectual outcome in these children relates to other adverse prenatal and postnatal factors. Infants born to these mothers are smaller and have smaller head circumferences (Kandall et al 1976). However it is difficult to be certain about the exact causes of any long-term harmful effects because so many factors are involved all of which are interlinked. These include:

- the effects of the drugs themselves on the developing fetus
- the use of other harmful substances by mothers who use drugs (e.g. cigarettes and alcohol)
- the effect of pregnancy complications
- the effect of the withdrawal syndrome on the developing neonate
- the effect of treatment to prevent withdrawal symptoms
- the effect of the home environment of the chaotic drug-user for the developing child
- genetic effects
- reporting bias means that negative associations with drug taking are more likely to be reported (Koran et al 1989).

REFERENCES

Chasnoff I J, Griffith D R, Freier C et al 1992 Cocaine/-polydrug use in pregnancy: two year follow up. Pediatrics 89:284–289

Collins J W Jr, Hoppe M, Brown K et al 1991 A controlled trial of insulin infusion and parenteral nutrition in extremely low birth weight infants with glucose intolerance. Journal of Pediatrics 118(6):921–927

Committee on Drugs, American Academy of Pediatrics 1983 Neonatal drug withdrawal. Pediatrics 72:895–902

Committee on Drugs, American Academy of Pediatrics 1989 Transfer of drugs and other chemicals into human milk. Pediatrics 84:924–936

CEMACH (Confidential Enquiry into Maternal and Child Health) 2005 Pregnancy in women with Type 1 and Type

2 diabetes in 2002–2003, England, Wales and Northern Ireland. CEMACH, London

Edmondson M B, Stoddard J J, Owens L M 1997 Hospital admission with feeding related-problems after early postpartum discharge of normal newborns. Journal of the American Medical Association 278:299–303

Finnegan L P, Kron R E, Connaughton J F et al 1975 Assessment and treatment of abstinence in the infant of the drug dependent mother. International Journal of Clinical Pharmacology 12:19–32

Fisher D A, Dussault J H, Foley T P et al 1979 Screening for congenital hypothyroidism: results of screening one million North American infants. Journal of Pediatrics 94:700–705

Fulroth R, Phillips B, Durand D 1989 Perinatal outcome of infants exposed to cocaine and/or heroin in utero. American Journal of Diseases of Children 143:905–910

Green A, Keffler S 1999 Neonatal biochemical reference ranges. In: Rennie J M, Roberton N R C (eds) Textbook of neonatology, 3rd edn. Churchill Livingstone, Edinburgh, p 1408–1414

Hadeed A J, Siegel S R 1989 Maternal cocaine use during pregnancy: effect on the newborn infant. Pediatrics 84:205–210

Herzlinger R A, Kandall S R, Vaughan H G 1977 Neonatal seizures associated with narcotic withdrawal. Journal of Pediatrics 91:638–641

Hawdon J M, Ward Platt M P, Aynsley-Green A 1992 Patterns of metabolic adaptation for pre-term and term infants in the first neonatal week. Archives of Disease in Childhood 67:357–365

Hughes I A, Houk C, Ahmed S F et al LWPES/ESPE Consensus Group 2006 Consensus statement on management of intersex disorders. Archives of Disease in Childhood 91:554–563

Kandall S R, Albin S, Lowinson J 1976 Differential effects of maternal heroin and methadone use on birthweight. Pediatrics 58:681

Koh T H H G, Eyre J A, Aynsley-Green A 1988a Neonatal hypoglycaemia – the controversy regarding definition. Archives of Disease in Childhood 63:1386–1388

Koh T H H G, Aynsley-Green A, Tarbit M et al 1988b Neural dysfunction during hypoglycaemia. Archives of Disease in Childhood 63:1353–1358

Koran G, Graham K, Shear H et al 1989 Bias against the null hypothesis: the reproductive hazards of cocaine. Lancet ii:1440–1442

Lifschitz M H, Wilson G H, Smith E O et al 1985 Factors affecting head growth and intellectual function in children of drug addicts. Pediatrics 75:269–274

Lucas A, Morley R, Cole T J. 1988 Adverse neurodevelopmental outcome of moderate neonatal hypoglycaemia. British Medical Journal 297:1304–1308

Lucas A, Fewtrell M S, Morley R et al 1996 Randomized outcome trial of human milk fortification and developmental outcome in pre-term infants. American Journal of Clinical Nutrition 64:142–151

Oddie S, Richmond S, Coulthard M 2001 Hypernatraemic dehydration and breast feeding: a population study. Archives of Disease in Childhood 85:318–320

Rivers R 1999 Infants of drug-addicted mothers. In: Rennie J M, Roberton N R C (eds) Textbook of neonatology, 4th edn. Churchill Livingstone, Edinburgh, p 443–451

Skuza K A, Sills I N, Rapaport R 1996 Prediction of neonatal hyperthyroidism in infants born to mothers with Graves' disease. Journal of Pediatrics 128:264–267

Srinivasan G, Pildes R S, Cattamanchi G et al 1986 Plasma glucose values in normal neonates: a new look. Journal of Pediatrics 109:114–117

Sutton L R, Hinderliter S A 1990 Diazepam abuse in pregnant women on methadone maintenance. Implications for the neonate. Clinical Pediatrics (Philadelphia) 29:108–111

Teng C S, Tong T C, Hutchinson J H et al 1980 Thyroid stimulating immunoglobulins in neonatal Graves' disease. Archives of Disease in Childhood 55:894–895

Theis J G W, Selby P, Ikizler Y et al 1997 Current management of the neonatal abstinence syndrome: a critical analysis of the evidence. Biology of the Neonate 71:345–356.

van Dommelen P, van Wouwe J P, Breuning-Boers J M et al 2007 Reference chart for relative weight change to detect hypernatraemic dehydration. Archives of Disease in Childhood 92:490–494.

Wraith J E, Walker J H 1996 Inherited metabolic disorders diagnosis and initial management. Willink Biochemical Genetics Unit, Royal Manchester Children's Hospital, Manchester

Zuckerman B, Frank D A, Hingson R et al 1989 Effects of maternal marijuana and cocaine use on fetal growth. New England Journal of Medicine 320:762–768

7

Section 7
The context of midwifery practice

SECTION CONTENTS

49 Pharmacology and childbirth

Jane M. Rutherford

CHAPTER CONTENTS

Most women are exposed to drugs of one type or another during pregnancy. The drugs may be prescribed or bought over the counter. They may be given as part of the management of the pregnancy itself or that of a coincidental medical problem. However, when considering the use of any drugs in a pregnant or breastfeeding woman, it is important to consider the effects of the drug not only on the woman herself, but also on the fetus or neonate. Many drugs have undesirable effects on the fetus and should therefore be avoided during pregnancy. On the other hand, some drugs are given to the woman because of their therapeutic effects on the fetus. For example betamethasone or dexamethasone are given to women at risk of preterm birth because of their effects on fetal lung maturation. It is therefore important to have a working knowledge of the issues surrounding the use of drugs in pregnancy and the puerperium so that women can be correctly informed and advised regarding the potential benefits and risks.

The chapter aims to:

- outline how pregnancy can influence the effects of drugs and their pharmacodynamics
- explain how drugs can affect pregnancy, and the developing embryo and fetus
- detail the use and effects of the commonly used drugs in pregnancy
- discuss the use of drugs in lactation
- outline the legal aspects of midwives' administration and prescription of drugs.

Effects of drugs in pregnancy

Transfer of drugs across the placenta and breast

A drug administered to a pregnant woman or a breastfeeding mother will, in most cases, be present in the blood circulating around her body. Exceptions are certain types of drugs that are not absorbed from the area where they are administered – for example some (but not all) skin creams. The maternal blood circulation will then take the drug to the placenta or breast, which are organs designed to allow the passage of substances from maternal blood into either fetal blood or milk, respectively. Drugs will pass across into the fetus or neonate in greater or lesser quantities depending on the characteristic of the drug molecules themselves. Some drugs will not pass across into the fetus or milk at all, whereas others will pass freely. The factors influencing passage across the placenta and breast are the size of the molecule, the ionization of the molecule, the lipid or water solubility and the protein binding. In general, large molecules do not cross the placenta and small molecules cross very easily.

Influence of pregnancy on drug dose

There are many physiological changes in pregnancy that influence the way in which the mother's body handles the drugs administered to her. These can result in differences in the circulating concentrations of the drug compared with those in a non-pregnant woman. The transit time in the gut is prolonged compared with that in the non-pregnant woman and this may result in changes in absorption of orally administered drugs (Parry et al 1970). The circulating plasma volume is increased and this results in an increased volume in which a defined dose of drug is distributed which leads to a decrease in the plasma concentration of the drug. Because there is an increase in the blood flow to the kidneys (Dunlop 1976), which are responsible for the elimination of many drugs, there may be an increase in the rate of excretion of a drug. The amounts of total body water and fat are increased (McFadyen 1989) and this may alter the distribution of the drug. Some metabolic pathways in the liver increase and therefore may result in quicker metabolism of a drug. There are also major changes in the levels of plasma proteins to which some drugs bind and this may affect the amount of drug that is available to exert its effect on the body.

Adverse effects of drugs in pregnancy

Many drugs have adverse effects during pregnancy. These vary depending on the stage of pregnancy. One of the major problems in giving advice to women is the paucity of information available regarding the effects of drugs in pregnancy and breastfeeding.

In most cases it is not ethical to perform randomized trials of drugs in pregnancy where their effects are unknown. Drug companies are also reluctant to promote or to license the use of their drugs because of the potential problems and the cost of subsequent litigation. Therefore, most evidence regarding the safety or otherwise of drugs in pregnancy and breastfeeding is accumulated through inadvertent use, or use in unlicensed circumstances. Indeed, many of the drugs that are now commonly used in pregnancy are still not licensed for use. Because of the way information is accumulated, there is a bias towards reporting of adverse events. In general, when choosing a drug to use in pregnancy, clinicians should use those agents that have been available for longest and about which most information has been collected. New agents should be avoided if possible.

Teratogenesis

The word 'teratogen' refers to a substance that leads to the birth of a malformed baby. Organogenesis occurs between approximately 18 and 55 days' post-conception (i.e. 4–10 weeks of pregnancy). A drug can cause a structural abnormality in a fetus only if it is present in the body during this time. This is an important consideration since it is a stage of pregnancy when a woman may not be aware that she is pregnant or may not have attended her midwife or doctor for advice. It is often the case, therefore, that exposure to a potentially teratogenic drug may have already happened before the woman is seen for the first time.

Identifying teratogenic drugs is not an easy process. It is unethical to expose human fetuses to drugs with unknown effects as part of a trial. Drug companies will often try to overcome this by performing animal studies. However, this will neither confirm nor refute that a drug is teratogenic in humans since there is wide interspecies variation. A well-known example of this is the drug thalidomide, which was marketed in the 1960s for sickness in pregnancy. Some 10 000 cases of limb abnormalities were reported before thalidomide was identified as a teratogen. No toxic effects had been noted in animal experiments because thalidomide is a teratogen only in primates.

Because prospective research on teratogenicity in humans is unethical, we rely on case reports and case studies. These can be misleading, however. If a woman has a baby with an abnormality and she took a certain drug in the first trimester, inevitably an association would be drawn. However, there is a background rate of fetal abnormalities of around 2–3% and an association cannot exclude a chance relationship. Larger cohort studies of several women exposed to the same drug who have offspring with the same abnormality are more reliable indicators.

Some of the commonly used drugs known to be teratogens are detailed in Table 49.1.

Other types of drug effect on pregnancy

Drugs may also exert other adverse effects on pregnancy. Any process that occurs during development of the fetus can be affected. For example β-blockers affect fetal growth (Butters et al 1991), angiotensin-converting enzyme (ACE) inhibitors cause fetal renal failure (Kreft-Jais et al 1988) and iodine affects fetal thyroid function. Some drugs may not cause a problem at one stage of pregnancy but may do so at another. For example, there is a risk that the commonly used antibiotic, trimethoprim, is teratogenic when given in the first trimester because it interferes with folate metabolism; however, it is safe in later pregnancy. On the other hand, non-steroidal anti-inflammatory drugs (NSAIDs), such as ibuprofen and diclofenac may be relatively safe if used in the first trimester but can cause premature closure of the ductus arteriosus and oligohydramnios if used in the third trimester. The most difficult effects to quantify are those which relate to neurodevelopment and behaviour. There is growing concern about the relationship between some drugs taken in pregnancy and neurodevelopmental and behavioural problems in later childhood.

Table 49.1 Commonly used drugs that are teratogens

Drug	Effect
Lithium	Cardiac defects
Warfarin	Facial anomalies, CNS anomalies
Sodium valproate	Neural tube defects
Phenytoin	Craniofacial abnormalities
Retinoic acid derivatives	Craniofacial, cardiac and CNS anomalies

Where possible, drugs should be avoided in the first trimester. Obviously, this is not always possible, and in some women it is imperative that a drug that is known to be teratogenic is not stopped abruptly during pregnancy. For example, a woman with epilepsy who is controlled with sodium valproate should not stop her medication abruptly despite the risk of neural tube defects as a prolonged seizure could have devastating effects on both her and her fetus. Where a woman on long-term medication is planning a pregnancy it is advisable for her to attend for pre-pregnancy counselling where plans can be made to minimize the risk.

If a new drug is to be started in pregnancy, one should be chosen that is 'safe'. Women should be informed about the potential risks of any medication they are prescribed. Where a woman is exposed to a teratogen during the first trimester then discussion with an appropriate consultant should be offered to explore the possible outcomes and allow the woman to make informed choices about her pregnancy.

Drugs used in pregnancy

Many drugs are prescribed for therapeutic reasons in pregnancy. It is therefore useful for the midwife to have a working knowledge of the drugs, their possible side-effects and contraindications. In the following sections, where specific references are not given, much of the information is gained from Briggs et al (2005) and Weiner and Buhimschi (2004).

Folic acid

It is recommended that all women planning a pregnancy should take folic acid in a dose of 400 µg daily and that this should continue throughout the first trimester. Folic acid is a vitamin that is involved in the process of cell growth and division. Demand for folate increases in pregnancy. It has been shown that peri-conception folic acid supplementation reduces the risk of neural tube defects (Lumley et al 2000). In addition, folic acid deficiency can lead to maternal anaemia so folic acid supplementation in later pregnancy can also be beneficial. The recommended dose in the general population is 400 µg daily, but women at risk of neural tube defects (e.g. with a previously affected fetus, or on carbamazepine or sodium valproate) should receive 5 mg daily. There are no risks associated with folic acid at this dose.

Iron preparations

Iron deficiency anaemia is common in pregnancy and iron preparations are frequently prescribed. There are many preparations on the market based on either ferrous sulphate or ferrous gluconate. Some are combined with folic acid. Commonly experienced side-effects are constipation (occasionally diarrhoea) and indigestion. Stools are coloured black. When side-effects are a problem, it may be worth trying a different preparation. It should be noted that absorption of iron is reduced by antacids and by some foods (e.g. tea).

Antacid drugs

Antacids are alkalis that act by reducing the acidity of stomach acid. Modern antacid drugs are mostly based on calcium, magnesium and aluminium salts, which are relatively non-absorbable. They are often combined with alginates, which coat the lining of the oesophagus and stomach and therefore reduce contact with stomach acid. Because they are relatively non-absorbable, they are safe for use in pregnancy. Older antacids such as sodium bicarbonate can cause systemic alkalosis and should be avoided.

Antiemetics

Nausea and vomiting may be particularly troublesome in the first trimester but may occur at other times in pregnancy. Where possible, women with mild 'morning sickness' should be encouraged to try non-pharmacological methods of controlling nausea such as eating small amounts frequently. If vomiting is a significant problem then it is preferable to use an antiemetic drug rather than risk dehydration and, in the most severe cases, malnutrition. Most of the commonly used antiemetics are considered safe to use in pregnancy and, as always, the older preparations have a longer established safety profile.

The drugs fall into four main categories:

Antihistamines

The most common side-effect is drowsiness, e.g. cyclizine.

Anticholinergic drugs

Rarely, in young people these, e.g. prochlorperazine, may cause a dramatic side-effect known as a 'dystonic' reaction or 'occulogyric crisis', where there is uncontrolled spasm of the muscles of the face and neck.

Antidopaminergic drugs

These, e.g. metoclopramide, may also cause dystonic reactions.

5HT3 receptor antagonists

This is a relatively new class of antiemetics, e.g. ondansetron. There is now one reasonable sized study of its use in pregnancy without any increase in fetal abnormalities (Einarson et al 2004). However, it should be used with caution, only in those whose vomiting fails to respond to other drugs.

Antibiotics

Antibiotics are one of the most commonly prescribed groups of drugs in pregnancy. They are a diverse group of compounds and have different indications and risks. There are definite indications for the use of antibiotics, but care should be taken as some are safe and others are contraindicated. Table 49.2 indicates some of the antibiotics with which caution should be exercised. Table 49.3 indicates those antibiotics considered safe for use in pregnancy.

Analgesia

It is relatively common for a pregnant woman to require analgesia during pregnancy. This may be for something as simple as a headache, a more significant problem such as rheumatoid arthritis, or for a pregnancy-related condition, such as pelvic girdle pain. However, many of the available analgesics, including 'over-the-counter' preparations, are not considered safe in pregnancy, so it is often difficult to control chronic pain satisfactorily.

Table 49.2 Antibiotics that can cause adverse effects in pregnancy

Antibiotic group (examples)	Risk
Tetracyclines (tetracycline, oxytetracycline, doxycycline)	Discoloration and dysplasia of fetal bones and teeth when used in second and third trimester
Aminoglycosides (gentamicin, netilmicin)	Risk of ototoxicity but often used in serious maternal infection where benefit outweighs risk
Chloramphenicol	'Grey baby syndrome' when used in second and third trimester
Nitrofurantoin	Haemolysis in fetus at term – avoid during labour and birth but safe at other times
Quinolones (ciprofloxacin, ofloxacin)	Arthropathy in fetus – most of this evidence has been obtained from animal studies

Table 49.3 Antibiotics that are considered safe in pregnancy

Antibiotic	Notes
Penicillins (benzyl penicillin, phenoxymethyl penicillin, ampicillin, amoxicillin, co-amoxyclav, flucloxacillin)	Alternatives if allergic
Cephalosporins (cephradine, cephalexin, cefuroxime, cefotaxime)	
Erythromycin	
Clindamycin	
Trimethoprim	Avoid in first trimester

Paracetamol

This is one of the drugs which has a long and unblemished safety record when taken in therapeutic doses. It should be the recommended first-line analgesic agent in pregnancy. However, in overdose it can be potentially lethal to the mother or fetus, or both, as it causes liver failure.

NSAIDs

Ibuprofen is widely available as an over-the-counter preparation. These drugs may be relatively safe in the first trimester but have the potential to cause fetal renal dysfunction, premature closure of the ductus arteriosus, necrotizing enterocolitis and intracerebral haemorrhage (Norton et al 1991). Indomethacin has been used on a short-term basis as a tocolytic agent and to reduce liquor volume in polyhydramnios, but should not be used in the long-term because of the above risks. These drugs are safe in breastfeeding.

Opiate analgesics

When used in analgesic doses, there is no clear evidence of teratogenesis with these drugs, e.g. pethidine, morphine, diamorphine, codeine, dihydrocodeine. For acute episodes there is probably little risk with the use of these drugs. However, with long-term use there is a risk of neonatal withdrawal after birth, in a similar pattern to the withdrawal symptoms seen with opiate abuse. This neonatal withdrawal can be demonstrated even in women using relatively moderate doses of codeine such as those available in over-the-counter preparations. When given in large doses in labour there is a risk of respiratory depression.

Aspirin

In analgesic doses, aspirin has been shown to increase the risk of maternal, fetal and neonatal bleeding because of its effect as an antiplatelet agent. Aspirin at an analgesic dose is therefore contraindicated in pregnancy. A common analgesic dose is 600 mg every 6 hrs. Aspirin in these doses is present in many commercially available cold remedies and analgesic preparations.

However, in *low* doses (75 mg daily) aspirin is used in pregnancy for treatment of women with recurrent miscarriage, thrombophilias (inherited risk of thromboembolism), and prevention of pre-eclampsia and intrauterine growth restriction. In low dose, there is evidence to suggest that there is no increased risk of maternal or neonatal haemorrhage (CLASP Collaborative Group 1994). Aspirin exerts its antiplatelet effect for around 10 days after administration and may prolong the bleeding time. Some clinicians therefore prefer to discontinue aspirin 3–4 weeks prior to birth to prevent complications as a result of this.

Antihypertensives

Antihypertensive drugs may be prescribed in pregnancy for pre-existing hypertension, pregnancy-induced hypertension or pre-eclampsia. Several of the drugs which are used in young women outside pregnancy are contraindicated in pregnancy and it is therefore important to recognize this and arrange for alternative medication if necessary.

Antihypertensives that are contraindicated in pregnancy

ACE inhibitors

These drugs, e.g. captopril, enalapril, lisinopril, are known to cause oligohydramnios, fetal anuria and stillbirth when used in the second and third trimester and are therefore *contraindicated* in the second part of pregnancy. Many young women are on these drugs and until now have been informed to stay on them until they are confirmed to be pregnant and change thereafter to a different agent. However, recent evidence suggests that there is an increased risk of fetal abnormalities when they are taken in the first trimester (Cooper et al 2006) and therefore, ACE inhibitors should be used only with caution even in the first trimester.

Diuretics

Diuretics, e.g. furosemide (frusemide), bendroflumethiazide (bendrofluazide), cause a reduction in circulating blood volume. This may potentially compromise uteroplacental circulation and these drugs are therefore not recommended in pregnancy.

Antihypertensives that may be used in pregnancy

Methyldopa

This drug has been available for many years. There is extensive experience with its use in pregnancy and there is no evidence of adverse effects on the fetus. It is one of the first-line antihypertensive drugs for use in pregnancy. The disadvantage is the maternal side-effect profile, which includes lethargy, drowsiness and depression. These side-effects may be dose dependent. It is given in 2–4 divided doses from a starting dose of 250 mg three times daily up to a total of 3 g daily. The onset of action is slow and it is therefore not suitable for acute blood pressure control. Caution should also be taken when stopping methyldopa in women who have been taking it for several weeks as sudden withdrawal may cause insomnia and anxiety symptoms. It should therefore be stopped gradually. It is safe in breastfeeding.

Beta-blockers

β-blockers, e.g. propranolol, atenolol, labetalol (which also has some α-blocking activity), act by reducing heart rate and stroke volume and therefore reducing cardiac output. Although they cross the placenta and may slightly reduce fetal heart rate, there is no significant change in variability. If commenced before 28 weeks' gestation they have been shown to cause a reduction in fetal growth in up to 25% of cases (Butters et al 1991). They are therefore good antihypertensive drugs for use in the third trimester, but caution should be taken earlier in pregnancy. β-blockers are contraindicated in women with asthma as they may cause bronchoconstriction. β-blockers are excreted into breastmilk and some (e.g. atenolol) may actually be concentrated in breastmilk. However, there are no reports of adverse effects on neonates and they are therefore considered safe in breastfeeding.

Calcium channel blockers

These, e.g. nifedipine, nicardipine, reduce blood pressure mainly by vasodilatation. Nifedipine is increasingly used as an agent in pregnancy. Nifedipine can be given in a rapid release formulation orally to reduce blood pressure quickly in acute situations. However, care should be taken as serious hypotensive reactions have been reported, especially in association with magnesium sulphate (Waisman et al 1988). In general, nifedipine should be given in slow release formulations as these have a more gradual onset and longer period of action. The major side-effect is a headache, which may cause difficulty when determining symptoms of pre-eclampsia. Nifedipine is considered safe in breastfeeding.

Hydralazine

This is a useful drug for management of hypertension in the acute situation. It can only be administered intravenously. It is given either by slow bolus injection or by infusion. It acts as a vasodilator. It is safe in pregnancy and breastfeeding.

Drugs for diabetes mellitus

Sulfonylureas (oral hypoglycaemic agents)

These drugs, e.g. glibenclamide, gliclazide, should be avoided since they cross the placenta and exert an effect on the fetus.

Metformin

This is occasionally used in infertility treatment in women with polycystic ovarian syndrome (PCOS). It is usually discontinued in pregnancy and is not generally used for diabetic control during pregnancy, although it is said not to cross the placenta.

Insulin

This is the mainstay of diabetic treatment in pregnancy. It is a naturally occurring hormone and most of the available preparations of insulin, which are synthetic human insulins or pork-derived insulins, are safe in pregnancy. Bovine insulin should be avoided, however.

Drugs used in asthma

The drugs commonly used in the treatment of asthma include: inhaled bronchodilators (e.g. salbutamol, salmeterol, ipratropium), inhaled chromoglycate, inhaled and oral corticosteroids and theophyllines. All of these drugs are considered safe. Indeed, in either an acute asthmatic attack or in an exacerbation of asthma, the benefits of the medication outweigh the risks to mother and fetus.

Anticoagulants

A degree of anticoagulation may be required in some women in pregnancy in several situations, such as a history of a previous thromboembolic problem, an acute event, a known thrombophilia or heart valve replacement. There are two main anticoagulant drugs: heparin and warfarin.

Warfarin

This drug crosses the placenta and is a teratogen, the critical time of exposure being 6–9 weeks' gestation. The risk of 'fetal warfarin syndrome' is around 10% of those exposed but there is also an increase in central nervous system abnormalities. The characteristics of fetal warfarin syndrome are: nasal hypoplasia, epiphyseal abnormality, eye defects, shortening of the extremities, deafness, developmental retardation, congenital heart disease and scoliosis. Women on long-term warfarin should therefore be aware of the risks and should be asked to inform their doctor immediately they become pregnant. In the second and third trimester, there is a risk of fetal intracerebral haemorrhage.

Generally, women on warfarin should be converted to heparin as soon as they become pregnant and will continue on heparin throughout pregnancy. The exception may be women with metal prosthetic heart valves who have an extremely high risk of thromboembolic complications and in whom the maternal risks of stopping treatment may outweigh the fetal risks of continuing on warfarin.

Warfarin is safe in breastfeeding and may be safely commenced in postpartum women.

The drug has a very gradual onset of action and requires a loading dose to be given over 2 or 3 days. The dose required is very variable and it is judged by monitoring the INR (international normalized ratio) in the blood. This gives an index of the prothrombin time in the patient compared with a standard control, which indicates how much longer it takes for certain coagulation pathways to be activated. In other words, it indicates how quickly or slowly the blood is clotting. Also, many other drugs can interact with warfarin so care should be taken when prescribing to women on warfarin.

Heparin

This does not cross the placenta and it is not excreted into breastmilk. It is therefore safe in pregnancy and breastfeeding. In its 'unfractionated' form, which can be given either intravenously or subcutaneously, it is a mixture of large molecules of differing sizes. Because of the variability of the molecular size, the anticoagulant activity can vary. The effectiveness of heparin is monitored by measuring the activated partial thromboplastin time (APTT); this is a measure of the activity of the intrinsic coagulation pathway, which is where heparin exerts its effect. The dose can be altered to keep it within a set level. Heparin is used in pregnancy both for prophylaxis of thromboembolic disease (subcutaneous) and for acute treatment (usually intravenous).

Side-effects of heparin include bleeding, and bruising at the injection site. Some patients have allergic reactions to heparin, which are usually skin rashes. There is a rare but potentially life threatening adverse reaction: heparin-induced thrombocytopenia, so all patients who are commenced on heparin should have a platelet count after 7–10 days of treatment. Long-term heparin therapy is associated with osteoporosis, and this in particular is a reason to weigh up the benefits versus the risk of treatment.

Heparin is now also available in low molecular weight (LMW) preparations, such as enoxaparin, dalteparin, tinzaparin. LMW heparins have a more predictable anticoagulant response and are usually given by once or twice daily subcutaneous injection. For most situations they are replacing unfractionated heparin. In pregnancy they are useful in prophylaxis and in treatment of an acute event. There is now a reasonable amount of evidence to support their use and LMWHs' are the recommended first line treatment (RCOG 2007). There is a lower incidence of thrombocytopenia and osteoporosis than with unfractionated heparins (Lin & Hu 2000). Some clinicians monitor the effectiveness of LMW heparin by measuring the anti-Xa activity about 4 hrs after a subcutaneous dose. (LMW heparins exert their greatest effect on the coagulation pathway by affecting factor Xa.) One of the disadvantages in pregnancy is that, because of the long duration of action of the drug, most anaesthetists are not happy to site epidural or spinal blocks within 8–12 hrs of an injection because of the risk of haematoma formation.

Antidepressants

There is an increasing number of women taking antidepressant drugs during pregnancy (see Ch. 36, Part B). Where possible, as with all drugs, the dose should be minimized or the drug stopped. There is increasing evidence that paroxetine and possibly other SSRIs (selective serotonin reuptake inhibitors) may be associated with fetal abnormalities (Wogelius et al 2005). In addition, there may be withdrawal effects in the neonate if the drugs are taken in the third trimester. These effects may include respiratory distress, jitteriness, cyanosis, hyperreflexia, irritability and sleeping problems. Paroxetine should therefore only be used with caution.

Older tricyclic antidepressant drugs are generally preferred in women who require them.

Tocolytics

At present, there are no 'perfect' agents for abolishing uterine activity in women in pre-term labour. No agents have been shown to prolong pregnancy significantly. However, tocolytic agents are beneficial for short-term use, either for transfer to a centre with neonatal facilities or for allowing 48 hrs for corticosteroids to be given. All of the following agents have been shown to be effective for short-term use.

Beta sympathomimetics

These drugs, e.g. ritodrine, terbutaline, salbutamol, are associated with significant maternal side-effects such as palpitations, tremor, nausea, vomiting, headaches, thirst, restlessness, chest pain and breathlessness. Tachycardia is common. The serious complication of pulmonary oedema is a risk but is usually associated with fluid overload. Blood sugar levels may rise and should be monitored; this is a particular risk in women with diabetes where the serious complication of diabetic ketoacidosis may follow. Serum potassium may also fall and urea and electrolytes should also be monitored. Because of these significant side-effects, great care should be taken when administering these drugs and the minimum dose required should be given. For example, ritodrine is given as an intravenous infusion and should be titrated down to the lowest possible rate to abolish uterine activity.

NSAIDs

Maternal side-effects of NSAIDs, e.g. indomethacin, include gastrointestinal bleeding, peptic ulceration, thrombocytopenia and allergic reactions. Renal function may also be impaired. Fetal side-effects when used in the long term include oligohydramnios, fetal renal impairment, premature closure of the ductus arteriosus, intraventricular haemorrhage and necrotizing enterocolitis.

Calcium channel blockers

These drugs, e.g. nifedipine, have the advantage of oral administration and fewer side-effects than some of the other agents. Profound maternal hypotension is a risk (Tsatsaris et al 2001).

Magnesium sulphate

This is commonly used in North America. Flushing, nausea, vomiting, palpitations and headaches are common maternal side-effects. Pulmonary oedema and acute respiratory distress syndrome (ARDS) are rare complications. Magnesium levels need to be monitored because of the risk of hypermagnesaemia, which may cause respiratory depression.

Oxytocin antagonists

This is a new class of drugs, e.g. atosiban, that appear to have fewer side-effects than other agents, but with similar efficacy.

Corticosteroids

Corticosteroids may be administered in pregnancy for pre-existing maternal disease such as asthma, rheumatoid arthritis and other inflammatory diseases. In such patients the most usual agent is prednisolone, which crosses the placenta in relatively small quantities. It is considered safe for use in pregnancy as there is no clear evidence of adverse effect on the developing fetus. As the drugs are generally used for significant maternal disease the benefits of administration far outweigh the risks.

If corticosteroids are administered, even in moderate doses throughout pregnancy, there is a risk of maternal adrenal suppression. This results in a failure of the normal mechanism of increased endogenous corticosteroid production in labour. Women who are on long-term steroid treatment should therefore receive extra corticosteroids in labour to compensate for this. This is usually given as intravenous hydrocortisone.

Corticosteroids are used in pregnancy for fetal lung maturation in actual or threatened preterm birth. Betamethasone or dexamethasone are used, both of which cross the placenta in higher concentrations than prednisolone. Betamethasone and dexamethasone are generally given as intramuscular injections in divided doses over 24–48 hrs. Different units use widely differing regimens. Treatment with antenatal corticosteroids has been shown to be associated with a substantial reduction in the incidence of respiratory distress syndrome (Crowley 2007). The most significant effect is noticed if 48 hrs has elapsed between administration of the drug and birth. There is a significant reduction in perinatal mortality and intraventricular haemorrhage. With a single course of corticosteroids, there is substantial benefit to the fetus/neonate. However, there is increasing evidence of possible adverse effects with multiple courses.

Magnesium sulphate

Magnesium sulphate has been used in the treatment of eclampsia in North America for many years. Following a study that produced convincing evidence of its effectiveness (Eclampsia Trial Collaborative Group 1995), it has become widely used in the UK for the treatment of eclampsia. It probably exerts its effect by acting as a cerebral vasodilator, thereby reversing cerebral vasospasm and increasing cerebral blood flow. Magnesium sulphate can be given intramuscularly or intravenously. There is no consensus as to the dosing regimen, but care should be taken to avoid magnesium toxicity. Because of this, some units monitor serum magnesium levels and aim to keep them below the threshold for toxicity, which is around 5 mmol/L. The clinical signs of magnesium toxicity are loss of the patellar reflexes, a feeling of flushing, somnolence, slurred speech, respiratory difficulty and, in extreme cases, cardiac arrest. The 'antidote' to magnesium sulphate is calcium gluconate, which is given intravenously when there is evidence of magnesium toxicity.

Some principles for managing drugs during pregnancy are listed in Box 49.1.

Box 49.1 Principles of managing drugs in pregnancy

- Avoid drugs where possible in the first trimester
- Provide pre-pregnancy counselling where feasible
- Do not stop long term drugs abruptly without medical advice
- Choose safe options where possible
- Inform women of the possible risks (if any) when starting new drugs
- When a woman has been exposed to a teratogen in the first trimester give as much information as possible about outcome to enable informed choice.

Drugs used in labour and the immediate puerperium

Prostaglandins

Prostaglandins are lipid molecules responsible for multiple physiological subcellular reactions. They also play a part in some pathological processes. The prostaglandins important in labour and the puerperium are PGE and PGF. They can be administered by any route but have significant side-effects when given orally.

Prostaglandin E_2

This is generally given by the vaginal route because of the relative lack of side-effects from this route. It is used for induction of labour and acts on both the cervix and the myometrium. The action on the cervix is not completely understood, but there is probably an alteration in the composition of the cervix as occurs in cervical ripening (Arias 2000). It is given in the form of gel or tablets that are modified-release preparations. Repeat doses should not be given within the time interval determined by the preparation because of the risk of uterine hyperstimulation. There is a potentiation of myometrial stimulation with oxytocin; therefore oxytocin should not be given within at least 3–6 hrs of prostaglandin because of the risk of uterine hyperstimulation.

Misoprostol

Misoprostol is a prostaglandin E analogue. It is now widely used for cervical ripening and for management of postpartum haemorrhage. For these purposes it is usually administered vaginally. It is a useful drug world-wide because it is relatively cheap and does not have to be refrigerated. However, it is not licensed for obstetric indications.

Prostaglandin $F_2\alpha$

This is used for the treatment of postpartum haemorrhage. It acts on the myometrium as a powerful contractile agent. The available preparation is carboprost, which is an analogue of $PGF_2\alpha$. This is given either intramuscularly or intramyometrially in cases of uterine atony.

Oxytocin

Oxytocin is a naturally occurring hormone that exerts a stimulatory effect on myometrial contractility. The effect of oxytocin on the myometrium is mainly dependent on the concentration of oxytocin receptors present. Receptors are not present in non-pregnant myometrium; they appear at around 13 weeks of pregnancy and increase in concentration until term. The highest concentration is in the uterine fundus. Synthetic oxytocin is given antenatally to aid uterine contractility, either in induction of labour or in augmentation of labour, or postpartum for prevention or treatment of uterine atony.

Oxytocin can be given by any parenteral route. In labour, it is generally given by intravenous infusion in order that the amount given can be titrated against its effect. It takes 20–30 min for oxytocin to reach a steady state and the rate of infusion of oxytocin should therefore not be increased at time intervals <30 min. The half-life of oxytocin is 10–12 min (Arias 2000). For treatment and prevention of postpartum haemorrhage, larger doses of oxytocin can be given either by intravenous or intramuscular bolus or by intravenous infusion. Care should be taken when administering intravenous bolus doses, which should be given by slow injection.

The major side-effect of oxytocin is water retention and hyponatraemia, which is particularly relevant in women with pre-eclampsia. This effect is compounded when the vehicle for administration of oxytocin is 5% dextrose.

Ergometrine

This is used in the treatment and prevention of postpartum haemorrhage. It is a powerful constrictor of smooth muscle and therefore causes myometrial contraction. It does, however, have the significant side-effects of nausea, vomiting and hypertension. In women with pre-eclampsia it is generally considered to be contraindicated except in exceptional circumstances because of the risk of severe hypertension.

It can be given intramuscularly (i.m.) or intravenously (i.v.). One of the benefits of ergometrine is that it has a sustained action, up to 2–3 hrs. In many areas Syntometrine (oxytocin 5 IU/mL with ergometrine 0.5 mg) is given i.m. for the third stage of labour. This has the advantage of the speed of action of oxytocin (within 3 min) and the sustained action of ergometrine. The disadvantage is the side-effect profile of the ergometrine (see Ch. 29).

Drugs and breastfeeding

It is important to remember that the concerns with drugs do not cease after birth. This applies not only to healthcare professionals but also to the women themselves who may be more relaxed about what they take after the baby has been born.

Most drugs will pass into breastmilk in greater or lesser concentrations. This is not, however, the most important factor in determining the potential effect on the baby – it is the concentration in the infant's serum that matters. This in turn will depend on the metabolism of the drug within the infant, which will be different to that in the adult.

The amount of a substance passing into breast milk will also depend on the timing of dosing in relation to feeds. Whether the drug is water or fat soluble will determine whether there are higher concentrations in foremilk or hindmilk, and the feeding pattern of the infant will affect how much of the drug is received. Thus a mother taking a largely fat-soluble drug will pass more to an infant that feeds for prolonged periods than to one who feeds little and often because of the relative amounts of the hindmilk consumed.

A detailed list of drugs and whether or not they are safe in breastfeeding is outside the scope of this chapter. Details can be found from the Further reading list, below.

Drugs that may affect milk production

Some drugs may adversely affect milk production and are therefore not recommended in breastfeeding. The most commonly encountered drugs that have this effect are:

- oestrogen: the combined contraceptive pill is therefore contraindicated
- bromocriptine and cabergoline
- large doses of thiazide diuretics (e.g. bendroflumethiazide (bendrofluazide)), although the normal pharmacological doses are probably safe
- ergotamine (used in treatment of migraine).

The law, midwives and medicines

Midwives are subject to legislation relating to prescriptions, supply and medicines management (NMC 2007) and to the Midwives rules (NMC 2004, rule 7). Midwives are also expected to comply with the NMC Code (2008).

The Medicines Act 1968

In the UK, the legislation relating to the prescribing, supply and administration of medicines is set out in the Medicines Act 1968 and in subsequent secondary (amendments) legislation. Medicines are divided into three categories:

- prescription-only medicines (POMs)
- pharmacy medicines (P)
- general sale list (GSL).

Specific drugs, including those normally available only on a prescription, may be supplied to midwives for use in their practice. Midwives are therefore recognized as being exempt from certain restrictions on the sale or supply of medicines under this Act. The products that a midwife can supply and administer have to be from an approved list and include:

- antiseptics
- aperients
- sedatives and analgesics
- local anaesthetic
- oxytocic preparation
- approved agents for neonatal and maternal resuscitation.

The Misuse of Drugs Act 1971

This Act covers drugs liable to misuse. Drugs subject to the Act's control are termed 'controlled drugs' and are separated into three classes, A, B or C, depending upon their level of control. Medicinal products containing controlled drugs are still subject to the Medicines Act and are all listed as POMs. They are divided into five schedules which relate to the safe custody, documentation, keeping of records and procedure for destruction.

The Misuse of Drugs Regulations

The Misuse of Drugs Regulations 1973, the Misuse of Drugs (Amendment) Regulations 1974, the Misuse of Drugs Regulations 1985, 2001 and the Misuse of Drugs (Northern Ireland) Regulations 2002, have permitted registered midwives to possess and administer controlled drugs in their professional practice. Subsequent POM Orders specify the list of drugs that can be supplied to midwives for administration without a doctor's prescription. The Health Act (2006) clarifies regulations for governance and monitoring of controlled drugs (see: http://www.dh.gov.uk/en/Publicationsandstatistics/Legislation/Regulatoryimpactassessment/DH 074272).

Supply order procedure and standing orders

Midwives in community practice must use the supply order procedure. With an increase in the illicit use of controlled drugs and the reduction in home births, midwives may prefer not to store and carry controlled drugs themselves but instead ask individual women planning to birth at home to seek a prescription for diamorphine, morphine, pethidine or pentazocine from their GP. In circumstances where a woman is transferred to hospital, drugs obtained under the supply order procedure may not be used. In-hospital local policies, although not required under legislation, have been developed as they provide clear guidelines as to best practice. These policies have traditionally been called 'standing orders' but it is now recommended that these are converted to Patient Group Direction (PGD) where the medication is not already subject to Exemption Order legislation.

Patient group directions and non-medical prescribing

In 1989 the first Crown report (DoH 1989) was published. This extended the power of prescribing a very limited set of medicines to district nurses and health visitors. It also recommended the supply of certain medicines under group protocols.

In 1998 a report (DoH 1998) was published to tighten regulations relating to group protocols. As a consequence the POM Amendment Order 2000 came into force clarifying the meaning of a 'patient group direction' (PGD), which replaced the use of group protocols. In England a Health Service Circular was issued (DoH 2000) to instruct Chief Executives to 'ensure that any current or new patient group directions comply with new legal requirements' (p 2). This circular also clarified that midwives are already exempt from certain requirements of the Medicines Act and this was further clarified by an NMC Circular (NMC 2005) entitled 'Medicine legislation, what it means for midwives'. This includes an explanation that whilst 'Standing Orders' is not a legal definition they have often been used to provide local guidelines.

The 1999 Crown report (DoH 1999) recommended extending the authorized list of prescribers, which includes midwives, and establishing two new categories of prescribers:

Independent prescribers

Midwives who have successfully undertaken an approved programme are permitted to make a diagnosis and prescribe the appropriate medication. This includes all POMs including some controlled drugs but must be within their field of expertise and competence.

Supplementary prescribers

Midwives may, where a doctor has made the initial assessment, go on to review the medication and make changes if appropriate to the woman's clinical care plan.

The formulary used by non-medical authorized prescribers was initially limited but is now so extensive that it is essential that prescribers' pharmacology knowledge and expertise is kept updated and regular reference made to the British National Formulary (see: http://www.bnf.org/) and Department of Health policy and guidance websites.

Administration of medicines and record-keeping

It is vital that, for the safety and well-being of the woman, all prescriptions for medication are legible and clear in their instruction. It is equally important that prescribed medicines are given at the appropriate time. This may be crucial in achieving the correct concentration of drug in the circulation. When drugs are administered this should be recorded in a legible fashion. Clarity and legibility are essential for safety. Where women are self-medicating, care should be taken to explain to the woman the importance of dosage and timing and ideally she should record her own medications.

To minimize the risk of human error in the administration of medicines, employers will normally have written policies, protocols and procedures. It is essential that midwives comply with these, and if in doubt about a drug or its dosage prescribed by another practitioner then advice should be sought before it is administered. The consent of the recipient, or parent of a baby, must be obtained before any medicine is given. As well as carefully checking that the drug and dosage are correct, the midwife must also check the expiry date.

The NMC emphasizes the importance of accurate record keeping. Midwives must adhere to the rules, standards, codes and local policy in relation to record keeping. Each midwife's supervisor of midwives will periodically audit records to maintain and improve standards of practice.

REFERENCES

Arias F 2000 Pharmacology of oxytocin and prostaglandins. Clinical Obstetrics and Gynecology 43:455–468

Briggs G G, Freeman R K, Yaffe S J 2005 Drugs in pregnancy and lactation, 7th edn. Lippincott, Baltimore

Butters L, Kennedy S, Rubin P C 1991 Atenolol in essential hypertension during pregnancy. British Medical Journal 301:587–589

CLASP Collaborative Group 1994 CLASP: a randomised trial of low dose aspirin for the prevention and treatment of pre-eclampsia among 9364 pregnant women. Lancet 343:619–629

Cooper W O, Hernandez-Diaz S, Arbogast P G et al 2006 Major congenital malformations after first-trimester exposure to ACE inhibitors. New England Journal of Medicine 354:2443–2451

Crowley 2007 Prophylactic corticosteroids for preterm birth. Cochrane Pregnancy and Childbirth Group Cochrane Database of Systematic Reviews, Issue 3

DoH (Department of Health) 1989 Report on nurse prescribing and supply. Advisory group chaired by Dr June Crown. HMSO, London

DoH (Department of Health) 1998 Review of prescribing, supply and administration of medicines: a report on the supply and administration of medicines under group protocols. Stationery Office, London

DoH (Department of Health) 1999 Final report on the prescribing, supply and administration of medicines. Chaired by Dr June Crown. Stationery Office, London

DoH (Department of Health) 2000 Health service circular 2000/026. Patient group directions [England only]. Stationery Office, London

Dunlop W 1976 Investigations into the influence of posture in renal plasma flow and glomerular filtration rate during late pregnancy. British Journal of Obstetrics and Gynaecology 83:17–23

Eclampsia Trial Collaborative Group 1995 Which anticonvulsant for women with eclampsia? Evidence from the Collaborative Eclampsia Trial. Lancet 345:1455–1463

Einarson A, Maltepe C, Navioz Y et al 2004. The safety of ondansetron for nausea and vomiting of pregnancy: a prospective comparative study. British Journal of Obstetrics and Gynaecology 111:940–943

Kreft-Jais C, Plouin P F, Tchobroutsky C et al 1988 Angiotensin-converting enzyme inhibitors during pregnancy: a survey of 22 patients given captopril and 9 given enalapril. British Journal of Obstetrics and Gynaecology 95:420–422

Lin R, Hu Z-W 2000 Hematologic disorders. In: Carruthers S G, Hoffman B B, Melmon K L et al (eds) Melmon and Morelli's clinical pharmacology, 4th edn. McGraw-Hill, New York, p 737–797

Lumley J, Watson L, Watson M et al 2000 Periconceptional supplementation with folate and/or multivitamins for preventing neural tube defects. Cochrane Database of Systematic Reviews, Issue 1. Update Software, Oxford

McFadyen I R 1989 Maternal changes in normal pregnancy. In: Turnbull A, Chamberlain G (eds) Obstetrics. Churchill Livingstone, London, p 151–171

Medicines Act 1968 HMSO, London

Misuse of Drugs Act 1971 HMSO, London

Misuse of Drugs Regulations 1973, 1974, 1985, 1986 HMSO, London

NMC (Nursing and Midwifery Council) 2004 Midwives rules and standards. NMC, London

NMC (Nursing and Midwifery Council) 2005 Circular 1. Medicine legislation, what it means for midwives. NMC, London

NMC (Nursing and Midwifery Council) 2007 Standards for medicines management. NMC, London

NMC (Nursing and Midwifery Council) 2008 The Code: standards of conduct, performance and ethics for nurses and midwives. NMC, London

Norton M E, Merrill J, Cooper B A B et al 1991 Neonatal complications after the administration of indomethacin for preterm labour. New England Journal of Medicine 329:1602–1607

Parry E, Shields R, Turnbull A C 1970 Transit time in small intestine in pregnancy. Journal of Obstetrics and Gynaecology of the British Commonwealth 77:900–901

RCOG 2007 Green top guideline No. 28. Thromboembolic disease in pregnancy and the puerperium: Acute management. RCOG, London

Tsatsaris V, Papatsonis D, Goffinet F et al 2001 Tocolysis with nifedipine or beta-adrenergic agonist: a meta-analysis. Obstetrics and Gynecology 97:840–847

Waisman G D, Mayorga L M, Camera M I et al 1988 Magnesium plus nifedipine: potentiation of hypotensive effect in pre-eclampsia? American Journal of Obstetrics and Gynecology 171:417–424

Weiner C P, Buhimschi C. 2004. Drugs for pregnant and lactating women. Churchill Livingstone, Edinburgh

Wogelius P, Nørgaard M, Munk E M et al 2005. Maternal use of selective serotonin reuptake inhibitors and risk of adverse pregnancy outcome. Pharmacoepidemiology and Drug Safety14:S72–S73

FURTHER READING

Rubin P C, Ramsay M 2007. Prescribing in pregnancy, 4th edn. Wiley Blackwell, London.

A short, readable text discussing the use of drugs in pregnancy.

50 Complementary therapies in midwifery

Denise Tiran

CHAPTER CONTENTS

The use of complementary therapies has become more widespread and therefore it is essential that midwives have an understanding of the principal complementary therapies in use and their possible application to the care of pregnant and childbearing women.

This chapter aims to:

- provide an introduction to complementary therapies and their application to the care of pregnant and childbearing women
- debate professional accountability issues for midwives wishing to implement complementary therapies in their practice
- discuss cautions, precautions and contraindications of using complementary therapies during pregnancy, labour and the puerperium
- explore selected symptoms and conditions of pregnancy and childbirth which may respond to complementary therapies.

Introduction

Complementary therapies (CTs) are increasingly popular with both consumers and professionals and are based on a philosophy of holism and an interaction between body, mind and spirit in which it is believed that all components in combination contribute to the whole. Within midwifery, use of CTs has been driven by mothers looking for strategies to help them cope with pregnancy and labour discomforts and to aid relaxation. It is thought that as many as three quarters of women may self-administer substances such as herbal, homeopathic, aromatherapy or Bach flower remedies (Refuerzo et al 2005), and it has previously been estimated that over a third of midwives use CTs in their practice (NHS Confederation 1997), although this figure is likely to have been exceeded in the last few years.

Classification of complementary therapies

There are in excess of 200 therapies considered complementary – or perhaps, alternative – to mainstream healthcare, the top 20 or so most commonly in use in Britain being classified by the House of Lords (2000) into three main groups.

Group 1 therapies are professionally organized, complete systems of healthcare with national standards of education, statutory or voluntary self-regulation, disciplinary codes of practice and a reasonable body of research evidence.

Osteopathy has been statutorily regulated since 1993 by the General Osteopathic Council and is based on the principle that misalignments of the neuromusculoskeletal system adversely affect homeostasis; treatment aims to re-align and re-balance the whole person. *Craniosacral therapy*, or *cranial osteopathy*, a branch of osteopathy, uses gentle manipulation of the bones of the skull, meningeal membranes and nerve endings in the scalp to re-balance the cranial rhythmic impulse, running throughout the body, and has been used effectively to treat infants with colic (Hayden & Mullinger 2006).

Chiropractic has been statutorily regulated since 1994 by the General Chiropractic Council and is similar to osteopathy. The main difference is that osteopaths are concerned with mobility of joints whereas chiropractors deal with relative positions of joints. Different manipulative techniques are used and many chiropractors use more X-rays to aid diagnosis (although not during pregnancy). Osteopaths also use more soft tissue massage prior to manipulation than chiropractors. Both osteopathy and chiropractic can be useful techniques for pregnant women with musculoskeletal problems such as backache, sciatica, symphysis pubis discomfort and carpal tunnel syndrome, as well as soft tissue disorders including hyperemesis, heartburn, indigestion and constipation

(Lisi 2006, Wang et al 2005). In addition, obstetric conditions such as breech presentation are thought by these practitioners to result from misalignment of the spine and bony pelvis, causing an accentuated angle of inclination of the pelvic brim, which may be corrected with either osteopathy or chiropractic.

Acupuncture, regulated by the British Acupuncture Council (BAcC), works on the principle that the body has energy lines (meridians) running through it which pass through a major organ, after which they take their name, e.g. Bladder meridian, Kidney meridian, linking one part of the body to another. In optimum health, the energy flows freely around the body, but physical, mental, emotional or spiritual disorder causes blockages or excesses of energy. Acupuncture, the insertion of needles, attempts to correct this imbalance. Sometimes thumb pressure is applied to the points (acupressure); on other occasions, heat is used to stimulate deficient energy via moxa sticks (see moxibustion for *breech presentation*) or suction can be used to draw out excess energy by covering the points with special cups (cupping). Acupuncture needles may also be stimulated with mild electrical pulsations, similar to transcutaneous nerve stimulation. Certain points are contraindicated antenatally as they may trigger contractions, but acupuncture can be used to treat many pregnancy conditions including hyperemesis, backache and varicosities, while intrapartum use may facilitate progress and ease pain, anxiety and tension.

Herbal medicine: Most practitioners are registered with the National Institute of Medical Herbalists (NIMH) or the European Herbal Practitioners' Association (EHPA). Herbal medicine involves the therapeutic use of plants in various forms, which work pharmacologically. There is a common misconception that because herbal remedies are natural they are automatically safe but there is now a growing body of evidence about the risks of possible interactions between herbal and conventional medicines. Many herbal remedies should be avoided during the preconception and antenatal periods and when breastfeeding, because they may induce uterine bleeding or other systemic effects on the mother or because fetal effects are unknown, e.g. St John's wort, blue cohosh and kava kava, and others which should be used with caution, including raspberry leaf (Tiran 2003a, 2005a) (see Box 50.1).

Box 50.1 Safe use of herbal remedies in pregnancy

- Ask at booking if the mother is taking any herbal remedies
- As a general rule, avoid herbal remedies in the first trimester unless on expert advice
- Culinary use of herbs and herbal teas are generally safe in normal amounts
- Herbal remedies act *pharmacologically*, therefore may interact with prescribed medications
- Do not take herbal remedies routinely as a prophylactic or for prolonged periods of time as side-effects may occur
- Avoid *all* herbal remedies if there is a history of clotting disorders or bleeding, e.g. APH, or if taking anticoagulants or NSAIDs
- Avoid *all* herbal remedies if there is a history of diabetes, epilepsy, cardiac disease, hypertension
- Avoid *all* herbal remedies with pre-eclampsia, multiple pregnancy, IVF pregnancy or other major obstetric complication
- *Discontinue all* herbal remedies at least 2 weeks before elective caesarean or other surgery
- Aromatherapy essential oils are herbal substances and should also be used with caution
- Herbal remedies are *not* the same as homeopathic medicines
- If in doubt seek expert advice.

Adapted from Tiran 2005a with permission from Expectancy Ltd.

Homeopathy: Homeopathy is not the same as herbal medicine but is a form of 'energy' medicine which uses minute, highly diluted doses of substances that, if given in the full dose, would actually cause the symptoms being treated. For example, a highly diluted form of arsenic is used to treat certain types of severe vomiting and diarrhoea, yet ingesting arsenic could actually cause these symptoms. Most homeopathic medicines are in tablet form but do not work pharmacologically and will not interact with prescribed drugs, although certain drugs may inactivate the homeopathic remedies, since they are chemically fragile. Homeopathy treats the whole person and takes into account the personality of

the individual, as well as any factors which increase or reduce the symptoms. It is not however, completely 'harmless' since it can be very powerful; inappropriate or prolonged use of an incorrect remedy can cause a 'reverse proving' in which the person starts to develop the symptoms for which the remedy is intended. It is therefore important to inform women how to take homeopathic remedies correctly (Box 50.2). Medically-qualified homeopaths are registered with the Faculty of Homeopathy; lay or classical homeopaths are primarily registered with the Society of Homeopaths.

Group 2 therapies are complementary or supportive to other healthcare, with less available evidence; many therapies are in the process of regulatory development but it is not yet mandatory to be nationally regulated; most organizations have chosen voluntary self-regulation. Many group 2 therapies are practised by midwives, nurses and physiotherapists, as they lend themselves to incorporation alongside

Box 50.2 Advice on correct administration of homeopathic remedies

- Take only one remedy at a time
- Remedies must be chosen according to the *precise* nature of the individual's symptoms
- Use the 30C strength in pregnancy unless advised differently by a qualified homeopath
- Tip the tablet into the lid of the bottle – do not allow anyone other than the patient to handle it
- Do not use a metal spoon, as metal inactivates the remedy
- The mouth should be clear of food, drink, toothpaste (and cigarettes) for 15 min before and after taking each remedy
- Tablets should be dissolved under the tongue, not swallowed
- Normal dose is one tablet 3–4 times a day
- To increase the dose tablets should be taken more *frequently*, *not* by taking more tablets each time
- If there is no improvement after 5 days, *stop* the remedy and consult an expert.

Adapted from Tiran 2005b with permission from Expectancy Ltd.

conventional care, but these therapies are not normally classified as discrete systems of treatment.

Aromatherapy, regulated by the Aromatherapy Council, involves the use of highly concentrated plant essential oils administered via the skin (massage, water or compresses), via the respiratory tract (inhalations and vaporizers), via mucous membranes (pessaries and suppositories) and, occasionally, via the gastrointestinal tract (orally). Clinical aromatherapy combines the therapeutic properties of the oils' chemical constituents with mood-enhancing effects of the aromas and relaxation effects of the administration method, particularly massage. Essential oil molecules enter the body when the aromas are inhaled, reaching the limbic centre in the brain, the circulation and major organs: this is important to remember when essential oils are used in the maternity unit, as all people exposed to the aromas will be inhaling the chemicals and could, theoretically, be adversely affected, e.g. pregnant staff or epileptic relatives. All essential oils act in the same way as pharmaceutical drugs, being absorbed, metabolized and excreted via similar biochemical pathways, and may therefore theoretically interact with prescribed medications. Essential oils are largely assumed to be safe in pregnancy because there is no real evidence to the contrary, but midwives should continue to be cautious when advising expectant mothers about their uses (Tiran 2007). Inappropriate or inaccurate use may cause dermal irritation, photosensitivity, or changes in blood pressure, temperature or fluid balance. There are many oils which should not be used in pregnancy, although some may be used in labour and postnatally (see Tiran 2000, 2004a). Essential oils should not be used on neonates: the universal antibacterial action of essential oils may adversely affect the baby's extrauterine immunological development, the aromas may interfere with the mother–infant 'bonding' process which relies partly on odour recognition and some chemical constituents may cause skin irritation. Antenatal aromatherapy treatments can aid relaxation, thereby reducing the possible adverse effects of maternal anxiety on the fetus (Bastard & Tiran 2006).

Reflexology/reflex zone therapy involves precise pressure point manipulation, sedation and stimulation and is based on the principle that one small part of the body represents a map of the whole, such as the feet, hands, back, face, tongue or ear; it is not simply foot massage. Reflexology is widely thought to work via acupuncture meridians, although there are several other theories regarding its mechanism of action, and the zones may have a part to play in facilitating identification of changing physiopathology, aiding diagnosis (Tiran & Chummun 2005). Reflexology is a powerful therapy that can be very effective when used appropriately, but there are some contraindications, precautions and possible side-effects and complications of treatment (see Tiran 2002). Pregnant women often have very rapid and very profound reactions to reflexology so midwives should advise women to consult practitioners who have relevant training and experience to treat expectant mothers. Small scale research studies suggest it may be useful towards term to improve labour outcomes, and for oedematous ankles (McNeill et al 2006, Mollart 2003). Reflexology is not yet formally regulated.

Massage is the applied use of touch – there are many different forms, including traditional Swedish massage, lymphatic drainage, Hawaian lomi lomi and specific deep techniques, such as Rolfing. It is not yet formally regulated. Massage has been shown to be very relaxing, reducing blood pressure and increasing excretory processes, however it is also not without risks (Box 50.3). In labour it assists in reducing pain, aiding relaxation and easing fear and tension (Chang et al 2006, McNabb et al 2006).

Shiatsu is a Japanese variation of acupressure which originated in the 1950s. It utilizes the same meridians as acupuncture and focuses on re-establishing internal energy or 'Ki'. Shiatsu is very relaxing, helping to relieve anxiety, tension and pain in pregnancy and childbirth and useful for headaches, sickness, insomnia and depression. The therapy is not yet formally regulated.

Hypnotherapy/hypnosis uses advanced 'day dreaming' and deep relaxation, incorporating techniques relating to inner consciousness to heal core causes of problems in life such as habitual behaviour. It has been successfully used to reduce pain in labour, termination of pregnancy and infertility treatment (Cyna et al 2006, Levitas et al 2006, Marc et al 2007). *Note*: Some methods of maternity hypnotherapy are referred to by trade names which are almost synonymous with the concept of childbirth

> **Box 50.3** Precautions and contraindications to massage in pregnancy
>
> - First trimester sacral and suprapubic massage
> - Brisk heel massage in pregnancy – this corresponds to the reflexology zone for the pelvic area
> - Acupressure points contraindicated in pregnancy (Gall Bladder 21, Large Intestine 4, Spleen 6, Sacral plexus points)
> - Abdominal massage if history of antepartum haemorrhage/placenta praevia
> - Severe hypotension or fainting episodes; take care when sitting up after massage
> - Caution with pre-existing medical conditions
> - Maternal wishes
> - Professional doubt.

Adapted from Tiran 2004b with permission from Expectancy Ltd.

hypnosis, in the same way that Hoover™ has become synonymous with 'vacuum cleaner'; it is important for midwives to use the generic terms 'hypnosis' or 'hypnotherapy' when advising mothers, unless they can vouch for a particular commercial method from professional experience.

Bach flower remedies encompass the healing properties of flowers used to treat disease by relieving mental and emotional symptoms thought to be its cause. Rescue Remedy is a universal anti-stress remedy and is safe to take in pregnancy, although studies of its effectiveness have been inconclusive (Armstrong & Ernst 2001, Pintov et al 2005, Walach et al 2001).

Other therapies in Group 2 include *yoga*, which focuses on harmony between the mind and body using movement, breath, posture, relaxation and meditation; *Reiki*, an holistic form of non-touch 'laying on of hands'; the *Alexander technique*, which involves adjustment and correction of habitually misaligned body posture, to relieve muscle tension and allow the body to move with greater ease and efficiency; *nutritional therapies and stress management*.

Group 3 therapies are alternative, largely unregulated therapies with little or no body of evidence, divided into two sub-groups:

Group 3a – traditional systems, e.g. Traditional Chinese Medicine (TCM), Indian Ayurvedic medicine, Tibetan medicine, Japanese kampo, anthroposophical medicine, naturopathy

Group 3b – diagnostic therapies, e.g. crystal therapy, dowsing, iridology, kinesiology, radionics.

It is not the intention of this chapter to discuss these therapies as they currently have little or no direct application or evidence base in relation to maternity care; interested readers are referred to the sources of further reading and resources at the end of the chapter.

Use of complementary therapies in maternity care

Women are the most frequent users of complementary therapies and it is natural that they should wish to continue to use different therapies once pregnant (Thomas et al 2001), although many do so without informing their midwife or doctor (Ranzini et al 2001). It would be wise for midwives to ask routinely, at booking, if the mother is using any complementary therapies or self-administering any natural remedies, in the same way as enquiring about use of prescribed and over-the-counter drugs. Expectant mothers are keen to use complementary therapies because they provide a range of additional strategies for dealing with symptoms of pregnancy at a time when drugs are largely contraindicated, especially since physiological discomforts are often dismissed by the medical profession as 'minor disorders'. Also, many women wish to achieve as natural a birth as possible without recourse to drugs for pain relief in labour and some may request the presence of a complementary practitioner at the birth. Demand for and interest in natural remedies is high and their use may empower mothers to retain control of their bodies. General dissatisfaction with many aspects of conventional maternity care and its dependence on technology, the continuing 'conveyor belt' approach to antenatal care, lack of time to individualize care and staff shortages often prevent the allocation of quality interactions with each mother for the provision of holistic care.

The integration of CTs into midwifery is well publicized (Ager 2002, Mousley 2005, Tiran 2001) and there is an increasing body of CTs research-specific to maternity care (Burns et al 2000, Ingram et al 2005, McNabb et al 2006) although the National Centre for Health and Clinical Excellence (NICE) has so far failed to recognize this and has recommended that women should be actively discouraged from using natural remedies during pregnancy (National Collaborating Centre 2003), even though many will do so despite professional advice to the contrary, possibly compromising maternal or fetal well-being (Tiran 2005c).

Professional accountability of the midwife

Midwives wishing to incorporate CTs in their practice must work within Nursing and Midwifery Council (NMC) guidelines. The NMC cannot regulate CTs practice except when it is used in conjunction with midwifery, nursing or health visiting registration, but various documents provide guidance on the use of CTs by its registrants. The Midwives Rules and Standards (NMC 2004) advise the midwife to 'look to the best available evidence' of safety and efficacy in order to provide women with appropriate advice and discuss with the mother if the use of substances such as essential oils, herbal or homeopathic remedies is inappropriate (Rule 7, p 21). In the UK, the NMC (2008) requires registrants to ensure competence in both knowledge and skills to provide safe, effective and lawful practice and to acknowledge personal professional boundaries. The midwife must be able to demonstrate that she is 'adequately and appropriately' trained to use the therapy, although this does not necessarily mean that she must be a fully qualified practitioner (Tiran 2006a). It is permissible, for example, to learn to use a small selection of aromatherapy essential oils without being a trained aromatherapist, but the individual remains accountable for her midwifery practice and must be able to justify her actions. The use of CTs must not be at the expense of normal midwifery responsibilities, but rather should be considered an adjunct to other care. Informed maternal consent is essential, although this can be verbal consent. Women have the right to use and self-administer natural remedies, and midwives should try to act as the mother's advocate, but if there is doubt regarding the appropriateness of using a particular remedy, midwives should consult an expert practitioner for advice. In units where midwives wish to implement the use of a therapy alongside their existing practice, policies and protocols should be developed, even if there is only one midwife practising, for example acupuncture, and it is recommended that midwives' use of CTs should be monitored via the annual supervisory review (Tiran 2007). Communication and liaison with colleagues are vital to avoid conflict and attempt to dispel scepticism (see Box 50.4).

Box 50.4 Case scenario 1: Adequate education and training of midwives using complementary therapies is essential

I recently met with a small group of midwives who were implementing the use of reflexology into their practice. During discussion, I heard that the midwives were using a reflexology technique to turn breech presentation fetuses to cephalic. On further questioning, however, it transpired that the midwives had attended a study day organized by a beauty therapy school and that a male therapist, who did not specialize in caring for pregnant women, had shown them how to perform a simple technique on the little toes, which he said would cause the fetus to turn.

I asked the midwives to explain further and was concerned to learn that what they were doing was not, in fact, reflexology but was *acupressure*, based on the Bladder 67 point, as used in moxibustion. The midwives were totally unaware of this fact and, indeed, were not even able to identify exactly which *reflexology* points they thought they were stimulating. They had happily returned to their unit and started to use the 'reflexology' (an assumption made presumably because they were working on the feet) on women with breech presentations. There were no guidelines outlining parameters for their practice and, because of her own lack of knowledge, the manager/supervisor was allowing them to pursue a potentially unsafe practice.

The midwife's responsibilities when caring for women receiving complementary therapies from an independent practitioner

The Nursing and Midwifery Order (2001) forbids anyone other than a midwife or doctor, or one in training under supervision, from taking sole responsibility for the care of a childbearing mother, except in an emergency, therefore any therapies used at this time must be complementary, rather than alternative, to conventional maternity care. Where women choose to consult independent complementary practitioners the midwife should advise them to ensure that the therapist has a thorough understanding of pregnancy physiopathology and the therapist's role within conventional maternity services. Access to private therapists should preferably be through recommendation, although midwives would be wise to refrain from naming individuals unless they can vouch for their expertise. Mothers wishing to find a therapist should be advised to ask, when making the first appointment, for evidence of appropriate qualifications, relevant experience of treating pregnant women and professional indemnity insurance cover. Any therapist who is unwilling to disclose this information should be rejected.

If a therapist is to be present during labour, s/he must acknowledge that the midwife and/or doctor, legally retains overall responsibility for the woman's care. Many units ask the therapist to sign a disclaimer form stating that they will not rely on the hospital's vicarious liability insurance cover and that they agree to discontinue treatment if requested to do so by the midwife. The midwife should ensure that she is aware of any natural remedies administered, especially those which work pharmacologically such as essential oils and herbal remedies, and record this in the notes and on the cardiotocograph tracing as appropriate, even though she may not understand the mechanism of action. She cannot, of course, take responsibility for the actions of others but should ensure that all care is in the best interests of the mother and baby.

Complementary therapies for pregnancy and childbirth

Nausea and vomiting

Ginger is a well-known traditional herbal remedy for sickness and there is considerable research to demonstrate that it is an effective antiemetic (Jewell & Young 2003, Vutyavanich et al 2001, Willetts et al 2003), although other studies have disputed these claims (Arfeen et al 1995, Visalyaputra et al 1998). However, ginger is not suitable or safe for all women and may exacerbate nausea and cause heartburn (see Box 50-5). Ginger biscuits, an almost universal 'tip', should not be advised as any temporary improvement in nausea is attributable to the sugar, since there is insufficient ginger for any real therapeutic effect; furthermore, the sugar is likely to trigger peaks and troughs in serum glucose levels, making symptoms worse. There is increasing professional concern over the safety of herbal remedies in general (Marcus & Snodgrass 2005) and ginger in particular (Portnoi et al 2003, Tiran & Budd 2005), especially in relation to its effects on clotting times. Women who require ginger continuously for more than 3 weeks should be advised to request an investigation of blood clotting factors; those on prescribed medications, notably anticoagulants, antihypertensives and non-steroidal antiinflammatories should avoid ginger. An alternative remedy to ginger is peppermint, although this should not be taken by those with cardiac disease, epilepsy or concomitantly with homeopathic remedies.

Certain homeopathic remedies may be effective but need to be prescribed according to the precise symptoms of the individual mother. Examples include nux vomica, for women whose symptoms are worse in the morning and who tend to be 'workaholics'; ipecacuanha in severe cases with incessant vomiting and heartburn; cocculus, the remedy of choice when nausea is made worse by movement; colchicum for women who feel nauseated by odours; and pulsatilla for those whose symptoms and moods keep changing. There is no real evidence for the effectiveness of homeopathic remedies for nausea and vomiting in pregnancy, but anecdotal reports suggest that, when the remedies are prescribed appropriately, they do produce positive results, although whether or not this is a placebo effect is difficult to ascertain.

Many women are familiar with travel sickness wristbands, which work on the Pericardium 6 (PC6) acupressure point on the wrist. The PC-6 point is found by measuring, with the mother's own fingers, three fingers' width up from the inner wrist crease where the hand joins the arm, approximately where

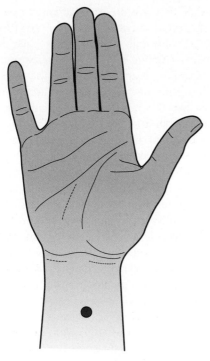

Figure 50.1 Diagram to show how to locate Pericardium 6 acupressure point. Use mother's own fingers to measure three finger widths up from the crease where the hand and the wrist meet, between the tendons on the inner wrist.

the buckle of a watch strap might rest (Fig. 50.1). The point is between the tendons and there should be a slight dip and some sensation of tenderness or bruising when the point is pressed, which is worse the more severe the sickness. The bands should be placed on both wrists prior to rising in the morning and should remain in position for the duration of the symptoms. This is a simple means of relieving sickness for many women, but acupuncture can also be effective; a qualified acupuncturist would take into account all imbalances within the body and may need to work on additional points, for example those on the Stomach, Spleen or Conception Vessel meridians. There are numerous research studies which have shown that P6 acupressure and/or acupuncture can be effective for reducing or eliminating nausea and vomiting, not only in pregnancy but also for sickness of other aetiology. For a comprehensive exploration of complementary therapies for nausea and vomiting in pregnancy, see Tiran 2003b.

Box 50.5 Case scenario 2: A little knowledge is a dangerous thing

The complementary therapy (CT) midwife saw Jean in her clinic for the treatment of severe nausea and vomiting persisting to 19 weeks' gestation. Jean knew about certain possible natural remedies for the problem and had thought that ginger may help, but found that this had made the sickness worse. The CT midwife advised her about acupressure to the PC-6 point. However, the midwife was horrified when Jean said that her sister had told her about the acupuncture point in the webbing between forefinger and thumb (LI-4 point) – and started to demonstrate by stimulating the point vigorously. Jean was unaware of the fact that stimulation of this point could potentially trigger uterine contractions and also, like most women, had not known that ginger may exacerbate sickness if used inappropriately.

Breech presentation

The use of moxibustion for breech presentation is gaining popularity in the UK. In this technique, a stick of dried mugwort herb is used as a heat source over the Bladder 67 acupuncture point on the outer edges of the little toes. This is thought to stimulate adrenocortical output, resulting in increases in placental lactogens and changes in prostaglandins, increasing myometrial sensitivity and contractility, which in turn increases the fetal heart rate and movements, causing the fetus to turn to cephalic. The procedure is normally done around 34–35 weeks' gestation and performed for 15 min on both feet, twice daily for up to 5 days (10 treatments). The mother can be taught to do this at home with help from her partner but must be advised that, if she believes the fetus may have turned during the course of the treatment, she should refrain from doing further treatments until the presentation has been checked by the midwife.

Several trials have shown statistically significant results ranging from 66% to 87% (Cardini et al 2005, Cardini & Weixin 1998). The number of cephalic births at term is greatest in the moxibustion group in these trials, despite the number of spontaneous versions and reversions, and appears to be more successful than external cephalic version (ECV). One

Japanese study, rather unrealistically, achieved a 92% success rate, but this was from 28 weeks' gestation, when it can be assumed that some apparently successful versions would revert spontaneously (Kanakura et al 2001). Although a few midwives now offer moxa to turn breech presentations, this is worthy of further development within midwifery practice for it provides a cost-effective alternative to caesarean section, is possibly safer than ECV and enables the mother to feel in control of her situation, although a Cochrane review (Coyle et al 2005) found insufficient evidence of effectiveness and safety to advocate its use within conventional maternity care. A multicentre moxibustion trial amongst acupuncturists is ongoing at the time of writing (Grabowska 2006), but it is of concern that acupuncturists do not receive adequate training to ensure that the presentation is still breech prior to the procedure, nor do they appreciate the exclusion criteria, which are similar to those for ECV. Needling by acupuncturists may also be effective in turning a breech presentation to cephalic. Moxibustion in conjunction with acupuncture has, however, shown some promising results in converting the breech to cephalic (Neri et al 2007, 2004), without any apparent adverse effects in the fetus.

Other methods of converting the breech include ginger paste, a Chinese 'hot' remedy used instead of burning moxa sticks (Tiran 2004c), homeopathic remedies such as pulsatilla or natrum muriaticum, the chiropractic Webster technique (Pistolese 2002) or hypnosis (Mehl 1994). The exaggerated Sim's, or knee chest position, has not been found to be statistically significant in isolation for turning the breech to cephalic, but may improve the success rate of other methods if done immediately before procedures such as moxibustion or even ECV (Hofmeyr & Kulier 2002, Smith et al 1999) as may fetal acoustic stimulation (music) (Annapoorna et al 1997).

Use of complementary therapies for labour

CTs offer an excellent adjunct to the midwife's normal labour care, with the nurturing therapies such as massage, aromatherapy and reflexology really coming into their own. One of the largest studies in aromatherapy was undertaken by midwives at the John Radcliffe Hospital, Oxford over a 9-year period, where they used 12 essential oils on self-selected labouring women, for pain relief, to ease fear and anxiety, facilitate uterine action and reduce nausea (Burns et al 2000). Although this was not a randomized controlled trial and, as such, has been excluded from the NICE guidelines on caring for women in normal labour (NICE 2006), over 8000 women received intrapartum aromatherapy; results showed a reduction in analgesia use, increased maternal and staff satisfaction and a <1% incidence of side-effects. A more recent pilot study on the neurophysiological effects of massage on pain in labour (McNabb et al 2006) has shown promising results and a full scale trial is pending (Kimber, pers comm). Reflexology performed in late pregnancy appears to have positive effects on labour duration and outcome (McNeill et al 2006), although this study lacked rigorous methodology as the sample size was very small and the number of occasions of antenatal reflexology performed on each woman was variable, with some women receiving only one session as late as 39 weeks' gestation, which in no way can be said to have influenced intrapartum progress.

Acupuncture has been shown to be effective for intrapartum pain relief, reducing analgesia requirements (Kinge 2003, Nesheim et al 2003) and shortening labour duration (Gaudernack et al 2006, Ramnero et al 2002, Skilnand et al 2002); it may, conversely, prolong pregnancy in cases of threatened pre-term labour (Pak et al 2000). Recent research shows promising results for selected acupoints, stimulated either by needling or with the thumbs (acupressure), both for induction and acceleration (Ingram et al 2005, Lee et al 2004, Rabl et al 2001). These points can easily be learnt by midwives and could be incorporated into practice, potentially reducing the use of oxytocics in post-dates women.

Raspberry leaf is a popular herbal remedy long advocated for preparing the uterus for birth. It is thought that certain constituents within the leaves of the raspberry bush affect uterine muscle making it more efficient, possibly preventing postmaturity, easing discomfort in labour and enhancing uterine action. Very little research has been carried out to test this theory; investigations in Australia appear to suggest that women who take raspberry leaf products are less likely to have pre- or post-term gestation, and may be less likely to require ARM, caesarean section, forceps or ventouse delivery than those in control groups (Parsons et al 1999, Simpson et al 2001), although it is acknowledged that further research is necessary. Qualified medical herbalists occasionally use raspberry leaf to treat threatened miscarriage but midwives should advise women not to take it until the third trimester. The tea, made from dried raspberry leaves, is more effective than tablets, although some brands of capsules can be opened to release the dried leaf from within, so that a tea can be made.

There is a current trend among some midwives, who do not have sufficient knowledge to advise women appropriately, to suggest that they delay taking raspberry leaf until 36 or even 37 weeks' gestation, in the belief that it will prevent pre-term labour, but as it takes time to take effect it should normally be started earlier than this. The remedy is thought to facilitate normal uterine action so in theory it should not over-stimulate the myometrium. However, it could be argued that it is not necessary to take raspberry leaf routinely, especially for multiparae who have had previous normal labours. They should, instead, be advised to allow their bodies to work normally and spontaneously. It is worth remembering that all herbal remedies act pharmacologically, so they may not be 'harmless' if used inaccurately or inappropriately. Furthermore, pregnancy and labour are normal physiological events, therefore any herbal preparation used should be viewed as a possibly unnecessary intervention which is simply an alternative to a conventional medical intervention.

Expectant mothers should commence taking raspberry leaf at about 30–32 weeks' gestation, starting with just one cup of tea or one tablet daily, giving themselves a few days to become accustomed to the effects before increasing the dose, to a maximum of four cups or tablets daily. Occasionally, strong Braxton Hicks contractions occur when taking raspberry leaf and although there is no evidence that these are harmful to the fetus, the mother may experience considerable discomfort and the dose of raspberry leaf should be reduced accordingly. The tea can be drunk during labour, as long as uterine activity is normal and no hypertonic contractions occur; it is best avoided if medical augmentation (e.g. oxytocin)

is administered. Any tea or tablets that the mother may have left after the birth can be taken postnatally to aid involution (Box 50.6).

Homeopathic remedies can also be useful in labour, and many women purchase homeopathic 'birthing kits' to bring with them into hospital or to use at home. If the midwife is caring for a woman in possession of one of these kits, she should enquire as to her knowledge and previous use of homeopathic remedies. The NMC advises midwives to act as the mother's advocate and to facilitate those who wish to self-administer natural remedies, but suggests that, in the event of uncertainty as to the appropriateness or safety of a particular remedy, midwives should contact a relevant experienced practitioner and record in the notes if the mother continues to use remedies against advice (NMC 2004). The problem for the midwife is that she

---

Box 50.6 Advice to women on safe use of raspberry leaf tea

- It is *not* necessary for a multipara to take raspberry leaf routinely if the uterus has worked efficiently in previous labours
- *Raspberry leaf* should be used, not raspberry fruit; the tea is more effective than the tablets
- Do not start before the third trimester: ideally commence at about 30–32 weeks' gestation
- Increase the amount gradually over several weeks from 1 cup/tablet daily to maximum of 4 cups/tablets daily
- If very strong Braxton Hicks occur, reduce the amount or frequency
- *Avoid* if previous caesarean section or other uterine scar, or if an elective caesarean is planned
- *Avoid* if there is a history of pre-term or precipitate labour, antepartum haemorrhage or low lying placenta
- *Avoid* in cases of multiple pregnancy, hypertension, breech presentation, grande multipara
- *Avoid* if the mother is anaemic or taking iron, calcium, magnesium supplements or is on antidepressants.

Adapted from Tiran 2005b with permission from Expectancy Ltd.

> **Box 50.7** Case scenario 3: Professional boundaries must be identified
>
> A mother books a home birth with her community midwife, and wishes to be accompanied in labour by her homeopath who has been providing care during the pregnancy. Labour progresses so rapidly that a second midwife is unable to reach the house in time before the baby is born. The virtually pre-cipitate birth causes the baby to have a very low Apgar scores and the midwife attempts resuscita-tion, to no avail. Suddenly, the homeopath pushes her out of the way and proceeds to administer to the baby a white powder which she calls the 'death remedy'. Almost immediately, the baby starts to gasp and the Apgar score rises to 9.
>
> It is not possible to know why the baby suddenly started to breathe – it may have been a delayed effect of the midwife's resuscitation, or a sponta-neous resolution, the homeopathy may have been effective or the powdery substance may simply have caused the baby to gasp and inhale air. However, when an independent practitioner is present, it is important that discussion takes place with the midwife so that individual boundaries can be identified before an emergency occurs.

may not be aware of the indications for use, nor understand the mechanism of action of homeopathy and will therefore be unable to assess whether or not the proposed remedy is correct (see Box 50.7). The difficulty for the mother in labour is that she may be unable to assess objectively which remedy is required, possibly administering the wrong remedy or continuing to administer a remedy which is no longer relevant, with the risk of a 'reverse proving'.

Some women appear to believe that homeopathic *caulophyllum* is suitable for inducing labour (some-times starting it before the due date in an attempt to expedite delivery (Tiran 2006b). However, inappro-priate use of this particular remedy can trigger mas-sive prostin-like contractions in which the mother experiences considerable pain but there is little, if any, cervical dilation and uterine contraction and retraction. Alternatively, if the remedy is used when the mother is in early, but not fully established labour, caulophyllum can cause contractions to stop.

There is no evidence from systematic reviews that caulophyllum has any value in initiating labour in the majority of women (Smith 2003), although one reputable placebo-controlled study on intrapartum use of homeopathy suggested that a combination of *arnica* and *bellis perennis* may have a positive effect on mild postpartum bleeding (Oberbaum et al 2005).

Postnatal discomforts

Many women are aware of the homeopathic remedy *arnica*, thought to combat shock, trauma and reduce bruising, available in both tablet and cream form and useful for post-episiotomy discomfort. Although some studies on the effectiveness of arnica have been inconclusive (Hart et al 1997, Ramelet et al 2000, Ste-vinson et al 2003), there are some promising contem-porary results suggesting that it may assist in trauma management (Brinkhaus et al 2006, Seeley et al 2006, Tveiten & Bruset 2003). It can be also used in conjunction with homeopathic *hypericum* for wound healing, e.g. after caesarean section. Mothers can buy arnica tablets in health stores; the 30C strength is pref-erable; they should be advised to start the tablets within 1 hr of the birth, and to take 1 tablet 4-hourly for up to 5 days, then stop. If a mother has had an instrumental delivery, she should increase the fre-quency, taking 1 tablet every 2 hrs for the first 3 days, then 4-hourly for the final 2 days. Arnica cream should not be applied directly to an open wound but is useful if the mother has very bruised buttocks. Homeopathic arnica, in combination with *bellis per-ennis*, may be effective for mild postpartum bleeding (Oberbaum et al 2005). Homeopathic remedies do not interfere with breastfeeding, nor do they adversely affect the baby, and indeed, some breastfeeding pro-blems may respond to homeopathy, although the research done to date has been in the veterinary use of remedies such as phytolacca in cows with mastitis (Holmes et al 2005, Varshney & Naresh 2005). *Laven-der aromatherapy oil* may also ease the discomfort of perineal wounds following childbirth (Dale & Corn-well 1994).

Inadequate lactation can be stimulated with reflex-ology, working on the foot zones corresponding to the breasts and pituitary gland. A simple technique which mothers can do for themselves is to massage firmly between the knuckles of each hand, as this relates to the hand reflexology zones for the breast; there is a theory that women who have an intravenous cannula inserted in the back of the hand could, theoretically, have impaired lactation. However, it is possible that the relaxation effect achieved with reflexology may contribute to facilitating lactation, since it is known that stress adversely affects milk production (Sobrinho et al 2003, Tipping & Mackereth 2000).

Cabbage leaves are well known to midwives as a method of easing breast engorgement, although it is of concern that the majority do not give accurate advice to women, since they fail to understand the mechanism of action and to appreciate that, as a form of herbal remedy, they should have adequate knowledge to advise their use correctly. It is thought that dark green cabbage leaves are the most effective as a chemical in the chlorophyll aids the process of drawing off excess fluid, although one non-English abstract, found when searching the literature, appears to suggest that white cabbage is more effective (Waas 2003). The leaves should be wiped clean, not washed, as this interferes with the process of osmosis, by which they work. Most women prefer to cool them in the refrigerator, simply for comfort, although Roberts et al (1995) found no therapeutic differences between chilled and room temperature leaves. The leaves should be placed inside the brassiere and left until damp, then replaced with new leaves; this process is repeated until relief is obtained. Evidence on effectiveness is inconclusive to date (Nikodem et al 1993, Roberts et al 1998). For those who choose not to breastfeed, there has previously been some suggestion that the application of *jasmine* flowers could act as a herbal means of suppressing lactation (Shrivastav et al 1988).

Conclusion

It can be seen that there are many complementary therapies, many of which can be applied to the care of pregnant, labouring and postnatal mothers, although they are not always without risk and must be used accurately and appropriately. Midwives must acknowledge women's wishes to use natural remedies and act as their advocate, while bearing in mind the health and well-being of both mother and fetus/baby. Enquiries should be made about women's use of CTs and self-administration of natural remedies before and during pregnancy. It is preferable that advice and/or treatment are integrated into the care provided by midwives and others in the conventional maternity services, or by independent therapists who have been adequately trained to treat pregnant women. Some therapies may be incorporated into midwifery practice relatively easily, avoiding the fragmentation that might result from being administered by independent practitioners. CTs enhance the nurturing aspects of midwifery care and may offer potentially less-invasive alternative options for women to help them cope with pregnancy and labour discomforts or to treat specific problems.

Midwifery has, however, become such a diverse profession that maternity complementary medicine (CT) should now be considered a specialist area of expertise, both by midwives and by therapists. It is not feasible for every midwife to have sufficient applied, comprehensive, contemporary evidence-based knowledge on the subject, although an awareness is vital, irrespective of the attitudes and beliefs of the individual. A specialist midwife in each Trust would be able to facilitate the availability of consistent accurate information for mothers and act as a resource for midwives and obstetricians (Tiran 1995, 2007). Complementary medicine can no longer be viewed as an 'alternative' but should be accepted as a fundamental and now well-established component of normal maternity care.

REFERENCES

Ager C 2002 A complementary therapy clinic – making it work. RCM Midwives' Journal 5(6):198–200

Arfeen Z, Owen H, Plummer J L et al 1995 A double-blind randomized controlled trial of ginger for the prevention of postoperative nausea and vomiting. Anaesthesia and Intensive Care 23(4):449–452

Armstrong N C, Ernst E 2001 A randomized, double-blind placebo-controlled trial of a Bach Flower Remedy. Complementary Therapies in Nursing and Midwifery 7(4):215–221

Annapoorna V, Arulumaran S, Anandakumar C et al 1997 External cephalic version at term with tocolysis and vibroacoustic stimulation. International Journal of Gynecology and Obstetrics 59(1):13–18

Bastard J, Tiran D 2006 Aromatherapy and massage for antenatal anxiety: Its effect on the fetus. Complementary Therapies in Clinical Practice 12(1):48–54

Brinkhaus B, Wilkens J M, Ludtke R et al 2006 Homeopathic arnica therapy in patients receiving knee surgery: Results of three randomised double-blind trials. Complementary Therapies in Medicine 14(4):237–246

Burns E, Blamey C, Ersser S J et al 2000 The use of aromatherapy in intrapartum midwifery practice: an observational study. Complementary Therapies in Nursing and Midwifery 6(1):33–44

Cardini F, Lombardo P, Regalia A L et al 2005 A randomised controlled trial of moxibustion for breech presentation. British Journal of Obstetrics and Gynaecology 112(6):743–747

Cardini F, Weixin H 1998 Moxibustion for correction of breech presentation: a randomized controlled trial. Journal of the American Medical Association 280(18):1580–1584

Chang M Y, Chen C H, Huang K F 2006 A comparison of massage effects on labor pain using the McGill Pain Questionnaire. Journal of Nursing Research 14(3):190–197

Coyle M E, Smith C A, Peat B 2005 Cephalic version by moxibustion for breech presentation. Cochrane Database System Reviews, Issue 2:CD003928

Cyna A M, Andrew M I, McAuliffe G L 2006 Antenatal self-hypnosis for labour and childbirth: a pilot study. Anaesthesia and Intensive Care 34(4):464–469

Dale A, Cornwell S 1994 The role of lavender oil in relieving perineal discomfort following childbirth; a blind randomized clinical trial. Journal of Advanced Nursing 19 (1):89–96

Gaudernack L C, Forbord S, Hole E 2006 Acupuncture administered after spontaneous rupture of membranes at term significantly reduces the length of birth and use of oxytocin. A randomized controlled trial. Acta Obstetrica et Gynecologica Scandinavica 85(11):1348–1353

Grabowska C 2006 Turning the breech using moxibustion. RCM Midwives 9(12):484–485

Hart O, Mullee M A, Lewith G et al 1997 Double-blind placebo-controlled randomized clinical trial of homeopathic arnica 30C for pain and infection after total abdominal hysterectomy. Journal of the Royal Society of Medicine 90 (2):73–78

Hayden C, Mullinger B 2006 A preliminary assessment of the impact of cranial osteopathy for the relief of infantile colic. Complementary Therapies in Clinical Practice 12(2):83–90

Hofmeyr G J, Kulier R 2002 External cephalic version for breech presentation at term (Cochrane Review). The Cochrane Library, Issue 4. Update Software, Oxford

Holmes M A, Cockcroft P D, Booth C E et al 2005 Controlled clinical trial of the effect of a homoeopathic nosode on the somatic cell counts in the milk of clinically normal dairy cows. Veterinary Record 156(18):565–567

House of Lords Select Committee on Science and Technology 2000 Report of the sixth committee on complementary and alternative medicine. HMSO, London

Ingram J, Domagala C, Yates S 2005 The effects of shiatsu on post-term pregnancy. Complementary Therapies in Medicine 13(1):11–15

Jewell D, Young G 2003 Interventions for nausea and vomiting in early pregnancy. Cochrane Database System Reviews, Issue 4:CD000145

Kanakura Y, Kometani K, Nagata T et al 2001 Moxibustion treatment of breech presentation. American Journal of Chinese Medicine 29(1):37–45

Kinge R 2003 Acupuncture during labor can reduce the use of pethidine (Norwegian). Tidsskrift for den Norske laegeforening 123(20):2920.

Lee M K, Chang S B, Kang D H 2004 Effects of SP6 acupressure on labor pain and length of delivery time in women during labor. Journal of Alternative and Complementary Medicine 10(6):959–965

Levitas E, Parmet A, Lunenfeld E et al 2006 Impact of hypnosis during embryo transfer on the outcome of in vitro fertilization-embryo transfer: a case-control study. Fertility and Sterility 85(5):1404–1408

Lisi A J 2006 Chiropractic spinal manipulation for low back pain of pregnancy: a retrospective case series. Journal of Midwifery and Women's Health 51(1):e7–10.

Marc I, Rainville P, Verreault R 2007 The use of hypnosis to improve pain management during voluntary interruption of pregnancy: an open randomized preliminary study. Contraception 75(1):52–58

Marcus D M, Snodgrass W R 2005 Do no harm: avoidance of herbal medicines during pregnancy. Obstetrics and Gynecology 105(Part 1):1119–1122

McNabb M T, Kimber L, Haines A et al 2006 Does regular massage from late pregnancy to birth decrease maternal pain perception during labour and birth? A feasibility study to investigate a programme of massage, controlled breathing and visualization, from 36 weeks of pregnancy until birth. Complementary Therapies in Nursing and Midwifery 12 (3):222–231

McNeill J A, Alderdice F A, McMurray F 2006 A retrospective cohort study exploring the relationship between antenatal reflexology and intranatal outcomes. Complementary Therapies in Clinical Practice 12(2):119–125

Mehl L E 1994 Hypnosis and conversion of the breech to the vertex presentation. Archives of Family Medicine 3 (10):881–887

Mollart L 2003 Single-blind trial addressing the differential effects of two reflexology techniques versus rest, on ankle and foot oedema in late pregnancy. Complementary Therapies in Nursing and Midwifery 9(4):203–208

Mousley S 2005 Audit of an aromatherapy service in a maternity unit. Complementary Therapies in Clinical Practice 11 (3):205–210

National Collaborating Centre for Women's and Children's Health 2003 Antenatal care: Routine care for the healthy pregnant woman. RCOG Press, London

Neri I, Airola G, Contu G et al 2004 Acupuncture plus moxibustion to resolve breech presentation: a randomized controlled study. Journal of Maternal-Fetal and Neonatal Medicine 15(4):247–252

Neri I, De Pace V, Venturini P et al 2007 Effects of three different stimulations (acupuncture, moxibustion, acupuncture plus moxibustion) of BL.67 acupoint at small toe on fetal behavior of breech presentation. American Journal of Chinese Medicine 35(1): 27–33

NICE (National Institute for Health and Clinical Excellence) 2006 Guidelines for consultation: Intrapartum care: care of healthy women and their babies during childbirth. Online. Available: http://www.nice.org.uk/page.aspx? o=334322 11 September 2007

Nesheim B I, Kinge R, Berg B et al 2003 Acupuncture during labor can reduce the use of meperidine: a controlled clinical study. Clinical Journal of Pain 19(3):187–191

NHS Confederation 1997 Complementary medicine in the NHS: managing the issues. NHS Confederation, Birmingham

Nikodem V C Danziger D Gebka N et al 1993 Do cabbage leaves prevent breast engorgement? A randomized controlled study. Birth 20(2):61–64

NMC (Nursing and Midwifery Council) 2004 Midwives Rules and Standards 05–04. NMC, London

NMC (Nursing and Midwifery Council) 2008 The Code: standards of conduct, performance and ethics for Nurse and Midwives. NMC, London

Nursing and Midwifery Order 2001 The Stationery Office, London

Oberbaum M, Galoyan N, Lerner-Geva L et al 2005 The effect of the homeopathic remedies Arnica montana and Bellis perennis on mild postpartum bleeding; a randomized, double-blind, placebo-controlled study – preliminary results. Complementary Therapies in Medicine 13(2):87–90

Pak S C, Na C S, Kim J S et al 2000 The effect of acupuncture on uterine contraction induced by oxytocin. American Journal of Chinese Medicine 28(1):35–40

Parsons M, Simpson M, Ponton T 1999 Raspberry leaf and its effect on labour: safety and efficacy. Journal of the Australian College of Midwives 12(3):20–25

Pintov S, Hochman M, Livne A et al 2005 Bach flower remedies used for attention deficit hyperactivity disorder in children: a prospective double blind controlled study. European Journal of Paediatric Neurology 9(6):395–398

Pistolese R A 2002 The Webster Technique: a chiropractic technique with obstetric implications. Journal of Manipulative and Physiological Therapeutics 25(6):E1–E9

Portnoi G, Chng L A, Karimi-Tabesh L et al 2003 Prospective comparative study of the safety and effectiveness of ginger for the treatment of nausea and vomiting in pregnancy. American Journal of Obstetrics and Gynecology 189(5):1374–1377

Rabl M, Ahner R, Bitschnau M et al 2001 Acupuncture for cervical ripening and induction of labor at term – a randomized controlled trial. Wiener klinische Wochenschrift 113 (23–24):942–946

Ramelet A A, Buchheim G, Lorenz P 2000 Homeopathic Arnica in postoperative haematomas: a double-blind study. Dermatology 201(4):347–348

Ramnero A, Hanson U, Kihlgren M 2002 Acupuncture treatment during labour: a randomised controlled trial. British Journal of Obstetrics and Gynaecology 109 (6):637–644

Ranzini A, Allen A, Lai Y 2001 Use of complementary medicines and therapies among obstetric patients. Obstetrics and Gynecology 97(Suppl 4):S46

Refuerzo J S, Blackwell S C, Sokol R J et al 2005 Use of over-the-counter medications and herbal remedies in pregnancy. American Journal of Perinatology 22(6):321–324

Roberts K L, Reiter M, Schuster D 1995 A comparison of chilled and room temperature cabbage leaves in treating breast engorgement. Journal of Human Lactation 11 (3):191–194

Roberts K L, Reiter M, Schuster D 1998 Effects of cabbage leaf extract on breast engorgement. Journal of Human Lactation 14(3):231–236

Seeley B M, Denton A B, Ahn M S et al 2006 Effect of homeopathic Arnica montana on bruising in face-lifts: results of a randomized, double-blind, placebo-controlled clinical trial. Archives of Facial Plastic Surgery 8(1):54–59

Shrivastav P, George K, Balasubramaniam N 1988 Suppression of puerperal lactation using jasmine flowers. Jasminum sambac. Australia and New Zealand Journal of Obstetrics and Gynaecology 28(1):68–71

Simpson M, Parsons M, Greenwood J et al 2001 Raspberry leaf in pregnancy: its safety and efficacy in labour. Journal of Midwifery and Women's Health 46(2):51–59

Skilnand E, Fossen D Heiberg E 2002 Acupuncture in the management of pain in labor. Acta Obstetrica et Gynecologica Scandinavica 81(10):943–948

Smith C A 2003 Homoeopathy for induction of labour. Cochrane Database System Review, Issue 4:CD003399

Smith C, Crowther C, Wilkinson C et al 1999 A RCT in knee-chest position for breech presentation. Birth 26(2):71–75

Sobrinho L G, Simoes M, Barbosa L et al 2003 Cortisol, prolactin, growth hormone and neurovegetative responses to emotions elicited during an hypnoidal state. Psychoneuroendocrinology 28(1):1–17

Stevinson C, Devaraj V S Fountain-Barber A 2003 Homeopathic arnica for prevention of pain and bruising: randomized placebo-controlled trial in hand surgery. Journal of the Royal Society of Medicine 96(2):60–65

Thomas K J, Nicholl J P, Coleman P 2001 Use and expenditure on complementary medicine in England: a population based survey. Complementary Therapies in Medicine 9(1):2–11

Tipping E, Mackereth P 2000 A concept analysis: the effect of reflexology on homeostasis to establish and maintain lactation. Complementary Therapies in Nursing and Midwifery 6(4):189–198

Tiran D 1995 Complementary therapies education in midwifery. Complementary Therapies in Nursing and Midwifery 1:41–43

Tiran D 2000 Clinical aromatherapy for pregnancy and childbirth, 2nd edn. Churchill Livingstone, London

Tiran D 2001 Complementary strategies in antenatal care. Complementary Therapies in Nursing and Midwifery 7:19–24

Tiran D 2002 Using reflexology in pregnancy and childbirth. In: Mackereth P, Tiran D (eds) 2002 Clinical reflexology: a guide for health professionals. Elsevier Science, London, Ch. 7, p 133–146

Tiran D 2003a The use of herbal remedies in pregnancy: a risk-benefit assessment. Complementary Therapies in Nursing and Midwifery 9(6):176–181

Tiran D 2003b Nausea and vomiting in pregnancy: an integrated approach to care. Elsevier Science, Edinburgh

Tiran D 2004a Midwives' enthusiasm for complementary therapies: a cause for concern? Complementary Therapies in Nursing and Midwifery 10(2):77–79

Tiran D 2004b Implementing aromatherapy in maternity care: a manual for midwives and managers. Expectancy Ltd, London

Tiran D 2004c Breech presentation: increasing maternal choice. Complementary Therapies in Nursing and Midwifery 10(4):233–238

Tiran D, Budd S 2005 Ginger is not a universal remedy for nausea and vomiting in pregnancy. MIDIRS Midwifery Digest 15(3):335–339

Tiran D, Chummun H 2005 The physiological basis of reflexology and its use as a diagnostic tool. Complementary Therapies in Clinical Practice 11(1):58–64

Tiran 2005a Safety of herbal remedies in pregnancy. Expectancy Ltd, London

Tiran D 2005b Complementary therapies in pregnancy: downloadable information leaflets for expectant mothers. Expectancy Ltd, London

Tiran D 2005c Complementary therapies in maternity care: NICE guidelines do not promote clinical excellence. Complementary Therapies in Clinical Practice 11(2):50–52

Tiran D 2006a Complementary therapies in pregnancy: midwives' and obstetricians' appreciation of risk. Complementary Therapies in Clinical Practice 12(2):126–131

Tiran D 2006b Late for a very important date: complementary therapies for post-dates pregnancy. Practising Midwife 9(2):2–6

Tiran D 2007 Complementary therapies within midwifery: time to act? Practising Midwife 10(3):14–19

Tveiten D, Bruset S 2003 Effect of arnica D30 in marathon runners. Pooled results from two double-blind placebo controlled studies. Homeopathy 92(4):187–189

Varshney J P, Naresh R 2005 Comparative efficacy of homeopathic and allopathic systems of medicine in the management of clinical mastitis of Indian dairy cows. Homeopathy 94(2):81–85

Visalyaputra S, Petchpaisit N, Somcharoen K, et al 1998 The efficacy of ginger root in the prevention of postoperative nausea and vomiting after outpatient gynaecological laparoscopy. Anaesthesia 53(5):506–510

Vutyavanich T, Kraisarin T, Ruangsri R. 2001 Ginger for nausea and vomiting in pregnancy: randomized, double-masked, placebo-controlled trial. Obstetrics and Gynecology 97 (4):577–582

Waas R 2003 Cabbage leaf wrap. White cabbage works better. [in German] MMW Fortschritte der Medizin 145(41):14

Walach H, Rilling C, Engelke U 2001 Efficacy of Bach-flower remedies in test anxiety: a double-blind, placebo-controlled, randomized trial with partial crossover. Journal of Anxiety Disorders 15(4):359–366

Wang S M, DeZinno P, Fermo L et al 2005 Complementary and alternative medicine for low-back pain in pregnancy: a cross-sectional survey. Journal of Alternative and Complementary Medicine 11(3):459–464

Willetts K E, Ekangaki A, Eden J A 2003 Effect of a ginger extract on pregnancy-induced nausea: a randomised controlled trial. Australia and New Zealand Journal of Obstetrics and Gynaecology 43(2):139–144

FURTHER READING

Tiran D 2007 Teach yourself positive pregnancy. Hodder Headline, London

Focuses on using natural remedies and complementary therapies to achieve a satisfying pregnancy and prepare for the birth and parenthood, aimed at parents.

Tiran D, Mack S (eds) 2000 Complementary therapies for pregnancy and childbirth, 2nd edn. Baillière Tindall, London

Comprehensive introduction to the subject with chapters on the main therapies in use today, written either by midwives actively using the therapy within midwifery or by practitioners who specialize in treating pregnant and childbearing women.

USEFUL WEBSITES

British Acupuncture Council:
www.acupuncture.org.uk

Governs qualified acupuncturists and promotes research.

Aromatherapy Council:
www.aromatherapycouncil.co.uk

Newly formed regulatory body to maintain standards of aromatherapy education including regular reviews of the National Occupation Standards.

European Herbal Practitioners Association:
www.ehpa.eu/index

Represents medical herbalists within the European Union, sets standards of training and practice of therapists and quality of herbal medicines.

Expectancy Ltd. Expectant Parents' Complementary Therapies Consultancy:
www.expectancy.co.uk

Education and consultancy services for midwives; information and advice for mothers on safe use of complementary therapies in pregnancy.

General Chiropractic Council:
www.gcc-uk.org

Statutory regulatory body for chiropractors, responsible for standards of education, practice and conduct.

Society of Homeopaths:
www.homeopathy-soh.org

Registers professionally qualified, non-medical homeopaths.

British Medical Acupuncture Society:
www.medical-acupuncture.co.uk

Association for doctors, dentists and veterinary surgeons interested in or practising acupuncture.

National Centre for Complementary and Alternative Medicine:
www.nccam.nih.gov/research

Database of complementary medicine research with good abstracts.

National Institute for Medical Herbalists:
www.nimh.org.uk

Primary professional organization of medical herbalists in the UK, maintains standards of education and practice.

General Osteopathic Council:
www.osteopathy.org.uk

Regulates osteopathy in the UK, responsible for standards of education, practice and conduct.

Reflexology Forum:
www.reflexologyforum.org

Developing regulatory body for reflexologists, aiming to set standards for education, training, practice and conduct of therapists and to promote research.

Faculty of Homeopathy/British Homeopathic Association:
www.trusthomeopathy.org

Promotes academic and scientific development of homeopathy education, training and practice by doctors, midwives, nurses, dentists, pharmacists, veterinary surgeons and other statutorily registered healthcare professionals.

51

Community, public health and social services

Chris McCourt

CHAPTER CONTENTS

A midwife needs knowledge of community health and social services for three main reasons: to appreciate better the social context of health and how this impinges on the role; to be able to advise a woman about other services that may be helpful for her, and to refer appropriately to other services when their input would be beneficial.

The chapter aims to:

- discuss community health and social services in the context of a broad theoretical understanding of health and illness
- provide information that will be useful for midwives in key areas of these services
- discuss the principles, structures, policies and practices that influence the character of each
- discuss the role of the midwife in public health and health promotion
- provide a framework for continuing learning, updating of relevant information and developing local knowledge and networks.

Introduction

The factors influencing the health of mothers and children are broad and complex. Their impact begins long before pregnancy and will continue long after a woman's discharge from the maternity services. Community health and social services, therefore, play an important role in the cycles of family life in many societies. Social services, community- and hospital-based health services have been through several phases of integration and separation in the UK since their establishment in the early part of the twentieth century. Currently, they are provided under quite separate institutional arrangements but much of recent health policy has focused on developing more 'seamless' and community-based models for providing care and this has been particularly evident in the field of children's services. To some extent, these separate arrangements and the structures described in this chapter are products of our tendency to view health within a narrow and mechanistic framework. In consequence, health, social

and other personal services, hospital- and community-based services are categorized separately, so that effort is then needed to piece them back together. The recent development of Children's Centres in the UK is a key example of that effort. The boundaries in many of the issues discussed in this chapter are fuzzy and should be so, since that is the way health and illness are influenced and experienced by people, as part of their lives.

The importance of viewing maternal and child health in its social context

It is a common but misplaced assumption that it is provision of healthcare that is mainly responsible for our health. Evidence from a range of research disciplines, including epidemiology, social science and natural sciences, indicates that health should be viewed much more as an ecological concept; it is a product of many factors, including living environment and conditions, nutrition, occupation and education, and is profoundly influenced by maternal health. The health of mothers receiving maternity care, and of their babies, is most likely to be influenced by such issues as their nutritional status, their housing and working conditions and the level of social support available. This means that the role of maternity services is additional and relatively short term. However, it is important for midwives to remember that the effects of the short-term transition of pregnancy and birth are long-term and profound, as shown by increasing weight of evidence of the effects of maternal and fetal well-being on health in later life and between generations.

The importance of the social context on women's health is reflected particularly clearly in the different social class patterns of health (Acheson 1998). A key example of this is birthweight; this is a useful indicator, since it is readily measurable, and is an important predictor of future health status (Oakley 1992) and low birthweight is strongly associated with poverty, inequality and lack of social support. The physical health of the mother will have been influenced by similar factors, which have a very long-term effect. Birthweight is a good example of the multifaceted nature of health, as well as the importance of social context on health (Barker 1998, Richards et al 2001, Roberts 1997).

What is meant by community?

'Community' is a very broad term that is currently widely used in policy developments in Euro-American societies. Generally, community is identified along three dimensions: place, relationships and sentiment or sense of belonging (Turton & Orr 1993). All contribute something to the concept, but the degree of importance attached to each is variable. When discussing health and social services, these aspects of community are all relevant, but community tends to be defined by service providers very much in service terms (i.e. the location of a service, the way in which it is delivered and its scale). Popular images of community care often take it to mean care provided at home, rather than in an institution of some type, and provided by family, friends or neighbours, rather than professionals or paid workers. To clarify these different concepts of community care – with very different implications for social policy – Bulmer (1987) drew a distinction between care 'in' the community and care 'by' the community, mostly care provided unpaid by friends, kin or neighbours, which is also referred to by service providers as 'informal' care.

The different areas of health services

Historically, the role of medicine has in many respects been peripheral to the concerns of public health, since it is mainly responsive to disease and concerned with the diagnosis and treatment of ill health (McKeown 1979, Stacey 1988). This is reflected in the separation of different health-related activities into the institutional spheres of social services, hospital services and community (or primary) health services.

Maternity care, and particularly midwifery, occupies a different role from much of conventional healthcare, since childbirth is an important life event and transition and pregnant women are generally understood to be healthy people, requiring care and observation for possible problems, rather than curative treatment. Nevertheless, in the latter half of the twentieth century, maternity services in the UK and other industrialized countries were organized increasingly along the lines of acute medical services, based mainly in hospitals, with women routinely referred to them by their General Practitioners (GPs) or family physicians (Hunt & Symonds 1995). Women were generally categorized into those deemed high or low risk on an agreed set of medical indicators. Care for women classified as of 'low risk' was then in many cases referred back to community health services – the GP and midwife – for shared care.

Following the 'Changing Childbirth' report (DoH 1993), a number of services in the UK moved towards greater integration of community- and hospital-based midwifery, for example through caseload practice (McCourt et al 2006) or community-based group practice (Sandall et al 2000). Additionally, during the 1990s, UK government attempts to shift appropriate areas of healthcare back into a community base led to a renewed emphasis on primary care (DoH 1997a,b; see also Ch. 4). Since 2000 in the UK, acute hospital services have become increasingly centralized. As many local communities questioned centralization of maternity services, a number of stand-alone midwife-units (Community Maternity Units in Scotland) were developed to offer care to women of low medical risk. Similar patterns of centralization, accompanied by development or re-opening of small community units have been evident in a number of countries with complex healthcare systems. In 2007 the Department of Health England offered a guarantee that by 2009, women would again be able to choose their place of birth: a home birth, birth in a local facility, including a hospital, under the care of a midwife, or birth in a hospital supported by a local maternity care team including midwives, anaesthetists and consultant obstetricians (DH 2007a).

The structure and role of community health and social services

As indicated in the introduction to this chapter, the structure of these services has been subject to a number of policy changes and varies from one country to another. The structure of the health service is described in more detail in Chapter 54.

The origins of the current system in the UK

Prior to 1946 in the UK, health and social services were largely privately paid for or charitable. The Poor Law had been the main instrument for caring for people who were disabled, chronically ill or destitute, and its operation had become punitive over time in order to discourage people from claiming relief. The nineteenth century, with rapid industrialization and urbanization, saw the growth of hospitals as places to provide healthcare, but it was not until the twentieth century that hospitals came to be seen as a desirable option in care for women giving birth (Donnison 1988). The foundations of the current welfare and health system were set down in the years following the Second World War responding to the enormous social changes taking place at that time. The NHS Act 1946 created the National Health Service, with free healthcare provided according to need, while the National Assistance Act 1948 replaced the Poor Law with a system of means-tested welfare benefits and a duty for local authorities to provide residential care for those in need. At this point, the emphasis was very much on creating the institutional structures for welfare; relatively little attention was given to community-based services – that is, support to people living in their own homes (Clements 1996).

Health services

Between 1974 and 1993 in the UK, health authorities were the main providers of health services, incorporating hospitals and some community services such as community midwifery. After the NHS and Community Care Act 1990, their role became mainly one of planning and contracting for care on behalf of the local population. Hospitals, and some community-based services such as those for people with long-term care needs, developed NHS Trust status, working independently within the health service and, in theory at least, competing with other service providers.

Following the 1997 government White Paper, 'The new NHS, modern, dependable' (DoH 1997a), this system was reformed again to remove the concept of an 'internal healthcare market' and to devolve organization of care as far as possible to a community level. The new policy introduced Primary Care Trusts (PCTs) (see Ch. 54) to commission services for their local population on behalf of the local health authority (Carnell & Kline 1999, DoH 1997a,b). After much discussion of the need for structural reform to address maternity care as a community-based service, in 2007, a report on the organization of services in London proposed four possible models of service, managed by maternity/perinatal networks, with a higher proportion of women giving birth in 'stand-alone' or 'co-located' midwife units, or at home (NHS London 2007).

Local authorities

Local authorities in the UK have a key role in planning, monitoring and developing services for the needs of the local community in a range of departments, including education, social services, housing and environmental services. All these areas have an influence on health, giving the local authority a potentially powerful role in enhancing the health and welfare of its population. In practice, the different departments have not always worked together effectively in a health-promoting role, partly because the health implications of such public services have been under-recognized. Following the NHS and Community Care Act 1990, these authorities, like health authorities, were given a more strategic role in planning services for local needs and purchasing these from independent service providers as well as continuing to provide them where appropriate. Knowledge of local authority social services is the most relevant for midwives, since social services departments have legal duties to assess people's needs for support in the community and to provide or arrange for services assessed as being needed. The local authority social services are responsible for assessing overall community health and care needs and producing regular community care plans. They also take a lead role in child protection issues.

New structures for collaboration across community health and social services

During the late 1990s in the UK, government policy responded to research exploring the complex links between social conditions and health and the need for broad social policies to tackle these. Critical research on health education indicated that attempts to change individual knowledge and behaviour were ineffective without attention to the context of people's lives. This was reflected in the publication of a health promotion strategy, 'Our healthier nation' (DoH 1998) and in new policy schemes such as Sure Start (see: www.surestart.gov.uk) and the New Deal for Communities (see: http://www.neighbourhood.gov.uk/page.asp?id=617). In 2007, the government extended the Sure Start scheme as part of an initiative to integrate and develop services for children across health and social care (DH 2004a, DES 2004) and children's centres were developed to provide such integrated services. In some areas these are based on educational premises, and some include community-based midwifery teams or practices.

The Sure Start scheme focuses on the importance of the early years and maternal and infant health for future health, development and well-being. A number of projects were developed in areas of social and economic deprivation, and following evaluation these were extended more widely. Sure Start projects work with all families with young children but focus particularly on supporting socially disadvantaged families, with the intention of 'breaking the cycle of disadvantage' in the important early years of development. Examples of Sure Start schemes include family support, nutritional advice, play facilities and provision of support workers in the community (see Box 51.1, Carnell & Kline 1999, DES 2004).

Schemes such as the New Deal for Communities are more broadly based regeneration schemes applied to areas with high levels of, often multiple, disadvantages and low levels of 'social capital': informal and other social resources for communities to build on. Following the lessons of earlier attempts to ameliorate the negative effects of poverty with single measures, these projects integrated areas such as health, housing, employment, leisure, child care, education and nutrition or food access schemes – all areas of disadvantage that tend to have a cumulative or 'spiral' effect.

The midwife's role in relation to community health and social services

Midwives are in a good position to provide general care and support to the woman during a period of great personal and social adjustment as well as physical change. In addition to clinical skills, midwives provide information and advice and, in many cases, social support. Such a role has the potential to

---

Box 51.1 Sure Start scheme to support new mothers (Beake et al 2005)

Midwives working in West London teamed up with a local Sure Start programme to develop ways of promoting maternal and infant health. The Coningham Sure Start programme pioneered a scheme to increase breastfeeding and reduce smoking in new mothers by providing hands-on support from an Infant Feeding Support Worker. She works closely with midwives and health visitors, visiting women at home and running groups, on a long-term basis, from pregnancy to the months following birth. Developing the project brought together midwives who work with a personal caseload of women in a socially deprived area and health visitors who work with a strong public health focus as part of the Sure Start team. Previously, contact was limited, despite the overlap of roles and interests in promoting the health of mothers and babies, due to the handover of care at about 10–28 days following birth, and by working for different organizations. Community-based schemes like this one, with midwives able to follow women across traditional boundaries such as hospital–community or high–low risk and to plan and provide care around their needs, may be one basis for midwives to develop the more health-promoting focus that has always been seen as an ideal.

The aim of Sure Start

To work with parents-to-be, parents and children to promote the physical, intellectual and social development of babies and young children – particularly those who are disadvantaged – so that they can flourish at home and when they get to school, and thereby break the cycle of disadvantage for the current generation of young children.

provide a positive impact on the general health and wellbeing of women and their families during a period of change and development. Midwifery care is relatively short term but interventions during certain critical periods may have a long-term impact, however small. A good example of this is the midwife's role in health promotion and in supporting women in feeding their babies (Crafter 1997).

When a woman needs more general sources of advice and social support than those provided through the maternity services, midwives can still play a key role in providing relevant information and advice and in referring her to other professionals and organizations for support. This role is underpinned by:

- developing and updating broad health knowledge
- developing local community knowledge and contacts
- reflection and awareness of one's own impact as a practitioner.

Public health role of midwives

Government policy has recognized the difficulties caused in practice by the institutional split between health and social and community services and advocated returning maternity services towards a more seamless model of care. The National Service Framework (NSF) for Children, Young People and the Maternity Services (DH 2004a) advised a stronger public health role for the midwife, through changing the organization of care and expanding the scope of the midwife's roles and responsibilities. Although it did not set out the precise nature of this expanded role, or how it would be achieved, it recommended more integrated models of care, with midwives working across hospital and community service boundaries, for example, with personal or group practice caseloads, or with specialist roles. The framework also advocated a stronger public health role, in collaboration with other primary care practitioners, with an increased focus on health promotion and additional support to socially disadvantaged women. This emphasis was reinforced by the findings of successive reports on maternal and infant health, which (e.g. Lewis 2007) indicated that contributory causes of maternal death in the UK were social exclusion,

deprivation, social and mental health related problems. The health promotion role advocated for midwives was particularly through health education for women and through focusing care more effectively on women with particular needs for support arising from problems such as domestic violence or substance abuse.

Although much of midwives' work is primary, preventive healthcare, to date there has been little involvement of midwifery in this new focus on primary and preventive health services. Development of more integrated, child and family-centred services, such as children's centres, may help to support more public health-focused roles. Similarly, while health visitors and midwives have tended to work separately in recent years, one following on from the other, such community projects and the proposals for extended public health roles for midwives may involve them in more collaborative ways of working together (e.g. Box 51.1).

The legal framework

Community health and social services operate within a legal framework (Acts of Parliament) set out by government. Local and health authorities are provided with guidance to follow in interpreting and implementing the legislation. Guidance is normally mandatory, for example Executive Letters issued by the Department of Health, whereas guidelines are advisory (e.g. good practice guides), to assist with the complexities of putting policy into practice. UK legislation also operates within the framework of European (EU) legislation and policy directives and is increasingly expected to develop in line with this framework. The relevant frameworks in other countries will differ, but it is important for all midwives to become familiar with the legal framework in their own country of practice.

Relevant legislation

The main relevant legislation in the UK at the time of writing is shown in Box 51.2 The central pieces of legislation for practitioners in the UK are the Health and Social Care Act 2001 (DH 2001), which set out a newly combined framework for health and social services – the National Health Service Act

---

Box 51.2 The UK legal framework for community health and social services

- Department of Health, Health and Social Care Act 2001 and the National Health Service Act 2006
- The Housing Act 1977 – which established local authority housing departments with a duty to provide housing for homeless people in certain circumstances (and as amended by subsequent Housing Acts)
- The Disabled Persons Services, Consultation and Representation Act 1986 – which set out the rights of disabled people to receive assessment for community services
- The Race Relations Act 1976 (and Amendment Act 2000), the Sex Discrimination Act 1975 and the Disability Discrimination Act 1995 – which established rights for people of different ethnic groups and people with disabilities and protection against discrimination based on ethnicity, disability or gender, including pregnancy
- The Children Act 2004 and related policy guidance
- The Mental Health Act 2007 – which provided a framework for services for people with mental health problems, including community services and the terms under which people in distress can be admitted to hospital or treated without their consent and the rules and procedures for discharge from compulsory admissions
- Mental Capacity Act 2005 – provides a statutory framework to protect vulnerable people, carers and professionals. It makes it clear who can take decisions in which situations and how they should go about this. It starts from the fundamental point that a person has capacity and that all practical steps must be taken to help the person make a decision.

Guidance

- Department of Health, National Services Framework for Children, Young People and Maternity Services (2004)
- Department for Education and Skills, Every Child Matters: Change for Children (2004).

2006 and the Commissioning Framework – which operationalized its principles (DH 2006a). The key aims were to integrate the different services better and to improve organization of services for people with care needs, particularly since many services are now community based. Many health problems are not easily divided into health and social care needs.

Care management

In the UK, anyone who comes to the attention of the local authority or health service as having possible needs for support is entitled to an assessment, followed where appropriate, by a plan for care, which should include an integrated 'package' of services. This is referred to as a 'personal health and social care plan' (DH 2006b). The principle is that the needs of the person should be central and services should be sought to respond to these needs, rather than fitting people into the services. A midwife can request or assist a woman or family in requesting a care assessment. The needs for support – and the possible solutions – can be quite wide-ranging, including 'home help' and additional childcare. Assessment should involve the woman, her family where appropriate, and all relevant professionals, who may include the community midwife. If she, or her child, is considered to have care needs, a care manager will be appointed to ensure that adequate and suitable support services are arranged. Care managers are often social workers but they may be other professionals (including home care organizers, community nurses or midwives) according to the nature of the individual's needs. In 2006 the UK government introduced a plan for joint health and social care managed networks and/or teams for people with complex needs and in 2007, they introduced the role of Community Matron, with the aim of improving case management of people with long-term health or social care needs, and improving integration of services across boundaries such as primary and secondary health services, health and social care.

As Community Matrons are appointed it will be useful for midwives to familiarize themselves with their developing roles, and to establish contact, since midwives may care for women in pregnancy who have other, often complex health and social care needs. It is also important to try to anticipate needs (such as a woman needing home help after birth or an infant needing support for physical impairments) well in advance and encourage and support the woman to seek additional support when needed. Some services may be charged for on a means-tested basis and there is considerable variation in provision according to where people live. Needs for care are not tightly defined because they are meant to be broad, but generally the policy is aimed at people (adults and children) who have physical, sensory or intellectual impairments, chronic health problems or mental health problems, or who care for people with such problems. Pregnant women and those who have recently given birth are included. Those who are providing regular and substantial care for friends or relatives, informal carers, are also entitled to an assessment of how they are affected by their caring responsibilities (Clements 1996, Dimond 1997).

Maternity rights and benefits

In most countries, women are entitled to a series of benefits and have particular rights during pregnancy and childbirth regarding employment. In EU countries these have increased in recent years. Midwives are in an ideal position to advise women of their general rights and entitlements and to respond in a timely fashion to requests for information on rights and benefits and on where to go for further help.

The Benefits Agency (BA)

The Benefits Agency works at national level on behalf of the UK government's Department of Work and Pensions (formerly the Department of Social Security). It assesses needs for financial support, in line with national legislation, and provides payments, exemption certificates and loans where appropriate. It is responsible for the administration of maternity benefits of various types. Local offices and telephone lines are provided for information and enquiries.

Although the overall framework of rights and benefits is relatively stable, details may change from year to year. A checklist of sources of information and advice is important, as is regular renewal of the forms and information leaflets provided by the BA. For these reasons, it is crucial not to rely on a textbook; however, the following section summarizes the system of rights and benefits in the UK in operation in 2007.

Maternity rights

Women's rights at work are set out in UK law and in EU directives. Where the two differ, UK law is generally expected to comply with EU directives, unless it provides for greater rights. Maternity rights also operate within the broader framework of employment and discrimination law (IDS 2007). They include employment protection, health and safety, paid time off for healthcare, rights to maternity and parental leave and rights to return to work (Box 51.3). Detailed but clear and accessible information on maternity rights is available in the following leaflet:

- Pregnancy and Work. What you need to know as an employee (DTI/Pub 8541/250K/06/07/NP – 1st April 2007).

This and other useful guidance can be accessed at: www.direct.gov.uk

For those with computer access – at home, at work or perhaps through a local library or community centre – the government has set up an interactive website that can be used for general information and more personalized advice: www.tiger.gov.uk. This will be an excellent resource for midwives as well as for pregnant women. It can be used by women to get a good idea of the benefits they are be entitled to.

Maternity benefits

These include monetary and non-monetary benefits (benefits in kind or exemptions). The key monetary benefits related to maternity are set out in Box 51.4. The changes in family circumstances due to childbirth may also mean changes in entitlement for families that rely on housing benefit, working families tax credit or income support because of low incomes. Generally, each additional child increases entitlement and may sometimes mean the difference between qualifying for a benefit and not. Since

Box 51.3 UK maternity and employment rights at 1 April 2007 – key points

Protection of employment

A woman with a contract of employment cannot be dismissed from her job for being pregnant or on maternity leave. She maintains general employment rights including protection against discrimination. Further advice can be obtained from the ACAS helpline on 08457 474747.

Health and safety

Employers are responsible for ensuring health and safety at work for women who are pregnant or breastfeeding, or, if not practicable, must provide suitable alternative work or suspension on full pay. Detailed advice can be obtained from //www.hse.gov.uk or the health and safety information line on Tel: 0845 345 0055.

Leave

A woman is entitled to paid leave for antenatal-health-care, including home visits and parent education or preparation classes. An employer may request verification of appointments. All employees are entitled to maternity leave for up to 52 weeks, and a minimum 2-week period is compulsory (4 weeks in factories). Fathers are also entitled to take up to 2 weeks paid paternity leave.

Right to return

A woman has a right to return to her previous job, on no less favourable terms, provided she complies with limited conditions of notice and returns within the statutory periods of leave. There are some limited exceptions to this rule. Parents may also request more flexible working arrangements and provisions for time off for care for dependents.

Box 51.4 Monetary maternity benefits in the UK – at April 2007: key points

Statutory Maternity Pay (SMP)

This is payable to women in continuous employment and earning above the statutory limit for National Insurance contributions before the pregnancy started. Payment is for up to 39 weeks at a level equivalent to 90% of earnings for 6 weeks followed by a lower flat rate, set annually, and can commence at any time from 11 weeks before the expected week of confinement (EWC), or earlier if the baby has been born. It is administered by employers, who should be given 15 weeks' notice of the intended date for taking leave (although the date can be amended up to 28 days before leave). Women continue to be liable for tax and national insurance, and employers must continue to pay pension contributions.

Many employers, especially large organizations, operate more generous schemes than the statutory minimum. The woman should check these terms and whether they apply to her with her employer or human resource department in good time.

Maternity Allowance

This is paid to women not entitled to SMP but who have paid National Insurance contributions during the qualifying period. It is paid weekly for up to 39 weeks, at a flat rate or 90% of earnings, whichever is lower. Application must be made on form MA1 accompanied by forms MATB1 and SMP1 (which is issued by the employer) from 26 weeks of pregnancy and before leaving work. Women not entitled to either SMP or MA may be able to claim Incapacity Benefit or Income Support during their leave period.

Sure Start Maternity Grants

Women who receive income support, income-based jobseekers allowance, working families or disabled person's tax credit can claim a single payment to assist in the costs of a new baby. The grant is payable from 29 weeks of pregnancy and must be claimed before the baby is 3 months old or within 3 months of adoption.

Child Benefit

All primary carers of children under 16 (or in full-time education until 19) are entitled to Child Benefit. It is payable for each child, with a higher rate for the first child and for lone parents. The Child Benefit claim form must be accompanied by the child's birth certificate.

women may seek advice on any of these benefits, or general advice about coping with new economic demands, it is important to obtain a full set of advice leaflets. Entitlements and benefits are liable to change from one year to another owing to legal and policy changes as well as inflationary increases in benefit levels, so it is important to update all leaflets, and one's own information sources, annually. Detailed information on maternity benefits can be found in the information booklets NI 17A Guide to maternity benefits and BC1 Children and benefits, which are available from local BA offices and most post offices.

Checking entitlements

Up-to-date details of benefits and entitlements can be obtained by using the local BA office or an independent advice agency. Some local authorities employ welfare rights advisors, who have in-depth knowledge of rights and benefits and who can undertake casework where needed.

Pregnant and childbearing women are also entitled to a range of non-monetary benefits, such as vitamins, some of which are universal (i.e. all are entitled) while others are available only to those who are entitled to income support or family credit. The previous 'welfare foods' provision is now referred to as Healthy Start, and vouchers available for young mothers and those on low incomes can be exchanged for a range of healthy foods (see: www.healthystart. nhs.uk).

Forms and certificates to be supplied by the midwife or GP

Midwives or GPs are responsible for providing the certificates that the woman will need to exercise her employment rights and claim relevant benefits. These include:

- form MATB1: proof of expected date of confinement
- form MATB2: certificate of confinement
- form MA1: for application for statutory maternity pay or maternity allowance
- form FW8: for exemptions from prescription and related charges.

Box 51.5 Advice and information checklist

- Benefits Agency helpline
- Benefits Agency local office
- Citizens' Advice Bureau (local office)
- Welfare Rights Officer
- Law Centre
- Local authority social services/neighbourhood office
- Sure Start local office
- Interpreting or language advice service.

Complete the checklist given in Box 51.5, to function as a ready reminder of where to go for information.

The community health services

Community health services encompass what is generally known as primary healthcare. They include community-based services for health promotion, such as child health clinics and school health services, and for longer-term health needs, such as mental health centres. The philosophy of the 2006 policy paper 'Our health, our care, our say' (DH 2006b) relates closely to the reality of health needs, which do not fit easily into professional or organizational categories and it attempts to put the person at the centre of services. The development of Children's Centres will also see greater opportunities for integration of services for families of young children. Children's Centres will be based mainly in Sure Start schemes or other local services, such as schools, and will offer a base for antenatal services, early years care, parent support and other services relevant to young children and their parents. A range of professionals will be based in these centres, or use them as a sessional base, so facilitating greater contact between different professionals as well as easier access for families.

The GP and the GP practice

In the UK, GPs provide much of the everyday healthcare for families and act as the key gatekeepers for secondary healthcare. GPs are independent professionals, who contracted into the health service after its inception in 1948, while maintaining much of their independent status (see Ch. 54).

GPs and maternity care

In the early part of the twentieth century GPs had little involvement in maternity care, since birth was largely managed by midwives. Many women could not afford a doctor's fees and some doctors, in any case, had arrangements with local midwives, delegating care for uncomplicated births (Leap & Hunter 1993, Robinson 1990). After increasing in importance during the century, the role of GPs in childbirth declined from the 1970s. The Peel report (MoH 1970) and the Short report (House of Commons 1980) had advocated a shift of all maternity services to consultant-led hospital units and the closure of small GP-led units or cottage hospitals, despite lack of research evidence that they were less safe (Tew 1990). More recently, centralization of care into larger obstetric units has taken place, but Midwife Units or Community Maternity Units have been developed to provide more local care for women of low obstetric risk. Similar patterns of development have been evident in many countries with 'developed' healthcare systems.

Except where a GP has a particular interest in birth, GPs are now mainly involved in antenatal care, which they may share with a practice-linked community midwife, group practice or caseload midwife. A 2007 review of services advocated a set of models appropriate to women with different levels of obstetric or social risk, including a more primary care-based pathway for women of low obstetric risk, with choice of birth at home, in Midwife Units, or an obstetric unit (NHS London 2007), reflecting the direction of development set out in Maternity Matters (DH 2007a).

Health visitors and child health services

Health visitors are registered nurses or midwives who specialize in health promotion and advice for families with children under 5 years and, sometimes, older people. The health visitor's role can, however, be applied to the positive or preventive health needs of the local community in general in that it focuses on health education and prevention of ill health rather than responding to illness and so is proactive – looking for health needs – rather than reactive. Four key principles of health visiting were outlined in 1977 and confirmed by the Health Visitor's Association and the Standing Conference on Health Visitor Education in 1992:

- the search for health needs
- stimulation of awareness of health needs
- influence on policies affecting health
- facilitation of health-enhancing activities (Turton & Orr 1993).

While health visiting means working with communities and taking political action, in addition to working with individuals and families, in practice, the collective aspects of their role have been less well developed. However, the Sure Start initiative provides a route through which health visitors are increasingly becoming involved in such community-oriented, health promotion work (Cowley 2002). The pathfinder Children's Trusts, for example, set up to implement principles of Every Child Matters (DES 2004), are focused in areas of social deprivation, and aimed to provide more integrated and accessible support services, and health visitors have a key role in these. An initial evaluation of these has suggested positive potential (UEA/NCB 2007) and the UK government plans to roll-out their development more widely, often based in Sure Start Children's Centres.

Health visiting in the UK had its origins in the nineteenth century social reform movement that was a response to the problems of rapid industrialization, urbanization and poverty (Robertson 1988). Concerns about public health also led to improvements in general sanitation (especially sewerage and water supply) and housing conditions. The most important moves towards improving public health and decreasing the high mortality due to infectious diseases were, therefore, set in place as a result of careful observation of living conditions, before the precise mechanisms of infection were understood (McKeown 1979). Modern health visitors continue this public health role and increasingly focus on psychosocial care and on the health effects of inequality as well as the more traditional concepts of public health.

Health visitors visit families to give advice or support and run health clinics. In some areas health visitors visit women during pregnancy to offer health advice and preparation for parenthood, or provide parent education classes jointly with community midwives. They may also play a role in providing preventive support or referral for problems such as postnatal depression.

After a baby's birth, in the UK, the parents are given a child health record book to keep, along with general information about community health services, and are invited to visit the child health clinic regularly.

The broad remit of health visitors, including screening, health education and prevention roles for the local population, gives them a less clearly defined professional identity than some other health professionals, and their roles are likely to change with the advent of integrated Children's Centres and moves towards development of more integrated professional roles. They are increasingly encouraged to work with existing or potential social support networks, rather than to attempt to provide all support themselves or adopt the role of experts. This connects to a wider debate about the nature and effectiveness of health education and promotion programmes. This is reflected in their roles within Sure Start projects, or developing links with wider regeneration projects that reflect a broad health promotion role and a renewed emphasis on tackling the problems of poverty and social exclusion (see Box 51.1, also Cowley 2002). However, like other professionals, health visitors also have to balance potentially conflicting roles of providing support and monitoring or surveillance of families. Such dilemmas are faced most acutely when considering child protection issues.

Health education and preventive healthcare

While community health services such as health visiting and midwifery aim to focus on preventive healthcare, they also encounter the basic problems confronting health professionals in attempting to provide health education and preventive care as some women may also view it as an unwarranted interference in their lives.

Preventive healthcare has been described as operating on three levels:

- *primary:* before a disease process starts (e.g. immunization or advice on nutrition)
- *secondary:* to alleviate or arrest disease (e.g. screening, diagnosis and treatment)
- *tertiary:* to limit or alleviate the effects of disease or illness (e.g. rehabilitation).

Pregnancy and adaptation to parenthood are important life changes and a time when adults are particularly responsive to information and often seek it out actively. Nonetheless, health education, as traditionally conceived, has the important limitation of tending to focus on individual lifestyles and desired behavioural changes, outside the context of the constraints on people's lives and the ways in which such conditions affect health. For example, the 'Health of the Nation' document (DoH 1992) sets out clear priority areas and targets for reduction of morbidity and mortality, but was criticized for its emphasis on altering individuals' behaviour in the absence of structural changes to promote healthy lifestyles or increase individual choices. The following government document 'Our Healthier Nation' (DoH 1998) responded with a far greater emphasis on the conditions that produce ill health and this is also reflected in more recent government policies for health and social care, as described above.

Crafter (1997) distinguished health education, which largely involves working with individuals or groups to enhance or change knowledge, with the aim of helping people to make informed and positive health choices, from health promotion, a broader concept that recognizes the importance of social and environmental influences on health. To promote positive health, it is increasingly acknowledged that health education must work hand in hand with efforts to change the structural and environmental factors influencing health, either directly or through the choices people feel able to make. Principles for health education are set out internationally by the World Health Organization and these have shifted since the 1980s towards involving individuals and communities in planning and implementing healthcare. The Ottawa Charter, for example, states:

health promotion works through effective community action in setting priorities, making decisions, planning strategies and implementing them to achieve better health. At the heart of

this process is the empowerment of communities, and the ownership and control of their own endeavours and destiny.
(WHO 1986, p 1, quoted in Jones & Sidell 1997.)

Immunization

Immunization is an important aspect of preventive healthcare globally. There are different forms of immunization, but they all function through stimulation of the immune system in order to enhance resistance to a particular mechanism of infection.

Vaccines are available for a range of diseases, some of which have severe symptoms (e.g. polio), whereas others are important for protection against congenital defects. Immunization against rubella (German measles) is a good example of protecting a vulnerable group, namely pregnant women, by means of protecting the general population. While the disease produces only mild symptoms in children and adults, it has severe implications for early fetal development. Immunization thus has a dual role in public health:

- *population protection*: decreasing the incidence of an infectious disease
- *individual protection*: decreasing the individual's likelihood of contracting a disease or the severity of symptoms experienced where protection is not complete.

Although population protection is arguably the most important function of immunization, epidemiologists have pointed out that, historically, its role in improving public health and decreasing mortality has been overestimated in relation to more general measures such as improved nutrition and sanitation (McKeown 1979).

A series of immunizations focusing on the most common and the most potentially damaging childhood illnesses is offered to all children in the UK from about 8 weeks of age. Since women may ask for advice about immunization during their postnatal care, it is important for midwives to increase their own knowledge of its benefits and limitations, recommended practice and contraindications for certain individuals.

Since immunizations can, rarely, have serious side-effects, parents should always be advised about contraindications and precautions when they are encouraged to take up immunization. Parents are particularly likely to raise questions about vaccinations that have been subject to controversy. The pertussis vaccine, which protects against whooping cough, was a focus of concern regarding severe side-effects during the 1970s, which led to a significant fall in take-up rates. Subsequent studies have failed to confirm the level of risk conclusively and policy documents have emphasized the high level of risk from the disease itself in relation to possible vaccination risks. The combined measles, mumps and rubella vaccine (MMR), introduced during the 1990s as a mass immunization programme, has also been controversial, with some professionals arguing that the programme was speculative and unnecessary in view of possible side-effects and others arguing that considerable research has shown few ill-effects and considerable benefits, and that the seriousness of some diseases are now easily overlooked by modern populations. Currently, although a number of parents may enquire about separate vaccinations, Department of Health advice is that combined immunization is safer, and separate vaccines are not provided by the NHS (DH 2004b). In all such cases, the complexity of influences on public health means that definitive evidence on the benefits and risks of immunization is hard to obtain. Current policy remains that, on the balance of evidence, the benefits to public and individual health greatly outweigh possible risks. Up-to-date advice on immunization and current versions of schedules can be obtained from the NHS at www.immunization.org.uk

Social services

The local authority social services departments hold the main responsibility for community care arrangements, liaison with health services and support for specific needs and problems such as childcare and protection, although the services arranged to meet such needs may be provided by a range of organizations. Facilities provided or contracted for by social services include home care, respite care, and day and residential childcare.

Social workers

Social workers play a key role in community care and also have specific statutory duties with respect to mental health and child protection. They also act as gatekeepers to other services, such as home help or assistance with child care. They may also provide direct support to clients, using a casework approach. Most social workers have a generic role that is concerned with a range of client groups although some work as specialists. This is more common in mental health social work, where some qualify as Approved Social Workers and are obliged to carry out statutory assessments under sections of the Mental Health Act 1983 and in child protection.

Social work, like health visiting, has its origins in social reform movements. The approach of social work in the UK today was laid out when local authority social services departments were created following the Seebohm report in 1970 (Clements 1996). The main areas of social work relevant to midwives' work are their childcare and protection and their mental health roles. These roles operate within the frameworks of the Children Act 2004 and the Mental Health Act 2007.

Child protection and families needing support

In general, the aim of social services is to provide support to families that will help them to manage their situation and prevent the need for more extensive services or interventions. A good example of this would be the provision of respite care (care for short breaks), home care, and aids and adaptations in the home for parents whose child has a disability, which may avoid the need for residential care. These aims are not always met in practice owing to funding shortfalls or simply because of problems in coordination of services. Midwives can promote good practice by advising women of their rights to apply for assessment for services and supporting them in the assessment process.

The Children Act 2004 in the UK focused on the needs of the child and emphasized that childcare services or proceedings should always consider their welfare and interests as paramount. For example, it states that court orders should be made only where it is in the interests of the child to do so. The policy aims to support families so that they can remain together where possible and provides guidance on appropriate social service responses where this may not be in the interest of the child.

The Children Act 2004 provided the legal underpinning to the policy guidance Every Child Matters (DES 2004). Its focus was on children's well-being and defined five key outcomes, which were developed more fully in the Every Child Matters guidance: Be healthy; Stay safe; Enjoy and achieve; Make a positive contribution; Achieve economic well-being. This policy was also intended to work in close synergy with the health policy priorities set out in the NSF (DH 2004a) to ensure that children's services are truly integrated. The 2004 Children Act replaced a 'needs' focused approach with a more child- and family-centred approach that regards all children as having positive needs for development and well-being and Every Child Matters aims to help professionals to form a view of what children need to thrive, whatever their social or cultural background. When a child has particular needs by virtue of disability or other problems, social services departments have a duty to respond. Since midwives have close contact with women and their families in the perinatal period, they may have an important role in identifying where families need additional support and advising those with special needs (DES 2004).

Child protection procedures

However, positive its intended focus, such legislation has to clarify professional responsibilities and actions in cases where there is concern that children's well-being is not being protected. The Act established Local Safeguarding Children Boards (LSCBs) to be set up by each Local Authority, as part of the wider context of Children's Trust arrangements, and details are set out in the Working Together to Safeguard Children document (HM Govt. 2006). This guidance (and Section 11 of the Children Act 2004) made clear that all agencies have shared responsibilities and duties to make arrangements to safeguard and promote the welfare of children and emphasized the importance of joint working to achieve this. Although the primary duty is with each local authority, all professionals who come into contact with children have duties to promote its general principles:

- aim to ensure that all affected children receive appropriate and timely therapeutic and preventative interventions

- those professionals who work directly with children should ensure that safeguarding and promoting their welfare forms an integral part of all stages of care they offer

- those professionals who come into contact with children, parents and carers in the course of their work also need to be aware of their safeguarding responsibilities

- ensure that all health professionals can recognize risk factors and contribute to reviews, enquiries and child protection plans, as well as planning support for children and providing ongoing promotional and preventative support through proactive work (HM Govt. 2006).

Midwives need to be aware of child protection procedures (Fig. 51.1) since they are likely to be in contact with families that pose serious concerns about the child's welfare. The Working Together to Safeguard Children document provides detailed advice on actions to be taken and routes of referral for any professionals who develop concerns about the welfare of a child. It advises that all health professionals who work with children and families should be able to:

- understand the risk factors and recognize children in need of support and/or safeguarding

- recognize the needs of parents who may need extra help in bringing up their children, and know where to refer for help

- recognize the risks of abuse to an unborn child

- contribute to enquiries from other professionals about children and their family or carers

- liaise closely with other agencies, including other health professionals

- assess the needs of children and the capacity of parents/carers to meet their children's needs, including the needs of children who display sexually harmful behaviour

- plan and respond to the needs of children and their families, particularly those who are vulnerable

- contribute to child protection conferences, family group conferences and strategy discussions

- contribute to planning support for children at risk of significant harm, e.g. children living in households with domestic violence or parental substance misuse

- help ensure that children who have been abused and parents under stress (e.g. those who have mental health problems) have access to services to support them

- play an active part, through the child protection plan, in safeguarding children from significant harm

- as part of generally safeguarding children and young people, provide ongoing promotional and preventative support, through proactive work with children, families and expectant parents

- contribute to serious case reviews and their implementation.

The guidance, therefore, or equivalent guidance in other countries, should be read and retained for reference by all midwives.

The distinction between the need for support and the need for child protection is a difficult one and, in many situations, adequate and timely support for a family can prevent the need for child protection measures. The transition to parenthood is an important life event for all parents, and life events, even where they are wanted and viewed positively, can be major sources of stress and emotional distress (McCourt 2006). Childcare and adjustment to parenthood present a challenge to most parents and there is no clear and simple line between those who are able and those who are unable to cope with the demands of a new baby. However, there are circumstances that have been shown to be strongly associated with parents' capacity to care for a child, in particular families with multiple problems (Cleaver et al 1999).

Compulsory intervention is advised in cases where there is concern about significant harm to the child (Children Act 2004, HM Govt. 2006). Where midwives are concerned about possible significant harm, they should normally contact the relevant Local Authority, or their Local Safeguarding Children Board (LSCB). In the first instance, concerns can be raised with the supervisor of midwives or with the named senior midwife with responsibility for child protection, who should ensure that the appropriate social services officers are contacted. Each Primary Care Trust is responsible for ensuring that health service providers have clear policies in place, and each PCT and NHS Trust should

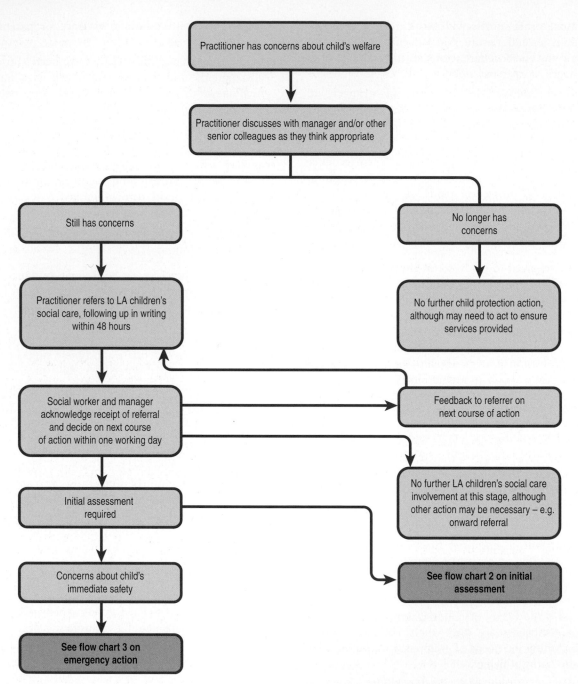

Figure 51.1   The child protection process: initial referral. (© Crown copyright. Working together to safeguard children 2006).

appoint a lead nurse or midwife and a lead doctor for child protection. Each midwife in the UK should be familiar with these policies and key contacts. In emergencies out of hours, police child protection teams may be involved or an Emergency Protection Order may be sought. The midwives code of practice also provides basic guidelines to appropriate conduct.

Midwives may become concerned about potential child abuse antenatally, influenced by factors in the woman's history, her current mental state or her living situation. This may include concerns about domestic abuse towards the woman herself, and research has shown that there are strong associations between situations of domestic abuse and child abuse (Cleaver et al 1999). Antenatal care is a good point at which to work with a woman and to provide support, or assist the woman in obtaining the support she needs, in order to prevent possible problems arising after the baby is born. Indeed many of the family problems that are often associated with higher levels of abuse are those where parents, mothers in particular, would benefit from high levels of ante- and postnatal support. Interventions to support women with mental health problems, substance abuse problems and those who suffer from social isolation, poor support or domestic abuse are important preventive and health promoting measures (DH 2004a). In cases of concern about significant harm, a Child Protection Conference may be called regarding an unborn child, and midwives are particularly likely to be involved in such cases (HM Govt. 2006).

Identifying possible child abuse

Abuse is difficult to define and even more difficult to judge. The incidence of abuse is difficult to measure since it depends on reporting or detection; that is likely to be related to social awareness and policy as much as anything else.

Recent UK research has shown that, although abuse is very widespread and is by no means confined to particular social groups, when child protection cases reach court proceedings, high rates of identifiable parental problems such as mental illness, domestic or substance misuse are found. Domestic abuse is an important issue in its own right and is also associated with increased risk of child abuse and it is estimated that one-third of domestic abuse commences or escalates

during pregnancy. For both reasons, it is important for health professionals to respond to signs of possible domestic abuse. Women may often present problems but in an indirect rather than overt manner, such as repeated visits to health providers complaining of vague illness symptoms, or through self-harm or symptoms of mental distress (NCB 1995, Turton & Orr 1993). Rates of child abuse are particularly high where families are experiencing multiple problems. None the less, the majority of mothers with such problems are able to care for their children well, particularly if they have support from their partner or family, and supportive services to turn to (Cleaver et al 1999).

This evidence lends further weight to the current emphasis in child protection on prevention and efforts to work with families. It is helpful if problems are not seen as resulting from a dichotomy in parenting styles but as occurring on a continuum from calm and confident parenting through the normal range of most parents to those who have great difficulties and potential for abuse. It also highlights the potential value of appropriate midwifery support in pregnancy. It is important for midwives to respond to early signs of stress or distress in pregnant and postnatal mothers and their families, by being ready to listen and to provide advice and information or referrals to other sources of support, including self-help groups.

Robertson (1988) argued that health visitors dealing with child protection should work within a framework of cross-cultural and societal violence and should maintain a focus on prevention. By this she meant understanding that child abuse is not just an individual issue but takes place within the framework of social and cultural conditions and values. Professionals should focus on the basic needs of the child and on the child *per se* and avoid relying on subjective judgements about what constitutes good or appropriate parenting, which are strongly influenced by cultural norms (Cloke & Naish 1992, Narducci 1992). It is tempting to believe, particularly as a service provider, that one's own knowledge and values are naturally right or superior.

Child abuse can be identified in various forms and, although problems tend not to fall into neat categories, in practice these may be of use in assessing possible abuse. The categories used in government policy are listed in Box 51.6.

Box 51.6 Categories of child abuse (HM Govt. 2006, p 37–38)

Physical abuse

May involve hitting, shaking, throwing, poisoning, burning or scalding, drowning, suffocating, or otherwise causing physical harm to a child. Physical harm may also be caused when a parent or carer fabricates the symptoms of, or deliberately induces, illness in a child.

Emotional abuse

The persistent emotional maltreatment of a child such as to cause severe and persistent adverse effects on the child's emotional development. It may involve conveying to children that they are worthless or unloved, inadequate, or valued only insofar as they meet the needs of another person. It may feature age or developmentally inappropriate expectations being imposed on children. These may include interactions that are beyond the child's developmental capability, as well as overprotection and limitation of exploration and learning, or preventing the child participating in normal social interaction. It may involve seeing or hearing the ill-treatment of another. It may involve serious bullying, causing children frequently to feel frightened or in danger, or the exploitation or corruption of children. Some level of emotional abuse is involved in all types of maltreatment of a child, though it may occur alone.

Sexual abuse

Involves forcing or enticing a child or young person to take part in sexual activities, including prostitution, whether or not the child is aware of what is happening. The activities may involve physical contact, including penetrative (e.g. rape, buggery or oral sex) or non-penetrative acts. They may include non-contact activities, such as involving children in looking at, or in the production of, sexual online images, watching sexual activities, or encouraging children to behave in sexually inappropriate ways.

Neglect

The persistent failure to meet a child's basic physical and/or psychological needs, likely to result in the serious impairment of the child's health or development. Neglect may occur during pregnancy as a result of maternal substance abuse. Once a child is born, neglect may involve a parent or carer failing to: provide adequate food, clothing and shelter (including exclusion from home or abandonment); protect a child from physical and emotional harm or danger; ensure adequate supervision (including the use of inadequate care-givers); ensure access to appropriate medical care or treatment. It may also include neglect of, or unresponsiveness to, a child's basic emotional needs.

The UK policy guidance notes that there are no absolute criteria for judging significant harm but advises that:

Consideration of the severity of ill-treatment may include the degree and the extent of physical harm, the duration and frequency of abuse and neglect, the extent of premeditation, and the presence or degree of threat, coercion, sadism and bizarre or unusual elements. Each of these elements has been associated with more severe effects on the child, and/or relatively greater difficulty in helping the child overcome the adverse impact of the maltreatment. Sometimes, a single traumatic event may constitute significant harm, e.g. a violent assault, suffocation or poisoning. More often, significant harm is a compilation of significant events, both acute and long-standing, which interrupt, change or damage the child's physical and psychological development. Some children live

in family and social circumstances where their health and development are neglected. For them, it is the corrosiveness of long-term emotional, physical or sexual abuse that causes impairment to the extent of constituting significant harm. In each case, it is necessary to consider any maltreatment alongside the family's strengths and supports.'

(HM Govt. 2006, p 36)

Signs and symptoms of abuse are not always clear. Bruising, for example, may be the result of a range of causes and suspicion of abuse is more likely if the bruising forms a particular pattern. The signs are more likely to be taken seriously if a number of symptoms are found together or where inconsistent accounts of accidents are given and where there are delays in seeking care (Robertson 1988).

Fostering and adoption

Midwives often provide care for women whose pregnancy was not planned. This is more common than many professionals may realize and it is important not to make assumptions about the woman's feelings about her pregnancy. For example, in a study of women's experiences of maternity services, between 22% and 40% of women in the groups studied had mixed or negative initial feelings about the pregnancy (McCourt & Page 1996). In many cases women will be happy about an unplanned pregnancy, whereas others may be ambivalent and need support and possibly non-directive counselling to assist them in making decisions and plans for the future. For some women, this may involve relinquishment of the child for adoption. It is important to remember that such women share ordinary needs for information and support in pregnancy and childbirth, as well as having additional needs for support around relinquishing their child. Midwives can make a difference to how women feel in quite simple ways, such as avoiding judgmental or insensitive comments or approaches to care, by offering women a chance to discuss their situation privately but openly, and by providing advice on where they might find more specialized support.

Adoption procedures were reformed by the Children Act 1989 and 2004 so that there is now a greater emphasis in the UK on open adoption where possible, so that relinquishing mothers may remain in agreed forms of contact with their children. Practice in childcare agencies has also developed in recent years so that children who are adopted, fostered or placed in residential care are given more opportunity to understand and talk about their personal history. Fostering (on a short- or long-term basis) may be a consideration for mothers who are unable to care for their babies after birth but who do not wish to relinquish their children for adoption. The Children Act also increases flexibility for family members to care for children or remain in contact with them where mothers are unable to do so.

Other community services

Childcare services

Childcare services may be important in providing support to families experiencing stress, for example due to poor or temporary housing, caring responsibilities or postnatal depression. Childcare services for children under 5 years old are mainly the responsibility of social services, although education departments may manage local authority provision for children aged between 3 and 5. They generally provide a limited number of places but are responsible for the registration and inspection of all other facilities for the under 5s in their local area, including privately owned nurseries and individual childminders. Some services, often run by voluntary agencies, are also geared to the needs of families under stress. These include family centres, where parents and children can attend together and receive parenting support, and schemes such as Homestart or Newpin (Family Welfare Association) and Sure Start Children's Centres.

Social services departments often provide under-5s advisors. Local authorities often publish guides to local child care facilities, not only day care but resources for parents and small children to use together, such as playgroups or toy libraries and crèche facilities linked to adult education or sports activities. The UK government's Sure Start website gives some useful and regularly updated information on finding and using childcare.

Interpreting, advocacy and link workers

Women and families from minority ethnic communities have two closely related sets of needs from maternity and other community health and social services (see Ch. 3). First are the ordinary needs, which they share with women of all backgrounds but which are often attended to more poorly owing to language or cultural barriers or to discrimination. Second are the particular needs resulting from their minority status, which may include language access and more specialized services. In practice, both are likely to be related. For example, women in a small-scale study of a refugee community in West London voiced concerns about lack of information, advice, choices and sensitive personal care. These concerns were widely shared among local women but they were experienced as far more severe problems by women from ethnic minorities (Harper-Bulman & McCourt 2002).

Women who are refugees may also be socially isolated and need practical support in adjusting to life in a new country. Many will have come from situations of fear and conflict, only to meet with the difficulties of the asylum process on arrival. There is debate around the psychological health status of refugees, between those who emphasize the likelihood of post-traumatic stress and the need for psychological interventions such as counselling, and those who argue that medical approaches to the needs of refugees are not necessarily or always appropriate. Sensitive care from midwives that provides good levels of support, tuned in to the woman and family's self-perceived needs, may make a difference. In addition minority groups (particularly refugees and asylum seekers) will benefit particularly from continuity of care and carer (McCourt & Pearce 2000).

Housing

Housing is important for both the physical and psychological health of parents and children. Local authorities in the UK have a statutory duty to provide housing for families who are homeless, including pregnant women, but this may involve temporary accommodation that is not well suited to caring for a child. The duty to provide accommodation for those in unsuitable housing is less clear cut and many families join long waiting lists, with priority given to those with the highest 'points' for several categories of need. Local authorities may also nominate families to the waiting lists of housing associations, trusts and cooperatives, some of which also operate their own application systems. Midwives may be asked to support applications for housing or improved housing, usually by writing letters.

Accommodation with support may be available or offered for mothers and babies in certain circumstances, including refuges for women experiencing domestic abuse and supported accommodation for mothers of school age, or those experiencing depression or other mental health problems. Shortage of specialist mother and baby facilities, however, may limit what can be offered to women who need such support. The emphasis is, where possible, on providing care for mothers and babies together or,

when children need accommodation without their mothers, on gaining support from the wider family if possible or providing foster care.

Voluntary and independent services

Voluntary organizations have been a major influence by showing what can be done and by campaigning for particular interest groups or services. They are linked to a long tradition of charitable work undertaken before the advent of the modern welfare state and were traditionally often linked with religious groups, as were the early hospital services in many countries. Voluntary organizations have shifted over time from being primarily charitable to a mutual or self-help focus, with many organizations founded by relatives of people in need of long-term services and, more recently, service user organizations. Government policy since the 1980s in the UK has strongly encouraged broadening the range of organizations providing services, including private companies. Voluntary and private providers of care are often referred to in policy terms as 'the independent sector'.

Voluntary organizations have generally combined two rather different roles effectively: that of campaigning or providing information and advice and that of providing community health or social services. Services provided were often innovative, or responded to a gap in provision, which would, if effective, gradually be adopted by the statutory service providers. Following the NHS and Community Care Act 1990, they were encouraged to take on a far greater role in service provision and in some areas are now key providers of essential services such as residential and day childcare (Box 51.7).

Services for mothers with disabilities

A range of services are provided by local authorities and voluntary or mutual support groups for women with disabilities, including those who are mothers. Although many are informal, and benefit from being so, it is important to remember the framework of rights and procedures provided by the NHS and Community Care Act 1990 and subsequent Disability legislation. In addition to service information, it is important for midwives to enhance their own

---

Box 51.7 Voluntary organizations relevant for pregnant women and families with young children

- Informal and mutual support groups – often locally based or focused on a particular issue, e.g. local postnatal support groups facilitated by health visitors or community workers, or developing from formal parent education classes
- Parent and baby or toddler groups and clubs – these are generally locally, informally run and play an important part in preventing social isolation
- Childbirth groups which combine campaigning with practical and social support, e.g. National Childbirth Trust
- Breastfeeding support groups, which provide practical and moral support to women establishing breastfeeding, e.g. La Leche League
- Postnatal depression and women and mental health groups
- Minority ethnic community groups, refugee organizations and women's groups, which play a valuable role for women and families who may need practical and social support, including language services
- Groups for people who have suffered pregnancy loss or bereavement including mutual support, advice and counselling organizations, e.g. the Stillbirth and Neonatal Death Society (SANDS) or the Foundation for the Study of Infant Deaths (FSID)
- Groups for families under stress or needing support, e.g. Family Welfare Association, Homestart
- Groups for parents of children with disabilities or chronic health problems
- Support and counselling for relinquishing mothers and those whose children are in residential or foster care – such support is often now provided by voluntary adoption and fostering agencies, e.g. British Association for Adoption and Fostering (BAAF)
- Groups for parents with baby crying problems, e.g. Cry-Sis
- Groups for single parents, e.g. Parentpack, Gingerbread
- Groups for fathers e.g. Fathers Direct.

A number of directories of local and national organizations are published and will be valuable to keep to hand for reference. (See also links on the website: www.tiger.gov.uk)

---

awareness of disability issues, in order to provide a good service to all women whatever their needs. Issues for mothers with physical disabilities are considered in Chapter 3.

Learning disability

Midwives need awareness of learning disability issues both to support parents who may have some form of learning disability but also, increasingly, to provide information and support to all pregnant women offered screening for different disabilities. The issues surrounding parents with learning disabilities are particularly sensitive since social policy in the UK and other industrialized societies has historically been strongly influenced by eugenic ideas and focused on preventing people with disabilities from reproduction or parenthood. Many individuals are still sterilized, if not through force then by persuasion, or are encouraged to terminate pregnancies. In this context,

disabled activists and academics have argued that the availability of screening and termination for impairments reflects and contributes to assumptions that physical or intellectual impairment is always and only a negative thing. Such a cultural environment is likely to impact on the feelings of people with such impairments, particularly when approaching the issue of parenthood. A number of theorists have, therefore, identified three different models of disability: the medical (or individual deficit model), the religious (or moral) model and the social oppression model. The last of these models recognizes that disability occurs as a result of social forces rather than simply because of the person's impairment. What may be disabling for particular individuals with impairments are features of that environment, for example emphasis on literacy, design of buildings, or stigmatizing attitudes (Barnes et al 1999, Oliver 1996).

The category 'learning disability' covers a wide span and includes people who will need very high levels of support in becoming parents. Professional knowledge of learning disability, like 'lay' knowledge, is often very limited, partly because of the history, before recent philosophical and policy changes, of keeping people with disabilities socially segregated. 'Mental handicap' hospitals were built in the UK in the early part of the twentieth century (rather like the psychiatric asylums built before them) as geographically isolated institutions that functioned rather like self-sufficient communities (Alasewski 1986). Midwives need to learn more about learning and other disabilities to provide education and support for mothers with disabilities and to advise and counsel parents about antenatal screening and diagnostic tests (Dixon 1997).

Mental health and illness

The prevalence of mental health problems among women is acknowledged to be high, and mental health problems are far more widespread within the population than many people imagine, since mental illness is often associated with distorted media-based images of psychosis or violence. The importance of midwives' attention to mental health issues is discussed in Chapter 36B. The public health emphasis in the National Service Framework (DH 2004a) is particularly focused on social deprivation as a major predisposer to mental health problems, on maternal mental health problems and their potential impact on the whole family. As with other community health and social care issues, therefore, midwives have great potential, as well as responsibility, to support women and families during this critical time of transition and development for women and families.

Conclusion

This chapter has highlighted key areas of community health and social services with which midwives need to be familiar. Some are important for general awareness and some for more specific roles such as providing advice, support or referral. A textbook can only provide an introduction and these areas have seen radical and rapid change in recent years. The references and further reading suggestions below will provide some pointers for developing further knowledge.

REFERENCES

Acheson D 1998 Independent enquiry into inequalities in health. The Stationery Office, London.

Alasewski A 1986 Institutional care and the mentally handicapped. Croom Helm, London

Barker D J P 1998 Mothers, babies and health in later life. Churchill Livingstone, Edinburgh

Barnes C, Mercer G, Shakespeare T 1999 Exploring disability, a sociological introduction. Polity Press, Cambridge

Beake S, McCourt C, Rowan C 2005 Evaluation of the role of an infant feeding support worker in the community to support breastfeeding in disadvantaged women. Maternal & Child Nutrition 1(1):32–43.

Bulmer M 1987 The social basis of community care. Allen & Unwin, London

Carnell J, Kline R (eds) 1999 Community practitioners and health visitors' handbook. Radcliffe Medical, Abingdon

Cleaver H, Unell I, Aldgate J 1999 Children's needs – parenting capacity. The impact of parental mental illness, problem alcohol and drug use, and domestic violence on children's development. The Stationery Office, London

Clements L 1996 Community care and the law. Legal Action Group, London

Cloke C, Naish J (eds) 1992 Key issues in child protection for health visitors and nurses. Longman, London

Cowley S 2002 Public health in policy and practice. A sourcebook for health visitors and community nurses. Baillière Tindall, Edinburgh

Crafter H 1997 Health promotion in midwifery. Principles and practice. Arnold, London

DES (Department for Education and Skills) 2004 Every child matters: change for children. The Stationery Office, London

DoH (Department of Health) 1992 The health of the nation. HMSO, London

DoH (Department of Health) 1993 Changing childbirth: report of the expert maternity group. HMSO, London

DoH (Department of Health) 1997a The new NHS: modern, dependable. Cm 3807. The Stationery Office, London

DoH (Department of Health) 1997b NHS (Primary Care) Act. DoH, London

DoH (Department of Health) 1998 Our healthier nation. A contract for health. Cmd 3852. The Stationery Office, London

DH (Department of Health) 2001 The Health and Social Care Act. TSO, London.

DH (Department of Health) 2004a National Services Framework for Children, Young People and Maternity Services. The Stationery Office, London.

DH (Department of Health) 2004b MMR information pack. Online. Available: www.dh.gov.uk

DH (Department of Health) 2006a Health Reform in England: update and commissioning framework. The Stationery Office, London

DH (Department of Health) 2006b Our health, our care, our say: a new direction for community services. The Stationery Office, London

DH (Department of Health) 2007a Maternity matters: choice, access and continuity of care in a safe service. The Stationery Office, London

DH (Department of Health) 2007b Commissioning framework for health and well-being. The Stationery Office, London

Dimond B 1997 Legal aspects of care in the community. Macmillan, London

Dixon K 1997 Practical tips for supporting pregnant women with learning disabilities. MIDIRS Midwifery Digest 7 (1):40–42

Donnison J 1988 Midwives and medical men. A history of the struggle for the control of childbirth. Historical Publications, Barnet

Harper-Bulman K, McCourt C 2002 Somali refugee women's experiences of maternity care in west London: a case study. Public Health 12:365–380

HM Government 2006 Working together to safeguard children: A guide to inter-agency working to safeguard and promote the welfare of children. The Stationery Office, London

House of Commons Social Services Committee 1980 Perinatal and neonatal mortality (the Short report). HMSO, London

Hunt S, Symonds S 1995 The social meaning of midwifery. Macmillan, London

IDS (Incomes Data Services) 2007 Maternity and parental rights, employment law handbook. IDS, London. Updated annually. Online. Available: www.incomesdata.co.uk/studies/maternity.htm

Jones L, Sidell M 1997 The challenge of promoting health. Exploration and action. Macmillan/Open University, Basingstoke

Leap N, Hunter B 1993 The midwife's tale: an oral history from handy women to professional midwife. Scarlett Press, London

Lewis G (ed.) 2007 The Confidential Enquiry into Maternal and Child Health (CEMACH). Saving mothers' lives: reviewing maternal deaths to make motherhood safer 2003–2005. The seventh report on Confidential Enquiries into Maternal Deaths in the United Kingdom. CEMACH, London

McCourt C 2006 Becoming a parent. In: Page L, McCandlish R (eds) The new midwifery. Science and sensitivity in practice, 2nd edn. Churchill Livingstone, Edinburgh

McCourt C, Page L 1996 Report on the evaluation of one-to-one midwifery. Centre for Midwifery Practice, Thames Valley University, London. Online. Available: www.health.tvu.ac.uk/mid

McCourt C, Pearce A 2000 Does continuity of carer matter to women from minority ethnic groups? Midwifery 16:145–154

McCourt C, Stevens T, Sandall J et al 2006 Working with women: continuity of carer in practice. In: Page L, McCandlish R (eds) The new midwifery: science and sensitivity in practice, 2nd edn. Churchill Livingstone, Edinburgh

McKeown T 1979 The role of medicine: dream, mirage or nemesis? Blackwell, Oxford

MoH (Ministry of Health) 1970 Domiciliary midwifery and maternity bed needs: the report of the standing maternity and midwifery advisory committee (the Peel report). HMSO, London

Narducci T 1992 Race, culture and child protection. In: Cloke C, Naish J (eds) Key issues in child protection for health visitors and nurses. Longman, London, Ch. 2, p 12–22

NCB (National Children's Bureau) 1995 Children and domestic violence. NCB, London NHS and Community Care Act 1990. HMSO, London

NHS London(2007)Report of the Maternity and Newborn Clinical Working Group. (Part of the review led by Darzi A. Healthcare for London: a framework for action. Online. Available: www.healthcareforlondon.nhs.uk

Oakley A 1992 Social support and motherhood. The natural history of a research project. Blackwell, Oxford

Oliver M 1996 Understanding disability: from theory to practice. Cassell, London

Richards M, Hardy R, Kuh D et al 2001 Birth weight and cognitive function in the British 1946 birth cohort: longitudinal population based study. British Medical Journal 322(7280): 199–200.

Roberts H 1997 Socioeconomic determinants of health: children, inequalities and health. British Medical Journal 314(7087):1122–1125

Robertson C 1988 Health visiting in practice. Longman, Edinburgh

Robinson S 1990 Maintaining the role of the midwife. In: Garcia J, Kilpatrick R, Richards M (eds) The politics of maternity care. Clarendon, Oxford

Sandall J, Davies J, Warwick C 2000 Evaluation of the Albany midwifery practice. Kings College, London

Stacey M 1988 The sociology of health and healing. Unwin & Hyman, London

Tew M 1990 Safer childbirth? A critical history of maternity care. Chapman & Hall, London

Turton P, Orr J 1993 Learning to care in the community, 2nd edn. Edward Arnold, London

UEA/NCB (University of East Anglia & National Children's Bureau) 2007 Children's Trust Pathfinders: innovative partnerships for improving the well-being of children and young people. National Evaluation of Children's Trust Pathfinders, Final Report. Online. Available: www.everychildmatters.gov.uk/resources-and-practice/IG00209

FURTHER READING

Texts on health visiting are useful for midwives since they focus on relevant areas of work such as health advice, preventive care and monitoring, and child health and development. Read some introductory texts to increase your understanding of health visitors' aims and ways of working and explore how these relate to the approach of midwives.

Social science textbooks will also be useful, as will those more directly related to analysis of maternity care, the health of mothers and babies and accounts of research into health beliefs, practices and social conditions. For example:

Cornwell J 1984 Hard earned lives. Tavistock, London

Oakley A 1993 Essays on women, medicine and health. Edinburgh University Press, Edinburgh

Stacey M 1988 The sociology of health and healing. Unwin & Hyman, London

It is also important to obtain a good and up-to-date range of local and national directories of organizations and services. For example:

MIDIRS Directory of Maternity Organizations. MIDIRS, Bristol.
Updated regularly by means of the addition of inserts when new information is received.

Whitfield C (ed.) People who help. A guide to voluntary and other support organizations. Profile Productions, London.
Updated regularly. A number of guides to the legislation, aimed at health professionals, are published. For example:

DH 2003 What to do if you're worried a child is being abused. DH, London

DH 2003 Responding to domestic abuse: a handbook for health professionals. DH, London
It is important to check that they reflect the most up-to-date guidance and legislation that is still in force.

USEFUL WEBSITES

UK government publications, policy and guidance in general:
www.direct.gov.uk

The Department of Health:
www.dh.gov.uk

The Department of Trade and Industry – employee rights:
www.dti.gov.uk

The Department of Work and Pensions (formerly Department of Social Security) – rights and benefits:
www.dwp.gov.uk

Sure Start and Every Child Matters:
www.surestart.gov.uk

52 Midwifery supervision and clinical governance

Jean Duerden

Supervision of midwives empowers midwives to work within the full scope of their role, provides professional support for midwives, promotes good midwifery practice and protects the public by providing a framework for scrutiny of professional standard practice (NMC 2002). It facilitates a non-confrontational, confidential, midwife-led review of a midwife's level of knowledge, understanding and competence (ENB 1999). The philosophy of midwifery supervision and the standards it develops, reflect the key themes of clinical governance described in NHS First Class Service (DH 1998). These themes are:

- professional self-regulation
- clinical governance
- life-long learning.

This chapter aims to:

- describe the supervision of midwives and how it supports the clinical governance framework
- review the various aspects of clinical governance
- promote the supervision of midwives as a mechanism for quality assurance, sensitive to the needs of mothers and babies
- assist midwives in using supervision effectively.

Supervision of midwives

A short history of the supervision of midwives

Supervision of midwives was introduced in Edwardian times with the passing of the Midwives Act in

1902. Under the Act, the Central Midwives Board (CMB) was established and through that Board, the inspection of midwives. The inspectors of midwives so created were not practising midwives, as the supervisors of midwives are today, but middle class women, 'ladies', used to supervising subordinates (Kirkham 1995), and who had domestic standards much higher than those of the working class midwives. As a result, they were extremely critical of the poor environments in which many of the midwives then lived. These lady inspectors attempted to impose their middle class standards on the midwives, and had little understanding of the needs of midwives who had to undertake the domestic work in their own homes themselves. They expected the midwives to 'use plenty of clean linen' (Kirkham 1995) despite the fact that the women they attended could not afford such linen. Similarly, the midwives struggled to comply with the Midwives Rules that instructed them to summon medical aid even though there was no possibility of the family paying the doctor's fee. It was not until 1918 that this matter was resolved when a further Midwives Act required midwives to notify the Local Supervising Authority (LSA), via the supervisor of midwives, that they had summoned medical aid. If summoned by a midwife the GP could be paid.

The LSA Officers were the Medical Officers of Health. They passed on the bulk of their LSA work to non-medical inspectors who were at liberty to inspect the midwives in any way they felt appropriate. They could follow them on their rounds, visit their homes, question the patients they had cared for and even investigate their personal lives (Kirkham 1995), in addition to inspecting their equipment. Records could not be checked; they were rarely made as many midwives were illiterate, notwithstanding their immense practical knowledge and independence. Midwives who disobeyed or ignored the rules would be disciplined. The Midwives Act also called for the LSA to investigate midwives who were guilty of negligence, malpractice or misconduct, personal or professional, and to report these midwives to the CMB for disciplinary action. The LSA Officer had to report any midwife convicted of an offence, suspend a midwife from practice if likely to be a source of infection, report the death of any midwife and submit a roll of midwives annually to the Board.

The roll of midwives was introduced with the 1902 Act that demanded the registration of midwives. Midwives must have their names on the roll of midwives, in order to continue practising. Training for midwives was established at the same time, but it was not until the 1910 Act that registration was permitted only on successful completion of an approved training course for midwives. Despite the training, it was not until 1936 that another revision of the Midwives Act led to the LSA being required to provide a salaried midwifery service. The amended Act empowered the CMB to set rules requiring midwives to attend refresher courses. It also determined the qualifications required to be a supervisor. Medical supervisors had to be medical officers, and non-medical supervisors, midwives, the latter under the control of the former. By 1937, the Ministry of Health had recognized the difficulties that midwives were experiencing by not having been supervised by midwives, and these changes were detailed in a Ministry of Health letter (MoH 1937), changing the title from inspector of midwives to supervisor of midwives, and requiring the supervisors to be experienced midwives. For some reason, it was thought appropriate that they should not be engaged in midwifery practice. A real change of heart had taken place since the 1902 Act, as the letter referred to the supervisor of midwives as 'counsellor and friend' rather than 'relentless critic' and expected the supervisor to display 'sympathy and tact'.

Further revisions of the Midwives Act took place and in 1951 the most significant change wrought was for supervisors of midwives to ensure that midwives attended statutory refresher courses and to supply the names of those midwives who should attend. This statutory requirement continued until 2001 when rule 37 of the Midwives Rules (UKCC 1998) was superseded by Post-Registration Education and Practice (PREP) requirements (UKCC 1997). The PREP requirements detailed a gradual programme of change that would be completed in 2001.

Supervision of midwives did not move away from the auspices of the Medical Officers of Health until 1974 when the National Health Service (Reorganization) Act nominated Regional Health Authorities as LSA, and District Health Authorities nominated supervisors of midwives for appointment by the

LSA. In 1977, the medical supervisor role was finally abolished and all supervisors were required to be *practising* midwives. The reorganization also led to supervision being introduced into the hospital environment as well as in the community. In 1979 the framework for the United Kingdom Central Council for Nursing, Midwifery and Health Visiting (UKCC) and the National Boards of England, Scotland, Wales and Northern Ireland was established. The National Boards were required to provide advice and guidance to the LSA, leading to the abolition of the Central Midwives Board (CMB) in 1983.

Courses for supervisors of midwives were not introduced until 1978 when induction courses became a requirement for any supervisor of midwives appointed after 1974. The CMB introduced the first induction course that year; it was a 2-day course to be undertaken within the first year of appointment by the LSA. Today, these courses are much more rigorous and undertaken at first degree or masters level. Midwives must complete the course successfully before being eligible for appointment as a supervisor of midwives. The requirement for training as a supervisor of midwives *prior* to appointment did not exist until as recently as 1992 when the English National Board for Nursing, Midwifery and Health Visiting (ENB) developed an Open Learning Programme (ENB 1992). In 1993, the revised Midwives Rules (Rule 44(2) UKCC 1993) stipulated that this preparation take place prior to appointment, meaning that all four UK countries had to introduce training for supervisors, but only England and Wales used the ENB Open Learning Programme with associated study days. Scotland and Ireland had a less structured training which has become more rigorous over recent years.

In 1994, the Midwives Code of Practice (UKCC 1994) was revised to include a section which emphasized the relationship between midwife and supervisor of midwives as a partnership, rather than as one of controlling. In 1998 the UKCC amended the Midwives Rules and Code of Practice, now a combined document, changing rule 44 to address both preparation and updating for supervisors of midwives (UKCC 1998).

The Nursing and Midwifery Council (NMC) was established in 2002 when the UKCC ceased to exist and the National Boards were abolished. New 'Midwives rules and standards' (NMC 2004) were produced, dropping the 'Code of Practice' for midwives. Within these rules, supervision is addressed much more robustly, demonstrating greater commitment to the supervision of midwives. Although these revised rules did not provide much new detail about the preparation and updating of supervisors of midwives, a new publication, 'standards for the preparation and practice of supervisors of midwives', (NMC 2006a) covers both of these matters in great detail.

The introduction of supervision of midwives in 1902 resulted in improvement in standards in midwifery and created a situation in which women were exposed to safe practitioners. Midwives were obliged to notify their intention to practise each year so that the roll of midwives was regularly updated and monitored. The midwifery inspectors could report to the LSA Officer midwives whose standards were considered unsatisfactory and who were considered dangerous to the public. In such cases, the LSA Officer could suspend the midwife from practice. Many of these functions continue today, although in a much more supportive fashion. The principal function of supervisors of midwives continues to be the protection of the public, but the main ethos is support for midwives. Midwives still have to notify their intention to practise midwifery each year to the LSA, and each LSA office maintains a database of all midwives practising within the LSA area. Information from the notifications of intention to practise is added to the details of registration on the NMC register.

Supervision of midwives in the twenty-first century

Midwives today enjoy the benefits of having a named supervisor of midwives to whom they can relate and look to for support, and with whom they can share their concerns. Among the competencies for a supervisor of midwives listed in the 'standards for the preparation and practice of supervisors of midwives' (NMC 2006a) is 'working in partnership with women'. This endorses the need for midwives and supervisors of midwives to work towards a common aim of providing the best possible care for mothers and babies and there is a mutual responsibility for effective communication between them.

There is always a supervisor of midwives on call at any time who can be contacted if there are any practice concerns, or if there has been a critical incident. There are certain times when a supervisor of midwives must be called, such as in the event of an unexpected stillbirth, although this is no longer listed as a requirement in the Midwives rules and standards (NMC 2004). This is still an expectation and appears within most LSA Guidelines. There is more than one reason for this. From a regulatory point of view, the supervisor of midwives needs to be sure that there was no sub-standard practice leading to the unexplained stillbirth. Equally important is the supervisor of midwives' role in supporting the midwife who has been through this very sad and traumatizing experience.

Record-keeping in midwifery must be accurate, contemporaneous and provide a good account of care planning, treatment and delivery (NMC 2005). Supervisors of midwives are responsible for ensuring good record-keeping standards. They regularly check the midwifery records at their Trust, and feed back to midwives on their standards of record-keeping. This assists midwives in perfecting their notes and helps them to avoid problems which could lead to litigation.

The Midwives rules and standards (NMC 2004) still refer to the inspection of equipment and premises, but much less heed is paid to inspecting the bags of community midwives than was the case in earlier years. Much more emphasis is placed on discussion, support and professional development needs and being there for the midwives when they are in need, providing a confidential framework for a supportive relationship. A comprehensive list of the activities of a supervisor of midwives appears in Box 52.1.

Supervisory reviews

The annual supervisory review provides dedicated time for midwives to sit down with their supervisors of midwives and reflect on their practice over the preceding year. If midwives are concerned about any aspects of

---

Box 52.1 Activities of a supervisor of midwives

- Are approachable and accessible to midwives to support them in their practice
- Act as a source of sound practical advice on all midwifery matters
- Support best practice and ensure women-centred, evidence-based midwifery care
- Are available for advice, guidance and support
- Offer guidance and support to women accessing maternity service
- Act as a confident advocate for midwives and mothers
- Act as effective change agents
- Provide professional leadership
- Act as role models
- Undertake the role of mentor
- Empower women and midwives
- Facilitate a supportive partnership with midwives
- Support midwives through dilemmas
- Assist midwives with their personal and professional development
- Facilitate midwives' reflection on critical incidents
- Support midwives through supervised practice
- Maintain an awareness of local, regional and national NHS issues
- Give advice on ethical issues
- Liaise with clinicians, management and education
- Maintain records of all supervisory activities
- Are accountable to the LSA for all supervisory activities.

---

their practice they can discuss this frankly with their supervisor within the confidential environment of the supervisory review knowing that they will be offered support and guidance, rather than criticism.

Although it is customary for only one supervisory review a year, this is not fixed in tablets of stone and midwives are able to access their supervisor of midwives as, and when, they need or want to. As many supervisors of midwives hold clinical posts, they often work alongside the midwives they supervise and have more regular contact on an informal basis.

Critical incidents

If midwives have been involved in critical incidents, they will be encouraged to meet with their supervisor and reflect on the incidents, the events leading up to the incidents and the outcomes. The named supervisor of midwives is there to support the midwife, and acts on behalf of the LSA, not the Trust. If the incident is sufficiently serious, another supervisor of midwives may be asked to carry out a supervisory enquiry, again on behalf of the LSA, but a midwifery manager might undertake a management enquiry on behalf of the Trust. The named supervisor will support the midwife throughout the enquiry and will help to identify any weaknesses in practice and ascertain if there were any knowledge gaps. Such gaps can then be addressed through appropriate learning, and a learning contract can be prepared to address these deficiencies, supported by the supervisor of midwives. The contract will have a specific time frame, and regular meetings with the named supervisor to monitor progress will be accommodated. An appropriate mentor of the midwife's choice will be allocated to support the midwife in the work area and there will be liaison with the head of midwifery education at the local university if academic input is required. These are the only individuals who need to be aware of the difficulties that the midwife has experienced, and every effort will be made by these people to maintain confidentiality at all times to protect the integrity of the midwife concerned.

Local supervising authorities

A practising midwife, with experience as a supervisor of midwives, performs the local supervising authority midwifery officer role in every LSA. Following reorganizations of health authorities in England earlier (DOH 2001A) on 1 July 2006, the number reduced to 10 strategic health authorities. There are, at the time of writing, just 10 LSAs in England with one LSAMO for each.

Until recently, in the other UK countries the LSA responsible officer was not necessarily a midwife. In Scotland, there were 16 link supervisors of midwives who performed much of the LSA function for the health board LSA officers who were not midwives,

as well as carrying out their substantive posts, which were usually head of midwifery. In 2006, this changed with LSA midwifery officers being appointed in accordance with the Nursing and Midwifery Order (2001) (DH 2001b). There are now three LSA midwifery officers covering the health boards which have been grouped into three consortia of local supervising authorities for Scotland.

In Wales, the health authorities had appointed practising midwives, similar to the Scottish system, but the midwives were referred to as 'lead supervisors of midwives'. There were four senior midwives appointed as lead supervisors of midwives to cover the LSA function in five health authorities, with one of the lead midwives taking responsibility for two health authorities. In 2002, the health authorities were abolished and the National Assembly for Wales designated Health Professions Wales as the local supervising authority. Two LSA midwifery officers were appointed to be responsible for the LSA standards in Wales. In 2006, the Welsh Assembly Government abolished Health Professions Wales and the functions of the LSA were transferred to Health Inspectorate Wales where the two LSA-MOs continue their roles covering the whole country.

In Northern Ireland, the four health boards had link supervisors of midwives to carry out the LSA function on behalf of the non-midwife LSA officers at the health boards. The LSA officers were, in fact, directors of nursing. The link supervisors were from a Trust in each health board area (Duerden 2000a). This changed in 2005 with the appointment of an LSA midwifery officer to cover three of the health boards. At last, dedicated time is given to the LSA role in Northern Ireland, but still on a part-time basis. The fourth health board is still awaiting cover at the time of writing.

The LSA role has no management responsibility to Trusts, but it acts as a focus for issues relating to midwifery practice (ENB 1999) and its strength lies in its influence on quality in local midwifery services. All LSAMOs have to be aware of the wider NHS picture and contemporary issues. The UK wide National Forum of LSA Midwifery Officers meets every 2 months to ensure a national framework in which the midwifery officers can contribute informed advice on issues impacting on midwifery, such as structures for local maternity services and post-registration education for midwives.

The Nursing and Midwifery Order (2001) states that each LSA shall:

a. exercise general supervision over all midwives practising in its area

b. where it appears to it that the fitness to practise of a midwife in its area is impaired, report it to the Council

c. have power in accordance with the rules made under Article 42 to suspend a midwife from practice.

All of these aspects are clarified within the Midwives rules and standards (NMC 2004) and make much easier reading and comprehension. There is also further detail within this chapter to assist the reader and a list of the duties of an LSA midwifery officer in Box 52.2.

Box 52.2 Duties of the LSA midwifery officer

- Ensures that supervision is carried out to a satisfactory standard for all midwives within the geographical boundaries of the LSA
- Provides impartial, expert advice on professional matters
- Provides a framework for supporting supervision and midwifery practice
- Operates a system that ensures midwives meet statutory requirements for practice
- Selects and appoints supervisors of midwives and deselects if ever necessary
- Ensures the supervisor of midwives to midwives ratio does not normally exceed 1:15
- Provides a formal link between midwives, their supervisors and the statutory bodies
- Implements the NMC's rules and standards for supervision of midwives
- Provides advice and guidance to supervisors of midwives
- Provides a framework of support for supervisory and midwifery practice
- Ensures each midwife meets the statutory requirements for practice
- Participates in the development and facilitation of programmes of preparation for prospective supervisors of midwives
- Provides continuing education and training opportunities for supervisors of midwives
- Provides advice on midwifery matters to health authorities

- Works in partnership with other agencies and promotes partnership working with women and their families
- Manages communications within supervisory systems with a direct link between supervisors of midwives and the LSA
- Conducts regular meetings for supervisors to develop key areas of practice
- Investigates cases of alleged misconduct
- Determines whether to suspend a midwife from practice, in accordance with Rule 5 of the Midwives rules and standards (NMC 2004)
- Conducts investigations and initiates legal action in cases of practice by persons not qualified to do so under the Nursing and Midwifery Order (2001)
- Receives reports of maternal deaths
- Leads the development of standards and audit of supervision
- Maintains a list of current supervisors
- Receives notifications of intention to practise
- Facilitates inter-Trust activities, such as provision of cover by supervisors of midwives from other Trusts
- Prepares an annual report of supervisory activities within the report year, including audit outcomes and emerging trends affecting maternity services for the NMC, health authorities and Trusts
- Publishes details of how to contact supervisors
- Publishes details of how the practice of midwives will be supervised
- Publishes the local mechanism for confirming any midwife's eligibility to practise.

Risk management and the supervision of midwives

Chapter 53 specifically relates to risk management. All of the functions of a supervisor of midwives could be considered to have a risk management element as the framework for supervision is based on safety and good outcomes. The supervisor of midwives acts as an advocate for the consumer by monitoring the professional performance of midwives; thereby ensuring a safe standard of midwifery practice and enhancing the quality of care for a mother and her family. Supervision is a separate function from the management of the midwifery service and, although some supervisors may have responsibility for both, their responsibility for supervision is to the LSA.

Supervisors of midwives, in fulfilling their role of protecting the public, must be aware of the current safety culture in their units and be prepared to inform Trust executives of the risks being taken by staffing their maternity unit both inadequately and inappropriately.

The safety culture of the midwifery profession is bound by the Midwives rules and standards (NMC 2004) and the NMC Code (2008), by which all midwives must abide. The NMC code requires registrants to only undertake practice and accept responsibilities for activities in which they are competent. It is not always easy to refuse when there is no one else to carry out the tasks, especially if this means that clients' needs will not be met, but the onus is placed on the individual by the code. The supervisor of midwives has to ensure that the rules and the code are honoured, and take action in the event of breach of any of them. Supervision should, through its development and use, enable practitioners to make a real contribution to any organization's ability to manage risk effectively.

It is impossible to be a supervisor of midwives without practising risk management. Supervisors can ensure the best outcome for mother and baby by influencing how midwives practise. When supervision is carried out effectively, with a particular regard to the monitoring of midwives' practice and competence, the perceptions of risk can be related to midwifery practice, as can the principles of risk management.

Supervision and management

These two entities are often confused and yet they are distinctly separate. This confusion is probably a legacy from the introduction of supervision of midwives into hospitals in 1974 when the midwifery managers became supervisors of midwives. To many midwives the positions appeared synonymous; indeed many of the supervisors themselves failed to distinguish between the two roles (RCM 1994). There are many more supervisors of midwives in clinical posts than in management, so the differences are much clearer to midwives today. Much work has been done in recent years to educate midwives, and supervisors of midwives, about the different roles and to increase awareness of the benefits of statutory supervision. There is now a trend for any midwifery managers who are also supervisors of midwives, not to supervise the midwives they manage.

There is no hierarchy within supervision; from the moment of appointment, supervisors of midwives have full supervisory responsibilities. They will be preceptored into their role by more experienced supervisors, but there is no seniority or ranking of supervisors.

There should not be any conflict between supervision and management as, when acting in either capacity, the objectives are clear and separately defined. The aims of supervision are to ensure the safety of mothers and babies and support midwives in order to achieve high standards of practice, while the aim of management is to achieve a high quality service to meet contract specifications and make the best use of resources. If there is a critical incident to be investigated, the same one person cannot act as both manager and supervisor, as the former is acting on behalf of the Trust and the latter as advocate for the midwife with responsibility to the LSA (Duerden 2000b). Despite this, confusion continues to exist, particularly considering suspension (Shennan 1996) and the difference between suspension from duty, a management procedure, and suspension from practice, a recommendation to the LSA by a supervisor of midwives.

To assist the reader, a list of responsibilities of a supervisor of midwives is given in Box 52.3.

Box 52.3 Responsibilities of a supervisor of midwives

Each supervisor of midwives

- Receives and processes notification of intention to practise forms from midwives on their caseload
- Ensures that midwives have access to the statutory rules and guidance, and local policies to inform their practice
- Investigates critical incidents and identifies any action required, while seeking to achieve positive learning and appropriate experience for the midwives involved, liaising with the LSA as appropriate
- Reports to the LSA serious cases involving professional conduct where the NMC Rules and Codes have been contravened and when it is considered that local action has failed to achieve safe practice
- Contributes to activities such as Confidential Enquiries, risk management strategies, clinical audit and clinical governance

- Provides guidance on maintenance of registration and PREP requirements
- Monitors standards of midwifery practice through audit of records and assessment of clinical outcomes
- Monitors local maternity services to ensure that appropriate care is available to all women and babies
- Arranges regular meetings with individual midwives, at least once a year, to help them to evaluate their practice and identify areas of development
- Participates in the identification and preparation of new supervisors of midwives
- Identifies when peer supervisors are not undertaking the role to a satisfactory standard and takes appropriate action.

Clinical governance

Clinical governance was defined in First Class Service (DH 1998, p 33) as 'a framework through which NHS organizations are accountable for continuously improving the quality of their services and safeguarding high standards of care by creating an environment in which excellence in clinical care will flourish.' This systematic approach to maintaining and improving the quality of patient care continues in the NHS. Since 1998 the Government has published a further three white papers on the reform of professional regulation and clinical governance: (DH 2007a,b,c).

Professional self-regulation and life-long learning are key themes within clinical governance and these have all been integral to the supervision of midwives for some time past. The philosophy for the supervision of midwives and the standards it develops thus reflect the key themes of clinical governance.

Supervision of midwives promotes and develops safe practice and ensures the dissemination of good, evidence-based practice and innovation (LSAMO & NMC 2008). Since 1955, supervision of midwives has ensured a statutory framework for continued professional development, and compulsory refreshment of midwifery

knowledge has led to a life-long learning programme for midwives throughout their careers. Supervision has provided a formal focus of support and reflection with a confidential review of professional development needs. It is evident, therefore, that the supervision of midwives contributes to an effective framework of clinical governance, minimizing risk, reducing patient complaints, and contributing to a multidisciplinary collaboration in producing practice guidelines (ENB 1999).

The government has set clear national standards backed by consistent monitoring arrangements. The LSA Midwifery Officers, through their supervisory audit visits to each maternity unit, regularly monitor standards of practice against documented evidence such as that produced by the Confidential Enquiry into Stillbirths and Deaths in Infancy (CESDI) and the Confidential Enquiry into Maternal Deaths (CEMD). National standards are also developed through National Service Frameworks (NSF) and the National Institute for Health and Clinical Excellence (NICE). The implementation of the Maternity Standard of the NSF for Children, Young People and Maternity Services (DH 2004) can also be monitored in this way.

Where there are unacceptable variations in clinical midwifery practice, or care is inappropriate for women's needs, the LSA Midwifery Officer, as an outside assessor, is in a position to recommend remedial action (Duerden 2000a). Similarly, the LSA can contribute to the dissemination of information from NICE to ensure the implementation of the most effective care.

The clinical governance framework

First Class Service (DH 1998) described a clinical governance framework (3.11) to:

- modernize and strengthen professional self-regulation and build on the principles of performance
- strengthen existing systems for quality control, based on clinical standards, evidence-based practice and learning the lessons of poor performance
- identify and build on good practice
- assess and minimize the risk of untoward events
- investigate problems as these arise and ensure lessons are learnt
- support health professionals in delivering quality care.

All of these aspects of clinical governance are covered within the ambit of supervision of midwives. Supervisors of midwives monitor midwifery practice and they are able to discuss with midwives the regulation of midwifery practice and ensure full understanding of accountability to themselves, to the Nursing and Midwifery Council and to the Trust that employs them.

The principles of life-long learning are deep rooted in supervision with its history of regular refresher courses.

Systems for quality control, based on clinical standards, evidence-based practice and learning the lessons of poor performance, are met through supervisory audit. Evidence-based practice is a term which might be considered to be over- and inappropriately used, but it is crucial to the Government's programme of quality improvement activities within clinical governance: 'Evidence-based practice is supported and applied routinely in everyday practice' (DH 1998, p 36). Supervisors of midwives have a responsibility to monitor midwifery practice. Not only must they ensure that the practice within their own clinical area

is evidence-based, but they must also challenge areas of practice which are carried out, out of a sense of tradition, and without any evidence for maintaining them. They must also ensure that the midwives concerned understand not only the meaning of evidence-based practice, but that they also know where and how to find evidence and evaluate it adequately, being able to differentiate between poor and high quality studies.

Supervisors of midwives are in an excellent position to identify good practice and also to learn of examples of good practice in other maternity units which can be adopted within their own Trust, as such examples are shared through the supervisory network. Where midwives have ideas for changing and improving practice, supervisors of midwives should be able to empower the midwives to introduce such change and support them in their initiatives acting as their advocate with senior staff. A supervisor of midwives should be among the membership of every labour ward forum (RCOG-RCM 1999) providing a useful opportunity for the sharing of new ideas and encouraging midwives to attend in order to promulgate their suggestions for changing practice.

Through regular monitoring of midwifery practice, especially by supervisors of midwives who work in the clinical environment, areas of risk can be identified and addressed. Critical incident analysis is a crucial part of the supervisor's role. Following any untoward event or 'near miss', some sort of incident form will be completed. All untoward events involving midwives are recorded, investigated and monitored by supervisors. An illustration of how the statutory supervision of midwives sits within clinical governance is shown in Figure 52.1.

Quality

Most hospitals have regular perinatal audit meetings, designed to review the outcomes of clinical care and identify possible areas for improvement. These are excellent arenas for supervisors of midwives to monitor midwifery practice and take appropriate action where suboptimal care has been demonstrated.

The results of research should inform our decisions about healthcare. It is, however, evident from the conclusions of Enkin et al (2000) that research

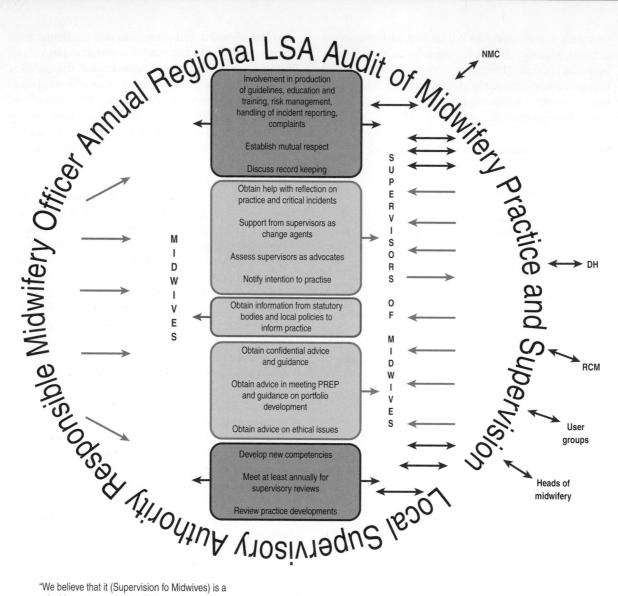

Figure 52.1 The link between clinical governance and statutory supervision of midwives devised by supervisors. (Original model devised by supervisors of midwives at Airedale Hospitals NHS Trust. Permission to reproduce from Carol Paeglis, when Practice Development Nurse/Midwife, Airedale Hospitals NHS Trust and Rachel Wilson, Medical Illustrator, Airedale Hospitals NHS Trust.)

findings appear often to be only slowly and incompletely reflected in practice. Many journals available to midwives provide a great deal of up-to-date information on research findings relevant to practice, but access to information alone does not always influence putting research findings into clinical practice. Research reports can also be from very small studies where the findings are not sufficiently significant or robust to put into general practice. Support and advocacy from a supervisor will often be necessary to make relevant changes to practice and to avoid implementing unsubstantiated practice.

Another body that, through the Government's Modernization Programme, monitors quality and performance in Trusts is the Healthcare Commission. With the regular monitoring visit of the LSA responsible midwifery officer, plus a visit by the Healthcare Commission, it is understandable if midwifery staff can sometimes feel overwhelmed and over-inspected. In addition to these visits there will be visits from the Royal Colleges to assess the practice area for medical staff training. The NMC periodically assesses the practice area for the education and training of student midwives. This rigorous monitoring means that, from a clinical governance perspective, there can be confidence in the standard of care provided in each maternity unit.

The National Institute for Health and Clinical Excellence (NICE) is a government-appointed body which sets standards and guidelines for clinical practice in all specialities. There are now many sets of guidelines published by NICE which dictate practice for midwives and obstetricians and supervisors of midwives have a role here in ensuring that midwives implement these guidelines. The electronic fetal monitoring guidelines (NICE 2001) created problems for some midwives who felt insecure if they did not monitor every woman admitted in labour for at least 20 min, and supervisors of midwives have had to support midwives through a change of practice which can enhance woman-centred care, rather than medicalizing a problem-free labour.

Policies, protocols and guidelines

Many maternity units will have protocols, policies and guidelines in place to govern the way in which care should be provided. These terms sometimes lead to confusion, and may be used interchangeably. The word protocol now has many different meanings in different professions, especially in information technology and mathematics. Within healthcare research it is an action plan for a clinical trial, but generally a *protocol* is a written system for managing care that should include a plan for audit of that care. Baillière's Midwives' Dictionary (Tiran 2007) describes a protocol as 'protocol agreement between parties; multidisciplinary planned course of suggested action in relation to specific situations'. Protocols determine individual aspects of practice and should be researched using the latest evidence. Most protocols are binding on employees as they usually relate to the management of consumers with urgent, possibly life-threatening, conditions. A protocol may exist for the care of women with antepartum haemorrhage, but not for the care of women in labour without complication. If midwives work outwith a protocol they could be considered to be in breach of their employment contract.

Guidelines, or procedures, are usually less specific than protocols and may be described as suggestions for criteria or levels of performance that are provided to implement agreed standards.

Policies are general principles or directions, usually without the mandatory approach for addressing an issue, but might be considered mandatory in some Trusts. They are often set at national level, such as the Maternity Standard, National Service Framework for Children, Young People and Maternity Services (DH 2004).

It is essential that supervisors of midwives ensure that midwives clearly understand the different definitions.

Midwives' contribution to clinical governance

The Midwifery Action Plan (DH 2001c), written in response to Making a Difference, a strategy for nursing, midwifery and health visiting (DH 1999), gives suggestions (p 13) as to how midwives can contribute to clinical governance:

- auditing and reflecting on own practice
- identifying issues and participating in critical incident reporting

- reviewing and applying the outcomes of risk management reviews to own practice
- making best use of available support from supervisors of midwives.

Using supervision effectively

Partnership

To benefit from supervision, mutual respect between supervisors of midwives and midwives is essential. Midwives should work in partnership with their supervisors and make the most of supervision (LSAMO & NMC 2008), so that it can be effective for not only themselves but also for the mothers and babies for whom they care. When supported by a supervisor of midwives, a midwife can practise safely with confidence.

The primary responsibilities of a midwife are to ensure the safe and efficient care of mothers and babies; maintain personal fitness for practice and maintain registration with the NMC. The supervisory relationship enables, supports and empowers midwives to fulfil these responsibilities. In Figure 52.2 the reader can see how a midwife can make the most of the supervision and the benefits of a professional relationship with the named supervisor of midwives.

Accountability and advocacy

Accountability of midwives means that midwives are answerable for actions and omissions, regardless of advice or directions from another professional. There will be occasions when midwives have difficulty appreciating their own accountability, especially when carrying out the instructions of medical staff, but it is clear from the NMC Code (2008) that accountability cannot be either delegated to or borne by others; it simply rests with the practitioner. A registered midwife is accountable to the NMC as well as to the employing Trust. The dilemmas that this might create can be discussed with a supervisor of midwives for greater clarity and understanding.

When acting as advocates for women exercising their choice, which might not be in keeping with Trust policy, midwives may wish to seek the help of their supervisor or the supervisor of midwives on call. The supervisor can help by supporting midwives in caring for women, giving advice about documentation and even initiating a review of the policy in light of new evidence.

Just as Trust policies can inhibit a woman's choice, so can the availability of services. Examples of this are home births and water births. Women may demand either of these services when the Trust either cannot or does not provide them. Home birth services are occasionally temporarily withdrawn during staffing crises, and some Trusts will not support women giving birth in water. Women will sometimes opt for a home birth when their obstetric history would place them outwith the criteria. Situations such as these will challenge a midwife's responsibilities both as a midwife and as an employee. This is another useful time to seek out the support of a supervisor of midwives to talk through the issues.

Choice

Midwives are able to choose their supervisor of midwives, usually from a list provided by the contact supervisor. A midwife should consider carefully with which supervisors an open and honest relationship could be formed and whether or not there would be mutual respect. The supervisor should also be able to appreciate the environment in which the midwife is currently practising.

Midwives prioritized the qualities required in a supervisor during an audit of supervision (Duerden 2000b). The results in priority order were: approachable; clinically experienced; in touch and up-to-date; willing to take action; a good listener; a good role model; a good advocate; wise; empathetic and sympathetic. In Modern Supervision in Action (LSAMO & NMC 2008, p9) the qualities of a supervisor of midwives are listed as approachable; committed to woman-centred care; a source of professional knowledge and expertise; visionary and inspiring; able to resolve conflict; motivated and thorough; articulate trustworthy; sympathetic and encouraging; and, finally, fair and equitable. These lists make a supervisor of midwives sound like the perfect being, but realistically it is impossible for one person to have all these qualities. It is, however, important for a midwife to judge which qualities are important in a supervisor of midwives and to consider the qualities of each supervisor on the proffered list.

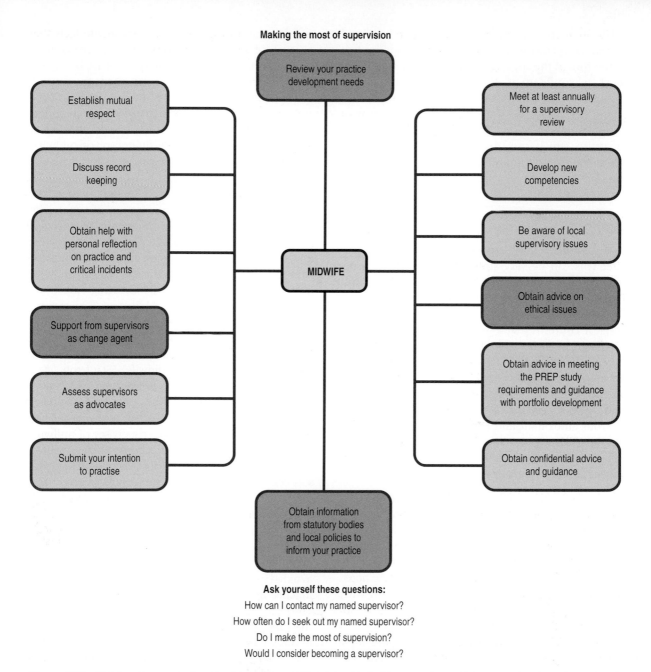

Figure 52.2 Making the most of supervision. (From Supervision in Action ENB 1999, with permission from English National Board for Nursing, Midwifery and Health Visiting.)

The ability to maintain confidentiality is not listed among the qualities described above, but it is implicit in the role of the supervisor of midwives. A midwife must feel confident at all times that discussions with a supervisor of midwives will remain confidential. There will always be times when the supervisor of midwives may need to take action in the interest of safety, in which case discussion would take place about the need to share the information. Similarly, the midwife might be encouraged to take the initiative to raise the issue with the midwifery manager.

Support

In the modern NHS, change occurs at an alarming rate. This can be very stressful for midwives, especially if it means a change in practice or the work area. The supervisor of midwives is well placed to advise and guide midwives who are challenged by change and any concerns that a midwife might have, should be shared with the named supervisor. Similarly, the supervisor can act as advocate for the midwife in debate among professional groups, especially if the practice being suggested is not evidence-based. At all times, the supervisor of midwives' responsibility is to protect the public and ensure the highest standards of care and professional practice by midwives.

Supervisory reviews

The annual supervisory review should be used by midwives to reflect on their midwifery practice in a confidential arena where aspirations and goals for the future can be shared. Both midwife and supervisor should value the meeting, as this is the opportunity to take time out and consider personal learning needs and professional development requirements in order to achieve goals. Midwives are responsible for meeting their own PREP requirements before re-registering with the NMC (NMC 2006b) and these requirements can be discussed with the supervisor of midwives during the review. The supervisor will probably have information about the Trust professional development budget and will be able to guide the midwife if further academic study is being considered.

This secure environment should provide an opportunity to evaluate practice, and share any practice issues causing concern. If it is felt necessary, the supervisor will investigate the matter in confidence

and take appropriate action. If a midwife feels that, because of allocation to one practice environment for a protracted time, midwifery skills are being lost, the supervisory review can be used to consider mechanisms for gaining relevant experience in other areas and receiving the necessary professional update.

A midwife may have a particular interest in research or audit. Using the supervisor of midwives as a sounding board can assist greatly in making decisions, and guidance can be obtained.

There cannot always be a perfect supervisory relationship, but to get the most out of supervision the relationship must have the essential elements of mutual respect and confidentiality. Research (Stapleton et al 1998) clearly demonstrated that midwives who feel empowered by their supervisor of midwives feel able to empower their clients. Being valued and supported by supervisors and having achievements recognized will enhance professional confidence and practice. The supervisory decisions perceived as empowering are those made by consensus between the supervisor and the midwife (Stapleton et al 1998). If this relationship is not recognized by either midwife or supervisor, then the opportunity to change supervisor should be taken by the midwife, possibly with the encouragement of the supervisor of midwives who will know that there can be no success without the necessary rapport and confidence in the supervisory relationship. It benefits some midwives to change their supervisor every few years, while others feel the need for a longer-term relationship.

An over-secure relationship should also be avoided as the supervisor is not there to attend to the midwife's every need. At all costs, dependency should be avoided. Midwives are accountable for their own practice and continuous professional development. They should not be seeking out their supervisors all the time, but should recognize that all supervisors of midwives have substantive posts to which supervision is an addendum. For many, this means that much of supervision is carried out in personal time, so demands made on the supervisor should be considered, and arrangements made to meet at mutually convenient times. When the named supervisor of midwives is not available, there is always an on-call supervisor to deal with emergencies. A helpful list of ways to get the best from supervision is provided at Box 52.4.

Box 52.4 Getting the best from supervision

- Respond to invitations to meet from your supervisor of midwives
- Make yourself known to your supervisor of midwives if the supervisor does not contact you first
- Make sure you know the local arrangements to contact your own supervisor and/or the supervisor of midwives on call
- Make sure you know each supervisor's specific areas of expertise. Consider who, for example, you would approach for advice on research evidence or ethical considerations
- Discuss with your supervisor any ideas you may have for new approaches or developments within the service. Explore together the feasibility and opportunities for implementation
- Alert your supervisor to potential problems at an early stage, so the supervisor is aware of the action you intend to take and can support you

- Enlist the help of your supervisor to open doors which may be closed to you; for example, when the care you are giving requires cooperation or authorization by personnel or departments with which you do not normally have contact, such as the Chief Executive of the Trust or the Primary Care Trust
- Discuss with your supervisor your preferences for your professional development, after you have identified what you feel would best enhance your practice
- Be aware of the value of discussing complicated issues in clarifying your thoughts and drawing upon your pooled knowledge and experience
- If you feel unhappy with the advice or action taken by your supervisor, ask to discuss the issue again, or approach another supervisor
- Remember that mutual respect is the key to a successful relationship with your supervisor of midwives. If this is not possible within your supervisory relationship you might want to consider changing your supervisor.

Conclusion

With the support of supervisors of midwives, midwives can expect to practise confidently and competently, but they must value supervision in order to gain its maximum benefit and to receive the empowerment it can provide. The changing role of the midwife, described in this book, highlights the need for support through the change programme.

REFERENCES

DH (Department of Health) 1998 First Class Service. HMSO, London

DH (Department of Health) 1999 Making a difference: strengthening the nursing, midwifery and health visiting contribution to health and healthcare. HMSO, London

DH (Department of Health) 2001a Shifting the balance of power: launch of the NHS modernization agency speech by Secretary of State, 24 April

DH (Department of Health) 2001b Establishing the new Nursing and Midwifery Council, April. DH, London

DH (Department of Health) 2001c Making a Difference – the nursing, midwifery and health visiting contribution. The Midwifery Action Plan. DH, London

DH (Department of Health) 2004 Maternity standard, national service framework for children, young people and maternity services. DH, London

DH (Department of Health) 2007a Trust, assurance and safety: the regulation of health professionals in the 21st century. Online. Available: http://www.dh.gov.uk/assetRoot/04/14/31/43/04143143.pdf

DH (Department of Health) 2007b Safeguarding patients. Online. Available: http://www.dh.gov.uk/assetRoot/04/14/32/48/04143248.pdf

DH (Department of Health) 2007c Learning from tragedy: keeping patients safe. Online. Available: http://www.dh.gov.uk/assetRoot/04/14/32/49/04143249.pdf

Duerden J M 2000a The new LSA arrangements in practice. In: Kirkham M (ed.) Developments in the supervision of midwives. Books for Midwives, Hale

Duerden J M 2000b Audit of supervision of midwives. In: Kirkham M (ed.) Developments in the supervision of midwives. Books for Midwives, Hale

ENB (English National Board for Nursing, Midwifery and Health Visiting) 1992 Preparation of supervisors of midwives: an open learning programme. ENB, London

ENB (English National Board for Nursing, Midwifery and Health Visiting) 1999 Advice and guidance to local supervising authorities and supervisors of midwives. ENB, London

Enkin M, Keirse M (eds) 2000 Effective care in pregnancy and childbirth, 3rd edn. Oxford University Press, Oxford

Kirkham M. 1995 The history of midwifery supervision. Supervision Consensus Conference Proceedings. Books for Midwives, Hale

LSA Midwifery Officers National (UK) Forum & Nursing and Midwifery Council (2008) *Modern Supervision in Action - a practical guide for midwives* NMC, London

MoH (Ministry of Health) 1937 Circular 1620 Supervision of midwives. MoH, London

NICE (National Institute for Health and Clinical Excellence) 2001 Electronic fetal monitoring: The use and interpretation of cardiotocography in intrapartum fetal surveillance. NICE, London

NMC (Nursing and Midwifery Council) 2002 Preparation of supervisors of midwives. NMC, London

NMC (Nursing and Midwifery Council) 2004 Midwives rules and standards. NMC, London

NMC (Nursing and Midwifery Council) 2005 Guidelines for records and record keeping. NMC, London

NMC (Nursing and Midwifery Council) 2006a Standards for the preparation and practice of supervisors of midwives. NMC, London

NMC (Nursing and Midwifery Council) 2006b The PREP handbook NMC, London

NMC (Nursing and Midwifery Council) 2008 The NMC Code: Standards of conduct, performance and ethics for nurses and midwives. NMC, London

RCM (Royal College of Midwives) 1994 Supervision of midwives and midwifery. Practice Paper 6: Future practices of midwifery. RCM, London

RCOG/RCM (Royal College of Obstetricians and Gynaecologists and Royal College of Midwives) 1999 Towards safer childbirth – minimum standards for the organization of labour wards. RCOG, London

Shennan C. 1996 Midwives' perception of the role of a supervisor of midwives. In: Kirkham M (ed.) Supervision of midwives. Books for Midwives, Hale

Stapleton H, Duerden J, Kirkham M 1998 Evaluation of the impact of the supervision of midwives on professional practice and the quality of midwifery care. English National Board, London

The Nursing and Midwifery Order 2001 (Transitional Provisions) Order of Council 2004 (SI 2004/1762)

Tiran D 2007 Midwives' dictionary, 11th edn. Baillière Tindall, London

UKCC (United Kingdom Central Council For Nursing Midwifery and Health Visiting) 1993 Midwives rules. UKCC, London

UKCC (United Kingdom Central Council for Nursing Midwifery and Health Visiting) 1994 Midwives code of practice. UKCC, London

UKCC (United Kingdom Central Council For Nursing Midwifery and Health Visiting) 1997 Midwives Refresher Courses and PREP. UKCC, London

UKCC (United Kingdom Central Council for Nursing Midwifery and Health Visiting) 1998 Midwives rules and code of practice. UKCC, London

FURTHER READING

LSA Midwifery Officers National (UK) Forum & Nursing and Midwifery Council (2008) *Modern Supervision in Action - a practical guide for midwives* NMC, London

This useful little book helps midwives to get the most out of supervision. It is very user friendly and explains the supervision of midwives very succinctly from the perspective of the midwife rather than the supervisor of midwives.

Kirkham M (ed.) (1996) Supervision of Midwives. Books for Midwives, Hale

This book contains a comprehensive examination of the supervision of midwives beginning with a fascinating history of supervision and also giving some examples of good practice within supervision.

Kirkham M (ed.) 2000 Developments in the supervision of midwives. Books for Midwives, Hale

Following on from the previous book, this edition explores how the supervision of midwives has developed in recent years, describing research and audit of supervision, changes in practice and education and training for supervisors of midwives.

53 Risk management in midwifery

Robina Aslam   Susan Brydon

Midwives work in an environment that entails risks to mothers, to babies, to their employer and to themselves. They must understand the basic principles of risk management and how it applies specifically to their practice.

Although its original application in healthcare lay in an attempt to reduce litigation, risk management is now seen by most practitioners and NHS Trusts as a vehicle for enhancing the quality of client care as part of modern clinical governance.

The chapter aims to:

- discuss the origins and approaches to risk management
- describe the role played by risk management in clinical governance
- outline the practice of risk management in a clinical setting
- give an overview of reporting procedures associated with risk management and, most particularly, untoward incident and near-miss reporting
- briefly review the role of the Clinical Negligence Scheme for Trusts.

Introduction

The various meanings of 'risk management'

In the context of healthcare in general and midwifery in particular, the term 'risk management' can be used in a number of senses.

- *In its narrow sense,* it is strongly associated with litigation avoidance. When it was originally introduced into the NHS in the mid-1990s, the central aim of risk management was to reduce litigation risk.

1015

- *In a broader sense*, risk management in maternity services means a formal process for identifying, assessing and responding to risk so that the decisions taken about childbirth and its associated care lead to the elimination (insofar as is possible) of undesired outcomes and the promotion of desired outcomes. This is the sense in which the term is used in an industrial context, where risk management is typically used as part of a company's overall strategy to enhance the quality of the service offered. An airline, for example, needs to ensure that the service it offers is as safe as is humanly possible – in other words, that the risks of harm to passengers are minimal; but it also has to offer a service that is attractive, convenient, comfortable and affordable. Because of the need to strike the right balance between safety, quality and price, risk management is necessarily integrated with other facets of the management process such as quality management.

In this chapter, risk management will be examined both as a broad philosophy and in the more restrictive sense in which it is sometimes used in the NHS. As will be seen, these two approaches are rapidly converging – or, more correctly, the narrower approach is largely giving way to the broader approach. The practice of care in the NHS is becoming much more client/patient orientated. Furthermore, it is becoming clearer to clinicians and litigation-funders alike that the best way to achieve the goals of the Health Service as a whole and, at the same time, to reduce litigation risk is to use the available resources to provide the best possible service to the client – risk management should be used positively to deliver that service rather than seeking primarily to counter the threat of litigation.

Risk and the midwife

In the publication 'Engaging Clinicians', the National Patient Safety Agency (NPSA) (2005) puts risk management at the heart of the process of ensuring patient safety:

Everyone who works in the NHS contributes to the systems which deliver healthcare ... Patient safety is therefore everybody's business. The process by which an organisation makes patient care safer should involve:

- *risk assessment*
- *identification and management of patient-related risks*
- *reporting and analysis of incidents*
- *the capacity to learn from and follow up on incidents and implement solutions to minimise the risk of incidents occurring*

(NPSA 2005, p 3)

While childbirth is reasonably safe in the developed world, there are aspects which demand proper risk management. Risk in maternity is getting ever greater attention; for example, the Healthcare Commission (HCC), the watchdog on delivery of NHS services and NPSA jointly held a conference entitled 'Safe Delivery – Reducing Risk in Maternity Services'. At the conference, Lord Patel, Chairman of the NPSA, identified what he described as a new paradigm in healthcare:

The identification, analysis and management of patient-related risks and incidents in order to make patient care safer and to reduce harm.

(Patel 2007)

The standard Maternity Care Pathway set out in Maternity Matters (DH 2007) describes the first key activity as a 'standardized risk and needs assessment'. Midwives will be called on to weigh risks at all stages of the process, for example in discussing with women whether provisional pathway choices need to be reconsidered – a woman who has provisionally opted to have a home birth may need to review this in the light of later information, e.g. detection of raised blood pressure, and it will fall to the midwife to discuss the risks with the woman.

While supervisors of midwives are required to promote childbirth as a normal, physiological event they must also 'demonstrate the ability to undertake assessments of practice to identify potential/actual risks and mitigate where possible' (NMC 2006).

It is essential that midwives take their responsibilities in respect of risk seriously, but midwives must interpret these responsibilities within their own professional context. Although childbirth is a relatively safe and natural process, a number of factors have, in recent years, amplified the perceived risks:

- *Screening tests* – pregnant women were once simply congratulated on the happy circumstances in which they found themselves. Now they are assessed for various risks and offered various screening options. The results of these tests are often expressed in the language of risk (see Ch. 18).

- *Litigation statistics* – although midwives work in a field with the highest litigation risk, statistics need to be put in perspective. It does not mean that there are any more incidents in maternity than other services. What it does mean is that the compensation payable (which can include round-the-clock care for the claimant over a lifetime) is likely to be much greater than, say, for an accident in a healthcare of the elderly department.

- *The medicalization of childbirth* – medical practitioners tend to apply a medical model of care whereby pregnancy is defined as a potentially dangerous condition requiring close monitoring.

Midwives must use risk management responsibly. In particular, midwives must be aware that the terminology of risk can be disempowering. Women may see themselves no longer as independent actors but as reliant on 'medical' professionals to steer them safely through a dangerous condition. Thomas (1998) advises midwives:

> ... to use risk management as a tool in the planning and provision of safe systems of care, while at the same time supporting the view that pregnancy and birth is a safe process for the majority. To do this the midwife will need to understand the risks, using the evidence as it becomes available, and to put those risks into proper perspective. This will enable the midwife to explain risks to the mother in a way that allows constructive debate and decision making without creating anxiety, which in itself can lead to unnecessary intervention.

A brief historical review of risk management in midwifery

The original view of risk management: a response to litigation risk

The NHS pays out almost £600 million annually in litigation costs (NHSLA 2006). Some 30% of this vast cost to the NHS arises from midwifery/obstetric work although this proportion is difficult to assess because obstetric-related claims tend to be delayed. Analysis also shows (DH 2000) that the vast majority of

mistakes – probably >75% – are caused by 'systems failures'. This means that no one individual can be said to have caused the incident. The real cause of the mistake was a failure of one or more of the following: communication, supervision, checking, staffing levels, equipment, etc.

As a result of such statistics, it was clearly seen that the most significant improvement in healthcare outcomes could be produced not by new medicines or treatments, but by tightening up on the management of the system, particularly in midwifery and maternity departments.

Those who developed the early ideas were clinical negligence lawyers and medical practitioners with experience of reviewing legal claims. A consequence of this was that 'risk management' was seen in these early days almost entirely in terms of minimizing litigation risk. For example, Clements (1995) suggested: 'Risk management is the reduction of harm to the organisation, by the identification and as far as possible elimination of risk'. Dineen (1997) explicitly links 'risk management' with clinical negligence litigation.

The development of a broader view of risk management: enhancement of client care

Many people – both policy-makers and employees of the NHS – were uneasy about risk management which was designed to protect the 'organization' (i.e. the Hospital) against the 'patient'. As a consequence, an alternative approach to risk management developed – the 'enhancement of client care' model. Aslam (1999, p 42), for example, says: 'enhancement of client care, rather than litigation avoidance, should be the principal driving force in implementing risk management procedures'. This alternative approach places little direct emphasis on saving the hospital from litigation; rather, it takes as its starting point the provision of a quality service in the interests of all parties, but especially mothers and babies. It involves balancing risks against opportunities in clinical decisions so that – like an airline company – it provides a safe, satisfying and convenient service.

This latter approach is now broadly supported by the professional institutions as well as the Government. For example, the Royal College of Obstetricians and Gynaecologists (RCOG 2005) advise that risk management should promote reflective practice and be used to improve subsequent care.

The more common use of the term 'risk management' in its wider sense does not mean that the use of the term to describe processes that are exclusively aimed at reducing litigation risk has disappeared. Indeed, it will not disappear because Trusts must, of course, take reasonable precautions to safeguard themselves from spurious litigation; and they have an obligation to ensure that funds are used for the benefit of all.

The clinical negligence scheme for Trusts

One of the most significant changes in the structure of the NHS took place in the early 1990s with the establishment of NHS Trusts. The legislation that established the Trusts also required them to meet the considerable litigation costs. In order to manage this most effectively, a system of pooled insurance – known as the Clinical Negligence Scheme for Trusts (CNST) – was established in 1994 and came into effect in 1995/6. It is administered by a special health authority, the NHS Litigation Authority (NHSLA).

Although membership of the CNST is optional, the vast majority of Trusts did in fact join and so the CNST requirements were, in essence, requirements placed on all Trusts. These requirements were published as standards that participating Trusts are required to meet. The standards were expressed in terms of processes, most of which clearly fell within the general realm of 'risk management'. Thus, risk management was no longer an optional extra for Trusts striving for excellence, but was now a core activity. Indeed, because discounts on the insurance premiums are available for improved compliance with the standards (level 1 is the basic requirement for cover, 2 is good and 3 is the top level of attainment), risk management has become an activity with significant funding implications.

The CNST publishes a general set of standards for Trusts and also a special standard for maternity services as maternity claims account for a significant proportion of those reported to the NHSLA (2007).

The CNST standards for maternity services are contained in eight categories: organization, learning from experience, communication, clinical care, induction, training and competence, health records, implementation of clinical risk management and staffing levels.

The modern context of risk management: a strand within clinical governance

The Government has actively promoted a view of risk management that begins to resemble that used in many other industries: risk management as part of the overall provision of a quality, customer-focused service.

As a result of the Health Act 1999, Trusts are obliged to implement, maintain and improve quality. This is achieved under the banner of clinical governance, the essential features of this are the integration of all those processes that improve client care, including improving clinical quality by building on good practice, development of clinical risk reduction programmes, the promotion of evidence-based practice and the detection and open investigation of adverse incidence and near misses.

The formal system of clinical governance places a responsibility on all to have the appropriate systems in place and to ensure that such systems are effective. However, even prior to the introduction of the current system of clinical governance, midwifery already had systems that operated in that spirit. These include statutory supervision, the setting of standards, evidence-based policies and protocols and research and audit. The professional institutions have all welcomed clinical governance. The Royal College of Midwives' paper, Assessing and managing risk in midwifery practice (RCM 2000) says, for example: 'Clinical governance is to be integrated with risk management to raise standards of care. The fundamental aims of this process are to raise standards of care and define best practice, thereby improving quality outcomes. It also has the potential to reduce medical negligence claims'.

The risk management process

A generic model

Many of the principles of risk management are generic; the basic principles apply equally to operating a

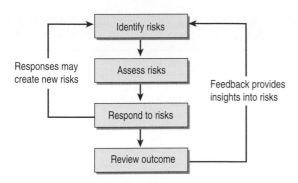

Figure 53.1 Simple generic risk management model.

passenger airline as they do to midwifery. Risk management is often described using a 'process model' such as that shown in Figure 53.1. This model can be described as follows.

Identifying risks

Risks are those factors that may affect our prospects of achieving an optimal result. The types of question that need to be asked are: 'what could go wrong?', 'what are the chances of it going wrong and what would be the impact?', 'what can we do to minimize the chance of this happening or to mitigate damage when it has gone wrong?' and 'what can we learn from things that have gone wrong?' (RCOG 2005, section 3.2). Personal experience is a relatively uncertain form of data acquisition, despite reflective practice models (e.g. Clements 2000). More reliable will be incident reporting and Confidential Enquiry reports (e.g. Lewis 2007).

Assess risks

Those factors that generate the greatest risk need to be assessed in order to gain some indication of how high those risks are. The risk of an outcome is generally considered to be the product of the probability of that outcome multiplied by the severity of that outcome if it were to occur. Thus, life-threatening outcomes must be kept at very low levels of probability to be acceptable, whereas outcomes such as vaginal/perineal lacerations and short term discomforts may be tolerated at much higher levels of probability.

Respond to risks

In the most dangerous situations, such as a compromised fetus, risk response may be dramatic – for instance by opting for an emergency caesarean section. In less risky situations, monitoring may be required. Responses must be guided by the need to minimize the risks without sacrificing the aspirations of the client; for example, if a client expresses a sincere desire to have a natural childbirth, the midwife should refer to the possibility of medical intervention only when this is becoming increasingly advisable.

Review outcome

As part of an ongoing commitment to improving service, performance is reviewed in order to improve the service provided.

There are two 'feedback loops' in the model. The first (emanating from 'respond to risks') requires the midwife to identify whether the response to existing risk itself has created any new risks. For example, if a drug is administered to control one problem, it may have side-effects, which also need to be risk managed. The second feedback loop involves an input from experience into the way that the individual and team as a whole identify, assess and respond to risks for future clients.

Reactive and proactive risk management

Reactive risk management involves learning from one's mistakes. However, the generic model presented in Figure 53.1 encourages a more proactive approach. The aim is to identify and manage risks before they occur so as to avoid harm rather than to learn from it. It is sometimes said that proactive risk management helps us to learn from our mistakes without having to make them.

Of course, all midwives should aspire to proactive risk management by continually striving to develop new and better forms of care, subjecting each to a rigorous risk assessment before implementation. But it is necessary also to be realistic and to recognize that many risk factors are well understood only after having caused adverse outcomes. In practice historical data are relied upon to identify, assess and respond to risk. But it is essential always to be alert to identify new risks and to manage them before they become unfortunate statistics.

Guidelines and protocols

Although the generic model applies to every situation, and although proactive risk management is desirable, it is nevertheless unrealistic and indeed inappropriate for each midwife (or other health professional) to consider the application of the generic model in each and every clinical situation. Not only is there not usually enough time to carry out detailed individual assessments in most routine cases, but the individual carer is unlikely to have a sufficient in-depth knowledge of the relevant data to enable them to make full assessments. Therefore, in order to assist carers in their choice of care, guidelines are developed for day-to-day use. These provide a much more efficient and effective way of ensuring that staff act in line with acceptable evidence-based practice.

Guidelines are now drawn up in most maternity units for most critical or common conditions. For those Trusts subscribing to CNST, guidelines are mandatory. The CNST standards for maternity services (NHSLA 2007) require that:

4.1.1 There are referenced, evidence-based multidisciplinary guidelines/pathways of care, for the management of all key conditions or situations on the labour ward. These are prominently placed in all ward areas

4.1.2 The Trust has a guideline on the use of antenatal and intrapartum fetal monitoring which includes guidelines on performing fetal blood sampling

4.1.3 There are clear guidelines for when high dependency care for the mother is necessary

4.1.6 There are clear multidisciplinary guidelines, which ensure that whenever mothers or babies move between care settings or professionals there is effective transfer of information.

Some aspects of practical risk management

Identifying risks in a clinical setting

Risks occur in many forms. Table 53.1 sets out one way of classifying these risks.

Risks arising from medical, obstetric, social conditions, client choices and professional mis-interpretation are covered in other chapters. This chapter explores 'systems failures'. Box 53.1 gives an example of a problem arising which cannot be ascribed to the failure of any specific individual. It may, in reality, be that almost all situations can be seen as part of a systems failure if for example skills drills for potential emergency situations are not regularly practised.

Table 53.1 Classification of sources of maternity service risks

Class of risk	Specific examples
Pre-assessable Medical, obstetric or social complications	Diabetes
	Obesity (BMI 30 kg/m^2 or above
	Hypertension, cardiac disease
	Smoking, alcohol or drug abuse
	Maternal age ($\geq$40, teenagers)
	Breech presentation
	Psychiatric disorders
Client choice risks	Home birth when risk factors
	Elective caesarean
	Refusal or acceptance of interventions
Systems failures	Ineffective communications
	Inadequate training for emergencies
	Faulty or ineffective equipment
	Poor or inappropriate staffing
Professional Misinterpretation risks	Mis-diagnosis
	Inappropriate response – insufficiently rapid, or without checking
Emergency situations	Shoulder dystocia
	Maternal haemorrhage

Risk management is not just for 'risk managers', but for everyone. The following principles may assist in correctly identifying and managing risks in practice.

Involving women in decision-making

The central importance of women's informed choice is consistently underlined by all recent government policies, including Maternity Matters (DH 2007).

An example which raises difficult questions when midwives are faced with seeking to offer women their preferred pathway, but at the same time to promote childbirth as a natural and reasonably safe process, is the question of caesarean delivery. For example, NICE Clinical Guidance 13 (NICE 2004) speaks in terms of risk: 'When considering a caesarean section (CS), there should be discussion on the benefits and risks of CS compared with vaginal birth specific to the woman and her pregnancy'.

Identifying risks at an early stage

This is emphasized by Maternity Matters (DH 2007) which proposes a standardized 'risks and needs assessment' as the first stage of maternity care. This

---

Box 53.1 Systems failures in maternity care

General management and staffing

Following unexpectedly high rates of maternal deaths (10 deaths in 3 years) at an NHS Trust, 'Special Measures' were imposed by the Secretary of State. The structure of the unit was visibly altered with clinical leadership becoming more visible and supported by senior Trust staff. Staffing levels were raised generally to the levels in other similar hospitals and consultant obstetrician presence was raised by 50%. Revised protocols and guidelines were issued, coupled with better risk management processes, audits and multidisciplinary learning. Following marked improvements, 'Special Measures' were lifted in 2006. The Healthcare Commission report in August 2006 identified the following issues: 'difficult decisions often left to junior staff ... failure in a number of cases to recognize and respond quickly where a woman's condition changed unexpectedly ... inadequate resources to deal with high risk cases ... failure to learn lessons on the unit ... failure by the Trust's Board to appreciate the seriousness of the situation'.

(Adapted from NPSA Case Histories No. 4, 2005)

---

will essentially build on the system in place at present for carrying out:

- a booking history
- screening tests, as appropriate and as selected by the woman.

Dealing with risks when they arise

(see Box 53.2) This includes:

- properly educating, training and updating midwives
- basing practice upon evidence rather than tradition
- guidelines being made available for all critical and common situations
- ensuring there is a system in place for referring developing situations to senior staff (e.g. a consultant midwife).

A system of feedback

This includes:

- proper reporting of practice whether or not there is any untoward event, together with proper investigation of serious incidents
- audit and review of records
- a fair and responsive system for dealing with possibly unsafe practitioners

- staff reflecting upon and sharing experiences in a no-blame environment so as to create a self-reflective organization with memory.

A means of managing women who have experienced an untoward incident

This includes:

- full, timely and open response to any enquiries by the women.

Evidence-based practice and communication

It is important that decisions concerning the management of an individual woman's care are made with their full and informed consent (except, of course, in unavoidable emergencies). This frequently means that the risks must be fully and clearly explained to her. For example, if the woman's inclination is to have a totally natural childbirth, but the fetus is in a breech presentation, the risks and contingency plans need to be explained in a way that:

- addresses all the key issues (i.e. does not simply deal with the carer's preferred plan)
- provides clear advice on the benefits and risks of each option
- supports the decision of the woman, whatever that decision might be.

Box 53.2 Scenario 1

J. was an experienced midwife and worked part-time, usually on the wards. She was allocated to work on the labour ward for a nightshift and was caring for Mrs W., who was in labour following induction for suspected intrauterine growth restriction and raised blood pressure. When she took over the care, the on-call medical team had made an assessment as part of the routine labour ward round and there were no concerns about fetal or maternal well-being. There was no specific plan in the clinical notes. An epidural was in place and Syntocinon was being used to stimulate uterine activity. Midwife J. knew that continuous monitoring was required, in accordance with the unit protocol.

Midwife J. was finding it difficult to keep her records up-to-date as she was not used to caring for a woman with an epidural and Syntocinon and was kept very busy giving care and support to Mrs W. and assessing fetal and maternal condition. Over time, a pattern of shallow decelerations were seen on the trace and midwife J. was aware of this and noted it in the clinical records. She was able to assess that these were early/variable and therefore consistent with cord compression and advancement of labour. Midwife J. considered that this may be a sign of the onset of the second stage. The baseline rate of the fetal heart rose from 130 b.p.m. to 155 b.p.m. and midwife J. was not concerned, as she was aware that the normal fetal heart rate should be within the range of 110–160 b.p.m. When the variability reduced to below 5 b.p.m. midwife J. was not concerned, as she was aware that it needed to be reduced for a period of more than 40 min for there to be any concern.

Several hours after the shift started, the coordinator sent midwife B. to relieve midwife J. for a break. On entering the room, midwife B. observed that the CTG trace showed evidence of late decelerations, almost absent variability and a baseline rate at the top of the normal range. The coordinator was informed and medical assessment led to a fetal blood sampling. The result indicated significant fetal acidosis and an emergency caesarean section was performed. The baby was born in poor condition and required some resuscitation and transfer to the neonatal unit. The baby subsequently developed cerebral palsy. As the antenatal and early labour CTGs had been reassuring and there was evidence of slowly developing fetal heart rate abnormalities during several hours of labour, it was concluded that the damage to the baby probably occurred during labour.

Midwife J. was very upset, as she considered that she was totally responsible for the events and the outcome.

Issues

Education: The Unit had a system in place that ensured that all staff received yearly training and updating in CTG interpretation. Midwife J. had attended a session 9 months earlier. She had not cared for a woman in labour with a CTG since the day of training, as her only allocation to the labour ward had been to care for low-risk women who required intermittent monitoring.

Allocation: There was no attempt to ascertain whether midwife J. felt competent to care for a high risk woman in labour.

Midwife J. felt anxious about the allocation as she had not worked on the labour ward for some time but felt unable to communicate this to the coordinator, as the Unit was busy and as an experienced midwife, she was expected to be able to perform a full range of duties.

The coordinator was aware that midwife J. was not frequently allocated to the labour ward but was aware that she was an experienced midwife.

The coordinator was aware that there had been changes on the CTG trace as midwife J. had informed her that there had been some decelerations. She did not think it appropriate to assess the CTG for herself as midwife J. was an experienced midwife and should not require supervision.

Through the risk management system, another case had been identified in the previous year, whereby midwife J. had failed to inform the medical staff of a fetal bradycardia until it had been in progress for 6 min. In that case, an emergency caesarean section had been performed and the baby had been born in good condition. As there was no adverse outcome, no support or education was provided and no further action was taken. The coordinator was not aware that there had been concerns about midwife J.'s ability to interpret CTG traces in the past.

Findings and recommendations

There were several system failures:

- The Unit did not ensure that midwife J. was adequately prepared for labour suite duties as her allocation to the labour suite was infrequent
- The staff rotation was poorly organized
- CNST require that all staff received a 6-monthly update in CTG interpretation and this was not provided
- Midwife J. was known to have had problems in the past with CTG interpretation and this was not communicated confidentially to the coordinators. A period of supported practice had not been provided for midwife J. and she had not had the opportunity to enhance her skills
- The risk management system had identified a skills gap but adequate support and training to prevent further incidents was not put in place
- The coordinator made no attempt to ensure that midwife J. was confident with the allocation, despite being aware that she was infrequently allocated to the labour suite
- There were other midwives available who worked more regularly on the labour suite and who could have cared for Mrs W. or provided support for midwife J. and this was not acted upon

- The coordinator made no attempt to review the condition of Mrs W., despite being aware that there were decelerations on the CTG trace some hours earlier. No update was obtained and no support was offered
- Midwife J. did not communicate with the coordinator about her concern regarding her ability to care adequately for Mrs W.

Recommendations

- The provision of 6-monthly CTG updates for all staff should be provided
- All incidents that highlight gaps in skills and or education should be fully investigated and a package of support and education put in place as required, regardless of whether the incident led to an adverse outcome or was a near-miss
- The rotation for staff should be improved and updating provided for all staff as required
- When midwives have had a serious problem with CTG interpretation, this should be communicated confidentially to all coordinators in order that support and supervision can be provided
- Coordinators to be provided with leadership training.

Clearly this not only involves good communications skills, but also requires that the midwife must fully understand the risks before attempting to communicate them to the client. Understanding of risks requires the midwife continually to update herself and to take a critical interest in research as published to ensure that the information being given is up to date, balanced and appropriate to the context.

The midwife needs also to be able to put risk data into perspective for the woman. For example if, following screening, the risk of the baby having a particular condition is '1 in 200', some women may consider this a remote risk, whereas others may consider it a high risk. Some clients may wish to have a second, more invasive test, which carries a new risk of damaging the fetus and that new risk may also be expressed as a probability, say '1 in 50'. It is difficult for many people to comprehend these probabilities, and to decide what

to do. The problem becomes even more acute when the woman is in a state of emotional shock; significant communication skills are required by the midwife to ensure not only that the risk data are presented but that their significance is fully understood.

Untoward incidents: reporting and staff issues

Reporting of untoward incidents

Reporting of untoward incidents is a key part of the risk management process and forms part of the drive to create organizations with a memory and reflective practice (DH 2000). The National Patient Safety Agency was established to develop a national framework for reporting incidents in a no-blame setting; it has set out 'Seven Steps to Patient Safety' (NPSA 2004), which supports blame-free reporting as part of an integrated risk management process. Reporting of incidents also forms an essential element of the CNST standards (see below).

In broad terms, incident reporting is designed to:

- identify the frequency of and the correlated factors associated with adverse incident
- identify systems failures with a view to rectifying them so as to reduce risk
- ensure that teams of clinicians reflect critically on their own performance and that of their team
- develop 'an organization with a memory' (i.e. one in which common lessons are learned by all and past mistakes inform future action).

The reporting framework

Effective management requires feedback on performance and, over recent decades, most maternity units have operated reporting systems – with a greater or lesser degree of formality. CNST 'standard 2: Learning from experience' (NHSLA 2007) sets out the requirements of a reporting system:

> *2.1.1 Adverse incidents and near misses are reported in all areas of the maternity service by all staff groups*
> *2.1.2 Summarised adverse incident reports are provided regularly to the maternity services risk management group (or equivalent) for review and action*
> *2.1.3 The maternity service considers and applies the recommendations made in the national confidential enquiries*
> *2.2.1 The maternity service has a strategic approach to the management of adverse incidents that might lead to a claim.*

Incident report forms

Incident reporting forms have developed considerably over recent years. Added impetus comes from the requirements of CNST and Building a safer NHS for patients. Most Trusts have come to the view that a single Trust-wide form is appropriate, not least because it creates a sense of a common interest in reducing risk. Features of incident report forms include:

- the form is in a common style for use across the Trust and is not specifically used for midwifery
- the incident types are classified
- some of the incident types are 'non-clinical' (e.g. thefts and assaults)

- the risk management department assesses whether non-clinical departments need to be informed (e.g. the health and safety advisor, fire safety officer, etc.) and whether 'further action is required'.

This action may include:

- recommending new procedures or the enhancement of existing procedures
- general training for staff or specific retraining for the individual involved.

There is a growing body of literature on the analysis of incident report forms to which reference may be made (e.g. Vincent et al 2002).

Incident reporting: concerns of midwives

Risk management procedures such as adverse event and near-miss reporting may cause concern to staff, including midwives. Some may see it as a means for fostering rivalry and distrust among staff. However, the Government guidance has been at pains to promote a blame-free approach to reporting.

Adverse incident reporting is, first and foremost, a device for learning about the *system* and seeking to prevent systems failures. For example, Building a safer NHS (DH 2001) quotes Saul Weingart who says: 'Improvement strategies that punish individual clinicians are misguided and do not work. Fixing the dysfunctional system, on the other hand, is the work that needs to be done'. Many Trusts are now seeking actively to allay the concerns of staff members about the effect of reporting an adverse incident in which they have been involved.

Nevertheless, no Trust can say categorically that no action will be taken. That is simply unrealistic – indeed, a Trust Chief Executive's legal obligation (as part of his or her general clinical governance obligations) is to have appropriate procedures in place for dealing with staff whose performance needs correction.

Disciplinary action should not result from a report of an adverse incident, except in one or more of the following cases:

- where there have been repeated incidents involving the same individual despite training or other intervention
- where there is evidence of breaking the law

- where in the view of the professional registration body the action causing the incident is far removed from acceptable practice
- where there is a failure to report an incident in which a member of staff was either involved or about which they were aware.

Conclusion

Midwives have traditionally seen childbirth as a reasonably safe and natural process. The advent of risk terminology and widespread screening has thrown the issue of risk into sharper focus. Risk is now a key factor to be considered in midwifery practice.

Risk management was first introduced into the NHS as a device for reducing litigation risk. The emphasis has changed over the past decade and the term 'risk management' is now largely used to mean risk reduction processes for the enhancement of client care.

The CNST was formed in the mid-1990s as a funding body for clinical negligence. Most Trusts have joined the CNST. They must therefore abide by the CNST standards, which contain detailed rules about the risk management processes that the Trust must operate. Maternity services are unique in having their own set of standards.

One of the most visible areas of risk management is that of 'incident reporting'. In this chapter, we have examined some of the requirements laid down by the CNST and the involvement of central government through the National Patient Safety Authority. 'Reporting' is to be done within a culture that focuses on improving the system rather than blaming the individual.

The precise direction risk management will take in the future is somewhat uncertain. One thing that is certain, however, is that risk management will continue to play an important role in delivering a quality health service and that midwives will continue to play a key role in managing risk to provide enhanced client care.

REFERENCES

Aslam R 1999 Risk management in midwifery practice. British Journal of Midwifery 7(1):41–44

Clements C 2000 Critical incident analysis of the third stage of labour. British Journal of Midwifery 8(8):500–504

Clements R V 1995 Essentials of clinical risk management. In: Vincent C (ed.) Clinical risk management. BMJ publishing Group, London, p 335–349

Dineen M 1997 Clinical risk management and midwives. Modern Midwife 7(11):9–13

DH (Department of Health) 2000 An organisation with a memory. HMSO, London

DH (Department of Health) 2001 Building a safer NHS for patients. HMSO, London

DH (Department of Health) 2007 Maternity Matters: Choice, access and continuity of care in a safe service, DH London Health Act 1999 HMSO, London

Lewis G (ed.) 2007 The Confidential Enquiry into Maternal and Child Health (CEMACH). Saving mothers' lives: reviewing maternal deaths to make motherhood safer 2003–2005. The seventh report on Confidential Enquiries into Maternal Deaths in the United Kingdom. CEMACH, London

NHSLA (NHS Litigation Authority) 2006 Report and accounts, NHSLA, London

NHSLA (NHS Litigation Authority) 2007 Clinical negligence scheme for Trusts: clinical risk management standards for maternity services. NHS Litigation Authority, London

NICE (National Institute of Health and Clinical Excellence) 2004 Caesarean sections. Clinical Guideline 13. NICE, London

NMC (Nursing and Midwifery Council) 2006, Standards for the preparation and practice of supervisors of midwives. NMC, London

NPSA (National Patient Safety Agency) 2004 Seven steps to patient safety. NPSA, London

NPSA (National Patient Safety Agency) 2005 Engaging clinicians. NPSA, London

Patel Lord Narem 2007 Making maternity care safer. Presentation at the joint Healthcare Commission and NPSA Conference. Safe Delivery: Reducing Risk in Maternity Services , 26 June, London

RCM (Royal College of Midwives) 2000 Assessing and managing risk in midwifery practice (RCM clinical risk management paper). RCM Midwives Journal 7:224–225

RCOG (Royal College of Obstetrics and Gynaecology) 2005 Clinical risk management for obstetrics and gynaecology – clinical governance advice No. 2

Thomas B G 1998 The disempowering concept of risk. Practising Midwife 1(12):18–21

Vincent C, Taylor-Adams S, Chapman J et al 2002 How to investigate and analyse clinical incidents. British Medical Journal 320:771–781

FURTHER READING

Clements R V (with specialist contributors) 2001 Risk management and litigation in obstetrics and gynaecology. Royal Society of Medicine Press in association with the Royal College of Obstetricians and Gynaecologists. London

A comprehensive review of risk management in its narrower sense of being specifically related to litigation risk. The first section focuses on the law, and considers the duties of the obstetrician, with respect to liability and causation in clinical negligence claims. The second section considers the principles of clinical risk management and includes an analysis of adverse outcomes, the basic principles of risk management, and how they relate to obstetrics and gynaecology. In the third and fourth sections, a variety of specialist clinical topics are dealt with.

Symon A (ed.) 2006 Risk and choice in maternity care: an international perspective. Churchill Livingstone, Edinburgh

This book explores the relationship between risk and choice in maternity care. It contains a collaboration that sheds an international perspective with chapters on maternity care in the UK, USA, Australia and Ireland contributed by midwives, obstetricians, risk management experts and sociologists. The aim of this book is to illustrate the changing reality of risk management as it relates to maternity care, and to highlight risk management concerns that may limit the choices available to pregnant women.

USEFUL WEBSITES

Healthcare Commission:
www.healthcarecommission.org.uk

National Health Service Litigation Authority:
www.nhsla.com

National Institute for Health and Clinical Excellence:
www.nice.org.uk

National Patient Safety Agency:
www.npsa.nhs.uk

54 Organization of the health services in the UK

Lindsay Reid

CHAPTER CONTENTS

The United Kingdom of Great Britain and Northern Ireland (UK) has different systems of governance to respond to the needs of the UK's four countries: England, Wales, Scotland and Northern Ireland. The distinct characteristics of the people of each of these countries require the provision of appropriate health services. This chapter aims to explore some aspects of the health services in the UK. Today the primary source of health services is the National Health Service (NHS). A relatively small independent sector also exists but as the NHS is the main provider of UK health services, this chapter will concentrate on the NHS. It is appropriate also to highlight areas where the NHS in its early years, and latterly, affected midwifery and maternity services.

The chapter aims to:

- give an overview of the background to the NHS
- demonstrate differences which are apparent between the countries and cultures of the UK
- highlight aspects of the new NHS from 1948
- show how the new NHS affected midwifery and maternity services
- look at the reorganization of the NHS in 1974
- examine further changes and new plans
- explore the position of midwives in the twenty-first century NHS.

The NHS: background and history

The story of the NHS has a long beginning. In the early twentieth century, the UK contained extremes of circumstances, which affected the population's health: poverty and deprivation on the one hand; on the other, great wealth. Healthcare varied: some people paid medical expenses by weekly subscription to Friendly Societies; some attended dispensaries, out-patient departments of voluntary hospitals, or, often generous, general practitioners (GPs); some used folk remedies or patent medicines; others went without (Brotherstone 1987a, p 36).

Within the aims of this chapter, it is appropriate to conduct a brief exploration into the recent past. Since the early 1900s, development of the UK health services, while differing depending on the mores of each home country, has shown universal progression. As part of social history, this has had an impact on the health and well-being of all members of society (McLachlan 1987, p xi).

Modern healthcare is a huge complicated web of personal services. Its background lies in the Victorian era's pressures for social justice, Chadwick's seminal report (1842) and succeeding wars which highlighted the need for improved health and other services. For instance, the growing acknowledgement of the poor physical stature of children of Britain, highlighted by the rejection of army recruits for the Boer War (1899–1902), further stimulated the growing interest in maternal and infant welfare.

In 1908, Poor Law medical relief represented the biggest public commitment to medical care. However, Labour politicians started pushing for a comprehensive health service for everyone. In 1905, the Conservative government appointed a Commission to investigate the Poor Law and recommend reforms (Brotherstone 1987a, p 43). However, consensus on increased State involvement in the promotion of health was hard to achieve: the Commission's impact was minimal. Nevertheless, their reports advocated a coming together of concerned individual services to form a health service. This was to be at the heart of much of the subsequent development of public medical care (Brotherstone 1987a, p 47).

National health insurance

Early twentieth century healthcare provided by the Friendly Societies was inadequate, unsatisfactory and unfair. Excluded from membership were: chronic invalids; 'high-risk' people; and members' wives and children. Chancellor of the Exchequer at that time, David Lloyd George, believed that a state-supported health insurance scheme was necessary and in 1911 his National Insurance Act was passed (Brotherstone 1987a, p 48).

The National Insurance Act aimed to relieve poverty among manual workers when off work through illness and to provide a minimum healthcare service. There was a recognized ongoing need to extend the Act. However, in practice, mainly due to costs, little difference in the health services was seen at the time (Pater 1981, p 4–6).

Highlands and Islands Medical Service

There was a need for a special health service in the Highlands and Islands of Scotland, a wide sparsely populated area. For the self-employed crofters who lived barely above subsistence level, with no money to spare for healthcare, the National Insurance Act was of little relevance. Within 2 years of the Act, Parliament acknowledged the special case of the Crofting Community, allocated funding, and the Highlands and Islands Medical Service (HIMS) was set up. This was 'Britain's first comprehensive state medical service'. It 'provided ... necessary pointers towards a full and comprehensive health service in Scotland' and demonstrated a 'system of co-operative effort' (McCrae 2003, p 1–29) which can be seen in some multi-professional team working of today.

The idea of public medical care

In the 1920s and 1930s, the trend towards public policy for the organization of medical services grew (Fox 1986). There was a growing public sense of need. Charitable agencies existed but were not enough to meet the needs of the very deprived; slowly public services became involved (McLachlan 1987, p xii). In addition, voluntary donations attempted to keep hospitals afloat. Anne Bayne recalled:

> *[When I was four] my mother ... took me to visit my aunt in Aberdeen Royal ... when it was all voluntary donations (mid 1930s). The nurse ... [had] to go round with the plate ... and she came and handed me the plate to take round [the visitors].*

(Reid Archival Collection 1997–2002:91)

Change across the UK was required. In 1936, the Department of Health for Scotland (DHS) recognized the need for a national health policy and laid the foundation of a State medical service (DHS 1936; Brotherstone 1987a, p 75). A decade later, an NHS for the UK was about to become a reality.

In the early 1940s, cross-UK debate regarding future health service policy was energized by the publication of a wide-ranging scheme for reconstructing social security; the term 'welfare state' was born and 'a comprehensive health service would be made available to all' (Brotherstone 1987a, p 88; Department of Health and Social Security [DHSS] 1942). Thus, this was to be a 'national health service for prevention and comprehensive treatment' (Webster 1998, p 7). Early in 1943, the National Government committed itself to this ideal; the finer details remained for participating bodies to bring slowly and sometimes acrimoniously to a conclusion.

The 'appointed day' for implementation of the NHS acts

The long-awaited 'appointed day', 5 July 1948, saw the implementation of two separate Acts in Britain: the 1946 NHS Act for England and Wales and the 1947 NHS (Scotland) Act. At this time, since 1922 Northern Ireland had already had considerable legislative autonomy with its own Parliament at Stormont, outside Belfast (Davies 1999, p 917, Levitt et al 1999, p 84). Thus, Northern Ireland's 'appointed day' was heralded by the 1946 Health Services Act (Northern Ireland) (O'Sullivan 2001, p 95–101).

In instigating this huge change in health policy and establishment of political accountability, Aneurin Bevan, the Minister of Health predicted that a 'dropped bed-pan would resound through the corridors of Whitehall' (Talbot-Smith & Pollock 2006, p 1). The changes have kept coming: the bedpan has never really come to rest.

Three central values formed the core ideology of the NHS:

1. It would provide a universal standard of healthcare across the UK

2. It would cover all health needs, making it completely comprehensive

3. It would be free at the point of delivery and available to all on the basis of need, not ability to pay.

Funding for this 'new institution' was to be mainly through central taxation (Talbot-Smith & Pollock 2006, p 2). Other sources of funding were local rates and public contributions to a national insurance scheme (Brotherstone 1987b, p 106).

Administratively, the NHS was originally designed to be run on a tripartite scheme: first, Regional Hospital Boards; second Executive Councils which administered general medical services, including dentistry and pharmacy (under the NHS, GPs retained their status as independent contractors); third, there were Local Health Authorities (LHAs) responsible for providing maternity services, child welfare, midwifery (but not including hospitals), health visiting and home nursing (Brotherstone 1987b, p 106).

The early days

The Beveridge Report (DHSS 1942) assumed that 'there was a fixed quantity of illness in the country'. This would gradually grow less with the new NHS. The cost of healthcare would level off, become stable, and perhaps, as people became healthier, it would even decline (Ham 1992, p 17). The cracks in this prediction soon showed as people's expectations grew along with the spiralling costs of medical care (McCrae 2003, p 242).

No-one in the UK has remained untouched by 'one of the greatest social constructions of the twentieth century' (Christie 1998). The general public, hitherto unable to afford treatment, now used the new NHS to the full. One doctor recalled:

> There was a colossal amount of unmet need that just poured in . . . women with prolapsed uteruses literally wobbling down below their legs . . . [and] hernias . . . men walking around with trusses holding these colossal hernias in . . . they couldn't afford to have it done.
>
> (Christie 1998, p 4)

Now they could 'have it done'. However, expanding waiting-rooms and lengthening queues soon demonstrated that the NHS was a victim of its own success. In addition, along with their consultation, patients expected a free prescription. The rising cost of new drugs and the demand for free false teeth and spectacles added to the total expenditure. In 1949, the government imposed a charge of 1 shilling (5 pence) per prescription and in 1951, further charges on spectacles and false teeth. However, by 1953, costs were prejudicing necessary NHS developments (McCrae 2003, p 244). A subsequent review of NHS finances 'revealed the potentially unlimited demand for healthcare and the necessity of containing that demand within a finite budget' (Brotherstone 1987b, p 148).

The new NHS: effect on midwives

The new NHS affected midwifery services and midwives' practice. Although the NHS did not directly alter the Central Midwives Boards (CMBs) or their responsibilities, its tripartite administrative structure fragmented maternity services. This led to the possibility of overlapping, confusion and a diminishing role for the midwife (Johnstone 1953, Robinson 1990, p 73). First, pregnant women could now go to their GP free of charge to 'book'. Midwives were thus no longer the first point of contact. Second, GPs began to perform an increasing amount of antenatal care. This, exacerbated by the NHS, caused conflict between some GPs and midwives and signalled an 'unwelcome trend which could wreck the structure of the midwifery services' (Ministry of Health [MoH] et al 1949, p viii; Robinson 1990, p 72). Extra payment for undertaking maternity care saw GPs' proportion of antenatal care rising quickly, diminishing the midwife's role and experience for pupil midwives (Robinson 1990, p 73–74). Third, the NHS brought problems of safety and continuity of care: 'In some cases, midwives are not seeing patients until they go to deliver them' (MoH et al 1949, p viii). Fourth, the NHS reinforced the existing trend towards hospital births. The new policy of centralization of obstetric care matched an increasing demand for hospital births with a corresponding increase in medical involvement in normal maternity care (Robinson 1990, p 75, Tait 1987, p 420). From the mother's point of view hospital births sometimes made economic sense; they also gave many mothers a welcome rest (Williams 1997, p 200). Nevertheless, although the number of hospital maternity beds was rising there were not

enough to meet the rising demand (Reid 2003, p 138). Some mothers took for granted the availability of a hospital bed and did not book. Mary McCaskill recalled:

> ... a relative would phone in ... Mrs A was in labour ... could she go into hospital? ... [If there was no bed] ... I had to go out ... as a municipal midwife ... and ... tell them [this] ... and the baby was going to be born in the house ... [We] often got a hostile reception ... because a family was unprepared ... for a home confinement.
>
> (Reid 2003, p 138, Reid Archival Collection 1997–2002:27)

Nevertheless, hospital births were on the increase and some midwives in the district began to feel very vulnerable. Mary McCaskill continued:

> [By 1952] the home deliveries had ... started to decline ... Older midwives ... probably in their fifties ... didn't have so many bookings and they were wondering ... what was the future ... would they be diversified into some other duties?
>
> (Reid 2003, p 138, Reid Archival Collection 1997–2002:27)

Thus the early NHS played a part in diminishing the role of the midwife, and the move towards hospitalization of birth. This also affected midwifery training, the viability of training institutions, and eventual changes in the midwifery curriculum (Reid 2003, p 139).

Reorganization

Successive government reviews of the NHS culminated in a reorganization of the NHS in 1974 following the 1973 NHS Act for England and Wales and the 1972 NHS (Scotland) Act. These Acts abolished the tripartite structure and integrated all health services under a single management structure with a three-tier system through regional, area and district health authorities (Brotherstone 1987b, p 130, NHS 1972). The new structure for England is summarized in Table 54.1 (Ham 1992, p 27).

The new NHS structures in Wales, Scotland and Northern Ireland differed from that in England. In Wales there were no RHAs. The Welsh Office had the dual role of central government department and RHA (Ham 1992, p 28). The 1972 Scottish Act

Table 54.1 NHS: structure in England 1974–1982

Name	Members appointed by	Function
Regional Health Authority (RHA)	Secretary of State for Social Services	Planning of health services
Area Health Authority (AHA) (parallel to FPCs below)	RHAs; local authorities; Members of non-medical and nursing staff	Planning and management; development of services
Family practitioner committees (FPCs)	AHA, local professionals and local authorities	Administered contracts of GPs, dentists, pharmacists, opticians
District management team (parallel to CHCs below)	Formed from areas	Administration of health districts (divisions of areas)
Community Health Councils (CHCs)	Drawn from public	To represent views of public to HAs

aimed for a fully integrated service. Instead of RHAs, 15 health boards (HB), were to unite the organization and management of Scottish health services with Local Health Councils (LHCs) equating with CHCs (Brotherstone 1987b, p 132–135). In Northern Ireland four health and social services boards, each split into districts, responsible for personal and social services and health, were in direct contact with the DHSS (Northern Ireland). District Committees functioned as CHCs (Ham 1992, p 28).

Reorganization and midwifery

The 1974 reorganization brought more cohesion between hospital and community but with it, problems associated with integration of midwifery between the community and hospital. This affected midwifery practice. Many midwives were administered by senior hospital nurses often without a midwifery qualification; similar problems arose in midwifery education (Reid 2003, p 149, 151). Administrative change was spurred on by the 1966 Report of the Salmon Committee with concerns over nursing and midwifery structure, status and standards (Davies & Beach 2000, p 3). The timing and thinking behind the implementation of 'the Salmon Structure' in the 1970s fitted with Reorganization of the NHS. However, it was the Briggs Committee (DHSS et al 1972) in its review of nursing and midwifery which examined in depth the needs of an integrated health service. Thus, it started changes signaling the end of the existing statutory bodies (Reid 2003, p 166–181).

Integration of the maternity services after 1974 was part of the wider NHS reorganization. By the mid-1960s the service remained disjointed with neither mothers nor midwives achieving continuity. Government attention turned to integration of maternity services but brought with it, without supporting evidence, further hospitalization of birth (Reid 2003, p 159).

Overall, this first major reorganization of the NHS had good intentions. However, integration resulted in the unpopular closure of many small units accompanied by administrative difficulties. To make matters worse the British economy was plunged into a recession following the Middle East Oil crisis and NHS expansion slowed. Staff demonstrated their frustration in unrest and increasing militancy (Brotherstone 1987b, p 146).

The Thatcher influence

In 1979 the Conservative Party was returned under Margaret Thatcher and remained in power for 18 years. The Thatcher administration made NHS spending more ruthless. A change in general management introduced a new breed of hospital managers, business trained and disciplined. Outsourced cleaning and catering services initiated the private sector into the NHS (Talbot-Smith & Pollock 2006, p 7).

This was the beginning of the transition of the NHS to a market. Over the years, wide-ranging disagreement over all aspects of funding undermined the NHS's initial powerful consensus of public ownership and control (Talbot-Smith & Pollock 2006, p 7). Aware of conflict, the government was reluctant to embark on another total reorganization (Levitt et al 1999). However, in England, for financial efficiency and improved patient care, the government removed one tier of administration and set up District Health Authorities (DHAs). It retained FPCs and CHCs and ordered strict cost limits (DHSS 1979; Ham 1992, p 29).

Change was also evident elsewhere. In Wales, a system of unit management similar to the English one replaced the district level. The Scottish approach created a system of unit management in 1984 (Kinnaird 1987, p 266) and called for increased provision of long-term care (Brotherstone 1987b, p 149, SHHD 1980). In Northern Ireland the basic structure remained. All agreed the importance of delegating power to local level (Ham 1992, p 30).

The new structures were ineffective, lacking in leadership and led to another Report (DHSS 1983): general managers should be appointed throughout the NHS. This would provide leadership and a more dynamic management approach, motivate staff and bring about change and improve costs. The Report did not cover Wales, Scotland nor Northern Ireland; nevertheless, the principles of the Report were adopted there (Ham 1992, p 32, Kinnaird 1987, p 266).

The introduction of NHS general managers reflected governmental preoccupation with analogies of industrial line management. However, to equate the health service with industry was seen as less than satisfactory. It was possible that general managers (sometimes lacking a health service background) could become pre-occupied with the minutiae of management and financial control (Brotherstone 1987a, p 149).

The 1980s saw an overriding concern developing: to maintain financial control. Consumer responsiveness and quality of care took second place. Managers were expected to be actively interested in clinical work; in reality tension remained between professional and managerial values for a long time (Ham 1992, p 35).

Internal market

In 1991 the government instituted what was imprecisely called an 'internal market' within the NHS (Webster 1998, p 202). Hospitals, groups of hospitals and other bodies became Trusts and started behaving like businesses in a market place (DH et al 1989). Health authorities and boards became 'commissioners' or 'purchasers' of health services and the trusts were 'sellers'. This changed the way

that NHS resources and funding were accounted for and the term 'purchaser-provider split' came into use (Talbot-Smith & Pollock 2006, p 6). The change was designed to improve the service by allowing the purchaser to choose and buy care. However, the proposed hasty reorganization, caused the 'biggest explosion of political anger and professional fury in the history of the NHS' (Webster 1998, p 194). Nevertheless, regardless of NHS staff feelings of insecurity, alienation and status reduction to an insignificant element in the market mechanism, the reforms went ahead (Webster 1998, p 197). A sense of crisis in the NHS escalated in the 1990s: a 'decade of turmoil' which neither tackled nor solved the problems (Webster 1998, p 205).

There were other changes relevant to the internal market. Now all NHS service providers had to pay to the Treasury an annual 'capital charge' from what they earned on the value of their land and equipment: paying for their use would make trusts more economical with their assets. An alternative way of drumming up capital for public investments was introduced in 1992: the Private Finance Initiative (PFI). In the PFI a consortium of big businesses join together to 'design, build and operate NHS premises in return for an annual charge paid by the NHS over the lifetime of a contract, usually 25–30 years'. Thus, Trusts lease back their own facilities from the PFI consortium (Talbot-Smith and Pollock 2006, p 7).

Midwifery in the 1990s

There was also unrest in the maternity sector. The background to the need for change was UK-wide and engendered several significant documents including DH 1993a, NIDHSS 1994, SHHD 1993, Welsh Office 1996. Each of these documents called for change, for more informed choice and control for women, for more continuity of care and/or carer and a better way of working for midwives. The much discussed term 'woman-centred care' came into vogue (Hillan et al 1997).

Partners with the public

While managerial turmoil continued, the thinking behind patient care began to change. There was an acknowledgement that there were priority groups, including maternity care, with wide variations in clinical care and the provision of services. Watchdog bodies voiced concerns. Public health, at the root of the NHS, had a new dynamic importance: the public was invited to be involved with their own care; schemes were afoot to target causes of early death; good health could be for everyone; education of the public was encouraged; partnership between patient and professional was an achievable goal; the NHS should deliver services responsive to user-need including projected improvements in waiting times. In addition there was a universal commitment to improve and maintain standards of all aspects of care across the NHS (DH 1993b, SHHD 1991).

Change of government: change of plan

In 1997 the Labour party achieved a landslide electoral victory. Initially, the incoming Labour government introduced a few NHS changes and maintained that clinical services would not be privatized (Levitt et al 1999, p 256, Talbot-Smith & Pollock 2006, p 7). However, the *NHS Plan* (DH 2000) turned this commitment on its head only to change again as policy-makers acknowledged that a significant volume of private services was not feasible without recourse to NHS staff (Talbot-Smith & Pollock 2006, p 7). The systems which emerged demonstrated a new way of setting and enforcing standards through monitoring, inspections, auditing and legal challenges.

In 1999 devolution of government led to the establishment of a Scottish parliament in Edinburgh, a Welsh assembly in Cardiff and the continuation of Northern Ireland's assembly in Belfast (although from 2002–2007 suspension of devolution in Northern Ireland caused the responsibility for Northern Ireland departments to be passed to the Northern Ireland Office in London). Differences in the health services across the UK now became more significant. Committees and consultations across the UK led to an NHS plan for each country, commensurate with the needs of its population and demographic spread (DH 2000, DHSSPS 2000, SEHD 2000, WAG 2001).

The *Plans* in each country agreed with each other in their philosophies for better financial management,

greater professional working together, partnership with patients, improved health of each population, better overall statistics on a global scale and improved patient experience. However two main areas where they diverged lay in ideas of structure and finance. Constraints of space preclude a full examination and comparison of the *Plans*. In addition, plans and minds change as time and thinking move on. Therefore this section will include: a brief description of the current NHS structure in each of the UK countries; comments on differing methods of how the NHS is financed; reference to standards in the NHS and current ways of developing and maintaining them; and, Agenda for Change, a programme that affects every member of staff in the NHS.

Structure

The Secretary of State for Health and the DH have ultimate responsibility for the NHS in England. Accountable to the DH are strategic health authorities which along with the DH are classed as organizations with strategic roles. Commissioners of care, accountable to strategic health authorities, are known as primary care trusts (PCT) and (social) care trusts. Below this level in the structure are providers of care:

- primary care: GPs; dentists; opticians; pharmacists
- walk-in centres
- independent sector comprising primary care, treatment centres and hospitals
- NHS treatment centres
- NHS trusts (accountable to strategic health authorities) moving to foundation status. Foundation trusts are accountable to an independent regulator: Monitor (Talbot-Smith & Pollock 2006, p 8).

Thus, we can see that the line of responsibility runs directly through the levels of the structure to the Secretary of State for Health. Even foundation trusts are ultimately accountable to parliament but they are directly accountable only to Monitor (established 2004), the independent regulator of NHS foundation trusts (Talbot-Smith & Pollock 2006, p 112).

NHS Wales is administered by the Welsh Assembly Government. The Welsh Assembly has executive powers and can determine policy through secondary legislation and implementation of primary Westminster legislation. The current structure of NHS Wales goes from the level of the Welsh Assembly Government through the NHS Wales department, to three regional offices. They are the organizations with strategic roles. These lead to the organizations commissioning services: 22 local health boards in partnership working with local authorities. This level leads to organizations providing services: 15 NHS trusts and, for example, GPs, opticians, pharmacists and dentists (Talbot-Smith & Pollock 2006, p 165).

The Minister of State for Health and Community Care at the Scottish government heads the structure of NHS Scotland and the Scottish Executive Health Department (SEHD). These are the organizations with strategic roles. They are followed by organizations planning and delivering services comprising 15 NHS boards, divided into two operating divisions: hospital services and, primary, community and mental health services. The latter division leads on to community health partnerships forming a joint futures body with local authorities and the voluntary sector (Talbot-Smith & Pollock 2006, p 158).

The Minister of Health and Personal Social Services heads the organization of the NHS in Northern Ireland and leads the Department of Health, Social Services and Public Safety (DHSSPS) in its strategic role. Organizations commissioning services follow: four health and social services boards. Then come organizations providing services: 19 health and social services trusts including hospital services and social care services; and, five local health and social care groups encapsulating primary care, other family health services and community care (Talbot-Smith & Pollock 2006, p 171).

Finance

Funding for the NHS in the UK is complex and varied, depending on the country. In general, funding for the NHS comes as before from general taxation, national insurance contributions and charges and is allocated to different parts of the service.

In England, recent legislation allowed the formation of Care Trusts. This permitted voluntary partnerships between PCTs and local authorities, thus giving PCTs access to local authority funding. PCTs

may also generate additional funds through marketing activities, forming companies either alone or in partnership with the private sector, or selling clinical services. NHS funding can also come from capital allocation to buy and replace, for instance, buildings and equipment. Most assets are now owned by NHS trusts and PCTs. However, PFIs are now a major source of funding for new capital investment in the NHS. In addition some NHS Hospital trusts have become foundation trusts operating under a different framework (Talbot-Smith & Pollock 2006, p 78–103). Thus the *Plan* allows for different market strategies to take place. In addition there is a new financial framework, 'payment by results' which is intended to provide incentives to increase the efficiency and quality of services. There will be competition and contracts, conditions and penalties. The intention/hope is to have efficient, good quality services with choice for the patients (Talbot-Smith & Pollock 2006, p 109).

The Scottish government through the SEHD is responsible for developing health policy, allocating resources and delivering services. The Scottish government's plan for the NHS (SEHD 2000) has moved forward through legislation and structural reform (SEHD 2005) to do away with the purchaser-provider split and self-governing trusts in Scotland (Talbot-Smith & Pollock 2006, p 157). NHS Scotland is an integrated system with unified health boards funded by annual budgets and responsible for planning and delivering services. Within the health boards local health plans specify how services will be provided; operating divisions take the responsibility for providing services. All primary care services are provided under the title of 'primary medical services'. Foundation trusts have not been introduced in Scotland. However, being introduced are alternatives to traditional models of secondary healthcare which the SEHD funds. These include 'special health boards', for example, NHS 24, NHS Education for Scotland (NES) and the Scottish Ambulance Service (Talbot-Smith & Pollock 2006, p 158).

In Wales, as in England, the 'purchaser-provider' split is still employed. Local organizations commission or purchase hospital and community services on behalf of their populations. Yet, Wales has not introduced the policy of foundation status, nor the payment by results financial framework. Neither has it introduced the independent sector as a mainstream provider of NHS services (Talbot-Smith & Pollock 2006, p 166).

In Northern Ireland, health and social services are integrated under a single central ministry. Like England and Wales, Northern Ireland also employs the purchaser-provider split; like Wales, it has not gone down the foundation status, payment by results routes. Although the DHSSPS 'has no immediate plans' to use the independent sector as a major provider, it has declared its intention of watching and learning from what happens elsewhere (Talbot-Smith & Pollock 2006, p 174).

Flying standards

Since the 1990s a plethora of related words and terms have come into fashion. Words like: targets; national standards; accountability; clinical performance; performance rating systems; professional regulation; appraisal and revalidation; and, life-long learning. There are many more but these words will do as examples. They are not necessarily new but in the current atmosphere of a rapidly changing NHS, with the added transition in some areas from a public to a market based system of mixed public and private provision it is important to remember that alongside the changes, the patients/users are still coming through the doors and require an ongoing high level of safety and standards of care. So, these terms are on the lips of NHS personnel much more readily than hitherto. They all have something in common and a similar aim: best practice.

Best practice is difficult, perhaps impossible to measure (Reid 2007, p 9–29). In addition, perceptions and opinions of best practice will vary depending upon who is the practitioner, the era under discussion, or, whether or not the best practice is individual or collective. However, it is generally agreed within the NHS that standards which aim towards best practice are better to be discussed, agreed, formalized, written down and disseminated at both local and national levels.

Each government and health department within the UK may decide its process of setting, implementing and monitoring standards. In practice there is some co-working. For instance, the National Institute for Health and Clinical Excellence (NICE) is a mechanism overseen by the DH. Its role is 'to provide health professionals and the public (in England) with authoritative and reliable information on evidence-based best practice'. NHS organizations are expected to abide by NICE's recommendations (Talbot-Smith & Pollock 2006, p 113). While NICE applies to England, its remit also extends to NHS Wales. In Scotland, Quality Improvement Scotland (QIS), one of Scotland's special health boards, ensures quality of services. Within its duties of appraising and advising on treatments and medicines, QIS disseminates NICE guidelines and comments on them regarding their appropriateness for use in Scotland. QIS also funds and supervises the work of the Scottish Inter-Collegiate Guidelines Network (SIGN). This multidisciplinary working group produces evidence-based national clinical guidelines for the management of specific conditions (Talbot-Smith & Pollock 2006, p 161–162). In Northern Ireland, the DHSSPS also uses NICE as a resource and advises health boards and trusts on its appropriateness. In addition there is a multiprofessional advisory committee: the Clinical Resource Efficiency Support Team (CREST) which equates to SIGN in Scotland (Talbot-Smith & Pollock 2006, p 175).

A vital component of the effort towards collective and individual best practice is clinical governance. Clinical governance was introduced for all NHS organizations in April 1999. It is a framework to enable NHS organizations to be accountable for constant improvement of the quality of services and safeguarding of high standards, by making the NHS a service of excellence. So, it is about expanding courses of action that support the continual improvement of standards, services and patient involvement (Proctor 1999, Pulzer 1999, Talbot-Smith & Pollock, 2006, p 114).

Agenda for change

Moving to a 'market mind-set' called for changes in terms of service of NHS staff. In 2004, under the title Agenda for Change (AfC), pay restructuring arrived and the requirement for most NHS staff to undergo annual development reviews. This involves: discussions with a line manager; a demonstration of staff members' ability to apply their knowledge and skills against the requirements of their posts; identification of how to maintain current levels of knowledge and skills; and, how to improve where these are lacking (Talbot-Smith & Pollock 2006, p 126). Thus AfC is a key factor of the pay modernization agenda within the NHS. It reinforces the need for articulation between skills frameworks and career pathways and offers opportunities for new ways of collaborative working (NES 2004).

Knowledge and skills for each post are identified through the Knowledge and Skills Framework (KSF). Thus, there is a KSF outline for every post in the NHS (Talbot-Smith & Pollock 2006, p 126) Also, in October 2004 new contracts for hospital consultants and GPs were introduced. The new consultants' contract enabled foundation trusts in England to vary their conditions of service and the GPs' contract withdrew GPs' monopoly over provision of primary care (Talbot-Smith & Pollock 2006, p 10). Regardless of differences in policy across the UK, AfC also applies in Scotland, Wales and Northern Ireland (Talbot-Smith & Pollock 2006, p 163, 169, 176).

Midwives and the new NHS: discussion

As we have seen above, midwives have been involved with, and affected by the NHS since its inception. On one occasion in the 1950s an enterprising midwife was shown where she stood. At the time, mothers in the postnatal ward were kept in bed for five days unless they had an infected episiotomy when they were allowed up for a shower. The midwife thought that it would prevent infection in the first place if all the mothers were allowed up for a shower and suggested this to the senior midwife. She recalled, 'I was told I wasn't paid to think' (Reid 2003, p 281; Reid Archival Collection 1997–2002: 116).

Today midwives who are prepared to think about, embrace and promulgate innovative practice, are the norm rather than the exception. The Nursing and Midwifery Council (NMC) reproduces the globally-recognized definition of a midwife (NMC 2004, p 36), which gives a wide range of skills that a midwife may employ in pursuit of her profession. However it implies a freedom to practise that not all

enjoy. Most midwives in the UK practise within the NHS and midwifery practice is therefore conditional upon NHS legislation, restriction, protocol and policy which exist at both governmental and local levels. A strong element of midwifery leadership is needed here, and in the creation of midwifery guidelines. At the same time all midwives, from the most to the least experienced, need to have a part to play in formulating and disseminating best practice. Thus, schemes to improve maternity care across the UK are evolving from a multiprofessional standpoint with professional groups cooperating with others on an equal basis. This brings parity and respect for the opinions and practice of others.

Two examples of multiprofessional cooperation come from Wales and Scotland. In Wales under the auspices of a multiprofessional steering group the All Wales Normal Labour Pathway is flourishing. 'The intention of the Pathway was to reduce unnecessary intervention in labour and to give midwives the freedom to practise based on evidence and partnership'. It has made an impact on midwifery care all over Wales (Kirkman & Ferguson 2007, p 115).

In Scotland, the Scottish Multiprofessional Maternity Development Group (SMMDG) comprises representatives of all professions with a part to play in the maternity services. The group is working on writing, producing and organizing a continually evolving evidence-based programme of courses (Reid 2007, p 250). Again, the impact has been felt across midwifery care in Scotland.

Yet, all is not well with the challenge of change. In her Zepherina Veitch Lecture, Appleby (2006) highlighted some issues of NHS reforms: foundation trusts; payment by results; modernization and redesign; involvement of patients; the commissioning process; further restructuring. Midwives have not been involved enough with the dialogue and have been asked to do 'more and more with less and less' (Appleby 2006). And, financial shortfalls in some NHS Trusts have created further economic restraints in maternity services (Magill-Cuerden 2007).

Some issues, like patient or user involvement, are very commendable. But many midwives feel they cannot provide the service they would like and that families expect because of economic constraints. Yet midwives can make changes: the protest to stop the closure of the maternity unit at Stroud is an example (Magill-Cuerden 2007). Another is the work to prevent the closure of three small maternity units in north-east Scotland and the continuing work to create 'new' birth units there (Anonymous 2007a).

The new NHS is not going to go away. Midwives need to accept new ideas and challenges and be a part of the professional team showing the way to reform as succeeding governments struggle to redraw the NHS. As Appleby (2006, p 305) says: 'Engage with the modernization and redesign agenda ... Find out what your services are planning to do ... Challenge them ... Your service [must] engage with the reforms ...You can always ask for pump-priming money or a loan to get your project off the ground'. Even if borrowing is not your style, health professionals in general need to accept change in order to provide safe high-quality care. More specifically, there is a clinical case for change in maternity care with an acceptance that a midwife should be the first point of contact for a pregnant woman leading to earlier entry into the maternity care system (Anonymous 2007b, Shribman 2007). And, the government is committed to developing a high quality, safe and accessible maternity service promising a new national choice guarantee for women (DH 2007).

The NHS is in transition (Talbot-Smith & Pollock 2006, p 1): Bevan's dropped bedpan (page 1029) is still rolling. There are changes happening within this transition that many find unattractive and unacceptable alongside changes that are necessary and good. This is so across the NHS as well as in the maternity services. But in the maternity services, midwives have the knowledge, the evidence and the will to make change for the better. Stephens (2007, p 159) says 'there is no place for silence'. Midwives at all levels, for the sake of mothers and babies, the profession of midwifery and the NHS as a whole need to support each other, apply research evidence, talk openly with other professionals in maternity care – and all the while keep looking after our mothers and babies.

REFERENCES

Anonymous 2007a Scottish birth units get the go-ahead. The Practising Midwife 10(3):10

Anonymous 2007b New focus for maternity services. The Practising Midwife 10(3):7

Appleby S 2006 Engaging with the challenge of change. Midwives 9(8):302–305

Brotherstone J 1987a The development of public medical care 1900–1948. In: McLachlan G (ed.) Improving the common weal: aspects of Scottish Health Services 1900–1984. Edinburgh University Press, Edinburgh, p 35–102

Brotherstone J 1987b The National Health Service in Scotland 1948–1984. In: McLachlan G (ed.) Improving the common weal: aspects of Scottish Health Services 1900–1984, Edinburgh University Press, Edinburgh, 103–159

Chadwick E 1842 Report on the sanitary condition of the labouring population of Great Britain. This edition Flinn M 1965 Edinburgh University Press, Edinburgh

Christie B 1998 An historical perspective on the NHS. In: Scottish Office, The NHS in Scotland 1948–1998. NHS 50, Glasgow, 4–5

Davies N 1999 The Isles: a history. Macmillan, London

Davies C, Beach A 2000 Interpreting professional self-regulation: A history of the United Kingdom Central Council for Nursing, Midwifery and Health Visiting. Routledge, London

DH 1993a Changing childbirth, Parts 1 and 2. Report of the Expert Maternity Group. HMSO, London

DH 1993b The patients' charter. HMSO, London

DH 2000 NHS Plan. HMSO, London

DH 2007 Maternity matters: choice, access and continuity of care in a safe service. DH, London. Online. Available: http://

www.dh.gov.uk/en/Publicationsandstatistics/Publications/PublicationsPolicyAndGuidance/DH_073312 2 July 2007

DH, DHSS, DHSSPS 1989 Working for patients. London, HMSO

DHS 1936 Report of the Committee on Scottish Health Services, (Cathcart). Cmnd 5204, Edinburgh

DHSS 1942 Report of the Committee on Social Insurance and Allied Services (Beveridge). Cmnd 6404, HMSO, London

DHSS 1979 Patients first. HMSO London

DHSS 1983 NHS management enquiry. (Griffiths) HMSO, London

DHSS, SHHD, Welsh Office, 1972, Report of the committee on nursing (Briggs). Cmnd 5115, HMSO, London

DHSSPS (Department of Health, Social Services and Public Safety) 2000 Investing in Health. DHSSPS, Belfast

Fox D 1986 The National Health Service and the Second World War: the elaboration of concensus. In: Smith H (ed.) War and social change: British society in the Second World War. Manchester University Press, Manchester, p 32–57

Ham C 1992 Health policy in Britain, 3rd edn. Macmillan, Basingstoke

Hillan E, McGuire M, Reid L 1997 Midwives and woman-centred care. University of Glasgow and Royal College of Midwives, Scottish Board, Edinburgh

Johnstone R 1953 Chairman's Review of the Board's Progress since 1915. National Archives of Scotland (NAS) CMB(S), 1/7, CMB Minutes, Edinburgh 26 February, 3–4

Kinnaird J 1987 The hospitals. In: McLachlan G (ed.) Improving the common weal: aspects of Scottish

Health Services 1900–1984, Edinburgh University Press, Edinburgh, p 213–275

Kirkman S Ferguson P 2007 Does being a principality with an Assembly government help midwives in Wales to be free to practise? In: Reid L (ed.) Midwifery: Freedom to practise? Elsevier, Edinburgh, p 102–120

Levitt R, Wall A, Appleby J 1999 The reorganised Health Service, 6th edn. Stanley Thornes, Cheltenham

McCrae M 2003 The National Health Service in Scotland: origins and ideals. Tuckwell Press, East Linton

McLachlan G (ed.) 1987 Improving the common weal: aspects of Scottish Health Services 1900–1984. Edinburgh University Press, Edinburgh

Magill-Cuerden J 2007 Change is up to us to achieve. Midwives 10(1):4

MoH, DHS, Ministry of Labour and National Service 1949 Report of the Working Party on Midwives. HMSO, London

NHS Reorganization: England 1972 White Paper (Joseph) HMSO, London

NHS Education for Scotland (NES) 2004, Midwifery leadership in Scotland: a competency framework, NES Edinburgh

Northern Ireland Department of Health and Social Services (NIDHSS) 1994 Delivering choice. Report of the Northern Ireland Maternity Unit Study Group, Belfast

Nursing and Midwifery Council (NMC) 2004 Midwives Rules and Standards. NMC, London

O'Sullivan J 2001 The history of obstetrics in Northern Ireland 1921–1992, Ulster Medical Journal 70(2):95–101. Online. Available: http://www.users.zetnet.co.uk/jil/ums/umj070/070_095.pdf 7 Mar 2007

Pater J 1981 The making of the National Health Service. London: King Edward's Hospital Fund for London

Proctor S 1999 Clinical governance: the new black. RCM Midwives Journal 2(7):204

Pulzer M 1999 Clinical governance and the midwife. RCM Midwives Journal 2(8):250

Reid L 1997–2002 Archival collection of oral testimonies between these dates. Cited as1–128

Reid L 2003 Scottish Midwives 1916–1983: The Central Midwives Board for Scotland and Practising Midwives. Unpublished PhD thesis for the University of Glasgow

Reid L 2007 Normal birth in Scotland: the effects of policy, geography and culture. In: Reid L (ed.) Midwifery: freedom to practise? Elsevier, Edinburgh, p 242–262

Robinson S 1990 Maintaining the independence of midwives. In: Garcia J, Kilpatrick R, Richards M (eds) The politics of maternity care. Clarendon Press, Oxford, p 61–91

SEHD 2000 Our National Health: a plan for action, a plan for change. SE, Edinburgh

SEHD 2005 Building a health service fit for the future: a national framework for service change in the NHS in Scotland (Kerr). SE, Edinburgh

SHHD Scottish Health Authorities 1980 Priorities for the eighties. A report by the Scottish Health Service Planning Council. HMSO, Edinburgh.

SHHD National Health Service in Scotland 1991 Framework for Action. HMSO, Edinburgh.

SHHD 1993 Provision of Maternity Services in Scotland – A Policy Review. HMSO, Edinburgh

Shribman S 2007 Making it better: for mother and baby. DH, HMSO, London.

Stephens L 2007 Midwifery led care. In: Reid L (ed.) Midwifery: freedom to practise? Elsevier, Edinburgh, p 146–165

Tait H 1987, Maternity and child welfare. In: McLachlan G (ed.) Improving the common weal. Edinburgh University Press, Edinburgh, p 411–440

Talbot-Smith A, Pollock A 2006 The new NHS: a guide. Routledge, London

Webster C 1998 The National Health Service: a political history. Oxford University Press, Oxford

Welsh Assembly Government (WAG) 2001 Improving health in Wales. A plan for the NHS with its partners. WAG, Cardiff

Welsh Office 1996 Welsh Maternity Services Review, Cardiff

Williams A S 1997 Women and childbirth in the twentieth century. Sutton Publishing, Stroud

USEFUL WEBSITES

NES:
www.nes.scot.nhs.uk

NHS:

www.nhs.uk

Scotland:
www.show.scot.nhs.uk

Wales:
www.wales.nhs.uk

Northern Ireland:
www.n-i.nhs.uk

RCM:
www.rcm.org.uk

SEHD:
www.scotland.gov.uk

SMMDG:
www.scottishmaternity.org

55 International midwifery

Della Sherratt

CHAPTER CONTENTS

The chapter outlines the issues and agendas facing midwifery from an international perspective. Its focus is on the major events and global issues that have helped raise the profile of midwives and their profession.

The chapter aims to:

- consider the issues facing midwifery in different cultural settings and the practicalities of midwives working outside their own country
- describe the major international events and organizations relevant to midwifery, in particular the International Confederation of Midwives (ICM), the global Safe Motherhood Initiative (SMI) and the Baby Friendly Hospital Initiative (BFHI)
- outline some of the issues facing midwives in other countries, their education and working conditions and highlight some of the main barriers to providing quality midwifery care.

In such a short chapter it is not possible to give an in-depth analysis of the global situation, nor describe in detail midwifery in every country. When reference is made to the situation in a named country, it is done so as an example to assist understanding and not to criticize the midwives working there. The aim of this chapter is to increase understanding of the midwifery context globally and foster a sense of unity and respect for a shared philosophy that underpins the profession, despite the different models of health or education systems in use throughout the world.

Introduction

Today, the effects of globalization, including advances in technology and use of the internet, as well as ease of travel, mean that the issues and problems of the world are finding their way into both the workplace and our homes. Health has to some extent always been considered a global issue, especially in relation to communicable diseases. However, renewed interest as a result of the increased commercialization of health as a commodity, is making many countries, such as the UK, invest in developing a specific global health strategy (see UK Dept of Health website at: http://www.dh.gov.uk). In addition, widening socioeconomic differentials, failures of the global market place, demographic shifts and ageing populations have contributed to workforce shortages, especially in the public sector and acutely so in the health sector. One of the strategies used to fill such shortages, especially by the richer OECD countries (organization for economic cooperation and development), has been to recruit health workers from other countries, often from countries that can ill afford to lose such a valuable resource. Finally, the last decade has uniquely seen unprecedented massive population shifts and displacements for economic or humanitarian reasons due to natural disasters or conflict and across Europe, due to opening of borders, especially between East and Western Europe. The rise in migration of peoples across nations is seen as one of the major issues currently facing health service planners in a number of countries, particularly low-income countries in Africa (Awases et al 2004, Mensah et al 2005, WHO 2006a).

Therefore, for all the above reasons it is likely that at some time in their working career all midwives will find themselves working in another country with different cultures, traditions and resources, or working alongside midwives from other countries, or providing services to women and families from other countries with vastly different cultures and traditions. As such, more than ever, midwives need to have an acute sense of the global village we live in and the issues facing midwifery globally. This chapter will first try to explore some of the issues as well as practicalities of working in another country, as well as working in an international setting. It will then try to outline some of the relevant international health agendas and initiatives that impact on midwifery. In one chapter it is not possible to cover all aspects of international midwifery in depth, but rather the main aim is to give some insights to the various issues with the aim of benefiting those who wish to explore this field of practice, as well as those who are just interested in what is happening in relation to midwifery globally.

The practicalities of working in another country

Before departure

One of the first practical issues to address for those wishing to work outside their own country is obtaining permission to work and ensuring that they have the correct visa. This can be difficult, as many countries have stringent regulations for issuing work visas and it may be necessary to produce an official letter of invitation from the employing agency or company. Without the correct documents and letter of invitation, it can be complicated to gain entry into the country and obtain permission to stay and work there; therefore it is always advisable to check the requirements carefully before departure. Most embassies or consulates will provide the necessary information and advice on the documentation needed to apply for a work visa.

Attention to health and personal safety is another essential practicality that must be taken care of before departure. In particular, it is essential to have adequate medical insurance cover. Where possible, always ensure insurance cover will allow an unscheduled return home to deal with personal difficulties, as trying to arrange this very quickly from another country can be traumatic. Many agencies or employers will be sympathetic and may include this as a benefit in the recruitment package or terms and conditions of the contract, if one exists. When responding to advertisements for a specific post, these details should be clarified before accepting the position. Critically it is vital to have up-to-date vaccination cover. Information on necessary immunizations, health precautions and so on is readily available from the WHO. Many countries also have a national travellers' help-line or institution and professional association that will also be able to offer advice.

The issues that are frequently least easy to deal with are the actual feelings and psychological practicalities of working in another culture. Adaptation to working in a different country with different customs, beliefs and traditions can be difficult, even when anticipated. Midwives may find such feelings difficult to accept, as they conflict with their internal view of themselves as a capable, flexible practitioner. A great deal of illness however, can result from the stress of working in such conditions. The potential for such illness needs to be acknowledged by those going to other countries to work, as well as those recruiting staff from other countries. Therefore speaking to and if possible spending some time with someone who has worked in the same area can be very helpful and rewarding. One of the difficulties of preparing for such stress is that it is not easy to predict how well an individual will cope in a given situation at any specific time. The factors that help adaptation are different in every situation. Experience of working in different cultures and countries can help, but each situation is new and must be seen as such.

Increasingly, organizations are providing courses or workshops for health workers who would like to consider this work, to help explore some of these issues before making a definite decision. The International Health Exchange in the UK and the International Red Cross are two such organizations and they provide excellent courses for those intending to work internationally and those wishing to consider it. Information on such courses is often available in quality primary or international healthcare journals. Also there is an increase in the number of university programmes that include elective periods where a short time can be spent in another country undertaking a small project or work experience. Finally The Royal College of Midwives (RCM), the Royal College of Nursing (RCN) and the British Medical Association all have printed materials to help health practitioners who wish to work overseas.

One factor that can influence adaptation to working in another country is the careful consideration of the motives for doing so. As with all career choices, there are varied and complex reasons why someone would choose this particular path. There is no one valid reason for embarking on such a career move, only an issue of individual choice. However in doing so, midwives must apply a certain level of objectivity to ensure the right choice is being made about the suitability, type, as well as place of work that is appropriate for them. It is all too easy to become quickly disillusioned with the new environment if the main motive for seeking this type of work was travel, but the project or place chosen makes travel difficult or impossible.

Clarification of motives is also helpful when faced with unfamiliar, frustrating or difficult situations. Working in another country in a culture that is unfamiliar, is very different from visiting on holiday or for pleasure or interest. However, such work does have its rewards. It can help to develop a wider view of midwifery, motherhood and health. It offers the opportunity for reflection and seeing one's own practice through different eyes. Most midwives who have done such work feel that it allows them to develop greater flexibility, innovation and self-confidence. Of course, much will depend upon the type of work undertaken, but the advantages and the friendships that develop while undertaking such work often outweigh the difficulties.

Working in a different culture

The requirement to provide culturally sensitive care is embodied in the International code of ethics for midwives (ICM 1999). The main issue facing midwives from another country developing culturally sensitive care is often around difficulties with language and being unable to listen to women's voices; often transmitted through traditional songs and folklore. Also, in some countries, particularly in Asia, beliefs and taboos surrounding pregnancy and birth can make listening to women's stories particularly difficult, as they are usually not spoken about directly, for fear of evoking bad spirits or bringing bad luck. Just to acknowledge the pregnancy might be viewed as dangerous. This raises obstacles to both provider and recipients of midwifery care. For example, encouragement of antenatal care, promotion of health in pregnancy, or even advice on planned pregnancies is problematic in a culture where to do so is seen as culturally unacceptable.

One way to overcome such cultural barriers is to work with the local community, especially women's groups and community or religious leaders. Where such leaders are usually men however, this can raise other gender-laden issues. Gender training or gender sensitivity courses may help the midwife to find a way to work with or through male leaders in a way that will empower women, although it is always essential to first identify, together with the women, what strategies women currently use for dealing with such issues. Assisting the male leaders and the community to consider general household practices and beliefs, and the effects that these may have on childbearing women, is possible, and where this approach has been used it has had positive results (Mullay 2006).

When working on empowerment issues it is important to remember that notions of empowerment are also culturally bound (Portela & Santarelli 2003). Women from different cultures have different ideas about what they see as empowerment (Chitnis 1988, Collins 1994, Dawit & Busia 1995). Given the opportunity however, women from all cultures have clear ideas about what they think would assist them to give birth in a way that is safe and yet culturally sensitive.

Use of appropriate technology

In addition to adopting the right approach to providing such care, midwives also need to concern themselves with the appropriate use of technology. Careful consideration is necessary when taking new technology from one country to another. For example, in many industrialized settings it is no longer considered essential to give iron supplementation routinely to well-nourished pregnant women. In under-resourced countries however, haemorrhage before, during and after birth remains the major cause of death owing to poor nutrition and social deprivation (WHO 2005a). In these situations, faced with high maternal mortality and high levels of under nutrition, it is clearly appropriate to have a protocol that promotes routine iron supplementation to all pregnant women.

Importing systems, technologies and tools without ensuring they get appropriately adapted can adversely affect the quality of care. Although in themselves the tools may be good, if they are not adapted to meet the cultural complexity of the country, they may be ineffective, or used in an inappropriate way. For example, there is almost universal acceptance that the partograph is a useful and effective tool, yet in some countries or cultures the counting of time is not in units of minutes or hours, and even the idea of charting events on a graph can be very difficult. Midwives working in an international arena therefore, need to ensure that the technology they take with them is appropriate and that correct training and systems are provided for its effective implementation and use.

The role of the consultant midwife

Beware the 'expert'

Although the above practicalities of working in a different country are of concern for all midwives, it is particularly problematic for those working as international midwifery consultants or expatriate project workers, trainers or managers. The temptation to allow oneself to be seen as the 'expert', the one who knows all, is sometimes difficult to avoid. In the eyes of the new community, women and local midwives, there is a serious risk of being perceived as the expert who knows all. Such views can leave the midwife seen as an outsider, precluded from being accepted into the local community and therefore denied access to their knowledge and cultural systems.

The issue of being viewed as an outside expert is particularly problematic when working in countries that do not have recent experience of personal autonomy or personal responsibility. In countries that have a particular political tradition of being controlled from the centre, women may feel more comfortable seeing the consultant midwife as an 'expert', dictating the actual activities of care to be provided. Those not familiar with democracy or participation in decision-making may feel slightly afraid or unsure when introduced to participatory approaches. Therefore locals may initially resist or misinterpret requests for their views and opinions, or may not respond to opportunities to share their ideas with the newcomer.

Equally, for the consultant faced with enthusiastic individuals eager for change, tight work schedules, needs that often far outweigh resources or expectations that they will be the one to sort out the problems, can be daunting. In such situations it can be difficult to hold firm to principles of facilitation and participatory approaches to decision-making. In these situations, advocacy can easily stray into paternalism (or maternalism) and then only the voice of the 'expert' midwife is heard. The midwife's role is always to encourage women to find their own voice and as far as possible ensure that it is the local women's voice that is being heard; for the international consultant this includes the voices of the local midwives. The key skills for the consultant midwife are listening, supporting and participating in the daily lives and tasks of those they work with, be they receivers of care, or working colleagues.

Finally, the role of the consultant midwife can be lonely; therefore anyone taking on this role should ensure that they have a good personal support system from family, friends or long-standing colleagues (preferably ones with similar experiences).

International issues

International Confederation of Midwives (ICM)

One of the main actors in the global arena working to improve maternity services by empowering of midwives, especially through strengthening professional associations and promoting good practice, is the International Confederation of Midwives (ICM). ICM, a non-governmental organization (NGO), was started by midwives in Belgium in 1919 as the International Midwives' Union. The purpose of the union was to 'improve the services available to childbearing women through campaigning for a stronger, better educated and properly regulated midwifery profession' (ICM 1994, p 1).

In the early 1960s ICM gained accreditation by the United Nations (UN) as a NGO in official relations, which means it can be part of official UN consultations. ICM works closely with UN organizations especially World Health Organization (WHO) and United Nations Population Fund (UNFPA) as well as with United Nations Fund for Children (UNICEF). ICM now has more than 85 member associations that cover approximately 72 countries.

ICM Council admits new members on demonstration they meet the criteria for membership and payment of a membership fee, calculated against the number of midwives in the association and taking into account the economic situation of the country.

ICM has a small but friendly office that relocated from the UK to the Netherlands in 1999. The office welcomes both visitors and enquiries from midwives and midwifery organizations from anywhere in the world. Information on the history of the ICM, along with other information and leaflets, is obtainable from ICM HQ (see Useful addresses). The ICM also produces a regular newsletter free to its member associations, but is available to individuals on payment of a modest subscription.

ICM accomplishments

In recent years, the ICM has been proactive in a variety of global initiatives. By working collaboratively with other agencies, ICM has contributed to the increasing acceptance of the midwife as the key provider of quality maternity care. Working with WHO and the International Federation of Gynaecologists and Obstetricians (FIGO) ICM developed the International definition of the midwife. Having been first devised in 1966 and later revised in 1992, the latest revision was adopted by ICM Council in Brisbane during the 2005 Triennial Congress.

Most recently, ICM has been a significant actor in the establishment of the global Partnership for Maternal, Newborn and Child Health (PMNCH) the secretariat of which is housed in WHO HQ Geneva. PMNCH is the successor to the Inter-Agency Group on Safe Motherhood (IAGSM) established at the beginning of the Safe Motherhood Initiative in 1987. PMNCH aim is to bring together all constituent groups working on safe motherhood, newborn and child health. For more information on the work of PMNCH, see their website at: http://www.who.int/pmnch. In addition, ICM is working with both WHO, the United Nations' Population Fund (UNFPA) and other partners such as The White Ribbon Alliance, to increase global, regional and national advocacy for investing in midwives and midwifery. The focus of the work is to accelerate progress to reach the Millennium Development Goals (MDG), in particular for improving maternal health (MDG Goal 5), as well as contributing to improving child health (MDG-4) and increasing gender equity (MDG-3). Information on and progress reports on achieving the MDGs can be found on many of the UN websites.

In addition to the development of the International Code of Ethics for Midwives (ICM 1999), other ICM achievements include instituting and coordinating of the International Day of The Midwife (annually on 5 May). Each country and midwifery organization may choose to devise the programme for celebrating this day. However, ICM Board draws up the major theme each year, with the intention to assist midwives and midwifery associations unite under a central banner to promote the role and responsibilities of the midwife.

By far, one of the most rewarding accomplishments of ICM, is the bringing together of groups of midwives from different countries for workshops, seminars and the triennial congress. The meetings, particularly the triennial congresses, are valuable not only for allowing midwives internationally to meet, debate and network, but also have been a useful vehicle for promoting midwives and midwifery in the host country. For example, the opening ceremony of the triennial congress is usually attended by high-ranking political officials of the host country and remains a favourite and often moving spectacle for all who attend.

Immediately prior to the congress, ICM often hosts a workshop, usually for 3 days on a theme related to safe motherhood; these too have been extremely beneficial for those attending and for raising certain issues related to midwifery in the international arena. A report of these workshops, which usually include useful background papers or information and material for the midwives attending the workshops, is always published. The action orientation of these workshops has allowed midwives from a variety of countries to develop plans and activities for improving the midwifery services to women nationally and globally.

The global Safe Motherhood Initiative

The global Safe Motherhood Initiative (SMI) was officially launched in Nairobi in February 1987. WHO, UNICEF and the World Bank as well as many NGOs, associations and multi- and bilateral aid agencies and ICM, have supported the global programme from the beginning. The impetus for this initiative was the outrage that many maternal deaths are preventable and that MCH programmes, at that time, focused mainly on the child and ignored the health and well-being of the pregnant woman. The slogan used in the early days being: 'where is the M in MCH?'

The aim of SMI was to achieve a reduction of 50% in the global number of maternal deaths by 2000. Initially, SMI advocates envisaged that the goals of SMI would be achieved through empowerment of women. This point was further strengthened following the International Conference on Population and Development in Beijing and the UN Conference on Women Platform of Action, Cairo 1995, both of which called for the rights of women to be further strengthened and respected. Since 1987, various strategies have been employed to achieve the goal of safe motherhood and more attention has been given to the right to health and adoption of a rights based approach to health policy (Cook & Dickens 2001). Consequently there was an increase in strategies that focused on improving the sociopolitical and legal status of women, increasing their access to wealth and ending gender discrimination, especially in education and access to healthcare. However, the target set for 2000 was not achieved.

In 1997, to mark the tenth anniversary of SMI a technical review was held in Colombo, Sri Lanka to consider and document lessons learned (Starrs, IAGSM 2000). At this review a number a key messages were agreed – as a call for action. One of the major key messages was a call for ensuring all women have access to a 'skilled attendant' at birth (WHO UNFPA UNICEF World Bank 1999). A skilled attendant is a professional health provider with midwifery skills (Box 55.1) (WHO 2004a); to most people this is a professional midwife, someone who has the competency for provision of normal care, is able to manage or initiate first-line care for emergencies and is linked to a facility where specialist obstetric and neonatal care is available for management of complications and cases that fall outside the midwife's scope of practice.

The call for 'skilled attendants' for all women came about as a result of perceived failure to reduce maternal deaths by employing a 'risk approach' to

---

Box 55.1 Definition of a skilled attendant

A revised version (from the original that appeared in the 1999 statement on maternal mortality reduction by WHO, UNFPA, UNICEF, and the World Bank) was developed in 2004 by WHO ICM and FIGO to clarify that all skilled birth attendants must be able to provide life saving skills and offer pregnancy and post-natal, including newborn, care. It stated that:

A skilled attendant is an accredited health professional – such as midwives, doctor or nurse – who has *been educated and trained to proficiency in the skills needed to manage normal (uncomplicated) pregnancies, childbirth and the immediate post-natal period, and in the identification, management and referral of complications in women and newborns.*

(This definition has been endorsed by UNFPA, The World Bank and ICN 2004.)

(From: WHO 2004a Making pregnancy safer: the critical role of a skilled attendant. A joint statement by WHO, ICM FIGO.)

---

antenatal screening, whereby pregnant women identified as having risk factors were provided with specialist obstetric care. Criticism of the risk approach strategy for reducing maternal mortality focused around the lack of specificity, sensitivity and predictability of the risk factors used. Even though it is known that some women with certain histories and medical conditions have a potentially higher risk than others for developing a pregnancy-related complication, research shows that a significant proportion of life-threatening problems occur in women identified as being at low risk when using most of the risk-scoring systems. The failure of the risk approach and risk scoring to directly reduce maternal deaths does not mean that antenatal care does not play a significant role in maternal healthcare and identification of problems. Indeed much research has been undertaken that shows the effectiveness of a more focused approach to antenatal care.

Current SMI strategies: skilled care for all pregnant women

Based on the lessons learnt at Colombo and supported by historical evidence around maternal mortality reduction, the prevailing consensus of the maternal and newborn health community is that safe motherhood can only be achieved if all pregnant women have access to a continuum of care throughout pregnancy, childbirth and the postnatal period; in particular have access to a skilled attendant and emergency obstetric care, especially at and around the time of childbirth. (Campbell & Graham 2006, De Brouwere & Van Lerberghe 2003, Koblinsky 2003, Koblinsky et al 2006, Loudon 2000, WB 2005, WHO 2005a). The same is true when considering reductions in perinatal mortality and morbidity. The WHO considers almost a half of all perinatal deaths could be avoided if all newborns were assisted at birth by a skilled birth attendant (WHO 2006b). As testimony to the commitment to women and recognizing their importance in development and health, the compact agreed by 189 Heads of States towards poverty alleviation resulted in the MDGs. Included as one of the targets to be achieved by 2015, requires governments to increase access for all women to skilled care, especially at the time of birth, by including a target of 95% of all births to be attended by a skilled attendant, of which the figure of 85% was set for developing countries (see the MDG website: http://www.un.org/millenniumgoals).

The evidence shows however that the skilled attendant alone is not sufficient and, that minimally skilled attendants must work in an enabling environment where systems are in place to allow the practitioner to provide skilled care. These systems include among others, a regular safe supply of drugs and equipment, as well as supportive supervision and close links for easy referral to a facility able to offer higher level medical obstetric and neonatal services (Graham et al 2001). Recent estimates however suggest that in 2006 only between 40% and 60% of all pregnant women globally had access to a skilled attendant at birth (Stanton et al 2007).

Although the initial focus of SMI was only maternal mortality, in recent years this focus has shifted slightly and is now on the broader women's health and reproductive health for all, especially adolescents. Also, using a human rights lens, there is also concern for morbidity. Studies in India and Bangladesh give morbidity rates as high as 15–16 times that of mortality rates (Goodburn 1995, WHO 2005a). A great deal of the morbidity was found to be due to unsafe and unhygienic practices based on superstitions and taboos, such as putting mustard oil into the vagina to try to hasten cervical dilatation and ensure a speedy exit through the birth canal, or use of excessive fundal pressure to deliver the placenta, in the belief that it is the placenta that harbours or attracts the evil spirits. Access to sexual and reproductive health services has now been added to the indicators for monitoring MDG-5.

At the twentieth anniversary of SMI, the number of maternal deaths worldwide remains similar to when it began in 1987, although analysis of data on maternal mortality, using 2005 data, shows there has been a slight reduction of MMR at the global level of 1% per annum since the late 1980s, however this is far below the 5.5% annual reduction needed to achieve the MDGs (WHO 2007).

Major global actions under the Safe Motherhood banner

1987 – The Safe Motherhood Initiative was launched in Nairobi.

1989 – The first global study on maternal mortality was published (Royston & Armstrong 1989) and WHO's global factbook on maternal mortality (WHO 1991). The factbook is a compendium of data collected from all over the world. Both are available from WHO, Geneva.

1990 – The partograph, a tool for effective monitoring of labour, was launched, following a large multicentre trial to review the effectiveness of this tool. The results concluded that the tool had potential benefits for the timely management of prolonged labour (WHO 1994a).

1990 – The ICM triennial congress was preceded by a workshop to discuss 'midwifery education for safe motherhood' (WHO, UNICEF, ICM 1991). One of the recommendations from this workshop was a call to countries to make the midwifery curriculum more community based and include management of selected obstetric emergencies.

1994 – WHO produced the mother–baby package: a practical guide to implementing safe motherhood in all countries (WHO 1994b). In this package it is recognized that the key to successful safe motherhood is 'appropriately trained midwifery personnel living and working in the community'. The package makes strong recommendations for countries to give priority to developing the midwifery skills of their health personnel, especially those providing community-based care.

1996 – WHO launched the midwifery education modules for safe motherhood. Initially there were five modules, which include teachers' and students' notes. Each module deals with a specific aspect of maternal mortality. The Foundation Module – the Midwife in the Community, is unique in that it covers how to understand the community, how to measure maternal mortality and how to work with the community to devise culturally and locally applicable solutions to preventing maternal mortality. The other four modules deal with the major causes of maternal mortality: obstructed labour, pre-eclampsia and eclampsia, postpartum haemorrhage and puerperal sepsis. A new module (bringing total to six) on incomplete abortion has been included in the revised second edition (WHO, ICM 2007).

1996 – saw the first global technical meeting on practices for care during normal birth (WHO 1996a). This was also the first technical working group held by WHO where equal numbers of internationally accredited obstetricians and midwives sat together to review the evidence for all the current practices and interventions used throughout the world in caring for women having a normal uncomplicated birth.

1997 – Safe Motherhood 10-year review, held in Colombo, Sri Lanka.

2000 – International Conference on Skilled Attendants in Tunis, organized by the IAG and co-chaired by ICM and the World Bank. The same year, WHO launched its new initiative for safe motherhood, 'Making Pregnancy Safer'.

2006 – The global maternal, newborn and child health constituencies joined together in an attempt to build on the interest generated by the World Health Report 2005 (WHO 2005a) and the report of the Task Force set up for the Millennium Development Goals by forming the new global Partnership for Maternal, Newborn and Child Health (PMNCH). Whether or not these constituencies can work together for the benefit of all mothers, newborns and children is yet to be seen, as in the past they have held very different, and at times opposing views, on how resource-poor countries should address these priority areas.

2007 – To celebrate 20 years of global action on safe motherhood, a global conference entitled 'Women Deliver' was held in London. Political leaders, scientists, researchers, practitioners and women's health activists worldwide joined together for a global advocacy for greater investments into the health of women, to stop the estimated 10 million women lost in every generation due to failure of health policies and systems. Materials and background paper are available on the 'Women Deliver' website: http://www.womendeliver.org

Other global events significant to Safe Motherhood

1990 – World Summit on the Health of the Child. This summit put the child on the world's agenda and paved the way for the signing the Convention on the Rights of the Child (UN 1990) at the UN General Assembly in the same year. Both at the World Summit and by signing The Convention on the Rights of the Child, governments agreed that they would take steps to improve the health of children throughout the world. Article 6, which deals with survival and development, lays down the need for effective prenatal care and the right to have the delivery conducted by appropriately trained health personnel. Other Articles deal with non-discrimination (effectively outlawing practices such as gender selection, female fetocide and discriminatory feeding practices based on gender), the best interests of the child, separation from the family and family reunification. By 1997, The Convention on the Rights of the Child had been ratified by all members of the UN, except for the Cook Islands, Oman, Somalia,

Switzerland, the United Arab Emirates and the USA (UNICEF 1997a).

1994 and 1995 – Many interesting meetings were held including the International Conference on Population and Developments in Cairo 1994, the World Summit for Social Democracy, Copenhagen 1995 and the Fourth World Conference on Women in Beijing 1995. They all had safe motherhood as an integral issue. At all these conferences, governments from all over the world declared intent to improve the health of women. This included provision for strengthening the health services to women, particularly in and around childbirth.

2000 – The international agreement by 189 Heads of State to Eliminate Poverty and achieve significant progress in this by 2015 made in the Millennium Declaration gave rise to agreements about specific goals and targets to monitor progress towards this agreement. The goals MDGs addressed were the major constraints to poverty alleviation: lack of education, especially for girls; gender inequity; poor health, especially of mothers and children, but also the continuing pandemics of infectious diseases such as malaria, TB and HIV; as well as the environmental factors such as lack of access to safe drinking water, safe sanitation and a clean environment. The MDGs have created a new impetus and sparked a renewed wave of actions towards achieving safe motherhood through skilled care for all women and newborn wherever they lived. Evidence shows that in all countries poverty was a major barrier to accessing skilled care, with huge differentials in access between the richest quintiles and the poorest (Kunst & Howlling 2001). Consequently, more recent work has been focused on achieving access of poor and vulnerable populations to skilled care at and around the time of birth – the time when most maternal and perinatal deaths take place.

2005 – The publication of the World Health Report 2005, the theme of which was maternal, newborn and child health, was launched on the World Health Day (7 April). This was the first time that the World Health Report was launched on the day the world celebrated the creation of WHO; it thus added to the international interest in the facts and figures presented in the World Health Report 2005 – 'Make every mother and child count' (WHO 2005a).

One other important initiative, which has undoubtedly helped focus global attention on the continuing need to develop safe motherhood programmes, has been the WHO, UNICEF and UNFPA partnership around monitoring Maternal Mortality Ratios (MMR) across the globe and developing a new way to estimate MMR (WHO 1996b, 2001a). The revised estimates for 1990 for example demonstrated unequivocally that the figures for maternal mortality had been drastically underestimated, with some 8000 more deaths than was initially thought. Subsequent estimates of MMR demonstrate that the anticipated decline in maternal mortality set at the beginning of the Safe Motherhood Initiative has not occurred. In some countries there had been either a levelling off, or even a rise in MMR (WHO 2005a, WHO 2007). A recent systematic review of national reports show that variability of national maternal mortality estimates remain large across regions and within sub-regions (Gülmezoglu et al 2004). This is, or at least should be of concern to all involved in safe motherhood. It underlines the fact that there is no room for complacency in the attempts to make motherhood safer, if not completely safe. Therefore, efforts to recruit, train and deploy health personnel with midwifery skills is an urgent, continuing and priority need, especially in countries with high levels of maternal mortality.

Safe motherhood means more than surviving pregnancy and childbirth

The Safe Motherhood community is not just concerned with maternal mortality. Recently more attention has been given to morbidity and to the newborn health, although some would say not yet adequately. Increasingly, newborn health and reduction of perinatal mortality and morbidity is being highlighted in national maternal and child health and/or Safe Motherhood plans. Safe Motherhood advocates are also highly concerned with adolescent health and maternal morbidity, including access to family planning and safe abortion care. In addition to the estimated 530 000 women who die each year from complications of pregnancy and childbirth, with over 90% occurring in South-Asia and sub-Saharan Africa, there are in the region of 10–20 million each year who suffer severe morbidity following childbirth, of which obstetric fistula is probably the most debilitating and devastating. To highlight this, UNFPA in 2002 with WHO and others partners, launched a global advocacy programme on obstetric fistula (Donney & Weil 2004).

To summarize, safe motherhood is not just about ensuring that women do not die in childbirth. It is also about empowering women to take control over their own bodies to enable them to achieve optimum health. This must include being empowered to make effective and informed choices about if and when they will embark upon pregnancy. If they choose to become pregnant, then they should have access to all services, education and support (including community support) needed to achieve a healthy outcome; this may include access to safe abortion in countries where abortion is not against the law. It also includes the need for women, families and society to be assured that the newborn can reach healthy adult maturity; without this the pressures on women to conceive many babies will not be reduced and family planning strategies will be impeded. Above all it requires empowerment of women to demand services and to demand quality. Midwives as women (for the vast majority are usually women in many countries), also need to be empowered, both as women and as healthcare providers. They too need to be able to demand better services, better training, improved supportive supervision and support. Moreover they need and must be able to demand, better human resource policies – to ensure they can not only function effectively and provide quality midwifery care where and when women need it, but so they are able to earn a basic living wage and receive appropriate remuneration for their work.

The strategies required to achieve all of the above will vary from country to country. In most countries this will require addressing the sociological perspectives of women's health, as well as the management and provision of effective health services. As Thompson & Bennett (1996) outline in their ICM pre-congress paper, 'the provision and access to healthcare has only a small effect on the overall determinants for the health of women'. It would appear that by far the most important strategy for improving women's health, are changes in the cultural practices, eliminating gender inequalities and improving the environment in which the woman lives – which include elimination of poverty and improved nutrition. This inevitably means that, in addition to developing appropriate technical midwifery skills, midwives must also involve themselves in political action to address these issues, as increasingly it is acknowledged that they have a direct effect on improving women's health (Gill et al 2007).

The role of the midwife in Safe Motherhood

Much has been written and discussed in the various symposia, conferences, events, books and articles on the contribution midwives can make to the Safe Motherhood Initiative and safe motherhood programmes. However, what all midwives must remember is that safe(r) motherhood, in its broadest and narrowest sense, is still not an option for many thousands of women across the world (WHO 2005a). Although women in highly industrialized countries are subject to a different lack of control over their own bodies from women in developing or transitional market economy countries, both are frequently denied their rights related to pregnancy and childbirth. They are denied the right to choose and denied their right to exercise control over their own birth processes. Some Western countries however are making progress in this field, in particular New Zealand along with The Netherlands and the UK are in the forefront of ensuring that women have the right to choose what type of assistance they want during pregnancy and childbirth and where and when they want it. Yet other countries are seeing an acute rise in medicalization and medical dominance over pregnancy and childbirth care.

It is clear there is urgent need for strengthening the evidence-base for many safe motherhood interventions in low-income and resource-poor countries and in some countries for more effective scale up of midwifery (Miller et al 2003). For this reason, midwives must become more pro-active and learn to relate to, work with and seek to influence the leaders and major decision makers, both at the local and at the national level. They must also work more collaboratively with other professions, specifically their obstetric colleagues, to advocate for increased commitment to ensure skilled care for all women and newborns regardless of where they live, or of their socioeconomic situation.

Global Initiatives including Breastfeeding and Baby Friendly Hospital Initiative (BFHI), Saving Newborns Lives (SNBL)

Baby Friendly Hospital Initiative (BFHI)

Since the launch of the Safe Motherhood Initiative, there has been a number of related global activities of which the Baby Friendly Hospital Initiative (BFHI), driven by UNICEF and WHO is now considered to be one of the most effective mechanisms for creating strong political commitment to breastfeeding. The BFHI was launched in 1991 following the joint WHO/UNICEF statement on breastfeeding made in 1989, which outlined the 'ten steps to successful breastfeeding' (WHO, UNICEF 1989). The 'ten steps' have become the management tool and criteria for awarding BFHI status. According to recently published materials from WHO the BFHI has been implemented in 152 countries (WHO, UNICEF 2006). A training package for hospitals that wish to work towards the award of the status 'baby friendly hospital' can be downloaded from: http://www.who.int/nutrition/topics/bfhi

Unfortunately, despite the reported success of BFHI, global indicators demonstrate that the decline of breastfeeding, which began in the 1950s, and the trend towards bottle-feeding continues to date in many countries, including low-resource countries. This is despite of the research supporting the promotion of exclusive breastfeeding in the first 4–6 months, particularly for the control of diarrhoeal disease and upper respiratory tract infections. Understandably, the HIV pandemic and the findings that the virus can be found in breastmilk has given rise to concerns and debate regarding recommendations for replacement feeding in high HIV areas. The most recent WHO guidelines however, suggest that the risk of HIV transmission must be weighed against the risk of bottle-feeding in many low-resource countries (WHO 2001b) and others support this view (Latham & Prebble 2000). The WHO also suggest that mothers who are HIV-seropositive and where replacement feeding is not optimal and therefore choose to breastfeed, should continue to do so exclusively for the first few months. They should then, over a period of days and weeks (rather than abrupt cessation), change to replacement feeding, providing the conditions for safe replacement feeding are in place (WHO 2004b).

Difficulties to be overcome to achieve exclusive breastfeeding

Despite these global initiatives, the lack of exclusive breastfeeding for 4–6 months and the practice of discarding the colostrum remain the two major difficulties yet to be overcome in many countries. Very often, such practices, influenced by strong cultural superstitions and belief systems, cannot be overcome by simply presenting mothers with scientific evidence. Despite almost universal agreement that it is unacceptable and immoral to import and promote formula feed to countries where the water supply is not safe, violations of the code that governs marketing of formulae feeds continue, much as was highlighted by UNICEF more than a decade ago (UNICEF 1997b). Consequently, the International Baby Food Action Network (IBFAN) and others must continue to advocate for vigilance as well as identifying violations of the International Code of Marketing of Breastmilk Substitutes.

The newborn

In recent years, more attention has been given for the need to ensure that safe motherhood includes care for the newborn. Not only does each newborn, as a sovereign being, have the right to a safe start in life under the UN Convention on the Rights of the Child agreed in 1990, (UNICEF website: http://www.unief.org/crc), but governments have a responsibility to newborns. Moreover it is also recognized that attempt for parents to limit their fertility and avoid the cycle of rapid childbirths, which too often ends in maternal death, is undermined if the newborn does not survive. One of the leading advocates on newborn health has been Save the Children, who in 2000 launched a global Saving Newborns Lives (SNBL) initiative, which not only addresses policy issues, technical issues and advocacy, but also works with countries, as partners, to integrate better the issue of essential care of newborns (see: www.savethechildren.org/health/healthsavingnewbornlives).

International agenda

Midwifery identities

Listening to midwives at many and varied conferences and meetings worldwide, it would appear that the global concerns of midwives and the constraints they face have changed little since Kwast & Bentley published their paper in 1991 (Kwast & Bergström, 2001, Odberg-Pettersson et al 2007, Sherratt 2007). Their seminal paper, presented at the ICM pre-congress workshop in 1990, detailed the constraints and problems facing midwives worldwide, which include both the shortage and maldistribution of midwives, as well as the economic and training problems facing midwifery in many countries.

Midwives need specific policies and legislation to practise

One of the most common and urgent needs facing midwives in many countries is the need for specific (if not separate) policies and legislation to enable them to practise. This was highlighted most recently during the first International Forum on Midwifery in the Community organized by UNFPA, ICM and WHO in collaboration with partners. At this pivotal meeting, a Call to Action was made (Hammamet Call to Action) for increased investments in midwifery. Participants at this forum agreed, where separate policies and practices for midwifery are not identified, midwives can be hampered if they have to practise under nursing protocols and legislation, which too often do not cover the midwife's right to practise essential life-saving skills for pregnancy, childbirth and newborn care.

Also of common concern, as expressed at this Forum, was the continuing issue that faces many midwives internationally, the lack of acceptance that they have a right to practise as autonomous practitioners. The manifestations of this issue will vary depending on the country concerned. For many, the domination of the medical profession will be the most difficult barrier to overcome. However, it is heartening to recall that, as far back as 1985, the

WHO and some obstetricians recognized the pivotal role of the midwife in providing quality maternity care (Wagner 1994). Moreover, as evidenced by the increasing number of joint statements and joint action between the professional associations representing obstetricians and those for midwives, including at the international level, this mutual respect is growing and more is being translated into action. Nevertheless, too often the relationship between the two professions in some countries remains contentious and leads to the fragmentation of care and services for women and babies, as well as placing barriers for the delivery of broader public health interventions (de Bernis et al 2003).

It is true to say however, that the unique nature of midwifery practice, as separate and distinct from nursing, is still not universally accepted. In many countries in Africa and elsewhere, there are logical and rational reasons for having a multi-professional provider such as a nurse-midwife, where the provider has competencies of both professions. Moreover, 'midwifery' can appropriately be a qualification obtained after training as a nurse, especially where the nurse-midwife may be the only healthcare person available in a rural setting (Box 55.2). However, what is unequivocal, yet still needs highlighting, is that the two professions each have a distinctive, if overlapping, body of knowledge and practice. As such they both need valuing for their individual contribution to a nation's health. It is also clear that legislation

and structures must reflect these differences, as well as the similarities. Legislation must be drafted in such a way that it respects and assures each profession as to the right to practise. While legislation must be sensitive to the particular situation in a country, it must permit the midwife the responsibility to provide quality care – including care during labour and birth, as well as delivery of certain interventions necessary for saving life.

Another issue requiring urgent attention is 'licence to practise'. Although licence to practise is an issue of safeguarding the public and therefore a matter for government concern and good stewardship and governance, mechanisms to support licensure are too often absent or weak. In many resource-poor countries there is a lack of professional standards, including competency-based standards for education and training, as well as the rigorous systems and mechanisms to ensure that such standards are not just set, but complied with. As such, the mechanisms used to ensure licence to practise, including re-registration and mandatory continuing professional updating are compromised. Good governance however, must not be confused with political interference or dominance in the determination of professional standards. It is the responsibility of governments to ensure that frameworks exist that will demonstrate that individual health practitioners have received appropriate education – but not necessarily their role to execute such systems – this being the prerogative of the profession.

Box 55.2 Tanzania

Many women in our country still live in rural areas, whereas most skilled attendants (midwives) work in urban areas. Therefore many births are still attended by TBAs (Traditional Birth Attendants) or family members. The reasons why midwives prefer working in urban areas include: lack of infrastructure, lack of incentives, high workload in rural areas where the midwife must do more than midwifery, poor safety and professional isolation. Not only is there a need to address these issues, there is also a need to strengthen the skills, knowledge and attitude among the skilled providers. Women are reported to have preference for TBAs' services rather than skilled midwifery services because of the bad attitudes of those skilled attendants (midwives) and that, although trained, many woman feel the midwives still have insufficient and inadequate skills. There is also lack of updating of skills specifically for those few in the rural areas. Recently many actions including the White Ribbon Alliance in Tanzania is taking steps to redress this situation.

(Report of Tanzanian midwifery representative at WHO technical meeting on strengthening midwifery services to support Making Pregnancy Safer, November 2001.)

Education of midwives

The education of midwives has been a matter of long-standing debate and concern in many countries, for a variety of reasons. While education and in-service training for midwives in some countries is weak, it must be remembered that education and training is only one element to ensuring that providers are competent; there must also be adequate and appropriate supportive supervision. Moreover, there must also be a functioning health system to support service providers and create an environment where midwives are able to carry out their function correctly, including ensuring their safety and proper remuneration and career pathways.

As previously stated, in some countries, the preparation of midwives may follow on from nursing. While there may be good reasons for this in some situations, there are also a number of disadvantages, particularly where nursing does not have a sufficiently strong public health basis. In some situations, the midwifery-following-nursing model can result in midwifery being seen as an adjunct to nursing. The consequence of this can be that midwifery is too often afforded very little time within the nursing curriculum, as happens in both resource-poor countries and highly industrialized ones.

Increasingly, because of the global shortage of human resources, as outlined in the World Health Report 2006 (WHO 2006a), many countries are or have turned to semi-skilled or multi-purpose workers to fill their human resources for health gaps, especially for provision of healthcare at the community level. Where multi-purpose providers exist, there can be role confusion, as well as overlaps or even gaps in continuity of care for pregnant women and their newborns. For example, sometimes community health workers, or multipurpose public health workers provide the prenatal services work completely separately from midwives who offer intranatal care. Often these multipurpose workers have minimal midwifery input into their curriculum. Some midwifery experts agree the move to increased use of multipurpose workers, coupled with incorporating midwifery into nursing curricula, has led to an ever-spiralling decrease in midwifery standards. The teaching of midwifery being weak, leads to practitioners who have limited midwifery competencies who eventually find themselves as teachers, ill-equipped for developing midwifery competencies in others. For Kwast and Bergström, midwifery, as a specialization, has in many low-income and resource-poor countries become reduced to maternal and child healthcare, or obstetric or maternity nursing (Kwast & Bergström 2001); many others would echo this. These multipurpose practitioners are often unable to perform the full range of midwifery competencies, in particular the essential life-saving skills. Given the short time the curriculum allows for developing midwifery competencies, coupled with the low case-loads because of low utilization of healthcare professionals and/or health facilities, it is little surprise that many of these multipurpose and community healthcare workers also lack confidence and are unable to perform midwifery skills outside of the hospital environment, or without supervision. This issue becomes even more problematic as less and less time is available for developing specific midwifery competencies due to increasing demands on their curricula for additional content related to HIV AIDS and other relatively new public health concerns, such as SARS and avian flu.

Everyone will agree training must be skills-based. However, many training programmes in the past have failed to take account of the fact that midwifery is essentially a practical profession, where practice is underpinned by evidence, scientific principles and knowledge coupled with sound practical application using critical thinking skills (Penny & Murray 2000). The skills required by the midwife may vary from country to country, depending on the specific needs of the country. However, ICM (2002) have now developed a list of international evidence-based core competencies – essential competencies (Fullerton & Thompson 2005). During the First International Forum on Community Midwifery, participants agreed that the ICM competencies should be used as the international benchmark for assessing midwifery competence (Odberg-Pettersson et al 2007). It must be remembered however that in some situations additional core competencies, that may not be seen as usual for midwives in the UK, are required as standard (essential) for all midwives in many resource-poor countries. For example, being able to undertake a manual removal of the placenta or being able to

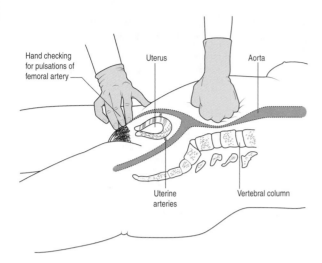

Figure 55.1 Aortic compression. (Based on WHO 1996a.)

apply aortic compression competently as shown in Figure 55.1 and outlined in the WHO manual Managing Complications of Pregnancy and Childbirth (WHO 2000) may be the only way to save a woman's life in some countries. Midwives from industrial countries therefore should be aware that, in some resource-poor settings, midwives may find themselves in a situation where knowledge and skills alone are all that are available to save the woman's life. Training for these and other life-saving skills must therefore focus on achieving competence, which implies use of critical thinking skills, as well as sufficient opportunity for hands-on-practice. Very often in some countries, although the theoretical knowledge may be taught well in the initial pre-service programmes, there is too often little or no opportunity to practise the skills in the clinical situation. As a result, all too frequently, newly trained midwives find themselves lacking in confidence and competence in many of the core midwifery competencies.

With the above in mind, many countries including Western countries such as the USA, Canada and New Zealand, have successfully introduced direct entry programmes into midwifery, while others are exploring the issue. Direct entry programmes have been well established in some countries such as France, the UK, and Holland as well as Chile and Indonesia to mention but a few, for many decades. Some feel that such programmes offer a greater opportunity for midwives to be acknowledged as autonomous practitioners and true partners in the team required for safe pregnancy and childbirth (Box 55.3). Such programmes would also allow developments based on a fitness-for-purpose model (Fig. 55.2). The fitness-for-purpose approach to curriculum planning looks

---

Box 55.3 Midwifery in Canada: an autonomous direct entry profession by Bridget Lynch from the Canadian Midwives Association

In Canada, midwifery is legislated and regulated at a provincial rather than federal level. Since the early 1990s, six of ten provinces have legislated midwifery as a direct entry health profession, with legislation pending in two more provinces. Midwives in Canada are independent practitioners who provide primary care to low risk women and their newborns from conception to 6 weeks' postpartum. Midwives are required by provincial regulation to attend women, as appropriate, in a woman's choice of birthplace, whether in the home, in a birth centre, or in hospital. The midwives' scope of practice includes admitting and discharge privileges in the hospital setting. Continuity of care, with a small group of midwives known to a woman providing care throughout her pregnancy, birth and the postpartum, is fundamental to the Canadian model of midwifery.

The route of entry to the profession is through a Bachelor of Science in Midwifery, offered in both francophone and anglophone university settings. There is also a process offered by provincial colleges, the regulators of the profession, to assess and register midwives who have been educated in jurisdictions outside of Canada. In several provinces, aboriginal midwives and the practice of aboriginal midwifery are recognized and protected through legislation. Midwifery services are funded through the public health-care system.

(For more information on midwifery in Canada, visit the website of the Canadian Association of Midwives at: http://www.canadianmidwives.org)

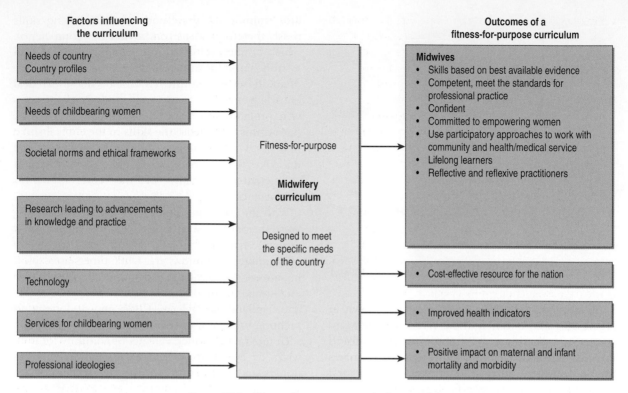

Figure 55.2   Fitness-for-purpose curriculum model.

at the required competencies of a midwife for that particular situation or country, and helps countries develop innovative and tailor-made programmes to suit the specifics of their own nation; as for example done by Canada, to address the specific midwifery needs of their First Nation's (aboriginal) population (NAHO 2004).

Attempts are being made to strengthen the skills of midwives in many countries. However, this is complicated by the fact that identification of who is a midwife is not always easy. For example in a survey across the 10 countries that make up the WHO South-east Asia Region, there were approximately 18 different categories of worker providing maternity services, of which only seven had the word 'midwife' in their job title (WHO SEARO 1996). Some, such as the border midwives in Bhutan, had only 3 months' training in midwifery and provide delivery (intra-partum)-only care, while others had 1-year mid-wifery after nursing programme and in Indonesia, midwives follow a 3-year direct entry diploma

programme. At a recent regional meeting on nursing and midwifery, from data presented in the various country reports it would appear the situation has not changed and there remains a lack of clarity as to which cadres of maternity workers are truly competent in midwifery.

As outlined in the recent International Forum on community midwifery, one of the main difficulties facing the preparation of midwives is the lack of sufficient numbers of appropriately trained midwife teachers (Odberg-Pettersson et al 2007). Many countries, including some European countries, are currently without a standardized approved preparation for their midwife teachers. This is not new however and has been recognized as a problem for many years. It was partly the debate about strengthening midwifery education and in recognizing the needs of midwive teachers in some countries for additional teaching material, which led WHO to fund the development of the midwifery modules for safe motherhood.

Finally, issues around the omission of research from the midwifery curriculum also remain hotly debated. The lack of research appreciation and research skills in the formal curriculum in many countries is recognized as being detrimental to the preparation of critically thinking midwives. Lack of research training hampers development of the needed documentary evidence from operations research to show how best to strengthen midwifery and midwifery practice in under resourced countries. Midwives must have the capacity to be both pro-active and responsive to the needs of individual mothers and babies. Without midwives who are active researchers, not simply research assistants or data gatherers for medical research, engaging upon midwifery research is difficult. Yet without such endeavours it is impossible to build up a sufficient evidence-base to midwifery practice. It is imperative therefore that each country has a mechanism by which some midwives are able to receive adequate preparation not just as expert clinicians and teachers, but also as researchers. Such research is not only essential for midwives and their clients, but is also needed by governments and other decision-makers, to assist with improving maternity services and care. What is needed to bring this to fruition however, yet lacking in too many under-resourced countries, is strong midwifery leadership coupled with sufficient management capacity, including and especially workforce planning, to be able to build an effective midwifery workforce.

Employment and the need for a positive practice environment

Another major problem facing many midwives worldwide includes issues surrounding employment and the environments in which midwives work. Changes such as the rise in HIV and demographic changes and increasing migration to city dwellings (bringing with it the demise of family support networks for childbearing women) will require different approaches to the provision of maternity services.

Mass urbanization, with its overcrowding, increased poverty and deprivation often leading to higher crime and violence, has resulted in an increased concern for the safety of midwives at work. Civil conflict, an increasing phenomenon in many parts of the world,

also brings specific issues for midwives and the provision of quality midwifery care. Coupled with the likelihood of poor nutrition, poverty, and other factors that usually accompany civil conflict (the lack of access to medical care), the health of women and their newborns are at greater risk and so the midwife's role becomes even more crucial. Sometimes the midwife is the only professional healthcare provider that women and their families have access to. However in these situations, both holding and obtaining equipment and drugs become a major issue for the midwife. Midwives in some places have been subject to violence against them because militia have thought they have drugs, which they need for their fighters. Such violence against midwives however is not just a feature of resource-poor countries or in conflict situations. Midwives working in large urban and periurban areas in almost any country of the world where there are high levels of drug-related crime, face such risks on a daily basis.

Demographic changes due to internal migration and increasingly to displacements of populations from conflict areas and/or natural disaster areas, bring with them an explosion of demands on the health services. The resulting economic burden laid on communities means that obtaining adequate remuneration for all public sector workers is a major issue. South Africa for example is facing such problems since the move to free healthcare following the political changes that marked the end of apartheid. Coupled with the effects of mass urbanization and the rise in HIV AID, South Africa is struggling with an overstretched health service, where demand exceeds hospital and district budgets. Midwives working in similar situations are being faced with many of the same problems (Box 55.4).

Finally, in many countries, despite the challenges placed on public services, setting up of independent community practice is difficult and is often devalued. Even some Western countries, including the UK and some states in the USA and Canada and Norway, are facing similar problems with independent midwifery as insurance companies can be reluctant for a variety of reasons to pay for this type of service. Often the reason for these problems relates to the close association of insurers with the medical profession, who are not always supportive of midwifery-led care. As funding of healthcare becomes

---

Box 55.4 Midwives in Zimbabwe

Midwives in Zimbabwe have a long tradition and have done a great deal to strengthen midwifery care to ensure they meet the changes in society. One of the greatest challenges Zimbabwe has had to face in recent years has been the incredible rise in HIV/AIDS. The midwifery curricula have been revised to take on board HIV/AIDS and counselling. Currently, the country is busy strengthening midwifery education and services through offering a master's degree with specialization in MCH and midwifery. However, these gains are being wiped out due to the current crisis, namely increased migration of midwives to other countries that are offering better salaries and packages including improving safety. Due to the staff shortage, the need for capacity building is greater than ever in the country. Sometimes even in the large hospitals there are not sufficient midwives and nurses and others are left to assist the woman during birth. The midwife then becomes a supervisor of staff rather than carrying out the skills she has been trained to do.

(Report of Zimbabwe midwifery representative at WHO technical meeting on strengthening midwifery services to support Making Pregnancy Safer, November 2001.)

---

increasingly reliant on insurance scheme, this is likely to become an increasing problem.

The success of the midwives in The Netherlands, Canada and New Zealand to have their services recognized as a legitimate option for pregnant women, does however offer hope (Donley 1989, Donley 1995, Smulders & Limburg 1995), but it should be remembered that these successes were as a result of hard-fought battles. In each case, although circumstances may be different, the force of medical opposition was enormous and the midwifery profession had to unite and work in partnership with women to achieve success. In both Canada and New Zealand the force of women's support was paramount. This can be achieved only if women are free and able to offer this support – free in that they are not excessively burdened with malnutrition, ill health and poverty. Unfortunately in some countries, women's status is low and many women are still being denied freedom to demand what should be a basic human right – the right to access care during pregnancy, childbirth and for the important months after, from a competent professional midwife.

Scope of midwifery practice increased in some countries

Increasingly, turbulence, war and political upheaval are posing new problems for midwifery. Violence against women is more than ever on the international agenda, despite the UN Convention on the elimination of all forms of discrimination against women (UN 1979) and the Declaration on violence against women (UN 1993). According to a large-scale scientific study conducted in collaboration with WHO it was revealed that between 10% and 50% of all women reported they had been subject to physical abuse by an intimate partner in their lifetime, much of the violence beginning in and around pregnancy (WHO 2005b).

Female genital mutilation is still a concern in many countries, as is the damage inflicted on women as a result of lack of appropriate healthcare in pregnancy and childbirth. Morbidity, especially pelvic floor problems, incontinence and vesico-vaginal fistulae, and the provision of appropriate and safe reproductive healthcare for refugees and displaced persons, are perhaps the most pressing concerns for research and innovations by midwives. Such occurrences call for midwives in those countries to extend their practice into the broader sexual reproductive health and rights' arena. Midwives in some of these countries are being trained to undertake limited surgical procedures such as performing a caesarean section and repairing vesico-vaginal fistulae, as well as carrying out medical abortions and menstrual regulation. Therefore, despite the catalogue of challenges facing midwifery and midwives worldwide, there are signs that midwives are increasingly being seen as key workers and the current climate is favourable for strengthening and making midwifery more visible.

Conclusion

It is not possible to reflect all the issues or the different approaches being made by midwives in different countries in one short chapter. What is possible though, is to heighten all midwives' awareness that today, more than ever, globalization does have an impact on the work of individual midwives in many countries, including those who practise only within their own country. Midwives must become more politically active if they are to bring about safe(r) motherhood in their own and other countries. It is clear that what is required to bring about safe motherhood in most countries is sufficient well-trained midwives and the resources to provide holistic quality care, including emergency obstetric care, which includes care of newborns with life-threatening conditions. Such care must be available close enough for all women to gain access to it. Equally, women must be able to influence the provision of care to ensure it is culturally acceptable. This requires action by community leaders, policy makers and politicians. Therefore midwives must become active in political debates concerning structures of society, especially the rights of women and women's empowerment. In addition, if they are to be true advocates for mothers and newborns, midwives must also be able to identify and influence local leaders and key decision-makers in the community.

With this in mind there is a need to re-think the skills required in midwives seeking work experience and job opportunities in low income and resource-poor countries. It is no long sufficient to be a competent clinical midwife, but there is a need for midwives looking for such opportunities to have additional broader skills in leadership, management, especially in human resource planning and in teaching and research.

Finally, if midwives are to provide appropriate effective care anywhere in the world, they must always listen to and respect the women they seek to serve. For midwives working at an international level or working outside their own country, this means ensuring that it is the voices of women, including the midwives they work with (regardless of the gender of the midwife) that are heard and that it is their voice leading actions to strengthen midwifery.

REFERENCES

Awases M, Gabary A, Nyoni J et al 2004 Migration of health professions in six countries: A Synthesis Report for World Health Organization Regional Office For Africa, Division of Health Systems and Services Development. WHO AFRO, South Africa

Campbell O, Graham W 2006 Strategies for reducing maternal mortality: getting on with what works. Lancet 368 (9544):1284–1299

Chitnis S 1988 Feminism: Indian ethos and Indian convictions. In: Ghandially S (ed.) Women in Indian society: a reader. Sage, London

Collins P 1994 Shifting the centre: race, class, and feminist theorizing about motherhood. In: Glenn E, Chang G, Forcey L (eds) Mothering ideology, experience, and agency. Routledge, New York

Cook R, Dickens B 2001 Advancing safe motherhood through reproductive rights. World Health Organization, Department of Reproductive Health and Research, Geneva. Online. Available: http://who.int/reproductive-health/publications/RHR_01_5_advancing_safe_motherhood

Dawit S, Busia A 1995 Thinking about culture: some programme pointers. Gender development. Oxfam Journal 5(1):7–11

de Bernis L, Sherratt D R, AbouZhar C et al 2003 Skilled attendants for pregnancy and childbirth. In: Rodeck C, ed. Pregnancy, Reducing maternal death and disability. British Medical Bulletin; 67: 39–57. Online. Available: http://www.bmb.oupjournals

De Brouwere V, Van Lerberghe W eds 2003. Safe motherhood strategies: a review of the evidence. Studies in Health Service Organization and Policy 17: 7–33

Donley J 1989 Professionalism. The importance of consumer control over childbirth. New Zealand College of Midwives Journal September:6–7

Donley J 1995 Independent midwifery in New Zealand. In: Murphy-Black T (ed.) Issues in midwifery. Churchill Livingstone, Edinburgh

Donney F, Weil L 2004 Reproductive health and rights. Obstetric fistula: the international response. Lancet 363 (9402):71–72

Fullerton J, Thompson J 2005 Examining the evidence for The International Confederation of Midwives' essential competencies for midwifery practice. Midwifery 21(1):2–13

Gill K, Pande R, Malhotra A 2007 Women deliver for development. Lancet 370(9595):1347–1357

Goodburn E 1995 Maternal morbidity in rural Bangladesh: an investigation into the nature and determinants of maternal morbidity related to delivery and the puerperium. Bangladesh Rural Advancement Committee, Dhaka

Graham W, Bell J, Bullough C H W 2001 Can skilled attendance at delivery reduce maternal mortality in developing countries? In: De Brouwere V, Van Lerberghe W V (eds) Safe motherhood strategies: a review of the evidence. Studies in Health Services Organization and Policy 17:97–130

Gülmezoglu A M, Say L, Betrán A P et al 2004 WHO systematic review of maternal mortality and morbidity: methodological issues and challenges. BMC Medical Research Methodology 5 (4):16. Online. Available: http://www.biomedcentral.com/1471–2288/4/16

ICM (International Confederation of Midwives) 1999 International code of ethics for midwives. Online. Available: http://www.interntionalmidwives.org

ICM (International Confederation of Midwives) 1994 A birthday for midwives: seventy five years of international collaboration. The International Confederation of Midwives 1919–1994. ICM, London

ICM (International Confederation of Midwives) 2002 Essential competencies for midwives. ICM. Online. Available: http://www.interntionalmidwives.org

Koblinsky M (ed.) 2003 Reducing maternal mortality: learning from Bolivia, China, Egypt, Honduras, Indonesia, Jamaica and Zimbabwe. Human Development Network. Health, Nutrition and Population Series. The World Bank, Washington, DC

Koblinsky M, Matthews Z, Hussein J et al 2006 Going to scale with professional skilled care. Lancet 368(9544):1377–1386

Kunst A, Howlling T 2001 A global picture of poor-rich differences in the utilization of delivery care. In: De Brouwere V, Van Lerberge W (eds) Safe motherhood strategies: a review of the evidence. Studies in Health Services Organization and Policy 17:297–315

Kwast B, Bentley J 1991 Introducing confident midwives: midwifery education – action for safe motherhood. Midwifery 7:8–19

Kwast B, Bergström S 2001 Training professionals for safe motherhood In: Lawson J B, Harrison K A, Bergström S (eds) Maternity care in developing countries. RCOG Press, London

Latham M C, Prebble E A 2000 Appropriate feeding methods for infants of HIV infected mothers in sub-Saharan Africa. British Medical Journal 328:1656–1659

Loudon I 2000 Maternal mortality in the past and its relevance to the developing world today. American Journal of Clinical Nutrition (1S):241S–246S

Mensah K, Mackintosh M, Henry L 2005 The 'skills drain' of health professionals from the developing world: a framework for policy formation. Medact, London

Miller S, Sloan N L, Winikoff B et al 2003 Where is the 'E' in MCH? The need for evidence-based approach to safe motherhood. Journal of Midwifery Women's Health 48(1):10–18

Mullay B 2006 Barriers to and attitudes towards promoting husbands' involvement in maternal health in Katmandu, Nepal. Social Science and Medicine 62(11):2798–2809

NAHO (National Aboriginal Health Organization) 2004 Midwifery and Aboriginal midwifery in Canada. NAHO, Ottowa

Odberg-Pettersson K, Sherratt D R, Mayo N T. 2007 Midwifery in the Community: lessons learnt. International Forum on training and scaling up midwives. Final Report. UNFPA, New York

Penny S, Murray S 2000 Training initiatives for essential obstetric care in developing countries: a 'state of the art' review. Health Policy and Planning 14(4):286–393

Portela A, Santarelli C 2003 Empowerment of women, men, families, and communities: true partners for improving maternal and newborn health. In: Rodeck C (ed.) Pregnancy, reducing maternal death and disability. British Medical Bulletin 67:59–72. Online. Available: http://www.bmb.oupjournals

Royston E, Armstrong S 1989 Preventing maternal deaths. WHO, Geneva

Sherratt D R 2007 Towards MDG 5: Scaling up the capacity of midwives to reduce maternal mortality and morbidity. In: Odberg Pettersson K, Sherratt D R (eds) Midwifery in the community: lessons learnt. International forum on training and scaling up midwives. Final Workshop Report. UNFPA, New York, 21–23 March

Smulders B, Limburg A 1995 Obstetrics and midwifery in the Netherlands. In: Kitzinger S (ed.) The midwifery challenge. Pandora, London

Stanton C, Blanc A K Croft T et al 2007 Skilled care at birth in the developing world: progress to date and strategies for expanding coverage. Journal of Biosocial Science 39(1):109–120

Starrs A, IAGSM 2000 The Safe Motherhood Action Agenda: Report on the Safe Motherhood Technical Consultation, 18–23 October 1997, Colombo, Sri Lanka. Inter Agency Group for Safe Motherhood, New York

Thompson J, Bennett R, 1996 Women are dying: midwives in action. Background paper for ICM/WHO/UNICEF Pre-Congress Safe Motherhood Workshop. WHO/ICM, Oslo, May

UN (United Nations) 1979 Convention on the elimination of all forms of discrimination against women. UN, New York

UN (United Nations) 1990 The convention on the rights of the child. UN, New York

UN (United Nations) 1993 Declaration on violence against women. UN, New York

UNICEF (United Nations Children's Fund) 1993 The progress of nations. UNICEF, New York

UNICEF (United Nations Children's Fund) 1997a The state of the world's children: 1997 summary. UNICEF, New York

UNICEF (United Nations Children's Fund) 1997b Cracking the code (code no. 16027). UNICEF, Essex

Wagner M 1994 Pursuing the birth machine: the search for appropriate birth technology. Ace Graphics, Camperdown

WB (World Bank) 2005 World Development Report 2004. Making services work for poor people. World Bank, Washington DC

WHO (World Health Organization) 1991 Maternal mortality: a global factbook. WHO, Geneva

WHO (World Health Organization) 1994a The application of the WHO partograph in the management of labour. Maternal Health and Safe Motherhood Programme, Division of Family Health, WHO, Geneva

WIIO (World Health Organization) 1994b Mother–baby package: a practical guide to implementing safe motherhood in countries. Maternal Health and Safe Motherhood Programme, Division of Family Health, WHO, Geneva

WHO (World Health Organization) 1996a Normal birth. Safe Motherhood Programme. Maternal Health and Safe Motherhood Programme, Division of Family Health, WHO, Geneva

WHO (World Health Organization) 1996b Revised 1990 estimates of maternal mortality: a new approach by WHO and UNICEF. WHO, Geneva

WHO (World Health Organization) 2000 Management of complications in pregnancy and childbirth: guidelines for midwives and doctors. WHO, Geneva

WHO (World Health Organization) 2001a Maternal mortality in 1995: Estimates developed by WHO, UNICEF, UNFPA. WHO, Geneva

WHO (World Health Organization) 2001b New data on the prevention of Mother-to-Child Transmission of HIV and their policy implications. Technical consultation: UNFPA/

UNICEF/ WHO/UNAIDS Inter-Agency Team–Conclusions and recommendations. WHO Department of Reproductive Health and Research, Geneva

WHO (World Health Organization) 2004a Making pregnancy safer: the critical role of the skilled attendant. A Joint Statement by WHO ICM FIGO. WHO, Geneva

WHO (World Health Organization) 2004b HIV transmission: a Review of Available Evidence. WHO Department of Child and Adolescent Health and Development and Department of Nutrition, Geneva

WHO (World Health Organization) 2005a World Health Report 2005. Make every mother and child count. WHO, Geneva

WHO (World Health Organization) 2005b Multi-country study on women's' health and domestic violence against women. WHO Department of Gender and Women's Health, Geneva

WHO (World Health Organization) 2006a World Health Report 2006. Working together for health. WHO, Geneva

WHO (World Health Organization) 2006b Neonatal and perinatal mortality – country, regional and global estimates. WHO, Geneva

WHO (World Health Organization) 2007 Proportion of births attended by a skilled attendant – 2007 updates. WHO Department of Reproductive Heath and Research, Geneva. Online. Available: http://www/who.int/ reproductive-health/global_monitoring/skilled_attendant_atbirth2007

WHO, ICM 2007 Midwifery education modules: education for safe motherhood, 2nd edn. WHO Department of Making Pregnancy Safer, Geneva. Online. Available: http://www/who.int/making_pregnancy_safer

WHO SEARO (World Health Organization South-East Asia Regional Office) 1996 Standards for midwifery practice for safe motherhood. Working Paper 1: An inter-country consultation. WHO/SEARO, New Delhi, India, November

WHO, United Nations Children's Fund 1989 Protecting, promoting and supporting breastfeeding: the special role of maternity services. WHO, Geneva

WHO, United Nations Children's Fund 2006 Baby-friendly hospital initiative: Revised, updated and expanded for integrated care: Section 1: Country Implementation. Online. Available: http://www.who.int/nutrition/topics/BFHI_Revised_Section1.pdf

WHO, United Nations Children's Fund, International Confederation of Midwives 1991 Midwifery education action for safe motherhood: report of a collaborative pre-congress workshop, Kobe, Japan, 5–6 October 1990. WHO, Geneva

WHO/United Nations Population Fund/United Nations Children's Fund/World Bank. 1999 Reducing maternal mortality. WHO, Geneva

FURTHER READING

Berer M, Sundari Ravindran T K (eds) 1999 Safe Motherhood Initiatives: critical issues. Blackwell Science, London

Devries R, Benoit C, Van Teijlingen, Wrede S (eds) 2001 Birth by design pregnancy, maternity care, and midwifery in North America and Europe. Routledge, New York

A good review of the policies and development of maternity care in Europe and North America.

Jeffrey P, Jeffrey R, Lyon A. 1988 Labour pains and labour power: woman and childbearing in India. Zed Books, London

Although now dated, a very useful read for those wishing to gain an appreciation of the taboos and cultural issues surrounding pregnancy and childbirth in India. Many of the same taboos can also be found in neighbouring countries.

Klien S, Miller S, Thomson F. 2004 A book for midwives. Care for pregnancy, birth and women's health. The Hesperian Foundation, Berkeley

A very useful textbook for those who are working in low-resourced countries. Contains many useful simple line diagrams and explanations to assist when teaching midwifery staff in situations where there are few resources.

Murray S (ed.) 1996 Midwives and safer motherhood. Mosby, London.

A useful collection of interesting scholarly works on midwifery and maternity care from a wide range of countries. The accompanying textbook dealing more specifically with breastfeeding and attempts to bring about mother-friendly quality care is also useful.

Murray S (ed.) 1996 Baby friendly/mother friendly: international perspectives on midwifery. Mosby, London

USEFUL ADDRESSES AND WEBSITES

World Health Organization
1211 Geneva 27 Switzerland
website: www.who.int

International Confederation of Midwives HQ
Laan van Meerdervoort 70, 2517 AN The Hague, The
Netherlands
Tel: +31703060520; Fax +31703555651
website: www.internationalmidwives.org

Save the Children SNBL initiative:
www.savethechildren.org/health/healthsaving
newbornlives

United Nation's Population Fund:
www.unfpa.org

56 Maternal and perinatal health, mortality and statistics

Alison Miller

It is a woman's basic right to achieve optimal health throughout pregnancy and childbirth for themselves and their newborns. (WRA 2007)

In the UK, the lifetime risk of a mother dying as a result of pregnancy or childbirth is approximately 200 times less than the lifetime risk for women in developing countries; 99% of the world's maternal deaths occur in developing countries (WHO 2004) and similarly 98% of perinatal deaths, the majority of which could be prevented (WHO 2006a). However, despite the increased maternal and perinatal survival in the industrialized world, many of the deaths that do occur are due to substandard care given by clinicians and midwives and thus may be avoided.

The chapter aims to:

- provide an introduction to maternal health in the UK
- provide an introduction to maternal and perinatal mortality in the UK
- provide an introduction to how on-going surveillance and topic-specific research can identify risk factors which contribute to poor maternity outcomes
- provide an introduction to the need for on-going local and national audits to ensure care is provided at an optimal level
- provide an introduction to an international perspective on maternal and perinatal mortality.

Maternal health in the UK

The changing profile of the national population impacts on the services that are required to provide the maternity population with the most appropriate care. Specific changes both in areas of public health and culture have been widely documented in recent years. It is important that midwives are aware of these changes as they may contribute to the reason why outcomes, both maternal and perinatal have not improved for pregnant women over the past 20 years.

Three of the issues identified as increasing risk of poor pregnancy outcome are the changing age distribution, increasing obesity and changing ethnicity profiles within local populations, including inward migration of women in the childbearing age group. Although these factors do not in themselves cause poor outcomes, maternal and perinatal mortality data show that all three lead to an increased risk for these women.

In 2004, the fertility rate in women aged 30–34 increased by nearly 5% to 99.4/1000 women since the previous year. This meant that for the first time women in this age group had a higher fertility rate than those in the 25–29 age group. It was also the highest fertility rate recorded in any age group since 1998 (ONS 2005). This trend is also mirrored in the 40–44 year age group; in 2004 15.3/1000 women had a pregnancy resulting in childbirth whereas this figure was only 7.6 in 1994. The maternal mortality rate is seen to increase for women over 35 years of age (Lewis 2007, Lewis & Drife 2004). Similarly perinatal mortality was shown to increase for women at both extremes of age groups; <20 and >40, when compared with other age groups (CEMACH 2007b).

Obesity is also observed to increase maternal and perinatal mortality (CEMACH 2007b, Lewis 2007). The increase in body mass index (BMI) in the general population is reflected in the maternal population and will therefore be an increasing issue in the provision of maternal care. Taking a BMI of >30 as a definition used by the Information Centre's Health Survey, obesity in women has increased from 16.4–24.8% between 1993 and 2005 (The Information Centre 2006). This is most prevalent in women of Black African, Black Caribbean and Pakistani ethnicity. The same survey identified an increase in obesity in female children of 12–18.1% between 1995 and 2005, which has implications for the future childbearing population.

Obese women are also 13 times more likely to develop type 2 diabetes which increases their risk of poor pregnancy outcome, as discussed later in this chapter (CEMACH 2007a).

Ethnicity of the population in the UK is changing over time. More recently, with the opening up of the European Union, there has been an inward migration of women in the childbearing population. Between 1995 and 2005 there has been a two-fold increase in the percentage of live births to women from other European Union countries, from 1.7% to 3.2%. The total percentage of live births to women from outside the UK has increased from 12.6% to 20.8% in the same period (National Statistics 2005).

Maternal mortality in the UK

The tenth revision of the International Classification of Diseases, Injuries and Causes of Death (ICD10), defines a maternal death as 'the death of a woman while pregnant, or within 42 days of termination of pregnancy, from any cause related to, or aggravated by the pregnancy, or its management, but not from accidental or incidental causes'.

Maternal deaths are routinely classified into a number of categories as defined below.

Direct deaths

Deaths within 42 days of delivery, termination or abortion resulting from obstetric complications of the pregnant state (pregnancy, labour and puerperium), from interventions, omissions, incorrect treatment or from a chain of events resulting from any of the above, e.g. thrombosis. This 42-day limit is an internationally recognized standard.

Indirect

Deaths within 42 days of delivery, termination or abortion resulting from previous existing disease, or disease that developed during pregnancy and which was not due to obstetric causes, but which was aggravated by the physiological effects of pregnancy, e.g. cardiac disease.

Coincidental (fortuitous)

Deaths from unrelated causes which happen to occur in pregnancy or the puerperium. The term 'coincidental' is now preferred to 'fortuitous' as being more appropriate and sensitive, e.g. road traffic accidents.

Late

Deaths occurring between 42 days and 1 year after delivery, termination or abortion, that are due to *Direct* or *Indirect* causes.

There are two routinely used measures of maternal mortality; maternal mortality rate and maternal mortality ratio. There are important differences in their definitions. The international definition of maternal mortality ratio is *Direct* and *Indirect* deaths per 100 000 live births.

In the UK, when discussing rates of maternal death, they are defined as *Direct* and *Indirect* deaths per 100 000 maternities. Maternities encompass the number of pregnancies that result in a live birth, at any gestation, and stillbirths occurring at or after 24 weeks of completed gestation (required to be notified by law). The latest published maternal mortality ratio in the UK is 13.8 ($n = 295$) per 100 000 live births, while the UK maternal mortality rate is 13.9 ($n = 295$) per total births (Table 56.1) (Lewis 2007).

The UK maternal mortality rate dropped considerably in the mid-1990s before reaching a plateau towards the end of the decade. However, there has been a small increase in the number of deaths since 1999 (Lewis 2007). These changes in trend have been attributed to a number of factors:

- Increased awareness among medical staff of the need to notify maternal deaths. This would lead to improved *ascertainment* of maternal deaths.

- The linkage programme set up by the Office for National Statistics to identify all women who have died in a given calendar year and who appear on the registration of a birth that occurred in the 12 months preceding the death. This would lead to improved *ascertainment* of maternal deaths.

- An increase in the number of newly arrived immigrants, refugees and asylum seekers who did not access care. This would lead to an increase in the *number* of maternal deaths (Lewis & Drife 2004).

- An increase in the number of women receiving substandard care (Lewis & Drife 2004). This would lead to an increase in the *number* of maternal deaths.

The main causes of *Direct* death have remained very much unchanged over the past 50 years. These deaths were predominantly due to thrombosis and thromboembolism, hypertensive disease of pregnancy, haemorrhage and amniotic fluid embolism (Table 56.2). The main causes of *Indirect* death are those related to cardiac conditions and deaths associated with psychiatric illness (see Ch. 36B).

Avoidable factors identified through the confidential enquiries into UK maternal deaths during 2003–2005 (Lewis 2007) were in many cases assessed to have been due to healthcare professionals failing to recognize and manage common medical conditions or potential emergencies outside their immediate area of expertise. In addition, resuscitation skills were considered to be unacceptably poor in some cases.

It is the responsibility of the midwife to maintain and update her skills and knowledge to ensure she can appropriately recognize deviations from normal and act and refer appropriately (NMC 2004, 2008).

Table 56.1 Direct and Indirect maternal mortality rates/100 000 maternities as reported to the Registrars General (ONS) and to the Enquiry: UK 1997 2005

	1997–1999[a]		2000–2002[b]		2003–2005[c]	
	n	**Rate (95% CI)**	**n**	**Rate (95% CI)**	**n**	**Rate (95% CI)**
Direct deaths	106	5.0 (4.1, 6.0)	106	5.3 (4.4, 6.4)	132	6.2 (5.3, 7.4)
Indirect deaths	136	6.4 (5.4, 7.6)	155	7.8 (6.6, 9.1)	163	7.7 (6.6, 9.0)
Total direct or indirect deaths	242	11.4 (10.1, 12.9)	261	13.1 (11.6, 14.8)	295	13.9 (12.4, 15.6)

All Rates are given per 100 000 UK maternities.
[a]Total number of maternities in UK for 1997–1999 is 2 123 614.
[b]Total number of maternities in the UK for 2000–2002 is 1 997 472.
[c]Total number of maternities in the UK for 2003–2005 is 2 114 004.

Table 56.2   Major Direct and Indirect causes of maternal deaths reported to the Enquiry: UK 1997–2005

	1997–1999[a]		2000–2002[b]		2003–2005[c]	
	n	Rate (95% CI)	*n*	Rate (95% CI)	*n*	Rate (95% CI)
Thrombosis and thromboembolism	35	16.5 (11.9, 22.9)	30	15.0 (10.5, 21.4)	41	19.4 (14.3, 26.3)
Hypertensive diseases of pregnancy	15	7.5 (4.6, 10.6)	14	7.0 (4.2, 11.8)	18	8.5 (5.4, 13.5)
Haemorrhage	7	3.3 (1.6, 6.8)	17	8.5 (5.3, 13.6)	14	6.6 (3.9, 11.1)
Amniotic fluid embolism	8	3.8 (1.9, 7.4)	5	2.5 (1.1, 5.9)	17	8.0 (5.0, 12.9)
Cardiac disease	35	16.5 (11.9, 22.9)	44	22.0 (15.5, 28.5)	48	22.7 (16.7, 29.6)
Indirect psychiatric causes	15	7.1 (3.5, 10.6)	16	8.0 (4.1, 11.9)	18	8.5 (5.4, 13.5)

All rates are given per 1 000 000 UK maternities.
[a]Total number of maternities in UK for 1997–1999 is 2 123 614.
[b]Total number of maternities in the UK for 2000–2002 is 1 997 472.
[c]Total number of maternities in the UK for 2003–2005 is 2 114 004.

A satisfactory healthcare system should include maternity and peripartum services such as to ensure that every pregnant woman emerges from the birth as a healthy mother with an equally healthy term baby. Indeed, such an outcome is vital since mother–child bonding is more likely to occur successfully when both are physically and mentally healthy. An inability to bond is not only a personal tragedy for the family, but could precipitate later problems which may result in health-related complications. Furthermore, where a pregnancy results in death of the mother, child or both, this has repercussions not only for the family and friends, but also healthcare professionals involved in the care. Moreover, it is almost impossible to estimate the effect of losing a mother on any older children. Thus, despite the perceived small number of maternal deaths, their impact should not be underestimated, and it is imperative that efforts to reduce this number further are not diminished.

Providing healthcare during pregnancy

There have been a number of government initiatives set up to try to identify and address some of the issues for women accessing maternity services with the aim of maternal health and outcomes for pregnant women in the UK. These include: the National Service Framework for Children and Young People (NSF) (DH 2004), Changing Childbirth (DoH 1993), and Maternity Matters (DH 2007).

Some of the risk factors for poor maternal outcomes which have been identified by these initiatives and also the reports on confidential enquiries into maternal deaths in the UK (Lewis 2007, Lewis & Drife 2004) are listed below:

- social deprivation or disadvantage
- being a member of a minority ethnic group
- late booking or poor attendance
- substandard clinical care.

There has been much investigation into the role of substandard care in maternal morbidity and mortality, since this is the most obvious factor that can be practically addressed in improving services. Substandard care can be divided into two categories: (1) *Major substandard care* where substandard care contributed significantly to the death of the mother, and thus the death was likely to be avoidable, and (2) *Minor substandard care* where the standard of care was a relevant contributory factor to the death, but the mother's survival was unlikely in any case. In their investigation of all maternal deaths occurring in 2003–2005, the confidential enquiry reported that 55% of mothers who died from *Direct* causes were assessed to have had major substandard care (Lewis 2007). This is not only a disturbing indictment on a small minority of healthcare professionals, but also demonstrates the comparative ease with which significant decreases in maternal deaths could be made.

Perinatal and neonatal mortality

Recent studies suggest over 1 in 200 pregnancies end in stillbirth and around 1 in 300 babies die in the first 4 weeks following birth (CEMACH 2007b). While a number of these deaths may not be preventable, it is imperative that thorough surveillance systems remain in place to allow identification of trends and problem areas.

Perinatal mortality includes all stillbirths and deaths of live born babies in the first week of life.
  Definitions:

- *stillbirths*: babies born with no signs of life from 24 completed weeks of gestation
- *early neonatal deaths*: live born babies whose death occurs in the first week of life
- *late neonatal deaths*: live born babies whose death occurs between seven and 28 days following birth.

The rates of neonatal deaths are commonly calculated per 1000 live births, while rates for stillbirth are given per 1000 live births and stillbirths total births.

Since 1992 the stillbirth rate has remained largely unchanged. However, the neonatal mortality has declined significantly (Fig. 56.1).

While there has been an increase in the neonatal survival rate of very pre-term babies, no progress has been made in reducing the overall stillbirth rate (CEMACH 2007b).

In looking for explanations of long-term trends it is important to take account of a wide range of factors such as the establishment of the NHS in 1948. The passing of the Abortion Act 1967 has resulted in the termination of many pregnancies for congenital abnormalities and thus the removal of deaths from these causes from the perinatal mortality statistics.

The re-definition in 1992 of the age of legal viability of a fetus as being 24 weeks' instead of 28 weeks' gestation has brought more babies within the definition of stillbirth. Consequently, there has been an increase in perinatal mortality figures over this time period. However, more recent guidelines for stillbirth have been released in an effort to provide health professionals with advice on how to interpret

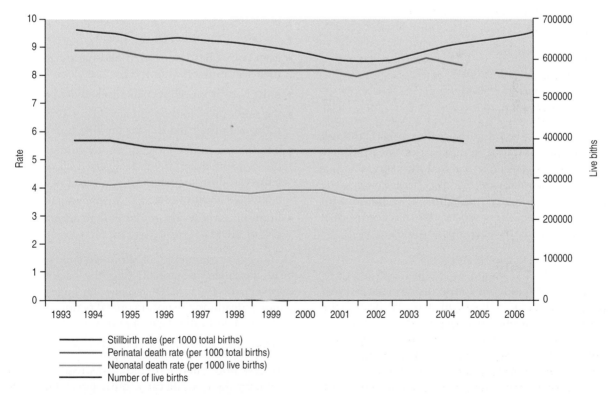

Stillbirth rate (per 1000 total births)
Perinatal death rate (per 1000 total births)
Neonatal death rate (per 1000 live births)
Number of live births

Figure 56.1 Stillbirth and neonatal mortality, England and Wales 1993–2006. (From ONS and CEMACH.) *Note:* Stillbirths were defined using the RCOG Guidance from 2005.

the current law, particularly around the issue of a fetus that has died *in utero* before 24 weeks, but delivered after 24 weeks (RCOG 2005). This has led to a slight decrease in the published stillbirth rates from 2005 (CEMACH 2007b).

Causes of mortality which have occurred at a relatively consistent rate over the last 5 years include low birthweight, (pre-term and small-for-gestation babies), intrauterine hypoxia, respiratory depression at birth, intracranial injury and congenital abnormality. However, the cause of death in around 50% of stillbirths is not identified (CEMACH 2007b). The main causes of early neonatal death are congenital anomaly and immaturity, and the causes of late neonatal death are immaturity and infection.

It may be impossible to attribute a perinatal death to any one of the listed causes, but a combination of predisposing factors increases the risk of death. These include:

- socioeconomic disadvantage
- poor maternal health (including effects of smoking, alcohol consumption, drug abuse and poor diet)
- multiple pregnancy
- antepartum haemorrhage
- pre-eclampsia
- breech presentation.

Thus it can be seen that issues that increase the risk of perinatal mortality, in many cases, unsurprisingly mirror those listed for maternal mortality. Furthermore, suboptimal care has also been found to be an issue in perinatal mortality. In common with many other conditions, social class has been shown to be an important determinant of outcome.

Infant mortality

An infant death is defined as occurring in the first year of life. Thus this includes all neonatal deaths; the remainder are termed post neonatal deaths (28–364 days). The infant mortality rate is calculated per 1000 live births. This rate is taken as an important measure of the health of the population of a nation.

Some of the essential causes that a midwife should be aware of are non-accidental injury, infection and, in older babies, accidents in the home. Sudden

Infant Death Syndrome (SIDS) is also significant; these are unexpected deaths in which no cause is identified.

In a study investigating sudden unexpected deaths in infancy (SUDI) between the ages of 1 and 52 weeks (Fleming et al 2000), a total of 418 infant deaths were examined. A total of 93 were explained, and nearly half of these showed signs of illness severe enough to need medical attention in the 24 hrs preceding death, using the criteria of the Cambridge Baby Check (Morley et al 1991).

Investigation into the causes of post-neonatal death has led to a number of key points and recommendations to be made, based on evidence presented in a number of studies. These have been produced as a leaflet by the Foundation for the Study of Infant Death (FSID):

- cut smoking in pregnancy – this should include fathers
- do not let anyone smoke in the same room as the baby
- place the baby on the back to sleep
- do not let the baby get too hot
- keep baby's head uncovered and place baby with their feet to the foot of the cot
- if the baby is unwell seek medical advice promptly
- the safest place for baby to sleep is in a cot in the room with the parent(s) for the first 6 months
- bed sharing can be dangerous after drinking alcohol or using drugs, if you feel very tired or your baby was born prematurely, was small at birth or is under 3 months old
- immunization decreases rather than increases the risk of SIDS.

Fleming et al comment that, although sudden infant death has fallen substantially since the 'back to sleep' campaign in 1991, SUDI remain the largest single group of deaths in the post-neonatal period (Fleming et al 2000). Robinson (1996) points out the international success of the campaign, but also stresses the continuing adverse influence of poverty.

The key points above should be discussed with the parents by the midwife early in the postnatal period and should be included within the programme for parent care classes.

The role of the midwife

Midwives can contribute towards optimizing the care given to each woman on two levels: ensuring a positive experience for the mother of childbirth as a crucial life-event, and more broadly, by reducing maternal and perinatal morbidity and mortality. These have been discussed in previous chapters, and opportunities to improve care are given in the key recommendations and those specifically for midwives in the Confidential Enquiry Reports (Lewis 2007, Lewis & Drife 2004).

Caring for the bereaved family, as discussed in Chapter 38, is also part of the midwife's role. Often, the only link for the family with the deceased, whether it be a mother or the baby, is through the place where the death occurred and with the staff involved at the birth.

The Confidential Enquiry into Maternal and Child Health (CEMACH)

CEMACH is commissioned by the National Patient Safety Agency (NPSA) to carry out surveillance and confidential enquiry topic-work with the aim of improving the health of mothers, babies and children. CEMACH operates throughout England, Wales and Northern Ireland. NHS Quality Improvement Scotland (NHS QIS) has participated fully in the maternal health aspects of the enquiry work since 2006.

There are two streams of work: (1) surveillance of maternal, perinatal and child mortality and (2) confidential enquiry work into specific topics in mortality and/or morbidity.

The continuation of reporting of maternal and perinatal surveillance is important for the following reasons:

* to provide long-term trend data on maternal and perinatal health
* to provide comparative data for national and local level health targets
* to aid in the identification of factors which have increasing impact on the mortality rates.

The enquiry work includes the confidential enquiry into maternal deaths, plus project work on topics which have been identified as impacting negatively on maternal or perinatal mortality and morbidity rates. This enables further exploration of maternal and perinatal health issues as they arise and evolve, allowing for the formulation of appropriate public health initiatives.

Reporting responsibilities following a maternal death

There is a statutory requirement for all maternal deaths (occurring up to 42 days postpartum) to be notified to the Strategic Health Authority (SHA) within the area where the death occurred. This action is the responsibility of the designated supervisor of midwives (SoM) within the Trust whose SHA relationship is directly with the local supervising authority midwifery officer (LSAMO). The SoM also informs the CEMACH regional office of the maternal death. Once a death has been notified to CEMACH, the confidential enquiry is initiated. A proforma is sent to the Trust which requests information about the mother and the care provided to her during her pregnancy, the birth of her baby and in the time leading up to her death. The CEMACH team also seek other sources of information from the GP, specialist services and post mortem. If relevant, the coroner's report is also obtained.

The case then undergoes regional and central assessment. A crucial role of the assessment procedure is to ascertain which, if any, of these deaths were avoidable and identify those factors which directly resulted in the poor outcome. This review also seeks to identify both substandard and good practices. Analysis and aggregation of all maternal and perinatal deaths in the UK provides a means of identifying trends by which recommendations for service provision, clinical practice and other public health initiatives are derived.

There are a number of other department leads who must be notified including the clinical risk manager of the Trust. It is their responsibility to ensure that a serious untoward incident is recorded and an internal review of the circumstances around the death carried out as promptly as possible.

Notification of perinatal death

All deaths of babies from 24 weeks' gestation to 28 days postpartum should be reported to CEMACH as soon as possible using the perinatal death notification (PDN) form (most units have an allocated midwife responsible for ensuring all perinatal deaths are notified to CEMACH). This surveillance system is also used to inform future topic-specific work due to the significant contribution each makes to the perinatal and neonatal mortality rates.

As data are analysed both nationally and on a local level, it is possible to identify and feedback emerging trends specific to a locality. On-going surveillance and production of trend data are essential for identification of topics for future research.

Recent projects

Outcomes for babies born at 27–28 weeks' gestation (Macintosh 2003)

The Confidential Enquiry into Stillbirths and Deaths in Infancy (CESDI) carried out a study looking at outcomes for babies born at 27–28 weeks' gestation. The main issues identified were substandard care or lack of current guidelines: this was observed more frequently in babies who died. Two key points where midwives could make a difference when caring for women in pre-term labour were:

1. Thermal requirements

   Finding: Poorer outcomes were seen in babies whose temperature was recorded to be below 36°C on admission to Neonatal Unit (NNU).

   • Recommendation: temperature of 25°C should be maintained in the labour room.

2. Attendance of skilled staff at birth of pre-term infants

   Finding: Issues with intubation skills were more frequent in babies who died than in babies who survived.

   • Recommendation 1: The midwife caring for a woman in pre-term labour should alert the neonatal unit and ensure the staff caring, and in attendance at birth, are appropriately trained

   • Recommendation 2: staff responsible for the immediate care of a baby born at 28 weeks' gestation or less should be trained in neonatal life support. At least one should be skilled in tracheal intubation

   • Recommendation 3: The conduct of a vaginal birth of a baby at 28 weeks' gestation or less

should be performed or supervised by a member of the high-risk team.

CEMACH diabetes programme

The purpose of this programme was to audit the provision of services and care for women with type 1 or type 2 diabetes during pregnancy.

There were three modules:

1. A survey of diabetes services for women with type 1 and type 2 diabetes in pregnancy (CEMACH 2004).

2. An audit of care provided to women with type 1 and type 2 diabetes in pregnancy (CEMACH 2005).

3. A confidential panel review of women with type 1 and type 2 diabetes in pregnancy (CEMACH 2007a).

The standards used for the audit were those set out in the National Service Framework for Diabetes (DH 2001).

The main findings were:

1. Women with type 1 or type 2 diabetes have a five-fold increased incidence of stillbirth, three times the risk of neonatal death and twice the risk of their baby having a major congenital anomaly than women in the general population.

2. Women with type 2 diabetes have the same risk of poor outcome as women with type 1 diabetes in pregnancy compared with the general population.

The key findings and recommendations were divided into clinical issues, aimed at improving practice and policy, and social and lifestyle issues recommending how service providers could engage and empower women by educating them to better understand the importance of managing their diabetes prior to, during and after pregnancy.

Maternal and perinatal mortality: an international perspective

Maternal mortality and perinatal mortality rates remain the highest in the developing world; 95% of maternal deaths occur in Africa and Asia with only 1% in developed countries. Indeed, both maternal and perinatal mortality rates are increasing in some less developed countries (Lawn et al 2005, WHO 2004). The perinatal mortality rate in Western Africa is almost 10 times that seen in North America. A total of 30% of global births occur in South-Central Asia and this region accounts for almost 40% of perinatal deaths. This gives a clear indication that the majority of maternal deaths are avoidable or preventable.

Reasons for the inequitably high maternal mortality rates in developing countries are attributed mainly to the lack of skilled healthcare available to these women, particularly teenagers who are less likely to access care if available (Magadi et al 2007). Maternal mortality occurs more frequently around the time of birth due predominantly to the result of haemorrhage, infections and hypertensive disorders and in some countries, unsafe abortion. Thus, both a lack of resource and background social and cultural circumstances can be seen to have a role in the international disparity.

Although overall mortality rates are much lower when investigating developed countries, important differences occur between them. 'Western' countries commonly report better outcomes with maternal mortality of between 7 and 13/100 000 live births in Western Europe; the UK rate is 13.9 and France 9–13 in 2001 (Bouvier-Colle et al 2001). Similarly, the USA report a rate of 12.9/100 000 live births 2001 (Berg et al 2003). However, Eastern Europe displays a differing picture with rates ranging from 50/100 000 live births in Georgia to 18 in Azerbaijan in 2003 (WHO 2006b). However, these figures may be an underestimate in some countries. It has been suggested that under-reporting may range from 22% in France to 93% in Massachusetts. This may also be an issue in developing countries as births may take place at home and mortality may not be registered or reported. It is very difficult to identify comparative international maternal and perinatal mortality rates as each country collects and presents its data in differing ways and for different years.

While the mortality rates for developed countries are favourable as a whole when compared with those from the developing world, it must be remembered that there still may be wide disparity within countries with regard to pregnancy outcomes, with key groups more likely to have a poorer outcome. For example, it has been clearly shown that babies born to parents with lower socioeconomic status are more likely to have low birthweight compared to babies born to parents from higher socioeconomic backgrounds. It has also been shown that the indigenous Aboriginal and Torres Strait Islander women have a maternal mortality rate greater than that of the general Australian population during 2000–2002 (AIHW 2006). Thus many of the resource, training, social, economic and cultural issues must still be addressed within countries. However, these issues can be very different to those previously discussed; e.g. the increased availability of fertility treatment resulting in multiple pregnancy and/or pre-term birth.

Programmes addressing the issues of treatable infectious diseases, such as malaria, have helped to improve the underlying health of women across the world, with particular effects on women from regions where these conditions are endemic. Furthermore, there is a greater understanding of appropriate nutrition, including the availability of vitamin and other supplements. The subsequent increased health of women of childbearing age has resulted in increased positive outcomes in pregnancy.

To attempt to address global maternal mortality 189 countries pledged support to the Millennium Development Goals (MDGs) in 2000 (UN 2000).

However, to be effective in meeting these goals there has to be political commitment (Filippi et al 2006) (see Ch. 55).

Notification of birth

In 1915, it became a statutory requirement for the early notification of a birth. It is the duty of the father or any other person in attendance, or present within 6 hrs of the birth, to notify the appropriate medical officer within 36 hrs. It is usually the midwife who carries out this responsibility as notification of birth in the UK is now electronic. Notification applies to the birth of all live and stillborn babies but not those born before 24 completed weeks of pregnancy. The birth information is made available to the Registrar of Births and Deaths in the district in which the birth took place and also to the primary healthcare services to enable appropriate care to be planned.

Registration of birth

Under the Births and Deaths Registration Act 1953 all births must be registered within 6 weeks (3 weeks in Scotland). If the father or mother fails to do so then the Registrar will request any other person present or at the birth to complete the registration details. If the father and mother are not married then, if attending above, the father must take with him a Statutory Declaration made by the mother that he is the father of the baby.

The choice of surname needs to be carefully considered by the mother as it is only possible to change surnames in particular circumstances, e.g. if she later marries the father and she wants the father's surname.

Stillbirths

A baby born after the 24th week of pregnancy and 'which did not at any time after being completely expelled from its mother, breathe or show any other sign of life' is called a stillbirth under the Births and Deaths Registration Act 1953 (as amended by the Stillbirth [Definition] Act 1992). A medical practitioner, or a midwife present at the birth, may write and sign a stillbirth certificate. If the parents wish to have the baby cremated, rather than buried, then the signature must be that of a medical practitioner.

Registration of stillbirth has to be undertaken by the parents before the Registrar will issue a certificate for burial or cremation (see NMC 2004).

Registration of deaths is the responsibility of the family. If the baby died shortly after birth, both the birth and death have to be registered.

Summary

The role of the midwife is central to the care and successful outcome for mothers accessing maternity care in the UK. It is therefore crucial that all midwives follow the NMC Code (2008) and rules (NMC 2004) and participate in local and national surveillance, audit and research. Midwives should not underestimate their essential role in these processes and must be aware that any recommendations and new initiatives should directly inform their work.

REFERENCES

AIHW 2006 Maternal deaths in Australia 2000–2002: Maternal deaths, Series No. 2. The Australian Institute of Health and Welfare National Perinatal Statistics Unit, Canberra

Berg C J, Chang J, Callahan W M et al 2003 Pregnancy-related mortality in the United States. Obstetrics and Gynaecology 101(2):289–296

Bouvier-Colle M H, Pequignot F, Jougla E J 2001 Maternal mortality in France: Frequency, trends and causes. Journal de gynécologie, obstétrique et biologie de la reproduction 30 (8):768–775

CEMACH 2004 Maternity Services in 2002 for women with type 1 and type 2 diabetes in pregnancy. Confidential Enquiry into Maternal and Child Health. RCOG Press, London

CEMACH 2005 Pregnancy in women with type 1 and type 2 diabetes in 2002–2003, England, Wales and Northern Ireland. Confidential Enquiry into Maternal and Child Health. CEMACH, London

CEMACH 2007a Diabetes in Pregnancy: Are we providing the best care? Findings of a national confidential enquiry: England Wales and Northern Ireland. Confidential Enquiry into Maternal and Child Health. CEMACH, London

CEMACH 2007b Confidential enquiry into Maternal and Child Health. Perinatal mortality 2005: England, Wales and Northern Ireland. London, CEMACH

DoH (Department of Health) 1993 Changing childbirth. HMSO, London

DH (Department of Health) 2001 National Service Framework for Diabetes: standards. DH, London

DH (Department of Health) 2004 National Service Framework for Children, Young People and Maternity Services, Standard 11. Maternity Services. DH, London

DH (Department of Health) 2007 Maternity Matters: choice, access and continuity of service in a safe service. DH, London

Filippi V, Ronsmans C, Campbell O M et al 2006 Maternal health in poor countries: the broader context and a call for action. Lancet 368:1535–1541

Fleming P, Blair P, Bacon C et al (eds) 2000 Sudden unexpected deaths in infancy: the CESDI SUDI studies 1993–1996. The Stationery Office, London

Lawn J E, Cousens S, Zupan J and the Lancet Neonatal Steering group team 2005 4 million neonatal deaths: When? Where? Why? Lancet 365(9462):891–900

Lewis G, Drife J (eds) 2004 Why Mothers Die 2000–2002; sixth report of the Confidential Enquiries into Maternal Deaths in the United Kingdom. RCOG, London

Lewis G (ed.) 2007 The Confidential Enquiry into Maternal and Child Health (CEMACH). Saving mothers' lives: reviewing maternal deaths to make motherhood safer 2003–2005. The seventh report on Confidential Enquiries into Maternal Deaths in the United Kingdom. CEMACH, London

Macintosh M 2003 Project 27/28: An enquiry into quality of care and its effects on the survival of babies born at 27–28 weeks. CESDI. The Stationery Office, London

Magadi M A, Agwanda A O, Obare F O 2007 A comparative analysis of the use of maternal health services between teenagers and older mothers in sub-Saharan Africa; evidence from demographic and health surveys (DHS). Social Science and Medicine 64(6)1311–1325

Morley C J, Thornton A J, Cole T J et al 1991 Baby check: a scoring system to grade the severity of acute illness in babies under six months old. Archives of Disease in Childhood 66:100–106

National Statistics 2005. Birth statistics: Review of the Register General on Births and patterns of family building in England and Wales. Series FM1, No. 34. Online. Available: www.statistics.gov.uk/downloads/theme_population/FM1_34/FM1_no34_2005.pdf 18 May 2007

NMC (Nursing and Midwifery Council) 2004 Midwives Rules and Standards. NMC, London

NMC (Nursing and Midwifery Council) 2008 The Code: Standards of conduct, performance and ethics for nurses and midwives. NMC, London

ONS (Office for National Statistics) 2005. Online. Available: www.statistics.gov.uk/pdfdir/birthstats1205.pdf 18 May 2007

RCOG 2005 Registration of stillbirths and certification of pregnancy loss before 24 weeks' gestation. Good Practice No. 4. RCOG, London

Robinson J 1996 The emperor's new clothes. British Journal of Midwifery 4(11):609–610

The Information Centre 2006. Statistics on obesity, physical activity and diet: England. Online. Available: www.ic.nhs.uk/webfiles/publications/opan06/OPAN%20bulletin%20finalv2.pdf 21 May 2007

UN 2000 United Nations Millennium Development Goals. Online. Available: www.un.org/millenniumgoals 20 May 2007

WHO 2004 Maternal mortality in 2000: Estimates developed by WHO, UNICEF and UNFPA. Online. Available: www.who.int/reproductive-health/global_monitoring/index 12 May 2007

WHO 2006a Neonatal and perinatal mortality: country, regional and global estimates. World Health Organization, Geneva

WHO 2006b Highlights on health: Georgia. Online. Available: www.euro.who.int/eprise/main/WHO/Progs/CHHGEO/cis-mortality/20060209_1 18 May 2007

WRA 2007 The White Ribbon Alliance for Safe Motherhood. Online. Available: www.whiteribbonalliance.org/About/default.cfm?a0=mission 17 May 2007

Glossary of selected terms

Abortion Termination of pregnancy before the fetus is viable, i.e. before 24 weeks' gestation in the UK.

Abruptio placenta Premature separation of a normally situated placenta. Term normally used from viability (24 weeks).

Acardiac twin One twin presents without a well-defined cardiac structure and is kept alive through the placental circulation of the viable twin.

Acridine orange A stain used in fluorescence microscopy that causes bacteria to fluoresce green to red.

Aetiology The science of the cause of disease.

Amenorrhoea Absence of menstrual periods.

Amniotic fluid embolism The escape of amniotic fluid through the wall of the uterus or placental site into the maternal circulation, triggering life-threatening anaphylactic shock in the mother. (The word 'embolism', denoting a clot, is a misnomer.)

Amniotomy Artificial rupture of the amniotic sac.

Anterior obliquity of the uterus Altered uterine axis. The uterus leans forward due to poor maternal abdominal muscles and a pendulous abdomen.

Antigen A substance which stimulates the production of an antibody.

Anuria Producing no urine.

Atresia Closure or absence of a usual opening or canal.

Augmentation of labour Intervention to correct slow progress in labour.

Bandl's ring An exaggerated retraction ring seen as an oblique ridge above the symphysis pubis between the upper and lower uterine segments, which is a sign of obstructed labour.

Basal body temperature The temperature of the body when at rest. In natural family planning, it is taken as soon as the woman wakes from sleep and before any activity occurs or after a period of at least 1 hour's rest.

Beneficence To do good.

Bicornuate uterus A structural abnormality of the uterus.

Bioavailability The degree to which or rate at which a drug or other substance becomes available to the target tissue after administration.

Bioequivalent Acting on the body with the same strength and similar bioavailability as the same dosage of a sample of a given substance.

Birth centres These may be freestanding (away from hospital) or in hospital grounds or in the hospital. The emphasis is on providing a less medical environment and supporting normal birth.

Bishop's Score Rating system to assess suitability of cervix for induction of labour.

Burns Marshall manoeuvre A method of breech delivery involving traction to prevent the neck from bending backwards.

Calendar calculation The fertile phase of the menstrual cycle is calculated in accordance with the length of the woman's 6–12 previous cycles.

Cardiotocograph Measurement of the fetal heart rate and uterine contractions on a machine that is able to provide a paper print of the information it records.

Caseload practice Generally this refers to a personal caseload where named midwives care for individual women.

Central venous pressure line An intravenous (i.v.) tube which measures the pressure in the right atrium or superior vena cava, indicating the volume of blood returning to the heart and by implication, hypovolaemia.

Cephalopelvic disproportion Disparity between the size of the woman's pelvis and the fetal head.

Cerclage Non-absorbable suture inserted to keep cervix closed.

Cervical eversion Physiological response by cervical cells to hormonal changes in pregnancy. Cells proliferate and cause cervix to appear eroded.

Cervical intra-epithelial neoplasm (CIN) Progressive and abnormal growth of cervical cells.

Cervical ripening Process by which the cervix changes and becomes more susceptible to the effect of uterine contractions. Can be physiological or artificially produced.

Cervicitis Inflammation of the cervix.

Choanal atresia (Bilateral) membranous or bony obstruction of the nares; baby is blue when sleeping and pink when crying.

Choroid plexus cyst Collection of cerebrospinal fluid within the choroids plexi, from where cerebrospinal fluid is derived.

Coloboma A malformation characterized by the absence of or a defect in the tissue of the eye; the pupil can appear keyhole-shaped. It may be associated with other anomalies.

Colposcopy Visualization of the cervix using a colposcope.

Commensal Micro-organisms adapted to grow on the skin or mucous surfaces of the host, forming part of the normal flora.

Conjoined twins Identical twins where separation is incomplete so their bodies are partly joined together and vital organs may be shared.

Couvelaire uterus (uterine apoplexy) Bruising and oedema of uterine tissue seen in placental abruption when leaking blood is forced between muscle fibres because the margins of the placenta are still attached to the uterus.

Cryotherapy Use of cold or freezing to destroy or remove tissue.

Deontology Duty-based theory.

Deoxyribonucleic acid (DNA) The substance containing genes. DNA can store and transmit information, can copy itself accurately and can occasionally mutate.

Diastasis symphysis pubis A painful condition in which there is an abnormal relaxation of the ligaments supporting the pubic joint, also referred to as pelvic girdle pain.

Dichorionic twins Twins who have developed in their own separate chorionic sacs.

Diploid Containing two sets of chromosomes.

Disseminated intravascular coagulation/ coagulopathy A condition secondary to a primary complication where there is inappropriate blood clotting in the blood vessels, followed by an inability of the blood to clot appropriately when all the clotting factors have been used up.

Dizygotic (dizygous) Formed from two separate zygotes.

Doering rule The first fertile day of the cycle is determined by a calculation based upon the earliest previous temperature shift. This is an effective double check method to identify the onset of the fertile phase.

Dyspareunia Painful or difficult intercourse experienced by the woman.

Echogenic bowel Bright appearances of bowel, equivalent to the brightness of bone. Also associated with intra-amniotic bleeding and fetal swallowing of blood-stained liquor.

Echogenic foci in the heart Bright echoes from calcium deposits in the fetal heart, often the left ventricle. These do not affect cardiac function.

Ectopic pregnancy An abnormally situated pregnancy, most commonly in a uterine tube.

Embryo reduction (see Fetal reduction).

Endocervical Relating to the internal canal of the cervix.

Epicanthic folds A vertical fold of skin on either side of the nose which covers the lacrimal caruncle. They may be common in Asian babies, but may indicate Down syndrome in other ethnic groups.

Erb's palsy Paralysis of the arm due to the damage to cervical nerve roots 5 and 6 of the brachial plexus.

Erythematous Reddening of the skin.

Erythropoiesis The process by which erythrocytes (red blood cells) are formed. After the 10th week of gestation, erythropoiesis production rises and seems to be involved in red cell production in the bone marrow during the third trimester.

External cephalic version (ECV) The use of external manipulation on the pregnant woman's abdomen to convert a breech to a cephalic presentation.

False-negative rate The proportion of affected pregnancies that would not be identified as high risk. Tests with a high false-negative rate have low sensitivity.

False-positive rate The proportion of unaffected pregnancies with a high-risk classification. Tests with a high false-positive rate have low specificity.

Ferguson reflex Surge of oxytocin, resulting in increased contractions, due to stimulation of the cervix, and upper portion of the vagina.

Fetal reduction The reduction in the number of viable fetuses/embryos in a multiple (usually higher multiple) pregnancy by medical intervention.

Fetofetal transfusion syndrome (twin to twin transfusion syndrome, TTTS) Condition in which blood from one monozygotic twin fetus transfuses into the other via blood vessels in the placenta.

Fetus-in-fetu Parts of a fetus may be lodged within another fetus. This can only happen in monozygotic twins.

Fetus papyraceous A fetus that dies in the second trimester of the pregnancy and becomes compressed and parchment-like.

Fibroid Firm, benign tumour of muscular and fibrous tissue.

First pass effect Drugs given orally are absorbed in the small intestine, transported to the liver via the hepatic portal vein and metabolized prior to systemic circulation. As a result, oral administration leads to lower levels of the drug reaching the target tissue than other routes of administration.

Fraternal twins Dizygotic (non-identical).

Fundal height The distance between the top part of the uterus (the fundus) and the top of the symphysis pubis (the junction between the pubic bones). This assessment is undertaken to assess the increasing size of the uterus antenatally and decreasing size postnatally.

Group practice Generally refers to a small group of midwives who provide care for a group of women.

Haematuria Blood in the urine.

Haemostasis The arrest of bleeding.

Haploid Containing only one set of chromosomes.

HELLP syndrome A condition of pregnancy characterized by haemolysis, elevated liver enzymes and low platelets.

Herpes gestationis An autoimmune disease precipitated by pregnancy and characterized by an erythematous rash and blisters.

Homan's sign Pain is felt in the calf when the foot is pulled upwards (dorsiflexion). This is indicative of a venous thrombosis and further investigations should be undertaken to exclude or confirm this.

Homeostasis The condition in which the body's internal environment remains relatively constant within physiological limits.

Hydatidiform mole A gross malformation of the trophoblast in which the chorionic villi proliferate and become avascular.

Hydropic vesicles Fluid filled sacs, or blisters.

Hypercapnia An abnormal increase in the amount of carbon dioxide in the blood.

Hyperemesis gravidarum Protracted or excessive vomiting in pregnancy.

Hypertrophy Overgrowth of tissue.

Hypovolaemia Reduced circulating blood volume due to external loss of body fluids or to loss of fluid into the tissues.

Hypoxia Lack of oxygen.

Hysteroscope An instrument used to access the uterus via the vagina.

Induction of labour Intervention to stimulate uterine contractions before the onset of spontaneous labour.

Intraepithelial Within the epithelium, or among epithelial cells.

Intrahepatic cholestasis of pregnancy (ICP) An idiopathic condition of abnormal liver function.

LAM A method of contraception based upon an algorithm of lactation, amenorrhoea and 6 months' time period.

Lanugo Soft downy hair which covers the fetus *in utero* and occasionally the neonate. It appears at around 20 weeks' gestation and covers the face and most of the body. It disappears by 40 weeks' gestation.

Løvset manoeuvre A manoeuvre for the delivery of shoulders and extended arms in a breech presentation.

Macrosomia Large baby.

Malposition A cephalic presentation other than normal well-flexed anterior position of the fetal head, e.g. occipitoposterior.

Malpresentation A presentation other than the vertex, i.e. face, brow, compound or shoulder. (Breech may be included in this category.)

Mauriceau–Smellie–Veit manoeuvre A manoeuvre to deliver a breech which involves jaw flexion and shoulder traction.

McRoberts manoeuvre A manoeuvre to rotate the angle of the symphysis pubis superiorly and release the impaction of the anterior shoulder in shoulder dystocia. The woman brings her knees up to her chest.

Midwife-led care Midwives or a midwife take the lead role in care of a woman or group of women.

Miscarriage Spontaneous loss of pregnancy before viability (see Abortion).

Monoamniotic twins Twins who have developed in the same amniotic sac.

Monochorionic twins Identical twins who have developed in the same chorionic sac.

Monozygotic (monozygous) Formed from one zygote (identical twins).

Multifetal reduction (see Fetal reduction).

Naegele's rule Method of calculating the expected date of birth.

Natural Family Planning (NFP) Methods of contraception based on observations of naturally occurring signs and symptoms of the fertile and infertile phases of the menstrual cycle.

Neoplasia Growth of new tissue.

Neutral thermal environment (NTE) The range of environmental temperature over which heat production, oxygen consumption and nutritional requirements for growth are minimal, provided the body temperature is normal.

Non-maleficence Do no harm.

Oedema The effusion of body fluid into the tissues.

Oligohydramnios Abnormally small amount of amniotic fluid in pregnancy.

Oliguria Producing an abnormally small amount of urine.

One-to-one midwifery One midwife takes responsibility for individual women. A partner backs up the named midwife. It integrates a high level of continuity of caregiver and midwifery-led care. It is geographically based and includes women who are both 'high risk' and 'low risk'.

PaCO$_2$ Measures the partial pressure of dissolved carbon dioxide (CO_2). This dissolved CO_2 has moved out of the cell and into the bloodstream. The measure of a PaCO$_2$ accurately reflects the alveolar ventilation.

PaO$_2$ Measures the partial pressure of oxygen in the arterial blood. It reflects how the lung is functioning but does not measure tissue oxygenation.

Paronychia An inflamed swelling of the nail folds; acute paronychia is usually caused by infection with *Staphylococcus aureus*.

Peak mucus day A retrospective assessment of the last day of highly fertile mucus which is seen or felt around ovulation.

Pedunculated Stem or stalk.

Pemphigoid gestationis (see Herpes gestationis).

Perinatal Events surrounding labour and the first 7 days of life.

pH A solution's acidity or alkalinity is expressed on the pH scale, which runs from 0–14. This scale is based on the concentration of H^+ ions in a solution expressed in chemical units called moles per litre (mol/L). When the fetus is hypoxic the increased acid produced raises the acidity of the blood and the pH falls.

Pill-free interval The 7 days when no pills are taken during combined oral contraceptive regimen.

Placenta accreta Abnormally adherent placenta into the muscle layer of the uterus.

Placenta increta Abnormally adherent placenta into the perimetrium of the uterus.

Placenta percreta Abnormally adherent placenta through the muscle layer of the uterus.

Placenta praevia A condition in which some or all of the placenta is attached in the lower segment of the uterus.

Placental abruption (see Abruptio placenta).

Polyhydramnios An excessive amount of amniotic fluid in pregnancy. Also referred to as hydramnios.

Polyp Small growth.

Porphyria An inherited condition of abnormal red blood cell formation.

Postnatal period The period after the end of labour during which the attendance of a midwife upon the woman and baby is required, being not less than 10 days and for such longer periods as the midwife considers necessary.

Postpartum After labour.

Pre-eclampsia A condition peculiar to pregnancy, which is characterized by hypertension, proteinuria and systemic dysfunction.

Primary postpartum haemorrhage A blood loss in excess of 500 mL or any amount which adversely affects the condition of the mother within the first 24 hours of birth.

Progestogen Synthetic progesterone used in hormonal contraception.

Prostaglandins Locally acting chemical compounds derived from fatty acids within cells. They ripen the cervix and cause the uterus to contract.

Proteinuria Protein in the urine.

Pruritus Itching.

Ptyalism Excessive salivation.

Puerperal fever/pyrexia A rise in temperature in the puerperium. This is poorly defined in the textbooks but is assumed to be based on the definition of pyrexia which is a rise above the normal body temperature of 37.2°C. Where pyrexia is used as a clinical sign of importance, the elevation in temperature is generally taken as being 38°C and above.

Puerperal sepsis Infection of the genital tract following childbirth; still a major cause of maternal death where it is undetected and/or untreated.

Puerperium A period after childbirth where the uterus and other organs and structures which have been affected by the pregnancy are returning to their non-gravid state. Usually described as a period of up to 6–8 weeks.

Quickening First point at which the woman recognizes fetal movements in early pregnancy.

Retraction Process by which the uterine muscle fibres shorten after a contraction. Unique to uterine muscle.

Rubin's manoeuvre A rotational manoeuvre to relieve shoulder dystocia. Pressure is exerted over the fetal back to adduct and rotate the shoulders.

Sandal gap Exaggerated gap between the first and second toes.

Secondary postpartum haemorrhage An 'excessive' or 'prolonged' vaginal blood loss which is usually defined as occurring from 24 hours to 6 weeks after the birth.

Selective fetocide The medical destruction of an abnormal twin fetus in a continuing pregnancy.

Sheehan's syndrome A condition where sudden or prolonged shock leads to irreversible pituitary necrosis characterized by amenorrhoea, genital atrophy and premature senility.

Short femur Shorter than the average thigh bone, when compared with other fetal measurements.

Shoulder dystocia Failure of the shoulders to spontaneously traverse the pelvis after birth of the head.

Siamese twins Conjoined twins.

Speculum (vaginal) An instrument used to open the vagina.

Subinvolution The uterine size appears larger than anticipated for days postpartum, and may feel poorly contracted. Uterine tenderness may be present.

Superfecundation Conception of twins as a result of sexual intercourse with two different partners in the same menstrual cycle.

Superfetation Conception of twins as a result of two acts of sexual intercourse in different menstrual cycles.

Surfactant Complex mixture of phospholipids and lipoproteins produced by type 2 alveolar cells in the lungs that decreases surface tension and prevents alveolar collapse at end expiration.

Symphysiotomy A surgical incision to separate the symphysis pubis and enlarge the pelvis to aid delivery.

Symphysis pubis dysfunction (see Diastasis symphysis pubis).

Talipes A complex foot deformity, affecting 1/1000 live births and is more common in males. The affected foot is held in a fixed flexion (equinus) and in-turned (varus) position. It can be differentiated from positional talipes because the deformity in true talipes cannot be passively corrected.

Team midwifery Midwives are team-based rather than ward- or community-based. The team takes responsibility for a number of women. Teams may be restricted to hospital or community, or cover both.

Teratogen An agent believed to cause congenital abnormalities, e.g. thalidomide.

Torsion Twisting.

Trizygotic Formed from three separate zygotes.

Twin-to-twin transfusion syndrome (see Fetofetal transfusion syndrome).

Uniovular Monozygotic.

Unstable lie After 36 weeks' gestation, a lie that varies between longitudinal and oblique or transverse is said to be unstable.

Uterine involution The physiological process that starts from the end of labour that results in a gradual reduction in the size of the uterus until it returns to its non-pregnant size and location in the pelvis.

Utilitarianism Greatest good for greatest number.

Vanishing twin syndrome The reabsorption of one twin fetus early in pregnancy (usually before 12 weeks).

Vasa praevia A rare occurrence in which umbilical cord vessels pass through the placental membranes and lie across the cervical os.

Withdrawal bleed Bleeding due to withdrawal of hormones.

Wood's manoeuvre A rotational or screw manoeuvre to relieve shoulder dystocia. Pressure is exerted on the fetal chest to rotate and abduct the shoulders.

Zavanelli manoeuvre Last choice of manoeuvre for shoulder dystocia. The head is returned to its pre-restitution position, then the head is flexed back into the vagina. Delivery is by caesarean section.

Zygosity Describing the genetic make-up of children in a multiple birth.

Index

Page numbers in *italic* denote figures or tables.